MANUAL OF
EXOTIC PET
PRACTICE

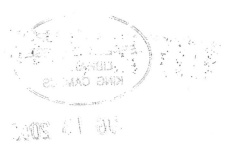

MANUAL OF
EXOTIC PET
PRACTICE

Mark A. Mitchell, DVM, MS, PhD

College of Veterinary Medicine
University of Illinois
Urbana, Illinois

Thomas N. Tully, Jr., DVM, MS, Dip. ABVP (Avian), ECAMS

School of Veterinary Medicine
Louisiana State University
Baton Rouge, Louisiana

SAUNDERS

ELSEVIER

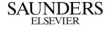

11830 Westline Industrial Drive
St. Louis, Missouri 63146

MANUAL OF EXOTIC PET PRACTICE   ISBN: 978-1-4160-0119-5
Copyright © 2009 by Saunders, an imprint of Elsevier Inc.

Library of Congress Control Number: 2007925165

Vice President and Publisher: Linda Duncan
Publisher: Penny Rudolph
Developmental Editor: Shelly Stringer
Publishing Services Manager: Pat Joiner-Myers
Senior Project Manager: Gena Magouirk
Design Direction: Julia Dummitt

Printed in China.

Last digit is the print number: 9 8 7 6 5 4 3 2 1

Contributors

Maya Bewig, DVM
Associate
Grey Wolf Veterinary Hospital
Sequim, Washington, USA

Wildlife

Deborah Carboni, DVM, MS
Ontario Veterinary College
Guelph, Ontario, Canada

Marsupials

M. Camille Harris, DVM, MS, BS
PhD Student (Ecology of Infectious Diseases)
Department of Biological Sciences
Virginia Polytechnic Institute and State University
Blacksburg, Virginia, USA

Hamsters and Gerbils

J. Jill Heatley, DVM, MS, Dip. ABVP (Avian)
Clinical Associate Professor, Zoological Medicine
Department of Clinical Sciences
College of Veterinary Medicine and Biomedical Sciences
Texas A&M University
College Station, Texas, USA

Hamsters and Gerbils
Hedgehogs

Megan Kirchgessner, DVM
Clinical Veterinarian
New England Wildlife Center
South Weymouth, Massachusetts, USA

Chelonians

Stephen M. Miller, DVM
General Curator
North Carolina Zoo
Asheboro, North Carolina, USA

Ornamental Fish

Mark A. Mitchell, DVM, MS, PhD
Associate Professor, Zoological Medicine
Department of Veterinary Clinical Medicine
College of Veterinary Medicine
University of Illinois
Urbana, Illinois, USA

History of Exotic Pets
Preparing Your Hospital for Exotic Pets
Invertebrates
Ornamental Fish
Snakes
Chelonians
Rabbits
Chinchillas
Wildlife

Natalie Mylniczenko, DVM, MS
Associate Veterinarian
Chicago Zoological Society
Brookfield Zoo
Brookfield, Illinois, USA

Amphibians

Javier Nevarez, DVM, PhD
Assistant Professor, Zoological Medicine
Department of Veterinary Clinical Sciences
School of Veterinary Medicine
Louisiana State University
Baton Rouge, Louisiana, USA

Crocodilians
Lizards

Shannon M. Riggs, DVM
Staff Veterinarian
International Bird Rescue and Research Center
Fairfield, California, USA

Guinea Pigs
Chinchillas

Thomas N. Tully, Jr., DVM, MS, Dip. ABVP (Avian), ECAMS
Professor, Zoological Medicine
Department of Veterinary Clinical Sciences
School of Veterinary Medicine
Louisiana State University
Baton Rouge, Louisiana, USA

Birds
Marsupials
Mice and Rats

Kristine M. Vennen, DVM
Clinical Veterinarian
Loftin Veterinary Clinic
Youngsville, Louisana, USA

Rabbits

Tiffany M. Wolf, DVM
Clinical Veterinarian
The Minnesota Zoo
Apple Valley, Minnesota, USA

Ferrets

Trevor Zachariah, DVM, MS
Veterinary Resident
Chicago Zoological and Aquatic Animal Residency Program
University of Illinois
Urbana, Illinois, USA

Invertebrates

Preface

Exotic companion animals are increasingly being recognized as a significant area of interest within veterinary medicine. For decades, veterinarians have been asked to consult on cases involving ornamental fish, rabbits, small rodents, birds, reptiles, or even an occasional spider or hermit crab. Many veterinarians have found it difficult to treat and consult on these cases because of a lack of published information; many are forced to make recommendations that are based on subjective or anecdotal information. Fortunately, the practice of exotic pet medicine has made great strides in the past two decades. Although there remains much work to be done, the current knowledge base regarding nontraditional pets has been improved through scientific discovery and communication among veterinarians. Historically, much of the exotic pet literature was based on an understanding of what was done with domestic species. Today, veterinarians have many more resources for information on the species mentioned in this book, including several peer-reviewed journals publishing exotic animal–specific articles that provide a scientific foundation to better treat and manage these species in captivity. It is from an expanded information base that the editors and authors have compiled this text.

This textbook is one of the first of its kind to include sections on all of the major exotic animal groups. As the editors of this text, we felt that there was a strong need for a general exotic pet textbook that could be used by veterinarians to manage any exotic animal that came their way. There is a large percentage of the veterinary profession practicing small or mixed animal veterinary medicine that has a small to moderate caseload of exotic pets. It is for this group of veterinarians that this text was written. There are certainly other excellent textbooks that go into extensive detail on the needs of each group of exotic pet animals and would certainly be beneficial to the veterinary practitioner. Unfortunately, to purchase each textbook on its own would require a significant monetary investment. Although initially intended as a general reference for those individuals looking for a general exotic pet text, this text will become an important reference for those individuals with more exotic pet experience.

Acknowledgments

We wish to thank each of the authors for their contributions to this text. Because of the spectrum of coverage this text provides, it would be difficult, if not impossible, to complete such a textbook without their contributions. We would also like to thank Ms. Verna Serra for her invaluable administrative assistance during the preparation of this text. We are also grateful to our publisher, Elsevier, for providing us an opportunity to bring to fruition a textbook that will provide an invaluable resource to so many in our profession. Our primary contact at Elsevier, Ms. Shelly Stringer, was most helpful with keeping us on track and guiding this much-needed book to completion.

Dedication

In life, it is important to find that which inspires you. For me, my inspiration comes from my wife, Lorrie, and daughter, Mary Yansheng. Lorrie and Mary, it is your love that serves as my source of energy and ensures that I can succeed at whatever endeavor I pursue. I love you both. To my coeditor, Thomas N. Tully, thank you for your mentorship, friendship, and guidance during my tenure at LSU. You will always be my chief. **(MAM)**

I dedicate this book with love to my parents, Donna and Thomas N. Tully, Sr. Their guidance and support have been invaluable assets to my professional development. I wish to extend a heartfelt thank-you to my wife, Susie, and two daughters, Claudia and Fiona, for their day-to-day patience and inspiration. To my coeditor, Mark Mitchell, thank you for being the best colleague, friend, and office mate one could ask for over the past 10 years. **(TNT)**

Contents

Mark A. Mitchell

CHAPTER 1

HISTORY OF EXOTIC PETS

■ WHAT IS AN EXOTIC PET?

The word *exotic* is used as an adjective to describe many different things in society. Generally, this term indicates something unique, dangerous, or exciting. In *Merriam-Webster's Collegiate Dictionary,* 11th edition,[1] the definition of exotic includes: "1. introduced from another country: not native to the place where found, 2. (Archaic) foreign, alien, and 3. strikingly, excitingly, or mysteriously different or unusual." Any of these definitions are applicable to the species of interest in this book. However, there are other adjectives commonly used to describe exotic animals too, including *nontraditional* or *nondomestic.*

Selecting the best adjective to describe the species addressed in this text can be difficult. For example, to call all of these pets *exotic* may not be correct, as certain species, such as box turtles *(Terrapene carolina)* or red-eared sliders *(Trachemys scripta elegans),* are kept as pets in the United States but are native to large regions of the country. The use of the term *nondomestic* or *nontraditional* would not necessarily be correct for certain species either, such as ferrets, as these animals have been associated with humans for over 2,300 years.[2] For purposes of simplicity, the editors have selected the adjective *exotic* to describe the species described in the text because they are certainly considered by most to fit the third dictionary definition for the term *exotic:* "strikingly, excitingly, or mysteriously different or unusual." There are those nonexotic (or traditional, domestic) species that the public acknowledges as common or usual, including the dog, cat, cow, horse, sheep, goat, pig, or chicken, and then there are those that are anything but common or usual, such as the goliath bird-eating spider *(Theraphosa blondi),* freshwater angelfish *(Pterophyllum scalare),* blue poison dart frog *(Dendrobates azureus),* blue-tongued skink *(Tiliqua scincoides),* hawk-headed parrot *(Deroptyus accipitrinus),* or chinchilla *(Chinchilla lanigera).*

History of Exotic Pets

Exotic pets have long held the interest of humans. During the early and mid-20th century, it was not uncommon for newly imported reptiles, birds, or mammals to stir the imagination of the public. The following is a brief historical review of how some exotic animals gained in popularity.

Ornamental fish represent one of the oldest groups of exotic pets. Evidence suggests that the Sumerians were the first to keep fish in captivity (2500 BC), but it was for food.[3] The Egyptians and Romans were likely the first groups to keep fish as something more than just a food source. However, it was the Chinese (Sung Dynasty: 960-1279) who were the first to actively keep and breed fish for their aesthetics. Goldfish were the first fish to be actively maintained for this reason. It was not until the 17th century that these ornamentals made their way to the Western world (Europe). A major problem encountered by those who did not have regular access to natural spring water was the inability to maintain the health of the fish. Losses were likely great in those days from elevated ammonia and nitrite levels in the water. Issues of water quality were first addressed by Robert Warrington in the 19th century. His theory for a successful aquarium was to use plants to produce oxygen for fish and snails to eat the detritus. It was not until the early and mid-20th century that the importance of aeration and filtration was acknowledged. Ornamental fish arrived in the United States in the late 19th century/early 20th century. The ornamental fish hobby grew with the advent of commercial travel. Fish could be moved globally by ship, railroad, or plane. The cost of the fish and equipment, although expensive, finally became affordable after the 1940s. Over the past 2 to 3 decades, significant advances have been made in filtration techniques, water quality standards, and fish nutrition. The ornamental fish industry remains an important contributor to the overall pet market; however, to date, veterinarians have not developed any significant inroads into this field.

Reptiles have only recently become popular as pets and something more than a "dime store" fancy. From the 1940s to the 1970s, the primary reptiles being sold in the United States were native species, such as the red-eared slider turtle and green anole *(Anolis carolinensis)*. In the earlier decades of the 20th century, hatchling turtles were collected from wild nests and offered for sale. Starting in the 1950s and 1960s, turtle farming became popular in the southern states (e.g., Louisiana). Green anoles and other native reptiles were also routinely captured from the wild for the pet retail trade. After the U.S. Food and Drug Administration instituted the 1975 regulation restricting the interstate and intrastate sales of chelonians under 10.2 cm (4″), turtle farmers began exporting the turtles. During the latter half of the 20th century, reptiles were imported from Australia, Africa, South and Central America, and Asia; however, it was not until the 1980s and 1990s that a real explosion in the pet reptile trade occurred. Much of the initial trade revolved around green iguanas, although boids (e.g., boa constrictor, *Boa constrictor*) and pythons (e.g., ball python, *Python regius*) were also being imported in large numbers. In 1997 alone, more than 566,000 green iguanas, 94,000 ball pythons, and 29,000 boa constrictors were imported.[4] During the 20th and into the 21st century, there has been a move toward captive propagation of reptiles. Many of the "designer" reptiles that are currently available, including corn snakes *(Elaphe guttata)*, leopard geckos *(Eublepharis macularius)*, bearded dragons *(Pogona vitticeps)*, and ball pythons, have been derived from the establishment of specialized genetic lines. With the current high dollar value of many of these animals (e.g., $5,000-$30,000 for ball pythons), individuals are often interested in obtaining veterinary care for their pets. The current status of the reptile trade in the United States is based on a combination of both wild-caught and captively propagated species. Wild-caught animals continue to be primarily distributed through retail pet stores, where the client's knowledge regarding the care of these animals is limited, whereas captive animals, especially high dollar animals, are trading hands by more experienced herpetoculturists.

Psittacines may represent the class of exotics that have been kept the longest in captivity. Records in Egypt suggest birds were kept in captivity for purposes in addition to food since 4000 BC.[5] With the advent of open water sailing during the 15th to 18th centuries, the movement of exotic birds became more commonplace. Many of the birds considered common, such as canaries *(Serinus canaria)*, parakeets *(Melopsittacus undulatus)*, and zebra finches *(Poephila guttata)*, have been bred in captivity since the 18th and 19th centuries. In the United States, aviculture became very popular with the turn of the century. With the advent of flight, it became even easier to transport birds across the country. Through most of the 20th century, a large proportion of birds being sold in the United States were wild-caught animals. These could be distinguished from captive-born birds by their open leg band. Fortunately, over the past 2 decades, the number of birds being imported has declined, and the majority of the psittacines offered for sale are captive-born (closed leg band).

Ferrets are one of the exotic species of animals that have a long and documented history with human civilization. Originally brought into captivity around 350 BC, these animals have held many roles in captivity, including hunting partner, vermin control, and companion animal. Ferrets are thought to have been introduced into the United States during the 1700s. These animals would have been brought over during the great migration to the New World. Their value for hunting and mousing certainly would have gained them favor among their caretakers. Today, these animals have a lifestyle that is very different from their past. Ferrets, no longer considered "working animals," spend the majority of their day slumbering and serve as companion animals. In certain parts of the world, such as the United Kingdom, ferrets remain active working animals, assisting hunters with the capture of rabbits.

Domestic rabbits, like ferrets, have been associated with human civilization for over 1000 years. *Oryctolagus cuniculus,* the domestic rabbit, was originally found on the Iberian Peninsula at the end of the Pleistocene era.[6] Historical records suggest that it was the Phoenicians who first exported rabbits to Spain in 1100 BC.[7] However, it was a group of French monks that were credited with domesticating and selectively breeding the rabbits that are consistent with the animals known today. Rabbits were prized by the Romans and English. There is little documentation regarding the landing of domestic rabbits in the United States before the 20th century. It is likely that animals were imported from Europe before this time, but not in any great numbers. The Belgian hare was the first rabbit to catch the American public's attention. This large breed was prized not only because of its aesthetics but also because it could provide meat and fur. The first organized rabbit association, the National Pet Stock Association, was formed in 1910. The organization, which has since changed its name to the American Rabbit Breeders Association, has over 37,000 members. Rabbits remain popular today in the United States for production of meat and fur, as research animals, and as companion pets.

Chinchillas remain exotic animals of interest in the United States. These animals, like ferrets, have served many different roles since being acknowledged by humans, including providing fur and meat, acting as research models for auditory research, and serving as companion pets. Chinchillas originallly served as a prey species, providing meat and fur to indigenous peoples of the Andes mountains. An international trade for chinchilla fur was founded in the 1500s, but by the late 1800s native populations had been decimated.[8] Chinchillas were originally introduced into the United States in 1923 by Mathias F. Chapman. This founder stock comprised 11 animals, 3 of which were females. Although chinchillas are still being raised for fur production, they are now very popular as pets.

WHY ARE EXOTIC PETS BECOMING MAINSTREAM?

A Survey of Exotic Pet Ownership

For veterinarians to be successful, they must have patients. When a veterinarian attempts to establish a site for a veterinary hospital, it should be based on the potential to have access to a sufficiently sized patient population. In some areas of the United States, animal populations can be estimated based on rabies vaccine registrations for dogs and cats or Coggin's test results for horses. Unfortunately, this is more difficult to do for exotic species. With the exception of vaccinating ferrets for rabies, there is no community-based method for identifying the number of exotic pets in a geographical area. Because of this, veterinarians must rely on larger, national surveys to identify the size of their potential caseload.

The American Veterinary Medical Association (AVMA) and the American Pet Product Manufacturer's Association (APPMA) are two national organizations that routinely survey the pet population landscape in the United States. Their surveys provide an estimate of the number of households that maintain companion pets in the United States and also attempt to estimate the number of animals in a given household. This information is derived primarily by these two organizations to provide their respective industries with the information they need to develop future strategies regarding the sale and care of pets in the United States.

The last published report by the AVMA was in 2002.[9] The results of the survey suggested that exotic pets are not uncommon in U.S. households. Interestingly, 60% of pet households owned more than one type of pet. As many as 65.4% and 49.4% of bird owners were likely to have dogs and cats, respectively. This is vital information for veterinarians attempting to decide whether to incorporate additional species (e.g., birds) into their practices, as many pet owners would likely prefer the convenience of visiting a single veterinarian rather than two or more veterinarians. Of all the exotic species included in the survey, fish represented the largest group being kept as pets (49.2 million). This is interesting because veterinarians play a limited role in providing health care for ornamental fish. Birds represented the second largest group of exotic animals being kept as pets (approximately 10 million); however, according to the survey, the number of birds kept as pets had decreased by almost 20% compared to the number found 5 years earlier (1996). Rabbits represented the third largest group of exotic

animals being kept as pets (4.8 million). Reptiles (lizards, snakes, chelonians, and others) accounted for approximtately 2.9 million animals in the survey. If all rodents were combined (e.g., hamsters, gerbils, guinea pigs, other rodents), then the total number of these animals being kept as pets was approximately 2.6 million. Ferrets represented the smallest number of animals being kept as pets (approximately 1 million); however, these animals are illegal to own in California, and the survey probably underestimated the true number of ferrets in the United States.

When attempting to derive estimates of a pet animal population from published surveys, it is important to recognize that these types of surveys can underestimate the actual number of cases. For example, the 2001 AVMA survey suggested that approximately 2.9 million reptiles were being kept as pets in the United States, whereas the 2000 APPMA survey suggested the number might be as high as 9 million.[10] This represents a 68% discrepancy in the number of proposed animals. With over 1 million animals being imported annually, it would suggest that more reptiles are being kept as pets than the AVMA survey suggests. Although it is arguable that many of the imported animals succumb during transport, these numbers do not account for the thousands of captive-born reptiles being sold in the U.S. market. Amphibians were also not included in the AVMA survey; however, they would not be expected to account for such a discrepancy between the studies.

REFERENCES

1. *Merriam-Webster's Collegiate Dictionary,* ed 11, Springfield, Mass, 2003, Merriam-Webster.
2. Fox JG: *Biology and Diseases of Ferrets,* ed 2, Baltimore, 1998, Lippincott Williams & Wilkins.
3. Aquarium, from Wikipedia, http://en.wikipedia.org/wiki/Aquarium, May 20, 2006.
4. U.S. Fish and Wildlife Service, Law Enforcement Management Information System, from www.fws.gov, 1997.
5. Rutgers A, Norris KA: *Encyclopedia of Aviculture, vol 3,* Dorset, UK, 1977, Blandford.
6. Grzimek: *Grzimek's Encyclopedia of Mammals, vol 4,* New York, 1990, McGraw-Hill.
7. Brown M: *Exhibition and Pet Rabbits,* Surrey, UK, 1982, Spur.
8. Chinchilla, from Wikipedia, http://en.wikipedia.org/wiki/Chinchilla, May 20, 2006.
9. Wise JK, Heathcott BL, Gonzalez ML: Results of the AVMA survey on companion animal ownership in US pet-owning households, *J Am Vet Med Assoc* 221(11):1572-1573, 2002.
10. American Pet Product Manufacturer's Association: *2001-2002 APPMA National Pet Owners Survey,* Greenwich, Conn, 2001, APPMA.

Mark A. Mitchell

CHAPTER 2

PREPARING YOUR HOSPITAL FOR EXOTIC PETS

◼ ADVANTAGES AND DISADVANTAGES OF INCORPORATING EXOTIC PETS INTO A VETERINARY PRACTICE

When considering whether to incorporate exotic species into a veterinary practice, veterinarians should first identify the potential advantages and disadvantages associated with such a change. Incorporating exotic pets into a veterinary practice can have multiple benefits (e.g., provide new challenges for veterinarians, provide clients a single hospital resource for all [most] of their pets, and increase hospital revenue). The potential disadvantages for adding these species to a practice include the additional time that will be required for acquiring continuing education, additional monies required to purchase equipment and literary resources for the veterinary library, and the time required to publicize the practice's entrance into the field of exotic pet medicine.

Veterinarians are an ambitious lot. The pursuit of a veterinary professional degree requires commitment, intelligence, and ambition. Because these are traits that are inherent to veterinarians, it is important that they continually challenge themselves to satisfy their intellectual and emotional needs. Upon graduation, veterinarians may find veterinary medicine challenging because of the "newness" of it all; however, after this "newness" wears off, many veterinarians find themselves not satisfying their desires for intellectual challenge. Working with exotic pets can provide veterinarians with this much needed challenge. Although mastering the majority of issues regarding dogs and cats would be feasible in a career, it is unlikely that anyone could become highly competent working with the thousands of exotic species that could be presented

to the veterinarian. Although many veterinarians call what they do "veterinary practice," it could not be any more true than with exotic animals. Some might argue that attempting to work with so many species would be difficult and that veterinarians should focus more on the types of animals they already work with. It is important that veterinarians understand their limitations. For example, if a veterinarian has limited orthopedic surgical experience, he or she should not attempt to place a dynamic compression plate on a femoral fracture in a poodle. The same logic applies in the case of exotic species too.

The 2001 American Veterinary Medical Association (AVMA) survey confirms that the majority of U.S. households with pets have multiple pets. This is an important consideration for veterinarians. Once a veterinary-client releationship has been established, it is easier for the client to maintain it for all of his or her pets. Using a single veterinary resource would be preferred by most clients, for both emotional reasons and convenience. Many clients would not hesitate to bring their dog or cat to the veterinarian for an annual examination but are unaware that their exotic pets need the same level of care. If the veterinarian is not making these types of recommendations, then the client's exotic pets will not be provided the same level of health care.

The inclusion of exotic pets into a veterinary practice can also be financially rewarding. Yes, there are those clients that will remind the veterinarian that their pet hamster can be replaced for $5, but there are also those who will pursue any level of care for their $5 hamster because of the human-animal bond they have developed with their pet. The same mentality is still held for "outdoor" cats and "pound" puppies. Until there is a real recognition of the responsibility associated with

TABLE 2-1	Professional Exotic Species Associations	
Organization	Contact Information	Journals
American Association of Zoo Veterinarians	http://www.aazv.org/	Journal of Zoo and Wildlife Medicine (Quarterly)
Association of Avian Veterinarians	http://www.aav.org/	Journal of Avian Medicine and Surgery (Quarterly)
Association of Exotic Mammal Veterinarians	http://www.aemv.org/	Journal of Exotic Pet Medicine (Quarterly)
Association of Reptilian and Amphibian Veterinarians	http://www.arav.org/	Journal of Herpetological Medicine and Surgery (Quarterly)
International Association for Aquatic Animal Medicine	http://www.iaaam.org/	IAAAM News (Quarterly)
National Wildlife Rehabilitator's Association	http://www.nwrawildlife.org/	Wildlife Rehabilitation Bulletin
Wildlife Disease Association	http://www.wildlifedisease.org/	Journal of Wildlife Diseases (Quarterly)

owning a pet, there will always be clients (e.g., dog, cat, horse, and exotic) who believe veterinary care is expensive and unnecessary. I will not focus on them in this chapter. Instead, I will focus on the fact that being a thorough diagnostician can be financially rewarding. Exotic animals have evolved to mask their illness to avoid predation. Therefore, to fully ascertain the status of an exotic pet requires the pursuit of diagnostic tests. A physcial examination alone will not suffice. At minimum, a database for exotic pets should include a complete blood count, plasma chemistry, urinalysis (mammals), and fecal examination. In many cases, radiographs, ultrasound, or endoscopy are also required. Veterinarians that successfully treat exotic pets are able to explain to their clients the necessity of these diagnostics for evaluating their patient's condition while, at the same time, generating income for their practice. Working with exotic pets requires more "client time" than does working with domestic pets. Often it is important to spend additional time with the client, covering husbandry and nutrition issues that would be unnecessary with a dog or cat client. Because of the additional time required to work with these animals, veterinarians should institute fees commensurate with the time allocated to the examination and consultation.

I, along with the other editor of this text, believe that the potential disadvantages associated with incorporating exotic pets into a practice are truly negligible. One of the potential disadvantages mentioned previously was the need to acquire continuing education and literature to expand the veterinarian's medical knowledge base. With the large number of available national and international continuing education opportunities (e.g., Central Veterinary Conference, Kansas City, MO; North American Veterinary Conference, Orlando, FL; Western Veterinary Conference, Las Vegas, NV) that incorporate both domestic and exotic species, the potential to obtain the necessary knowledge and hands-on laboratories to expand clinical skills in exotic pets while maintaining learning opportunities with domestic pets is great. Those interested in further expanding their opportunities to learn exotic pet medicine and remaining current on new trends and scientific

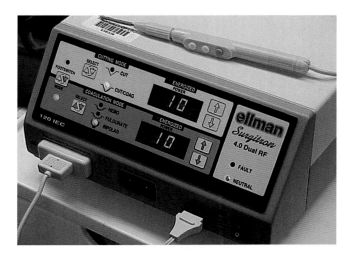

Figure 2-1 An Ellman radiosurgery unit can be used to perform surgery on exotic and domestic species. I find these units invaluable for hemostasis in all patients, regardless of size.

discovery in the field of exotic pet medicine can become members of the various exotic species professional veterinarian organizations (Table 2-1).

The argument that the inclusion of exotic pets into a practice will lead to significant expenses for equipment is not valid for high-quality small animal practices. The majority of the equipment that is used to treat and diagnose exotic pets is also invaluable for domestic cases. For example, a radiosurgery unit (Ellman International, Inc., Oceanside, NY) (Figure 2-1) is used extensively in my practice to manage hemorrhage and minimize tissue trauma for small patients. This same unit can, and in many cases should, be used by those working with domestic pets for the same inherent reasons. The VetScan (Abaxis Inc., Union City, CA) (Figure 2-2) chemistry analyzer provides the exotic animal veterinarian with the ability to analyze chemistries from 100 µL of whole blood or plasma. This is important when dealing with small patients, such as budgerigars or geckos. However, those of us who work with (or have worked with) domestic pets can certainly remember

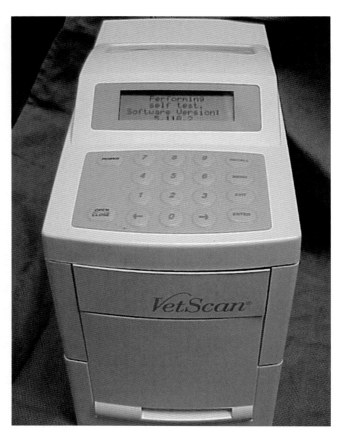

Figure 2-2 The VetScan chemistry analyzer can be used to perform whole blood or plasma chemistries on a variety of species, including both domestic and exotic species. Because of the light weight of the unit (11.2 pounds; 5.1 kg), it can easily be taken into the field to use with exotic or domestic species.

those times when no more than 100 µL of blood could be collected from a puppy or fractious cat. Again, the "proposed" expense would not only be useful for incorporating exotic pets but would simplify diagnostic testing for domestic species as well.

"If you build it, they will come" is the famous line from the 1989 movie *Field of Dreams.* Can the same be said for an exotic practice? By expanding a practice, will clients inherently come? If veterinarians promote the fact that their practices accept exotic pets to their current client base, and, their clients have both domestic and exotic pets,[1] veterinarians may realize an immediate expansion of their practices. A detailed history for domestic pets should include a question asking clients if they have other pets. This information can then be used to promote the practice's treatment of exotics. In addition to promoting exotic pets with established clients, veterinary practitioners can also pursue new clients by establishing relationships with local retailers and local specialty clubs. Pet retailers are generally the primary source of exotic animals in a community. It is worthwhile to schedule time with a local retailer to discuss the specific needs of the different exotic pets they have for sale. It also can be beneficial for the veterinarian to offer a training seminar for the pet retail employees. Provid-

ing these individuals with information about exotic pet care will help ensure that the pet retail employees make the appropriate recommendations to potential pet owners. Historically, veterinarians do not visit with a pet owner until after they have purchased the animal and the equipment. In many cases, veterinarians may have to educate the client on the incorrect purchases they made, which for many, is upsetting. A proactive approach of training pet retailers can prevent unnecessary animosity between the veterinarian and the pet retailer. By establishing a solid relationship with the pet retailer, the veterinarian can expect to receive referrals, which will expand his or her caseload and be financially rewarding.

■ DEVELOPING A KNOWLEDGE BASE

As was mentioned previously, there are numerous opportunities to obtain the knowledge required to work with exotic pets. From the standard continuing education meetings to the more specialized scientific meetings, every need can be met. Each of the professional organizations in Table 2-1 has an annual scientific meeting, which allows veterinarians to share information in both formal and informal venues. These professional organizations also publish quarterly, peer-reviewed journals that provide cutting edge information related to the specialty.

There are also learning opportunities through the Internet. Because there is a large amount of non–peer-reviewed and unregulated material on the Internet, veterinarians should be cautious and discerning. The two most accessible and useful Internet sources of information on exotic pets are the Veterinary Information Network (http://www.vin.com/) and the AVMA Network of Animal Health (http://www.avma.org/). Both of these networks provide veterinarians the opportunity to communicate with specialists in exotic pet medicine.

There is a wealth of other literature available to veterinarians too. To assume that this single text could provide all that is needed to practice exotic pet medicine would be shortsighted. This book is intended to provide its readers with a collective introduction to the numerous exotic species that may present to their practices. Veterinarians that develop a special interest should obtain additional texts that go into more depth regarding the husbandry, medicine, and surgery for a class of animals. Box 2-1 represents a list of individual texts that can provide more detail on exotic animals (by class).

Those interested in the ultimate pursuit of specialization in exotic pet medicine should consider advanced specialty training. Currently, there are two opportunities: board certification with the American Board of Veterinary Practitioners (AVBP)(Avian) and the American College of Zoological Medicine. Future certification opportunities in exotic mammal and reptile/amphibian medicine are being evaluated. There are two paths that can be followed to become board eligible: (1) Perform a residency at a certified institution, or (2) have at least 6 years of clinical practice in the field. For those interested in obtaining additional information regarding these programs,

BOX 2-1	Textbooks That Can Be Used to Further Pursue the Husbandry, Medical, or Surgical Needs of Exotic Pets by Class

Amphibians
Wright KM, Whitaker B, editors: *Amphibian Medicine and Captive Husbandry,* Malabar, Fla, 2001, Krieger, 499 pp.

Avian
Harcourt-Brown N, Chitty J, editors: *BSAVA Manual of Psittacine Birds,* ed 2, Gloucester, UK, 2005, British Small Animals Veterinary Association, 323 pp.
Tully TN, Lawton MPC, Dorrestein GM, editors: *Avian Medicine,* Boston, 2000, Butterworth-Heinemann, 411 pp.

Mammals
Harcourt-Brown F, *Textbook of Rabbit Medicine,* Boston, 2002, Butterworth-Heinemann, 436 pp.
Quesenberry KE, Carpenter JW, editors: *Ferrets, Rabbits and Rodents: Clinical Medicine and Surgery,* ed 2, St Louis, 2004, WB Saunders, 461 pp.

Ornamental Fish
Noga EJ, *Fish Disease: Diagnosis and Treatment,* Ames, 2000, Iowa State Press, 367 pp.
Stosskopf MK, editor: *Fish Medicine,* Philadelphia, 1993, WB Saunders, 882 pp.

Reptiles
Girling SJ, Raiti P, editors: *BSAVA Manual of Reptiles,* ed 2, Gloucester, UK, 2004, British Small Animal Veterinary Association, 383 pp.
Mader DR, *Reptile Medicine and Surgery,* ed 2, St Louis, 2006, WB Saunders, 1242 pp.

visit the following websites: http://www.abvp.com/ and http://www.aazv.org/.

PREPARING THE STAFF

The reception staff at a veterinary hospital is arguably the most important "face" of the hospital. Regardless of the veterinarian's reputation, an unimpressive first phone call or answer to a question can be sufficient to disuade a client from scheduling an appointment. Therefore, it is important to provide the reception staff the training necessary to guarantee their success in managing clients. The reception staff should be provided resources (e.g., veterinarian, veterinary technician, pet retailer, continuing education, and "cheat sheets") that they can use to promptly and accurately answer questions. The veterinarinan is likely the best resource but may not always be available. In those cases, an experienced veterinary technician could assist in answering any questions. When the questions are husbandry related, directing the client to a pet retailer would be appropriate. The pet retailer should be an individual with whom the

veterinary hospital has an established relationship. As mentioned previously, this type of relationship can be mutually beneficial. Regular staff meetings offer an opportunity to expand the knowledge base of the reception staff. Information from these meetings can be compiled for the staff and strategically placed near the phone for ready access.

Veterinarians are finally recognizing the true potential of employing a certified veterinary technician. A competent veterinary technician can do many of the tasks veterinarians have historically done (e.g., processing hematologic, parasitic, and radiographic diagnostic test materials), providing the veterinarian with the opportunity to address other concerns in the hospital. In many of the technician programs, exotic pet medicine is becoming available to those who are interested in the field. For many veterinary technician graduates, like veterinary graduates, experience with exotic pets can be an important consideration for prospective employers. The additional training provides the "something extra" that enables that applicant to stand out among other competent individuals. Hiring technicians with experience in exotic pet medicine can help expedite the incorporation of an exotic pet practice into a hospital.

There are now numerous continuing educational opportunities open for support staff. Many of the large continuing education meetings (e.g., Central Veterinary Conference, North American Veterinary Conference, Western Veterinary Conference) have tailored specific all-day programs for veterinary technicians, and exotic animal medicine is routinely a "track" offering. The major scientific meetings have also recognized the importance of providing training for veterinary technicians, and the meetings often have lectures and laboratories designed to meet the specific educational needs of these individuals.

PREPARING THE WAITING ROOM

Preparing a waiting room for the inclusion of exotic pets can take some forethought. First, it is important to realize that not everyone finds 6 foot (1.8 m) long boa constrictors something they want to examine up close. To ensure the comfort of all clients, it may be wise to establish two waiting rooms. If this is not possible, then scheduling appointments so that the exotic and domestic pet appointments are at different times may be useful.

By its very definition, the *waiting room* is not a place most people want to spend much time. Because people live busy lives and waiting is generally not a favorite pastime, it might be a good idea to change the name. It could be called the *educational room* or the *information room,* for example. Regardless of what the room is called, it should be set up to maximize clients' time before their pet is examined. The reception staff can initiate the educational experience by providing species-specific brochures (http://www.exoticdvm.com/index. cfm?fuseaction=books.showIcons&) that provide information regarding the client's pet. The provision of preliminary information can save the veterinarian and veterinary technician time later that otherwise would be used for client education.

The preexamination period is a good time to acquire initial historical information. Providing the client an easy-to-read and thorough history form to complete before the examination can again save time later for the veterinary staff and keep the client involved in thinking about his or her pet. The reception area should reaffirm the hospital's interest in exotic pet medicine. Information charts and appropriate exotic pet artwork can be used to generate a feeling of warmth for the client and provide additional educational information. Some veterinary hospitals will maintain live exotic pets in their waiting rooms. This can be used to reinforce the appropriate care of exotic pets. Easy-to-read signs that discuss husbandry and care of the animal can be placed around the animal's habitat. The placement of display animals reinforces that the veterinary hospital has an interest in caring for exotics and provides the veterinarian and his or her staff real-world experience in exotic pet management and husbandry. If live animals are kept in the hospital for display, it is important that the habitat be maintained to high standards.

■ NECESSARY EQUIPMENT

Most veterinary practices have the equipment (e.g., isoflurane anesthesia) needed to provide a high standard of veterinary care for exotic pets. The additional equipment that veterinarians may use will depend on the species they accept and the extent to which they plan to practice on exotic pets. If the clinician's desire is to provide basic health care and refer more complicated cases, then his or her equipment requirements will be minimal. If the clinician's desire is to offer a comprehensive exotic animal care service, then it may be necessary to acquire additional specialized equipment. The following is a general list of equipment that veterinarians practicing exotic pet medicine should consider obtaining. (For information on specific equipment recommendations for particular species, see other chapters in this book.)

Housing

Housing exotic pets in a veterinary practice is an important consideration. Many veterinary hospitals use stainless steel cages to hospitalize their dogs and cats. These cages can be used for some exotic mammal and avian patients, but they are generally less desirable for reptiles. I have used these cages for large reptiles, but had to use external heating sources to maintain an appropriate environmental temperature. Temperature-controlled incubators are a must for exotic animal practices (Figure 2-3). These incubators allow the veterinarian to hospitalize a range of exotic species, while meeting the specific environmental needs of these different animals. Environmental humidity can also be controlled in some incubators.

Diagnostics

A high-quality light microscope is an important tool to have in a veterinary hospital. Unfortunately, with the advent of national diagnostics laboratories, veterinarians have become less reliant on analyzing their own patients' samples. However,

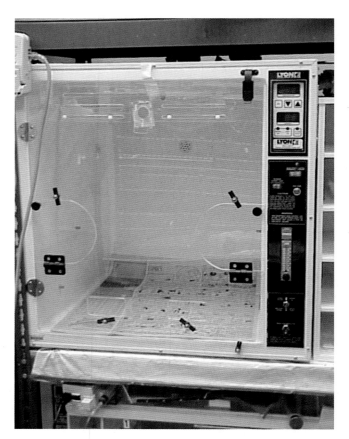

Figure 2-3 Temperature-controlled incubators can be used to provide exotic pets a thermally controlled environment.

there are certainly times when samples cannot be processed in a timely manner with a laboratory, and the clinician needs to be able to evaluate the sample. Hematologic samples provide important information regarding the health status of a patient. Veterinarians who regularly work with lower vertebrates (e.g., fish, amphibians, reptiles, and birds) and invertebrates realize that these animals have nucleated red blood cells, and to perform a complete blood count requires one of the estimation techniques (e.g., eosinophil unopette). A quality microscope capable of providing 400 to 1000 × magnification is required. The microscope can also be invaluable for interpreting fine needle aspirates, cytologic scrapings (e.g., skin scrape or gill biopsy in fish), and fecal examinations.

Biochemistry can also provide a significant amount of information regarding the health status of a patient. One of the major drawbacks for some hospitals is that their laboratory requires a sizeable volume (0.5-1.0 ml) of blood to perform a chemistry panel. The general recommendation for collecting blood from exotic species is that no more than 0.5-1.0 ml/100 grams (body weight) be collected. Based on these minimum requirements, it would be difficult to collect sufficiently sized blood samples on small psittacines (e.g., budgerigar, cockatiel), passerines (e.g., finch, canary), small reptiles (e.g., leopard gecko, Jackson chameleon), or fish to perform biochemistries. The VetScan (see Figure 2-2) is one tool that I have found useful for processing these small samples. In addition, the samples can be processed in less than 14 minutes, which is an important consideration when managing a critical case.

Radiographic imaging is a valuable diagnostic tool for the veterinarian. However, only high-quality radiographs are of any value. When considering radiographic equipment for a small and exotic animal practice, it is important to purchase equipment that can manage a range of patient sizes (e.g., canary to bullmastiff). I prefer a machine capable of a wide-ranging kVp (e.g., 40-100). Rare-earth cassettes and single-emulsion films should be used for taking radiographs of exotic animals. These films will enable the veterinarian to detect small changes in anatomy. Digital radiography is another consideration and would benefit the veterianrian when working on either exotic or domestic pets. Digital radiography enables the veterinarian to produce films quickly for interpretation, which is important when they have anesthetized patients.

Ultrasound is a diagnostic tool that has variable usage among species. For example, ultrasound has limited value for evaluating the coelomic cavity of avian species, because it is encased by the keel and ribs, whereas the same diagnostic tool can be used to readily evaluate the viscera of a reptile patient. For ultrasound to be useful, the veterinarian should pursue continuing education to fully understand the operation of the device.

Endoscopy has become an essential diagnostic tool for the exotic animal veterinarian. Both flexible and rigid endoscopes are routinely used. Rigid endoscopes (2.7 mm) are used to perform coelioscopies and cloacascopies in birds and reptiles. I have also found them to be invaluable for assisted tracheal intubation in rodents and lagomorphs. Flexible endoscopes are frequently used to assess the proximal and distal gastrointestinal tract and respiratory system. Veterinarians attempting to justify the purchase of an endoscope should also consider the many applications these tools can also provide for their domestic pet patients.

Pathology

Because exotic pets can mask their illness, many cases are presented to the veterinarian as "dead, but breathing." In those situations where the client has multiple animals, it is important to recommend having any dead animals necropsied or to sacrifice diseased animals to obtain a definitive diagnosis. There are a number of different pathology services available to the veterinarian, but not all of these services have pathologists who are competent with exotic species. There are two pathology services in the United States that have excellent track records working with exotic species: Northwest Zoopath (Monroe, WA; http://www.zoopath.com/) and Zoo/Exotic Pathology Service (West Sacramento, CA; http://www.zooexotic.com/html/who.html).

■ SURGERY

Loupes

Because many of the exotic patients we work with are small, magnifying loupes can be very helpful in characterizing small changes during an examination of blood vessels and nerves during a surgery. Basic head loupes are inexpensive and can be

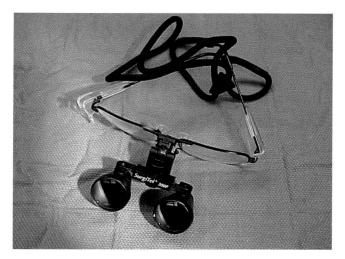

Figure 2-4 Magnification loupes can greatly enhance a veterinarian's visual field during surgery.

purchased for $30 to $50. For higher magnification, clinical magnification systems (Figure 2-4) should be used. These systems can be used with or without additional lighting. A variety of systems are available (http://www.surgitel.com/), and these systems can cost between $1,000 and $2,000. I find magnifying loupes extremely useful during surgical procedures.

Radiosurgery

When performing surgery on small patients, hemostasis is essential. What may appear as a small volume of blood in a larger animal can represent a significant blood loss in a smaller patient. For example, a 3-ml blood loss in a german shepherd would be considered unremarkable, while in a 100-g cockatiel it would represent 30% of the animal's blood volume. Radiosurgery can be used to minimize blood loss. I would recommend a dual frequency unit (http://www.ellman.com/) that enables the veterinarian to incise, incise and coagulate, and fulgurate. Again, this type of unit could also be used for domestic pet procedures (e.g., incision, mass removal).

■ THERAPEUTICS

Because of the small size of many of our exotic pet patients, it can be difficult to deliver therpeutics without significant dilution. For this reason, it is important to establish a relationship with a compounding pharmacy. A major benefit to using compounded drugs is that multiple concentrations can be created for the same drug. For example, I routinely have several concentrations of ivermectin (Merial Limited, Iselin, NJ) (stock 10 mg/ml; dilution 1 : 1 mg/ml, dilution 2 : 0.1 mg/ml) or butorphanol (Torbugesic, Fort Dodge Animal Health, Ft. Dodge, IA) (stock: 10 mg/ml, dilution 1 : 2 mg/ml, dilution 2 : 0.5 mg/ml) made to simplify dosing. The other benefit of using compounded drugs is that they can be flavored according to the animal's taste. For example, my pharmacy routinely flavors ferret compounds with meat-based flavoring agents and rabbit compounds with fruit-based flavoring agents. One potential drawback associated with compounded drugs is that the drug may not be evenly distributed throughout the carrier. To evaluate the concentration of a compounded drug, I suggest sending the medication to a private analytical laboratory for evaluation.

REFERENCE

1. Wise JK, Heathcott BL, Gonzalez ML: Results of the AVMA survey on companion animal ownership in US pet-owning households. *J Am Vet Med Assoc* 221(11):1572-1573, 2002.

Trevor Zachariah
Mark A. Mitchell

CHAPTER 3

INVERTEBRATES

Invertebrates represent the largest group of animals on Earth, with approximately 1 million species characterized to date. Additional species are being discovered all of the time, and it has been estimated that as many as 30 million invertebrates may reside on planet Earth. The diversity among invertebrates is enormous, with over 30 different phyla and myriads of subsequent taxa. Differences between the groups are so great that the only common feature among them is that, as their name implies, they do not possess a true vertebral column.

Though it is easy to overlook, invertebrates are vital not only to the natural world but also to the lives of humans. Many invertebrates play important roles in the fields of agriculture, ecology, biology, medicine, and commercial and industrial trades, to name just a few. Invertebrates have also become increasingly popular as pets and display animals in zoological collections. There are numerous reasons for this trend, including the "awe factor," relative inexpense of the animals, and their low-maintenance husbandry requirements. Because of their importance and increasing popularity, it is expected that invertebrate species will be presented to veterinarians with increased frequency. Unfortunately, like many other exotic pet species, little is known about the medical needs of these animals. To date, only a limited amount of research in this field has been published, and there is a strong need to expand the current knowledge base of invertebrate medicine. This chapter serves as an introduction to the biology and medicine of captive invertebrates.

■ COMMON SPECIES KEPT IN CAPTIVITY

The only unifying feature common to all invertebrates is an absence of a vertebral column. Both because of this fact, and the diversity of species, the taxonomy of invertebrates is dynamic. Because of the large numbers of invertebrate taxa, it is not possible to review all groups in this chapter. Instead, this chapter reviews those groups important to the captive pet trade or aquaculture.

Cnidarians

There are approximately 10,000 different species of cnidarians, and the majority of these animals are found in the marine environment. Cnidarians are classified either as polyps or medusae. The polyps include the corals (Figure 3-1), hydrae, and anemones (Figure 3-2). The medusae include the true jellyfish and the box jellyfish. Cnidarians can be found as individuals or colonies, depending on the group. Most are carnivorous, subduing and killing their prey with specialized cells called *cnidocytes* (see Anatomy and Physiology). Jellyfish are one species with cnidocytes, which also are venomous to humans.

Gastropods

There are approximately 60,000 different species of gastropods, and these animals are primarily aquatic, although terrestrial forms exist. Among the aquatic gastropods, the majority of animals are found in benthic habitats. Gastropods are the most numerous and diverse class within the phylum Mollusca and are the only group to have members that have evolved a terrestrial lifestyle (the Pulmonata). The gastropods are primarily represented by the snails (Figure 3-3) and slugs.

Arachnids

There are approximately 70,000 different species of arachnids, and more than 80% of the animals in this group are spiders

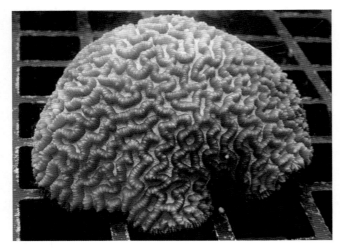

Figure 3-1 Maze brain coral (*Platygyra* sp.). These stony corals are popular in the aquarium hobby. (Photo by Trevor Zachariah.)

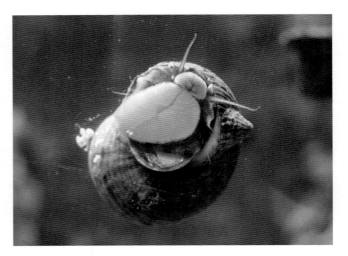

Figure 3-3 Turbo snail (*Turbo* sp.). These marine gastropods are commonly recommended for marine aquaria. In this image, note the dextral twist of the shell, the extended antennae, the oral opening between them, and the large foot. (Photo by Trevor Zachariah.)

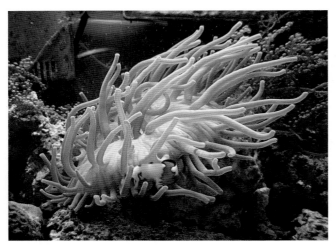

Figure 3-2 Bubble tip anemone *(Entacmaea quadricolor).* As indicated by this photo, these anemones are popular with clown fish. (Photo by Trevor Zachariah.)

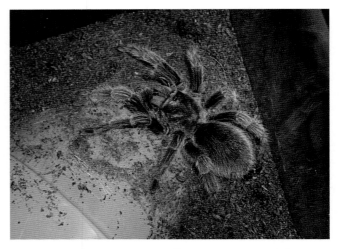

Figure 3-4 Chilean rose spider *(Grammostola rosea).* Because of its hardy and docile nature, this species of giant spider is commonly found in captivity. (Photo by Trevor Zachariah.)

and mites. The majority of arachnids (Figure 3-4) are terrestrial and carnivorous. The arachnids, like the cnidarians, may possess specialized tools (e.g., venom) to capture and kill prey. In some species (e.g., spiders and scorpions), the venom can also be harmful to humans. Certain species of arachnids, such as the mites and ticks, have evolved to live as parasites on vertebrate hosts.

Myriapods

There are approximately 13,000 different species of myriapods, all of which are terrestrial. Centipedes (≈3000 species) are from the order Chilopoda, and most of these animals are nocturnal predators. These invertebrates possess fangs, which they use to envenomate their prey or potential predators. Millipedes (≈10,000 species) are from the order Diplopoda, and

all of these animals are nocturnal detritivores (Figure 3-5). Diplopods possess more legs than any other animal. Unlike the chilopods, diplopods are secretive and prefer to hide from predators rather than challenge them. Diplopods do not pose any real danger to humans.

Insects

The insects represent the largest group of invertebrates, with over 900,000 described species. It is estimated that more than 75% of the animal species on Earth are insects. The greatest diversity among any group of living animals is seen with the insects. Most are terrestrial, but some have also developed the ability to fly. Some species of insects have developed parasitic

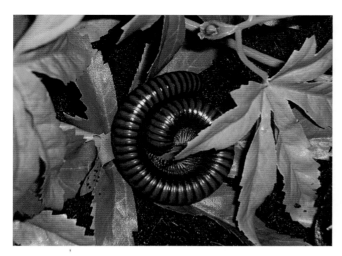

Figure 3-5 A fire millipede (*Aphistogoniulus* sp.). Millipedes of a variety of colors and sizes are available to hobbyists. (Photo by Trevor Zachariah.)

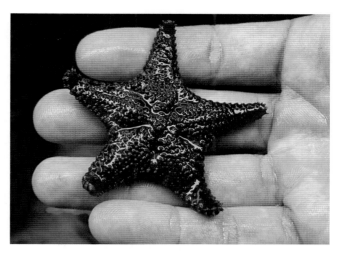

Figure 3-6 A common sea star found in the marine trade. These echinoderms remain quite popular with hobbyists. (Photo by Trevor Zachariah.)

life cycles, many of which include human involvement. Some species of insects can pose a danger to animals and humans through their defensive mechanisms (e.g., bees). Numerous species are of economic importance to humans as pests.

Crustaceans

There are approximately 42,000 different species of crustaceans, most of which are aquatic. The taxon is a diverse group, with many of the inconspicuous species playing a central role in ecologic webs. Some of the larger species are important to aquaculture.

Echinoderms

There are approximately 6,000 different species of echinoderms. Many of these animals are common to the commercial aquarium trade, including the sea stars, brittle stars, sea urchins, sand dollars, sea cucumbers, and sea lilies (Figure 3-6). All of these species are marine and benthic. The echinoderms share a five-part radial body plan, also known as *pentamerous symmetry,* and have the ability to voluntarily move connective tissue, known as *catch connective tissue* (see Anatomy and Physiology).

■ ANATOMY AND PHYSIOLOGY

Veterinarians working with any species must develop a basic understanding of the anatomy and physiology of that animal. This is no different with invertebrates. However, due to the great diversity of form and function among this large group, only a basic introduction to the anatomy and physiology of the invertebrates is presented here. For additional information, see the Suggested Readings at the end of the chapter.

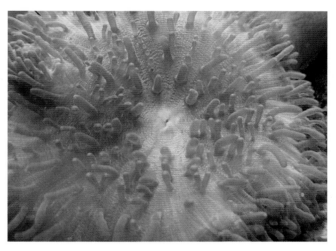

Figure 3-7 Sebae anemone (*Heteractis* sp.). In the center of the image is the slit mouth of the anemone, surrounded by a number of tentacles. (Photo by Trevor Zachariah.)

Cnidarians

Whether in the form of a polyp or medusa, all cnidarians have a basic body plan that is radially symmetric. There are two tissue layers: the epidermis, which lines the outside of the animal, and the gastrodermis, which lines the inside of the animal. These layers are separated by a nonliving layer of elastic, gelatinous material known as the *mesoglea,* which provides structure and buoyancy without metabolic cost. Tentacles ring the mouth, the single opening to the digestive system (Figure 3-7). All surface tissues perform direct gas exchange.

In the tentacles, and sometimes in the living tissue layers of the body, cnidocytes can be found. Cnidocytes contain a specialized, secreted organelle called a *cnida.* When stimulated by chemical or tactile cues, the cnidae use osmotic pressure to propel a hollow tube with great force out of the cell toward prey or predators. The tube can be used to physically subdue or inject venom into prey. The venom used in cnidae can be quite potent and may also be used for defense. Each cnida can be used only once, after which the cnidocyte must secrete a new one.

The nervous system is comprised of a web of neurons, and attached to it are sensory systems that belie the simplicity of this web. Statocysts assist with balance, ocelli sense light, and sensory lappets register tactile stimuli. Box jellies take this one step further and have complex eyes that may be capable of forming images.

The muscles of cnidarians are comprised of epitheliomuscular cells. Cnidarian muscles serve two purposes: (1) contractile functions to assist with locomotion, and (2) intracellular food digestion. The muscles are arranged in longitudinal and circular arrangements, allowing for a variety of types of movement. The most common locomotive movement for jellyfish is jet propulsion, and that is accomplished by contracting and releasing the body against the mesoglea, which acts as a spring.

The mouth opens into the coelenteron, a cavity that is lined with the gastrodermis. The coelenteron may be partitioned into pouches or canals to increase the surface area of the gastrodermis and distribute nutrients throughout the animal. Many species also harbor mutualistic algae, known as *zooxanthellae,* which provide another source of nutrition.

Cnidarians have an amazing ability to heal and regenerate. This is also reflected in the fact that asexual reproduction by budding or fission is common to cnidarians. Sexual reproduction also occurs, and most cnidarians are gonochoric. Fertilization is external and is followed by the development of a ciliated, planktonic, nonfeeding larva, known as the *planula.*

Gastropods

Many gastropod species are characterized by the presence of a shell. The shell of most species is coiled in a dextral manner (e.g., right-handed), whereas a few species possess sinistral shells (e.g., left-handed). The central axis of the shell is the *columella,* and the opening at the base of the shell is the *aperture.* The first revolution of the shell is known as the *body whorl,* and this is where most of the visceral mass of the animal resides. The remaining whorls are collectively known as the *spire,* which culminates at the peak, or *apex,* of the shell. There are also many species with reduced or nonexistent shells.

Gastropods are connected to their shells by a columellar muscle, which extends into the foot and to the operculum, if present. The foot is a mass of muscles and connective tissues, and it functions as the locomotory organ of the animal. Some species possess an operculum on the foot, which is a rigid disc that acts as a door to the aperture when the animal is retracted into its shell.

The internal anatomy of gastropods is determined by their development, which includes a 180-degree torsion of the body. This leaves the majority of the mass of the body (and the shell, in those species which possess one) atop the head and foot.

The process of torsion also causes a reduction or absence of some of the organs—ctenidia, osphradium, kidney, heart auricle—on the side corresponding to the direction of the torsion (e.g., left side for sinistral and right side for dextral).

The space within the body whorl created by the torsion process is known as the *mantle cavity.* As the name implies, the mantle cavity is lined with the tissue known as the mantle, which secretes the shell. In the terrestrial species, the mantle cavity is modified into a sac-like structure with increased vasculature and an opening called the *pneumostome.* Thus equipped, the mantle cavity functions as a primitive lung. In the aquatic species, the mantle cavity contains the *ctenidia,* or gills, adjacent to which is the *osphradium,* an organ specialized for chemoreception. The heart lies within the pericardial sac and is located within the mantle cavity. The heart is a single ventricle and supplies hemolymph to an open circulatory system. Some species possess an elongated siphon for intake of water into the mantle cavity.

Gastropods have a tubular digestive system that begins with a mouth and ends with an anus. The basic organs of the digestive tract include a buccal cavity, esophagus, stomach, intestine, and rectum. There are many variations on this theme, including a crop as part of the esophagus, a crystalline style, a gizzard, and a cecum. The crystalline style is found in the stomach of herbivorous species and provides mechanical and enzymatic assistance with digestion. The *nudibranchs,* or sea slugs, have a highly branched digestive tract. They prey upon cnidarians, and the digestive tract delivers undigested cnidocytes to the many tentacles that sprout from their bodies.

Some gastropod species possess a proboscis within which the buccal cavity resides. Within the buccal cavity is a specialized feeding organ known as the *radula.* The radula is a layer of chitinous teeth that lie over a mass of cartilage and muscle known as the *odontophore.* The odontophore supports and moves the radula, which has evolved into many different forms. In some species, the radula serves as a harpoon, whereas in others, it serves as a rasp. The function of the radula is based on the feeding mode of the gastropod. The teeth of the radula vary in number and are continually worn and replaced.

Gastropods sense the world through a variety of organs. Most gastropods have two eyes, which can be found on eyestalks or at the base of the cephalic tentacles. In a few species, the eyes may be capable of forming images; however, the majority of gastropods are able only to sense light through their eyes. Tentacles primarily serve chemoreceptive and mechanoreceptive purposes. The osphradium serves a chemoreceptive purpose. A pair of statocysts can be found in the foot and provide a sense of orientation. Also, a few species of gastropod appear to have magnetoreceptors.

Almost all gastropods reproduce sexually. Primitive gastropods are gonochoric and perform external fertilization. More evolved species, including those that are terrestrial, are hermaphroditic and rely on internal fertilization. The planktonic larval stage of gastropods is called a *veliger,* and it is characterized by a large, ciliated organ known as the *velum.* The velum is used for locomotion, food collection, and gas exchange.

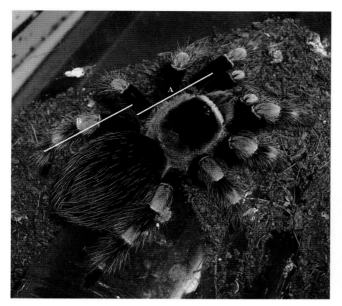

Figure 3-8 Mexican redknee spider *(Brachypelma smithi).* Line A delineates the region of the prosoma, and line B delineates the region of the opisthosoma. The pedicel is the narrowing that connects the two regions. (Photo by Trevor Zachariah.)

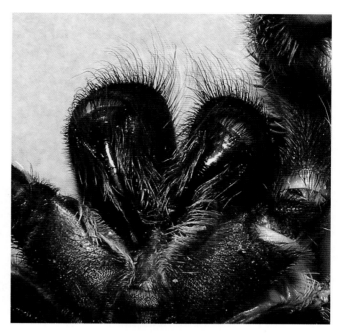

Figure 3-9 Mexican redknee spider *(Brachypelma smithi).* Note the large chelicerae and the attached fangs. The opening of the mouth is found between the bases of the chelicerae. (Photo by Trevor Zachariah.)

Arachnids

The body plan of the arachnids has two major components: the prosoma and the opisthosoma (Figure 3-8). The *prosoma* is comprised of a fused head and thorax that is covered dorsally by a carapace and ventrally by a sternal plate. The pleurae join the two and are flexible, which allows them to move relative to each other. The *opisthosoma,* or abdomen, contains the majority of the internal organs. In spiders, the prosoma and opisthosoma are joined by a narrow bridge called the *pedicel.* In scorpions, the two body segments are fused, and the opisthosoma is segmented and divided into two parts: the anterior mesosoma and the posterior metasoma, or tail. The metasoma is comprised of five to seven segments and, at its terminus, has a telson with a stinger.

Most of the appendages originate on the prosoma. The most cranial pair of appendages are called the *chelicerae.* The chelicerae help to grasp and tear prey and bear the fangs in those species that have them (Figure 3-9). After the chelicerae, the next pair of appendages are called the *pedipalps.* The pedipalps come in a variety of forms and can serve different functions. In spiders, the pedipalps are similar to the legs but lack the metatarsal segment, whereas in scorpions, they terminate with pincers. In both groups of arachnids, the pedipalps are used to grasp prey and assist with copulation. The remaining prosomal appendages are the walking legs, of which there are four pairs. Each leg has seven segments, including (proximal to distal) the coxa, trochanter, femur, patella, tibia, metatarsus, and tarsus. The distal end of each leg bears a tarsal claw and, in many species, *scopulae,* dense tufts of hair that allow the arachnid to climb. The last set of spider appendages originate on the posterior end of the opisthosoma and include the three

pairs of spinnerets. The spinnerets are variously modified to meet the needs of each species. Any of the appendages of arachnids may be autotomized, or voluntarily detached, and regenerated after several molts.

The external openings to the arachnid respiratory organs are found on the abdomen. In spiders, the small openings, or spiracles, allow air to enter the multilayered, internal book lung, so called because hemolymph and air spaces interdigitate and look like the pages of a book in cross-section. Scorpions have four pairs of book lungs, one for each anterior opisthosomal segment. Primitive spiders, like the giant spiders, or tarantulas, have two pairs of book lungs. More evolved spiders have branching, tubular tracheae, which perform gas exchange directly with the tissues. The book lungs are the site of gas exchange. Hemolymph is circulated throughout the body of arachnids by an open circulatory system. The heart is located on the dorsal midline of the opisthosoma, surrounded by a pericardium, and connected to an open-ended arterial system. The movement of hemolymph throughout the body is achieved by a combination of pressure and suction from the heart and its sac. Hemolymph is light blue in color due to the oxygen-carrying molecule *hemocyanin,* which contains two copper atoms rather than iron as in the hemoglobin of mammals.

The opisthosoma also contains the majority of the digestive system. This includes the extensive diverticula of the midgut where most of digestion takes place. Also in the opisthosoma are the Malpighian tubules and stercoral pocket, which are involved in excretory processes. The gonads and silk glands are also present in the abdomen.

The prosoma contains the anterior portion of the digestive tract, including the diverticula of the midgut, which extend through the pedicel; the sucking stomach; and the mouth, which is just posterior and ventral to the chelicerae. A pair of venom glands are also found in the prosoma of spiders. These glands are under voluntary control and are connected directly to the fangs. The prosoma is highly muscular and contains pseudoskeletal, cartilage-like structures called *endosternites,* which serve to anchor the muscles. The prosomal muscles maintain hemolymph pressure by contracting and relaxing the carapace and sternal plate, which in turn allows for extension of the appendages.

Sensory perception in arachnids is achieved through a number of specialized organs. Spiders are covered in different types of hairs that allow for sensing of tactile, seismic, and chemical stimuli. Scorpions possess paired *pectines,* which are paired comb-like organs used to detect chemical and seismic stimuli. The pectines are located caudal to the last pair of legs.[1] Both spiders and scorpions possess eyes, although the number (up to 12) varies. The visual acuity of arachnids can also vary among species. It is generally believed that giant spiders have poor vision, whereas jumping spiders (family Salticidae) can make well-developed images.

In many of the New World giant spiders, hairs are used as a defense mechanism. *Urticating hairs,* located on the opisthosoma, are small, barbed structures that can be discharged to ward off a threat. Giant spiders use their caudal pair of legs to rapidly kick these hairs into the air. When the urticating hairs settle on the body surfaces of a potential predator, they cause severe irritation. Individual spiders may have more than 1 million urticating hairs on their abdomen, at a density of approximately 10,000 hairs per square millimeter.[2] The urticating hairs are replaced after each successive molt.

Arachnids reproduce by internal fertilization; however, because of their predatory nature, copulation can be somewhat dangerous. Female spiders produce egg sacs, whereas female scorpions gestate their eggs internally and are ovoviviparous. Maternal care is rare among spiders, whereas scorpions invest significant energy into caring for their young. Female scorpions carry their newly delivered young on their dorsum to reduce predation.

The life span of some scorpion species may reach 25 years.[3] The most common species kept in captivity, the African emperor scorpion *(Pandinus imperator),* has a life span of 3 to 8 years.[1] Male giant spiders live only a short time after reaching sexual maturity and have a life span of 6 to 18 months, on average.[4] Female giant spiders, however, live significantly longer, with anecdotal reports of individuals surpassing 30 years of age. With proper captive care, it would not be uncommon for female giant spiders to live in excess of 20 years.

Myriapods

The myriapod body plan is elongated and composed of numerous segments (Figure 3-10). Each segment, except for the head and anal segments, bears either one (centipedes) or two (millipedes) pairs of legs, although the first few segments in milli-

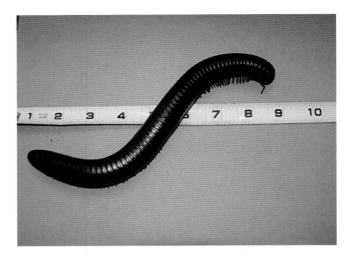

Figure 3-10 Giant African black millipede *(Archispirostreptus gigas).* Note the large size and long, tubular body form. (Photo by Trevor Zachariah.)

pedes bear only one pair of legs. Despite their names, centipedes and millipedes do not have 100 and 1000 legs, respectively. In actuality, these animals generally have 40-60 and 150-200 legs, respectively. Most of the body mass of the myriapod consists of the trunk. Millipedes are cylindrical in shape, with a hard, calcified exoskeleton. Centipedes are dorsoventrally flattened, with no waxy outer cuticle layer. Centipedes are built for speed when catching prey, whereas millipedes are slow and built for powerful digging.

Besides the legs, myriapods have other appendages that are important for their survival. A pair of antennae are located on the head and the jaws, providing sensory input. Centipedes also possess a pair of forcipules on the first body segment, which are essentially venomous fangs used for acquiring prey. On the anal segment of centipedes is a pair of anal legs. These structures can have various functions, including tactile, defense, and aggression, depending on the species.[3]

The digestive system in all myriapods is long and tubular. Centipedes have a pharynx and esophagus that represent the majority of the gut length, whereas the millipede gut consists primarily of midgut. Millipedes have salivary glands associated with the oral cavity, whereas centipedes have a variety of glands associated with the pharynx and esophagus.[3] The paired Malpighian tubules serve as the primary excretory organs. Millipedes have a layer of tissue that surrounds the midgut that has both energy storage (e.g., glycogen) and detoxification properties.[3]

The heart is a tubular organ that lies dorsally along the length of the trunk. Ostia act to move blood in and out of the heart. The dorsal pericardial sinus is formed by a horizontal membrane, as is the ventral perineural sinus. The perivisceral sinus is located in the middle of these other sinuses.[3] Myriapods have an open circulatory system.

In myriapods, gas exchange occurs via tubular trachea that delivers oxygen directly to the tissues. The trachae open to the environment through spiracles in the exoskeleton. In most species, the spiracles cannot be closed, which greatly hampers water conservation and results in the necessity of maintaining a humid, moist environment. The spiracles are located ventrally in millipedes and laterally in centipedes.

Sensory structures in myriapods consist mainly of the eyespots and antennae. The eyespots consist of a varying number of *ommatidia* (individual sensory units), depending on the species. In most myriapod taxa, the ommatidia are not clustered in densities high enough to form a true compound eye, such as is found in insects.[3] Myriapods are not believed to be capable of forming images. Instead, it has been suggested that these animals are limited to sensing light and movement.[3] The antennae are able to sense both tactile and chemical stimuli.

Myriapods are gonochoric and practice internal fertilization. In general, female centipedes are protective of their egg masses until the young hatch and disperse.[3] Centipedes generally have a life span of 4 to 6 years; millipedes live for 1 to 10 years.[3]

Insects

The diversity of insect morphological forms is astonishing. However, all the forms are derived from modifications of a basic plan. For purposes of brevity, those important to captive insects will be presented.

The insect body is divided into three body sections: the head, thorax, and abdomen. The head bears a single pair of dorsal antennae, a variable number of ocelli, a single pair of compound eyes, and the ventral mouthparts. The mouthparts are modified to reflect the feeding strategy of the taxa. For example, sucking mouthparts are found on moths and butterflies (order Lepidoptera); piercing and sucking mouthparts on aphids, cicadas, and assassin bugs (order Hemiptera); cutting and sponging mouthparts on flies (order Diptera); and chewing and sucking mouthparts on bees and wasps (order Hymenoptera).[3]

The insect thorax bears three pairs of legs and one or two pairs of wings. The legs each have six segments, including the coxae, trochanter, femur, tibia, tarsus, and pretarsus. Each leg ends in a pair of tarsal claws. The wings of an insect can be modified, even into different structures. Two extreme examples of this include the beetles (order Coleoptera), in which the cranial pair are hardened elytra (e.g., wing covers), and the flies (order Diptera), in which the caudal pair are reduced to gyroscopic halteres to aid in flight.

The abdomen of insects is segmented and relatively devoid of appendages. A terminal pair of cerci are usually present as are, in some species, external genitalia.[3] The abdomen is often the largest of the three basic body segments and houses the majority of the viscera.

The digestive system of insects is divided into three regions: the foregut, midgut, and hindgut. The foregut consists of the mouth, pharynx, esophagus, crop, and proventriculus. The midgut is the primary site for food digestion. Attached to the anterior end of the midgut are two to six ceca.[3] The hindgut is comprised of the intestine, rectum, and anus. A variable

number of Malpighian tubules (e.g., 2 to 250, depending on the taxon) are attached to the anterior end of the hindgut.[3] The hindgut serves as the major excretory center in the insect body and resorbs most of the water from the digestive system.

The circulatory system of insects is open, and the tubular, ostiate heart is found in the dorsal abdomen. The aorta extends cranially from the heart and is the only hemolymph vessel. An accessory heart is present at the base of most appendages, and facilitates the delivery of hemolymph to the tissues.

Oxygen is delivered directly to the tissues by tubular trachae, in a fashion that is similar to that of myriapods and some arachnids. Spiracles are found on the thorax and abdomen, but not on the head.[3] Unlike the spiracles of myriapods, those of most insects can be closed to prevent loss of moisture or water.

In insects, the perception of multiple types of sensory stimuli is performed by *sensilla,* or hair-like receptors. These structures are found all over the body, although the majority are found on the appendages.[3] Chemical, tactile, temperature, and humidity receptors are found on the antennae and tarsi. The abdominal cerci contain tactile and seismic receptors. The ocelli are used to detect changes in light intensity and aid in orientation.[3] Visual stimuli are detected by the compound eye, and each of the ommatidia has its own lens. Thus, contrary to popular misconception, the insect brain, similar to the brain of vertebrates, integrates the information from each ommatidium to form a mosaic image.[3] Many insects also have tympanic organs for the detection of sound.

Insects are gonochoric and practice internal fertilization. There are three types of development among the insects. Hemimetabolous development involves juveniles called *nymphs,* which are dissimilar from adults, are aquatic, and grow and molt until reaching a final molt into the adult form. Paurometabolous development involves juveniles that are also called nymphs; however, these are similar to adults and grow and molt into the adult form. Holometabolous development (e.g., metamorphosis) involves juveniles called *larvae,* which grow and molt until forming a pupa, from which the adult form emerges. Holometabolous development is a successful life strategy, as approximately 80% of insects (e.g., approximately 740,000 species) utilize it.[3]

Crustaceans

The crustaceans, like the insects, represent a diverse group of animals, with variable body forms. One of the most commonly recognized forms, the order Decapoda (e.g., crabs, lobsters, crayfish, and shrimps), will be described here (Figure 3-11).

The crustacean body is comprised of two sections: the head and trunk. The head is small relative to the trunk and, along with the anterior of the trunk, is covered by a carapace. Five pairs of appendages adorn the head: two pairs of antennae, a pair of mandibles, and two pairs of maxillae. The maxillae assist with feeding. The head also bears one pair of compound eyes that are located on movable stalks.

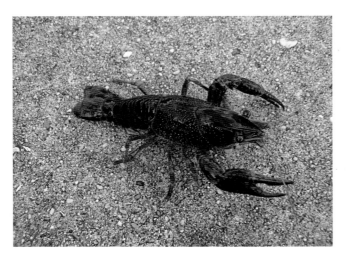

Figure 3-11 Louisiana red swamp crawfish *(Procambarus clarkii).* This species is a typical decapod crustacean. *P. clarkii* are farmed extensively for human consumption. (Photo by Trevor Zachariah.)

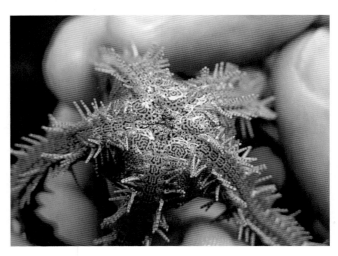

Figure 3-12 Bubble tip brittle star (*Ophiarachna* sp.). This is a view of the oral side of the central disc of a brittle star. In the center of the image is the opening of the mouth. (Photo by Trevor Zachariah.)

The anterior section of the trunk bears eight pairs of appendages. The anterior three appendages, or *maxillipeds,* assist with feeding, while the posterior five, *pereopods,* are used for walking. There are seven segments of the pereopods, including the coxae, basis, ischium, merus, carpus, propodus, and dactyl. In many species (e.g., crabs, lobsters, and crayfish), the first pereopod is modified into an enlarged cheliped or pincer that is used for defense, food acquisition, and courtship. Limb autotomy is a common occurrence in decapods and most often occurs as a result of combat with conspecifics or in defense against predators. The limbs regenerate with later molts.

The posterior of the trunk is comprised of a variable number of segments, depending on the taxon. The terminal end of the trunk bears a telson and paired uropods, and together, these form a tail fan. The tail fan helps to create the backward thrust of shrimp, crayfish, and lobsters. The five pairs of appendages arising from the posterior trunk are the pleopods. The pleopods are biramous and may be modified to serve a variety of functions, including swimming, burrowing, creating ventilating or feeding currents, brooding eggs, gas exchange, and copulating.[3] In crabs, the posterior abdomen and pleopods are reduced and found ventral to the carapace.

The digestive system begins with the cranial mouth and leads into a two-chambered stomach. In the stomach, both mechanical and chemical digestion of food occurs. Absorption of food occurs in the ceca, which are connected near the junction of the stomach and intestine. The intestine follows the length of the abdomen and terminates at an anus in the telson.

Decapods have a compact, ostiate heart. This organ is located dorsally under the carapace. The heart is connected to a system of arteries (seven main arteries leave the heart), capillaries, and venous sinuses.[3] Hemolymph is transferred through the circulatory system to the gills for oxygenation. The gills, of which they may have up to 24 pairs, are also responsible for

excreting nitrogenous wastes.[3] Ion balance in crustaceans is maintained primarily by the antennal glands (e.g., green glands), which are located in the cranial aspect of the head. Urine is created and stored in a bladder that opens near the base of the ventral pair of antennae.

Sensory perception in crustaceans is accomplished by the eyes, antennae, and appendages. The stalked eyes are somewhat mobile, and some crustaceans may be able to detect color.[3] *Setae* (hair-like receptors) are capable of detecting chemical stimuli and are primarily found on the antennae and appendages. *Aesthetascs,* or collections of setae, are located on the dorsal pair of antennae. *Statocysts* are found at the base of the dorsal antennae and assist with orientation. In some crustaceans, statocysts may also be found on other appendages.[3]

Crustaceans are primarily gonochoric, with a few (hermaphroditic) exceptions. Internal or external fertilization is possible, depending on the taxon. In most decapod species, females carry the eggs until they hatch. The egg masses are held on the ventrum by the pleopods. Decapods go through an indirect development, and there can be a number of larval stages. Other crustacean taxa may have direct or indirect development.

Echinoderms

The body plan of echinoderms follows pentamerous symmetry. Though a type of radial symmetry, the echinoderms are not closely related to the cnidarians. Pentamerous symmetry is based on a central axis around which five body regions aggregate. The body surfaces are described as oral and aboral (Figure 3-12). Sea cucumbers (class Holothuroidea) maintain pentamerous symmetry in an elongated body form, with the ends of the animals being described as oral and aboral.

Besides their recognizable body forms, another unique feature of echinoderms is the water-vascular system (WVS). The basic anatomy of this system starts with a *madreporite,* an eccentric, porous opening that is found on the aboral surface of sea stars and urchins and on the oral surface of brittle stars. The madreporite opens into a stone canal, which then leads to a circumoral ring canal. Leading perpendicularly from the ring canal are the radial canals and blind sacs known as *polian vesicles.* The radial canals reach into the arms of sea and brittle stars and along the inside to the aboral surface in sea urchins and cucumbers.[5] Multiple lateral canals direct water from the radial canals to ampullae, each of which is attached to a tube foot. The ampullae are used in a manner that is similar to the bulb of a turkey baster, increasing pressure to extend the tube feet and decreasing pressure to contract them. The function of the polian vesicles has not been fully determined, but it may serve in aiding maintenance of fluid pressures within the WVS.

The madreporite and stone canal function to maintain fluid pressure within the WVS. The stone canal is supported by calcareous ossicles and is lined with cilia, which beat to create water flow. The fluid within the WVS is essentially seawater, with increased cellular, protein, and potassium concentrations.[3,5]

The body wall of echinoderms is comprised of regions called *ambulacral* areas and *interambulacral* areas. Ambulacral areas represent those regions that bear the tube feet. These two types of areas generally alternate around the oral-aboral axis of sea urchins and cucumbers, whereas only ambulacral areas are found on the oral side of the arms of sea and brittle stars. The exoskeleton of echinoderms contains numerous ossicles, comprised of calcite microcrystals, embedded in the dermis. Ossicle structure can vary at the species level and is often a trait used to identify echinoderms. Some ossicles are modified for specific purposes, such as the paxillae of burrowing sea stars. In these animals, the ossicles form a protective shield for the aboral surface. *Pedicellariae* are specialized ossicles that occur on many different echinoderms. Pedicellariae are stalked or sessile ossicles that have a set of jaws and are used for defensive purposes. Sometimes these pedicellariae are equipped with poison glands (see Human Health Hazards).

Another unique feature of echinoderm anatomy is catch connective tissue. This tissue is mutable, which allows these animals to vary the rigidity of their bodies at will. The stiffness or softness of the dermis is due to the extracellular matrix, in which nerves have been found to terminate.[3] Research has found that calcium ion concentrations vary proportionally to the rigidity of the tissues.[3]

■ HUSBANDRY

Because of the enormity of invertebrate species, it is not possible to cover all of the husbandry needs of these animals in a single chapter. Instead, we will give a short review of the husbandry needs of the most common species; for a more detailed review, see Lewbart.[6] In considering the captive

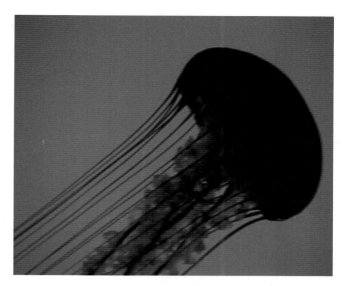

Figure 3-13 Cnidarians are dependent on constant circulating water flow. If these animals are placed into an inappropriate system they can be damaged. (Photo by Mark A. Mitchell)

care of an invertebrate, it is best to have some background knowledge of the particular species' natural history. Even though there is relatively little known about the needs of the myriad species of invertebrates, it is best to try to mimic the natural environment and diet as much as possible. Many times, it is best to maintain a simplistic approach, as more advanced attempts at maintaining these animals may have negative results.

Cnidarians

As with most aquatic species, water quality is the most important factor associated with the successful management of cnidarians in captivity. Stoskopf[7] recommends the following guidelines: ammonia levels less than 0.1 ppm, nitrite levels less than 1 ppm, nitrate levels less than 10 ppm, dissolved organic matter levels between 0.5 and 3.0 ppm, undetectable phosphate levels, calcium levels between 400 and 450 ppm for corals, pH between 8.2 and 8.4, alkalinity between 3.2 and 4.5 mEq/L, and a specific gravity (as a surrogate measure for salinity) around 1.025 to 1.027. Trace elements are another important consideration, and these animals depend on the water to provide these essential nutrients. Unfortunately, little is known regarding the specific needs of these animals, so attempts should be made to mimic natural levels of trace elements based on the natural body of water from which these animals are derived.

Water motion is particularly important for cnidarian species (Figure 3-13). Cnidarians are generally classified as being either mobile or sessile. Water motion is essential for both groups because it facilitates nutrient gathering and oxygenation. For mobile species, water motion is important also for transporting the organisms.[7] Because sessile species cannot move away from their wastes or accumulated organics, water motion serves to disperse potential toxicants. Cnidarians exposed to excessive water motion can be injured. The force of the water movement can push cnidarians into the walls of the aquarium or other fixed objects within the aquarium.[7] Even sessile cnidarians can be injured by excessive water movement, as the fixed organisms are battered by the substrate. Water motion can be provided by way of a power head, airstone, or wave maker. Water motion is generally measured in gallons of water moved per hour. Determining the most appropriate flow rate depends on aquarium size and volume. The authors generally look at the movement of the cnidarians in the aquarium to determine what is best. If the cnidarians appear to be moving too quickly or are being battered against the aquarium or substrate, then the flow rate should be reduced.

Due to their diversity, the cnidarians as a group are well adapted to a variety of temperature ranges; however, individual species may have a relatively narrow tolerance for temperature changes.[7] As a general guideline, tropical anemones and corals should be kept between 20° and 31° C (68°-87.8° F), with an optimal temperature being around 24° C (75.2° F).[7] For temperate species, a temperature range of 20° to 24° C (68°-75.2° F) is considered more appropriate.[7] Thermostatically controlled aquarium heaters are the best method to provide an appropriate temperature range within an enclosure. In larger aquaria, multiple heaters may be required to establish an appropriate temperature range. Thermometers should be placed in different areas of the aquarium to monitor temperature.

Many cnidarians derive a significant amount of their nutrients, sometimes up to 90%, from symbiotic algae (e.g., zoochlorellae or zooxanthellae) that are embedded in their tissues.[3] The loss of these organisms, due to improper lighting or water quality conditions, can be devastating for a cnidarian. Full spectral lighting that mimics the sun is considered ideal. The light should provide ultraviolet and visible light. Stoskopf[7] recommends photosynthetically active radiation (e.g., 400-700 nm) with more flux density between 400 and 550 nm than between 650 and 700 nm. The lighting should be maintained close to the water surface (<6 cm) to maximize its value.

In some cases, high-intensity lighting can overheat the water, and the lighting positioning may need to be altered. Certain components of full-spectrum lighting, such as ultraviolet radiation, are lost within the upper surface of the water. The photoperiod for cnidarians should be set on a 12-hour cycle. If animals are to be reproduced, the day may need to be lengthened (13-14 hours) for some animals. The intensity and diversity of light provided should be based on the cnidarians' natural position in an aquatic system. For example, animals found in deep-water benthic systems need less intense lighting than those found in shallow coral reef systems. Individuals working with potent full-spectrum lights should wear appropriate protective eyewear and minimize direct skin exposure to reduce the likelihood of developing secondary health problems.

The diet of cnidarians varies with the species of interest. In general, cnidarians are fed on a weekly basis.

Gastropods

Gastropods represent another diverse group of organisms. To simplify the captive care of these animals, it is best to separate them into one of two categories: aquatic or terrestrial. It is important to identify into which group a particular species fits to ensure that they are provided the most appropriate captive conditions.

Aquatic species of gastropods exhibit a great diversity in size, shape, and habits, but most can be kept by following the same basic husbandry practices used for other aquatic animals. The most important aspect of husbandry for aquatic gastropods is the water environment in which they live. The water parameters important to these animals are the same as those for other invertebrates and fish—that is, ammonia, nitrite, nitrate, pH, hardness, alkalinity, and temperature. Gastropods should be maintained in systems that have less than 0.1 ppm ammonia, less than 0.1 ppm nitrite, less than 10 ppm nitrate, a neutral pH, and moderate alkalinity and hardness. Hardness can be especially important to developing gastropods, as this is an important source of calcium and magnesium. The water temperature of an aquatic gastropod aquarium should be based on the animal's natural climate. Temperate species are more tolerant of temperature fluctuation (e.g., seasonal) and may require a reduction in temperature for aestivation. Most gastropods can derive sufficient oxygen from a nonaerated aquarium; however, aeration may be needed in systems with mixed species (e.g., gastropods and fish) when animal densities are high. Live plants may serve as an important substrate for some aquatic gastropods, especially for those species that lay their eggs on plant leaves.

Aquatic gastropods are generally opportunistic feeders. Most species will consume both animal and plant material. A number of species are detritivore specialists, which endears them to aquarists, whereas others are plant specialists and are not well liked. Invertebrate zoology or gastropod biology texts can provide specific foodstuff recommendations for particular species. Vegetable material, such as romaine lettuce, squash, and zucchini, or animal material (e.g., frozen-thawed silversides) are appropriate offerings.

Gastropods spend the majority of their time in contact with a fixed surface. Because of this, any substrate (surface) in an enclosure should be kept clean. Flat surfaces, both horizontal and vertical, are preferred for gastropod vivaria because they do not impede the movement of the animals. These surfaces are also easier to clean.

Terrestrial species are easily kept in terraria of different sizes; however, vertical enclosures are preferable for arboreal species and horizontal cages for terrestrial species. A moist substrate, such as damp sphagnum moss, should be used to provide moisture and will help to maintain a relatively high humidity level in the enclosure. The substrate should be changed periodically to reduce the likelihood of opportunistic pathogens. Gastropods left on "dirty" substrate are more prone to dermatitis and shell lesions. The frequency of substrate changes will depend on the number of animals, size of the vivarium, and frequency and types of food offered. Cork bark can be placed in the enclosure to provide hiding places for the animals. Because of gastropods' ability to climb perpendicular surfaces, a tight-fitting, solid lid is recommended (e.g., glass top). This will also help to maintain the high humidity level. Although humidity is important, it is just as important that the air in the enclosure does not become stagnant. Stagnant air can lead to the overgrowth of certain pathogens that can affect gastropods. Gastropods are most comfortable and active with low-intensity lighting. Temperature requirements will vary depending on species; for some species, temperatures exceeding 23° C (73.4° F) should be avoided.[8] Again, knowledge of where an animal originates can help a veterinarian determine the most appropriate temperature range.

The nutritional requirements for most terrestrial gastropods can be met by offering fresh fruits and dark green, leafy vegetables. These items can be fed to gastropods even if they have slightly passed their expiration point for human consumption; however, these food sources can be contaminated with opportunistic pathogens and should be offered only if the food is properly washed. Terrestrial gastropod diets can be supplemented with limited amounts of dry dog food, as well. Captive animals should be offered food ad lib, as these animals can consume large amounts of food on a regular basis.

Arachnids

The size of an enclosure for a giant spider does not need to be expansive, as most species are not large in size or extremely active. Also, they should not be kept communally, because cannibalism is possible. A 35.6 cm × 25.4 cm × 25.4 cm (14″ × 10″ × 10″) glass container can be used as a basic enclosure and provides ample space for all but the adults of the largest species of giant spiders (e.g., *Theraphosa blondi, Lasiodora parahybana, Pseudotheraphosa apophysis*). In addition to glass tanks, plastic storage containers, large plastic or glass bottles, and glass or plastic fish bowls can be used. A distinction can be made between arboreal and terrestrial species of giant spiders. With terrestrial species, care must be taken to keep the height of the enclosure to a minimum. All spiders are capable of climbing vertical glass and plastic surfaces and can suffer life-threatening injuries from short falls (see Common Disease Presentations). Arboreal species, however, should be provided an enclosure with a high vertical-to-horizontal ratio (e.g., 3 : 1) (Figure 3-14).

In many cases, the size of the enclosure should be commensurate with the size of the animal. This is especially true for young animals (e.g., breeders often sell spiderlings of approximately 1 cm in length), which could easily become lost in a large terrarium. If an enclosure is capable of accommodating substrate and the appropriate accessories, then it should be adequate in size.

Whatever type of enclosure is used, a secure lid is essential to prevent escape. A missing spider of considerable size can prove to be an uncomfortable situation! Many of the glass tanks and plastic containers made specifically for pets have appropriate lids and locking mechanisms. Other types of enclosures need to have their lids weighted down or specifically

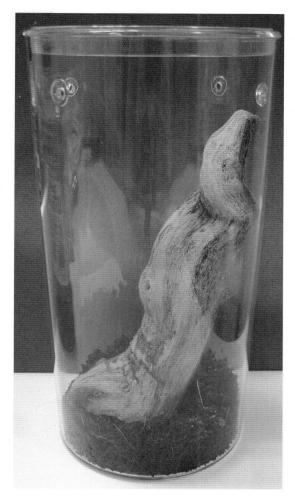

Figure 3-14 Basic arboreal spider habitat. Note the large vertical-to-horizontal ratio. (Photo by Trevor Zachariah.)

constructed for them. The lid should be safe for the animal contained within the enclosure (e.g., giant spiders can injure themselves by catching their claws in the wire junctions of woven screen mesh).

Temperature and humidity are important factors to consider in caring for giant spiders. Again, some knowledge of the animals' natural habitat is important. Enclosures should be monitored with a thermometer and hygrometer on a regular basis. Optimal temperature ranges vary; however, most fall between 21.1° and 32.2° C (70°-90° F). Therefore, most species can be maintained at ambient room temperature, with few exceptions. Most direct heating methods (e.g., under-tank heaters and heat lamps) are not needed and can reduce humidity levels to life-threatening levels.

For giant spiders, humidity must be closely regulated, even more so than temperature. Excessive humidity can lead to potentially harmful fungal and pest infestations within an enclosure. Insufficient humidity can lead to desiccation and dehydration. There are several ways to regulate humidity: change (1) the moisture in the substrate (e.g., higher water-to-substrate ratio), (2) the size of the water dish, or (3) the amount of ventilation of the enclosure. To increase humidity, the substrate moisture and the water dish size should be increased, while the amount of ventilation is decreased. To reduce the humidity within an enclosure, the opposite should be done. Lightly misting the enclosure with lukewarm water (24.4°-26.7° C, 76°-80° F) can also be done to increase humidity. For large vivaria, live plants can be used to increase humidity. For giant spiders, a general rule is that tropical species require 70% to 100% humidity, desert species 40% to 60% humidity, and temperate species 50% to 70% humidity.[9,10]

Giant spiders can vary in their daily periods of activity, and no broad generalizations can be made for this group. For most species of giant spider it is not known whether the animal is diurnal, nocturnal, or crepuscular; however, it is known that all species appear to be extremely averse to bright light.[10] For this reason, giant spiders should not be kept under a direct light source. Also, as stated earlier, direct light sources (e.g., incandescent bulbs) can desiccate an enclosure and its resident. Direct sunlight has the same effect and should be avoided. Low or ambient lighting works well for most species, and a 10- to 12-hour photoperiod is recommended.

There are a variety of substrates available, either commercially or naturally, for use in giant spider enclosures. Organic materials are usually preferred. Examples include topsoil, potting soil, peat moss, sphagnum mass, bark or mulch (except pine or cedar), ground coconut hull, and leaf litter. All of these substrates are good at enhancing humidity levels in an enclosure, but they are also prone to supporting fungal and pest infestations.[9-11] To reduce the likelihood of opportunistic infestations, the material should be dry or only slightly damp.

Nonorganic materials are also popular substrates for giant spiders. Examples include vermiculite, aquarium gravel, artificial turf, and sand. Compared to organic substrates, these materials are not as efficient at maintaining humidity. Sand and aquarium gravel are not recommended, as they can abrade the exoskeleton of a giant spider and provide unstable footing. Many of these nonorganic substrates can be mixed in various ratios to provide an appropriate environment. For burrowing species, the substrate should be packed well and be coarse enough that the risk of burrow collapse is minimized. For giant spiders, Marshall[9] recommends a substrate depth of 8 to 20 cm for terrestrial species and 2.5 cm for arboreal species. Substrates that are strongly contraindicated include cat litter (too dusty), carpet (potential injury from snagging), newspaper (pest and fungal problems), and wood chips (pest and fungal problems, pine and cedar toxicity).[10,11]

Accessories added to a giant spider enclosure can be essential for mimicking the animal's natural habitat and thus behavior, or can be used for decorative purposes. An essential addition for most species is a shelter of some kind. Types of materials that make good shelters include a flower pot on its side, a flat rock, a sturdy piece of driftwood, cork bark, a real or plastic log, a paper towel tube, an egg crate, or a plastic or live plant. Arboreal species need materials upon which they can climb. Terrestrial species will often dig their own shelter or adopt and modify materials to suit their needs.

Live plants are not essential components to making a vivarium. Although they add a decorative touch, they are not needed to properly maintain most species. Plastic plants can be used and are easier than live plants to disinfect. Live plants used in a giant spider vivarium must be relatively small in size and able to tolerate low light levels. Cacti, or plants with spines or sharp edges, should be avoided because they can be injurious to the spider.[9] Marshall[11] recommends snake plants (*Sansevieria* spp.), bromeliads (*Cryptanthus* spp.), peperomias (*Peperomia* spp.), and climbing plants (e.g., philodendrons (*Philodendron* spp.) or pothos (*Epipremnum* spp.) for giant spider enclosures.

Giant spider enclosures need to be cleaned and disinfected on a regular basis. The frequency of cleaning will depend on the amount of waste produced by the animal, the quantity of leftover prey, and the type of substrate used. Remaining food items should be removed after each feeding. A thorough cleaning is recommended if there is a visual buildup of waste material or whenever an animal molts. Dilute dishwashing detergent or bleach (0.2%-0.5%) can be used to disinfect an enclosure. The enclosure and all accessories should be thoroughly cleaned and rinsed before replacing the spider.

Crickets are the most common prey item offered to giant spiders.[11] Although crickets do not provide a balanced diet for vertebrates (e.g., inadequate calcium), they appear adequate for invertebrates. However, a varied diet comprised of different invertebrate and vertebrate prey species is still considered more appropriate.[9] Cockroaches, grasshoppers, mealworms, superworms, kingworms, wax moth larvae, earthworms, and neonatal mice may be used to vary the diet.[8,12] Small lizards, crayfish, goldfish, and raw meat have also been given to giant spiders but are less common and generally not recommended.[10] Captive-reared prey is preferred over wild-caught prey. Wild-caught prey can serve as a source of toxin exposure or infectious disease.[13] All prey items should be offered a high-quality diet before being offered to the spider. If the prey items are not promptly fed to the spider, they will be of limited nutritional value.

Many giant spider species are stimulated by movement of their prey, so it is usually best to feed live prey items when appropriate. Exceptions to this include vertebrate prey that may injure the spiders. When live prey items are offered, they should be monitored carefully to ensure that they do not harm the spider. This is especially true during the molting process, when the exoskeleton is more fragile; a giant spider should never be fed during a molt. Prey of appropriate size should be offered. A good rule of thumb to follow for spiders is that the prey should be no larger that the spider's opisthosoma,[10] or one third to one fourth the length of its body.[12] If any prey is left uneaten after 24 hours, it should be removed. The quantity of food offered to a giant spider should be based on the dietary habits of the particular species, its life stage, and the environmental conditions. For example, adult giant spiders should be fed on a weekly[9,12] or, at a minimum, monthly basis,[10] whereas spiderlings should be fed every 2 days.[12]

Water should always be made available to giant spiders, as they will actively drink water. Open water dishes should be

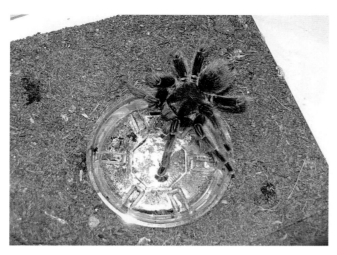

Figure 3-15 Haitian brown spider *(Phormictopus cancerides)*. This spider is drinking water. Note the position of the dish, the top of which is level with the surface of the substrate. The spider is able to tilt its mouthparts down to the water. (Photo by Trevor Zachariah.)

provided, though the depth should be limited to prevent drowning. Some sources recommend placing a soaked sponge or cotton in the water dish; however, this is not considered hygienic and can serve as a source of opportunistic bacterial infections for the spider.[10,13] For giant spiders, the water dish must be positioned so that the animal can tilt its mouthparts down to the surface (Figure 3-15).[8,10] The water dish should be cleaned and refilled regularly, or as often as it is soiled.

Scorpions can be kept in a manner similar to giant spiders, though most common captive species are adapted to desert conditions and the humidity can be maintained at a relatively low level (40%-60%). Although they are not quite as adept at climbing as spiders, scorpions can use their tail as a prop, so the sides of an enclosure should be kept smooth and relatively tall. The recommended substrate for scorpions, unlike that of giant spiders, is loam or coarse sand. The dietary requirements of scorpions are similar to those of giant spiders.

Myriapods

Millipedes and centipedes can be kept in a manner that is similar to that of terrestrial arachnids. However, there are certain facets of their captive husbandry that differ and deserve careful attention.

Most millipedes are tropical, burrowing animals that can be kept communally. Therefore, an adequate depth of substrate and a heating source are recommended. The best method of providing heat is through the use of a heating pad or under-tank heater placed at one end of the enclosure. This creates a thermal gradient, similar to what is recommended for many reptile species. Heating and light provided by a bulb are not recommended due to the risk of desiccation. The recommended temperature range is from 20° to 25° C (68°-77° F).[14]

Substrate should be relatively deep to provide sufficient burrowing space. Potting soil or peat moss can be used as the base substrate and should be kept at a depth of 8 to 10 cm. The base substrate can be covered with an additional 3 to 4 cm of leaf litter.[14] Leaf litter should be relatively clean and free of other visible animals. The substrate should be changed every 2 to 3 months, or more frequently if soiled or malodorous.[14] The substrate should be kept damp. To maintain soil moisture levels, use a solid lid, as it will help maintain humidity and limit the likelihood of escape.

A millipede's diet is similar to that of the terrestrial gastropods and should include dark green leafy vegetables, carrots, cucumbers, and some fresh fruits. Always offer fresh products, as old decaying material can lead to the introduction of pathogens. Millipedes should be fed a calcium supplement, as well. In the authors' experience, a simple method of providing calcium supplementation is to offer small pieces of plain blackboard chalk, which millipedes will consume.

Centipedes are primarily native to the tropics and can be kept in a similar manner as millipedes; however, they should not be housed communally, and their humidity levels should be kept at a higher level. Centipedes are more prone to dehydration and typically need 80% to 90% humidity. Exceptions include species from arid regions, which only require a small region of their enclosure to achieve such high levels of humidity.[14] Centipedes are adept at escaping unsecured enclosures, so use a solid, escape-proof lid on the enclosure for these animals. Secure, solid lids can also help to maintain the humidity level in the centipede habitat. The temperature range for temperate species should be between 20° and 25° C (68°-77° F), whereas tropical species like the temperature to be slightly higher (25°-28° C, 77°-82.4° F).[14]

Centipedes are aggressive animals and will consume practically anything offered. In general, centipedes can be offered a diet that is similar to that of the arachnids.

Insects

Insects are a widely diverse group. Most insect species are adapted to specific ecosystems, and are therefore susceptible to changes in their environment (e.g., drastic shifts in temperature or humidity). The focus of this discussion will be on those groups that are the most popular in the pet trade: stick and leaf insects, mantids, large beetles, and exotic cockroaches.

Stick and leaf insects do well in glass, plastic, or screened terraria furnished with real or artificial foliage. It is best if the foliage is the same or similar to the natural environment of the species. These species can be kept communally.

Most stick and leaf insects meet their fluid requirements through the consumption of their food. These insects are herbivorous and will generally accept a variety of different foliages. If their natural diet is unavailable, then they will usually eat commercially available vegetables, such as romaine lettuce and collard, radish, and turnip greens. Other commercial foliages, such as blackberry, raspberry, and mulberry leaves, are also readily accepted.[8]

Mantids can be kept in a similar manner to the stick and leaf insects; however, they cannot be kept communally. These insects are carnivorous and should be offered a variety of prey, such as grasshoppers, crickets, moths, houseflies, and fruit flies. The type of prey offered is generally based on the size of the mantid.[8]

Mantids and stick and leaf insects thrive at moderate temperatures (22.2°-25.6° C, 72°-78° F). Fortunately, these temperatures can be attained using indirect lighting. The enclosures of these insects should be misted regularly, as this will provide an additional source of fluid for consumption.

Large terrestrial beetles can be maintained in a manner similar to millipedes, although their substrate need not be as deep. Accessories should be used to provide hiding places. These species can be kept communally; however, care must be taken to avoid overcrowding because they have a propensity to combat with each other.[8]

Most of the large beetles obtain water through their food. These insects are omnivorous and require a diet comprised of both animal and plant matter. There are a number of different commercially available foodstuffs that can be offered to meet these animals' needs, including fruits (e.g., banana, apples [with seeds removed], cherries, berries), legumes, and dry kibble dog food.[8]

Of all the insect species maintained in captivity, it should be no surprise that exotic cockroaches are the easiest. Many types of enclosures are suitable; the only caveat is that they must be made escape-proof. An easy method to prevent their escape (especially for wingless species) is to apply a one-inch-wide continuous strip of petroleum jelly around the top of the enclosure. Though many species are able to climb vertical surfaces, they cannot pass the petroleum jelly. The authors even know of a successful colony that was maintained in a plain metal trash can by this method. Exotic cockroaches can be maintained on a variety of different substrates, but the authors prefer a substrate comprised of potting soil and leaf litter. These insects should be provided a large number of hiding spaces. Sheet or tubes of cardboard rested on the substrate provide excellent hiding places.

Exotic cockroaches are indiscriminate feeders and thus accept a variety of foodstuffs. The authors recommend a diverse diet comprised of green leafy vegetables, supplemented with occasional fruits and calcium-fortified cricket feed. Open water should be provided in a shallow dish and the water changed as it becomes soiled.

Crustaceans

Crustaceans represent another group of invertebrates that are much too diverse to be described in a single chapter. However, because the most common species offered commercially are the hermit crabs and crayfish, they will be the focus of this discussion.

Hermit crabs come in both terrestrial and arboreal species, both of which can be kept communally, if desired. Both can be easily kept in a simple enclosure (Figure 3-16), with gravel or sand as a substrate. For arboreal species, driftwood or other commercially sold accessories will provide a surface for climb-

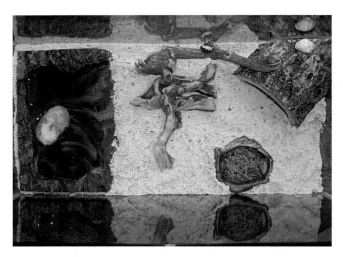

Figure 3-16 Basic hermit crab enclosure in a glass aquarium. Note the retreat in the upper right corner, the driftwood for climbing, and the water source on the left. (Photo by Trevor Zachariah.)

ing. Water should be provided in open pools that allow the hermit crab to get in and out easily. A miniature "beach" can even be made using the substrate. The water required is saline (specific gravity 1.018-1.023), though brackish water and freshwater are tolerated.[8] Aquarium salts sold for marine aquaria can be used to make an appropriate saltwater solution.

Hermit crabs are omnivorous. These animals thrive primarily as scavengers. A variety of commercial "crab foods" are available. It is best to evaluate these diets to determine their value to a crab. Diets primarily comprised of cornmeal and fillers are not recommended. These animals will readily accept a variety of vegetables, fruits, and dry kibble dog food. Hermit crabs will also readily accept dead fish, but this may result in exposure to infectious diseases (e.g., bacteria).

As they grow, hermit crabs discard their shells for larger ones. Because of this, they must be provided appropriate replacements. Crab shells are sold in a variety of sizes at pet supply stores. Shells can also be collected from nature; however, it is recommended that they be cleaned and dried thoroughly before introducing them into a hermit crab's environment. Empty shells that are larger than the one the animal resides in should always be made available to the animal in its enclosure.

Crayfish are freshwater crustaceans that can be kept in aquaria under conditions conducive to other freshwater aquatic species. Unlike hermit crabs, however, they are quite territorial, and a good rule of thumb is to provide at least 2 square feet of substrate per animal. Crayfish should be provided with an ample number of retreats for hiding. Similar to hermit crabs, crayfish are omnivorous and can be fed a variety of foods, including pelleted and staple fish foods and algal pellets. There are also diets available that are formulated specifically for aquatic invertebrates. Whatever diet is utilized, it should be fortified with calcium for proper maintenance of the exoskeleton.

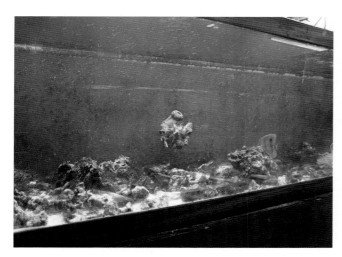

Figure 3-17 Pincushion sea urchin (*Lytechinus* sp.). The sea urchin is in the center of the image, slightly camouflaged by multiple pieces of debris stuck to its spines. Note the large amount of space in the aquarium in which the animal may roam. (Photo by Trevor Zachariah.)

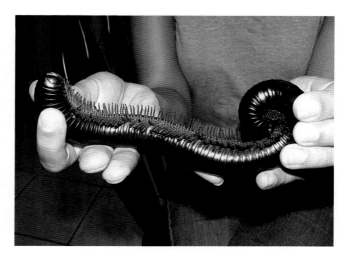

Figure 3-18 Giant African black millipede *(Archispirostreptus gigas).* Note that proper restraint of this animal includes a gentle but firm grip and support of its full length. (Photo by Trevor Zachariah.)

Echinoderms

Echinoderms should be kept in a manner similar to that of other marine aquatic species. As usual, care should be taken to optimize environmental conditions, including water quality, temperature, and lighting. These invertebrates are susceptible to the same poor water quality conditions of other invertebrates, so ammonia, nitrite, and pH should be monitored closely. Echinoderms are also susceptible to copper toxicity and should be removed from aquaria being treated with this metal.

Echinoderms can be kept at the same salinity as saltwater fish (1.018-1.023). These animals should be provided ample space in an aquarium, as they can be rather mobile (Figure 3-17). Echinoderms are susceptible to predation by fish and other invertebrates, and they should be housed in safe-community aquaria. Substrates that are appropriate for marine systems, including dolomite, crushed coral, and live rock, are appropriate for echinoderms. These invertebrates are omnivorous and readily accept a variety of commercially prepared invertebrate foods.

▪ PREVENTIVE MEDICINE

The development of a preventive medicine program for invertebrates should follow the same outline used for vertebrates. Clients should be encouraged to maintain records on feeding, ecdysis schedule (if applicable), and husbandry conditions. Food items being offered to invertebrates should be of the highest nutritional quality available. Hygienic conditions within the animal's habitat should be maximized by routine cleaning. Diagnosing a problem should follow a standard, thorough approach.[13] A postmortem examination should be done on any animal that dies. Autolysis can occur rapidly in invertebrates, so the necropsy should be done soon after the

animal expires (see Diagnostic Methods). Each specimen ideally should receive a thorough annual examination by a veterinarian. New acquisitions should be quarantined for no less than 4 to 6 weeks.[15]

▪ RESTRAINT

Invertebrate handling and restraint, although often necessary for examination and sample collection, should be kept to a minimum. This activity can be stressful, and poses a safety risk for the animal. The handler could also be at risk of potential injury, depending on the species of invertebrate (see Human Health Hazards). Many invertebrates are susceptible to injuries from falls or restraint that is too vigorous. When handling is required for an examination or medical procedure, there are two basic categories of restraint: manual or chemical. Regardless of the method of restraint employed, veterinarians should wear latex exam gloves, lightweight leather gloves, or both when dealing with invertebrates.

Techniques used to manually restrain invertebrates vary from species to species. Some species, such as snails, hermit crabs, millipedes, and cockroaches, are tolerant of being grasped and restrained by hand (Figure 3-18). Tame giant spiders can also be picked up by hand, but they should be gently nudged onto an open hand using a blunt object (e.g., the eraser end of a pencil). Some giant spiders tolerate being palmed,[10] and others cooperate when "pinched" by a gently placed thumb and index finger on either side of the prosoma between the cranial and caudal pairs of legs (Figure 3-19). Gentle pressure applied with a finger to the pedicel area can be used to pin the spider and reduce movement away from the handler.[12,16] Although these techniques can be used to capture and transport a specimen, they are not recommended for examination or diagnostic sampling because they provide minimal restraint.[17] Other manual methods for restraint include collecting the animal in a clear glass or plastic container, pinning the animal under clear

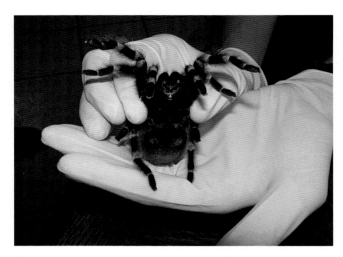

Figure 3-19 Mexican redknee spider *(Brachypelma smithi)*. Example of the pinching method for restraint of a giant spider. Note that the thumb and first finger are on either side of the animal, placed between the second and third pairs of legs. A gentle but firm grip is sufficient. Note also that the weight of the animal is supported from below. (Photo by Trevor Zachariah.)

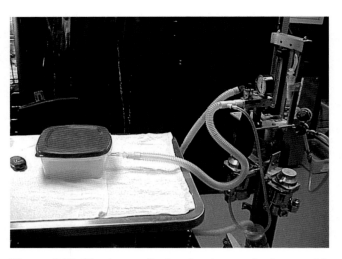

Figure 3-20 Simple anesthetic chamber made from a 3-L plastic food storage container. (Photo by Trevor Zachariah.)

plastic wrap, slinging the animal in gauze, or capturing it in an aquarium fish net.[17]

Chemical restraint for arachnids is accomplished using inhalant anesthetic agents.[17] This technique is preferred because it provides the anesthetist with the most control over the patient. The authors have used isoflurane exclusively for anesthetizing invertebrates. Halothane and sevoflurane can also be used, but we have no experience with them. Carbon dioxide may also be used, but it has a narrower margin of safety than the inhalant anesthetics.[17] For terrestrial invertebrates, the animals are placed into a sealed container that is filled with inhalant anesthetic and oxygen. The container should be sealed to prevent leakage and unnecessary exposure for the individuals working with the invertebrates. Applebee and Cooper[18] describe the construction of an elaborate anesthetic chamber, while the authors have had good success using a 3-L plastic food storage container (Figure 3-20). The authors generally induce the animals at 5% isoflurane (0.5-1.0 L oxygen) and maintain them at 2% to 3% isoflurane. Induction may take several minutes, and recovery several hours, but this is variable according to species, the animal's condition, and the ambient temperature.[17]

Terrestrial molluscs cannot be anesthetized with inhalant compounds; however, they can be anesthetized with a water-bath anesthetic solution. Tricaine methanesulfonate (MS-222) (100 mg/L), benzocaine (dissolved in acetone) (100 mg/L of water), and carbon dioxide dissolved in water have all been recommended.[17] The authors prefer MS-222. The animal must not be submerged in the anesthetic solution. The depth of the solution should be below the level of the head when it is extended. Repeated doses may be needed to achieve an appropriate level of anesthesia.

For aquatic invertebrates, gaseous anesthetics have been suggested, although they are difficult to regulate and control. The authors prefer MS-222 for aquatic invertebrates. The induction dose may vary from 100 to 250 mg/L. Iso-osmotic 7.5% wt/vol magnesium chloride ($MgCl_2 \cdot 6H_2O$) and eugenol (the active ingredient in clove oil) can also be used. These compounds can be slowly added to the water until the desired effects (e.g., loss of locomotion and righting reflex) are achieved.[19] The actual amount of anesthetic needed will vary according to the conditions of the situation and the species being anesthetized.

Hypothermia has been recommended and employed by some veterinarians as a method of restraint.[18,20-22] Lowering an animal's environmental temperature leads to a reduced metabolic rate and level of activity. However, these animals often remain responsive to noxious stimuli. Historically, hypothermia also has been recommended as a method of restraint for lower vertebrates (e.g., amphibians and reptiles) but now is considered inhumane.

Anesthetic monitoring of invertebrates is in its infancy. Generally, the presence or absence of movement and a righting reflex are measured. Monitoring respiration in terrestrial species is difficult because these animals respire through openings in their exoskeleton or body wall, and there is no body movement as is observed in vertebrates. The authors have been unsuccessful in identifying spider heart rates using a Doppler ultrasound, although this has been accomplished in an *Achatina* snail.[23] More invasive techniques to monitor heart rate have been employed[24] but are not practical. More research is needed to develop clinically relevant methods to monitor anesthetic events in invertebrates.

Recovery from an anesthetic event can be achieved by discontinuing the anesthetic agent and providing pure oxygen or room air and clean water. In some lower vertebrates (e.g., reptiles), recovery is faster in animals provided room air versus pure oxygen. This difference is related to the stimulus for respiration in these animals. Whereas higher vertebrates (e.g., birds and mammals) are stimulated to breathe by elevated concentrations of carbon dioxide, lower vertebrates appear to be stimulated by low oxygen levels. It is not known what the respiratory stimulus is for invertebrates, and research to answer this question should be pursued. In cases where there are prolonged recoveries, it may be difficult to ascertain whether or not an invertebrate is alive. If there are no signs of recovery 12 hours after the cessation of anesthesia, the animal may be presumed dead.[17]

HISTORY AND PHYSICAL EXAMINATION

A thorough and detailed history of an invertebrate can provide a great deal of information to guide the clinician in the management of the case. The history provides the veterinarian with an opportunity to determine the owner's knowledge regarding the care and maintenance of his or her pet. Because many of the disease problems encountered in invertebrate medicine are directly related to inadequate husbandry, the history can be as important as any diagnostic test in determining the diagnosis. The history should include questions pertaining to the care of the animal (e.g., enclosure type and size, environmental temperature and humidity, substrate, cage accessories, diet, water source, lighting and photoperiod, and hygiene protocol), the owner's knowledge of the animal (e.g., length of ownership, other animals in the collection, reference resources), and the reason(s) the animal is presented to the veterinarian (e.g., what the problem is, when the problem first occurred, whether the problem has occurred previously, whether there are any previous problems, and whether there are any previous treatments).

The veterinarian should approach the physical examination of an invertebrate with some knowledge of the normal state and behavior of the animal.[15] Examinations are limited in scope compared to vertebrate species, but care should be taken to note the turgidity of the body segments, position of the appendages, presence of ectoparasites, swellings, discolorations, and discharges.[15,16] The physical examination should be performed in a thorough, rapid manner and the animal returned to its enclosure immediately after the exam to minimize stress. Fractious or dangerous animals should be anesthetized for the physical examination.

DIAGNOSTIC TESTING

Diagnosing specific disease conditions in invertebrates is often difficult. This is most likely due to the fact that the accumulated knowledge of the normal state in these animals is limited. Given this fact, it is important for veterinarians to pursue diagnostics in these animals, accumulate more medical knowledge, and publish/share it with the veterinary community.

One of the easiest samples that can be collected from an invertebrate is a swab of the mouth or other orifice, lesion, hemolymph, exudate, or surface of the animal for bacterial and

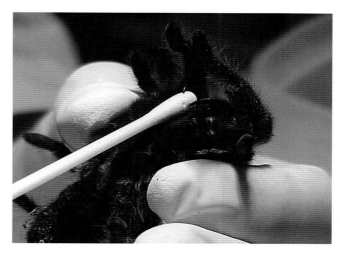

Figure 3-21 Swabbing of the mouthparts of a Chilean rose spider *(Grammostola rosea)* for bacterial culture. (Photo by Mark A. Mitchell.)

fungal cultures (Figure 3-21). It is important that the diagnostic laboratory to which the sample is submitted is aware of the fact that the sample was collected from an invertebrate (and must be provided the temperature of the animal's habitat). Certain pathogens, such as fungi, tend to be isolated at a higher frequency at ambient temperatures (25°-30° C). If the samples are only cultured at 37° C, then some potential pathogens may be lost. Bacteria are generally more tolerant of temperature extremes and can generally be grown at temperatures from 25° to 37° C. Veterinarians must consider, though, that invertebrates are poikilothermic, and culturing bacteriologic samples at high temperatures may not be as appropriate as culturing at the ambient temperature at which the sample was taken.[25] The media used for cultures can also affect the outcome. Media that have been used with success for isolating invertebrate pathogens include marine brain-heart infusion broth and agar, blood agar, MacConkey's agar, special sea-salt agars for marine species, and Sauboraud's dextrose agar for fungal cultures.[19]

Determining the significance of the organisms isolated from clinical samples can be difficult. Knowledge of "normal" flora versus "abnormal" flora is important. An invertebrate's environment can harbor many different organisms that can serve as potential pathogens. Often, sampling from affected and unaffected sites can yield useful comparisons.[19]

Swabs and scrapes of animal surfaces can also be taken for cytological examination. A wet mount of the sample can be made for direct microscopic examination. Wet mounts should be prepared with sterile saline or water, depending on the animal's environment.[19] Such slides can also be allowed to dry and stained with a variety of diagnostic stains (e.g., Diff-Quik, Gram stain, acid-fast stain) for further microscopic examination.[19]

Diagnosing parasitic infections in invertebrates is also difficult due to a lack of research. Parasitic, commensal, and symbiotic relationships among invertebrates are not always easy to separate.[25] Organisms found on or in an invertebrate should be saved and identified. Placing the specimen in 70% ethanol will preserve the sample. An exception is made for the mermithid nematodes, which are occasionally found to emerge from the opisthosoma of spiders. The parasite should be placed in a small petri dish with gravel and covered by water. Daily water changes should be made for approximately one month until the adult stage appears. The nematode can then be killed in 131° F water and placed in ethanol.[26] Mites are often associated with the Madagascar hissing cockroach *(Gromphadorhina portentosa)* and many species of millipedes and can actually be commensals.[25]

Fecal examinations can be performed to evaluate an invertebrate patient for the presence of biochemical analytes, excretory products, microorganisms, and parasites. A direct smear and fecal flotation should be performed to thoroughly assess the parasite status of an animal. Because parasites can be shed transiently, multiple fecal samples may be required. Fecal cultures may also be performed, but again, determining when an isolate is a pathogen may be difficult.

Hemolymph can be collected and analyzed for biochemical constituents, gas analysis, and cellular components. Reference values for these diagnostics have been determined in species of some taxa, most notably the molluscs, crustaceans, and arachnids.[25] In a review of the available literature, it quickly becomes obvious that there is a high degree of variability among the reference values for some species. Future studies are needed to refine the current reference ranges and to determine others for those species for which there are no data.

Hemolymph collection techniques vary depending on the species and taxa involved. Closed circulatory systems are rare in the invertebrate world, and knowledge of individual species is valuable.[19] Cnidarians have a completely open circulatory system, and collection of any fluids from these animals will be diluted with water from their environment. Hemolymph collection from snails and slugs is not commonly done but certainly can be done. Arachnid hemolymph is easily obtained from the heart or pericardial sac (Figure 3-22). Arachnid hemolymph can also be collected by inserting a needle through any number of the arthrodial membranes (the softer areas of cuticle that connect the hard sections of the exoskeleton) and into the hemocoel. This technique can also be done in most insects. When collecting samples from arachnid or insects, it is best to use the smallest gauge needle possible (25-30 gauge) to minimize hemolymph leakage. Sea urchin hemolymph can be collected by inserting a needle through the peristomial membrane (a flexible tissue that surrounds the oral opening). For sea stars, hemolymph can be collected by inserting a needle into the oral or aboral hemal ring via an arm tip.[5] Amputation as a means of collection of hemolymph has been recommended[5,19]; however, this is an extreme action and may not be suitable for individual animals that are kept as pets.

Hemolymph smears should be made immediately after collecting the sample. The slides should be coated with poly-*L*-lysine and the sample allowed to settle briefly before making the smear.[19] Samples can be preserved using ethylenediaminetetraacetic acid (EDTA) or a dilution of seawater (1 : 10).[19] For echinoderms, sodium heparin may be used.[5] The authors have

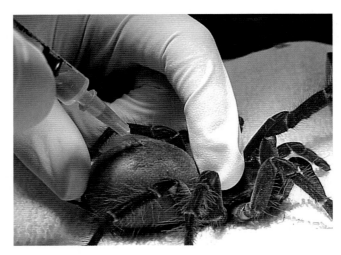

Figure 3-22 Collection of an intracardiac hemolymph sample from a goliath birdeater spider *(Theraphosa blondi)*. A 26-gauge needle attached to a 3-ml syringe is used for collection. The needle is inserted at a 45° angle through the midpoint of the dorsal midline of the opisthosoma. An insulin syringe may be used to collect hemolymph from smaller species. (Photo by Mark A. Mitchell.)

used lithium heparin to preserve giant spider hemolymph samples. Sodium citrate has also been recommended for giant spider hemolymph samples.[16] The efficacy of anticoagulants for invertebrate hemolymph is quite variable. More investigation is needed to determine the proper sample handling techniques for the various invertebrate taxa.

Diagnostic imaging modalities have been underutilized for assessing the health and disease of invertebrate species. The authors and Pizzi[4] have used radiography to assess giant spiders, although its application may be limited to the identification of foreign objects (e.g., surgical implants) and not the assessment of anatomic structures (Figure 3-23). Radiography is more useful for assessing the anatomic features and lesions of echinoderms.[5] Contrast radiography has been used to study the gastrointestinal tract of millipedes[14] and slugs.[8] Barium was used as the contrast agent. Magnetic resonance imaging has been used, to a limited extent, in cnidarians.[7] More investigations should be undertaken to explore the possible roles of different imaging modalities within invertebrate medicine.

A thorough necropsy should be performed on any recently expired invertebrate or a subset of a population (sacrificed) experiencing widespread mortalities. In general, invertebrate tissues deteriorate (autolyze) faster than those of vertebrate species, so it is recommended that necropsies be performed immediately after the animal expires.[19] Knowledge of an animal's normal anatomy facilitates the postmortem process. Photographs and good records should be taken during the necropsy and can be useful later, when summarizing a case.[19] Tissue samples, or even whole animals, may be preserved for later gross and histopathological examination using a variety of fixatives, including neutral 10% buffered formalin, greater than 70% ethyl alcohol, and other specific fixative formula-

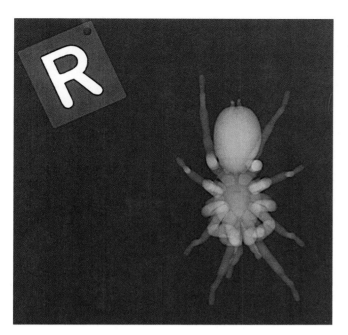

Figure 3-23 Dorsoventral radiograph of a Chilean rose spider *(Grammostola rosea)*. Survey radiographs of invertebrates are often not useful for assessing internal structures. (Photo by Trevor Zachariah.)

tions. See Berzins and Smolowitz[19] for detailed information on fixatives, sample handling, and sample preparation.

An invertebrate disease investigation may include sacrificing animals from an affected population. Both diseased and healthy animals should be sacrificed so that a comparison of tissues can be made. Euthanizing invertebrates and determining that an animal has expired can be difficult with these species. Murray[27] gives a concise list of the different methods considered acceptable for euthanizing and confirming the death of different invertebrate taxa. Although extreme hypothermia or hyperthermia is recommended by some veterinarians, the authors do not recommend this practice. Although the presence of pain perception in invertebrates is debated,[28] it has been demonstrated that invertebrates possess neuropeptides that are similar to those that are involved in pain responses in vertebrate species.[29] Invertebrates are also able to respond to stimuli in manners that are similar to pain responses in vertebrate species.[19] A conservative approach is best when the possibility of inflicting pain exists, as care must be taken to prevent unnecessary suffering in any animal species.

■ COMMON DISEASE PRESENTATIONS

The problems for which an invertebrate specimen is presented to a veterinarian can range from the simple (e.g., trauma) to the complex (e.g., poor water quality and bacterial overgrowth). In most cases, diseases of invertebrates are not well described, and a thorough investigation is needed. Diagnostic procedures that are commonly known to the veterinary profession should

be utilized (see Diagnostic Testing). Whatever the result of a disease investigation is, the potential for adding to the knowledge base is great.

Cnidarians

Any species of cnidarian is susceptible to trauma, and appropriate treatment (e.g., sharp debridement and prophylactic treatment) in captive situations can prevent secondary infections.[7] Jellyfish are particularly prone to trauma when they collide with any firm object, including the enclosure walls and life support equipment. Proper water circulation can prevent such collisions. Anemones are prone to serious, often fatal, trauma from tank accessories as well, including being pulled through mesh placed over pump intake pipes and thermal trauma from submersible heaters.[7] These items should be removed from the animal's environment or modified to protect the animal (e.g., foam baffles over intake pipes).[7]

Copper toxicity is a potential problem for corals. As little as 30 ppb (μg/L copper) can cause pathology.[7] Copper and other heavy metals, such as zinc and lead, may have deleterious effects on other cnidarian species too. Routine screening of aquatic systems can minimize the likelihood of problems. When cnidarians are housed in mixed exhibits with fish, it is important to remove invertebrates from the system if copper is used as a parasiticide for the fish.

Cnidarians are susceptible to a large number of infectious and noninfectious diseases in the wild. The most famous, or infamous, are the coral bleaching events. Coral bleaching is a complex problem involving interactions of multiple etiologies, including light levels, water temperatures, commensal zooxanthellae, and bacterial infections. Stoskopf[7] provides a concise review of cnidarian diseases.

Gastropods

Gastropods are susceptible to a number of parasitic diseases, including sporozoan, ciliate, turbellarian, trematode, annelid, and copepod infestations.[30] Bacteria can also pose a potential problem, though few specific diseases have been described.

Terrestrial species are susceptible to desiccation if they are not maintained in a humid, moist environment. Supportive care measures aimed at rehydration (e.g., placing the animal in a dish of very shallow water or misting the animal) may be tried in mild cases, but moderate to severe cases carry a grave prognosis.

Trauma is a problem most commonly associated with species that possess a shell. Defects in the shell can serve as a route for opportunistic bacterial or fungal infections. Proper care should be provided to avoid such infections and the shell repaired (see Surgery).

Arachnids

Arachnids are susceptible to opportunistic bacterial infections. In many cases, animals are presented for acute death, and necropsy confirms the diagnosis. Clinical signs for animals that present alive may include lethargy, anorexia, loss of body mass, open exoskeleton lesions, and drainage or discharge from a lesion or an orifice. Both Gram-negative and Gram-positive bacteria can serve as opportunistic pathogens in giant spiders. One of the difficulties with diagnosing bacterial infections in giant spiders, or any animal for that matter, is interpreting the culture results to distinguish indigenous flora from pathogens. Several authors have published the results of studies characterizing the microflora of giant spiders,[13,25,26] and a review of these lists suggest that many of them could serve as pathogens. To truly confirm an infection, histopathology and tissue culture are needed. Because this is not possible in most cases (antemortem), the authors generally refer to the growth on the plate. If a single type of isolate is found in pure culture, then it is pursued as a pathogen.

Bacterial infections should always be considered a differential diagnosis anytime there is evidence of pathology. A hemolymph sample should be collected and submitted for culture when a bacterial infection is suspected in a spider or scorpion.[21] Ideally, postmortem hemolymph samples are collected from the most distal leg joints, as these are affected last by postmortem invasion of intestinal flora.[13]

As with bacteria, it can be difficult to differentiate pathogenic versus indigenous fungi. Fungi from the Deuteromycetes (such as *Beauvaria bassiana*, which can affect over 500 species of insect), Ascomycetes (such as *Cordyceps* and *Gibellula* species), and others (such as *Hyphomycetes, Aspergillus,* and *Fusarium* species), can cause pathology in invertebrates.[25] However, fungal spores can be found on many healthy arachnids and cause no apparent harm.[25] Fungal infections of the exoskeletons of giant spiders and other invertebrates are commonly encountered, and if left untreated, these infections can breech the exoskeleton, become systemic, and lead to the demise of the animal. Inadequate husbandry, such as excessive humidity and poor hygiene, is often associated with fatal fungal cases, and these inadequacies must be corrected. Because fungal spores can be persistent in the environment, there is potential for recurrence.[13]

There are several groups of arachnid parasites that are of interest. The first is the parasitic insects, including flies of the family Acroceridae and wasps of the family Pompilidae. Acrocerid larvae infect giant spiders via the book lungs, enter a resting phase (which has been known to last up to 10 years), grow in size, and emerge from the host causing its death. Up to 14 larvae have been recorded to emerge from one host.[15] The pompilid wasps or "tarantula hawk wasps" are a well-known parasite of giant spiders.[10] The adult wasp stings and paralyzes a giant spider, transports it to a burrow, and lays an egg on it. The dead spider serves as the primary food source for the hatching larva.[15] These wasps have also been known to parasitize sun spiders.[8] Breene[20] has successfully treated several infested spiders using supportive care (e.g., fluids) and minimizing stress. These parasitic insects are not of great concern to captive animals but are mentioned here because of the serious harm they are able to inflict.

Nematodes from the family Panagrolaimidae have been reported to parasitize the oral cavity of various species of Old and New World giant spiders.[31] These infestations have been associated with secondary bacterial infections, are unresponsive to treatment (e.g., benzimidazoles and fluoroquinolones), and appear to spread easily in collections. Quarantine and/or euthanasia of affected individuals is recommended.[31]

Mites have long been considered an important parasite of giant spiders; however, there is some debate as to whether these organisms truly affect giant spiders.[20] It is known that larvae from the genera *Leptus, Trombidium, Isothrombium, Eutrombicula,* and *Pimeliaphilus* are parasites of various arachnid species.[32] The mites generally occur when there are unhygienic conditions in an enclosure.[13] A damp swab[26] or fine artist's brush[13,20] can be used to remove the mites from an anesthetized animal. Insecticides or pesticides should not be used to eliminate the mites, as they may also kill the host. Another method of removing the mites is to introduce a *Hypoaspis* species of predatory mite into the enclosure. These mites will consume the larval stages of the parasitic mites and then generally die out when the food source is eliminated.[20] Only one virus has been isolated from a spider. A baculovirus has been found that invades the hepatopancreas of *Pisaura mirabilis,* often leading to the demise of the spider.[13,26] Two viruses have been isolated from a scorpion, *Buthus occitanus,* and one, an icosohedral virus, was found to be pathogenic to the hepatopancreas.[26]

Anorexia is a common presentation for arachnids. This can be due to a disease process (e.g., parasitism, bacterial infection, trauma, toxicosis), incorrect husbandry (e.g., improper food items, high or low temperatures and humidity), or the result of normal circumstances (e.g., imminent molt, egg laying).[21] For example, the authors have observed spiders in their collection to remain anorectic for 4 to 6 weeks before an imminent molt. Indeed, giant spiders are able to endure long periods of starvation without apparent detriment because of their low rate of metabolism.[33] A good physical exam and/or correction of husbandry issues is recommended whenever an abnormal period of anorexia is noted.

Dehydration and hypovolemia are commonly encountered in wild-caught animals that are deprived of a water source during holding and shipping, after a significant loss of hemolymph (e.g., post trauma), or in captive situations where humidity is low and water is not provided.[10] As mentioned previously, animals should always have access to water. In spiders, severe dehydration or hypovolemia is characterized by a shriveled opisthosoma, general poor condition, and an inability to move.[22]

Dorsal opisthosomal alopecia is one of the most common presentations for New World giant spiders. When these spiders are disturbed or stressed, they can actively release urticating hairs from the dorsum of their opisthosoma as a defense mechanism. This presentation should not be mistaken for a pathological lesion but instead be an indicator of an unacceptable amount of stress in the animal's environment.[34] Urticating hairs are replaced when the spider molts.

Dysecdysis is a common problem in captive arachnids, especially giant spiders. Schultz and Schultz[10] have suggested that there are three primary reasons for this, including physical weakness due to old age or disease, previous injury and scar tissue, and mature males attempting a postultimate molt. Insufficient humidity has also been postulated.[13,34] Whatever the reason, if an animal has not been able to shed its entire exoskeleton within 24 hours, outside intervention is probably needed.[20] The relative humidity in the animal's environment can be raised by misting or adding a larger water dish.[12,16] Gentle traction on the retained piece of exoskeleton may be attempted, but excessive force should not be applied or damage to the underlying exoskeleton may occur. Glycerin applied to the affected area may help to lubricate or soften the shedding exoskeleton and facilitate removal.[10,20,21] In giant spiders, an amputation may have to be performed (see Surgery) if there is significant damage to the affected appendage(s).[10,13,20,33]

Toxicities in arachnids can occur as a result of the direct application of pesticide or insecticide on the animal or from feeding prey or other items that are exposed to these toxins.[13,21] Nicotine poisoning has been reported anecdotally, and it has been recommended that smoking be prohibited around these animals and that heavy smokers with nicotine-stained hands avoid handling spiders.[13,21] There are no known specific therapies for invertebrate toxicities. General supportive care should be instituted, including cleaning the environment,[21] optimizing temperature and humidity, maintaining adequate hydration, and feeding the animal by hand.[13] Neurologic disease is occasionally reported in giant spiders. The most common clinical signs include twitching, ataxia, and incoordination. Toxicity, infectious disease, and old age have been associated with neurologic deficits in spiders.[21] Treatment must be focused on providing supportive care and attempting to determine an underlying cause.

Traumatic injuries in arachnids occur most commonly as a result of falling, being attacked by prey, and experiencing difficulties during ecdysis.[26] When startled, many species can run at fast speeds and fall off of a hand, table, or the side of a container. Even a fall from a short height (e.g., 30 cm) can be disastrous for a giant spider.[13] The most common problems that occur as a result of traumatic injury are rupture of the exoskeleton and loss of hemolymph. Treatment should be focused on hemolymph stasis and the replenishment of lost fluids. The loss of a volume of hemolymph greater than 1% of body weight is considered severe and can be fatal.[15,35] There are several methods that can be used to provide hemostasis and repair the injury to the exoskeleton (see Surgery).

Myriapods

Bacterial and fungal infections are common among the myriapods and are usually opportunistic secondary invaders from the environment or gut flora of the animal.[14] Signs associated with such infections include discoloration of the exoskeleton, lethargy, and decreased feeding.[14]

Frye[8] reported finding rhabditiform nematodes and protozoa in the feces of healthy millipedes. However, it was not determined whether those organisms were parasitic. It is common to find mites on millipedes, and they are most likely harmless commensal organisms. Some may even benefit the millipedes in indirect ways.[14] There have been reports of possible harmful mites on millipedes. The presence of ectoparasites on centipedes is considered harmful.[14] Steps should be taken to remove the parasites without harming the host (see Therapeutics).

Myriapods are susceptible to problems with the exoskeleton. In young millipedes, wrinkling of the exoskeleton has been reported. The cause of this condition is not known, but may be associated with abnormalities in the chitin or the calcification of the exoskeleton.[14] Dysecdysis can also pose a significant problem for millipedes. Animals that are not treated can die. Dysecdysis may occur as a result of inappropriate environmental conditions, ectoparasites, infectious disease, or lesions resulting from trauma.

Traumatic injuries to myriapods generally occur from falls or dropping cage equipment on an animal. Injuries of the exoskeleton can lead to hemolymph loss. Severe injuries with the loss of a large volume of hemolymph can prove fatal. Attempts to repair the injury with cyanoacrylate glue can be made; however, the prognosis for these cases is often grave. Minor injuries to appendages may be successfully treated.[14]

Insects

Insects are susceptible to many of the same diseases as other invertebrates, including bacteria, fungi, protozoa, parasites, and environmental factors. Environmental factors are particularly important when dealing with captive animals. Husbandry conditions (e.g., temperature, humidity, nutrition, stress) are often specific or inhabit a narrow optimal range and, if not adequately provided, can lead to problems. Diagnosing diseases in insects should follow the same basic diagnostic protocols as for other invertebrates. Unfortunately, antemortem diagnostics are often limited for insects, and necropsy is required for diagnosis. Cooper[36] provides a good overview of the common infectious diseases of captive insects.

Neoplasia has been described in insects and can be found catalogued by the Registry of Tumors in Lower Animals.[36] Although these diseases are not considered clinically significant in the insects, they may be able to shed light on research into oncogenesis.[36]

Traumatic injuries represent the most common reason insects are presented to veterinarians. These injuries can be devastating to the insect, as their rigid exoskeleton can fracture. Fractures in the exoskeleton can lead to loss of hemolymph and a route of infection for opportunity pathogens. It is imperative that these injuries are repaired immediately. (See Therapeutics for a discussion of possible treatments.)

Most pesticides are developed for the sole purpose of killing insects, so toxicities are a common occurrence with even low dose exposure. Any chemicals with the potential to harm an insect should not be used within the immediate vicinity of the animal. This is especially important for aerosolized poisons. Products that are used for flea and tick control on dogs and cats are also harmful to insects, even from treated hairs that are shed by the animal into an insect's environment. Once a toxic episode ensues, death almost always occurs, despite supportive medical care.

Crustaceans

Few diseases specific to hermit crabs have been described. Proper husbandry is always important, especially when dealing with marine species. As with other aquatic species, it is imperative to optimize water quality.

Noga, Hancock, and Bullis[37] mention just two infectious diseases associated with hermit crabs. A fatal mycotic infection of the gills has been reported in marine hermit crabs (*Pagurus* sp.) in a laboratory setting due to *Fusarium solani*. Also, injury to the cecum of hermit crabs has been attributed to the plerocercoids of the dogfish cestode (*Calliobothrium verticillatum*).

Many more diseases have been described for crayfish, and this is only because of the widespread use of these animals in aquaculture. See Edgerton et al.[38] for a thorough overview of crayfish diseases. Noga et al.[37] note that some of the more serious diseases are systemic infections of Gram-negative bacteria, fungal (e.g., *Fusarium* sp.) infections, shell disease, and microsporidian infections. One of the most important crayfish diseases is crayfish plague, which is caused by a water mold, *Aphanomyces astaci*. Spores of this mold infect the crayfish shell and deeper tissues, causing 100% mortalities in susceptible species.[37] Most of the European crayfish are susceptible to this water mold, whereas the North American species are resistant. Resistant species can serve as carriers of *A. astaci*.[37] It is believed that *A. astaci* can only survive on live crayfish, thus depopulation and disinfection of affected captive environments may eliminate the organism.

Gas-bubble disease, which occurs when the water is supersaturated with atmospheric gases, has been reported in crustaceans. Air emboli enter the gills, leading to the death of the animal.[37] The animal should be removed from the system and placed into a "gas-free" aquarium. Air pockets can also form in the gills after a crustacean has been removed from and then replaced into water. In most cases, the crab can "burp" the air out, but if it can't, it can be fatal.[37] Traumatic injuries can also occur in crustaceans. Injuries to their rigid exoskeleton can lead to hemolymph loss and opportunities for secondary infections. If left untreated, these conditions can prove fatal.

Echinoderms

Systemic bacterial infections have been reported in echinoderms. Traumatic injuries and poor water quality can provide bacteria an opportunity to invade the normally sterile coelomic fluid.[5] A similar circumstance occurs when *Vibrio anguillarum* and *Aeromonas salmonicida* invade traumatized tissue of sea urchins. The resulting surface lesions form a ring of swelling and discoloration around a necrotic region where spines and tube feet have been lost, hence the name of bald sea urchin disease.[37] Recovery via sloughing and regeneration is possible if the lesions do not involve a large surface area (e.g., >30%).[37]

Multiple types of parasites affect echinoderms, including apicomplexans, amoebans, ciliates, algals, mesozoans, helminths, gastropods, and annelids.[37] Lesions resembling neoplastic growths have been reported in one species of brittle star (*Ophiocomina nigra*) and one species of sea cucumber (*Holothuria leucospilata*).[37] See Jangoux[39] for a complete review of echinoderm infectious diseases.

Evisceration is a defense mechanism practiced by some species and is a natural response to changing environmental conditions or a sequela to a pathological condition. Sea cucumbers are capable of forcefully discharging adhesive, sometimes toxic, Cuvierian tubules from their anus to entangle predators or intruders.[3] Many sea cucumber species are also able to discharge parts of their digestive tract in response to stress or as a natural seasonal process.[3] The Cuvierian tubules and digestive tract can be regenerated. Evisceration also occurs in severe cases of ulceration in sun stars (*Solaster* sp.). Sun star ulcers can also be much milder and are an idiopathic condition of captive individuals.[5]

General trauma occurs in echinoderms and will often lead to secondary infections. Regeneration is possible, even from severe injuries, although permanent defects may be present after healing.

■ THERAPEUTICS

Cnidarians

Treating cnidarians with chemical compounds can be a risky venture, as the accumulated knowledge and scientific research in this area are lacking. Whenever a treatment is attempted, it should be conducted, whenever possible, in a separate tank from the animal's main environment and the animal monitored carefully. Methods of drug removal or dilution (e.g., activated carbon filtration, conditioned replacement water) should be on hand in case of problems and the animal must be rinsed off before being returned to the main enclosure.[7]

Antibacterial treatments appear to be well tolerated by many cnidarian species.[7] In many species 5% Lugol's iodine solution (5-10 drops/L, 10-20 minute bath per day) can be used to provide broad-spectrum antisepsis and cauterize damaged tissues, but this should be evaluated on a species by species level, as some coral species do not tolerate Lugol's iodine well.[7] Tetracycline baths (10 mg/L) are safe for many corals; however, this antibiotic can be chelated by calcium in the water, lowering the effective dose.[7] In cases where the hardness of the water is high, the veterinarian may consider a higher dose of tetracycline. Chloramphenicol baths (10-50 mg/L) have been used with success.[7] The dosing frequency reported can be highly variable (24-72 hours). Chloramphenicol baths may be used in conjunction with a pretreatment or posttreatment Lugol's iodine bath.[7] Stoskopf[7] recommends inactivating chloramphenicol by adding 60 ml of chlorine bleach to every 20 L of treatment water several hours before discarding it.

Cnidarians can also be medically managed with topical therapeutics. Lugol's iodine (5%) can be applied topically with swabs to cauterize and disinfect wounds. Topical application should not be for longer than 20 to 30 seconds.[7] Pastes created from antibiotics, such as neomycin and kanamycin, or water-resistant compounding bases used by dentists have been used.[7] As with any topical therapy, only a small quantity of the therapeutic should be applied initially to determine if a reaction may occur.

Antiparasitic treatments against flatworms, protozoa, and metazoa generally follow similar plans for fish. Placing salt-water species in freshwater (1-3 minute bath) can be done with relative ease. Monitor the invertebrates closely for any obvious changes (e.g., color change), and remove immediately if they appear to be reacting negatively to the freshwater. Levamisole, an antiparasitic used regularly in vertebrates, can also be used as a bath treatment for cnidarians. Stoskopf[7] recommends an extended (8 mg/L, 24-hour) bath for cnidarians. Different species may react differently to these treatments, and the animals should be monitored closely during any treatment procedure.

When considering treatment plans for aquatic animals, it is important to think outside the box. Medicating a feed that is being offered to a patient is a common practice, although these foods are often commercially prepared. Instilling a medication into a live prey item, such as brine shrimp, may be more difficult. One of the most common methods for medicating difficult-to-treat live prey is to use osmosis. Placing brine shrimp, a salt-loving species, into freshwater will lead to the movement of water into these organisms. If a medication is placed in the freshwater, it will move into the brine shrimp, too. One potential drawback of this technique is that it is difficult to ensure the quantity of medication in these prey species. More research is needed to elucidate this information.

Gastropods

Delivery of antibiotics to gastropods can be achieved through several methods. Due to the porosity of the epithelium and gills of aquatic species, bath treatments are possible. The techniques described earlier will also work for these animals. Intramuscular injections via the foot, injection via the hemocoel in some species (e.g., opisthobranchs), and adding medication to the feed are other alternatives that can be used.[30]

Arachnids

Systematic analytical studies on the use of antibiotics in arachnids have not been attempted to the authors' knowledge. There are anecdotal reports, but most have varying results and are based on cases without a definitive diagnosis. Cooper[21] suggests the use of tetracycline solutions (e.g., 50 mg tetracycline in 25 ml fluid) for irrigating external lesions. Other preparations, primarily those used in the aquarium trade, have been used orally.[4] Enrofloxacin has been used in giant spiders at doses of 10 to 20 mg/kg PO q24h without apparent toxicity to the animal.[4] Trimethoprim-sulfonamides may be used topically or systemically,[4] but little is known about their effect or correct dosages. Both fenbendazole (10-200 mg/kg PO) and

oxfendazole (10-200 mg/kg PO q24h to biweekly) have been used safely in giant spiders, but they did not eliminate oral nematode infections.[4] When medicating arachnids, the drug may be delivered orally with a syringe or injected into a prey item before it is offered to the spider. Again, injecting the compound into the prey species may result in less than optimal dosing.

Mites are a common finding in imported arachnids. Most of the miticides used in veterinary medicine are toxic to all invertebrates, including arachnids. Although tedious, the method of removing mites with mineral oil on a cotton-tipped applicator is safe.

Treatment recommendations for fungal infections in arachnids are limited.[4,13] Pizzi has recommended the topical application of povidone-iodine (0.75% water-based solution) for giant spiders. Topical chlorhexidine can also be used to manage fungi on arachnids. The chlorhexidine or iodine can be placed on a cotton-tipped applicator and applied directly on the affected area of the exoskeleton. Other topical and parenteral medications may also prove effective, but further research needs to be performed to determine the efficacy of these treatments.

Invertebrates that are dehydrated or suffering from hypovolemia (e.g., trauma with loss of hemolymph) should be given fluids to replace any losses. Many arachnids will consume water offered directly from a syringe.[35] Animals that are active can be placed into a dish of shallow water and allowed to imbibe on their own will. It is important that the water not be too deep, as arachnids can drown if the water enters their respiratory openings.[10,13,35]

Giant spiders can be given parenteral fluids via the distal leg joint,[13] heart and pericardial sac,[22] and the opisthosoma.[10] When considering rehydrating a spider, veterinarians should base the selection of a fluid on the type of dehydration. The majority of cases presented to veterinarians will be associated with a hypertonic dehydration. Only one study has attempted to determine the osmolarity and electrolyte balance of giant spider hemolymph.[40] Based on that study, a "tarantula Ringer's solution" was recommended. Interestingly, the osmolarity of the solution was rather hypotonic (201 mOsm/L). Physiologic (0.9%) saline (273 mOsm/L) has been recommended as an alternative fluid for rehydrating giant spiders,[13] and we have been successful using this method. Pizzi[4] also reports the successful use of lactated Ringer's and Hartmann's solutions for fluid therapy. An alternative to replenishing hypovolemic spiders with commercial fluids is to use a transfusion of hemolymph from a donor spider using a small-gauge catheter, as described by Visigalli[16]; however, the effects this procedure would have on the transfused spider are not known.

The amount of injectable fluid that can be safely administered to a giant spider has not been clearly defined, but Stewart and Martin[24] were able to safely administer 0.5 ml (4% body weight) of fluid into a 12-g spider. Johnson-Delaney[22] has suggested that the fluid rate used for reptiles would be appropriate also for giant spiders. In a recent study by the authors, *Grammostola rosea* were given a single injection of physiologic saline into the opisthosoma representing up to 6% of their body weights, without any observed negative side effect. Additional research is required to determine the maximum volume and rate that fluids can be replenished in giant spiders and other arachnid species.

Myriapods

The information available for therapeutic use in myriapods is severely lacking. There is anecdotal evidence that fluid therapy and oral antimicrobials have been attempted. For millipedes, fluids may be replenished by placing the animal in a shallow dish of lukewarm water. This will only work for active, alert animals. For centipedes, placing them in an enclosure with a high humidity has been recommended.[14] This can be achieved by using dampened paper towels or moistened bedding.

Injecting oral antibiotics into prey items is an appropriate method for dosing both millipedes and centipedes.[14] Parenteral administration may also be attempted. Injection of water-soluble drugs into the hemolymph through the arthrodial membranes can be done, but dosing rates are empirical. The effect of parenteral antibiotics on the microbial flora of millipedes is unknown, but should be considered prior to administration.[14]

Insects

As with the myriapods, there is little information available regarding the use of therapeutics in insects. The most studied species is the honeybee *(Apis mellifera),* and Cooper[36] presents a limited formulary for insects in general (Table 3-1).

Crustaceans

Because most crustacean species are aquatic and most captive species are cultured for human consumption, the compounds used for these species in the United States are regulated by the Food and Drug Administration.[37] Animals that are not des-

tined for human consumption, such as pets or institutional specimens, may be treated with medications in an extra-label manner.[37] Table 3-2 provides a list of therapeutic agents and dosages used to manage penaeid shrimp. This formulary may be extrapolated for use in other crustaceans as well.

Echinoderms

Treatment of echinoderms, like other invertebrates, is in its infancy. Harms[5] has suggested that these animals can be treated with antibiotics via a bath or intracoelomic injection. He also suggested that chitin synthesis inhibiting parasiticides (e.g., lufenuron) might be applicable to these animals, although the dosing protocols, safety, and effectiveness of these compounds have not been described for these species.

■ SURGERY
Cnidarians

Surgical procedures of cnidarians are generally limited to debridement of lesions and fragmentation for propagation.[7] When treating cnidarians, veterinarians should use sharp dissection to remove damaged tissue(s). Debridement should take place ideally in an enclosure separate from the animal's primary enclosure to avoid contaminating the water system with debrided tissue, as this tissue can be infectious.[7]

There is a great deal of debate as to how to manage a defect that is created in a coral after debridement. Some veterinarians close the defect, whereas others manage the defect by second intention. Anecdotally, various substances have been used to fill defects with some success, including plasticine clay (with or without antibiotic impregnation), plaster of Paris, hydraulic cement, and specialized plastering compounds.[7] In addition to these products, Stoskopf[7] has also recommended several other substances that deserve investigation, such as dental compounding bases, methacrylates, cyanoacrylate gels, and underwater epoxies. For an overview of coral fragmentation, see Stoskopf.[7]

Gastropods

Gastropod shell injuries occur occasionally in captive collections. The gastropod shell can be repaired using the same basic concepts used for repairing chelonian shells. First, the shell should be disinfected. Dilute povidone-iodine or chlorhexidine and saline should be used for this purpose. It is important not to introduce these chemicals into the coelomic cavity, as they can be caustic to unprotected tissues. Dental acrylic, surgical epoxy/glue, and tape can be used to stabilize fractures. In severe, displaced fractures, cerclage wire can be used to reduce the fractures.

Arachnids

To the authors' knowledge, only one known elective surgical procedure has been described for arachnids. Passive integrated transponders were implanted into the opisthosomas of 12 giant

TABLE 3-1	Formulary for Insects	
Type	**Name**	**Route**
Fluids	Water	PO, nebulization
	Hypotonic saline* (0.2%-0.5%)	PO, nebulization, ICe
Antibiotics	Chlortetracycline	PO, topical
	Oxytetracycline	PO, topical
	Sulfadiazine	PO
Laxatives	Mineral oil	PO
Antimycotics	Povidone-iodine	Topical
	Ketoconazole or nystatin	Topical
	Fumagillin	PO
Antiprotozoals	Benomyl	PO
Antiseptics	Povidone-iodine	Topical

Adapted from Cooper JE: Insects. In Lewbart GA, editor: *Invertebrate Medicine,* Ames, Iowa, 2006, Blackwell, p 218.
*Do not use in stick and leaf insects.
ICe, intracoelomic; *PO,* per os.

TABLE 3-2	Formulary for Penaeid Shrimps	
Type	**Name**	**Dosage**
Antimicrobials	Benzalkonium chloride	0.6-1.0 ppm, 24 h
Antibiotics	Nitrofurazone	1-2 ppm
	Nifurpirinol	1-2 ppm
	Furazolidone	10-20 ppm, 24 h
	Oxytetracycline	40-60 ppm, 24 h
	Ormetoprim-sulfamethoxazole	50-100 mg/kg PO, 14 days
Antimycotics	Malachite green	0.5-0.8 ppm, 24 h
	Methylene blue	8-10 ppm, 24 h
	Trifluralin	0.01-0.1 ppm
Antiprotozoals	Copper sulfate	0.5-1.0 ppm, 10-12 h
	Zeolite	100-120 kg/m², applied to environment
Antiparasitics	Formalin	0.5-1.0 ppm, 24 h
	Potassium permanganate	25-30 ppm, 30-60 min

Modified from Noga EJ, Hancock AL, Bullis RA: Crustaceans. In Lewbart GA, editor: *Invertebrate Medicine,* Ames, Iowa, 2006, Blackwell, p 192.
PO, per os.

spiders, without complication, by Reichling and Tabaka.[41] Though this procedure was developed for research purposes, it may prove to have clinical application in the future.

Most surgical procedures performed on arachnids arise as a result of traumatic injury. Arachnids can naturally lose a limb through autotomy. When an arachnid suffers an injury to an appendage as a result of trauma or dysecdysis, the limb can be removed by the veterinarian with little damage, as the process is a natural response for the host.[13,35] It is important to remove injured limbs, as they can lead to excessive loss of hemolymph. To remove an injured leg or pedipalp, the appendage should be grasped with hemostats at the level of the femur and separated with a sharp upward tug on the leg. Several authors suggest that because autotomy is a voluntary act, arachnids should not be anesthetized during the procedure.[13,20] However, the process does result in tissue damage, which initially should mimic a noxious stimulus or aversion behavior. Some veterinarians take a similar approach with vertebrates (e.g., iguana tail autotomy, salamander limb autotomy).

Trauma to the exoskeleton of an arachnid requires immediate medical attention, as a significant loss of hemolymph is likely to be fatal. If not extensive, traumatic or iatrogenic (e.g., hemolymph collection, surgery, induced autotomy) exoskeleton defects can be repaired. There are various methods for doing this, including the application of cyanomethacrylate (e.g., surgical tissue adhesive), cyanoacrylate (e.g., super glue), or nail hardener.[4,13,20,35] Multiple applications may be needed depending on the extent of the lesion. Larger exoskeleton defects may be closed with 5-0 or 6-0 synthetic suture,[22] although Pizzi[4] discourages this practice as ineffective.

Myriapods

The only described surgical procedures for myriapods are wound repair and appendage removal. For both millipedes and centipedes, the application of adhesives may be done in a

manner similar to that described for arachnids. Large defects in centipedes may also benefit from closure with 5-0 to 8-0 synthetic suture.[14] Damaged appendages may be removed by sharp dissection and may be sealed with adhesive.

Insects

Although there are a number of surgical procedures described for insects, most of these are experimental in nature and not conducive to clinical medicine.[36] However, Cooper[36] does suggest that attempts at limb amputation, lesion removal and debridement, and wound repair (including suturing) be attempted in cases when deemed appropriate by the veterinarian.

Crustaceans

As with many of the taxa discussed in this chapter, little information exists regarding surgical procedures in crustaceans. However, this should not preclude attempts at minor surgical procedures such as amputation and wound repair. Presumably, these would be performed in a manner similar to what has been described for other arthropod species, with concern taken for the unique aspects of crustacean anatomy and physiology. For example, the autotomy reflex of decapod crustaceans, with a fracture plane between the basis and ischium segments, may serve as a method of amputating limbs.

Echinoderms

No surgical procedures have been described for echinoderms. Ophiuroids have an amazing ability to autotomize appendages, and this, along with their impressive regenerative capabilities, could be considered in cases where the animal suffers an injury.[5]

HUMAN HEALTH HAZARDS

Cnidarians

The cnidarians include some of the most venomous species of animals in the world. Certain species of box jellies, in particular, maintain highly potent nematocysts that are capable of inflicting extreme pain and even death in humans. The most notorious cnidarians are *Chironex fleckeri* (e.g., Australia's "sea wasp"), which is responsible for an average of two deaths each year, and *Chiropsalmus quadrumanus* (southeastern United States), which is responsible for at least one human fatality annually.[3] Other species of cnidarians are also capable of inflicting intense pain on humans; however, most are harmless. Although not intended to be injurious, the sharp edges of some corals are known to cause lacerations in humans.

Gastropods

Most gastropods are harmless. The family Conidae (e.g., cone snails), a group of carnivorous, marine snails, however, is an exception. Cone snails have a radula that is modified into a hollow harpoon that they use to envenomate prey. This weapon can also be used against humans. The venom of some species is toxic to humans and has been responsible for at least a few deaths.[3] Fortunately, these snails are not common in the commercial trade.

Arachnids

Arachnids are feared the world over, and this is unfortunate considering these animals prey on many of the insects considered to be pests or vectors for disease. One of the reasons that humans fear these animals is because of the perceived concern associated with their venom. With very rare exceptions, spiders possess venom. However, most are either unable to bite or their venom is not dangerous to humans. The World Health Organization lists four genera as exceptions: *Atrax, Latrodectus, Loxosceles,* and *Phoneutria.* The most common, from the standpoint of their relative abundance and popularity in the United States, are widow spiders (*Latrodectus* spp.) and recluse spiders (*Loxosceles* spp.). Widow spiders produce a neurotoxic venom that can cause abdominal and leg pain, high cerebrospinal fluid pressure, nausea, muscle spasms, and respiratory paralysis.[3] Death is infrequent, and signs usually resolve within 3 to 7 days after symptomatic treatment with or without antivenin therapy.[42] Recluse spiders produce cytotoxic venom that induces a necrotic ulcer at the site of the bite. It is rare that these envenomations become systemic.[42] Symptomatic treatment is usually sufficient, and reports of mortalities are uncommon.[42] Species from both of these genera are relatively common in captivity, although this practice is not recommended. Less commonly encountered, though particularly more potent in venom and aggressiveness, are the funnel web spiders (*Atrax* spp.) and the South American "banana spiders" (*Phoneutria* spp.).

Giant spider bites are not considered serious. In general, Old World species are believed to have more potent venom than New World species.[43,44] Most individuals envenomated by giant spiders develop mild to severe local pain, itching and tenderness, edema, erythema, joint stiffness and swollen limbs, burning feelings, muscle cramps, and temporary paralysis.[43] Schultz and Schultz[10] reported on the symptoms associated with the bites of various species of giant spider and found that all of them were mild and short-lived. Rather than toxicity, the real significance of giant spider bites may be the potential for mechanical injury. Fangs can be large, with those of adult *Theraphosa blondi* reaching up to 3 cm in length.[31]

As with any insult that compromises the skin, injuries from arachnid bites or stings have the potential to lead to secondary infections. Opportunistic pathogens may originate from the human or from the invertebrate. The microflora of the mouthparts of various captive giant spider species have been described, and a range of Gram-positive and Gram-negative bacteria found: *Staphylococcus aureus, Staphylococcus* spp., *Bacillus megaterium, B. subtilis, B. cereus, Pseudomonas diminuta, P. aeruginosa, P. fluorescens, P. cepacia, Pseudomonas* spp., *Aeromonas hydrophilia, Acinetobacter calcoaceticus, Micrococcus varians, M. mucilaginosus,* Coryneforms, and other Enterobacteriaceae.[29,45] At least three of these bacteria (*S. aureus, P. aeruginosa, A. hydrophilia*) are known human pathogens.[45] Infections with oral nematodes from the family Panagrolaimidae have been reported in giant spiders, and some species of this family are known to cause zoonotic disease.[31]

Giant spiders carry another potential risk to humans, their urticating hairs. As mentioned previously, New World species have urticating hairs on their opisthosomas. When alarmed, the spiders can brush off the hairs with their hind legs, which allows them to become airborne. Exposure to these hairs can occur from direct contact with the spider or indirectly from the animal's environment, especially when cleaning and replacing substrate. Each urticating hair is covered by hundreds of small hooks and can cause severe itching when it makes contact with the skin.[33] Cooke et al.[2] have shown that these hairs can embed themselves to a depth of 2 mm in human skin. A severe skin reaction has been observed by the authors in a colleague working with the *Theraphosa blondi* colony at the Louisiana State University School of Veterinary Medicine. This individual was changing the substrate in the cages and had indirect contact with the spiders. A severe, intense, pruritic cycle ensued that affected the hands and forearms (Figure 3-24). The reaction lasted for 14 days. A single case of papular dermatitis with edema resulting from urticating hair exposure has also been described.[46]

Although dermatologic exposure to urticating hairs is a self-limiting condition, urticating hairs can be much more harmful to the human eye. The hairs can penetrate the cornea and cause a multitude of symptoms, including panuveitis, iritis, anterior synechiae, vitritis, chorioretinitis, and keratitis. A review of the literature revealed more than a dozen case reports of ophthalmia nodosa (a granulomatous disease) caused by contact with a giant spider. Ocular disease caused by urticating hairs can be serious and chronic in nature. It is recommended that latex or nitrile exam gloves be worn whenever handling or cleaning the enclosure of a giant spider. Eye pro-

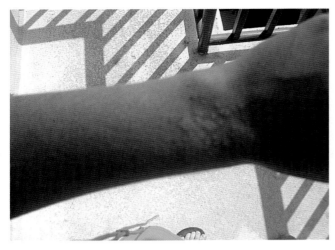

Figure 3-24 Human dermatitis resulting from giant spider urticating hairs. This colleague came into contact with airborne urticating hairs from a goliath birdeater spider *(Theraphosa blondi).* (Photo by Clare Guichard.)

tection may also be indicated. During the activity, it is best to avoid touching one's face or any area of skin. Washing one's hands afterward is also strongly recommended.

Most scorpions produce a venom that is painful but not dangerous to humans. The exceptions are found in the family Buthidae, which includes *Androctonus* and *Centruroides.*[3] Death from the neurotoxic venom is generally preceded by convulsions, paralysis of the respiratory muscles, and cardiac failure. Fortunately, some effective antivenins are available.[3] Veterinarians working with these species should be preemptive and have antivenins on hand. Clients should be made aware of the potential hazards to owning these animals.

Myriapods

Millipedes are generally slow, passive animals. However, many species are able to exude or squirt noxious substances from the glands found on the body segments.[14] These substances can affect the human skin by staining, irritating, or blistering and can cause potentially serious injuries if the human eye comes into contact with them.[14] As with arachnid species, latex exam gloves and/or eye protection is recommended when handling these animals.

Large centipedes have fangs of commensurate size, and their venom can be quite painful. Deaths resulting from the bite of a centipede are difficult to authenticate, although the potential for this may exist for *Scolopendra.*[3] Most species have the ability to move rapidly, so handling should be avoided if at all possible.

Insects

Insects pose a variety of health hazards to the humans that interact with them. The most obvious is through the physical injury (e.g., bite, sting, or pinch) that many species are able to

deliver. Various insects (e.g., bees, wasps, ants) are able to affect humans through chemical means (e.g., venom, acidic secretions) as well. However, barring allergic reactions or mass attacks, the effects of insects on humans are rarely more serious than the discomfort that they cause.

Wild-caught insects can serve as vectors for infectious diseases. Testing subsets of captive populations for those diseases of concern can be done to limit the likelihood for zoonotic disease transmission.

Crustaceans

The crustaceans in general do not pose much of a threat to humans. The most common injuries involve the pincing ability of the orders Decapoda and Stomatopoda (e.g., "mantis shrimps"). Such injuries may be severe when dealing with crustaceans of large size (e.g., lobsters). Grasping these animals at the cephalothorax can generally reduce the likelihood of being pinced.

Echinoderms

Sea urchins can inflict severe injuries to humans. The spines of these animals can cause both direct cell injury and, in some species, a toxin insult.[3] Delayed hazards include secondary opportunistic bacterial infections and chronic granuloma formation.[5] Some species also possess venomous pedicellariae, which are meant to protect the animal from predators and can produce a painful reaction in humans.[3]

SUGGESTED READINGS

Breene RG: *The ATS Arthropod Medical Manual: Diagnosis and Treatment,* The American Tarantula Society.

Breene RG: *Concise Care Guide for the 80 Plus Most Common Tarantulas,* The American Tarantula Society.

Brownell P, Polis GA: *Scorpion Biology and Research,* Oxford University Press.

Daly HV, Doyen JT, Purcell AH: *Introduction to Insect Biology and Diversity,* Oxford University Press.

Foelix RF: *Biology of Spiders* (ed 2), Oxford University Press.

Frye FL: *Captive Invertebrates: A Guide to Their Biology and Husbandry,* Krieger.

Hopkin SB, Read HJ: *The Biology of Millipedes,* Oxford University Press.

Keegan HL: *Scorpions of Medical Importance,* University Press of Mississippi.

Lewbart GA: *Invertebrate Medicine,* Blackwell.

Polis GA: *The Biology of Scorpions,* Stanford University Press.

Ruppert EE, Fox RS, Barnes RD: *Invertebrate Zoology: A Functional Evolutionary Approach* (ed 7), Brooks/Cole.

Schultz SA, Schultz MJ: *The Tarantula Keeper's Guide,* Barron's.

REFERENCES

1. Frye FL: Scorpions. In Lewbart GA, editor: *Invertebrate Medicine,* Ames, Iowa, 2006, Blackwell.
2. Cooke JAL, Miller FH, Grover RW, Duffy JL: Urticaria caused by tarantula hairs, *Am J Trop Med Hyg* 22(1):130-133, 1973.
3. Ruppert EE, Fox RS, Barnes RD: *Invertebrate Zoology: A Functional Evolutionary Approach,* ed 7, Belmont, Calif, 2004, Brooks/Cole-Thomson Learning.
4. Pizzi R: Spiders. In Lewbart GA, editor: *Invertebrate Medicine,* Ames, Iowa, 2006, Blackwell.

5. Harms CA: Echinoderms. In Lewbart GA, editor: *Invertebrate Medicine,* Ames, Iowa, 2006, Blackwell.

6. Lewbart GA, editor: *Invertebrate Medicine,* Ames, Iowa, 2006, Blackwell.

7. Stoskopf MK: Coelenterates. In Lewbart GA, editor: *Invertebrate Medicine,* Ames, Iowa, 2007, Blackwell.

8. Frye FL: *Captive Invertebrates: A Guide to Their Biology and Husbandry,* Malabar, Fla, 1992, Krieger.

9. Marshall SD: *Tarantulas and Other Arachnids,* Hauppauge, NY, 2001, Barron's Educational Series.

10. Schultz SA, Schultz MJ: *The Tarantula Keeper's Guide,* Hauppauge, NY, 1998, Barron's Educational Series.

11. Breene RG: *Concise Care Guide for the 80 Plus Most Common Tarantulas,* Carlsbad, N Mex, 1998, American Tarantula Society.

12. Cappelletti A, Visigalli G: What every veterinarian needs to know about giant spiders, *Exot DVM* 5(pt 6):36-42, 2004.

13. Pizzi R, Cooper JE, George S: Spider health, husbandry, and welfare in zoological collections. In *Proc Brit Vet Zoo Soc,* pp 54-59, 2002.

14. Chitty JR: Myriapods (centipedes and millipedes). In Lewbart GA, editor: *Invertebrate Medicine,* Ames, Iowa, 2006, Blackwell.

15. Williams DL: Invertebrates. In Meredith A, Redrobe S, editors: *BSAVA Manual of Exotic Pets,* ed 4, Gloucester, UK, 2002, British Small Animal Veterinary Association.

16. Visigalli G: Guide to hemolymph transfusion in giant spiders, *Exot DVM* 5(pt 6):42-43, 2004.

17. Cooper JE: Invertebrate anesthesia, *Vet Clin North Am Exot Anim Prac* 4(1):57-67, 2001.

18. Applebee KA, Cooper JE: An anaesthetic or euthanasia chamber for small animals, *Anim Technol* 40(1):39-43, 1989.

19. Berzins IK, Smolowitz R: Diagnostic techniques and sample handling. In Lewbart GA, editor: *Invertebrate Medicine,* Ames, Iowa, 2006, Blackwell.

20. Breene RG: *The ATS Arthropod Medical Manual: Diagnosis and Treatment,* Carlsbad, N Mex, 2001, American Tarantula Society.

21. Cooper JE: A veterinary approach to spiders, *J Small Anim Pract* 28(3):229-239, 1987.

22. Johnson-Delaney C: *Exotic Companion Medicine Handbook,* Lake Worth, Fla, 2000, Zoological Education Network.

23. Davies RR, Chitty JR, Saunders RA: Cardiovascular monitoring of an *Achatina* snail with a doppler ultrasound probe, *Proc Brit Vet Zool Soc,* Autumn Meeting:101, 2001.

24. Stewart DM, Martin AW: Blood pressure in the tarantula, *Dugesiella hentzi, J Comp Physiol* 88(2):141-172, 1974.

25. Williams DL: Sample taking in invertebrate veterinary medicine, *Vet Clin North Am Exot Anim Prac* 2(3):777-801, 1999.

26. Williams D: Studies in arachnid disease. In Cooper JE, Pearce-Kelly P, Williams DL, editors: *Arachnida: Proceedings of a Symposium on Spiders and Their Allies,* pp 116-125, 1992.

27. Murray MJ: Euthanasia. In Lewbart GA, editor: *Invertebrate Medicine,* Ames, Iowa, 2006, Blackwell.

28. Fiorito G: Is there pain in invertebrates? *Behav Processes* 12(4):383-388, 1986.

29. Stefano GB, Salzet B, Fricchione GL: Enkelytin and opioid peptide association in invertebrates and vertebrates: immune activation and pain, *Immunol Today* 19(6):265-268, 1998.

30. Smolowitz R: Gastropods. In Lewbart GA, editor: *Invertebrate Medicine,* Ames, Iowa, 2006, Blackwell.

31. Pizzi R, Carta RL, George S: Oral nematode infection of tarantulas, *Vet Record* 152(22):695, 2003.

32. Baker AS: Acari (mites and ticks) associated with other arachnids. In Cooper JE, Pearce-Kelly P, Williams DL, editors: *Arachnida: Proceedings of a Symposium on Spiders and their Allies,* pp 126-131, 1992.

33. Foelix RF: Biology of Spiders, ed 2, New York, 1996, Oxford University Press.

34. Williams D: Integumental disease in invertebrates, *Vet Clin North Am Exot Anim Prac* 4(2):309-320, 2001.

35. Cooper JE: Emergency care of invertebrates, *Vet Clin North Am Exot Anim Prac* 1(1):251-264, 1998.

36. Cooper JE: Insects. In Lewbart GA, editor, *Invertebrate Medicine,* Ames, Iowa, 2006, Blackwell.

37. Noga EJ, Hancock AL, Bullis RA: Crustaceans. In Lewbart GA, editor: *Invertebrate Medicine,* Ames, Iowa, 2006, Blackwell.

38. Edgerton BF, Evans LH, Stephens FJ et al: Synopsis of freshwater crayfish diseases and commensal organisms, *Aquaculture* (1-2):57-135, 2002.

39. Jangoux M: Diseases of echinodermata. In Kinne O, editor: *Diseases of Marine Animals, vol 3,* Hamburg, Germany, 1990, Biologische Anstalt Helgoland.

40. Schartau W, Leidescher T: Composition of the hemolymph of the tarantula *Eurypelma californicum, J Comp Physiol* 152(1):73-77, 1983.

41. Reichling SB, Tabaka C: A technique for individually identifying tarantulas using passive integrated transponders, *J Arachnol* 29(1):117-118, 2001.

42. Diaz JH: The global epidemiology, syndromic classification, management, and prevention of spider bites, *Am J Trop Med Hyg* 71(2):239-250, 2004.

43. Escoubas P, Rash L: Tarantulas: eight-legged pharmacists and combinatorial chemists, *Toxicon* 43(5):555-574, 2004.

44. de Haro L, Jouglard J: The dangers of pet tarantulas: experience of the Marseilles Poison Centre, *J Toxicol-Clin Toxicol* 36(1-2):51-53, 1998.

45. McCoy RH, Clapper DR: The oral flora of the South Texas tarantula, *Dugesiella anax* (Araneae: Theraphosidae), *J Med Entomol* 16(5):450-451, 1979.

46. Ratcliffe BC: A case of tarantula-induced papular dermatitis, *J Med Entomol* 13(6):745-747, 1977.

Stephen M. Miller
Mark A. Mitchell

CHAPTER 4

ORNAMENTAL FISH

Ornamental fish present an unusual paradox in that they are both well known and unknown to veterinarians. These animals are well known because they can be seen every day in the home aquarium, ornamental pond, pet store, and public aquarium,[1] while at the same time they are unknown because knowledge regarding their health care is limited (e.g., in the areas of antibiotic residuals, antibiotic resistance, emerging diseases, antiquated or undocumented diagnostic and surgical techniques, and pain management issues). The purpose of this chapter is to address some of the current and former issues related to the health and well-being of ornamental fish.

■ COMMON SPECIES KEPT IN CAPTIVITY

Fish represent the largest class of vertebrates, with more than 20,000 different species. This group also represents the largest number of species kept in captivity. While there may be tens or even hundreds of different species from another class of vertebrates kept in captivity, there are likely more than 1000 different species of fish that have been maintained in captivity. A visit to a local pet store will often reveal 50 to 100 different species of fish available for sale at any given time.

There are three major groups of fish kept in captivity: freshwater, brackish water, and saltwater. The fundamental difference among the three groups is the relative density of the water in which they live. Some fish can move between freshwater to brackish water or saltwater to brackish water, but relatively few fish can live in the two extremes (freshwater and saltwater). The various physiologic and anatomic characteristics among freshwater and saltwater fish will be addressed in the following sections.

■ FRESHWATER

It would be impossible and impractical to categorize every species of freshwater fish in a single book chapter, so we will present information about the two major groups of fish that are commonly kept in the captivity (freshwater temperate and tropical species) and refer to them as a general classification of bony fishes known as Actinopterygii. In addition, we will also provide more detailed information regarding three of the important groups of captive freshwater fishes: catfish, cichlids, and cyprinids.

Freshwater Temperate Fish

Most of the major taxonomic groups are represented by the freshwater temperate species.[2] For many, this group represents the species commonly considered as sport fish in the United States. The most common genera of freshwater temperate fishes maintained in captivity include the sturgeon (*Acipenser* spp.) (Figure 4-1), paddlefish *(Polyodon spathula),* eels (*Anguilla* spp.), pike (*Esox* spp.), bass (*Micropterus* spp.), sunfish (*Lepomis* spp.), walleye *(Sander vitreus),* mullet (*Mugil* spp.), spotted sea trout (*Cynoscion* spp.), salmonids, and cyprinids. Although many of these fish are raised by hobbyists, the majority of these species require much larger systems as might be represented in a public aquarium display. Consult an introductory ichthyology text for a more detailed description of the major taxonomic groups of freshwater temperate fish.

Freshwater Tropical Fish

Freshwater tropical fish represent the largest numbers of animals typically found in home aquaria. Generally, this group of fishes is readily available for a small to moderate investment and can be easily maintained by the novice aquarist or hobbyist. Families of freshwater tropical fish include characins (e.g., tetras: *Gymnocorymbus* spp., *Hemigrammus* spp., *Hyphessobrycon* spp., *Paracheirodon* spp., *Moenkhausia* sp.), cyprinids (barbs: *Barbus* spp.), catfish (e.g., *Corydoras* spp., *Pimelodus* spp.), killifish (e.g., *Aphyosemion* spp., *Fundulopanchax* spp.), rainbowfishes (e.g., *Iriatherina* spp., *Melanotaenia* spp., *Glossolepis* sp.), gouramies (e.g., *Colisa* spp., *Osphronemus* spp.,

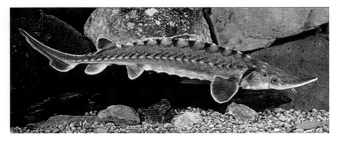

Figure 4-1 The sturgeon is a primitive freshwater temperate species. This genus has a wide range of species, representing relatively small sized animals to one of the largest freshwater species of fish. Although they are best known for their eggs (e.g., caviar), at least one species is offered for sale in the pet trade, and several others are routinely maintained in public aquaria.

Trichogaster spp.), livebearers (e.g., *Alfaro* spp., *Poecilia* spp., *Xiphophorus* sp.), and cichlids (e.g., *Pseudotropheus* spp., *Labidochromis* spp., *Iodotropheus* sp., *Dimidichromis* sp., *Copadichromis* sp., *Neolamprologus* spp., *Apistogramma* spp., *Microgeophagus* sp., *Aequidens* spp., *Cichlasoma* spp.).[2,3]

Catfish

Catfish (e.g., *Ictalurus* spp., *Lacantunia* spp., *Corydoras* spp., *Ancistrus* spp., *Pimelodus* spp., *Arius* spp., *Kryptopterus* spp., *Phractocephalus* spp.) represent one of the largest groups of freshwater fishes, with more than 2000 species. Catfish have a cosmopolitan distribution. Catfish are an important group because they serve many different roles, including as ornamentals (Figure 4-2, *A*), as food fish in aquaculture (Figure 4-2, *B*), as research animals, and for sport fishing. Most catfish are found in freshwater, although there are two families that contain saltwater species.[2,3] Although catfish have a cosmopolitan distribution, more than 50% of all catfish species are native to South America. There is a high degree of variability in the size and weight of these fish, with animals ranging from 10 cm to over 2 m in length and 10 g to over 300 kg in weight. Most species of catfish are nocturnal. Catfish are primarily benthic or bottom-dwellers. Because of their benthic lifestyle, catfish have sensory structures, barbels that assist them with characterizing food and nonfood items and substrate types in a low-light setting.

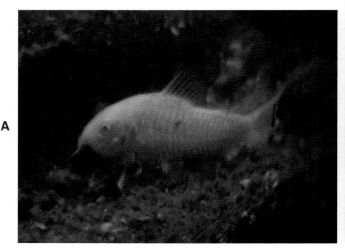
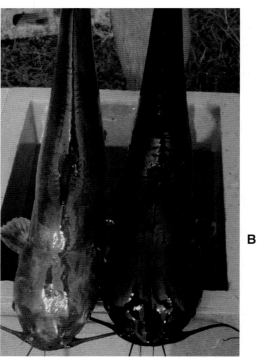

Figure 4-2 A, *Corydoras* sp. **B,** *Ictalurus* sp. Catfish represent a diverse group of fishes, with a significant amount of variability in morphology and physiology among genera. Although both are benthic, the catfish in **A** and **B** are shaped very differently.

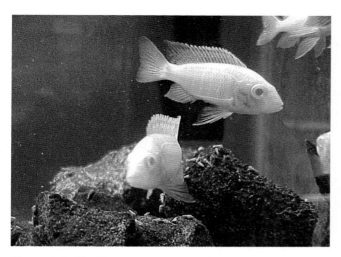

Figure 4-3 Cichlids represent one of the most popular groups of ornamental freshwater fishes kept in captivity.

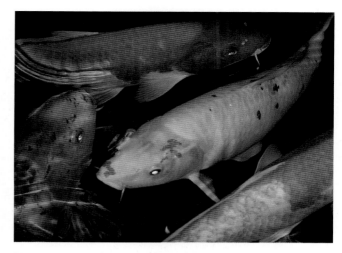

Figure 4-4 Koi (*Cyprinus carpio*) represent one of the most coveted groups of fish. These animals are prized for their color, size, and longevity. Their desirability is reflected in their value, with prized individuals selling for tens to hundreds of thousands of dollars.

Cichlids

The cichlids represent one of the most diverse groups of fish, with representation in North America, Central America, South America, and Africa. These fish are prized for their diversity in size, shape, and color. African lake cichlids are one of the most evolutionarily diverse groups in the world, as many different species have evolved within limited ecologic niches (Figure 4-3). With this rapid evolution have come highly variable morphology, feeding strategies, and dietary needs. Although cichlids can look highly variable from genus to genus, they all have a common "break" in their lateral line system. The lateral line is a mechanosensory structure that assists fish with interpreting events in their environment (e.g., shifts in water pressure suggesting a predator is approaching).

Cyprinids

Goldfish *(Carassius auratus),* koi *(Cyprinus carpio),* and carp (*Cyprinus* spp.) are members of the largest family (>2200 species) of freshwater fish, Cyprinidae. Cyprinids have the widest area of distribution of any of the freshwater fish. Southeast Asia is the center of origin for this family of fish; however, many species have been introduced around the world and have readily adapted to these new environments.[2] The carp are the largest species from this family and may hybridize with goldfish. Koi (Figure 4-4) are colorful domestic mutations of carp that are highly valued by hobbyists and the commercial pet trade. The koi can be divided into two major classifications: the nonmetallic koi and the metallic koi.[2] This division is based on typical color patterns, scale types, shape, and size. Goldfish are not koi but rather descendants of the Crucian carp *(Carassius carassius).*[2] Goldfish remain one of the most popular ornamental species and are often found in garden ponds and home aquaria. These fish generally do best if kept in cool waters (55°-68° F, 12°-20° C) with abundant plant life and adequate aeration. There are more than 30 varieties of ornamental goldfish available in the pet trade today.

■SALTWATER

Many marine fish species exist, and, again, it would be impossible to cover the diversity of these fishes in a single chapter. Therefore, this chapter will focus on the species most commonly seen in captivity, including marine tropical fish, marine coldwater fish, and the elasmobranchs (e.g., sharks, skates, and rays).[2-4]

Marine Tropical Fish

There are approximately 23 categories of marine tropical fish. These 23 groups can be arbitrarily divided into four major groups by their feeding attributes and compatibility with other species (Figure 4-5). Most of these groups are well represented in the aquarium trade and in public aquaria.

The first category of marine tropical fish is the "rapid eater" and includes the angelfish (e.g., *Pomacanthus* spp.), damselfish (e.g., *Amblyglyphidodon* spp.), squirrelfish (e.g., *Holocentrus* spp.), triggerfish (e.g., *Balistapus* spp., *Balistoides* spp.), and groupers (e.g., *Cephalopholis* spp., *Variola* spp.).[2] These fish do well if kept at low densities in the aquarium or if they are provided a large area where overcrowding is not an issue (e.g., large reef tanks in public displays). Hostile interaction is a major concern for these animals, as they can be very food aggressive.[2-4] These animals may be kept together quite readily if provided an abundance of food and a diverse diet. Often they are kept in live coral reef tanks with anemones and other species of animals from the same group.[2,3]

The slow eaters represent the largest subgroup of marine tropical fish. This group includes, but is not limited to, the

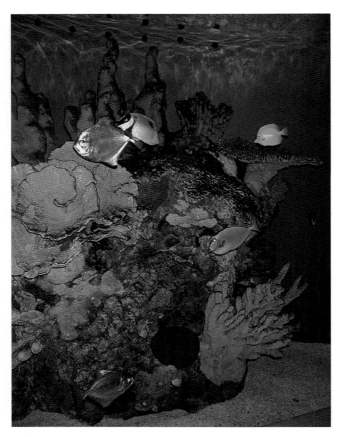

Figure 4-5 Marine tropicals should be housed based on their feeding strategy. This figure represents the typical setting for "rapid eaters."

anemone clown fish (e.g., *Amphiprion ocellaris*), parrotfish (e.g., *Sparisoma* spp.), puffers (e.g., *Carinotetraodon* spp., *Tetraodon* spp., *Colomesus* spp.), surgeonfish (e.g., *Acanthurus sohal*), wrasses (e.g., *Cheilinus* spp., *Halichoeres* spp., *Hemigymnus* spp., *Thalassoma* spp.), and trunkfish (e.g., *Aulostomus* spp., *Strophiurichthys* spp., *Ostracion* spp.). Compatibility is an issue with this group of animals, and they do best if maintained in large displays with a large amount of hiding area. Although these fish are grouped based on their feeding strategy, there remains a great deal of variability in the diets of these animals.

Another group extreme in feeding habits includes those animals that have difficulty competing for food. This group of animals includes some of the more unusual species, such as the seahorses (*Hippocampus* spp.), jawfishes (*Opistognathus* spp., *Stalix* spp., *Lonchopisthus* spp.), pipefish (*Stigmatopora* spp., *Lissocampus* spp., *Corythoichthys* spp.), and batfish (*Dibranchus* spp., *Halieutea* spp., *Halieutichthys* spp., *Malthopsis* spp., *Ogcocephalus* spp., *Zalieutes* spp.). Many of these fish are slow swimming and are easily outcompeted by faster swimming fish. Members of this group should be housed together with similar species and monitored closely to ensure that they obtain sufficient calories.

The last group of animals to be categorized as marine tropicals includes the snappers (e.g., *Lutjanus* spp., *Pristipomoides* spp., *Nemadactylus* spp., *Etelis* spp.) and grunts (e.g., *Haemulon* spp.). These are reasonably large, territorial schooling fish that are, for the most part, kept at public facilities. They can best be described as "gluttons," not only for the manner in which they feed but also for the almost insatiable hunger they exhibit. They are virtually fearless in their feeding habits and will attempt to remove food from the jaws of even large predators.[2]

Marine Coldwater Fishes

Although some of the smaller marine coldwater species are used for public display, many are too large to be accommodated in anything other than large aquaria. The majority of the species in this general category are used as commercial food fish. The first group, which represents approximately 70 different species, includes the gadids or cod (e.g., *Gadus* spp.), haddock (e.g., *Melanogrammus* spp.), hake (e.g., *Urophycis* spp.), and pollock (e.g., *Theragra* spp.). These species are valued as food and for their medicinal value. There are very few public aquaria that exhibit these large species, because they require systems in excess of 1 million gallons of seawater. Tuna (e.g., *Thunnus* spp., *Euthynnus* spp., *Katsuwonus* spp.) have become popular in large open ocean exhibits at public facilities, but only through improved and advanced life support technology and husbandry techniques has it been possible to exhibit this spectacular group of animals. By far the most common category of fish in this group is the flatfish. This group includes, but is not limited to, the flounder (e.g., *Platichthys* spp., *Scophthalmus* spp., *Limanda* spp., *Pleuronectes* spp., *Atheresthes* spp.), halibut (e.g., *Hippoglossus* spp.), and rock sole (*Lepidopsetta bilineata*). The sablefish (*Anaplopoma fimbria*) and lumpfish (*Paraliparis fimbriatus*) are also in this group of fish and are only occasionally represented in public displays.

Elasmobranchs

There are more than 350 species of sharks in the world, and only a small percentage are represented as display animals or kept by private aquarists and hobbyists. The species that are found occasionally in home aquaria include the carpet sharks (e.g., *Parascyllium* spp.) (Figure 4-6), catsharks (e.g., *Galeus* spp., *Scyliorhinus* spp.), and horned sharks (e.g., *Heterodontus* spp.). Most of the other species of sharks are much too large to be kept in anything less than a public aquarium or large commercial facility. Many public facilities display saw sharks (e.g., *Pristiophorus* spp.) and multiple species of ornamental sharks, including angel sharks (e.g., *Squatina australis*), dogfish (e.g., *Squalus* spp., *Scymnodon* spp., *Deania* spp., *Centroscymnus* spp.), and frilled sharks (e.g., *Chlamydoselachus* spp.).

Skates and rays are closely related to sharks; however, they are markedly different in appearance (Figure 4-7). There are both freshwater and saltwater varieties of stingrays. The skates and rays are dorsoventrally flattened animals and usually have at least one venomous spine on the dorsal caudal fin (tail).

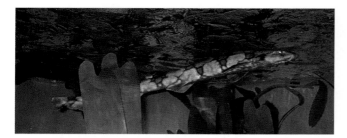

Figure 4-6 The carpet shark (*Parascyllium collare*) is one of the few species of elasmobranchs that can be kept in captivity by hobbyists.

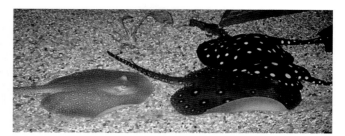

Figure 4-8 Freshwater stingrays are routinely found for sale in the pet trade. These animals originate from South America.

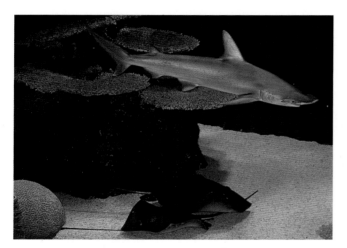

Figure 4-7 Sharks and stingrays have distinct morphologic features. Note the dorsoventrally flattened shape of the benthic (bottom-dwelling) ray compared to the streamlined pelagic (open water–dwelling) shark.

There are multiple freshwater species (Figure 4-8) that are small enough to be kept by the private aquarist; however, the majority of these animals are also found in public facilities. There are a number of ornamental species of saltwater rays, such as the guitarfish (e.g., *Rhinobatos* spp.), butterfly rays (e.g., *Gymnura* spp.), and cow-nose rays (e.g., *Rhinoptera* spp.), that have been maintained and successfully reproduced in public facilities. Many of the larger, saltwater rays, such as the southern stingray *(Dasyatis americana)*, Atlantic stingray *(Dasyatis sabina)*, eagle ray *(Myliobatis aquila)*, and giant manta ray *(Manta birostris)*, are also now being kept in public aquaria.

UNIQUE ANATOMY AND PHYSIOLOGY

When veterinarians begin to work with a new species of animal, it is imperative that they develop a basic understanding of the animal's anatomy and physiology. A background knowledge of anatomy and physiology will prove beneficial when collecting diagnostic samples or administering therapeutics. The following is a review of unique anatomic and physiologic features

of fish. (See other resources for additional information regarding this subject.[2])

Fish are covered with a mucous coat that is produced by cells in their integument. This mucous coat is an important component of the innate immune system and serves as the first line of defense against pathogenic organisms (e.g., bacteria, fungi, and viruses). The mucous barrier contains various sized proteins (e.g., immunoglobulins) that bind pathogens and prevent invasion. If this protective barrier is penetrated, fish have minimal protection against pathogens. To ensure that this barrier remains intact and undamaged, fish should be handled only when necessary.

The scales of a fish are located in the dermis and provide protection over the musculature. There are four types of scales found on fish: placoid, ganoid, cycloid, and ctenoid. Placoid scales are found on elasmobranchs, and ganoid, cycloid, and ctenoid scales are found on teleosts (e.g., bony fishes). The ganoid and cycloid scales are common on the more primitive species of teleosts, whereas the ctenoid scales are found on the more evolutionarily advanced fish. The scales serve as a protective armor, and damage or loss of the scales may result in the introduction of opportunistic infections. Handling should be minimized to avoid traumatizing the scales.

Teleosts typically have two sets of paired fins (e.g., pectoral and pelvic) and three unpaired fins (e.g., dorsal, anal, and caudal) (Figure 4-9). Fins are used for steering, balancing, and braking. Certain species have modified fins to adapt to certain niches. For example, the anal fin of the knifefish is a large, single fin located on the ventrum of the animal. This fins serves as the animal's primary source of locomotion. Spines may be associated with some fins and serve as a defense mechanism. The lionfish *(Pterois volitans)* produces venom that can be injected into a potential predator, causing significant pain and discomfort. Knowledge of the species that produce venom is essential to prevent injury to the handler. Fish may damage their spines when captured in a net. To prevent this, fish may be scooped into a plastic cup or bucket to facilitate removal from the aquarium.

The respiratory system of fish is vastly different from the respiratory systems of higher vertebrates (e.g., reptiles, birds, and mammals). Gills are the primary respiratory organs of most fish, although certain species use accessory organs to aid in the absorption of oxygen. Gills serve to absorb oxygen, excrete waste products (e.g., ammonia and carbon dioxide), and regulate ion and water balance. Teleosts have four pairs of gills; elasmobranchs can have five to seven pairs. The gills are attached to a bony gill arch, and each gill is comprised of primary and secondary lamellae. The secondary lamellae are the site of gas exchange (Figure 4-10). Exposure to parasites and toxic compounds, such as ammonia, results in excessive production of mucus, which can impede gas exchange. The presenting symptoms of affected animals include rapid opercular movements and gulping for air at the water's surface; among these animals sudden death may occur.

Fish have a simple, inline, two-chambered heart comprised of a single atrium and ventricle. The heart is located ventral to the pharynx and cranial to the liver. Unoxygenated blood is pumped from the heart to the gills, where it is oxygenated and distributed to the rest of the body. Fish possess two portal

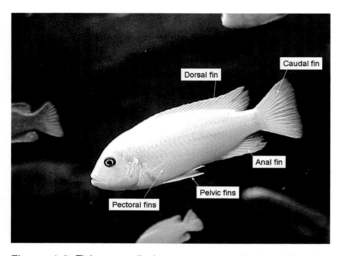

Figure 4-9 Fish generally have two sets of paired fins, the pectoral and pelvic, and three unpaired fins, the dorsal, anal, and caudal.

systems: a renal portal system, which drains blood from the caudal musculature, and a hepatic portal system, which drains venous blood from the digestive tract.

The lateral line is an important mechanosensory structure used by fish to detect changes in sound waves and water pressure. The lateral line originates on the head, around the eyes and nares, and extends along the lateral body wall. When maintained in captivity, certain groups of marine fish, including tangs and angelfish, may develop head and lateral line erosions. The specific causes of this syndrome have not been elucidated, but dietary deficiency, water quality, and infectious disease are all suspected.

Fish can be classified into three different feeding strategies: herbivore, omnivore, or carnivore. The length of the digestive tract can vary depending on feeding strategy. For example, the length of an herbivore's digestive tract is generally much longer than that of an omnivore or carnivore. The stomach is absent in some species, such as goldfish and carp. Pyloric cecae are found in some species of fish. These structures secrete digestive enzymes and increase the absorptive surface area of the digestive tract. Pyloric cecae are used as a taxonomic indicator in some species. The fish liver is a large structure and is located in the cranial coelomic cavity. The normal color of the liver should be red-brown; however, yellow, fatty livers are a common finding at necropsy. This finding is often the result of diets rich in fats and protein.

The fish kidney is a single structure that is comprised of two segments: anterior and posterior. The kidney is located dorsal to the swim bladder along the body wall. The fish kidney serves as both an osmoregulatory and a hematopoietic organ. The anterior kidney and the interstitium of the posterior segment serve as the primary sites for blood cell and immunoglobulin production in fish, as these animals do not have bone marrow. The posterior kidney primarily regulates electrolyte and urine output. Fish that are found in saltwater *(hypertonic)* environments tend to lose water and absorb salts.

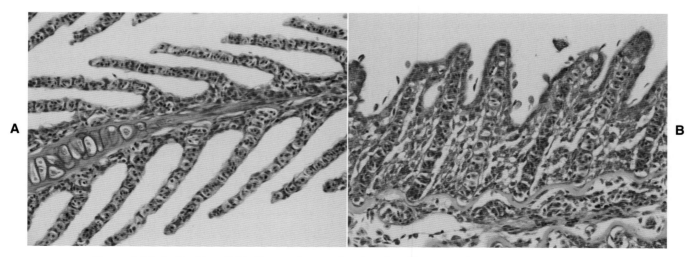

Figure 4-10 A, Healthy gill. **B,** Abnormal secondary lamellae. The secondary lamellae are the site of gas exchange and ammonia excretion in fish. Damage to these gills can result in reduced gas exchange, ammonia excretion, and death. (Courtesy Dr. Wes Baumgartner.)

To prevent dehydration, these fish must drink water and excrete excess electrolytes, such as sodium and chloride, through the kidney and gills. Fish that live in freshwater *(hypotonic)* environments constantly absorb water by osmosis. To prevent overhydration, freshwater fish excrete large volumes of dilute urine.

■ HUSBANDRY

Environmental Considerations

It is easy to recognize aquatic facilities (institutional or pet retail) that have the most disease problems on the basis of their appearance. There is usually an accumulation of trash, dirty exhibits, dead animals, and a general "unhealthy" appearance to the collection. This does not mean that a "clean" facility is free of disease but that they traditionally have fewer and less severe outbreaks of disease.[5] The general husbandry and maintenance of the aquatic facility and ecosystems have a direct relationship to the overall health of the animals. Maintaining clean areas behind the exhibits and nonpublic areas is essential to good health practices.[3,5] The same can be said for retail aquarium facilities. Accumulation of feces, excess food, and detritus are predisposing factors to poor water quality and can serve as substrates for facultative pathogens. Cleaning and disinfecting seines, nets, buckets, and tanks are imperative to maintain a high-quality health program at a facility. A dynamic team effort is required to maintain a clean facility and healthy animals, but a clean facility will pay dividends by providing a safer workplace, reduced disease incidence, increased production, and generally healthier fish.

Given ideal environmental conditions, ecosystems require a certain amount of space to fully develop, though quantitatively how much space is a debatable matter. Generally, to place an ecosystem in a very large aquarium or other holding space is not a major ecologic problem, although it might be considered an engineering endeavor. The difficulty arises when veterinarians attempt to scale down and include many components in a much smaller space than which would normally occur in the wild. To miniaturize an ecosystem and place it into a small space for observation, education, or research, veterinarians are immediately faced with a major dilemma, which is to scale the miniature so that it can still function as a reasonable facsimile of the wild ecosystem. This question is intimately related to the entire problem of how veterinarians affect wild environments and how they restore them, as well as how they construct their aquaria.[5,6]

Creating an Aquarium

There is little biologic reason for the traditional "box type" aquarium shape; however, the common reason for its existence is associated with availability and mechanical, aesthetic, and economic convenience (Figure 4-11). For many scientists and aquarists, the ease of purchase and setup of a ready-made tank outweighs all other factors when a water-based system is desired.

The presence of tank walls that can support benthic communities or allow excessive light is undesirable. A weakly translucent cylindrical tank that minimizes attachment surface for a given volume and has a rotating, cleaning mechanism to keep

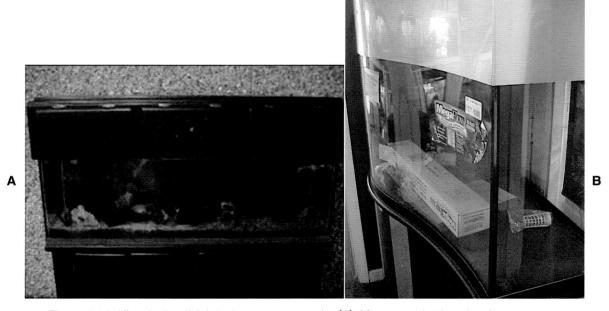

Figure 4-11 Historically, all fish tanks were rectangular **(A)**. More recently, there has been a movement by commercial tank manufacturers to create new tank shapes (e.g., bow front tank) **(B)**. These oddly shaped tanks do little for the aquatic ecosystem, and are primarily for aesthetics.

the surface free of sediment is highly desirable but very expensive.

For the hobbyist, aquarist, or scientist who wishes to construct an efficient model ecosystem, the materials (e.g., glass, plexiglass) are readily available to fabricate any shape or form of enclosure. Only after determining the ideal shape of the desired system, should one be concerned with the aesthetics, viewing, and construction of the aquarium.

TANK SIZE

Choosing the correct size of tank is an easy task. The main principle to remember is that bigger really is better. The smallest tank size we recommend is the commercially available 20-gallon tank (24″ × 12″ × 20″; 61 cm × 30.5 cm × 50.8 cm); however, the larger tanks provide an even more stable environment for fish. A larger tank also will offer the benefit of a much more liberal air-to-water surface area for the fish. However, with the advancements in life support technology today, it is possible to provide more than adequate life support to maintain large densities of fish in smaller aquaria while also maintaining a greater diversity of animals.[4,7,8]

TEMPERATURE

The term *tropical* places too much emphasis on the idea of "high temperature" for all exotic fishes. A number of these ornamental fish are not from the tropics, and quite a few from the tropics do not come from particularly warm water. It is important to recognize that a large number of exotic ornamental fish cannot thrive in cool, chilly water (<68° F or 20° C), because it affects their metabolic rate or immune function; other species cannot thrive in extremely warm water (>86° F or 30° C), because they need more oxygen than the water has the ability to carry. There is no exact degree of heat that is best suited to each species. Most fish tolerate a 10° F fluctuation over time and can stand a 5° F change in a short period of time (e.g., minutes) without consequence.[4,5] It is almost impossible to find a place in nature where the temperature falls into the controlled ranges that veterinarians try to achieve in the captive environment, and it would be reasonable to believe that temperature changes can be beneficial and stimulating to the animals. In practice, the aquarium environment should be geared toward the temperature needs of the species of fish that will inhabit the aquarium. It is best to create fish communities from similar ecosystems and attempt to maintain the temperature range as close as possible to the native waters of those particular species. Temperature changes will occur, but if they occur within the basic guidelines mentioned previously, these changes will be beneficial to the well-being of the animals.

FILTRATION

In nature, the waste products produced by fish are diluted into the vastness of the body of water and carried away by flowing water, reducing the potential dangers to fish. In closed systems (e.g., home or public aquarium), wastes and toxins can accumulate to levels that are harmful to fish. To avoid this problem, closed systems must be managed using some form of filtration. There are three primary types of filtration: mechanical, bio-

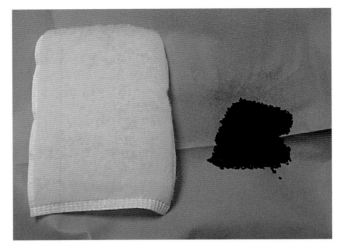

Figure 4-12 Mechanical filtration is used to remove detritus from an aquatic system. This type of filtration can be combined with the other methods to improve the overall water quality in a system. For example, this power filter cartridge is comprised of floss (mechanical) and carbon (chemical). Once in the system, it will also be colonized with nitrifying bacteria (biologic).

logic, and chemical. These different filtration mechanisms work independently of one another and can be used in combination.

Mechanical Filtration

Mechanical filtration represents one of the original forms of filtration used in the home aquarium. This type of filtration removes organic debris from the water by passing it through a filter material (e.g., floss, fiber, or paper cartridge) (Figure 4-12). The amount of filtration that can be accomplished using this type of filter depends on the type and size of the filter material and rate that the water is recirculated through the filter media. A densely packed fiber or small pore size will restrict the size of waste that can pass the filter media, resulting in less waste in the aquarium. Maintenance of these filters requires cleaning or replacement of the floss or cartridge. Mechanical filtration remains an important method of filtration in home aquaria, outdoor ponds, and public aquaria. This type of filtration is best used with other types of filtration (biologic or chemical) to improve the overall quality of water in the system. When a series of filters is used inline, it is best to place the mechanical filter first. This ensures that the heavy organic material will be removed before contaminating or clogging the other filters (e.g., chemical or biologic-sand filter). Mechanical filtration does have limitations; for example, it is not effective in trapping finite particles or chemicals.

Biologic Filtration

Ammonia is the primary end product of protein catabolism in fish. In a closed system, this waste product can be fatal to fish. It was the advent of biologic filtration that led to our ability to maintain large densities of fish in small volumes of water.

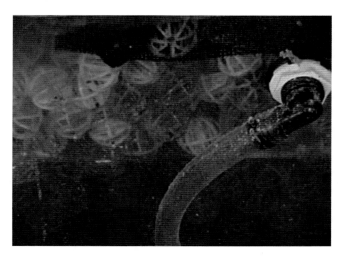

Figure 4-13 Biologic filtration is essential to maintaining fish in closed aquatic systems. There are many different ways to increase the overall surface area in a system to colonize nitrifying bacteria. This filtration method uses plastic balls as a surface for the bacteria.

Biologic filtration is the most common type of filtration used in the home aquarium and outdoor pond, and it comes in many different forms (e.g., under-gravel filters, bio-wheels, sand or bead filters, and wet-dry filters) (Figure 4-13). A biologic filter should be selected based upon the expected load on the system. If a large density of fish is going to be maintained in a system or the fish are going to be fed large quantities of food to ensure growth (e.g., aquaculture), then a large surface area for bacteria is needed.

The biologic filter is comprised of nitrifying bacteria. Although there are numerous types, the two most common genera discussed are *Nitrosomonas* spp. and *Nitrobacter* spp. *Nitrosomonas* spp. are important in denaturing ammonia, the primary waste product produced by fish, into nitrite. Both ammonia and nitrite are toxic to fish. *Nitrobacter* spp. are responsible for further reducing nitrite to nitrate.

Once an aquarium and biologic filter are colonized, the system becomes self-sufficient. However, there are several factors that can affect the function of a biologic filter, including temperature, oxygen content, and drugs/therapeutics. *Nitrobacter* spp. are not cold tolerant. Therefore, in outdoor ponds when the water temperature drops below 65° F (18.5° C), nitrite will not be converted into nitrate as rapidly. During those times when the water temperature may drop below 65° F, fish should be fed less food to reduce the load on the system. *Nitrosomonas* spp. and *Nitrobacter* spp. are aerobic bacteria. In the well-aerated home aquarium, oxygen levels are often adequate for the bacteria; however, in outdoor ponds, oxygen levels can become depleted on warm summer nights. To reduce the likelihood of biologic filter failure, it is recommended that outdoor ponds be aerated during warm, summer days and nights.

A biologic filter requires time to become established. The amount of time depends upon the temperature of the water

and the organic load on the system. New systems should be started slowly, adding only a small number of fish at a time. Closely monitoring the ammonia, nitrite, and nitrate levels on a daily basis is strongly recommended for new systems. Commercial microbial products (Fritzyme; Fritz Industries, Dallas, TX) are available that can expedite the establishment of the filter by seeding the system with bacteria. Water samples, filter pads, or aquarium substrates from established systems have also been used to seed a tank. However, the addition of these products to a new system may lead to the introduction of potential fish pathogens.

Chemical Filtration
There are numerous types of chemical filters in the pet trade. Chemical filtration refers to those filters that remove toxic compounds by binding them or converting them into nontoxic substances. The original form of chemical filtration was activated carbon. Carbon serves as a nonspecific binding agent for a number of different substances. When the binding sites on the carbon are full, they no longer act as filters and need to be replaced or cleaned. Other forms of chemical filtration are more specific, such as the resins that only bind ammonia. There are other forms of chemical filtration, such as ultraviolet (UV) sterilizers and protein skimmers, that alter or trap compounds. UV sterilizers expose compounds to short wavelength light, altering their form and rendering them harmless. UV sterilizers can be used to control certain pathogens and algae. A UV sterilizer has a UV bulb encased in a waterproof sheath within a cylinder. As water passes through the cylinder, the water is exposed to UV light, which can alter the DNA or RNA of the organism. The amount of time that it takes for the water to pass the bulb and the bulb wattage determine the effectiveness of the UV sterilizer. A low-wattage bulb in a short cylinder will have little effect on pathogens. These systems have also been used with great success at controlling algae and pathogens in outdoor ponds. Protein skimmers trap proteins in bubbles so that they can be separated from the water and removed. Chemical filtration, in combination with mechanical or biologic filtration, can improve the water quality dramatically, creating a "healthy" environment for fish.

LIGHTING
Correct lighting for the aquarium system depends on several factors, including the quality of the light emitted from the selected light source. Full-spectrum lighting is preferred. This type of lighting provides the three primary light spectrums: ultraviolet, visible, and infrared. The various spectrums can be affected by water depth, with certain spectrums (e.g., ultraviolet) being removed in the epilimnion (upper water level). Another important factor is the function of the system. If the tank is going to house deep-water African cichlids, lighting becomes less important; however, if the lighting system is needed for a reef tank that is going to be stocked with corals, a significant quantity of high-quality full-spectrum light will be required. The primary disadvantages associated with excess lighting are algae overgrowth and overheating the water in

smaller systems; otherwise, it is virtually impossible to have too much light in an aquarium system.[4] A 12 hour photoperiod is considered appropriate for most fish. For those individuals interested in breeding fish, the photoperiod should be lengthened to mimic a spring/summer season.

SUBSTRATE

Historically, aquarists have tended to ignore the substrate of an aquatic system, reducing it to a noninteracting element. In the aquaria of past decades, "clean," relatively inert gravel and under-gravel filters were used to provide environments for all but the most specialized natural situations. In nature, with the exception of gravel bottoms in relatively unproductive hard rock mountain streams or sandy beaches with sandstone composition, rarely is the substrate material neutral. In most aquatic and marine environments, soft substrates are rich in organic reservoirs and harbor a myriad of important invertebrates and microbes that support rich plant growth. Limestone substrates control water chemistry, and reef corals and rocks determine the very character of the organisms growing on the surface of the reef. The interest in so-called live rock in coral reef tanks in recent years is beginning a tendency to replace sterile environments with live ecosystems. The addition of "trickle trays" with calcium carbonate pebbles also shows a developing interest in further elucidating the carbonate cycle and control over the pH. Conversely, acid, black water streams are most likely to occur in granite or sandstone areas where the natural acidity of the rain and tannic acid from the forest litter cannot be neutralized. To recreate this environment, the aquarist is advised to use hard rock and silica sand. Coarse sand or gravel is perhaps the most difficult of benthic environments for organisms to adapt to, and within sand and gravel habitats there are relatively few common species. In a stream or small lake that is not large enough for significant wave activity, or in a bay or coastal lagoon along a sandy coast, the sediment becomes progressively finer from gravel, to sand and silt, to a soupy, silty-clay mud substrate. To remain sand, the bottom must stay in constant motion; therefore, special adaptations are required by any organism to adapt to it. Even bacterial numbers tend to be limited in sand and gravel because their organic substrates are often washed out.[9,10] It can be difficult to maintain a sandy, shore style substrate in a closed, captive system, as it can have a rather long profile in the energy regime required to maintain the sand. It would be impossible to recreate a wave-break, sandy scenario within a miniature system unless the benthic community is the only one desired.

Traditionally, the general approach to filtration followed by most aquarists was to avoid the natural detrital processes in an aquatic system and to keep bacteria in filters that mimicked the benthic community. However, in a filter, the variety, density, and capability of the bacteria are limited. Thus, aquarium procedures of the past have tended to short-circuit the natural cycling processes, which resulted in the loss of valuable energy to the many members of the community. Aquaria that do not have a fine sediment component should have a separate sediment trap that can be partially drained of sediment, especially if it is intended to drive a system faster than normal for scaling. For the aquarist, fine sediment bottoms should not be ignored. Given their full reign, with the proper environment and biota available, they can be important buffering systems and provide necessary stability for a healthy environment.

ACCESSORIES FOR AQUARIA

There are a myriad of commercial accessories available for aquaria today. These accessories range from simple items, such as heaters and aeration devices, to some of the most advanced biotechnology available in the field, such as chillers and wave machines. Most commercial accessories available on the market are well made, and the deficiencies have been minimized over the years. When choosing a particular item, selection should be based on function not brand. For example, with a heater, it is important to match the wattage of the instrument to the volume of water to be heated, taking into account the general temperature required for the environment in which the aquarium is to be located.[4] There are several types of heaters available, including basic submersible heating elements, solar units, flow through units, or a combination of similar systems.

Water filtration units should be selected based on desired type of filtration, the volume requirements of a particular system, and its intended use. For example, a sand filtration unit should be selected on the basis of the volume of water to be used, the turnover rate expected for that volume of water, and the frequency with which the sand filter must be backwashed. Sometimes it is preferable, if not necessary, to combine several methods of filtration (e.g., under-gravel filtration in combination with sand filtration and power filtration). This enables the water to be "cleaned" using multiple methods. The use of multiple filters inline is particularly important in a public facility where a large water volume and bioload are used.

Most saltwater aquaria utilize some form of ozonator in combination with a protein skimmer. Protein skimmers utilize the age-old technology that has been used by sewage treatment plants for years: Minute air bubbles are passed through water with a high organic waste content, and the protein is captured and trapped as foam at the surface of the water. The greater the degree of organic pollution there is, the more stable the foam will be. The skimmer collects the foam, and the foam is then collapsed to a liquid and removed from the aquarium without tainting the water.

WATER QUALITY ANALYSIS

The aquatic environment is a very complex system that is subject to constant physical and chemical changes. A water-assessment program should be devised for monitoring an aquatic ecosystem. Many factors need to be taken into consideration when designing a water quality monitoring program, including the volume of water in the aquarium/aquaria, the number and type of animals that will be present, the type of life support system, and the period of time the aquarium has been set up. Ideally, a water-assessment program should be established before designing and setting up a system, keeping in mind that most of the water quality analysis is done to keep its inhabitants healthy.[8]

Water testing should be done daily for new aquaria until the system has cycled. When collecting a water sample, it is important to collect a mid-water sample, as samples closer to the surface or substrate will reflect more extreme values.[2,3] Portable water analysis kits use premeasured reagents and simple analytic methods that may compromise the degree of accuracy. However, they are suitable for most private aquarists and small backyard ponds. Most large, public aquaria use more advanced analytic methods, such as mass spectrometry, saturometers, and sophisticated chemical analysis, for evaluating water quality. The acquisition and utilization of many of these processes and techniques are beyond the scope of what most private aquarists can afford. Commercial water quality laboratories can perform a complete water analysis for a modest price, and it may be a good idea to submit a sample to a laboratory for a baseline measurement. This method also offers the added benefit of comparing standardized values with the parameters derived from veterinarians' own testing methods.

Water quality is very important to the health of a fish, and poor water quality can prove fatal. There are two types of systems that can be used: open and closed. In open water systems, the water in the aquarium is continually replenished using a fresh water source. An individual who lives near the ocean may collect seawater for a home aquarium, although that is not recommended because of potential contaminants in the water. Open water systems are rarely used because they are labor intensive and require regular exchange of the entire system. The majority of home aquaria utilize closed recirculating systems, which recirculate the same water over and over again using a filter. In the closed system, fresh water is added only after evaporation or at the time of a water change.

Ammonia, Nitrite, and Nitrate

Ammonia is produced in fish as an end product of protein catabolism. This waste product is primarily excreted via the gills, although some excretion in the feces also occurs. Ammonia is also generated in the aquatic system from the breakdown of uneaten food and detritus. Ammonia nitrogen can occur in two forms: ammonium (NH_4^+) and ammonia (NH_3). Ammonia is the more toxic form for fish.[11] The relative concentration of each form varies with pH and water temperature.[12] Ammonia is soluble in water, and minimal amounts are lost through evaporation. In a closed system, such as an aquarium or backyard pond, ammonia levels can build up to toxic quantities (>1 ppm). Even low levels of ammonia can be toxic to the gills and skin, resulting in increased susceptibility to infections. Fish suffering from ammonia toxicity appear irritated, gasp at the water's surface, and rub against rocks in the aquarium as a result of the irritation caused by the toxin. Ammonia levels should be monitored closely in closed systems, especially those with high fish densities. Testing for ammonia should be done weekly using a standardized commercial test kit, which is available at local pet retailers. In an established system, ammonia levels should be zero. If the ammonia levels begin to rise, then the system should be reevaluated. Overfeeding and overstocking an aquarium can overburden the biologic filter. Severe temperature fluctuations and insufficient oxygen levels may

also result in a significant loss of the biologic filter. This is especially common in ponds that have significant summer algal blooms. New systems require time to become established, and new fish should be added gradually to prevent an overload of the biologic filter.

Because ammonia is a common waste product in the aquarium, most problems can be prevented by limiting the numbers of fish in the aquarium and regulating the amount of feed being offered. A general rule of thumb for feeding fish is to only offer what they can eat in a 2- to 5-minute period. In cases where ammonia levels are creating problems, the first recommendation is to remove 25% to 50% of the water from the system and replace it with fresh, dechlorinated water. There are commercial products available that can chelate the ammonia source, but they are only a temporary solution. The primary cause of the elevated ammonia levels must be diagnosed and corrected.

Ammonia is a colorless, odorless substance that can cause significant mortalities in a home aquarium. Most inexperienced aquarists tend to single out infectious diseases when they experience fish losses; however, poor water quality (e.g., excessive ammonia or nitrite) is often a primary/secondary cause of mortalities in these animals and should be tested on a regular basis.

The nitrogen cycle eliminates ammonia by converting it to less toxic compounds. The first step in the cycle is to convert ammonia to nitrite. *Nitrosomonas* spp. are the primary bacteria associated with this process. Unfortunately, nitrite is also toxic (>0.1 ppm) to fish and can be rapidly absorbed across the gills. Affected animals may develop a methemoglobinemia and have a characteristic "brown blood." This blood dyscrasia leads to reduced erythrocyte oxygenation and respiratory compromise. Fish with nitrite toxicity may behave similarly to fish with ammonia toxicity, and be found gasping for air at the water surface and die suddenly. When fish show clinical signs associated with nitrite toxicity, they should be removed from the toxic water and placed into a fresh, dechlorinated, well-oxygenated system. A significant water change (25%-50%) should be made in the original aquarium or pond and the biologic filter reestablished. Salt can also be used to diminish the toxicity associated with salt.

The second step of the nitrogen cycle occurs when *Nitrobacter* spp. oxidizes nitrite to nitrate. Nitrate levels less than 0.5 ppm are generally regarded as safe; levels less than 5.0 ppm are associated with stress and may predispose fish to opportunistic infections; levels greater than 10 ppm are considered toxic for some species. Reports of nitrate toxicity are rare in freshwater and saltwater fish, but at elevated levels they may be stressful and predispose the animals to opportunistic pathogens. Nitrate is utilized by plants and algae as a food source. Nitrate can be removed from an aquatic system by performing regular water changes.

Ammonia and nitrite levels in an aquatic system may rise soon after treatment of the water with antibacterial compounds or a reduction in water temperature. Antibiotics added to the water are nonselective and may kill both pathogenic and commensal organisms. If these compounds kill enough of the bacteria associated with the biologic filter, then oxidation of ammonia and nitrite may stop. *Nitrosomonas* spp. are more temperature tolerant and will recolonize before *Nitrobacter* spp., so ammonia levels should be expected to decrease before nitrites. Therefore, elevated nitrite levels are often detected soon after a reduction in water temperature.

"New Tank" Syndrome

"New tank" syndrome is a common occurrence with beginner aquarists and primarily occurs when fish are overstocked in a new aquarium. If large numbers of fish are added to an aquarium, and the biologic filter is not established, the system will be unable to eliminate the ammonia produced by the fish. In most cases, the owners report an acute mortality event with clinical signs consistent with ammonia and nitrite toxicity. These problems can be prevented if the new owner is patient and realizes the importance of providing a break-in for the filter (4-6 weeks). Fish should be stocked gradually, usually one to two fish per week. A standard rule of thumb for a freshwater stocking density is 1 to 1.5 inches of fish per gallon of water; in saltwater systems, the stocking density should be 2 to 2.5 inches of fish per gallon of water. With the advent of new filtration systems, stocking densities will continue to increase; however, if the filter becomes compromised or fails, the results would be disastrous.

Oxygen

In the aquatic system, oxygen diffuses into water at the surface when the surface tension of the water is broken. For home aquaria, this occurs regularly when external filters are used that "drop" the water back into the tank like a waterfall or when airstones are used. The amount of available or dissolved oxygen (DO) within the system can be measured using special equipment. In most cases, a DO greater than 5 ppm is sufficient to maintain fish. For the home hobbyist, oxygen depletion is generally only a major problem with outdoor ponds during the summer months. During the day, plants produce their own food (photosynthesis) by removing carbon dioxide from the water and using energy produced by the sun. As plants make their food, they release oxygen into the water. During the night when plants or algae cannot undergo photosynthesis, they actually consume oxygen. In ponds with a large number of plants or algae, the oxygen levels in the water can fall to dangerously low levels (<3 ppm) for the fish. Another factor that may affect oxygen levels in the water column is temperature. Oxygen is lost to the atmosphere more rapidly in warm water than cold water. The use of aerators or fountains, especially at night, will help maintain adequate levels of oxygen in a pond.

Water pH

The pH of water is measured by taking the negative logarithm of hydrogen ions in the water. In simplest terms, pH can de divided into three categories: acid, neutral, and basic. The range of pH values fits on a scale of 1 to 14. Values below 7.0 represent acidic water, values between 7.0 and 7.9 are neutral, and values above 8.0 are basic. The pH in most aquaria and ponds should fall between 6.5 and 8.5. In the extreme ranges (<4.0 or >10.0), water would be so acidic or basic that it would burn the fish. This means that the difference between 7.0 and 8.0 is much more significant than expected, because the pH values are based on a logarithmic scale. Therefore, if the pH is allowed to fluctuate, fish will become stressed and more susceptible to disease. The pH of natural bodies of water varies based on the substrate, water shed, and other environmental factors. Fish from Central America and South America thrive in water that is neutral or slightly acidic, whereas fish from Africa and Asia thrive better at neutral to alkaline water.

Water should always be tested before replacement into an aquarium. There are a number of factors that may affect the pH in an aquarium or pond, including the biologic filter, fish density, vegetation, and algae. Biologic filtration actually produces acid when ammonia is converted into nitrite. If the water has a low buffering capacity, and the aquarium or pond biologic filter is converting a large amount of ammonia, the pH could become very acidic. Fish produce carbon dioxide (CO_2) as a waste product. When an aquarium or pond is heavily stocked with fish, the amount of CO_2 can build up in the water. Carbon dioxide promotes acid production and can actually decrease the pH (acidic). Plants and algae, which use photosynthesis during the day to make energy, utilize CO_2. However, at night, plants and algae utilize oxygen (like fish) and expel CO_2 as a waste product. In a system with a large number of plants and a large amount of algae, the pH can drop to a dangerously low level. Fish die-offs in ponds are often associated with high CO_2, low pH, and low oxygen levels. When plants or fish die, they also release compounds that can lower the pH. To prevent this from becoming a problem, always immediately remove dead fish or plants.

Chlorine

Chlorine is an elemental gas that is added to municipal water as a disinfectant. Unfortunately, chlorine is also toxic to fish. Fish that are exposed to chlorinated water can develop life-threatening respiratory distress. Chlorine readily crosses the gills of fish and blocks the animal's ability to absorb oxygen. Fortunately, chlorine can be removed from the water by allowing it to de-gas for 48 to 72 hours or by adding a dechlorinator (e.g., sodium thiosulfate). Chlorine levels in municipal water can fluctuate with the season; thus, questions about the timing or the amounts of chlorine that are being added in a specific municipality should be directed to the local water company. Chlorine levels in a water sample can be tested using a commercial test kit purchased from a local pet retailer.

Chloramine

Chloramine represents another disinfectant that is routinely added to municipal water for sterilization purposes. Chloramines are a combination of chlorine and ammonia. Commercial dechlorinators can still be used to remove the chlorine from this molecule, but they do nothing to the ammonia. Because ammonia is toxic to fish, it is important that levels of this compound do not reach levels greater than 1 ppm. Fortunately, a functional biologic filter will prevent this from occurring.

Hardness

Hardness measures the quantity of divalent cations (e.g., calcium and magnesium) in the water. In natural waters, the divalent ions are derived from the limestone, salts, and soils. The general range for hardness in freshwater systems is 0 to 250 mg/L, whereas in saltwater systems, hardness can exceed 10,000 mg/L.[13] The divalent cations that represent hardness, calcium and magnesium, play an intricate role in water quality conditions. Calcium can alter osmoregulatory function in fish during times of low pH or elevated ammonia.[13] Calcium and magnesium are both important for growth and development in fish fry.[14] These minerals can also protect fish against heavy metals by competing for gill absorption sites. Copper is routinely used to treat parasites. Calcium and magnesium compete with the copper for absorption sites, reducing the effectiveness of the copper. Distilled water should never be used to replenish water in an aquarium because it is deficient in these essential cations.

Alkalinity

In natural aquatic systems (e.g., lakes, ponds, rivers, streams), fish are exposed to a relatively stable pH because of buffers. The most common buffers in aquatic systems are bicarbonate (HCO_3) and carbonate (CO_3^{2-}). Other buffers that may occur in water in lesser amounts include hydroxide (OH^-), silicates, phosphates, and borates. The quantity of buffers within a system depends upon the source of the water. Some municipal water supplies contain relatively low concentrations of buffers, whereas others may have large concentrations. In cases where the water has a low buffering capacity, commercial buffers can be purchased from a local pet store and added to an aquarium to create a more stable pH.

Total alkalinity can also play a protective role against potential heavy metal toxins. Heavy metals (e.g., copper and lead) in the water can be absorbed at the level of the gills, build up to toxic levels, and lead to the eventual death of an affected fish. Bicarbonate and carbonate can protect against heavy metals by chelating them in the water, rendering them harmless. This is important to remember when treating fish with nonchelated copper. If the alkalinity is high, the nonchelated copper may be bound and rendered useless.

MONITORING WATER QUALITY

New Tanks

Water should be tested daily for ammonia, nitrite, nitrate, and weekly for pH, alkalinity, and hardness. Testing should continue until the parameters show a consistent pattern. Allow 4 to 6 weeks for the biologic filter to become established. Only one to two fish should be added at one time to ensure that the biologic filter is not overloaded. If municipal water is being used, it is important to test it regularly to ensure that there is no major fluctuation in the various water quality parameters, especially chlorine and chloramines.

Established Tanks

Routine water changes are important to maintaining a healthy closed aquatic system. Approximately 10% to 20% of the water should be changed every 1 to 3 weeks. The frequency of the water change will ultimately depend on the load placed on the system. For example, smaller aquaria and highly stocked aquaria should have their water changed more frequently. Routine monitoring of the water (e.g., ammonia, nitrite, nitrate) is an excellent way to determine whether the frequency of water changes is sufficient for a system.

■ NUTRITION

Providing appropriate nutrition and good quality water are probably the two most difficult aspects of maintaining a successful aquarium. Because there are hundreds of different fish species in the aquarium hobby, ornamental fish nutrition is an art and a science that must be approached systematically and holistically. Examining species-specific anatomy and natural history are useful starting points.[15] Food fish research can be used to provide fundamental nutritional information, but food fish are not ideal research models for all confined species.

Dietary Requirements

Information on the nutritional requirements of many ornamental fish is still relatively unknown, as compared to the nutritional requirements of many cultured food fish. Examining the nutritional value of a diet being fed to confined fish, and comparing it with known nutritional requirements of the fish, can assist in the diagnosis of malnutrition related to disease processes.[15,16]

Natural diets of most fishes are rich in protein. The gross protein requirement for those fish in which the requirements have been established range from 25% to 56%. However, just measuring the protein quantity is not enough, as the protein quality, digestibility, and amino acid availability also must be considered to ensure that the protein content of a prepared ration is sufficient to meet the needs of the species being fed. Dietary fats represent a significant source of energy for fish. Phospholipids and steroid components of visceral organs rely on dietary lipids to synthesize specific fatty acids that are essential for health and growth. Optimal levels of dietary fats for ornamental fish have not been established at this time. Fish digest carbohydrates at a lower rate than do higher vertebrates. Natural diets of carnivorous fish are generally lower in carbohydrates. These fish utilize proteins and fats more efficiently than carbohydrates.[5,6,15,16] The carbohydrate molecular structure of prey species influences the digestibility of the feed stuff in carnivorous fish. Excess digestible carbohydrate in the diet of fish can increase blood sugar, liver glycogen storage, and liver mass, sometimes to pathologic levels.[6,17]

Little or no energy is expended by most fish to maintain their body temperature or position in the water, as the normal body temperature for most fish is about the same as the environmental temperature.

Vitamins essential to the survival of ornamental fish must be supplied in sufficient quantities and intervals to provide the minimum requirements for that particular fish species. Diets specifically formulated for ornamental fish should attempt to

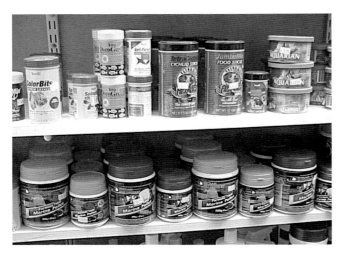

Figure 4-14 Foods depicted here represent only a sample of the commercially prepared foods that were available during a visit to a local aquarium store. It is important that veterinarians working with these animals carefully read the nutritional analysis and ingredient lists of these foods to determine their value for a specific population of fish.

incorporate a minimum quantity of essential vitamins (e.g., water soluble and fat soluble) and trace minerals. Veterinarians working with these species should make a habit of reading the nutritional analysis and ingredient lists of these diets (Figure 4-14). Ingredient lists should include natural components of the fish's diet. For example, fish meal would be an important ingredient for piscivorous fish, whereas cornmeal would not. Vitamin deficiencies may result in well-defined disease syndromes, with the possibility of high mortalities. Even partial deficiencies may result in increased susceptibility to disease.[16] Information on the quantitative vitamin and trace element requirements of specific species of fish that have been studied is often used to extrapolate dietary vitamin requirements for other fish that have a similar physiology.[3,6,18] Fish require the same mineral elements as higher animals, and each mineral has a similar function. Although dietary sources of vitamins and minerals are important for fish, their aquatic medium can also serve as an important source of the essential nutrients. This is especially true for fish fry. When fry are raised in water with a low hardness, they can develop calcium and magnesium deficiencies. Marine fish maintained in synthetic seawater can develop signs of hypovitaminosis or mineral deficiency because of a reduction or complete lack of vitamins and trace elements in the water. Routine diet and water analysis can alleviate problems associated with hypovitaminosis and mineral deficiency by monitoring for, and correcting, any deficiencies before the deficiencies become apparent in the fish.

■ PREVENTIVE MEDICINE

Preventive medicine is the concept of instituting preemptive measures for raising animals under conditions that optimize growth rate, feed conversion efficiency, reproduction, and survival, while minimizing problems related to infectious, nutri-

tional, and environmental diseases.[3-5] In an aquatic environment, there is a profound and inverse relationship between environmental quality and the disease status of the fish. As environmental conditions deteriorate, severity of infectious diseases increase; therefore, sound health maintenance practices can play a major role in maintaining a suitable environment where healthy fish can be raised. The application of preventive medicine programs is a positive concept that aids in disease prevention, emphasizes interruption of a disease cycle, and results in healthier, more productive animals. Its goal is to improve the health and well-being of animals that appear to be healthy. This is accomplished by several means, which include, but are not limited to, quarantine; routine diagnostic testing; and prophylactic treatment with dips, immersion baths, and/or parenteral treatment at acquisition and before release from quarantine. It also requires routine examination and review of acquisition and accession protocols. If sound health management and preventive principles are followed, the animals will be more productive and in better health.

Quarantine Essentials

An essential part of any preventive medicine program is a good quarantine system. All animals should be quarantined regardless of point of acquisition. However, the requirements for the length of quarantine may vary to a great degree. For example, wild-caught animals require a longer period of quarantine than captive-reared species. It makes sense that animals in the wild would have a much greater chance of being exposed to parasites and infectious diseases. Although there may be significant differences in protocols, a typical plan might recommend isolating animals in a clinical system for a minimum of 30 to 45 days. Before introducing fish to this clinical system, the animals should be closely examined and treated for external and internal parasites.

Stress plays a major role in the mortality rates of recent acquisitions. Fish can experience stress due to handling, transport, poor environmental quality, overstocking, mismatching species, and exposure to disease. The stress response exhibited by fish can cause several physiologic changes, resulting in an increased susceptibility to disease. Fish experiencing physiologic stress can have elevated corticosteroid and glucose levels, which can result in a depression of the immune response and increased susceptibility to disease. Most quarantined animals will show signs of disease shortly after transport in direct response to elevated stress levels. Some animals are more resistant than others in responding to the aforementioned stimuli and will not require any further attention. Animals that are showing clinical signs of disease should be treated accordingly.

Before release from quarantine, all animals should receive a second physical examination and series of diagnostic tests. Animals should only be removed from quarantine if they are found to be normal on examination and if the diagnostic tests are negative. We usually treat fish with a final immersion bath before introducing them into the resident population of the aquarium. This is a final step in reducing the likelihood of introducing pathogens into a display exhibit or home aquarium.

Preventive Measures

A preventive health maintenance program should be in place when an aquatic facility opens or when the home hobbyist acquires numerous aquaria. Health issues should be addressed on a daily basis, not just when a problem arises. When problems are encountered, a treatment regime should be implemented that identifies a short-term resolution to the problem with a long-range plan in mind.[3] Often a chemical can be added to the water and/or feed, which will result in a positive response and cessation of mortality. The effect of these treatments may be temporary, however, and disease may recur unless a commitment is made to seek and eliminate all predisposing factors.[5] The list of possible therapeutics can be found in Table 4-1. Although preventive health maintenance is important in controlling fish disease, it is not a "cure all." Some fish diseases are less preventable through environmental management than others, and for some there is no prevention or treatment at all. However, there is a large arsenal of treatments that are currently available and quite effective (see Table 4-1). No health maintenance program is perfect, but emphasis on disease prevention is well worth the effort.

Routine Examinations

The handling of aquatic animals both in and out of their natural environment almost always creates great difficulties. Struggle during capture, and even minimal handling, can have adverse effects on both the physiology and behavior of these animals. Consequently, it is often necessary to immobilize or chemically restrain animals for routine examination. For some procedures sedation may be necessary to eliminate or at least minimize stress or physical harm to the animal. Always determine before a procedure whether the benefit of the procedure outweighs the risk involved.[19] In many cases, a simple visual inspection of the animals is sufficient. For example, it might be beneficial to visually inspect small, schooling fish as a group to gain information about their general health.

■ RESTRAINT

Gross physical damage is a major concern when handling aquatic animals. The skin of a fish is very thin and easily damaged. There are also many delicate external appendages (e.g., fins) that may be easily damaged. This is a factor that is often overlooked, especially when the procedures are brief and the clinician believes it is void of consequences. In theory, if performing anything other than a visual inspection, sedation is advised.[3,19]

Manual Restraint

Manual restraint may be utilized if certain precautions are taken. It is feasible to move smaller animals with little or no direct contact with their skin. Nets, seines, buckets, acrylic transport containers, and plastic sleeves are all viable options.

Latex gloves should always be worn when there is a possibility of contact with the skin of aquatic animals. Bony fishes are extremely sensitive to contact with human skin, as are many species of aquatic invertebrates. Precautions should be taken to ensure that the latex gloves are thoroughly rinsed before having direct contact with the fish.

Chemical Restraint

An extensive range of drugs has been used for sedating and anesthetizing fish. However, describing all of the potential methods of aquatic animal restraint is beyond the scope of this chapter, and another text is recommended for that purpose.[19] Dose rates for sedating or anesthetizing fish can vary from one species to another, so it is important to be prepared for radically different dose responses from different species.

One of the most popular drugs used for fish anesthesia is tricaine methane sulfonate or MS-222 (Argent Laboratories, Redmond, WA). It is readily available, inexpensive, and very safe. MS-222 is an acidic compound and should be buffered (before use) to a neutral pH (7.0-7.5). A dose of 100 to 200 mg/L can be used for induction and 50 to 100 mg/L for maintenance. MS-222 can be conveniently stored as a 10 g/L (10,000 mg/L) stock solution.[20]

An alternative to MS-222 is eugenol, the active ingredient in clove oil. Eugenol is not completely soluble in water but may be diluted 1 : 10 in 95% ethanol for a 100 mg/ml stock solution. Eugenol produces similar effects to MS-222 at lower doses and can be administered at 40 to 100 mg/L (high end for induction, low end for maintenance).[20] One disadvantage associated with the use of eugenol is that it appears to have a narrower safety range.

There is very little information with supporting pharmacologic data on injectable anesthetics for fish; however, there has been some recent work in this area with selected species.

Transporting Fish to the Veterinary Hospital

Fish should be transported in a plastic, sealed container. The container should be used exclusively to transport fish and never reused to carry human food items. The container should be cleaned with warm, soapy water, and rinsed thoroughly after each use. Bleach should never be used to clean the container. The water used to transport the animal should come from the home aquarium. A separate container of aquarium water should also be brought to the veterinary hospital in case of spillage and for water quality testing. The fish should be transported immediately to the veterinary hospital. Special precautions should be made during the winter and summer to prevent water temperature fluctuations, such as preheating or cooling the transport automobile in the winter and summer, respectively. Signs of transport stress may not be apparent for several days after the move, so animals should monitored closely for 3 to 5 days following transport.[21]

TABLE 4-1	Compounds Commonly Used to Treat Fish	
Drug	**Dosage**	**Indication**
Acetic acid	0.5-2.0 ml/L, 30 s, every other day ×4 treatments	Protozoa, trematodes, nematodes
Acyclovir	25 mg/L, daily ×15 days	Antiviral
Amikacin	5 mg/kg, IM, q24h	Bacterial diseases
Amprolium	10 mg/L	*Eimeria* spp.
Aztreonam	100 mg/kg, IM, ICe, q48h ×15 days	*Aeromonas salmonicida*
Chloramphenicol	50 mg/kg, PO, IM once, then 25 mg/kg, q24h	*Aeromonas salmonicida* in goldfish
Chloroquine	10 mg/L, indefinite	Protozoa
Copper sulfate	2.3-4.0 mg/L, indefinite	Algae control
Enrofloxacin	5-10 mg/kg, IM, ICe, q48h ×15 days	Broad-spectrum antibacterial
Florfenicol	40-50 mg/kg, PO, q24h ×10 days	Broad-spectrum antibacterial
Formalin	37% solution only, 0.04 ml/L ×1 h	Protozoa, mycosis, good aeration, continuous monitoring during treatment
Freshwater	3-15 min	Ectoparasitism, marine fish only
Furazolidone	20-60 ppm, continuous, indefinite	Antibacterial, inactivated by light
Hydrogen peroxide	17.5 ml/L, 10 min	Protozoa
Iodine	7% tincture	Wound rinse
Itraconazole	1-5 mg/kg, q24h in feed 1-7 days	Systemic mycosis
Kanamycin	750 mg/L, 2 h, 4 times daily	Bacteria
Ketoconazole	2.5-10.0 mg/kg, PO, IM, ICe	Systemic mycosis
Malachite green	0.1 mg/L, every 3 days ×3 treatments	Freshwater fish protozoa, mycosis
Methylene blue	3 mg/L, prolonged bath	Mycosis
Metronidazole	50 mg/L, ≦24 h	*Hexamita* sp., other protozoa
Miconazole	10-20 mg/kg, PO, IM, ICe	Systemic mycosis
Nalidixic acid	13 mg/L, indefinite	Quinolone, Gram-negative bacteria
Neomycin	66 mg/L, every 3 days ×3 treatments	Bacteria
Nitrofurpyrinol	2 mg/L, 19 h	Antiprotozoan
Oxolinic acid	20-30 mg/L, indefinite	Quinolone
Oxytetracycline	10-50 mg/L, 1h bath	Topical bacterial infections
Potassium permanganate	5 mg/L, 30-60 min	Mycosis, freshwater bacterial infections, toxic high pH
Praziquantel HCl	2 mg/L, 5 days, repeat in 2 weeks	Monogenetic trematodes
Quinine HCl	10 mg/L, 3 days	*Cryptocaryon irritans*
Ribavirin	20 mg/L	Antiviral
Sarafloxin	10-14 mg/kg, PO, q24h ×10 days	Fluoroquinolone
Silver sulfadiazine	Topical q12h	Topical bacterial treatment, 30-60 s contact time required
Sodium chloride	1-3 mg/L, indefinite	Osmoregulatory stress
Sodium thiosulfate	100 mg/L	Chlorine exposure
Sulfamethazine	100 mg/L, 1 h ×7 days	Bacteria
Toltrazuril	50 mg/ml, 20 min, once	*Trichodina, Apiosoma*
Trichlorfon	0.25-0.5 mg/L, q12h ×3, 24 h between treatments	Trematodes, crustaceans
Trimethoprim-Sulfamethoxazole	28 mg/L, 6-10 h	Broad spectrum antibiotic
Virazole	400 mg/L, indefinite	Antiviral

HCl, hydrogen chloride; ICe, intracoelomic; IM, intramuscular; PO, per os.

■ HISTORY AND PHYSICAL EXAMINATION

A physical examination on a fish should follow the same procedure used to perform a physical examination on any other terrestrial animal. The exam should always begin with a complete history detailing the animal's husbandry and health problems. For fish, it is important to have the client submit a water sample from the animal's aquarium for a complete water chemistry analysis as part of the examination.

History

The history, or *anamnesis,* is the first attempt the veterinarian has to identify and organize the potential problems facing fish and their aquatic environment. Many of the problems that lead to disease in fish are directly related to their environment. There are four key areas that must be addressed in the history: the owner's general knowledge, the aquarium environment, the water, and the fish. Questions regarding the owners' general knowledge of aquarium management should include the length of ownership, if there are multiple aquaria, where the fish were obtained, the time spent viewing the fish, and the weekly maintenance program. The history of the aquarium environment should include questions about tank volume, tank placement, tank top, lighting, heating, filtration, substrate, and aquarium decorations (e.g., plants, rocks, logs, and toys). Tank volume is important because it allows the veterinarian to determine the relative stocking density of the aquarium. The placement of the tank within the home may provide insight into problems associated with algal overgrowth (e.g., direct sunlight exposure) or toxins (e.g., cleaning sprays). Some fish owners do not cover their aquaria with a top. Tanks without tops experience faster evaporation and are more prone to fish losses because of jumping. There are a number of different lighting systems available for the home aquarium. Owners should be asked whether they have fluorescent or incandescent lighting, the bulb wattage, and the amount of time the lighting remains on during the day. Incandescent lights exert radiant heat and are associated with increased water temperatures. Fluorescent lighting, especially full-spectrum lighting, is preferred for live aquatic plant systems. Most aquaria are heated with thermostatically controlled heaters. Questions regarding heater usage (yes or no), type, and wattage size should be asked. Owners should also be asked if they use a thermometer, and if so, the temperature in the aquarium. Fish are poikilotherms and must be provided an appropriate environmental temperature. Because there are a number of different types of filters, questions should be asked to determine the types of filters, length of usage, and the owners' general knowledge of filtration. Information should be ascertained regarding the aquarium decorations, such as plants, rocks, logs, and toys. The addition of new, live plants may serve as an introduction of disease.

Most aquarium clients have a limited knowledge of water chemistry. Questions regarding water quality should focus on the source of the water, the frequency with which the water is changed, and the water quality tests that have been performed. Veterinary hospitals that work with ornamental fish should have water quality test kits and should perform the appropriate water tests during the visits.

The final series of questions should focus on the fish. Questions related to the types and numbers of fish, the problem the fish are being presented for, and the duration of the problem are all important. Detailed information regarding the diet of the fish, including specific types of foods being offered, frequency food is offered, and whether dietary changes have occurred, should also be asked. Finally, information related to the preventive health program, previous treatments, recent

---

BOX 4-1 Calculations Used to Estimate the Body Weight of Fish

(Number of fingerlings) × (initial weight of fingerlings) = Initial total fingerling weight

(Total pounds of feed fed) ÷ 1.75 (approximate conversion ratio) = pounds of gain

(Initial total fingerling weight) + (pounds of gain) = Current weight of fish

(Current weight of fish) ÷ (number of fish) = Average current weight of fish

---

additions, and routine maintenance of the system (e.g., frequency of water changes) should be obtained.

Performing the Physical Examination

Fish presented to the veterinarian should first be visually inspected for physical and behavioral abnormalities. For a complete physical examination, the fish must be sedated. Once sedated, the animal may be weighed, measured, and examined for signs of external parasites. Box 4-1 provides a useful guide for estimating fish weight. While the fish is sedated, blood should be collected for analysis, biopsies of the skin and gills collected (if indicated), and a fecal sample collected. Radiographs and ultrasonography can also be performed at this time. A problem list should be made that prioritizes problems with regard to any immediate threat to life, primary disease considerations, and treatment options. An initial short-term plan for treatment should be identified and a long-term treatment and management plan developed.[3]

Common Abnormalities Found on Physical Examination

Sick fish often congregate, separating themselves from their healthier cohorts. Weak fish will often be found near a water outlet, skimmer box, or sump. They may also exhibit behavioral changes, such as staying near the surface if hypoxic, scraping their bodies because of external parasite infestation, and gill flashing. Color changes often occur in sick fish. Another common clinical sign observed in diseased fish is abdominal swelling, which is commonly found in fish with coelomitis regardless of etiology. Abdominal swelling may also be seen with morbidly obese fish, renal failure, and neoplasia. Abdominocentesis and cytology can be done to either confirm or rule out a diagnosis. Lesions of the eye, such as exophthalmia, are common in both infectious and noninfectious disease problems. Unilateral lesions often indicate a traumatic cause, whereas bilateral lesions are more typical of barotraumas or an infectious etiology. Cataracts are most often associated with either trauma or nutritional disease. Skeletal deformities are especially common in the vertebral column and are often seen in rapidly growing fish. Other skeletal lesions can be the result of a variety of disease entities, including infectious, nutritional, parasitic, and toxic insults.[3,6]

■ DIAGNOSTIC TESTING

Blood smears, fecal examinations, and skin scrapings should initially be reviewed in the veterinary hospital. With experience, the clinician will learn to identify many common problems with standard light microscopy. If detailed cellular or chemical analysis is required, it is best to collaborate with a commercial laboratory that is familiar with aquatic species and has specialized staining and culture capabilities. University and state aquatic diagnostic laboratories are also excellent resources for the aquatic animal veterinarian. Submitting specimens to specialized pathology services (Northwest Zoopath, Monroe, WA) for necropsy, histopathology, cultures, or special staining techniques should be considered when the clinician believes it is necessary or is beyond his or her level of expertise.

Special Diagnostic Tests

A gill biopsy can be performed to assess the gill status in animals maintained in poor water quality or to diagnose ectoparasites. Fish should be anesthetized for a gill biopsy to provide appropriate sedation and analgesia. MS-222 or eugenol can be used to anesthetize the patient. Once a fish is anesthetized, it can be removed from the anesthetic solution using a gloved hand and placed onto a dechlorinated, moist paper towel. A pair of fine iris scissors should be inserted under the operculum and gently lifted, enabling the handler to insert his or her thumb under the operculum to provide direct visualization of the gills (Figure 4-15). Iris scissors should be reinserted under the operculum and three to five gill filaments collected. The gill filaments should be placed onto a slide with 0.9%

saline and reviewed under a microscope. Once that procedure has been completed, the animals should be recovered in dechlorinated, fresh water.

A skin scrape can be performed to diagnose pathogens on the surface of a fish. Once again, the animal should be anesthetized to reduce stress. The animal may be restrained by hand or placed on a moistened paper towel. A microscope slide should be placed on the skin at a 45-degree angle caudal to the operculum and gently dragged in a caudal direction (Figure 4-16). The fish should be recovered in dechlorinated water.

A fin biopsy should be performed to evaluate specific lesions on the animal's fins. A fish undergoing this procedure should be anesthetized. A pair of iris scissors should be used to cut a sample of the affected fin between the fin rays, if possible (Figure 4-17). The sample should be mixed with 0.9% saline

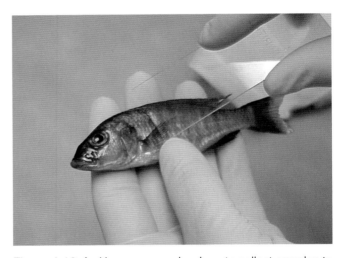

Figure 4-16 A skin scrape can be done to collect samples to evaluate bacteria and ectoparasite burdens on the skin. To collect the sample, place a glass slide on the skin surface and pull it in a cranial to caudal direction.

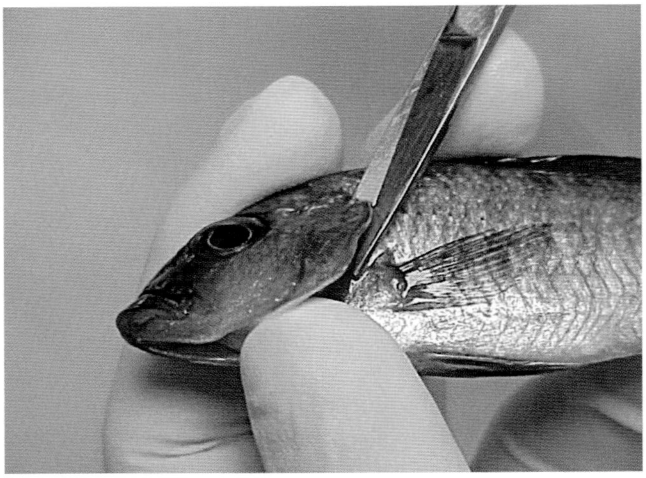

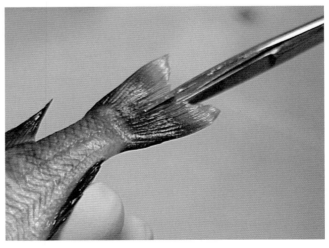

Figure 4-15 A gill biopsy can be used to collect samples to evaluate the condition of the gills. To collect the sample, insert a thumb under the operculum, expose the gills, insert a pair of iris scissors, and clip the gills.

Figure 4-17 A fin biopsy can be used to assess fin lesions. To collect a sample, excise a piece of fin that includes both the lesion and healthy fin.

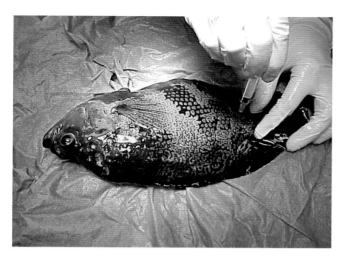

Figure 4-18 Blood samples can be collected from the ventral tail vein. This vein is located on the ventral aspect of the caudal tail vertebrae.

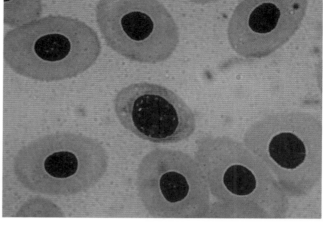

Figure 4-19 Mature and immature *(center)* erythrocytes from a bull shark.

on a microscope slide, covered with a cover slip, and evaluated under a microscope. The fish should be recovered in dechlorinated water.

Clinical Pathology

Fish have evolved to mask their illness; however, they can not hide abnormal conditions in their blood. Therefore, examining blood samples can provide insight into the general health of the animals, which might not otherwise be obvious on physical examination. The volume of blood that can be collected from a fish has been estimated to be similar to that of mammals, approximately 0.8 to 1.0% of the body weight.[2] Always preload the needle with heparin to prevent blood clotting. The primary site of venipuncture in the fish is the caudal tail vein, although the heart can also be used. The caudal tail vein is located ventral to the vertebral column and runs parallel to the spine (Figure 4-18). A 1-ml or 3-ml syringe with a 25- to 30-gauge needle is recommended for sample collection. The needle should be gently inserted at a 45-degree angle (between scales) into the caudal peduncle at the level of the lateral line and walked off the ventral edge of the vertebral column until a flash of blood is visualized in the needle. The blood sample from the caudal tail vein can also be collected from the ventral approach. The animal should be held in dorsal recumbency and the needle inserted in the ventral midline of the caudal peduncle at a 90-degree angle. The needle should be inserted to the level of the vertebral column and gently walked along the spine until a flash of blood is visualized.

The blood cells of fish are more closely related to lower vertebrates (e.g., amphibians and reptiles) than higher vertebrates (e.g., mammals). The erythrocytes of fish are oval shaped and have a pale cytoplasm and a centrally located nucleus (Figure 4-19). Fish leukocytes may be divided into two groups:

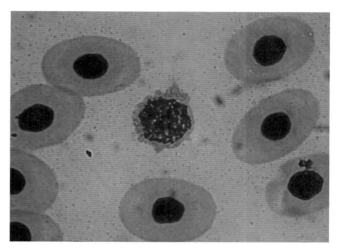

Figure 4-20 Lymphocyte from a bull shark.

agranulocytes (e.g., lymphocyte, and monocyte) and granulocytes (e.g., neutrophil/heterophil and eosinophil). Thrombocytes have a small nucleus and a spindle-shaped cell. These cells are analogous to platelets in mammals and are responsible for blood clotting. Lymphocytes are the most common cell type in fish and are morphologically similar to those found in mammals (Figure 4-20). Monocytes are the largest leukocyte and have a pale, blue-gray cytoplasm (Figure 4-21). Their primary role is to phagocytize pathogens and process the antigens for lymphocytes. Monocytes are commonly found with chronic inflammatory responses. Neutrophils/heterophils possess rod-shaped granules and are weakly phagocytic (Figure 4-22). These cells are primarily associated with acute inflammatory responses. Eosinophils exist in some species of fish, but their function is unclear (Figure 4-23). It is likely that they play some role in hypersensitivity and parasite control as in higher vertebrates. The existence of basophils is controversial.

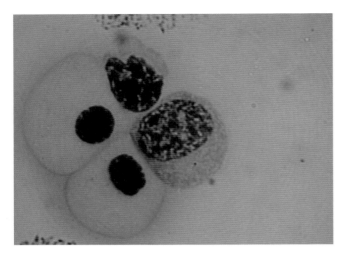

Figure 4-21 Monocyte from a bull shark.

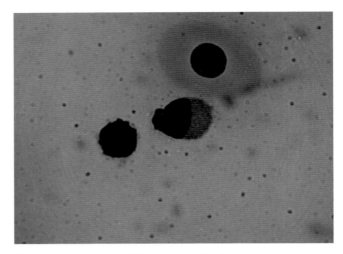

Figure 4-23 Eosinophil from a bull shark.

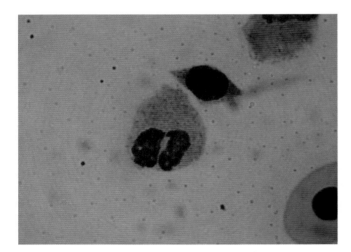

Figure 4-22 Heterophil from a bull shark.

Pathology

It is not intended that this chapter should encompass all aspects of pathology, as there are already many suitable medical and veterinary textbooks on this subject.[3,5,6] Many of the accepted clinical techniques currently in use for mammals require modification for use in fish pathology. However, there have been significant developments in many aspects of cellular biology, and new histologic techniques that until only recently were utilized by the mammalian pathologist are now available for the fish pathologist. For best results, only freshly dead or moribund fish should be considered for necropsy. Strict attention must be paid to handling biologic materials to be used for histology from fish. Fish have a very rapid rate of autolysis compared to mammals, and samples must be handled properly in order to avoid rapid degenerative changes.

Proper fixation is fundamental to satisfactory histologic preparation. If the fixation is unsatisfactory, the end product will reflect this. The primary objective of fixation is to preserve the morphology of the tissues to reflect the state of the tissues in the living animal. Formalin is the most widely used fixative. This fixative is not suitable for use in its concentrated form and therefore must be diluted to a 10% solution. Some pathologists will request special fixatives depending on the tissue being evaluated or a suspected etiology. We recommend contacting the laboratory before sample submission to obtain any specific guidelines for sample processing.

Diagnostic Imaging

For fish diagnostic imaging, the radiograph machines found in most veterinary clinics are adequate for routine examination. Portable units are beneficial if fieldwork is being done or if the ability to work at multiple sites is desired. The two major limiting factors associated with portable units are the ability to penetrate maximum thickness images on larger species and the lack of portability of the film processing unit. Recently, the technology in this area has developed more powerful, lightweight, and economically available radiograph machines and processor units. Portable digital units are also available and allow the veterinarian to review the image on a laptop computer. The radiograph films in use today are placed in cassettes, which must be adapted for use in a "wet" environment. This can be accomplished in a variety of ways. Smaller fish can be radiographed while being held in a small volume of water in either a glass or acrylic container placed on top of the film cassette. Larger species can be anesthetized and placed directly on a cassette for a brief period of time; however, advanced preparation is necessary for this method. Another technique for taking radiographs is to place the cassette in a watertight acrylic cassette case and place the cassette beneath the animal in a shallow pool or holding area. This has been an effective method for radiographing large predatory species.

Diagnostic ultrasound has become commonplace in human and veterinary medicine. Ultrasonography provides a safe, noninvasive method for visualizing the internal anatomy of many species. Ultrasound provides instantaneous results, and

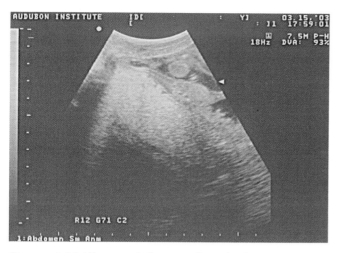

Figure 4-24 Ultrasound image of a freshwater stingray embryo.

protective apparel is not required.[22] Another advantage of using ultrasound is that serial views can be taken over time, and to date, there have not been any negative effects associated with this. There are a number of economic and efficient ultrasound units available that are capable of providing three-dimensional images and can operate off of a 12-volt direct current. Ultrasound imaging of aquatic species has become very popular in the past decade, from its initial use with marine mammals to its current applications with elasmobranchs and teleosts. Ultrasonography allows for the accurate measurement (e.g., width and depth) of structures by utilizing internal calipers and varying the orientation and penetration of the transducer. Many units can provide three-dimensional color images and perform volume and flow calculations. Ultrasound is useful in monitoring reproductive function, follicular changes, ovarian irregularities, sex determination, anatomic abnormalities, and monitoring embryonic growth rates (Figure 4-24). Since a fluid interface is required for quality imaging, it has been our experience that imaging procedures are easier to obtain and perform on animals that are already in an aquatic medium rather than utilizing gels or some other synthetic interface.

Microbiology

Microbiologic samples may be collected from a fish during an antemortem or postmortem exam. Antemortem samples are routinely collected from specific lesions on the skin, fins, or eyes. Contamination is a significant concern is these cases, and results should be interpreted accordingly. A sterile swab may be rubbed over the affected area to collect the sample. The sample should be refrigerated until it is plated, which should occur within 24 hours. Postmortem cultures routinely involve internal organs. To ensure sterility, the necropsy should be performed in a consistent manner. Seventy-percent ethyl alcohol should be applied to the ventral surface of the fish and the area flamed. Once the alcohol has burned off, samples

can be collected using either a sterile swab or sterile biopsy techniques.

There are many different options relative to the appropriate culture media and incubation temperatures to isolate bacterial pathogens from fish. A standard blood agar plate may be used as the initial plate, or other specialized plates may be used if a specific pathogen is suspected. Salt should be added to a plate when attempting to isolate pathogens from marine fish. Plates should be incubated between 20°-25° C and 37° C. Many fish pathogens can grow at a range of temperatures; faster growth can be expected at higher temperatures. Culture plates should be evaluated for growth at 24- and 48-hour time periods. A Gram stain should be performed on any isolate. Biochemical identification of the organism should follow standard microbiologic protocol.

Marine microbiology has evolved from a fringe discipline to one of the most exciting areas of aquatic animal medicine.[9] There has been a great deal of advancement in the field in the past decade, primarily in the area of diagnostic test development and emerging technology. New optics, radio tracing, and advanced molecular methods have enabled scientists to identify microbes that would have been impossible to detect a short time ago.

Early and accurate diagnosis of an infectious process is essential for maintaining healthy fish.[3] It is important to be able to recognize clinical signs of disease and have infected animals examined and treated as early as possible.[4] In most disease processes, mortalities are initially low but can be followed by a gradual increase in losses. As soon as the first moribund animal appears, an aggressive diagnostic plan should be implemented. Although early and accurate diagnosis is important for all infectious fish diseases, it is absolutely crucial in bacterial infections to implement treatment early. As with any disease situation, the earlier the diagnosis is made, the sooner corrective measures or treatment can begin and losses can be minimized.[3]

To be able to identify populations of bacteria in aquatic systems is of fundamental importance; however, there are several problems to overcome. Standard laboratory methods, or some variation of them, can often be applied, but in many cases, the method used will be determined, at least in part, by experimental design.[10] Dilution and plating is a relatively straightforward and technically simple method of swabbing surfaces or lesions and placing them into suitable diluents, serially diluting them, and plating for viable counts. This technique has been utilized successfully for a long time despite the obvious drawbacks of the technique. Light microscopy should be utilized to observe surface populations while advanced laboratory requests are pending. An even better method would be the use of phase contrast microscopy, as this would be suitable for rapid counts of organisms. Alternatively, Gram stains, Diff-Quick, and Wright's stain may be used to characterize the different types of bacteria present and other cellular anomalies. Photometric methods, which are routinely used in laboratories to estimate bacterial numbers in liquids, may also be used to determine surface densities of some substrata. After fixing samples and applying suitable staining, the optical density of liquid medium can be measured and the surface population can be estimated. Since the adenosine triphosphate (ATP) assay method was developed, extractable ATP has been used extensively to determine bacterial biomass in a variety of samples. ATP is rapidly lost from dead cells; consequently, any delay between sampling the population and performing the assay must be kept to a minimum. Therefore, the application of the method to surface populations is difficult unless the ATP can in some way be extracted in situ or if the experimental system is specifically designed around the ATP assay. The use of radioisotopes to perform bacterial counts has not attracted much attention. The reasons for this are self-evident. Dispersing labeled compounds into the environment is simply not acceptable, and this means that the technique can be applied only to closed laboratory systems.[18]

Many advances have occurred in the field of analytic biotechnology in recent years, including the use of biochemical methods for estimating microbial biomass. The rationale is that if a veterinarian can identify a key component for a particular group of organisms, then, provided a suitable assay is available, it should be possible to use that component as a means of assaying the biomass. The advantages of this type of approach to biomass estimation are that (1) microbial biomass can be estimated without the need for further microbial culture, and (2) as chemical extractions are performed, there is no requirement for the quantitative recovery of microorganisms from colonized surfaces. The disadvantages associated with this method are attributed to the limited sensitivities of the techniques used and the chemical extraction method.[10,18]

Parasitology

Wild populations of fish are usually infested with parasites. Although infested, the majority of fish species in the wild experience no serious disease effects as a result. However, in captive fish populations, parasites may cause disease outbreaks. Maintaining dense populations of fish in a particular ecosystem may promote very high levels of parasitic infestation. The number of parasites required to cause health issues in fish varies considerably with the size and health status of the host. Many parasites are host specific or are capable of infecting only one or a limited number of host species. There are many individual parasite species that have widely different effects on the host species. Life cycles of fish parasites demonstrate enormous diversity and may involve one or more intermediate hosts. These types of complex life cycles are necessary to disseminate the infective stages to the final host. Intermediate hosts often form part of the diet of the final host or the next intermediate host to ensure the parasites progress onto the next life stage. Free living stages may be released from the intermediate host to actively invade or be consumed by another host. Many fish parasites have a portion of their life cycle that is spent outside of the host as free swimming larvae. These particular parasite species have a direct life cycle and will infect other hosts by means of eggs, which are ingested. Knowledge of the life cycles of a particular parasite species is imperative to their control and/or eradication. Ectoparasites are frequently found on the gills, skin, and fins. Biopsies (e.g., fin or gill) or scrapings (e.g., skin) should be collected to confirm the presence or absence of ectoparasites. Endoparasites are generally found on fecal direct saline smears. Successful parasite control can be achieved by intervening in some aspect of the parasite life cycle. Fortunately, some parasite life cycles require an intermediate host, and these invertebrates are often not found in the captive setting. There are a variety of antiparasitics that can be used to treat parasites, and these are discussed elsewhere in this chapter.

Miscellaneous Diagnostic Tests

There are very few serologic tests that have been developed or are available for diagnosing infectious disease exposure in ornamental fish. Serologic studies have been performed on cultured food species and animals used in experimental studies to determine the presence of antibodies to specific pathogens, but these assays have limited value for ornamental fish. Nucleic acid probes can be designed with the specificity to differentiate between two antigenically related organisms, but they have differences in their nucleic acid sequences that alter the pathogenicity of the organisms. From a diagnostic perspective, probes are extremely valuable because they can be developed to characterize pathogens at the generic, species, or strain-specific level, depending on which portion of a nucleic acid sequence they are designed to detect.[10] Once a probe has been developed, it can be used to detect nucleic acid that is extracted from a sample and attached to a membrane, or it can be used to detect pathogen specific nucleic acid in a section of paraffin-embedded, formalin-fixed tissue that has been processed for histopathologic evaluation. In situ hybridization using pathogen-specific nucleic acid probes is particularly effective when a pathogen is present in relatively small numbers or produces a lesion that histologically resembles lesions induced by other pathogens.[18] In situ hybridization using viral-specific DNA probes can quickly and correctly determine which of these viruses induce histologic lesions (e.g., inclusion bodies). When compared with antibody staining techniques used for identifying pathogens in tissues, nucleic acid probes are more specific and more sensitive than other pathogen detection techniques. They also detect organisms that may have been antigenically altered during processing. In addition to confirming the presence of a pathogen in tissue, in situ hybridization can also be used to detect the type of cell infected and whether the pathogen's nucleic acid is present in the cytoplasm or nucleus of the host cell.[9,10,18] In infected tissues where high numbers of an organism are present, the use of DNA probes to detect the presence of an organism's nucleic acid is fairly straightforward. In contrast, detection of a pathogen in an excretion/sample where numbers of the organism may be small often requires further processing. To increase the likelihood of finding an organism in a diagnostic specimen, a sample to be tested is often subjected to a group of reactions that will amplify the number of pathogen DNA molecules in the sample, thus improving the ability of the probe to detect the organism.

Polymerase chain reaction (PCR) is the most commonly employed method for detecting portions of DNA by amplifying short nucleotide sequences within the DNA genome. PCR can be used for the detection of pathogens in cell culture, tissues, secretions, lavages, and other biologic samples. PCR requires oligonucleotide primers that are complimentary to the sequence being amplified.[18] Fortunately, there are a variety of generic level primers for many of the bacteria, fungi, and viruses that commonly infect fish.

■ COMMON DISEASE PRESENTATIONS

Disease can be caused by an etiologic (specific cause) or a nonetiologic (contributing cause) agent. Etiologic agents can be classified as either inanimate or animate. Inanimate etiologic agents are factors that can occur endogenously or exogenously. Endogenous, inanimate factors are those associated with genetic and/or metabolic disorders of the host. Exogenous, inanimate agents include trauma, temperature shock, electrical shock, chemical toxicity, and dietary deficiencies. These etiologic agents may serve as sublethal stressors that predispose fish to infectious disease.[3] Animate etiologies include living communicable infectious agents, such as viruses, bacteria, fungi, protozoa, helminthes, and copepods.[5]

Nonetiologic causes of disease are characterized as either extrinsic or intrinsic. Extrinsic factors are usually associated with trauma, environmental conditions, or dietary problems, whereas intrinsic factors include age, gender, heredity, and fish species. Both fish species and strain of fish are important because not all fish are equally susceptible to a specific disease organism. Feed quality, water quality factors, and water temperature extremes can be classified as either etiologic or nonetiologic extrinsic factors and can contribute to disease.[5]

Infectious Diseases

Fish diseases are caused by a wide range of infectious organisms, including viruses, bacteria, fungi, protozoan and metazoan parasites. Bacteria are responsible for the majority of the infectious diseases diagnosed in captive fish, with many acting as secondary opportunistic invaders that take advantage of diseased animals by overwhelming their natural host defense response. Opportunistic bacteria are widespread in the aquatic environment and represent a threat every time a fish is exposed to a stressful event (e.g., handling). However, their harmful effects rarely persist and generally cease with the removal of the original stressful event.

Bacterial Diseases

Many aquatic bacteria are facultative or obligate pathogens, and all fish culture systems suffer outbreaks of primary bacterial infections from time to time. The main groups of bacteria involved in fish mortalities in captivity are listed in Box 4-2.

Gram-negative bacteria are the primary pathogens isolated from fish. These pathogens are responsible for the majority of the acute, septicemic infections diagnosed in fish.[9] Chronic

| BOX 4-2 | Principle Bacterial Pathogens Isolated from Captive Fish |

Pathogen	Disease
Enterobacteriaceae (Gram-negative)	
Edwardsiella tarda	Red pest disease
E. ictaluri	Enteric septicemia in catfish
Yersinia ruckeri	Enteric red mouth
Vibrionaceae (Gram-negative)	
Vibrio anguillarum	Vibriosis
V. salmonocida	Hitra
V. viscossus	Winter ulcer disease
Vibrio spp.	Larval infections
Aeromonas salmonocida	Furunculosis
A. hydrophila	Septicemia
Pasteurellaceae (Gram-negative)	
Pasteurella piscida	Pseudotuberculosis
Pseudomonadaceae (Gram-negative)	
Pseudomonas anguilliseptica	Red spot disease
Flavobacteriaceae (Gram-negative)	
Flexibacter columnaris	Columnaris
Flavobacterium psychrophilium	Coldwater disease
Mycobacteriaceae (Gram-positive, acid-fast)	
Mycobacterium spp.	Tuberculosis
Nocardiaceae (Gram-positive)	
Nocardia kampachi	Nocardiosis
Nocardia spp.	Nocardiosis
Coryneforms (Gram-positive)	
Renibacterium salmoninarum	Bacterial kidney disease
Cocci (Gram-positive)	
Streptococcus spp.	Septicemia
Aerococcus viridans	Gaffkemia
Rickettsia-like organisms	
Piscirickettsia salmonis	Piscirickettsiosis

infections, which progress more slowly and may result in granulomatous internal lesions, are more commonly associated with Gram-positive bacteria (e.g., *Mycobacterium* spp.). Of the Gram positive bacteria, *Mycobacterium* spp. and *Nocardia* spp. are more often associated with chronic infections. *Mycobacterium marinum* has been associated with granulomatous lesions and zoonotic infections. Attempts at therapy of such infections are rarely reported. When considering treatment for Gram-negative or non–*Mycobacterium* sp. Gram-positive pathogens, it is best to base the therapeutic plan on the results of an antimicrobial sensitivity assay.

Mycotic Diseases

Mycosis is significant in all ornamental species. Fungi do not use photosynthetic pathways and are therefore considered saprophytic or parasitic. Oomycetes produce superficial infections in freshwater fish, particularly if under stressful conditions or where superficial wounds and abrasions occur. *Saprolegnia* spp. is a common water mold isolated from tropical ornamental fish and cold-water aquaculture species. Water molds are primarily opportunists; they often infect open wounds, although primary infections are also possible. Affected fish generally present with white, cotton-like lesions on fins and skin. A skin scrape or biopsy of an affected area can be used to confirm diagnosis of water molds, which are classified based on their branching nonseptate hyphae.

Such infections are susceptible to chemotherapy, such as malachite green. These infections are responsible for a broad range of serious and economically important diseases in fish. There are more than 100,000 species of fungi, and they are morphologically diverse. The ichthyoparasitic species are relatively few in number and difficult to classify.[10] Fungi considered important pathogens of fish are listed in Box 4-3.

Viral Diseases

The study of fish viruses has become important for wild and cultured fish. Diseases that were once attributed to bacterial diseases are now being found to be viral in origin. With the advent of comparative molecular biology for viruses, improved methods for virus detection, and experimental pathogenesis studies, emerging viruses can be expected to be diagnosed at an increased rate in the future.

Viruses multiply within the living cells of a host by utilizing the components of the host cell for their own reproduction. In the extracellular phase of the virus particle, or *virion,* the virus is metabolically inert. The virion carries the viral genome from the cell in which it had been produced to another cell where it can be introduced. Once the virus particle is inside the new cell, replication or infection occurs. Histologic changes associated with viral infection include cell swelling and loss of cytoplasmic detail, followed by irreversible changes and cell death.[10,18] If sufficient cell loss occurs, loss or damage to a particular physiologic function and/or transformation to a neoplastic state can occur. Infection may persist after early signs are evident or may be integrated into the genome with intermittent shedding.[6]

Once the virus spreads beyond a few host cells, a variety of nonspecific host defense responses will be elicited. The extent of disease experienced by a host depends on how effectively these responses contain the virus and minimize host cell and organ damage. Infected fish can develop either (1) clinical disease with morbidity (and mortality) that is recognized by the clinician or pathologist, or (2) infection with no clinical signs (e.g., a silent infection).

Viral diseases in ornamental fish are rare. The pathogenicity of viruses can vary with temperature. Most viral infections in fish are host specific. In many cases, young, naive fishes become sick and older animals become carriers. The most commonly reported virus in ornamental fish is lymphocystis, an iridovirus that infects fibroblasts.[23] Affected animals develop large, coalescing nodules that can occur anywhere on the body. The virus is self-limiting. In most cases, the fish resolves spontaneously; however, in cases where the lesions affect the eyes or mouth (e.g., its vision or the ability to eat), the animal may die. Lymphocystis can be diagnosed on gross examination or histopathology. There is no effective treatment, although the mass may be removed surgically if the tumor affects the animal's ability to eat, see, or swim. Box 4-4 represents a list of the major viral groups that affect ornamental and cultured fish species. For additional information regarding fish viruses, see other texts.[2,3]

Culture remains the most common and definitive method of diagnosing viral disease in fish.[6,18] Cytopathic effects in the cell culture represent the anticipated consequence of viral growth in the cell monolayer and form the basis of an initial positive diagnosis. However, positive culture of a virus should always be confirmed by a second diagnostic procedure. With the advent of advanced molecular diagnostic testing, there are now a number of other diagnostic tests available (e.g., polymerase chain reaction assays) that can be used to confirm a diagnosis of viral disease in fish.

Parasitic Diseases

Both ectoparasites and endoparasites are routinely identified on or in imported ornamental fish. When parasitized animals are added to an established aquarium, the parasites can quickly spread to the other tank inhabitants. To prevent the introduction of parasites into established systems, all newly acquired animals should be quarantine.

Protozoa are responsible for the majority of the opportunistic and obligate parasitic infections in fish. These parasites

---

BOX 4-3	Fungi Commonly Isolated from Captive Fish

Class	Order	Genus
Mastigomycotina		
Oomycetes	Saprolegniales	*Saprolegnia*
		Achyla
		Aphanomyces
		Branchiomyces
Chytridiomycetes	Chytridiales	*Dermocystidium*
Zygomycotina		
Entomophthorales		*Basidiobolus*
Deuteromycotina		
Hyphomycetes	Moniliales	*Exophiala*
		Aspergillus
Coelomycetes	Sphaeropsidales	*Phoma*

BOX 4-4   **Viral Diseases of Fish**

DNA Viruses
Iridoviruses
Lymphocystis
White sturgeon iridovirus disease
Redfin perch iridovirus disease
Rainbow trout iridovirus disease
Catfish iridovirus disease
Pike perch iridovirus disease
Red sea bream iridovirus disease
Cod ulcus syndrome
Turbot iridovirus disease
Eel iridovirus disease
Cichlid iridovirus
Viral erythrocytic necrosis
Cyprinid iridoviruses
Grouper iridoviruses
Large mouth bass iridovirus

Adenoviridae
Cod adenovirus
Sturgeon adenovirus

Herpesviridae
Channel catfish herpesvirus
Salmonid herpesviruses: Types I, II, and III
Cyprinid herpesvirus
Herpesviral hematopoietic necrosis
Acipenserid herpesvirus
Herpesvirus vitreum
Angelfish herpesvirus
Turbot herpesvirus
Pike epidermal proliferation
Smooth dogfish herpesvirus
Atlantic salmon papillomatosis
Japanese flounder herpesvirus
Pacific cod herpesvirus

RNA Viruses
Reoviridae
REO-respiratory-enteric-orphan disease

Aquareviridae
Not associated with any known disease

Birnaviridae
Picornaviridae
Salmonid picornavirus

Nodaviridae
Viral nervous necrosis
Striped skipjack nervous necrosis
Viral encephalopathy
Viral retinopathy

Togaviridae
Pancreas disease
Erythrocytic inclusion body syndrome

Orthomyxoviridae
Infectious salmon anemia

Rhabdoviridae
Infectious hematopoietic necrosis
Viral hemorrhagic septicemia
Hirame rhabdovirus disease

Lyssavirus-like group
Snakehead rhabdovirus
Eel virus B12
Carpione rhabdovirus

Vesiculovirus-like group
Spring viremia of carp
Pike fry rhabdovirus I
Pike fry rhabdovirus II
Ulcerative disease
Eel rhabdovirus EVA/EVX

Reverse Transcribing Viruses
Retroviridae
Walleye dermal sarcoma
Walleye discrete epidermal hyperplasia
Plasmacytoid leukemia of chinook salmon
Atlantic salmon swim-bladder sarcoma
Atlantic salmon papilloma
Esox sarcoma
Esocid lymphosarcoma
Pike epidermal proliferation
Damselfish neurofibromatosis
Xiphophorus sp. hybrid neuroblastoma
Hooknose fibroma/fibrosarcoma
Viral erythrocytic infection of seabass

can cause both external and systemic disease. The clinical signs associated with parasite infestation will vary depending upon the location of the parasite. Fish with gill flukes *(Dactylogyrids)* may become hypoxic with heavy infestations and may be found "gulping air" at the water surface. Fish infested with skin parasites, such as ich *(Ichthyopthirius multfiliis),* rub against hard surfaces, lose scales, and hemorrhage in the area of parasite attachment. Fish with endoparasites are often anorectic, in poor condition, and fail to thrive. Systemic protozoan infections (e.g., *Myxosporidia* and *Microsporidia*) in fish are responsible for the most serious losses. These parasites are generally refractory to treatment, and their practical significance is thus enhanced by the lack of effective chemotherapy. The life cycles of these parasites are often poorly understood, and only recently has it been recognized that one stage of their life cycles requires tubificid worms as alternate hosts.

TABLE 4-2	Antiparasitic Drugs Used to Treat Captive Fish	
Agent	**Dosage**	**Comments**
Chloroquine diphosphate	10 mg/L	*Amyloodium ocellatum*
Copper sulfate	100 mg/L, 1-5 min bath, maintain free ion levels at 0.15-0.2 mg/L tank water	Marine fish protozoa, trematode ectoparasites, must monitor copper levels daily; toxic to plants and invertebrates
Fenbendazole	2 mg/L water, every 7 days ×3 treatments; 50 mg/kg, PO, q24h ×3 treatments, repeat in 14 days	Nonencysted trematodes, nematodes
Formalin	37% formalin only, 0.4 ml/L, for up to 1h bath	Protozoa, trematode, and crustacean ectoparasites; potential carcinogen; keep tank well aerated and monitor continuously
Freshwater	3-15 min bath, repeat daily as needed	Marine fish, ectoparasites
Glacial acetic acid	2 ml/L, 30-45 s bath	Trematodes and crustaceans; safe for goldfish, but possible toxicity in smaller tropical fish
Hydrogen peroxide	17.5 ml/L, 4-10 min bath, once	Ectoparasites
Levamisole	50 mg/L, 1h bath	Ectoparasites, free living parasites; monitor closely, water change after 1 h
Malachite green	0.1 mg/L tank water, 3 treatments for 3 days	Freshwater fish protozoa
Praziquantel	2 mg/L, continuous treatment for 5 days, then repeat in 2 weeks	Monogenes
Trichlorfon	0.5-1.0 mg/L, every 3 days, 12 h intervals between treatments	Crustacean ectoparasites

PO, per os.

Many metazoan parasites of fish have been described, some having a multiple-host life cycle that cannot easily be completed under captive conditions. Some cause problems in culture systems; external parasites can proliferate in all environments where convenient fish species favor their development, and they present a constant threat in all kinds of facilities. Parasitic crustaceans find suitable conditions for their development in closed marine systems when naturally infected waters exist nearby. Under such conditions, sea lice can cause extensive damage and mortality.

To effectively control fish parasites and minimize losses, rapid diagnosis is essential. The diagnostic tests routinely used to identify ectoparasites include the skin scrape, fin biopsy, and gill clip. A fecal float and direct saline smear should be performed to evaluate endoparasite status. In some cases, only necropsy can be used to confirm the presence of an endoparasite infection.

There are a number of potential therapeutics that can be used to control and/or eliminate fish parasites; however, the range of effective treatments is limited by the margin of safety of the agent. Treatments can also be limited by environmental factors too (e.g., water temperature, hardness levels, pH). Table 4-2 represents a list of antiparasitic agents commonly used to treat captive fish.[6,9]

Nutritional Diseases

Nutritional diseases are uncommon in wild populations of fish. Although environmental factors may limit food availability and particular weather and geophysical phenomena may adversely affect the food chain, wild fish generally have the opportunity in their natural environment to acquire adequate levels of all their nutritional requirements.[15]

The same cannot be said for captive ornamental fish. There are many different types of diets available for ornamentals, including commercially prepared pelleted and flake foods, invertebrate-based foods (e.g., brine shrimp, daphnia, blood worms), and live vertebrate foods (e.g., goldfish and guppies), and the nutritional value of these foods is highly variable.

Most commercially prepared pelleted or flake foods are comprised of a combination of macronutrients and micronutrients. The levels of these different nutrients can vary between formulations, and this makes it extremely difficult to define nutritional disease in absolute terms because it is rare for a deficiency to be based on a single essential nutrient. Fish offered nutritionally deficient diets are often more susceptible to infectious conditions. The deficiency of a necessary component in the diet is only one aspect of nutritional disease, which has been defined as the deficiency, excess, or improper balance of the components present in a fish diet. The definition should also include the presence of noxious or toxic components within the food and/or endogenous antinutrient factors, as these have become increasingly significant and can also cause disease in fish.[15,16]

Although most dietary deficiencies are associated with a complexity of marginal or absolute deficiencies, confirming the specific role of a nutrient in the overall health of a fish requires detailed experimental study. In the clinical situation, however, nutritional deficiency is approached as a more general syndrome. Fish with this "syndrome" may display a range of clinical signs, including inappetence, weakness, lethargy, acute hemorrhage, infection, darkening skin color, and poor growth.[6] Artificial diets produced by major manufacturers and intended as a complete source of nutrients are usually of high quality, and it is rare that a particular mixture will be responsible for a nutritional deficiency. As a matter of fact, these commercial diets are more likely to cause problems associated with excessive nutrients (e.g., hepatic lipidosis) than a deficiency of nutrients. However, when feeding wet diets or frozen fish diets, the possibility of a nutritional deficiency or imbalance is much higher. Even high-quality diets are susceptible to nutrient loss during storage, especially if these diets are stored under conditions of high temperature and/or high humidity.

Fish are susceptible to both macronutrient (e.g., low protein, fat, carbohydrate, fiber) and micronutrient (e.g., vitamin and mineral) deficiencies or imbalances. In terms of macronutrients, most problems are associated with the lipid component of the diet. Excessive fat in the fish diet can lead to hepatic lipidosis. Among the micronutrients, any of a wide range of components can exert an effect, especially in fast-growing, younger fish.[6,16,18]

Starvation may occur in captive fish due to complete deprivation of food, inadequate feeding levels/frequency of a diet, offering a nutritionally deficient diet, or as a result of behavioral, physiologic, or mechanical limitations that prevent food intake. Inadequate feeding levels may be associated with inappropriate husbandry practices or to overstocking. The process of physiologic starvation is characterized, as might be expected, by a loss of weight and change in morphology. Affected fish become emaciated as a result of muscle loss, and the head becomes relatively larger in proportion to the body. Changes in skin color (e.g., darkened appearance) may also occur. Eventually the fish becomes anorexic. At necropsy, there is usually a general pallor (e.g., anemia) and serous atrophy of the fat and visceral organs.

Fish stocking densities, environmental water quality parameters (e.g., pH, temperature), transport, and handling all have a direct effect on the way stress affects captive fish.[5] The primary function of the aquarist is to maintain a system that is capable of minimizing the effects of these stressors. This has significant implications for growth and feed conversion, as well as susceptibility to infection. Stress induces catabolism, resulting in the breakdown of important energy reserves (e.g., fat, muscle). When this occurs, the energy required for such degradation and resynthesis is not available for growth. A number of other stressors that can play a role in determining the levels of nonspecific stress in fish are related to food and feeding. Inadequate or deficient diets, irregular feeding patterns, the presentation of feed, and buildup of detritus can contribute to the sum total pressures acting on the adaptive capacity of fish. The physiologic and biochemical changes that occur in the animal under the influence of environmental stressors, and which serve to moderate the negative effects of stressors, are termed the *general adaptive syndrome* (GAS).[6] They are neither species nor stressor specific, and are mediated by nervous and hormonal action. The end result, if the adaptive response is stimulated beyond physiologic levels and adaptive exhaustion is achieved, is that the fish are made increasingly vulnerable to infection. Opportunistic, obligate, or facultative pathogens extant in the animal's environment may cause infections in susceptible fish. Thus, many nutritional diseases in fish may be compounded by bacterial and fungal infection.[6,16]

Feeding activity is associated with a particular metabolic expenditure referred to as the cost of *specific dynamic action* (SDA).[6] The SDA is related to the metabolism associated with digestion, increased circulatory activity in the gut and related organs, production of enzymatic and other metabolic acids, and the excretion of nitrogenous metabolites. The exact process contributing to the metabolic oxygen demand created by SDA is well recognized, and at high temperatures when dissolved oxygen levels in water are reduced and the general resting metabolic oxygen demand by fish is high, feeding to satiation can result in such a high oxygen demand to satisfy SDA that oxygen starvation can occur. The clinical features associated with oxygen starvation in fish include death within 2 hours of feeding, a fixed, open mouth, and the presence of undigested food in the stomach and intestine. The likelihood for complications associated with feeding fish at high environmental temperatures is greatly exacerbated if there is underlying gill or blood pathology.[6,18] Hyperplastic or telangiectatic gill damage, which often occurs secondary to pollution, transportation, or handling, can result in a reduced ability of the gills to obtain oxygen and release carbon dioxide. It is frequently a feeding episode that places the final metabolic oxygen demand on compromised fish that leads to a mortality event.[6] Other conditions that can increase the susceptibility to SDA-mediated mortalities include fatty liver syndrome, chronic hemorrhagic conditions (e.g., warfarin toxicity), chronic viral septicemia, and infectious salmon anemia.

Neoplastic Diseases

Fish are subject to many of the same neoplastic conditions reported in higher vertebrates. The presence of neoplasms in fish can often be strongly correlated to environmental factors, which suggests that these animals can be important sentinels in aquatic ecosystems. The etiology of neoplasms is complex, and many of the factors that contribute to the growth and dissemination of tumors are unknown. Some of the contributing factors that have been identified include viruses, chemical or biologic toxins, physical agents, hormones, and the age, sex, and genetic predisposition of the animal.[6]

Neoplasms are classified on a histopathologic basis, according to cell origin (Table 4-3). Because the terminology used to classify tumors is based on the descriptions given for human neoplasia, the terms *benign* and *malignant* are routinely used to designate certain cell patterns. There is, however, no fine line of demarcation to separate these two types of descriptions in certain fish neoplastic conditions.

Miscellaneous Diseases

Gas-bubble disease (GBD) is a serious problem encountered in the captive fish setting. It was first described in aquarium

TABLE 4-3	Classification of Neoplasms Reported in Fish	
Tissue	**Benign**	**Malignant**
Epithelial	Papilloma (papillary folds, squamous cell, basal cell, odontoma)	Carcinoma (epithelioma, epidermoid)
	Adenoma	Adenocarcinoma
Mesenchymal (nonhematopoietic)	Fibroma	Fibrosarcoma
	Leiomyoma	Leiomyosarcoma
	Rhabdomyoma	Rhabdomyosarcoma
	Lipoma	Liposarcoma
	Chondroma	Chondrosarcoma
	Osteoma	Osteosarcoma
Mesenchymal (hematopoietic)	Lymphoma	Malignant lymphoma
Neural	Neuroma (neurilemmoma, ganglioneuroma)	
Pigment	Melanoma	Malignant melanoma
Embryonal	Teratoma, Nephroblastoma	

fish by Gorham in 1898 and is typically seen in most captive fish populations at some time or another. GBD appears under a wide variety of circumstances, so determining the etiology is not always a simple matter. In its simplest form, GBD is associated with the super saturation of the tissues with nitrogen or oxygen.[6] There are many factors that contribute not only to the initial inception of the disease but also to the severity of the disease. Some of the factors associated with the disease include temperature, mechanical failures of pumps or sumps, transport, and algal blooms.[6,18] The degree of supersaturation is the most important factor in relation to both the clinical picture and eventual outcome, but duration of exposure and subsequent treatment also affect survival. Fish should be removed from the affected system and placed into a separate, unaffected system. The affected system should be thoroughly evaluated and the inciting cause of the supersaturation corrected.

Low environmental temperature (hypothermia) can increase an animal's susceptibility to certain bacteria and decrease an animal's threshold to certain toxins. Saltwater fish from higher latitudes can develop severe abdominal distension if they become hypothermic. Affected animals can retain large quantities of water in their stomach, holding as much as 40% of their body weight in water. The principle mechanism of action associated with this pathologic event is an osmoregulatory stress associated with low temperatures and high salinity. Affected animals should be gradually warmed; however, mortalities are likely to be high. Prevention is the key, and this disease can be avoided by establishing appropriate environmental temperatures with appropriate heating devices.

There are many waterborne irritants that can adversely affect fish health. Each fish species has an optimum range for pH. Many of the factors that cause rapid changes in the pH are deleterious to the gills. Certain irritants, such as dust, silt, and ammonia, can also damage the gills but may not induce immediate clinical disease. This is because the gills initially have a delayed response to these irritants; however, over time the affected fish can become more dyspneic as a result of the reduced transfer of oxygen and carbon dioxide at the level of the gills. This dyspnea can be exacerbated by high environmental temperatures and low oxygen solubility.[3,6,18]

Color anomalies observed in cultured marine fish have a genetic origin and influence the basis for ornamental varieties or strains.[6] Pseudo-albinism, a frequent feature of flatfishes, is a husbandry-related developmental anomaly.[6] Partially pigmented or reverse-pigmented animals are also present to a significant level in confined species. The exact etiology for this color pattern is unknown; however, it has been suggested that it may be related to high levels of lighting and a lack of an essential trace nutrient during early development.

Physical deformities can be derived from multiple etiologies. Congenital malformations are not uncommon in cultured fish and may be influenced by multiple causative factors. Lesions associated with genetic factors, incubation temperature, or hormonal effects are apparent from early development, whereas lesions of husbandry or nutritional origin can occur at any stage of development.[5,6,16]

■ THERAPEUTICS

Therapeutics may be administered to fish in a water bath, per os (PO), intramuscular (IM) injection, intraperitoneal injection, or the intravenous (IV) route. Water bath treatment protocols to treat internal infections are of little value to freshwater fish but have been used with success to treat marine fish. Marine fish actually drink water, so any medication placed in the water will be ingested (Figure 4-25). Freshwater fish do not drink water and are not likely to receive the same benefit. Carbon filters should be removed when a bath or immersion treatment is used. PO medications can be placed into food and delivered to the fish during routine feedings. Unfortunately, many sick fish are anorectic and do not benefit from medicated food. PO medications can also be administered via a stomach tube. A red rubber feeding tube may be used for this procedure (Figure 4-26). The distance from the mouth to the mid-body should be measured and marked, thereby denoting the approx-

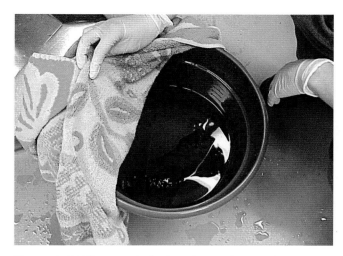

Figure 4-25 Therapeutic bath or immersion can be used to treat marine fish.

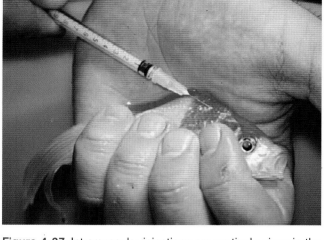

Figure 4-27 Intramuscular injections are routinely given in the epaxial muscles.

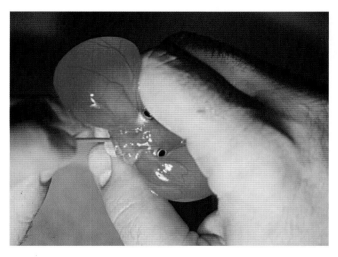

Figure 4-26 Fish that tolerate handling can be given medication per os via a tube.

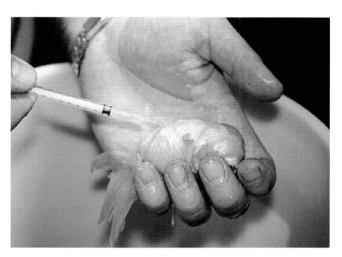

Figure 4-28 Intraperitoneal (intracoelomic) injections are an excellent method of delivering medications or fluids to fish. The fish should be placed in dorsal recumbency for the procedure.

imate location of the stomach. The tube should be inserted to the level of the mark and the medication delivered.

Parenteral routes are commonly used to treat fish. IM injections are administered into the epaxial muscles surrounding the spine (Figure 4-27). The needle should be inserted between the scales. Irritating compounds should not be administered IM because they can lead to muscle necrosis. Intraperitoneal injections are a rapid and effective method for administering different medications to fish (Figure 4-28). The fish should be held in dorsal recumbency, allowing gravity to drop the viscera, and the injection administered between the scales on the ventrum of the coelomic cavity. Again, irritating compounds should not be used. IV injections are not routinely used, but they may be useful during emergency situations.

Numerous factors can alter or mediate the efficacy of drugs used to treat fish. These factors can be divided into two general categories: biologic and environmental. Biologic factors that

can affect a therapeutic plan include species variation, physiologic and anatomic variation (e.g., ectotherms vs. endotherms), the presence of a renal portal system, vascular flow, high glomerular filtration rates, osmotic homeostasis, overall size/weight, sexual maturity, body condition, stress level, disease/immune status, seasonal patterns, nutritional status, and lipid content of the liver.[24] Species variation refers to body design and behavior, gill area to body-weight ratio, and positioning in the water (e.g., benthic vs. pelagic). Drug absorption, distribution, metabolism, and mode of excretion can affect each drug differently.[24,25] Environmental considerations address the specific parameters monitored in water quality, including temperature, pH, salinity, and hardness. Although it is useful to consider potential factors that may influence a response to a chemotherapeutic agent, it is not always possible to predict the clinical effect. Individual variation can create response variation within a species and may have dramatic affects on the outcome.[24]

In addition to trying to understand the effect physiologic, anatomic, and environmental influences have on fish therapeutics, it is important to consider the different properties of the drugs. Identifying certain characteristics about a drug, such as whether it is lipophilic (fat soluble) or hydrophilic (water soluble), protein bound (albumin in the blood) or not protein bound, and has specific binding sites, can influence the pharmacodynamics of a drug and whether it will or will not be effective.

The following factors should be considered when generating a therapeutic plan for a fish: (1) the pharmaceutical form of the drug, (2) the physical or chemical properties of the drug, (3) how quickly the onset of action should occur, (4) restraint of the animal, (5) behavioral characteristics of the animal, and (6) the nature of the particular condition being treated.[25] A drug is of no use unless it can be delivered to the patient in a form and at a site that is appropriate.

Fluid Therapy

Fluid therapy is a critical but inexact component of medical care for fish. Its application revolves around estimating the amount of fluid loss in a patient and, consequently, the amount of fluid that needs to be replaced. This determination can be estimated from the physical examination findings and laboratory tests (e.g., complete blood count and plasma biochemistries). There are three values that should be calculated to determine the volume of fluid to be administered: the hydration deficit, the maintenance requirement, and ongoing fluid losses. Fluids should be administered to restore the normal hydration status, replace electrolytes and nutrients, and administer medications that must be diluted in large volumes.

The type of fluid to be administered should be determined on a case-by-case basis. Estimating or calculating the plasma osmolality is the best method for determining the type of fluid to use for replacement. There are a variety of commercially prepared fluids available that fall into one of several basic categories. The primary categories of fluids used in veterinary medicine are the crystalloid solutions, colloid solutions, hypertonic solutions, fluid additives, and parenteral vitamin/mineral products. The amount, type, and method of administration should be determined by the clinician responsible for the animal.[24,25] Fluid replacement in fish is generally done PO or intracoelomically.

Therapeutics Used to Treat Infectious Diseases

No matter how effective an antimicrobial agent or parasiticide has been shown to be, it has no value if it is prohibited or not permitted by national or regional regulation. Regulatory controls that require veterinary medicines to be safe and effective before being approved for use have been in development over the past 30 years. A general lack of approved antimicrobial drugs for fish inevitably means an increasing reliance on off-label use.

Ideally, the selection of an antimicrobial agent should be based on the reliable diagnosis of the disease and pathogen involved, followed by determination of the most effective drug.[3] This decision should be made based on laboratory determination of the antibiotic sensitivity of the specific pathogen, taking into account factors such as the pharmacokinetic and pharmacodynamic properties of the drug.[25] Almost all treatments can be administered by parenteral injection; however, this is the most costly method in terms of labor, time, and associated stress. Therefore, if the parenteral route is excluded, then the most practical routes of administration are immersion bath and oral medications (see Table 4-1).[25]

Emergency Drugs

There are few pharmacokinetic data available on the use of emergency drugs in fish and even less on their use in specific species.[25] In our experience, the reaction of different species of fish to emergency drugs is completely unpredictable. Furthermore, these drugs may have dramatically varied responses in the same or similar species of fish. Table 4-4 represents a list

TABLE 4-4   Emergency Drugs Used to Treat Fish

Agent	Dose	Comments
Atropine	0.1 mg/kg IM, ICe, IV	Organophosphate toxicity, hydrocarbon toxicity
Dexamethasone	5 mg/kg IM, q24h to effect	Shock, trauma, stress
Doxapram	5 mg/kg ICe, IV, topical	Respiratory depression
Epinephrine (1 : 1000)	0.2-0.5 ml IM, IC, IV, ICe	Cardiac arrest
Furosemide	2-5 mg/kg IM q12-72h	Ascites, edema
Haloperidol	0.5 mg/kg IM	Dopamine blocking agent, use with LH to stimulate egg release
Hydrocortisone	1-4 mg/kg IM, ICe	Shock, trauma, stress
Hydrogen peroxide	0.25 ml/L water	Hypoxia
Oxygen (100%)	Titrate as needed	Hypoxia, stress
Sodium bicarbonate	30 g/L bath, 4% ICe	Acidosis, capture stress, euthanasia
Sodium chloride	1-3 g/L	Freshwater fish, stress
Sodium thiosulfate	10 mg/L	Neutralize chlorine

IC, intracardiac; ICe, intracoelomic; IM, intramuscular; IV, intravenous; LH, Lutenizing hormone.

of emergency drugs known to have some effectiveness in fish; however, precautions should be taken when using these drugs in a new species for the first time.

Nutritional Support

The provision of calories to a fish suffering from a negative energy balance can be the difference between treatment success and failure. In general, an acute weight loss of more than 10% of the optimal body weight, not related to dehydration, is sufficient evidence that nutritional support is needed. The likelihood of success increases dramatically if the nutritional support is initiated early.[16] The clinician should first correct fluid, acid-base, and electrolyte imbalances before implementing nutritional support.[25] Once this is done, then the clinician can choose the most practical and appropriate type of nutritional support. If the animal is still eating, than a diet rich in protein and fat may be appropriate. In some cases, providing nutritional support simply involves adjusting the diet to a common food source that may not have been previously offered to the animal.

The methods of providing calories via a gastrointestinal tube or force-feeding whole-prey items have had a moderate degree of success. If the animal is not eating or if tubing the fish and providing calories directly into the stomach is contraindicated, then options are limited to administering fluids either via the IV or intracoeloemic (ICe) route. If IV or ICe fluids are given, a mixture of aminoplex, electrolytes, and glucose may be administered with a high fluid component. A B-complex multivitamin should also be included in the mixture.[25] This type of supplementation will suffice for several weeks in the absence of severe metabolic abnormalities. Discontinuing the IV or ICe feedings must be done gradually over a 2- to 3-day period. Keep in mind that significant day-to-day changes in weight are usually caused by alterations in fluid content rather than by body mass. The clinical status of the animal should be monitored daily and additional laboratory tests done to address any abnormalities observed by the clinician.

Regardless of the feeding method used, unless specific contraindications exist, voluntary food consumption should be encouraged. Intensive intervention is often necessary to stimulate an anabolic response sufficient for the animal to begin eating voluntarily; however, it is preferable to avoid practices that may adversely affect the nutritional status of the patient.

Appetite stimulants have generally been found to have minimal effects in fish; however, the use of steroids and nonsteroidal antiinflammatory agents have been shown to work in some cases.[6] Providing B vitamins may also have some value as an appetite stimulant.[25]

Miscellaneous Drugs

Table 4-5 represents a list of miscellaneous compounds used in fish medicine.

■ SURGERY

Fish surgery is still in its infancy, and there is still much skepticism regarding its value.[20] However, surgical procedures are currently performed with regularity and reasonable success. This is a direct result of the improved anesthetic techniques available for aquatic species and an increased number of training opportunities to enhance the surgical skills of clinicians that perform specialized procedures on fish. Fish surgeries are performed in research, public facilities, and more recently, by private practitioners in their veterinary clinics. There are a number of reasons why the veterinary clinician may pursue a surgical option in a fish case, including an inability to manage the case using only internal medicine, the monetary value of the animal, to provide improved aesthetics for display animals suffering from a traumatic injury or disfiguring wound, or the emotional attachment of the owner.[20,26] There are multiple published resources available on the subject of fish surgery.[6,19,20,24,26]

Surgical site preparation for fish should follow the same standards set forth for higher vertebrates. Povidone-iodine (1 : 20) or chlorhexidine (1 : 40) can be used to reduce the gross contamination on the skin surface. Aggressive disinfection should be avoided, as it can cause significant damage to the integument. Clear plastic surgical drapes should be used to reduce the amount of contact with the protective mucous layer of the skin and to provide a moisture barrier for insensible water loss. The skin should be kept moist throughout the entire surgical procedure by continuous irrigation.

The benefits and risks of special diagnostic procedures should be considered before any surgical procedure is carried out. Conventional radiography works well for diagnosing gas

---

TABLE 4-5   Miscellaneous Agents Used to Manage Fish in Captivity

Agent	Dosage	Comments
Activated carbon	75 g/40 L	Removal of medications and organic waste
Carp pituitary extract	5 mg/kg, IM, q6h	Use with HCG to stimulate egg release
HCG	30 IU/kg, q6h	Stimulate release of eggs
LH-A	2 ug/kg, IM, q8h	Stimulate release of eggs, use with haloperidol or reserpine
Nitrifying bacteria	Use as directed for commercial products	Seed or improves development of biologic filtration
Reserpine	50 mg/kg, IM	Dopamine blocking agent

HCG, human chorionic gonadotropin; IM, intramuscular; LRH-A, luteinizing hormone.

trapping lesions and/or foreign body obstructions, but it is more limited when assessing soft tissue masses or lesions. If more advanced diagnostics are available, such as computed tomography or magnetic resonance imaging, and economically warranted, they may prove invaluable for assessing a soft tissue lesion and determining/confirming the value of a surgical approach.

Many of the same surgical instruments used to perform procedures in domestic mammals can be used for fish too. Modified spay-neuter surgical packs or ocular/microsurgical packs may be used for smaller species. Balfour or Gelpi retractors are useful for exploring the abdomen or extended gastrointestinal procedures. Radiosurgery is an invaluable tool for fish surgery. This surgical instrument can be used to make the initial incision, collect biopsy samples, and control hemorrhage. Magnification loupes are another important surgical tool. A magnification loupe can provide the surgeon with a significantly improved field of vision for a surgical procedure.

Skin closure in fish is optimized by the use of subcutaneous or subcuticular absorbable sutures. Closure may also benefit from the addition of a surgical adhesive such as Nexaband (Abbott Laboratories, North Chicago, IL). Localized dermatitis has been reported after the use of surgical adhesives; however, we have not noted any problems associated with this particular brand of adhesive. Fish skin heals very slowly in comparison to mammal skin. For fish, it is best to leave sutures in for a minimum of 4 to 6 weeks.

With ICe surgical procedures, it may be beneficial to irrigate the coelomic cavity postoperatively with an isotonic preparation of antibiotics. This has proven particularly beneficial when performing gastrointestinal procedures where there is a high risk of bacterial contamination. However, the efficacy of prophylactic antibiotic therapy being used in this manner in fish has not been rigorously evaluated and should therefore be pursued with caution.

Fish Anesthesia

The selection of a particular anesthesia for a fish procedure should be based on the procedure being done (e.g., length of procedure, amount of analgesia required, degree of immobility required) and anesthetic availability. Table 4-6 represents a list of commonly used anesthetics for fish.

Before an anesthetic event, the fish patient should be thoroughly evaluated to ensure that it is a good anesthetic candidate. Fish that are stressed are not considered good anesthetic candidates and may have inconsistent or rough anesthetic events. Food should be withheld for a minimum of 8 to 12 hours to ensure that a fish does not regurgitate and contaminate the anesthetic solution.

Traditional fish anesthesia was barbaric, and many "fish surgeons" would rely on "bruticaine" to restrain animals for physical examination and short surgical procedures. This technique is unacceptable, as there are a number of safe, reliable anesthetic agents that can be used to appropriately restrain or anesthetize a fish.

Monitoring fish during an anesthetic procedure can be difficult. In most cases, opercular movement, loss of equilibrium (e.g., absence of righting reflex), sensitivity to painful stimuli, fin color, and gill color are used to assess the patient. In larger specimens, a pulse oximeter, ECG, or crystal Doppler may be used to monitor heart rate, although the heart of fish may continue to pump for a period of time after the animal is dead.

TABLE 4-6	Anesthetic Agents Used in Fish	
Agent	**Dosage**	**Comments**
Atipamezole	2 mg/kg	Reversal agent for medetomidine
Butorphanol	0.05-0.10 mg/kg, IM	Analgesia
Carbocaine		Local anesthesia
Carbon dioxide	To effect	Euthanasia
Clove oil (eugenol)	40-120 mg/L	Stock solution 100 mg/L, 1 part clove oil to 9 parts 95% ethanol
Ethanol	1.0%-1.5% bath	Euthanasia
Halothane	0.5-2.0 ml/L	Bath or vaporize
Isoflurane	0.5-2.0 ml/L	Bath or vaporize
Ketamine	66-88 mg/kg, IM	Short procedures
Ketamine	1-2 mg/kg	Premedication
Medetomidine	0.5-0.1 mg/kg, IM	Reverse with atipamezole 0.2 mg/kg
Lidocaine	<5 mg/kg	Local anesthetic
MS-222	100-200 mg/L, induction, 50-100 mg/L, maintenance	Anesthesia, stock solution 10 g/L, buffered
Propofol	1.5-2.5 mg/kg, IV	Intravenous only
Quinaldine sulfate	50-100 mg/L, induction 15-60 mg/L, maintenance	Anesthesia, stock solution 10 g/L, buffered
Sodium bicarbonate	30 g/L, bath	Euthanasia

IM, intramuscular; IV, intravenous.

In the case of waterborne anesthetics, dechlorinated water may be used to irrigate the gills and "lighten" the plane of anesthesia.

Common Surgical Procedures

The most common surgical procedures performed on captive fish are biopsy collection (external and internal), exploratory laparotomy, and foreign body removal. Skin biopsies can be collected via an excisional (e.g., small section of tissue is removed for histopathology) or scraping procedure (see special diagnostic tests). Radiosurgery is recommended for excisional biopsies to minimize blood loss.

Exploratory laparotomy or laparoscopy is an excellent method for examining the internal organs of fish and collecting tissue biopsies for histopathology. This type of procedure can be done using a standard midline ventral approach or a laparoscope. In cases where the surgeon only expects to visualize the organs and collect biopsies, laparoscopy is preferred because it will cause minimal tissue damage. Another benefit associated with laparoscopy is that it is more aesthetically pleasing (e.g., small or no scar) and the patient can be returned to their display aquarium sooner. One limitation associated with laparoscopy in fish is the limited view that can be obtained in certain species or in obese animals. In these cases, a laparotomy is preferable.

Foreign body ingestion is a common occurrence in carnivorous fish. Diagnosing a foreign body in fish should follow the same diagnostic plan (e.g., diagnostic imaging) used for terrestrial vertebrates. In some cases, the foreign body can be removed using an endoscope or by direct visualization, whereas in others it requires a laparotomy. Before attempting a surgical procedure, it is important for the veterinarian to become familiar with the specific anatomy of their patient. The surgical procedure for removing a foreign body from a fish is similar to the procedure used for terrestrial vertebrates.

Preoperative and Postoperative Considerations

Preoperative and postoperative pain management in fish have not been studied in depth. However, butorphanol (0.1 mg/kg IM) has been used as both a preanesthetic and postanesthetic analgesic without adverse effects.[20] Fish being recovered from surgery should be placed in an isolated tank with nonanesthetic water taken from the animal's aquarium. The recovery water should be aerated to ensure appropriate dissolved oxygen levels in the water column. To prevent unnecessary trauma or accidental death, it is important to confirm that the fish has completely recovered before it is returned to a community system. External stimulation should be kept to a minimum during the recovery process to minimize stress (e.g., no excessive noise, movement, light). Some species exhibit a rebound effect to certain anesthetic agents. This is often more pronounced in cold-water species. The physiologic parameters monitored during the anesthetic event should continue to be evaluated

until the fish is deemed recovered (e.g., normal heart and respiratory rates, righting reflex returned, pain response [measured by fin pinch] returned).

ZOONOSES

Humans can be exposed to ornamental fish pathogens from direct contact with the fish or their water. Most of the zoonotic diseases attributed to ornamental fish occur as a result of microbes being introduced into open wounds or puncture wounds that occur during handling. Humans with a compromised immune system may be predisposed to opportunistic infections. Most cases of fishborne zoonotic diseases result in mild episodes of disease.[27] A number of opportunistic bacterial pathogens have been associated with human illness, including *Clostridium* spp., *Erysipelothrix rhusiopathiae*, *Mycobacterium* spp., *Staphylococcus* spp., and *Streptococcus* spp. Members of the family Enterobacteriaceae (e.g., *Edwardsiella tarda, Klebsiella* spp., *Salmonella* spp., *Yersinia* spp.) are routinely isolated from aquatic environments and have also been associated with human illness. Fish parasites and toxins have been found to cause human illness but are not generally a problem with ornamental fish because they are not eaten. To prevent the transmission of potentially zoonotic diseases, veterinary professionals should follow standard safety protocols and wear gloves.

REFERENCES

1. Adey HW, Loveland K: *Dynamic Aquaria,* San Diego, Calif, 1991, Academic Press.
2. Stoskopf MK: *Fish Medicine,* Philadelphia, 1993, WB Saunders.
3. Noga EJ: *Fish Disease: Diagnosis and Treatment,* St Louis, 1996, Mosby.
4. Axelrod HR, Burgess WE: *Saltwater Aquarium Fish,* Neptune, NJ, 1973, TFH.
5. Plumb JA: *Health Maintenance and Principle Microbial Diseases of Cultured Fishes,* Ames, 1999, Iowa State University Press.
6. Roberts RJ: *Fish Pathology,* Philadelphia, 2001, WB Saunders.
7. Cox GF: *Tropical Marine Aquaria,* New York, 1997, Grosset & Dunlap.
8. Axelrod HR, Burgess WE: *Atlas of Freshwater Aquarium Fishes,* Neptune City, NJ, 1997, TFH.
9. Paul JP: *Marine Microbiology,* San Diego, Calif, 2001, Academic Press.
10. Austin B: *Methods in Aquatic Bacteriology,* New York, 1989, Wiley.
11. Russo RC: Ammonia, nitrite, and nitrate. In Rand GM, Pertocelli SR, editors: *Fundamentals of Aquatic Toxicology,* New York, 1985, Hemisphere.
12. Emerson K, Russo RC, Lund RE et al: Aqueous ammonia equilibrium calculations: effect of pH and temperature, *J Fish Research Board of Canada* 32:2379-2383, 1975.
13. Tucker CS: Water analysis. In Stoskopf MK, editor: *Fish Medicine,* Philadelphia, 1993, WB Saunders.
14. Piper RG, McElwaine JB, Orne LE et al: *Fish Hatchery Management,* US Department of the Interior, Fish and Wildlife Service, Washington DC, 1982.
15. Halver JE, Hardy RW: *Fish Nutrition,* San Diego, Calif, 2002, Academic Press.
16. Yanong RP: Nutrition of ornamental fish, *Vet Clin North Am Exot Anim Pract* (1):19-42, 1999.
17. Post G: *Textbook of Fish Health,* Neptune, NJ, 1987, TFH.
18. Fudge AM: *Laboratory Medicine,* Philadelphia, 2000, WB Saunders.
19. Ross LG, Ross B: *Anaesthetic and Sedative Techniques for Aquatic Animals,* Malden, Mass, 1999, Blackwell.
20. Harms CA, Lewbart GA: Surgery in fish, *Vet Clin North Am Exot Anim Pract* 3:759-774, 2000.

21. Tomasso JR, Davis KB, Parker NC: Plasma corticosteroid electrolyte dynamics of hybrid striped bass (white bass × striped bass) during netting and hauling stress, *Proc World Mariculture Soc* 11:303-310, 1980.

22. Ackerman L: *The Biology, Husbandry and Health Care of Reptiles, vol 3, Health Care of Reptiles,* Neptune, NJ, 1997, TFH.

23. Dunbar CE, Wolf K: The cytological course of experimental lymphocycstis in the bluegill, *J Infect Dis* 116:466-472, 1996.

24. Stamper AM, Miller SM, Berzins I: Pharmacology in elasmobranchs. In Smith M, Warmolts D, Thoney D et al, editors: *Elasmobranch Husbandry Manual,* Columbus, OH, 2004, Ohio Biological Survey, Inc.

25. Lewbart GA: Fish. In Carpenter JW, editor: *Exotic Animal Formulary,* ed 3, Philadelphia, 2005, Elsevier.

26. Lewbart GA: *Ornamental Fish,* Ames, 1998, Iowa State Press.

27. Nemetz TG, Shotts EB: Zoonotic diseases. In Stoskopf MK, editor: *Fish Medicine,* Philadelphia, 1993, WB Saunders.

Natalie Mylniczenko

CHAPTER 5

AMPHIBIANS

■ COMMON SPECIES KEPT IN CAPTIVITY

The class Amphibia is divided into three orders: Anura (frogs and toads), Caudata (salamanders, newts, and sirens), and Gymnophiona (caecilians). There are over 4000 extant species, but very few (one tenth) are ever held in captivity.[1]

The frogs and toads are the most represented of these orders in captivity. The distinction between frogs and toads, according to most veterinarians, is whether the animals are found in or around water (frogs) or not (toads). Common species in captivity include the firebelly toads (*Bombina* spp.) (Figure 5-1), African clawed frogs *(Xenopus laevis),* dwarf clawed frogs (*Hymenochirus* spp.), ornate horned frogs (*Ceratophrys* spp.)*,* true toads (*Bufo* spp.), poison dart frogs (*Dendrobates* spp., *Phyllobates* spp., *Epipidobates* spp.), true frogs (*Rana* spp.), and tree frogs (*Hyla* spp.).

Newts and salamanders (grouped as caudates) have gained in popularity as vivarium pets in the past decade. The defining characteristic of a newt versus a salamander is that a newt maintains an aquatic lifestyle throughout both its larval and adult stages.[1] The redbelly or firebelly newt *(Cynops pyrrhogaster)* (Figure 5-2), water dog or tiger salamander *(Ambystoma tigrinum),* axolotl *(Ambystoma mexicanum),* mudpuppy *(Necturus maculosus),* rough-skinned newt *(Taricha granulosa),* red-spotted newt *(Notophthalmus viridescens),* and members of the *Triturus* genus are common to the pet trade. Sirens are a lesser known subset of this order and are not typically held in captivity except in some zoological facilities.

Caecilians are infrequently kept in amphibian collections. When observed in zoos or aquaria, the most common species found are the aquatic *Typhlonectes natans* (Figure 5-3) and the fossorial Mexican caecilian *(Dermophis mexicanus)* and Varagua caecilian *(Gymnopis multiplacata).*[1]

■ BIOLOGY

Amphibian body plans are consistent with those of other vertebrates. However, as with any exotic animal species, knowledge regarding the nuances of species variation for some anatomical and physiological traits can be helpful when developing a diagnostic or treatment plan for an amphibian patient. For example, amphibians do not have distinct thoracic and abdominal cavities. Instead, they have a single coelomic cavity. This information is important when considering surgery (e.g., no loss of negative pressure as would be the case with mammals). The following comments on anatomy and physiology will focus on salient clinical features. See other amphibian texts for greater detail.[2,3]

Unique Anatomy of Frogs and Toads[3,4]

MUSCULOSKELETAL

Four limbs are present, but there may be variable hindlimb lengths. The length depends on species locomotory modes; longer hindlegs occur in animals that jump (Figure 5-4). The forelimbs possess a fused radius and ulna (radioulna), whereas the hindlimbs have a fused tibia and fibula (tibiofibula). The forefeet possess four phalanges on each foot, whereas the hindfeet have five phalanges. The hyoid apparatus in some species is adapted to eject the tongue for prey capture. Vertebrae are separated into three fused regions: presacral, sacral, and postsacral (note that a sacrum is not present). The pelvic girdle is

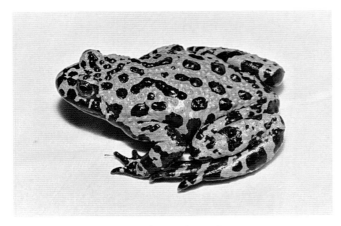

Figure 5-1 Firebelly toad (*Bombina* sp.).

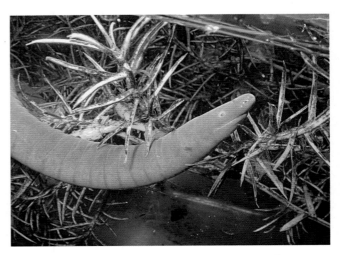

Figure 5-3 Aquatic caecilian *(Typhlonectes natans)*.

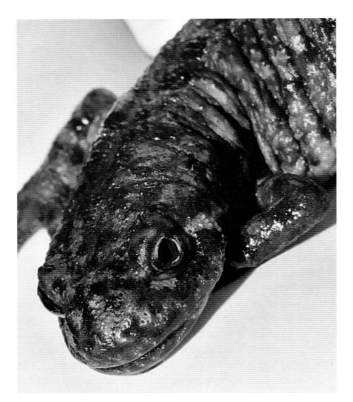

Figure 5-2 Firebelly newt *(Cynops pyrrhogaster)*.

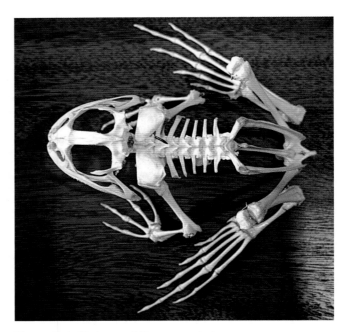

Figure 5-4 Skeleton of *Rana catesbeiana*.

fused with the last presacral vertebra, and a fused urostyle (or coccyx) is found caudal to the girdle. Some animals possess pigments that result in a blue coloration of the bones *(Phrynohyas resinifictrix)*. Amphibians do not have diaphragms.

INTEGUMENT SYSTEM

Anatomical modifications of the skin are highly variable among species, but the basic integument has a thin keratin layer (usually one cell layer thick) and a relatively thin basal epidermal layer (approximately eight cell layers thick). There is a significant subcutaneous layer that can accumulate fluid. In some species, this is normal (as a fluid reservoir); however, it

may also indicate a pathological condition. Ecdysis occurs regularly, and keratophagy (e.g., consuming the shed skin) may occur. The skin may contain venom glands for predator avoidance. In bufonids, the large parotid glands dorsocaudal to the eyes can produce noxious chemicals. Anurans have a patch of skin on the ventral pelvis that is highly water absorptive. Veterinarians may use this patch to facilitate fluid absorption in dehydrated amphibians.

RESPIRATORY SYSTEM

Three modes of respiration occur in anurans: buccopharyngeal, pulmonic, and cutaneous; the mode used depends on species variability and environment. Anurans have a short trachea, thus impacting clinical procedures such as tracheal intubation and washes. Two equally sized lungs are present.

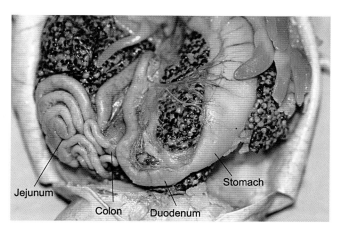

Figure 5-5 Gastrointestinal system (liver removed) of the frog (*Rana pipiens*).

The lungs of anurans are thin, sac-like structures. Care should be taken when positive pressure ventilating these animals to prevent pulmonary rupture.

CARDIOVASCULAR SYSTEM (ARTERIAL, VENOUS, AND LYMPHATIC)

Anurans have a three-chambered heart, and it is encased in the pectoral girdle. Both renal and hepatic portal venous systems are found in anurans. All amphibians possess lymph hearts, which beat in synchrony at about 50 beats per minute (bpm) independently from the cardiac system. Lymph accumulation typically implies illness. Fluid can be absorbed directly into the lymphatics and then into the kidneys, so some care must be used when administering drugs cutaneously or subcutaneously. The differences between lymph and blood are not well studied, but overall, the components (e.g., chemistries) are similar with the exception of the erythrocytes.

GASTROINTESTINAL SYSTEM

Teeth are absent in some frogs; others lack tongues (e.g., *Pipa pipa,* which uses negative pressure to create a vacuum to catch prey). Occasionally, frogs evert their stomachs in order to wipe noxious substances from their stomach mucosa. It is not unusual to see undigested insect skeletons, bones, or plant fibers in the feces of anurans. All amphibians (note: within this text, "all" amphibians will include caudates and caecilians) have a simple, short alimentary system that empties into a cloaca (Figure 5-5). A large bilobed liver (which can fill up to 50% of the coelom) encases the pericardium. There are typically two lobes, though a third will occur in some species. The color and shade varies from pale gray to brown to black. Melanomacrophages are present and can result in the dark coloration of the liver. In the larval amphibian, the liver is the primary hematopoietic organ, switching to bone marrow after metamorphosis. Anurans have a large gall bladder.

URINARY SYSTEM

The end products of protein catabolism in anurans may be ammonia, urea, or uric acid. Typically, aquatic anurans excrete ammonia (ammonotelic), because conserving water is not important. Urea-excreting animals (ureotelic), like toads, will have some contact with water. They produce dilute urine when they are in freshwater and typically do not urinate on land (thus, their plasma urea elevates). Uric acid–excreting animals (uricotelic) have the least contact with water (e.g., the tree frog).

Amphibians have mesonephric kidneys and cannot concentrate urine above the solute concentration of the plasma. The kidney is a dual filter for coelomic and vascular fluid (there are connections to the coelom via a nephrostome), and this has implications when administering drugs via the coelomic cavity.

REPRODUCTIVE SYSTEM

Some anuran species possess intromittent organs, but most do not. External fertilization is the primary reproductive strategy of anurans. However, internal fertilization may occur in some viviparous toads. Corpora lutea develop in some species. Males in the genera *Bufo* have a Bidder's organ, which is a rudimentary ovary. Sexual dimorphism may be seen in anurans and is usually characterized by color changes, size differences (males are typically smaller), and the presence of spines, tubercles, and tusks. Some males will have nuptial pads that develop during the breeding season or have larger toes than females.

HEMATOPOIETIC SYSTEM

All amphibians possess a thymus throughout their adult life. Terrestrial animals have functional bone marrow, but only lymphocytes and myelocytes are produced there. The spleen is the major site for erythropoiesis. Some red cell production can occur in the liver, kidney, and bone marrow in various species.

ENDOCRINE SYSTEM

Endocrine glands of all amphibians are similar to those of other vertebrates.

OTHER

Amphibians have two discrete lipid storage organs: coelomic fat bodies and inguinal fat bodies. Lipids are also stored in various cutaneous and subcutaneous fat deposits around the heart, in the liver, and in the tail of some plethodontid salamanders.

Unique Anatomy of Newts and Salamanders[3,4]
MUSCULOSKELETAL

Unique species features include the lack of a pelvic girdle in the sirens and greatly reduced limbs in *Amphiuma* spp. The vertebral column is not well differentiated in these animals, but it is not fused as with the anurans.

INTEGUMENT SYSTEM

In some species of aquatic salamander, there is no keratin cell layer. The dermis is firmly attached to muscle, and therefore there is no subcutaneous layer. Glandular secretions may contain toxic compounds. Folding of the skin and similar anatomical modifications may increase the available surface layer for respiratory purposes.

RESPIRATORY SYSTEM

There are four forms of respiration in caudates, and they are species dependent: branchial, cutaneous, buccopharyngeal, and pulmonic. Animals with gills may have short or long filaments depending on their natural environment. Animals with short gills are typically located in stream areas and thus have higher requirements for dissolved oxygen. Cutaneous respiration can occur in these animals because of a high surface area on the skin and a low metabolic rate; additionally, anaerobic glycolysis can occur. Behavioral responses, such as rocking, allow a current to run across the skin, optimizing contact with dissolved oxygen in the water. Most salamanders possess two lungs, with either single lobes (aquatic) or sacculated lobes (terrestrial). There is a lungless salamander. Costal grooves (skin folds along the ribs) also increase the integumentary surface area. Buccopharyngeal respiration technically is cutaneous respiration occurring within the oral cavity. The trachea of caudates is very short and should prompt the clinician to exercise caution when performing procedures like intubation and tracheal washes.

CARDIOVASCULAR SYSTEM (ARTERIAL, VENOUS, AND LYMPHATIC)

A three-chambered heart is found encased within the pectoral girdle. Renal and hepatic portal vein systems are present in these amphibians. Numerous lymph hearts are present, usually around 11 in the head and coelom and 4 caudal to the sacrum.

GASTROINTESTINAL SYSTEM

The liver is elongate and single lobed; it may have scalloped edges. The intestinal anatomy of newts and salamanders has no relevant clinical differences from other amphibians (Figure 5-6). The oral cavity hinges such that the maxilla is mobile while the mandible is static.

URINARY SYSTEM

Caudates possess secondary tubules in their kidneys, which attach to the primary tubules; however, they do not have many nephrostomes and thus rely heavily on vascular filtration. They possess variably shaped bladders (bilobate, bicornate, and cylindrical). The primary excretory product in the aquatic caudate is ammonia, whereas in the terrestrial animal it is urea.

REPRODUCTIVE SYSTEM

In the dorsal aspect of the female cloaca resides the *spermatheca* (site for sperm storage). Males produce a spermatophore, which is a gelatinous structure (e.g., sperm packet) that is taken into the female's cloaca. This is loosely considered "internal" fertilization (the male technically has no intromittent organ). External fertilization does occur in some species. Neoteny

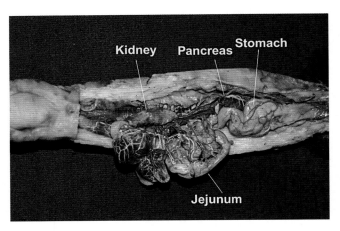

Figure 5-6 Basic anatomy of the caudate *(Ambystoma mexicanum).*

occurs (sexual maturity in juveniles); the adult form can be induced by using thyroxine or drying.

SENSORY SYSTEMS

Lateral lines are present; occasionally electroreceptors are also present. The lateral line is used to detect movement/motion in the water column (e.g., prey motion).

HEMATOPOIETIC SYSTEM

The ventral meninges in some species act as hematolymphopoietic tissue; otherwise, it is similar to that of anurans.

Unique Anatomy of Caecilians[2-5]
MUSCULOSKELETAL SYSTEM

Caecilians lack both a pectoral and pelvic girdle. Most of the ribs are double headed. Locomotion occurs by vertically directed musculature and hydrostatic motion.

INTEGUMENT SYSTEM

The skin has one layer of keratinized cells. Some species possess dermal scales. The glandular secretions of caecilians contain hemolysins and can prove to be very irritating to human mucous membranes, as well as to other caecilians. The skin is shed regularly and appears as thin strands of white mucoid material. Keratophagy may occur. As with salamanders, there is no subcutaneous area.

RESPIRATORY SYSTEM

Three forms of respiration occur in caecilians, and are again dependent on species variation and environment: pulmonic, buccopharyngeal, cutaneous. Some animals can use multiple modes. Caecilian lungs can have one or two (most aquatic animals) lobes, although one species, *Atretochoana eiselti,* does not possess any lung. Because the aquatic animals use pulmonic breathing as a primary means of respiration, care for depth of the animal's enclosure must be considered (especially with ill or neonatal animals).

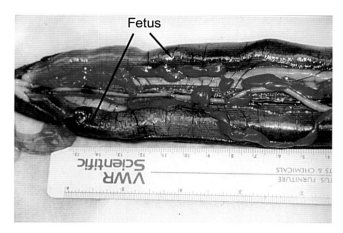

Figure 5-7 Caecilian *(Typhlonectes natans)* uterus with fetuses.

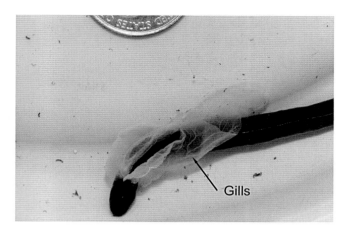

Figure 5-8 Caecilian *(Typhlonectes natans)* newborn with external gills.

CARDIOVASCULAR SYSTEM (ARTERIAL, VENOUS, AND LYMPHATIC)

Caecilians have a typical amphibian three-chambered heart. Caecilians can have over 200 lymph hearts. A renal portal system is presumed to exist, but it has not been documented.

GASTROINTESTINAL SYSTEM

Caecilians possess small sharp teeth that are positioned in two layers. The alimentary system tends to be elongated, as with snakes, due to their compact and long body size.

URINARY SYSTEM

Aquatic caecilians rely on the kidney for ammonia and water excretion, whereas terrestrial animals must excrete urea or uric acid. Caecilians have mesonephric kidneys, but they lack the secondary tubules found in caudates and anurans. Some caecilians have bilobate bladders.

REPRODUCTIVE SYSTEM

Male caecilians possess a phallodeum (intromittent organ), enabling them to practice internal fertilization. Caecilian ovaries are paired and are closely connected with the kidneys. Viviparous animals have an oviductal lining where embryos feed off the lining (Figure 5-7). Oviparity occurs in most caecilians, with some species-specific parental care occurring until hatching.

SENSORY SYSTEMS

There is a chemosensory and tactile tentacle between the eye and the nostril that is attached to the tear duct and the vomeronasal organ (Jacobson's organ). These animals rely heavily on this structure, as their vision is poor or absent. Audition is limited because many caecilians lack outer and middle ear cavities, but they are capable of detecting low-frequency vibrations.

HEMATOPOIETIC SYSTEM

Caecilians lack bone marrow and are thus dependent on the liver, spleen, thymus, and kidneys to produce red and white blood cells.

OTHER

Adipose color can vary from tan to very bright orange in *Typhlonectes natans,* and it should not be misclassified as abnormal.

Basic Premetamorphic Anatomy[2-5]
ANURANS

Tadpoles are markedly different from their postmetamorphic counterparts. They possess a large oval head and a laterally compressed tail. Gills are the primary respiratory organs for tadpoles. Most tadpoles have a very long digestive tract to accommodate a largely herbivorous lifestyle, although carnivory may occur in tadpoles either facultatively or in overcrowded conditions.

CAUDATES

Larvae possess large heads with external gills (three pairs). Terrestrial forms begin to resorb the gills as metamorphosis reaches completion. *Neoteny* occurs in some species (*Ambystoma mexicanum* and *Necturus maculosus*). This is the process in which the internal organs mature and allow reproduction while the external features remain larval.

CAECILIANS

Aquatic caecilians are viviparous. Larval animals are born fairly precocious, although they do have gills (Figure 5-8) present for the first day after birth. Oviparous caecilian larvae also have external gills that are quickly resorbed, but they also possess larval fins, which disappear shortly before hatching. The larval caecilian has a pronephric kidney that changes to a mesonephric kidney during metamorphosis. This change alters the kidney's function from a filtration system to a more complex excretory and water resorptive system.

General Clinical Physiology of Amphibians[3]

TEMPERATURE REGULATION

Amphibians are ectotherms. The ability of these animals to regulate their body temperature is highly variable among species but, overall, is regulated by behavior. Failure to maintain body temperature can result in failure to thrive. Hyperthermia can cause agitation, changes in skin color, inappetence, immunosuppression, and weight loss with good appetite. Hyperthermia is often rapidly fatal in amphibians. Hypothermia can result in lethargy, inappetence, bloating (decomposition of ingesta), immunosuppression, and poor growth. Hypothermia is more often associated with the development of chronic disease.

OSMOTIC BALANCE

Amphibian skin plays an important role in homeostasis. Significant water loss can occur through the skin. Because of this concern, the skin must be kept moist in order for gas exchange to occur (especially with lungless animals). Some amphibians, like tree frogs, have lipid glands that leave a waxy waterproof coating on their skin to prevent desiccation. Those amphibians with thicker skin, like toads, are more resistant to water loss. The gastrointestinal tract in most anurans does little to resorb water; thus, oral fluids are likely not as effective as intracoelomic or transdermal fluids. The pelvic skin patch of amphibians on the ventral abdomen can account for up to an 80% uptake of fluids. Because of this, it is possible to rehydrate animals by soaking them in appropriate fluids.

METABOLISM

In comparison to mammals and birds, amphibians have a relatively low metabolism. Amphibians typically rely on aerobic metabolism. However, when a burst of activity occurs, these animals can accumulate high concentrations of lactate. Sudden collapse has been reported once oxygen depletion occurs and fatigue sets in. Repeat handling may predispose an amphibian to collapse, especially in critically ill animals. Affected animals should be placed in a shallow quantity of dechlorinated and aerated water. Infusing oxygen into the water (e.g., by air pump or airstone) can lead to oxygen absorption via the ventral patch.

■ HUSBANDRY

Illness in captive amphibians is largely due to poor husbandry practices. It is outside the scope of this chapter to discuss the intimate details of building a successful vivarium for all the diverse species. Rather, the emphasis will be on general considerations for housing to educate the clinician in basic requirements and for designing hospital tanks. For information on captive amphibian husbandry, see Wright and Whitaker.[6,7] Additionally, examining natural habitat can be exceptionally useful in determining captive husbandry standards.

Environmental Considerations[4-8]

Amphibians can be aquatic, semiterrestrial, fossorial, terrestrial, or arboreal; thus, it is important for veterinarians to emphasize the importance of species-specific requirements.

AQUATIC

Animals that live in ponds versus streams have very different tolerance levels for water quality. Stream-dwelling animals generally have a greater need for more dissolved oxygen and higher quality water. In general, water quality should be maintained as for fish. Table 5-1 provides basic parameters to observe with most amphibians.

Dissolved oxygen should be greater than 80% (>5 mg/L) to maintain the biological filter (e.g., aerobic cycle). Water filtration (bacterial and mechanical) should be maintained as with fish. Under-gravel filters are acceptable if the tubing does not allow animals to get underneath the plates. Some amphibians do not tolerate vibration well; therefore, care should be taken to place filters away from the enclosure if possible. A 10% to 20% water change should be done every week or two with aged or dechlorinated water. For caecilians, water depth should be shallow enough to allow animals to obtain air without much effort, especially newborns. For most amphibians, there should be a basking/dry-out area where the animals can leave the water.

TABLE 5-1	Water Chemistry Parameters for Amphibians		
Parameter	Normal	Sublethal	Lethal
Dissolved oxygen	≥5 mg/L	2-4 mg/L	<2 mg/L
Ammonia (un-ionized)	<0.01 mg/L	0.5 mg/L	>1 mg/L
Nitrite	<0.1 mg/L	0.015-0.1 mg/L	>0.1 mg/L
Nitrate	0-5 mg/L	20-50 mg/L	Species dependent
pH	Species specific (~6.5-8.5)	5.5-6.5; 8.6-9.5	5.5-6.5; 8.6-9.5
Gas pressure	28 mmHg	28-78 mmHg	>78 mmHg
Hardness	75-150 mg/L	>150-250 mg/L skin lesions can occur	Unknown
Alkalinity	20-100 mg/L	>100 mg/L	Unknown
Chlorine (tadpoles)	0-2 ppm	2-4 ppm	>5 ppm

SEMITERRESTRIAL (STREAMSIDE ANIMALS)

Semiaquatic animals need standing water as well as areas to haul out. By providing this, it is possible to create humidity gradients that enable the animal to regulate its moisture. Aquaria can be tilted or accessories placed such that the bottoms have standing water and top layers are drier and well drained.

FOSSORIAL AND TERRESTRIAL

Fossorial and terrestrial vivaria are similar in every regard, except that there should be deeper soil for fossorial animals. Standing water receptacles are reasonable in these settings, but the water level should not be deeper than the animal is tall. Moisture gradients in the soil are very important for fossorial animals, and this is easily accomplished by tilting the aquarium to retain different levels of moisture. Leaf litter placed on the surface will allow the animal to forage while remaining covered. Live plants are not recommended for fossorial species, as the plants may be uprooted when the amphibian forages.

ARBOREAL

The enclosure should be tall with accompanying tall branches and plants. It is important to provide an adequate number of plants to provide ample hiding places.

Creating a Vivarium

Glass tanks are commonly used to house amphibians. They are well accepted because they allow excellent visualization of the amphibians, are relatively inexpensive, and hold moisture. The primary disadvantage associated with them is that they are not well ventilated. One way to improve ventilation is to have a secure, well-ventilated lid. The lid also helps prevent escape. Plastic tanks are also appropriate for making vivaria and may be more flexible for modification, though scratches can occur that obscure direct visualization of the animal. Lids that are hinged allow servicing to a portion of the enclosure while maintaining cover for the rest of the area. Solid plastic or glass lids should be considered when maintaining a high humidity is important. When these types of lids are used, it is important to still place some ventilation holes in them to prevent stagnant airflow.

Volatile organic compounds, such as those found in glues, need to be cured appropriately (under strict manufacturer conditions) before being used around amphibians; otherwise the fumes can leach into the environment and be irritating to the skin and respiratory epithelium.

Deionized water should not be used in an amphibian's vivarium, as it can disrupt osmolarity. Chlorinated tap water also is not recommended. Distilled water or reverse osmosis water is ideal.

ENCLOSURE SIZE

Enclosure sizes are highly variable and largely dictated by the environmental re-creation that is attempted. Arboreal species

BOX 5-1 Environmental Temperature Ranges for Amphibians Based on Natural Habitat

Tropical lowland	24°-30° C
Tropical montane (moist, cool, coniferous strata)	18°-24° C
Subtropical	21°-27° C
Temperate, summer	18°-24° C
Hibernation	10°-16° C
Aquatic, tropical lowland	24°-30° C
Aquatic, tropical montane	18°-24° C
Aquatic, subtropical	21°-27° C
Aquatic, temperate stream (summer)	16°-21° C
Aquatic, temperate pond (summer)	18°-24° C

should be provided vertical enclosures. Aquatic and fossorial species should be provided an enclosure with a large surface area (length × width).

TEMPERATURE

The environmental temperature range provided an amphibian should be based on its natural habitat (Box 5-1).[6,7] There should always be a gradient with a range of 5° to 8° C. When changing water, make sure the temperature matches the enclosure. Basking spots are necessary, and ceramic heaters (which produce no light) or spotlights can usually provide the necessary temperatures. Care and diligence are required for appropriate wattage and distance. Spot heaters are best placed outside of the enclosure to avoid trauma via thermal burns. Do not use heat rocks for amphibians.

Aquarium heaters may cause thermal burns for caecilians if they wrap around these devices. To prevent this, place mesh or PVC piping around the heater to prevent contact. It is ideal to use a thermometer that dually measures the warmest and coolest spot; the more advanced thermography units allow detection of temperature gradients as well.[9] Hibernation is important in some species for stimulating breeding, but it is unknown whether it is necessary for long-term health and success in captivity.[6] Many salamander species prefer cooler temperatures,[10] and some vivaria might require chillers.

HUMIDITY

A fine mist can be sprayed into the vivarium several times daily (manually or via misting systems). When doing so, distilled or aged water should be used. An air stone in a bowl of water or live plants can also be used to help maintain the environmental humidity. Relative humidity above 70% will suit most amphibians. Tree frogs have a natural behavior to adduct their heads and press against surfaces to retain water—if they do this exclusively, the environmental humidity is not adequate. Conversely, waxy tree frogs may develop dermatitis with excessive environmental humidity.[6]

LIGHTING

Full-spectrum lights are generally recommended for amphibians, but most do not provide radiation in the wavelengths consistent with vitamin D$_3$ synthesis. Ultraviolet B (UVB) (290-320 nm) radiation may be important for vitamin D$_3$ metabolism in amphibians, but the role of UVB radiation has not been fully examined. I prefer to be conservative and recommend the use of full-spectrum lights. Replacement of the bulbs is recommended every 9 months to ensure that the appropriate wavelength is emitted. UVB does not transmit through glass or plastic, and the depth at which it transmits is typically no greater than 9 to 18 inches away from the source. Care must be taken that the lighting does not adversely affect the animals. Low-level nocturnal lighting (moonlight simulation) may be useful for nocturnal species to ensure that the animals are not startled when the lights are turned on or off. Dimming lights gradually is ideal.

Amphibians should be provided with a natural photoperiod of 12 hours of light and 12 hours of darkness. If animals are going to be bred, the light cycle may need to be altered to mimic the normal reproductive season of the animal.

SUBSTRATE

Substrate selection is an important consideration for a vivarium. When considering different types of substrates, it is important to try to mimic an amphibian's natural habitat. Smooth or small pebble gravel may be used as a substrate, but it can become a gastrointestinal foreign body if it is ingested. This can be prevented by using large pieces of gravel (e.g., bigger than can fit in the oral cavity) or feeding animals away from such substrates. Soil substrates should be organically rich and pH balanced (neutral). For burrowing caecilians, soil depth should be 3 to 10 cm.[5] For fossorial species, there should be a moisture gradient and the soil should be loose enough to allow for tunnel formation. Soil should be replaced every 2 to 3 months. Substrates that need to be sterilized should be baked. Soil and leaf litter substrates should be sterilized to prevent arthropod and helminth infestation. To sterilize soil, bake at 200° F (95° C) in a thin layer (<2 cm) or place in direct sunlight for several hours. In general, soil substrates are very difficult to maintain. If sand is used, horticultural silver sand is recommended. Sphagnum moss is a useful substrate because it retains moisture, is soft and pliable, and is easily discarded. Sphagnum moss should be changed every 2 to 4 weeks to avoid compacting the substrate and breeding undesirable organisms. Living moss does not usually do well in amphibian vivaria because the water needs of moss cannot be met while maintaining a healthy amphibian. Certain substrates should be avoided. Rotting wood can be a good living substrate, but the risks of introducing disease may outweigh the benefits.[6] Vermiculite is not recommended because it can cause a gastrointestinal impaction. Peat moss and manure are not recommended because they are acidic and irritating to the skin. Mulch can be used, but aromatic woods (cedar, pine) should be avoided as they can be toxic and irritating.

ACCESSORIES

It is important to take time and consider what accessories are needed in a vivarium, as these items can be used to mimic an animal's natural habitat and reduce stress. Overplanting and overfurnishing a vivarium may make prey capture difficult for the animal. Plastic plants can be used to landscape a vivarium and are easily disinfected. Live plants can also be used and have the benefit of increasing environmental humidity. It is important to only use live plants that are known to be nontoxic, as prey being offered to amphibians may eat the live plants and transfer any toxin to the amphibian.[6] If live plants are chosen, the pet owner should check to see if harmful pesticides or fertilizers have been used. Live plants may be contaminated with parasitic ova (e.g., from Florida, where tree frogs live in the plants). Recently acquired live plants should be cleaned and their soil should be replaced to reduce the likelihood of contaminating the vivarium with unwanted pathogens. Aquatic plants can harbor snails, which can introduce parasites to a vivarium as they serve as intermediate hosts for a number of parasites.

"Furniture" considerations for a vivarium may include large rocks, branches, shelters, and waterfalls. Traumatic injuries may occur with such items if they are not secured, and all furnishings should have smooth edges. These items should also be conducive to sterilization or disinfection. Bear in mind that porous objects may retain disinfectants. Proper rinsing is critical. Shelter type will depend on the natural camouflage of the animal and should be provided. Such accessories are easily created (Figure 5-9).

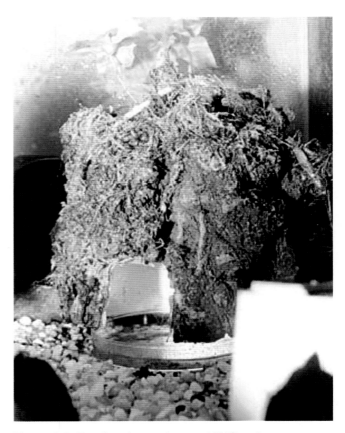

Figure 5-9 Frog housing made out of PVC and moss.

Hospital Tank

Veterinarians working with amphibians should maintain hospital tanks to treat cases presented to their facility. Smaller plastic containers with snap-on lids and small doors on the lid make access to the animal easy and safe. Bubble wrap placed on the bottom of the hospital tank provides a soft substrate, which stays moist and is atraumatic. Plastic wrap placed around the entire tank can be used to help maintain humidity, but the habitat should be serviced enough to provide adequate ventilation. This is not recommended for permanent or semipermanent housing, where the air may stagnate and predispose amphibians to conditions like pneumonia. Sphagnum moss, if used, should be thrown out weekly or when soiled, or more frequently if the patient has a known infectious disease. The hospital tank should be easily disinfected.

■ NUTRITION

Premetamorphic anurans are typically herbivorous, although obligate (e.g., poison dart frogs) and opportunistic carnivory occur. Once metamorphosis is complete, amphibians become carnivorous. Although primarily insectivorous, anurans may also consume fish, other amphibians, reptiles, rodents, and birds. In caudates and caecilians, larval and adult forms are carnivorous.

Recently imported animals may have difficulty converting from a live prey to pre-killed prey diet, and some animals never convert. Weighing animals and assessing body condition are useful for assessing whether an animal is eating. When live prey items are offered, they should be removed after the animal has stopped feeding, as prey can attack or feed on the amphibian.

Feeding Mechanisms

Larval anurans are filter feeders.[11] Water is pumped through the mouth, and then planktonic algae are extracted and entrapped by a mucus-covered filter in the pharynx and then directed into the esophagus. Adult, terrestrial amphibians use their tongues to capture prey. These animals have glands on their tongues, which produce a sticky substance that helps apprehend prey until it is securely placed in the mouth. Some anurans can shape their tongue into a tube to assist in feeding on ants, termites, and worms. Aquatic salamanders direct prey to their mouths by creating an inward flow of water into the oral cavity. *Pipa pipa* direct food and water into their mouth with hypobrachial pumping movements. Some aquatic amphibians use their long phalanges to direct the food into their oral cavity.

Feeding and Diet

Obesity can occur in amphibians. In captivity, there is a tendency to overfeed animals, either by offering too much food or offering food too frequently. As animals get older, the frequency with which food is offered can be decreased (e.g.,

ambush predators should be offered food every 2 weeks). Larval animals and smaller frogs should be fed daily. Nocturnal animals should be fed at night or late in the day; diurnal animals should be fed once a day, and sometimes twice daily, depending on species.

The list of possible invertebrates to offer amphibians is extensive.[12] In general, the most common food items offered to terrestrial amphibians include earthworms, red worms, mealworm larvae, waxworm larvae, crickets, fruit flies, other larvae, occasionally small reptiles (e.g., anoles), and amphibian eggs and larvae. For aquatic species, these same foods are offered, but bloodworms, blackworms, and crustaceans, such as crayfish and brine shrimp, may be offered as well. Some animals have very specific diets, like the termite-eating caecilian (*Boulengerula* spp.), and can be difficult to maintain in captivity.[5] Avoid brightly colored insects,[6] as they may be naturally toxic. Finally, although wild-caught invertebrates would provide enrichment and balance for an amphibian, caution must be exercised not to feed out organisms that have been subject to pesticides or other such toxins.

Feeding pelleted diets intended for fish or reptiles may not be appropriate for amphibians, as these diets may be intended for herbivores or omnivores and will not meet the fat, protein, and vitamin requirements of amphibians.[12] Rodents can be offered on occasion, but vitamin A levels are often too high in these prey items, and secondary nutritional hyperparathyroidism can occur without supplementation of vitamin D_3. On the other hand, oversupplementation with vitamin D_3 may cause mineralization of organs. Unfortunately our knowledge regarding vitamin D_3 metabolism in amphibians is limited.

Supplementing amphibian diets with vitamins and minerals is a questionable but necessary practice. With a truly well-balanced diet, supplementation is unnecessary and may even cause problems (e.g., hypervitaminosis A and D). Unfortunately, with the limited number of commercially available food items, providing a well-balanced diet is difficult. Based on this limitation, it is best to offer the largest variety (e.g., multiple prey species) of food types to provide the best nutrition. Most supplements target calcium and vitamin D_3 in an attempt to balance the Ca : P ratio (1.5 : 1 or 2 : 1). Contrary to that target, most invertebrates, with the exception of earthworms, have an inverse Ca : P ratio.[12] Invertebrates must therefore be "gut-loaded" with vitamins and minerals by feeding them a diet that is high in Ca and low in P (available commercially) in the 24 hours before offering that prey item. Some of these diets can result in death of the prey item if fed longer than 24 hours. Additionally, these diets are not balanced for invertebrates and should not be used long term. Another product used for increasing the nutritional value of invertebrates is to "dust" them with a supplement. Placing the supplement and invertebrates in a brown bag and gently shaking the bag will result in the invertebrate being covered with the supplement. Dusting can be used with small invertebrates where gut loading is not practical or lethal, and this should be done immediately before feeding.[12] Dusting larger invertebrates with these supplements does not successfully achieve the calcium levels that gut loading does. When feeding frozen fish, it is necessary to supplement the diet with thiamine as the fish produce natural thiaminases that destroy the thiamine in the tissues.

PREVENTIVE MEDICINE
Quarantine[13]

All new animals must be quarantined before being added to an extant collection of animals. Transporting animals and moving them into a new environment are exceptionally stressful events. Even though it is impossible to completely remove these stressors, they can be minimized once the animal is in quarantine. This can be accomplished by providing a quiet room, appropriate furniture in the new enclosure (e.g., a hiding spot, such as a film canister or plastic plants), and not overcrowding animals. Accessories must be easily disinfected. Partially covering the enclosure can also help reduce visual stressors. Multicolored papers (comic sections of newspaper) taped to the outside of the enclosure are excellent covers because a single color may not be easily perceived; avoid black, as it may act as a mirror and stimulate striking behavior.

Quarantine should last a minimum of 30 to 60 days for captive raised animals but should be extended to 90 days for wild-caught specimens. All in/all out principles should apply. Animals in quarantine should be serially examined for pathogens and parasites. A standard schedule may include three fecal examinations conducted a week apart. Prophylactic treatment is warranted when an animal is in poor body condition, has a normal appetite, and has a fecal exam that shows excessive numbers of flagellates, nematodes, trematodes, or cestodes. Whereas some of these organisms are normal or incidental flora, large numbers in a compromised patient may warrant a course of antiparasitics (e.g., metronidazole). Utensils used for an enclosure should not be shared with another group of animals.

Fecal samples can be collected by placing the animal into a disinfected and rinsed opaque, covered plastic container. The container should be well ventilated, and animals should not be kept in the containers longer than 12 hours. Several fecal samples should be collected to evaluate the status of the animal. It is important to remember that some parasites shed transiently, so multiple (serial) samples may be required to confirm a diagnosis. I perform the following exams when screening amphibian feces: fecal floatation with commercial hyperosmotic agent, direct saline smear, acid-fast stain, and Gram stain.

Routine Exams

A baseline examination on any amphibian presented to a veterinarian is recommended. In large colonies, or cases with exceptionally small animals, this may be impractical. The minimum database collected during an amphibian examination should include a physical exam, radiographs, weight, and, if possible, blood examination. Individual or group fecal examinations should be performed at least yearly. Visual examinations of every animal should be performed daily.

Disinfection and Sanitation

Utensils, accessories, enclosures previously occupied by amphibians, and enclosures with known disease entities, should be disinfected to prevent the spread of disease. Removal of all debris is necessary before application of a disinfectant, as some products are deactivated in the presence of proteins and other organics. Warm water and surfactants can be used to help break down organics during the cleaning process. Numerous classes of disinfectant are available, each with variable effectiveness against certain organisms (Table 5-2). Some products absorb the chemicals and can leach out while the amphibian is present (e.g., iodine products). Ammonia and chlorine bleach are good general disinfectants. With all chemical products, thorough and repeat rinsing is mandatory. For most disinfectants, a minimum contact time of 10 minutes is recommended. For more fastidious organisms, longer contact times are recommended. Porous objects should be discarded rather than reused, not only because they harbor pathogens but also because it is difficult to thoroughly rinse and remove the chemicals from these materials. Humidifiers should be disinfected weekly, as should any aerosolizing tools. Povidone iodine, chlorhexidine, isopropyl alcohol, and quaternary ammonium compounds are known to cause skin lesions and to be toxic in amphibians at high concentrations, and thus should be used with caution.[13]

In a healthy biologic environment (vivarium or aquarium) with normal microflora, the opportunity for pathogens to be a problem is minimal. To assist in maintaining a healthy biologic system, unnecessary organic loads can be reduced by spot-cleaning feces and other organic material in the enclosure and by changing out sections of soil, sand, and leaf litter regularly. Water changes of 10% to 20% should be performed weekly in aquatic systems to reduce both organic and inorganic loads on the system.

RESTRAINT

When handling amphibians, moistened, wet gloves should be worn to minimize the likelihood of damaging the animal's skin. If gloves are not worn, then hands should be rinsed with aged or dechlorinated water. As an indictment to the delicacy of amphibians' skin, smokers who handle smaller frogs can cause them to die, due to the nicotine residue on the smokers' skin.[14] Preparing water to use with amphibians is easily accomplished by retaining tap water in a bucket of water and aerating it with an air stone for an hour. The water can also be passed through charcoal to remove contaminants. Alternately, water can be dechlorinated by allowing it to degas in a nonaerated reservoir for 48 to 72 hours. After handling amphibians, clinicians should thoroughly wash their hands, as many species produce toxins that can irritate human skin and mucosa. Gloves should be changed between handling animals to decrease disease transmission and toxin transmission.

TABLE 5-2	**Disinfectants Commonly Used to Clean Amphibian Environments**				
Disinfectant	**Example**	**Target organism(s)**	**Contact time**	**Dilutions**	**Comments**
Ethyl alcohol	Ethanol	B, T, F, V, no spores	1-3 min	60%-90%	Evaporates rapidly (before disinfection is successful); hardens rubber, corrodes metal
Isopropyl alcohol	Isopropanol	B, T, F, some V, no spores	1-3 min	60%-90%	
Glutaraldehyde	Cidex (Johnson and Johnson)	B, M, F, V, no spores	45 min		2-week shelf life; good for *Pseudomonas* and *Mycobacterium*; removes debris from cleaning area
	Cidex Plus	B, M, V, T	20 min		
	Cidex OPA	B, M, V, T	12 min		
Formaldehyde	Formaldehyde	B, F, V, spores	1-15 min	37%	Carcinogenic
Chlorhexidine	Nolvasan solution	B, some V	10 min	0.2%-2%	Long residual action; not for *Pseudomonas* or *Mycoplasma*
Sodium hypochlorite	Bleach	B, F, V, P	Seconds to hours, depending on concentration	1 : 10-1 : 100	Corrosive to metal; organic matter decreases effectiveness
Iodine	Betadine	B, M, F, V, spores	15 sec	1%	Organic matter decreases effectiveness
			3 min	10%	
Phenols	Lysol	B, M, some V; no spores	Not listed	1 : 256	
	1-stroke Environ (Steris)	B, T, V	10 min	See below	
	Stat III (Ecolabs)	B, F, V, M	10 min	See below	
Quaternary ammonium (ammonia, benzalkonium chloride)	Roccal-D Plus (Pharmacia/Upjohn)	B, F, V	10 min	1 : 256	
	Unicide 256 (Brulin)	B, V, F, mildew	10 min	1 : 256	

B, bacteria; F, fungi; M, mycobacteria; P, protozoa; T, *Trichophyton*; V, viruses.

Manual Restraint[15]

Animals can be placed into containers for close visual examination without touching the animal. Suitable containers include small clear jars or boxes and plastic bags. Occasionally animals will feign death, but this must be distinguished from exhaustion. Under such a circumstance, place the animal in its traveling enclosure and wait. Avoid handling larval amphibians if possible.

Large frogs should be handled by firmly grabbing the animal around the inguinal region just cranial to the hindlimbs (Figure 5-10, *A*). Smaller frogs can be cupped into the palm of the hand for limited access or, while in this grip, gently restrained by the hindlimbs and caudal coelom using the opposing hand. When handling an animal in this way, it is important to take care not to squeeze or traumatize the animal (Figure 5-10, *B*). Expect anurans to urinate when handled, and be prepared to collect the sample if desired. Additional behavioral manifestations identified after handling may include breath holding or air sac insufflation, color change, and vocalizing.

Salamanders and newts should be handled at the pectoral girdle initially, then the hindlimbs (Figure 5-11). Tail

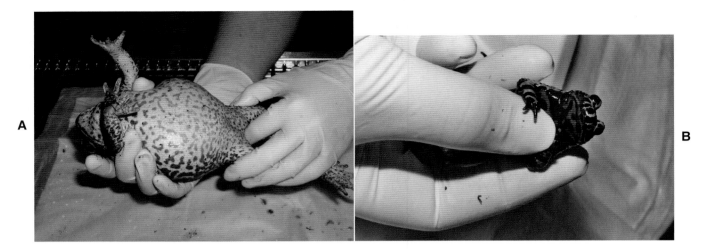

Figure 5-10 A, Handling technique for a large frog. **B,** Handling technique for a small frog.

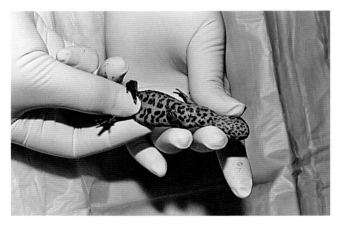

Figure 5-11 Two-hand technique for handling a newt.

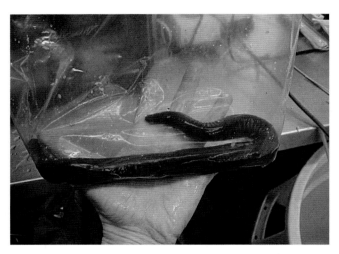

Figure 5-12 Handling technique for a caecilian using a sealed plastic storage bag.

autotomy can occur in these animals, and care should be taken to not hold the animal by its tail.

Caecilians are very difficult to manage with manual restraint. Clear tubing or a plastic bag can limit the mobility of these animals and facilitate examination (Figure 5-12). For a more thorough examination, the animal should be sedated.

Chemical Restraint

Before immobilizing an amphibian, fasting the animal is generally recommended to avoid aspiration pneumonia; however, this has not been described as a common complication. In an urgent situation, immediate anesthesia is recommended over delaying to fast the animal.

Local anesthesia can work very well on amphibians. Lidocaine can be injected or placed topically in the perimeter of a lesion. Emla cream (Astra Pharm, Westborough, MA) may also be used and can induce local anesthesia in minutes. Both may result in general anesthesia or death if caution is not exercised and too much product is used.

The most common general anesthetic agent used for amphibians is tricaine methane sulfonate (MS-222) (Finquel, Argent Chemical Laboratories, Redmond, WA). The drug comes in a powdered form and is usually reconstituted in distilled water. MS-222 acts by reverting transient sodium ion permeability and decreasing excitability and blocking conduction of nerve impulses.[16] This compound is very acidic and should be buffered with an equal volume of baking soda to stabilize the pH. Unbuffered MS-222 can be highly irritating to the amphibian, causing excitability and erythema. Unbuffered MS-222 can also result in a more rapid induction because uptake across the skin is more rapid in the ionized form. Although buffering the agent will result in slower uptake, it is far safer for the animal (e.g., hyperglycemia and tachycardia have been reported with unbuffered MS-222).[17] Induction at 100 to 200 mg/L will achieve steady state levels in most amphibians, but induction may be prolonged for more than 25 minutes. Higher doses (1-5 g/L) may induce anesthesia

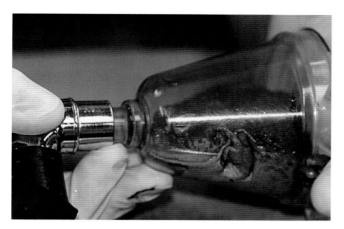

Figure 5-13 Anesthetic induction of a frog using a small animal facemask as a gas chamber.

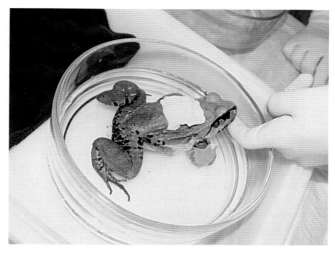

Figure 5-14 Anesthetic induction of a frog using a gauze soaked in isoflurane and water-soluble gel.

faster, but these levels are considered potentially lethal. Higher dosing levels can also prolong recovery. At induction, animals may try to jump out of the solution, as it can be irritating. Anesthetic deaths are rare with MS-222, but they are possible. Under MS-222 anesthesia, pulmonary ventilation is diminished or absent. Gas exchange across the skin is usually adequate to prevent hypoxia at low (<74° F) environmental temperatures. Once anesthetized, the animal's nares and oral cavity must be kept out of the water to avoid drowning. Keeping the animal at room temperature (74°-78° F) usually results in acidosis and hypercarbia. Oxygen can be aerated into the immersion solution, and this usually helps the animal compensate. MS-222 has been used intramuscularly (IM) and intracoelomically (ICe); however, I have not used these routes. When using these alternative routes, expect prolonged recoveries.

Gas anesthesia has been used in a variety of forms.[16-18] Using the vaporized form results in direct exposure to the inhalant, as with a face mask (Figure 5-13), and can induce hypothermia and/or dehydrate the animal. Therefore, when using this form of anesthesia, it is important to monitor the animal's hydration status and body temperature. Using direct exposure appears to be more successful in toad species than frog species. Dosing anurans percutaneously with topical isoflurane and halothane has also been successfully done, but it can induce a very deep plane of anesthesia and prolonged recoveries. Although some clinicians report that aerating an inhalant directly into water is useful, I have not had success with this method. Another potential complication with aerating the anesthetic into the water is that scavenging excess gas may not be possible, posing a human health risk. Finally, a gel mixture of a sterile KY jelly lubricant with isoflurane or sevoflurane and water mixed in a 3 : 3 : 1 ratio can be utilized. The mixture may be applied directly on the animal or via a gauze (Figure 5-14). This method results in rapid induction and recovery.

Clove oil (eugenol) has been used to anesthetize leopard frogs *(Rana pipiens)* and tiger salamanders *(Ambystoma tigrinum)*.[19,20] The dose required to induce surgical anesthesia in the salamanders (0.23 ml of 85% clove oil/500 ml dechlorinated water) is much higher than in the frogs (333 mg/L). Propofol was also evaluated in both species. Delivery in the frogs via the lingual vessels was difficult and produced only mild effects. When Propofol was administered intracoelomically in the tiger salamanders (35 mg/kg), surgical anesthesia was achieved in the majority (73%, 8/11) of test subjects.[20]

Monitoring the Anesthetized Patient

The amphibian heart rate can be monitored using a pulse oximeter, Doppler, or ultrasound. Respirations can be difficult to monitor. The best methods to use are to evaluate the excursion of the rib cage or the gular area. Oxygen supplementation is important, as hypercarbia and hypoxia are common during anesthesia. However, too much oxygen may limit respirations, based on the theory that these animals are stimulated to breathe based on low oxygen levels and not high carbon dioxide levels. Based on this, it is generally preferred to recover these animals on room oxygen (21%). Readings of 95% oxygen saturation or greater are expected in a normoxic patient.[15] If bradycardia occurs, reduce or end the anesthetic event. Atropine (IM or IV) can be used to increase the heart rate. If asystole occurs, begin cardiac compressions. Cardiac compressions can be used to re-stimulate the cardiac function. There are two methods that may be used: (1) Place the animal in dorsal recumbency. Then place an index finger on the cranioventral rib cage (e.g., level of the pectoral girdle) and compress downward. This will press the heart against the spine and act as a stimulus to restart the heart. (2) Grasp the lateral rib cage at the level of the pectoral girdle and squeeze inward. Epinephrine can be given intratracheally, intracardiacally, or intravenously to initiate cardiac function.

When monitoring the depth of anesthesia in amphibians, it is important to follow a consistent pattern and record all measurements. The following measurements are generally used: righting reflex, escape response, palpebral reflex, superficial pain response (e.g., pinch skin over dorsum of foot), and deep pain response (e.g., apply pressure to one of the rear digits). It is important to evaluate those reflexes before starting the anesthetic event, to provide a baseline for that animal. The generally accepted method for characterizing these reflexes is based on an ordinal scale: 0-present, 1-mild loss, 2-loss. Based on this scale, surgical anesthesia is achieved when all of the reflexes are recorded as a 2 (loss).

Recovery from water-bath–based anesthesia (e.g., MS-222, clove oil) can be accomplished by placing the animal into fresh, dechlorinated, anesthetic-free water or thoroughly rinsing the anesthetic off of the animal with the same type of water. When recovering the animal in a clean water bath, the animal should be monitored closely to prevent accidental drowning. The amphibian should be considered recovered when all of the reflexes have returned (0-present) and the heart rate and respiration rate are not different from the preanesthetic exam.

■ PERFORMING A PHYSICAL EXAMINATION

The amphibian patient should be evaluated from a distance before it is handled. An initial "hands-off" examination can provide significant information regarding the animal's well-being. Items to note include respiration rate and quality, animal posture and body position, ocular anatomy, and the presence of skin lesions. This may direct how the animal should be handled, if it is handled at all. Sloughing skin, large ulcers, fractures, tissue or organ prolapse, and extreme lethargy may warrant not handling the animal by traditional manual restraint methods.

Before handling an amphibian, it is important to consider the role of handling on the production and removal of lactate. If an animal is repeatedly handled, lactate may accumulate, and it can take a long time for this compound to be removed from the amphibian body.[3] In severe cases, an amphibian with excess lactate levels may collapse or develop a myopathy. To prevent this, restrict handling times, and be prepared to perform an examination and collect diagnostics at the same time.

Body weight should be recorded at the time of physical exam. Amphibian body weight may fluctuate due to hydration status and the volume of the urine in the urinary bladder, but establishing trends is important. Body condition should be noted. Animals with reduced muscle mass on the extremities and over the spine suggest a chronic course of disease. Evaluate the animal's symmetry, musculature, and posture. Obesity can be distinguished from fluid accumulation by the animal.

When performing a "hands-on" physical examination, it is important to be thorough and consistent to reduce the likelihood of misclassifying an exam finding. Amphibian skin may become hyperemic with handling, and dehydration is possible with prolonged examination, so it is important to keep the patient moist during the examination. Hyperemia needs to be distinguished from red-leg syndrome (see section titled Common Diseases). Evaluate the entire integument for any

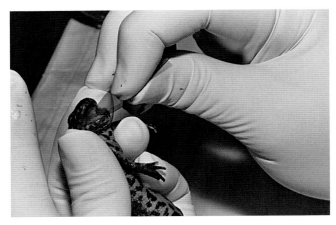

Figure 5-15 Oral examination of an amphibian using a piece of radiographic film.

lesions (e.g., ulcers, erosions, and lacerations). Damage to the integument opens an animal to opportunistic infections.

An ocular examination can be performed using an ophthalmoscope and slit lamp to examine the cornea, iris, and anterior and posterior chambers.[21]

Palpebrae are present in all amphibians except caecilians, where ocular examination is impossible in most species due to a lack of adnexa. Corneas of giant salamander species are vascularized. Amphibian pupils can take on various shapes, dependent on species, but are generally circular when dilated. Amphibians have voluntary control of their pupil size, so examination of pupillary light reflexes is not possible. Funduscopic exams are not rewarding in amphibians, as the pupils are usually not dilated. Given that the animal can control pupil size, mydriatics are generally unrewarding. Research to evaluate the effectiveness of topical or intracameral muscle paralysis on the iris needs to be completed.

An oral exam can be accomplished using a variety of tools as potential specula (Figure 5-15). Such tools may include radiograph film that is cut and rounded at the edge, standard metal bird specula, guitar picks, a rubber spatula, and credit cards.[22] Animals may bite, and therefore caution must be exercised when examining these animals. Salamanders use their maxilla to hinge upward rather than downward at the mandible, which is the opposite of what is observed in most amphibians. Overmanipulation of an amphibian's jaws can lead to fractures, so care should be exercised. The oral cavity of an amphibian should be moist and free of thick, ropy mucus. Excessive mucus often suggests dehydration. Look closely in the oral cavity for fractured teeth and oral abscesses.

Coelomic palpation can provide significant information regarding an animal's condition. Some animals will "puff up" when in a defensive mode, which can make palpation challenging, but patience will often result in success. After palpating the coelomic cavity, muscle tone and body condition should be assessed. With poor body condition, the clinician must examine the environment and the animal's caloric intake and pursue diagnostics for chronic infectious/parasitic diseases (recurrent bacteremia/septicemia, mycobac-

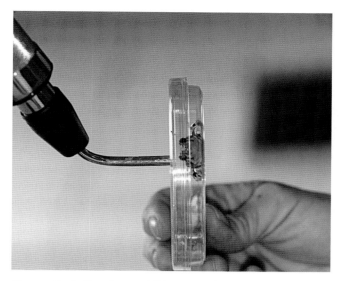

Figure 5-16 Female amphibians can be transilluminated to evaluate their reproductive status.

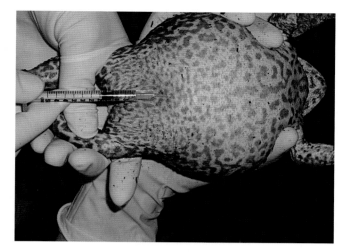

Figure 5-17 Blood draw from the ventral abdominal vein of an anuran.

teriosis, and parasitism). Skeletal confirmation should be evaluated and the long bones and rostrum palpated to assess for metabolic bone disease (e.g., secondary nutritional hyperparathyroidism).

Gender determination can be challenging, but it should be done at the time of physical examination. Sexual dimorphism can occur, but it is not present in most of the species found in captivity. Transillumination of the abdomen may reveal eggs (Figure 5-16). In male salamanders, the base of the tail may become enlarged.

Vital signs such as heart rate and rhythm can be evaluated using a Doppler and will help the clinician become aware of rate and quality. Though changes in rate can be anticipated during handling, a trend may be established for the clinician that can be used for preanesthetic evaluation. Auscultation of the lungs may be possible with larger animals.

A neurologic examination should be performed but is often limited to evaluating the palpebral blink reflex, superficial and deep pain reflexes, and the righting reflex.

■ DIAGNOSTIC TESTING
Clinical Pathology
SAMPLE COLLECTION

In frogs and toads, blood can be obtained from the ventral abdominal vein (Figure 5-17), lingual venous plexus, and the saphenous and femoral veins. Cardiocentesis may also be attempted but may be associated with asystole and death. Salamanders and newts can be bled from the ventral midline abdominal vein and the ventral caudal tail vein. Caecilians are most limited, and cardiocentesis is the only method available. Doppler can facilitate locating the heart when an apex beat cannot be found. A small volume of blood can provide useful information (e.g., hemoparasites, an estimated white blood cell count, hematocrit, and total protein). The approximate volume

of blood that can be safely collected from an amphibian is 1% of its body weight (1 ml/100 g body weight). In sick amphibians, a smaller volume (0.5 ml/100 g body weight) of blood should be collected.[23]

Once collected, blood is best placed in a lithium heparin microtainer. Microtainers are strongly recommended because they have an appropriate amount of anticoagulant for small blood volumes. Ideally, for blood cultures, there should be no anticoagulant. Wright-Giemsa or Diff-Quik stain can be used to evaluate amphibian white and red blood cells; I prefer the Wright-Giemsa stain.

Coelomic fluid can contain important information regarding the health state of an amphibian. A sample of coelomic fluid can be collected by placing the animal in dorsal recumbency. The area should be prepared using aseptic technique and a 25- to 26-gauge needle fastened to a 1-ml or 3-ml syringe inserted paramedially in the caudal coelomic cavity (avoiding the midline abdominal vein). The sample should be submitted for fluid analysis (total protein, specific gravity), cytologic exam, culture, and plasma chemistries. Amphibian coelomic fluid can be clear, blue, or green. The presence of blood urea nitrogen (BUN) in the fluid may suggest renal disease.[23]

Washes and lavages can be very valuable diagnostic tools. Tracheal washes can be obtained in the anesthetized animal by infusing a small volume of sterile 0.9% saline using a tomcat or IV catheter into the trachea and recollecting the fluid by aspiration. The trachea is short in anurans and caudates; therefore, care must be taken not to puncture the lungs. Gastric washes can be performed in larger animals by inserting an appropriate sized red rubber tube into the stomach, infusing sterile 0.9% saline, and then re-aspirating the infusion solution. Cloacal lavages can be attempted to collect feces by lubricating an appropriately sized red rubber tube and administering a small amount of 0.9% sterile saline (0.5-1.0 ml/100 g body weight). Examine all washes by performing a wet mount, cytology, and possibly culture.

Urine can be collected when the animal is handled or by rubbing the cloaca. Interpretation of the results is dependent on comparison with the same species, under the same environmental conditions, and at the same time of the year, as the composition of urine is greatly affected by many parameters.[24] Typically, amphibian urine is hypoosmotic (specific gravity: 1.001-1.008) and devoid of protein.

Cytologic examinations should be performed on all integumentary lesions. Additionally, cultures should be performed on chronic lesions or if multiple animals are affected. In non-healing wounds, acid-fast staining should be performed.

Although collected less frequently, lymph and joint fluid can be collected and analyzed. Lymph fluid is chemically equivalent to serum. The lymph hearts are located under the scapula and near the urostyles, and may become prominent with hydrocoelom. For joint fluid analysis, aseptically prepare the area as for a coelomic tap and collect the sample.[25] A 25- to 27-gauge needle fastened to a 1-ml or 3-ml syringe can be used to collect these samples.

Interpretation[23,26]

Complete blood counts (CBC) and plasma chemistries can be difficult to interpret. Significant species, gender, and seasonal differences can result in a high degree of variability among samples. Regardless, these tests should be performed and trends evaluated between individual animals' conspecifics under similar circumstances.

ERYTHROGRAM

Erythrocytes are typically nucleated, though a few amphibian species have plasmocytes that are enucleated red blood cells. Morphology is important. The majority of amphibian erythrocytes are nucleated with centrally located nuclei. Viral inclusions, bacteria, and parasites (e.g., trypanosomes, microfilaria) can be seen in diseased animals as well as nonclinical animals; therefore, the total clinical picture is important to establish a diagnosis. Hematocrit is highly variable, usually ranging from 20% to 40%. Amphibian thrombocytes are nucleated and highly variable in shape. They may appear similar to small lymphocytes. The primary distinctions are that thrombocytes have a pale clear cytoplasm and a higher cytoplasmic-to-nuclear ratio.

LEUKOGRAM

There is a general lack of information regarding changes in the amphibian leukogram with disease. Granulocytes in the amphibian include heterophils, neutrophils, basophils, eosinophils, and azurophils; however, their function may not be the same as in other species and using the terms should not lend to extrapolation or overinterpretation of the differential. Amphibian eosinophils have shown activity against trematode integument, but there is no evidence that they have a role in bacterial or fungal disease. Basophils may have a similar role; they tend to degranulate readily and may serve to recruit eosinophils to parasitic infections. Mast cells may represent a stage of the basophil cycle. Heterophils and neutrophils phago-cytize bacteria. Bands are not typically seen. Lymphocytes and monocytes are the common agranulocytes of amphibians. Lymphocytes are easily confused with thrombocytes and monocytes. Large lymphocytes can be distinguished from monocytes by evaluating the nuclear-to-cytoplasmic ratio. Lymphocytes have a higher nuclear-to-cytoplasmic ratio.

White blood cell (WBC) counts in amphibians can range from 4.5 to 13.0×10^3 cells/ml. Elevated WBC counts can result from stress and inflammation. Handling an amphibian may cause a specific increase in the monocyte count due to skin damage. Stress and glucocorticoids may result in a lymphopenia and neutrophilia (heterophilia and neutrophilia combined). The most important factor to consider when evaluating a hemogram is the cell morphology.

An unexplored aspect of amphibian blood is immunoglobulin (Ig) analysis. Three types of Ig are produced: IgM, IgY (IgG-like), and IgX. IgM increases with bacterial infections, whereas viral infections often produce IgM followed by IgY.

PLASMA BIOCHEMISTRIES

Highlights of plasma biochemical findings are included in this section; however, as with the hemogram, a high degree of variability can occur. Median glucose is typically around 50 mg/dl and may increase as much as 25% because of handling. The liver predominantly produces bilirubin, although small amounts of biliverdin may also be present. Most hepatic disorders diagnosed at necropsy suggest that a liver biopsy is more valuable than blood work for evaluating the liver. The enzymes generally used in other species to evaluate the liver, including gamma glutamyltranspeptidase (GGT), aspartate aminotransferase (AST), and alanine aminotransferase (ALT), do not appear to be specific for the hepatocytes in amphibians. GGT can fluctuate greatly with season. Bile acids have not been examined in amphibians. Standard renal parameters do not appear to be as significant in amphibians for evaluating renal disease. Ammonia can be measured in the plasma if there is a suspicion of ammonia intoxication, but as with small animal practice, the samples must be kept on ice and processed within 30 minutes. The plasma osmolality of amphibians should be greater than 200 mOsm/L.

Diagnostic Imaging[27]

Radiographs can be accomplished using a variety of techniques. Standard and dental radiography, as well as mammography, have all been utilized. Although mammography provides the crispest detail, most practices do not have access to such a tool. Standard radiography film can be adequate for even the smallest patients, as long as ultra detail film (single emulsion and high detail rare earth screens) is used. Dental films can be used with standard radiographic units or a dental unit. Animals can be placed directly on plates, within plastic bags, or in plastic boxes. A minimum of two views should be taken (Figures 5-18 and 5-19). Contrast radiography (Figure 5-20) can be accomplished using iodinated compounds or barium. These liquids can be administered orally or cloacally (e.g., enema). Pneumocoelograms and double contrast coelograms

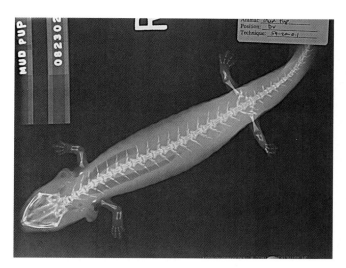

Figure 5-18 Radiographic dorso-ventral survey of an axolotl.

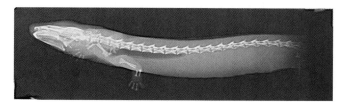

Figure 5-19 Radiographic lateral survey of an axolotl.

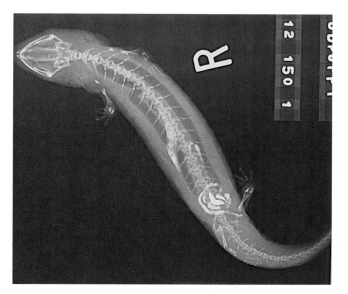

Figure 5-20 Radiographic barium contrast study of an axolotl.

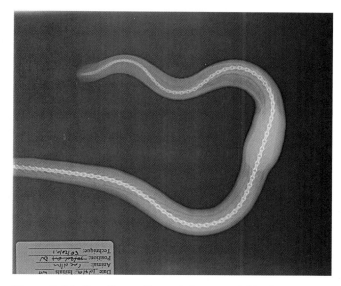

Figure 5-21 Caecilian radiograph for a caudal body mass that was diagnosed as a sarcoma.

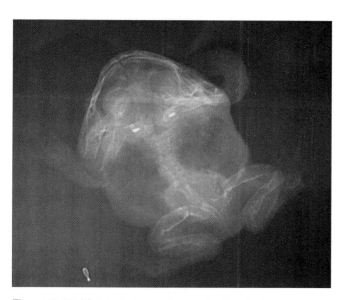

Figure 5-22 Metabolic bone disease in *Ceratophrys* sp.

(e.g., air and iodinated compound in coelom) can be used to further characterize disease processes. Various disease processes can be easily identified using radiography (Figures 5-21 through 5-25).

Advanced imaging techniques including computed tomography and magnetic resonance imaging may be used, but there are few comparisons for reference images, and they can be costly.

Ultrasound

Ultrasonography can be an invaluable tool for evaluating the heart, liver, gallbladder, stomach, gastrointestinal tract, reproductive organs, kidneys, and bladder of amphibians.[28] It can also be used to assess abnormal masses and fluid accumulation. Because of the small size of most amphibian patients, a 7.5- to 12-mHz translinear probe is generally required to thoroughly evaluate a patient. Note the image of a *Dendrobates terribilis* (Figure 5-26). A fluid-filled pocket can be visualized in the gular region of the animal; this pouch resolved within days,

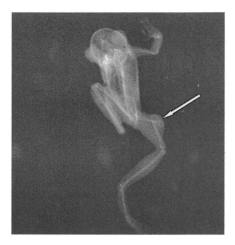

Figure 5-23 Fractured femur in a hylid frog.

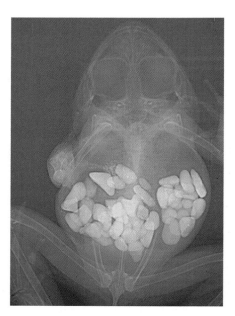

Figure 5-24 Gastric foreign body (rocks) in a leptodactylid.

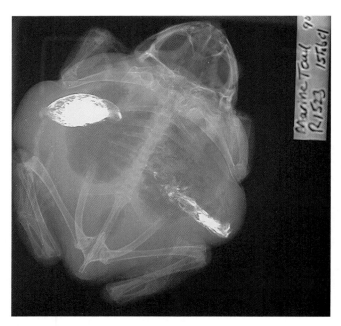

Figure 5-25 Gastric bezoar delineated by barium contrast material.

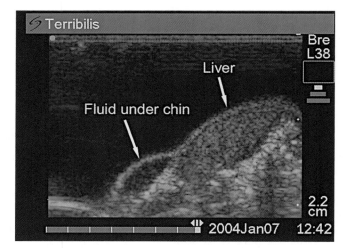

Figure 5-26 Ultrasound image showing fluid collection within the gular pouch.

suggesting a normal phenomenon (possibly stress). The larger ultrasound probes (2.5-5 mHz) may be used for larger animals, such as bullfrogs *(Rana catesbeiana)*. The benefit of this procedure is that it can be done without anesthesia, and most patients can be placed into a water medium to facilitate crisp images (Figures 5-27 and 5-28).

Microbiology

There is an excellent review of amphibian microbiology techniques; clinicians with a strong interest in pursuing in-house culturing should consult this resource.[29] For the practical clinician, collection of culture material into a culturette (Mini-tip culturette, Becton Dickinson Microbiology Systems, Cockeysville, MD) with transport medium is most versatile.

Thioglycollate broth may also be a good investment, as it will grow scant or fastidious microorganisms. To ensure growth of amphibian microorganisms, incubation should occur at 37° C despite originating from an ectotherm. Pathogenic bacteria will grow faster at high temperatures. Anaerobic cultures require special handling instructions and should be carried out as per the laboratory to which the specimens are being sent. Fungal culture can be accomplished with the same culturette system mentioned previously. Mycobacterial cultures should be pursued if there is a trend of acid-fast organisms being isolated or identified from animals within a given collection. Isolated cases of acid-fast organisms are not unusual, but certain myco-

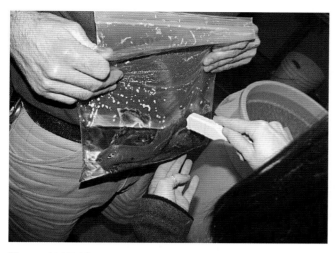

Figure 5-27 Ultrasound of a caecilian that is submerged in water within a plastic bag.

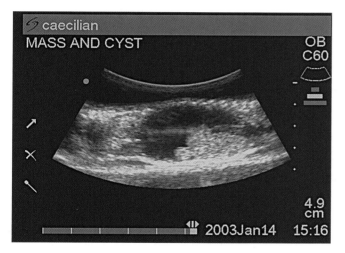

Figure 5-28 Ultrasound image of a caecilian neoplasm within a cyst.

bacterial species do pose a zoonotic risk and should be characterized.

Culture samples should be collected from any abnormal lesions or fluids, abnormal organs identified on postmortem, and for blood culture (tryptic soy broth or thioglycollate broth). Skin lesion cultures may lead to the characterization of an organism, although more commonly, superficial surface samples can be difficult to interpret as they are frequently overwhelmed by contaminants. Deep integumentary swabs are recommended. Avoid the perimeter of the skin when swabbing a lesion. Alternately, a second culture of normal skin can be taken as a comparison, but this may not be practical under some circumstances. Fecal culture is often unrewarding (unless it is a pure culture of a single organism) because the indigenous flora can include *Salmonella* sp., *Aeromonas* sp.,[24] and other bacteria considered to be opportunistic pathogens. If any bacterial epizootic occurs in a collection, consider culturing the soil, food, and water to identify a potential source of the infections.

Parasitology

A fecal parasitologic examination should include both a wet mount and a flotation. Protozoans can encyst with environmental change, so rapid evaluation is critical. Wright's-Giemsa stain, Gram stain, and acid-fast stains can also be used to thoroughly evaluate gastrointestinal disorders.

To assist in the collection of a fecal sample, assist-feed the animal with a prepared food slurry, like a pelleted food product mixed with water. Place the animal in a covered, well-ventilated plastic container and wait (a few hours) until a fecal sample is produced.

The normal microflora of amphibians includes flagellates, opalinids, ciliates, and nematodes. Distinguishing between pathogens and normal organisms is often difficult. Frequently, the clinician must rely on the relative numbers of organisms and on the clinical presentation of the animal. If there are numerous flagellates in an emaciated animal that is not behaving normally, treatment should be considered. Treatment should always be considered when abnormal feces are observed. Like the flagellates, nematodes can also be a component of the amphibian indigenous flora or act as obligate parasites. Separating these diagnostic guidelines can be difficult but can generally be done by characterizing the nematode to species and evaluating the health and condition of the host. For example, amoebiasis is generally distinguished by the presence of WBCs and amoeboid trophozoites in the feces.

Anytime leukocytes or erythrocytes are seen in the feces, there should be concern about mucosal damage and occult parasitism (such as apicomplexa).[30]

Cryptosporidium is not commonly found in amphibians, but it should be screened for during quarantine due to its potential risk to an animal collection and zoonotic potential. Acid-fast staining will accomplish this but has low sensitivity. A commercially available test may also be used, but this has not been generally applied.[13]

Miscellaneous Diagnostics

Electrocardiograms (ECGs) can be measured in amphibians, but are not generally done because of the animals' small size. There are some reviews of ECG results available to the interested clinician.[24] Endoscopy and laparoscopy are invaluable diagnostic tools that can be used to evaluate the internal organs and to collect biopsies antemortem. These diagnostic tools should be considered when more conventional diagnostic tools prove unremarkable.

Water Quality

Amphibians may display variable responses to poor water quality. In general, truly aquatic amphibians are more likely to suffer from the negative impacts of poor water quality than are semiaquatic amphibians. Any time multiple animals from a single enclosure are presented with similar clinical signs, water quality should be evaluated. Water testing for an amphibian vivarium should, at minimum, include ammonia, nitrite, pH, alkalinity, and temperature.

Testing methods frequently produce highly variable and sometimes inaccurate results. At-home testing kits may not provide results measured in fine units; therefore, to err on the side of caution, certain tests should read zero (e.g., as ammonia and nitrite). See Table 5-1 for reference values.

Supersaturation of different gasses can occur when there is a leak in a pipe fitting or a pump. In these situations, when air mixes with water under pressurization, the water becomes supersaturated and the gas can be absorbed by the amphibians. Affected animals will have obvious, grossly discernable bubbles under their skin. A saturometer is required to confirm gas saturation and is not readily accessible to most individuals. Clinical signs are usually sufficient to make a diagnosis. Supportive care should be provided, and the water source used for the vivarium corrected.

Dissolved oxygen levels in the water column of amphibians are a special concern for larval amphibians (e.g., gilled animals) and neotenic species that capture oxygen from the water. This becomes less important in amphibians that primarily respire with lungs. Animals that are maintained in water with low oxygen levels will often be seen gasping for air at the water's surface. Dissolved oxygen cannot be effectively measured with at-home kits, despite the availability of such tests. Aerating the water with air stones and making regular water changes are usually sufficient to provide appropriate oxygen levels.

Amphibians' water is best maintained at neutral pH (7.0-7.5). When the pH becomes strongly acidic (<5.5) or basic (>8.5), the water becomes very irritating to the amphibian, and it may attempt to leave the water. Affected animals may produce excess mucus on the skin as a protectant. It is important to pretest water being used for a vivarium. Water pH and alkalinity can vary between municipalities. There are a variety of methods that can be used to measure pH. Several different commercially available kits are readily available at local retail pet stores. All aquatic systems naturally start to lower their pH as buffers in the system are used. It is for this reason that it is important to measure alkalinity (buffering capacity). There are two common methods for altering pH in an aquatic habitat: (1) adding commercial buffers or (2) making water changes that have a good alkalinity (>100 ppm).

Hardness is a measure of cations (e.g., calcium, magnesium) in the water. These cations serve as the basic building blocks of minerals that amphibians can obtain from the water column, especially larval amphibians. Low levels of hardness (e.g., calcium) may result in nutritional deficiencies (e.g., metabolic bone disease, secondary nutritional hyperparathyroidism) in growing amphibians. Elevated levels of hardness (e.g., high mineral content) can be irritating to amphibians, especially caecilians. Commercial water testing kits routinely have hardness as one of their testing parameters. Hardness levels vary between water sources (e.g., municipalities). In areas where hardness levels are low, additional minerals can be added. In areas where hardness levels are high, the water can be diluted with deionized water.

Alkalinity measures the buffering capacity of a system. This is an important component of the water column because it can be used to predict the variability of the pH. Alkalinity can vary among water sources. Again, most commercial test kits measure alkalinity. If the alkalinity of the water is low (<60 ppt), then buffer can be added. Buffers are commercially available in local pet retail stores.

Ammonia is a natural by-product of protein catabolism and can be toxic when accumulated. Biological filtration, by way of the nitrogen cycle, removes ammonia from the water column by conversion into nitrite, then nitrate. The system is based on the presence of denitrifying bacteria. The most commonly discussed genera of this group are *Nitrosomonas spp.* and *Nitrobacter spp.* It is important to understand this cycle, and that it takes approximately 6 weeks for the filter to establish in a new system. (See Chapter 4, Ornamental Fish, to learn more about establishing these systems.) Ammonia is especially toxic to larval amphibians, because it is highly irritating to the gills. Microscopic examination of the gills of an affected animal often reveals inflamed swollen gill filaments. The natural response of the host is to produce mucus, which creates a barrier between the water and the gill. These different responses by the host lead to a reduced ability to transfer oxygen across the gill epithelium. Affected animals are often seen gasping for air at the water's surface. Ammonia can also be irritating to the integument. Again, the natural response of the host is to produce excess mucus as a protectant. Affected animals may be observed rubbing against various rough surfaces because of the irritation or pruritus generated by the ammonia. Treatment can be accomplished by moving the animal to an ammonia-free water source, establishing a biologic filter in the primary vivarium, and reducing ammonia loads on the system (e.g., reduce feeding, decrease animal density). In testing for ammonia, identify if the commercial kit being used measures total ammonia nitrogen (TAN) or un-ionized ammonia (NH_3). TAN is a measure of both the ionized (NH_4^+) and un-ionized (NH_4^+) forms of ammonia. NH_4^+ is the less toxic form and is found in higher concentrations at lower pH levels. Most kits measure TAN, and the actual value of the more toxic form (NH_3) can be identified based on pH and temperature. A chart showing this is available elsewhere.[8] Regardless, if a level of zero is targeted, it is irrelevant whether the clinician is measuring TAN or NH_3.

Nitrite, while not as critical as ammonia, can also be problematic in amphibians. Nitrite is primarily produced from the denitrification of ammonia by *Nitrosomonas* spp. Nitrite, like ammonia, can be readily absorbed across the surface of the gills. Amphibians affected with nitrite toxicity can develop methemoglobinemia (brown blood disease). Test kits are available to test for nitrogen. Methemoglobinemia results in a reduced carrying capacity for oxygen. Again, affected animals are often observed gasping for air at the water's surface. A diagnosis can be made by measuring nitrite levels in the water. A blood sample from the animal can be used, in addition to the water test, to confirm the presence of brown blood, or methemoglobinemia. Treatment is similar to that described for ammonia toxicity. Salting the water (100 ppm) is also protective. Commercial test kits are available that measure ammonia, nitrite, and nitrate.

Other Diagnostics

Serologic testing and advanced molecular testing (e.g., polymerase chain reaction assays) are currently not widely used or easily available to the exotic animal clinician. Rather, postmortem examinations provide the most valuable diagnostic tool. Necropsy must be performed shortly after death as autolysis occurs rapidly. Veterinarians should establish a good relationship with a pathologist who has experience interpreting the histopathology of amphibians.

■ COMMON DISEASE PRESENTATIONS

Infectious

BACTERIAL

In general, bacterial disease is very common in captive amphibians, and the majority of pathogens encountered in captivity are Gram-negative organisms. Bacterial disease can be focal (skin, liver) or systemic. The epidemiology of bacterial diseases in amphibians is highly correlated to environmental risk factors, including suboptimal environmental condition (e.g., low or excessive temperature, poor water quality, overcrowding), stress, and transport.

Disease: **Red-leg bacterial syndrome**[31,32]
Etiology: *Aeromonas hydrophila, A. aerogenes, A. aerophila, A. salmonicida, Citrobacter freundii, Flavobacterium* sp., *Klebsiella* sp., *Proteus* sp., *Pseudomonas* sp.
Clinical signs: hyperemia of the ventral skin (thighs, abdomen, digits), subcutaneous edema, full thickness cutaneous ulceration, petechial and ecchymotic hemorrhage, hypopion/hyphema, death (including mass mortalities in a population). Red-leg syndrome is a clinical presentation. Viral and fungal pathogens can also produce these clinical signs.
Diagnosis: culture from blood or tissue of the aforementioned organisms plus clinical signs. Note that many of these bacteria are indigenous florae and can be contaminants.
Differentials: historically considered only a bacterial disease; *Iridovirus, Ranavirus, Chlamydophila psittaci, Basidiobolus ranarum,* other bacteria, chytridiomycosis
General treatment scheme: fluid therapy, parenteral antibiotics based on culture and sensitivity, topical treatment on open wounds, improving environmental conditions

Disease: **Bacterial septicemia**
Etiology: any number of potential bacterial pathogens (primarily Gram-negative) and opportunistic organisms
Clinical signs: lethargy, anorexia, red-leg syndrome, death
Diagnosis: culture of blood and organ tissues, bacteremia on blood smear, histology

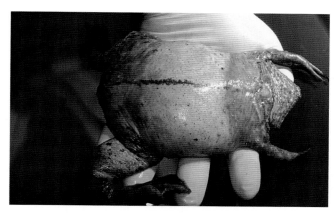

Figure 5-29 Hydrocoelom in a Surinam toad *(Pipa pipa).*

Differentials: historically considered only a bacterial disease; *Iridovirus, Ranavirus, Chlamydophila psittaci, Basidiobolus ranarum,* other bacteria, chytridiomycosis
General treatment scheme: fluid therapy, parenteral or bath antibiotics, improved environmental conditions

Disease: **Edema syndrome**[31]
Etiology: bacterial septicemia (esp. *Flavobacterium spp.*); renal, cardiac, or hepatic failure; toxic insult; poor water quality
Clinical signs: hydrocoelom (Figure 5-29), anasarca, or localized subcutaneous edema
Diagnosis: marked excess fluid subcutaneously and in coelom
General treatment scheme: furosemide, hypertonic amphibian Ringer's solution, correct underlying etiology if possible

Disease: **Chlamydiosis**[33]
Etiology: *Chlamydophila psittaci*
Clinical signs: as for red-leg syndrome
Diagnosis: histologic evidence of intracytoplasmic inclusion bodies, culture, PCR
Differentials: other systemic bacterial, viral, fungal diseases
General treatment: doxycycline, oxytetracycline
Other: Zoonotic potential is unknown but is probably limited. Another chlamydial organism that affects frogs is *Chlamydophila pneumoniae,* which causes skin sloughing and bloating.

Disease: ***Mycobacterium* spp.**[31,34-36]
Etiology: *Mycobacterium cheloniae* ssp. *abscessus, M. avium* complex, *M. ranae, M. marinum, M. fortuitum, M. thamnospheos, M. xenopi*
Clinical signs:
  Focal disease: nonhealing cutaneous lesion (Figure 5-30), granulomatous mass, occasionally liquefactive pus
  Systemic disease: chronic weight loss or wasting, nodules or granulomas in viscera and subcutaneously
Diagnosis: acid-fast staining of lesions (Figure 5-31), histologic evidence of acid-fast organisms, culture (not always rewarding). In my experience, a monocytosis or increased total white cell count does not always accompany systemic disease.

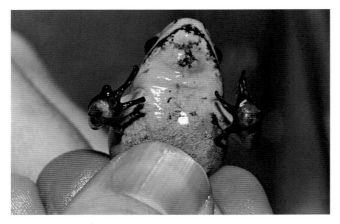

Figure 5-30 Ulcerative pododermatitis secondary to myco-bacteriosis.

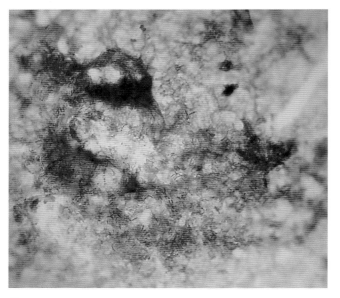

Figure 5-31 Acid-fast organisms on a skin smear from ulcerative dermatitis.

Differentials: neoplasia, chronic inflammatory disease

General treatment scheme: With systemic disease there is no effective treatment. Focal disease may be cured with complete surgical removal of the infected area (such as amputation); however, it may be impossible to determine whether the organism has been disseminated to other tissues, unless serial biopsies are taken. In these cases, the animal may still pose a health risk to other animals in the collection or to their human caretakers.

Other: zoonotic potential. Mycobacteria are ubiquitous in the aquatic environment, and the nonpathogenic strains can be found on the surface of the skin or in the feces.

VIRAL[36-38]

Diagnosing viral disease is not an easy or practical task. Although the prevalence of infection in captive amphibians is considered low, this may be misleading as there are few tests available to characterize these organisms today. The prevalence of viruses is considered higher in wild populations, and this is primarily based on diagnoses made during epizootics. Again, this could be misleading, because diagnosis of viral disease is more likely to be pursued in these cases. The following is a list of traditional viral diseases of amphibians:

Tadpole edema virus (TEV or Ranavirus type 3) results in edema, and skin, subcutaneous, and visceral hemorrhages. Basophilic intranuclear inclusions may be present.

Frog virus 3 (Ranavirus type 1) causes multifocal hemorrhages and basophilic intranuclear inclusions.

Bohle iridovirus (BIV) causes viral hemorrhagic septicemia of frogs resulting in multifocal necrosis of the liver, spleen, stomach, and lungs. Dermal hemorrhage and ulceration, systemic hemorrhage and ulceration, and systemic hemorrhage and gastroenteritis also can occur. Paralysis may occur secondary to neuronal degeneration. This disease is transmissible to fish.

Frog erythrocytic virus is associated with limited clinical signs but may not include anemia. Inclusions are visible in erythrocytes and leucocytes.

Herpes-like virus can cause small white to dark dorsal cutaneous vesicles and epidermal hyperplasia.

Lucke's disease is a herpes virus that causes a temperature-dependent renal adenocarcinoma (Lucke tumor herpes virus [LTHV]). Hypothermic animals shed more virus and are more likely to contract the disease. The virus is highly lethal in tadpoles, whereas most adults seem immune to new infection.

Cutaneous papillomas of Japanese newts can cause a single epidermal tumor; a virus is suspected as an etiological agent.

Pox virus–like particles have been found in European common frogs *(Rana temporaria)* and can cause a red-leg–like, hemorrhagic gastroenteritis.

Lymphosarcoma viruses are not well described but fairly well accepted.

FUNGAL[39,40]

The soils used in vivaria generally support many different types of fungi. In the healthy animal, these organisms do not pose a problem. However, in the compromised individual (e.g., stress, trauma, immunosuppression), ubiquitous organisms have the potential to become opportunistic pathogens. How and when an infection occurs is dependent on fungal species, individual host tolerance to disease, and presumably fungal load in the environment. Mycotic dermatitis should be suspected as a cause in any amphibian cases with ulcerative dermatitis. Systemic infections are less common than the fungal dermatitides, but should be considered when diseases are apparently refractive to antibiotic treatment. There are excellent reviews and photographs on mycoses in amphibians available.[39-40]

Disease: **Basidiobolomycosis**

Etiology: *Basidiobolus ranarum,* zygomycete fungus found in soil and amphibian gastrointestinal tract

Clinical signs: variable, but can be subtle as in slight paling of the skin. In one case series, dwarf African clawed frogs sought terrestrial areas. In other cases, the disease resembles red-leg syndrome.

Diagnosis: wet mount of lesions showing septate hyphae and fungal spherules with beaked zygospores, positive periodic acid-Schiff stain and negative Gomori's methenamine stain; histology shows spherules in outermost layers of epidermis, culture. Amphibians may be asymptomatic carriers.

Differentials: red-leg bacterial syndrome, other mycotic dermatitides, chlamydiosis

General treatment scheme: itraconazole

Disease: **Mucormycosis**

Etiology: *Mucor amphibiorum,* a zygomycete fungus from the soil; usually considered nonpathogenic

Clinical signs: multifocal red nodules on skin which can be raised and ulcerated; white, fuzzy material primarily on the ventral abdomen; lethargy, reluctance to move, lack of coordination, or emaciation, death

Diagnosis: uniform fungal spherules (diameter of spherules and length of hyphae) noted in granulomas, culture

Differentials: ulcerative bacterial dermatitis, red-leg syndrome

General treatment scheme: None has been attempted because clinical disease is uncommon and onset is very rapid (within days).

Disease: **Saprolegniasis**

Etiology: ubiquitous oomycete (water mold), opportunistic pathogen

Clinical signs: white cotton or fuzzy growth over open lesions; animal usually collapses when removed from water; rare systemic infection

Diagnosis: wet mount containing zoospores (flagellated oospore) and nonseptate branching hyphae; large numbers in a small section

Differentials: other oomycetes

General treatment scheme: benzalkonium chloride, sodium chloride. Treat skin lesions and correct for osmotic losses with appropriate fluid therapy.

Other: primary pathogen for amphibian eggs

Disease: **Chytridiomycosis**

Etiology: *Batrachochytrium dendrobatidis,* zoosporic fungus related to oomycete watermolds; ubiquitous in soil and water

Clinical signs: nonspecific, excess shedding, sloughing skin on ventral abdomen and legs, death (Figure 5-32)

Diagnosis: readily detected in wet mounts, spherical single-celled intracellular organism; positive for periodic acid-Schiff and positive for Gomori's methenamine stain

General treatment scheme: 1% itraconazole bath, trimethoprim-sulfa. Treat secondary skin lesions and correct for osmotic losses with appropriate fluid therapy.

Other: significant in global population declines in Australia, North America, and Central America. Some animals are carriers.[38] Can affect captive animals, including Dendrobatids and White's tree frogs.[41]

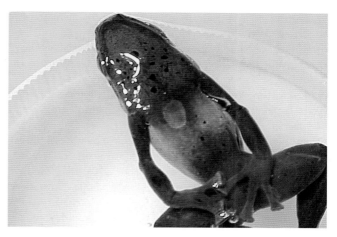

Figure 5-32 Skin lesions secondary to chytridiomycosis. (Photo credit Disney's Animal Programs, Deidre Fontenot).

Disease: *Ichthyophonus* sp.

Etiology: pleomorphic fungus, probably *Ichtyophonus hoferi*

Clinical signs: prominent swellings over body with normal skin over the nodules and lethargy

Diagnosis: histopathology, specific to muscle cells

General treatment scheme: none

Other: Free-ranging newts are susceptible.

Disease: **Chromomycosis (chromoblastomycosis)**

Etiology: brown or black pigmented septate fungal hyphae, including *Cladosporium* sp., *Phialophora* sp., *Exophiala* sp., and *Fonsecaea* sp.[42] They are saprophytes present in soil and decaying vegetation but can become opportunistic pathogens.

Clinical signs: nodular dermatitis that is slow growing. The lesions can be gray-black and associated with ulcers.

Diagnosis: histopathology and culture

General treatment scheme: None has been successfully treated. Consider amphotericin B (1 mg/kg intracoelomically [ICe] q24h).

Disease: *Dermocystidium* sp. (protozoan-like fungi)

Etiology: *Dermocystidium pusula* has been mistaken for a protozoan (12-14 µm).

Clinical signs: small white nodules less than 1 mm in diameter on skin and gills, possible increased respiratory rates, possible death as sequela

Diagnosis: skin scrapes and gill clips, cytologic and histopathologic review of samples

Differentials: miliary abscesses in integument

General treatment scheme: none developed, possibly mimicking behavioral fever by elevating temperature

PARASITIC[30]

Protozoa and nematodes can be both commensal and parasitic, depending on the species of the parasite and general condition of the host. It can be difficult to assess when endoparasites are causing problems. Numerous histopathologic reports suggest that mild to moderate loads of metazoans (nematodes) or trematodes can be found encysted in various tissues. Therefore, to confirm that a protozoan, trematode, or nematode is associated with disease, histopathologic changes should be confirmed. Chronic parasitism may have an overall negative effect on the host. Monitoring and surveying feces for microorganisms is a good way to characterize and understand the indigenous flora of amphibians. Knowledge of different life cycles of parasites is necessary to assess clinical disease and establish effective treatment plans.

The best time to treat amphibians against parasites is during quarantine, before they are introduced into a collection. When prophylactically treating for parasites, there is a risk of massive death caused by thromboemboli after a sudden kill-off of parasites or treatment toxicity. General treatment principles should be followed. After treatment, animals should be moved to a clean environment. Remove/eliminate any parasitic vectors, including live plants, substrates, or porous accessories.

ENDOPARASITES

Ciliates (*Nyctotheroides* spp., *Tetrahymena* sp., *Balantidium* sp., *Cepedietta* sp., *Trichodina* sp.)

Approximate size: variable 15-140 μm

Location: gastrointestinal tract (GI) (*Nyctotheroides*), skin, gills, urinary bladder (trichodinids)

Clinical signs: asymptomatic, stimulate excess production of mucus (irritant)

Life cycle: direct

Diagnosis: wet mount shows macronucleus and infundibulum, trichodinids in urinary bladder

Treatment: not usually required unless there is suspicion that the host is negatively affected. GI: metronidazole or paromomycin; skin/bladder: baths with saltwater or distilled water

Opalinids (*Opalina* sp., *Zelleria* sp.)

Approximate size: 20 × 150 μm

Location: gastrointestinal tract

Clinical signs: incidental finding on fecal exam

Life cycle: direct

Diagnosis: confused with ciliates; opalescent, have two nuclei that are the same size, no cell mouth

Treatment: none necessary

Flagellates (Trypanosomes, *H.* sp., *P.* sp., trichomonads)

Approximate size: ~20-80 μm

Location: skin/gills (dinoflagellates; *Ichthyobodo* sp. [*Costia* sp.]), gastrointestinal (*Giardia* sp. and *Trichomonas* sp.), and blood (trypanosomes, *Hexamita* sp.)

Clinical signs: asymptomatic, dermatitis, death caused by osmoregulatory imbalance, anemia

Life cycle: direct for most, indirect for trypanosomes

Diagnosis: wet mount of skin/feces or gastrointestinal washes and blood smear.

Treatment: Skin/gills—many are commensals: distilled water, saltwater, sodium chlorite. Trypanosomes: no treatments attempted, but suggestions include quinine baths (30 mg/L), oral quinolones 50 mg/kg PO once weekly. Gastrointestinal: metronidazole PO, bath for larval amphibians.

Amoeba

Approximate size: 10-60 μm.

Location: intestinal tract, liver, kidney (*Entamoeba ranarum*, most are nonpathogenic)

Clinical signs: anorexia, weight loss, diarrhea ± hemorrhage, dehydration, anasarca, ascites

Life cycle: direct

Diagnosis: Wet mount shows presence; if there are no clinical signs and no leukocytes or erythrocytes, then probably it is nonpathogenic.

Histopathology: organisms within organs

Treatment: metronidazole high dose 100 mg/kg PO every 14 days

Apicomplexa

Approximate size: ~20 × 30 μm

Location: blood (*Hemogregarina* sp., *Hepatozoon* sp.), tissues (*Isospora* sp., *Eimeria* sp.)

Clinical signs: asymptomatic, anemia rare with blood forms, weight loss, diarrhea

Life cycle: Hematologic organisms have an indirect cycle with invertebrate intermediate hosts (e.g., mosquito and leech). Direct life cycle occurs with tissue-invading species.

Diagnosis: Blood smears, uncommon finding on feces, sporulation can be induced in suspects with the potassium dichromate method.[30]

Histopathology: Generally found within cells with minimal response.

Treatment: none if there are no clinical signs (e.g., no anemia with high load of hemoparasites), amprolium unrewarding. Trimethoprim sulfamethoxazole places clinical disease into remission but does not cure.

Microsporidia

Approximate size: 5-20 μm

Location: striated muscle, connective tissue, oocytes, and Bidder's organ. Obligate intracellular organisms (*Pleistophora* sp., *Microsporidium* sp., *Alloglugea* sp.). Hypertrophied host cells are called *xenomas*.

Clinical signs: emaciation, muscle atrophy, death; one new case in *Phyllomedusa* sp. with ulcerative dermatitis

Life cycle: direct

Diagnosis: Transillumination of muscles may yield white streaks in striated muscles; these streaks will be seen on gross necropsy. Impression smears of lesions yield refractile pear-shaped organisms. Gram stain results in red-purple color (vs. other protozoa, which do not take up stain).

Treatment: depopulation, chloramphenicol injectable and topical oxytetracycline with polymyxin B sulfate for dermatitis, treatment not generally successful

Myxosporidia

Approximate size: 7-10 μm oblong

Location: gallbladder, urinary tract, kidneys, testes, ovaries

Species: *Chloromyxum* sp., *Leptotheca* sp., *Myxidium* sp., *Myxobolus* sp.; most nonpathogenic

Clinical signs: none usually; possibly organ specific

Life cycle: indirect and direct, depending on species (variable even within a genus)

Diagnosis: histology of affected organs; squash preps of organs. Pear-shaped or spherical refractile organism with two polar capsules.

Treatment: no treatments available, prevention with disinfection and good husbandry

Trematodes, Monogenea (flukes with hooklets, suckers, or clamps; *Gyrodactylus* sp.)

Location: skin, gills, urinary tract, intestinal tract

Clinical signs: irritation, increased mucus production, increased respiratory rate

Life cycle: direct

Diagnosis: skin scraping and transillumination of the bladder. Few organisms in an otherwise healthy individual are not generally considered a problem.

Treatment: praziquantel baths, consider diflubenzuron for at least 8 weeks in a system infected with the organism as the hooks of the parasite are made of chitin.

Trematodes, Digeneans (flukes)

Location: subcutaneous tissues, skin, heart, kidney, liver, intestine, lungs. Pathology is uncommon; however, encysted organisms can pose a later threat. Possible commensal in large intestine.

Clinical signs: melanophores surround the worms in the skin, renal damage associated with heavy infestations (*Gorgodera* sp., *Gorgoderina* sp.)

Life cycle: Indirect, larval, and adult digeneans can use amphibians as hosts. Intermediate hosts can be tadpoles, snails, and insect larvae; sometimes three or four hosts are required.

Diagnosis: heavy infestation witnessed usually postmortem; transillumination may visually display organisms in tissues

Treatment: usually unsuccessful; prophylactic treatment with corticosteroids 3 days before anthelminthic, then praziquantel PO, IM or ICe every 14 days × 3 treatments

Other: *Halipegus* spp. trematodes can be found in the oral cavity of frogs (*Rana* sp.) that are infected by the ingestion of dragonflies.[12]

Cestodes (tapeworms)

Location: Larvae can be found in muscle, skin, connective tissue, viscera, and coelom. Adults can be found in the intestine. Pathology is uncommon; encysted organisms can pose a later threat. *Nematotaenia* sp. may cause intestinal obstruction.

Clinical signs: possible proglottids hanging from cloaca

Life cycle: indirect

Diagnosis: proglottids and/or eggs observed in feces, possible verminous granulomas in the intestine on transillumination, incidental finding on necropsy

Treatment: Praziquantel can be used to eliminate adult worms in the intestine, whereas larvae are encysted and usually refractory to anthelminthics.

Nematodes (roundworms)

Location: lungs, gastrointestinal tract, skin. Larval forms may be found migrating through most tissues.

Species: *Rhabdias bufonis* (lung), *Strongyloides* spp., *Pseudocapillaroides xenopi* (capillarid nematode in skin, *Xenopus laevis*), *Foleyella* sp. (microfilaria in tissues, coelom, vessels, lymph sacs, and blood), others

Clinical signs: depends on affected organ system. Increased respiratory effort, ulcerative skin lesions, intestinal prolapse, weight loss, diarrhea, anemia, and failure to thrive are all possible signs.

Life cycle: indirect and direct (most)

Diagnosis: frequent finding on fecal examination, skin scrapes, tracheal washes, blood smears, and coelomic fluid. Determining pathogenicity is challenging. Always use fresh feces; active strongylid larvae may implicate *Rhabdias* sp., and Capillarids have bipolar plugs on the egg. Filaria generally observed in blood and coelomic aspirate.

Treatment: When clinical signs match a significant nematode load, fenbendazole, ivermectin, or levamisole may be used. Most treatments call for repeated treatments at least every 14 days for at least 3 treatments.

Other: Feeding live fish can be detrimental because it is the intermediate host for eustrongyloides.

Acanthocephala (thorny-headed worms)

Location: intestines; causes intestinal perforation, coelomitis, sepsis, weight loss

Clinical signs: weight loss, lethargy, hydrocoelom

Life cycle: indirect, crustacean or insect intermediate host

Diagnosis: fecal exam, spindle-shaped eggs in feces

Treatment: no effective treatment, consider loperamide 50 mg/kg PO q24h × 3 treatments

Other parasites include Pentastomids, common reptile parasites that may occur in amphibians. Characteristics are unmistakable: an oral region with a mouth and four retractine hooks and an annulated body with no true segments. On gross examination these parasites are more like crustaceans than helminths. *Monocystis* sp. and earthworm parasites can be found in the feces of amphibians that ingest invertebrates. *Monocystis* is a sporozoan that measures 60 × 200 μm and is not considered parasitic in amphibians.

ECTOPARASITES

As with other vertebrates, there are many types of amphibian ectoparasites. Protozoans (e.g., ciliates and flagellates) can be found on and in skin lesions and are most likely opportunistic pathogens or commensals. Crustacean parasites, such as trombiculid mites (chiggers) (1-2 mm orange-red vesicles), copepods, and lice (branchiurans, *Argulus* sp., a fish parasite), are large and easily identifiable. Leeches and ticks (Ixodidae) may be found on wild-caught specimens.

Insect problems can include bot flies that burrow subcutaneously, maggots that infest open wounds, and larval anurans that parasitize the nasal cavity (toadfly larvae, *Lucilia* sp.).

A diagnosis of ectoparasitism can be made by close examination of the skin, impression smears from skin scrapes, or biopsies. In cases of nasal myiasis, a nasal flush is required.

General treatment strategies for these patients include manual removal of large organisms, hypertonic baths (saltwater), anthelminthics, and diflubenzuron for crustaceans. Other baths, including formalin baths can be used, but they are considerably more irritating and potentially harmful to the amphibian host. In addition to treating the amphibian, the enclosure must also be treated to prevent reinfection.

Nutritional

Disease: **Nutritional secondary hyperparathyroidism (metabolic bone disease)**[43,44]

Clinical signs: skeletal deformity (Figures 5-33 and 5-34), abnormal posture, splay leg, fractures, tetany, bloating, hydrops, subcutaneous edema, gastrointestinal prolapses

Etiology: low calcium in diet or water, hypervitaminosis A, and/or fat and fatty acid imbalance. Hypocalcemia can cause tetany, reduce gastrointestinal peristalsis, and result in bloating.

Pathogenesis: Amphibians use lipoproteins as a transport mechanism for vitamin D_3; therefore, diets inappropriately

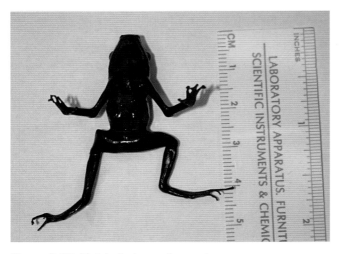

Figure 5-33 Metabolic bone disease in an anuran.

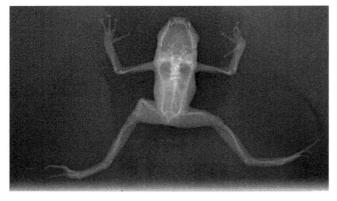

Figure 5-34 A survey radiograph of the frog with metabolic bone disease from Figure 5-33. Note the thin cortices and the folding femoral fracture.

balanced with fats and fatty acids (even with good levels of Ca, P, and D_3) may cause problems. The role of ultraviolet B radiation and vitamin D_3 is not well documented but may be a factor in some species.

Diagnosis: Plasma calcium levels are generally unremarkable because it is the tendency of the body to maintain available plasma levels of calcium. Radiographs are diagnostic. Affected animals will have a reduced cortical bone density.

Treatment: calcium supplementation, correction of diet, provision of ultraviolet B radiation

Disease: **Hypervitaminosis D_3**[32]

Clinical signs: anasarca, anorexia, weakness

Etiology: Comet goldfish prey fed to frogs that are fed a commercial fish flake food.

Pathogenesis: Calcium salts deposit in organs, causing multifocal soft tissue mineralization.

Diagnosis: usually a postmortem diagnosis

Treatment: none

Disease: **Hypervitaminosis A**[45]

Clinical signs: similar to metabolic bone disease

Etiology: rodent diet

Pathogenesis: Excess vitamin A interferes with absorption and utilization of vitamin D_3.

Diagnosis: correlates with radiographs and diet

Treatment: Supplement rodent diet with calcium and vitamin D_3 (2.7 µg/g of prey body weight). This treatment has not been tested, and its long-term safety is unknown. Feed fewer rodents.

Disease: **Hypovitaminosis A**[12]

Clinical signs: xerophthalmia, corneal lesions, inability to use tongue for prey capture

Etiology: deficiency in diet

Pathogenesis: keratinizing squamous metaplasia and secondary keratomalacia in mammals and birds; epidermal hyperplasia and hyperkeratosis also associated

Diagnosis: histopathology

Treatment: vitamin A supplementation to diet

Disease: **Corneal lipidosis**[21,44,45]

Clinical signs: cloudy haze to white tissue accumulation in the cornea(s)

Etiology: Commercial chows can contain high levels of cholesterol, which can be transferred through the food chain to captive amphibians.

Pathogenesis: Tree frogs are commonly affected, and females may be overrepresented in a diseased population.

Diagnosis: Visual examination of eye(s) will show raised and opaque, white corneal lesions, which are associated with high serum cholesterol (e.g., 1000 mg/dl for severely affected frogs).

Treatment: Surgical removal of one or both coelomic fat bodies may be warranted. Invertebrate diets should comprise only vegetables for 48 hours before offering them to amphibians. Topical ophthalmic antibiotic and antiinflammatory drops may be used, especially with keratotomy. Debulking the corneal lesions may cause an inflammatory response with increased infiltration of inflammatory cells in the local tissue. Enucleation may be required.

Disease: **Thiamine deficiency**[44]
Clinical signs: neuropathy, blindness
Etiology: a diet comprised of frozen-thawed fish
Pathogenesis: freezing results in leeching of vitamins from the food source. Fish have thiaminases that are not destroyed by freezing and therefore break down thiamine (a very labile protein).
Diagnosis: response to treatment
Treatment: Animals with neurologic dysfunction and a history consistent with thiamine deficiency can be given a dose of 250 mg thiamine/kg of fish.

Disease: **Iodine deficiency**[44]
Clinical signs: Tadpoles do not metamorphose; rather, they get very large.
Etiology: diets deficient in iodine or the consumption of excess goitrogens (e.g., cabbages and spinach)
Treatment: iodine and thyroxine

Disease: **Steatitis**[44]
Clinical signs: Abdominal discomfort is the presenting sign.
Etiology: Improperly stored or frozen fish or other whole prey may become rancid. Steatitic nodules develop in fat bodies.
Treatment: Removal of the fat body is recommended.[12] Treatment with vitamin E and selenium may be useful.

Other Diseases

Disease: **Acclimation and maladaptation syndrome (AMS)**[13]
Etiology: failure to thrive or adapt to captivity usually due to inappropriate husbandry, including unacceptable habitat, low environmental temperature and humidity, low-grade nutrition
Clinical signs: emaciated, anorexic, lethargic animal
Diagnosis: exclusion of other disease processes
Treatment: Provide supportive therapy until the animal can be acclimated. Screen for parasitic diseases and look for mycobacteria in animals that continue to suffer weight loss.

Disease: **Bloated animal**
Clinical signs: generalized enlarged body shape, focal enlargement around coelom
Etiology: (1) hydrocoelom, edema, anasarca (e.g., organ failure, metabolic derangement, sepsis, hypocalcemia, protein deficiency); (2) aerocoelom (gastrointestinal gas, subcutaneous emphysema [Figure 5-35], pulmonary bullous rupture[32]); and (3) gastric impaction
Diagnosis: ballotment, palpation, radiographs, ultrasound, laparoscopy with biopsy of liver and kidney, postmortem

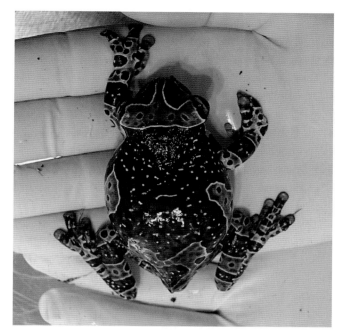

Figure 5-35 Gross appearance of a frog with aerocoelom.

evaluation. Blood work may prove to be useful in evaluating protein loss[12] and hypocalcemia.
Treatment: depends on initiating cause. Generally, make the patient comfortable by removal of impaction, decreasing air if excessive.

Disease: **Calculi**[44]
Clinical signs: lethargy, weight loss, hydrocoelom, edema
Etiology: (1) renal: oxalates in food items (terrarium plants that prey feed on) and (2) bladder (Figure 5-36): stones tend to occur in dehydrated uricotelic anurans. Both diseases may be exclusive to uric acid–producing organisms and are uncommonly seen.
Diagnosis: palpation (bladder stones), radiographs, postmortem finding
Treatment: cystotomy, diet change, supportive therapy

Disease: **Gastrointestinal impaction**
Clinical signs: lethargy, abdominal bloat, failure to pass feces; common problem in larger frogs
Etiology: consuming an overly large prey item or ingesting a foreign body (e.g., stones, coins, or accessories of the vivarium), bezoars (e.g., accumulated invertebrate skeletons). Large coelomic masses may cause decreased respiratory volume and consequent hypoxia and hypercarbia.
Diagnosis: Palpation may reveal the foreign body, and radiographs (with and without contrast) and ultrasound can be useful in confirming the location and origin of the foreign body.
Treatment: Removal of the prey or foreign item from the stomach may be relatively simple, as the stomach is a large organ, and anurans have a short esophagus. Manual removal

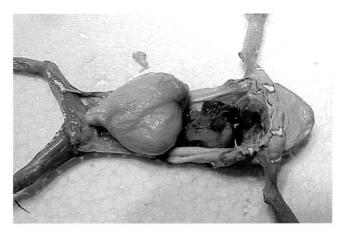

Figure 5-36 Bladder stones in a tree frog (Photo credit Disney's Animal Programs, Deidre Fontenot).

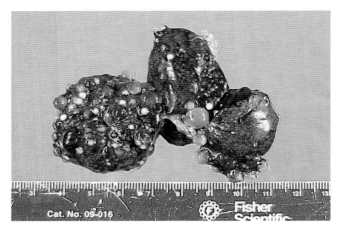

Figure 5-38 Liver cysticercoid.

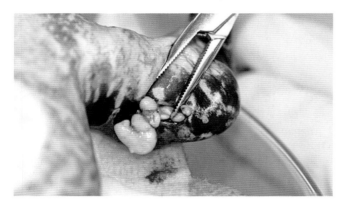

Figure 5-37 Mycobacterial abscess at the elbow of a frog.

or stomach lavage may be sufficient. For impactions in the intestinal tract, surgical intervention may be required. If there is evidence of normal peristalsis or the animal appears otherwise normal, mineral oil or laxatives may be attempted. If the animal is not defecating, or is obviously adversely affected by the impaction, surgery or endoscopy is warranted.

Disease: **Joint disease**
Clinical signs: swollen or painful joints
Etiology: Differentials for joint disease should include mycobacterial disease, sepsis, gout, neoplasia, articular infection (Figure 5-37), and arthritis.
Diagnosis: palpation of the affected joints, aspiration of joint fluid for cytologic examination, radiographs
Treatment: target inciting cause, amputation may be necessary

Disease: **Liver disease**[26]
Clinical signs: anorexia, lethargy, hepatomegaly, ascites, death
Etiology: Liver disease generally occurs as a sequela to other disease complexes (e.g., bacterial septicemia or parasitic

migrans) (Figure 5-38). Specific diseases that affect the liver include mycobacteriosis, chlamydiosis, chromomycosis (fungal hepatitis), recurrent septicemia, parasitism, trauma, and toxic insults (e.g., griseofulvin, chloroquine, primaquine, and aflatoxin [which can produce tumors]).
Diagnosis: radiographs, ultrasound, liver biopsy
Treatment: targeted to symptomatic treatment of clinical signs and disease process

Disease: **Ocular disease**[21,46,47]
Clinical signs: corneal haze, globe size change, anisocoria, visual deficits, lens opacity
Etiology: glaucoma, cataract, nematode migration, uveitis, panophthalmitis with septicemia, congenital abnormality (microphthalmia, anopthalmia, cyclopia) possibly linked to environment, corneal lipidosis
Diagnosis: impression smears, culture, postmortem analysis
Treatment: topical antibiotics, topical antifungals, enucleation. There are some concerns about swallowing difficulties after enucleation, though many animals do well. Therapy is often futile by the time ocular lesions develop.

Disease: **Paralysis**[48]
Clinical signs: flaccid paralysis of the hindlimbs, with some animals presenting with rigid paralysis
Etiology: frequently unknown etiology. There are no salient pathologic features. Some cases may be attributed to toxins; many zoological institutions have faced colony problems with no causative agent. The disease carries a poor prognosis unless there is a firm etiology (e.g., ivermectin overdose). There is a possible vitamin B/thiamine link. Botulism, hypocalcemia, and exposure to pesticides and other neurologic toxins should also be in the differential list.
Diagnosis: clinical signs. A full work-up should be performed if possible, and a complete postmortem examination performed if the opportunity presents itself.
Treatment: Vitamin B complex, corticosteroids, antibiotics, botulism antitoxoid, and calcium have been used as a "shotgun" therapy cocktail. Supportive care is sometimes

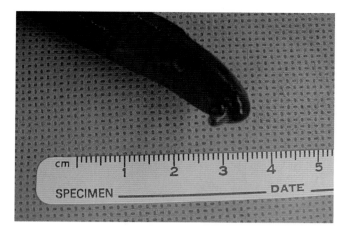

Figure 5-39 Cloacal prolapse in a caecilian.

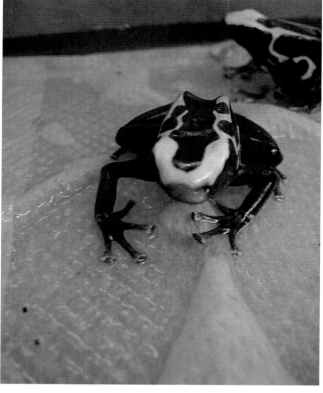

Figure 5-40 Rostral abrasions ("cage nose") in a dendrobatid.

the only treatment; some animals do survive, but the course of treatment can last for more than a month.

Disease: **Prolapse**

Clinical signs: obvious exposure of tissue (e.g., stomach) through the oral cavity or, more likely, the cloaca (e.g., rectum, oviduct, or urinary bladder)

Etiology: Gastric prolapse can be a transient occurrence in a healthy animal. It is not uncommon for anurans to evert their stomachs to expel noxious prey items. In the diseased animal it can be a terminal event. Gastric prolapse can also occur secondary to increased intraabdominal pressure (e.g., handling). Causes for cloacal prolapse may include hypocalcemia (decreased peristalsis), gastrointestinal impaction, parasites, toxins, unsuitable bulky diets, substrate-based foreign bodies, persistent parasitism or bacteremia, and as a result of anesthesia. Caecilians have been reported with cloacal prolapse (Figure 5-39) of unknown etiology.

Diagnosis: visual examination of the tissue. Knowledge of the normal anatomy is required to differentiate affected tissues.

Treatment: Resolution may occur uneventfully if the animal is kept quiet and moist. If the prolapse persists for more than a few hours, it should be further evaluated. Performing the evaluation under anesthesia is preferred. Treatment of a urinary bladder prolapse[32] requires disinfecting the bladder with 0.5% chlorhexidine (Fort Dodge Animal Health, Fort Dodge, IA), aspirating any urine to reduce the size of the the bladder, inserting an object into the bladder to replace it internally, and placing a suture to tack the bladder to the coelomic wall. Rectal or oviductal prolapse requires gentle cleaning and reduction of swollen tissue. This can be accomplished by liberally flushing the tissue with a hypertonic solution (e.g., sugar, honey, or ophthalmic saltwater drops). Reduction can be accomplished by applying gentle pressure with an atraumatic, blunt instrument and placing purse string or interrupted sutures around the vent. Again, this procedure should be done under anesthesia.

Disease: **Respiratory disease**[49,50]

Clinical signs: increased respiratory rate, open-mouth breathing, cyanosis

Etiology: Upper airway obstruction, pulmonary disease (bacterial or verminous pneumonia, *Rhabdias* sp.), pulmonary rupture and collapse, thoracic wound, and a space occupying coelomic mass will all cause respiratory disease. Gill damage can easily occur to neotenic caudates.

Diagnosis: radiographs, tracheal wash, gill clip

Treatment: must target specific disease process

Disease: **Rostral lesions**[51]

Clinical signs: "Cage nose" is an ulcerative dermatitis of the rostrum (Figure 5-40).

Etiology: May be observed with red-leg syndrome cases. More often it is caused by traumatic injuries sustained during escape attempts from an enclosure. It is frequently prompted by irritation (e.g., secondary smoke, avoidance of conspecifics, high temperature, loud noises, glue fumes, etc.). Lesions may take weeks to months to resolve.

Diagnosis: visual examination, impression smears to evaluate microorganisms, bacterial and fungal culture

Treatment: topical antibiotic and antifungal therapy. Debridement may be necessary and involves dissection of necrotic tissues.

Other: Wright[51] described a syndrome in captive redback salamanders *(Plethodon cinereus)* termed *atrophic mandibular stomatitis.* The injuries are caused by burrowing activity in

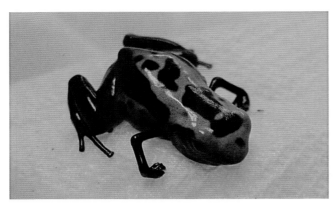

Figure 5-41 Spindly leg syndrome in a dendrobatid. (Courtesy Lincoln Park Zoo, Kathryn Gamble).

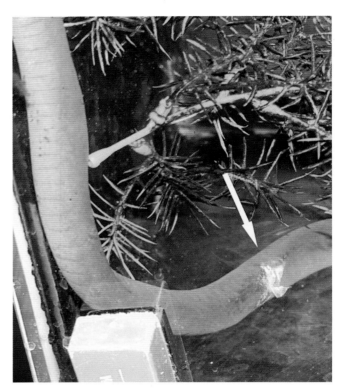

Figure 5-42 Caecilian with thermal burns secondary to contact with an aquarium heater.

an inappropriate habitat. Wright also described a similar condition in crocodile newts *(Tylototriton shanjing)* following shipment. Newts with mandibular fractures carry a poor prognosis because they are not able to suction feed. Pharyngostomy tubes have been used to allow supportive care during healing.[12]

Disease: **Skin lesions**
Clinical signs: discoloration of skin, ulcerations, increased mucus production, sloughing of skin
Etiology: numerous causes possible, including poor environment, bacteria, parasites (ectoparasites and larval migrans), fungus, trauma
Diagnosis: skin scrape and cytology, culture, evaluation of environment
Therapy: Fluid therapy is critical because of osmotic losses. After disinfection of lesion, consider application of liquid bandage or other covering. Appropriate therapy should be based on diagnosis.

Disease: **Spindly leg syndrome** (Skeletal and muscular underdevelopment [SMUD])[48]
Clinical signs: underdevelopment of forelimbs (Figure 5-41), when other anatomical features are normal
Etiology: nutrition (vitamin B deficiency), genetics, toxin, overcrowding, low oxygen levels, trauma
Diagnosis: physical examination, detailed history
Treatment: None. Feeding rich vegetation (algae) reduces incidence.

Disease: **Toxins**[52]
Clinical signs: irritation, hyperexcitability, neuropathies
Etiology: PVC glues (methyl-ethyl-ketone, tetrahydrofuran, cyclohexane), nicotine (injected into air pumps), pesticides, disinfectants, anthelminthics
Diagnosis: challenging; history of exposure, possible toxicologic analysis of organ tissue (limited samples). If there is a suspicion of toxicity, collect urine, feces, serum, and blood in ethylenediaminetetraacetic acid (EDTA). The urine,

feces, and serum should be frozen. Brain, liver, kidney, digestive tract contents, urine, and skin should also be collected for histopathology.
Treatment: Remove animal from source and rinse. A sodium thiosulfate soak (1% solution) can be used for halogen exposure. Assess heart rate and treat with atropine if necessary (0.1 mg/kg IM, SC, or ICe).

Disease: **Trauma**[51]
Clinical signs: skin lesions, hemorrhages, skeletal deformities, lethargy
Etiology: Crushing injuries can occur from human handling and the environment. Fractures can also occur with these events, and animals with MBD are more susceptible. Prey-induced trauma (e.g., crickets attacking amphibian) is common when leftover food items are not removed.
Diagnosis: history, physical examination, radiographs
Treatment: Limit the number of crickets fed so that the animals can consume them with no leftovers. Remove any uneaten live prey. Fractures can be stabilized in larger animals.[52]

Disease: **Other**
Ultraviolet A and metal halide lights may be too intense for amphibians, causing corneal opacities, erythema, excessive mucus production, and skin damage resulting in dermatitis. Sunburn may occur if direct sunlight is offered, resulting in ulcerative dermatitis. Thermal burns may also occur (Figure 5-42), secondary to direct or close contact with a heating

element. Clinical signs may include agitation, lethargy, ataxia, and death. Lesions may heal as white scars (fibrous tissue), but progressive dermatitis must be considered an outcome with severe wounds. Electric shock can occur if heating elements or other electrical gear break and have direct contact with animals. Death is a frequent outcome, and resuscitation may be attempted but is often unrewarding. Drowning can occur in animals kept in an inappropriate vivarium. Immediate clearance of the airways (e.g., massaging the animal, hold the head down) should be done to remove fluid. Articular and visceral gout[48] occurs, but the etiology is unknown. Dehydration and excessive dietary protein may play roles in the development of diseases, but these are speculative. Molchpest is a classic European newt disease associated with incomplete shedding and failure to consume a shed. Affected animals become hyperemic, and skin nodules may form. To some veterinarians, this is not considered a real disease.

Neoplasia[53,54]

The majority (50%) of all amphibian tumors are integumentary. Epidermal papillomas, also referred to as squamous papillomas, infectious warts, and epitheliomas, are described most frequently in urodelans. These papillomas are sessile, hypopigmented, and well demarcated with a folded or convoluted surface. Most are solitary lesions, pose little health concern, and are readily debulked or excised for diagnosis. Squamous cell carcinomas have also been reported in amphibians and are characterized grossly as hypopigmented, raised, sessile, or pedunculated masses, 0.3 to 1.5 cm in diameter. Surgical removal is recommended. Melanophoromas, also referred to as melanoma, melanocytoma, and melanosarcoma, are described in multiple species of urodelans and anurans. These neoplasms vary greatly in behavior and gross morphology, ranging from solitary to multicentric, hypopigmented to pigmented, nonpalpable to nodular, and regressive to invasive masses. Myxoma[32] (Figure 5-43) is a common, proliferative neoplasm in tree frogs, and recurrence is frequent after excision, but it is slow growing.

T-cell lymphomas in *Xenopus laevis* involve the thymus, resulting in a unilateral swelling in the cephalic area. Lymphoma may progress to leukemia. Diagnosis is made with a complete blood cell count and examination of a blood smear.

Lucke's renal adenocarcinoma of *Rana pipiens* is the best-known amphibian neoplasm. It is caused by a herpesvirus (Rana herpesvirus type 1 or Lucke's herpesvirus) and is prevalent under laboratory conditions where animals are maintained at high ambient temperatures.

Other tumors have been sporadically reported. In general, published treatments seem exclusively reliant on surgery.

Water Quality and Amphibian Disease[5,8,37]

Water quality has a huge impact on amphibian disease, especially semiaquatic or fully aquatic animals. Because there is free

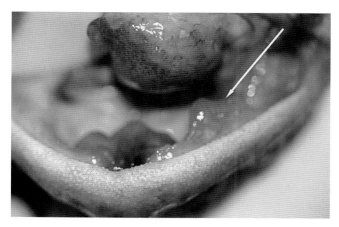

Figure 5-43 Oral myxoma in a Budgett's frog.

exchange of ions across the skin of amphibians, the components in the water are intimately involved with these animals. Treatments for all water quality problems involve improving dissolved oxygen levels by aerating the water and by performing water changes. Occasionally, supportive care and prophylactic treatments may be necessary depending on symptoms.

Low dissolved oxygen may cause an animal to gasp at the water's surface, and stagnation of the water may be evident. Conversely, high dissolved gasses (e.g., nitrogen and oxygen) can be forced into the water and supersaturate the system, causing gas bubble disease. Affected animals may have small, subcutaneous bubbles accumulating in their webbing, eyes, and skin. Occasionally, animals may succumb to air embolism.

Chlorine and chloramines are present in water from the tap. They are more toxic to tadpoles than adults. Sodium thiosulfate can be used to neutralize chlorine, as can aging the water for 72 hours or aerating the water for an hour.

Amphibians can generally tolerate shifts in pH; however, this can be a significant stressor. When the pH falls to less than 6.0, skin irritation can occur; when the pH increases to greater than 8.5, excess mucus production and hyperemia can occur. Long-term pH imbalance can also cause alterations in the acid-base status of the animal.[55,56]

Elevated ammonia can cause skin irritation (e.g., erythema), kidney damage, liver damage, and neurologic disease. Ammonia also can diminish the oxygen carrying capacity of the blood. Clinical signs can include hyperemia/erythema, gasping at the water's surface, excess mucus production, color change, and death.

Very little is reported on the effects of nitrite toxicity in adult anurans; however, methemoglobinemia can occur and be fatal. Nitrates, on the other hand, may cause developmental abnormalities in tadpoles. Although unusual in adults, nitrates may convert to nitrite and cause methemoglobinemia (brown blood disease).

◼ THERAPEUTICS

When considering a treatment regime, a holistic approach is necessary. Husbandry, behavior, diet, and specific treatments must be organized. With amphibians, it is also important to minimize stress, as this can lead to reduced immune function.

Temperature Change as a Therapy

Always provide an amphibian an optimal environmental temperature during convalescence. Behavioral fevers are not well explored, but they may prove useful under some circumstances. In these cases, placing the animal into the high end of its temperature range may provide a benefit toward healing and disease resolution.[57,58] Alternately, going outside the range of the organism (without detriment to the patient) may be a useful control mechanism, as with *Saprolegnia* sp., which prefers colder temperatures. Raising the temperature above 25° C[5] can help decrease the load of organisms in the system.

Administration of Medications[22,24]

The route by which a drug is administered is important. For example, the percutaneous uptake via a droplet or a bath is effective, but not as much as an injection. However, the former requires no handling. The clinician must make choices based on the patient, the diagnosis, and the ability to execute a treatment.

Oral treatment is most efficient when it can be administered with a food item and swallowed voluntarily. Invertebrate prey items can be injected with medications; however, this frequently renders them incapable of moving and the prey may be rejected. If necessary, medications can be administered by manual restraint and by gavage (Figure 5-44). Tools for assisting in the delivery of oral medications can include a micropipette, metal gavage tubes made for birds, intravenous catheters, and red rubber feeding tubes.

Topical treatment is a very effective and noninvasive method for administering medications to amphibians. The permeable skin of amphibians allows for percutaneous absorption via direct drops or via baths. Some drugs have irritating carriers, and their pH is a concern. Drops of medication applied topically on the animal require no handling. Ophthalmic drops frequently have high concentrations, and repeat dosing throughout the day may result in overdose.[24] To prevent this, the drops can be diluted. Baths are an excellent method for delivering fluid therapy and medicating an animal (Figure 5-45). When treating an amphibian via a bath, the ventrum must be immersed and care taken not to drown the animal. A covered container is ideal, and plastic bubble-wrap can be used to cover the animal and prevent jumping. The pH of a solution must be considered with any bath. The addition of chemicals to a vivarium to create a bath in the animal's habitat can be done, but large water changes must be performed that can disrupt the biologic filter and can stress the animal. Additionally, the drugs chosen for the treatment may kill or shock the bacteria in the filter. Activated carbon filters, protein skimmers, and sterilization tools will affect the drug in the water by deactivating it. Baths should be mixed in 0.5% saline and made fresh daily. Amphibian ringers can be used as well.

There are five parenteral routes for administering medication to amphibians: subcutaneous (SC), intramuscular (IM), intravenous (IV), intracoelomic (ICe), and lymph sac injection. In caudates and caecilians, the SC space is not present. In caecilians, IV actually means intracardiac (IC). ICe injections should be performed with the animal in dorsal recumbency, and the injection given in the caudal quadrant. Injection into the lymph sacs is rapidly absorbed (within minutes). IM is straightforward, given the existence of a renal portal system. IV injections can be difficult to administer in amphibians, and are generally not practical except for administering drugs for euthanasia (intracardiac).

Nebulization is a potential[22] treatment modality, but it is not routinely done to treat amphibians. It is possible that animals with pneumonia may benefit greatly from this modality. In one case, animals were nebulized with levamisole, and fatalities were recorded. However, it was not known whether the dose of levamisole or the nebulization procedure was responsible for the deaths.[59]

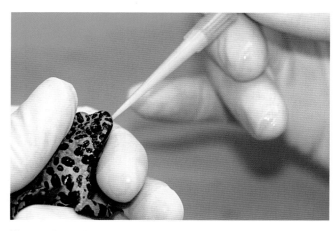

Figure 5-44 Administration of a prepared liquid food via a pipette.

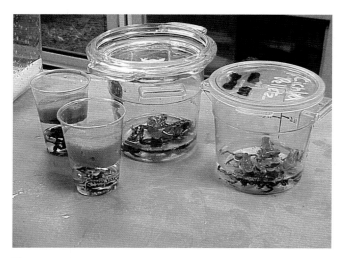

Figure 5-45 Medicating a large group of animals using a bath. (Photo credit Disney's Animal Programs, Deidre Fontenot).

Intratracheal and intrapneumonic infusion of therapeutics also could be used to treat pulmonic parasitism. Intraosseous catheters can also be used. Long-term use of catheters (IV or IO) has not been documented in amphibians, especially given the permeability and high success rate of delivery by bath.

Keep in mind that bioavailability and pharmacokinetic studies for amphibians are largely unavailable. Although amphibians have low metabolic rates and would be expected to require lower dosing levels compared to other vertebrates, they also have a high fluid turnover, which affects drug distribution and can increase a required dose. More research is needed to elucidate the therapeutic needs of these animals. Detailed formularies are available for amphibians,[58-60] but for rapid reference, a small formulary is provided in this text (Table 5-3).

TABLE 5-3 Formulary of Common Therapeutics Used to Treat Amphibians

Drug	Dosage	Route	Frequency	Duration
Bath or topical treatment				
Benzalkonium chloride	2 mg/L	Bath	q48h for 30 min	3 days, 5-day rest, retreat
Calcium glubionate (Neo-Calglucon)	2.3%	Bath	q24h for 1-2 h	
Chloramphenicol	10 µg/ml	Bath	q24h	
Ciprofloxacin	5-7 mg/L	Bath	q24h for 6-8 h	7 days
Dexamethasone sodium phosphate	0.1-0.5 mg/kg	Topical	q24h	3-5 days, then taper
Dimilin (diflubenzuron)	0.1 mg/L	Continuous immersion	Repeat with every water change or every 2 weeks	3 treatments
Enrofloxacin	10 mg/kg	Topical	q24h	10 days
Formalin 10%	1 ml/L	Bath	q48h for 10 min	To effect
Formalin/malachite green	0.007 ml/L	Bath	q48h, for 24 h	4 treatments
Gentamycin sulfate	8 µg/ml	Bath	q24h	
Itraconazole 1% suspension	0.01%	Bath	q24h for 5 min	11 days
Ivermectin	10 mg/L	Bath	Every 7 days, 60 min	
Ivermectin	0.2-2 mg/kg	Topical		
Ivermectin	2 mg/kg	Topical		
Levamisole	100-300 mg/L	Bath	q24h; repeat in 2 wk	3 treatments
Levamisole	10-100 mg/L	Bath in tank water; carbon filter at end of treatment	Continuous	3-5 days
Levamisole	10 mg/kg	Topical		
Levamisole (50 µl of 3.767 mg/ml)	94 mg/kg	Topical		Rinse 1 h
Levamisole in caecilians and *Pipa*	50-100 mg/L	Bath	q24h for 1-8 h (per animal tolerance)	Every 7 days
Metronidazole (50 µl of 1.008 mg/ml)	28 mg/kg	Topical	q24h	Rinse after 1 h
Morphine	20-160 mg/kg	Topical	As needed	
NaCl	1%-2.5%	Bath		
NaCl	20 mg/L	Bath	q24h for 6-8 h	
Nalidixic acid	10 µg/ml	Bath	q24h	
Nitrofurantoin	50 µg/ml	Bath	q24h	
Oxytetracycline	100 mg/L	Bath	q24h for 1 h	
Praziquantel	10 mg/L	Bath	3 h	
Praziquantel	8-24 mg/kg	Topical	Every 7-21 days	
Regranex	light coat	Topical	As needed	
Sodium chlorite (NaOCl$_2$)	20 mg/L	Bath	6-8 h	Once
Tetracycline hydrochloride	10 µg/ml	Bath	q24h	
Trimethoprim-sulfa	20-80 µg/ml	Bath	q24h	

TABLE 5-3	Formulary of Common Therapeutics Used to Treat Amphibians—cont'd			
Drug	**Dosage**	**Route**	**Frequency**	**Duration**
Injectable drug				
Amikacin	5 mg/kg	IM, SC, ICe	q24h, q48h	
Buprenorphine HCl	0.35-0.75 mg/kg	IM	q12h	
Butorphanol	0.05-1 mg/kg	IM, SC	q12h	
Calcium gluconate 10%	100 mg/kg	IM, IV, ICe	q4-6h	24 h
Calcium gluconate 10%	100 mg/kg	IM, IV, ICe	q4-6h	24 h
Ceftazidime	30 mg/kg	IM	q72h	
Dexamethasone sodium phosphate	0.1-0.5 mg/kg	IM, ICe	q24h	3-5 days, then taper
Enrofloxacin	5-10 mg/kg	IM	q24h	
Fentanyl	0.5 µg/g (ED$_{50}$)	IM		
Flunixin meglumine	1 mg/kg	IM, SC	q24h	
Furosemide	5 mg/kg	IM	As needed	
Ivermectin	0.2-0.4 mg/kg	IM		
Ketoprofen	2 mg/kg	IM, SC	q24h	5 days
Meperidine	200 µg/g	IM	q16h	
Morphine	20-160 mg/kg (as much as 100 µg/g)	IM, SC	As needed	
Oxytetracycline	50-100 mg/kg	IM	q48h	
Praziquantel	8-24 mg/kg	SC, ICe	Every 7-21 days	
Selenium	0.1 mg/kg	IM		
Thiamine	25-100 mg/kg	IM, ICe	Once; then PO	
Trimethoprim-sulfa	39 mg/kg	SC	q24h	
Vitamin D3	1000 IU/kg	IM		
Vitamin E	1 mg/kg	IM	Once; then PO	
Oral drugs				
Butorphanol	0.05-1 mg/kg	PO	q12h	
Calcium glubionate	1 ml/kg	PO	q24h	30 days
Doxycycline	5-10 mg/kg	PO	q12h, q24h	
Fenbendazole	100 mg/kg	PO	Every 7-14 days	
Fenbendazole	50 mg/kg	PO	q24h for 3-5 days	Repeat 2-3 wk
Itraconazole	2-10 mg/kg	PO	q24h	
Ivermectin	0.2 mg/kg	PO	Every 14 days	2-12 treatments
Metronidazole	50 mg/kg	PO	q24h	3 days, then reduce dose
Metronidazole	10 mg/kg	PO	q24h	5-10 days
Oxytetracycline	50 mg/kg	PO	q24h	
Paromomycin	50-75 mg/kg	PO	q24h	
Praziquantel	8-24 mg/kg	PO	Every 7-21 days	
Tetracycline	50 mg/kg	PO	q12h	
Thiamine	25 mg/kg	PO	Each meal	Until resolution of signs
Trimethoprim-sulfa	30 mg/kg	PO	q24h	
Trimethoprim-sulfa	15 mg/kg	PO	q24h	21 days
Vitamin B complex	0.1 ml/300 g	PO	q24h for 7 days, then q48h	
Vitamin D3	100-400 IU/kg	PO		
Vitamin E	100-400 IU/kg	PO	Every 7 days	

ICe, intracoelomic; *IM,* intramuscular; *IV,* intravenous; *PO,* per os; *SC,* subcutaneous.

Fluid Therapy[24]

Integumentary disease in amphibians is a very important condition, as the skin is an important organ in respiration and ion transport. When the skin is compromised, osmotic losses can be phenomenal. In cases of dehydration, amphibians may develop enophthalmia (sunken eyes), tacky mucous membranes, increased ropy mucus in the oral cavity, and wrinkled, discolored or tacky skin. Sometimes there is a "tightening" of the skin over the dorsum. Weight loss and a lack of urination during handling may also be indications of dehydration.

Aquatic amphibians rely on their kidneys for water excretion and solute retention. Should these organs fail, the animal cannot maintain ion, solutes, or fluid balances. In these cases, fluid therapy can be challenging. Replacement therapy may cause volume overload, which overextends the heart's capacity and can result in death. The key is to maintain electrolyte balance. The plasma osmolality should be greater than 200 mOsm/L. When the skin, kidney, or gills are damaged (as with infection), fatal electrolyte imbalances can occur. Fluid therapy is essential when there are obvious skin lesions or renal disease is suspected. Again, fluid overload is very common; therefore, isotonic solutions are critical. Freshwater is too hypotonic, whereas standard mammalian fluids are hypertonic. There are a number of amphibian isotonic solutions available, with the easiest for the clinician to make being amphibian ringer's solution (Box 5-2). When fluid overload is obvious (e.g., edema, ascites), then a more hypertonic solution is appropriate (Box 5-3). Wright[24] recommends keeping an amphibian no longer than 4 hours in a hypertonic solution without reassessment. In a pinch, a 3 : 1 nonlactated balance electrolyte solution using 5% dextrose and 0.9% sodium chloride can be used for ICe administration in life-threatening situations (e.g., very depressed, dehydrated animal; blood loss). Alternately, a 9 : 1 ratio (0.9% saline: sterile water) solution can be used but is not ideal.

BOX 5-2 The Recipe for Amphibian Ringer's Solution[62]

Distilled water	1 L
NaCl	6.6 g
KCl	0.15 g
CaCl$_2$	0.15 g
NaHCO$_3$	0.2 g

BOX 5-3 The Recipe for Hypertonic Amphibian Ringer's Solution[62]

Distilled water	1 L
NaCl	7.3 g
KCl	0.17 g
CaCl$_2$	0.17 g
NaHCO$_3$	0.22 g

Antimicrobials

There is not a great deal of pharmacokinetic data available for amphibians, and most doses are extrapolated from reptile medicine. Tetracyclines are not effective as a bath; ICe injection can cause local inflammation. The oral route is effective, but the drug is bitter and may not be accepted by the patient. Skin discoloration, irritation, and sloughing can occur with injection of enrofloxacin. In general, however, there are not many side effects reported at the published doses. Doses for antibiotics commonly used to manage amphibians can be found in Table 5-3.

Antiparasitics

The goal of treatment should not be to eliminate all protozoa, as many are considered indigenous flora; rather, when protozoa are considered a problem, treatment goals should be geared toward the reduction of protozoal numbers. Metronidazole is an effective drug for most protozoal infections. Paromomycin and sulfa drugs (SMZ-TMP) may be useful, especially with coccidia. Topical protozoal infections can be effectively dealt with using immersion baths in saltwater, dyes, and formalin (e.g., though this can be toxic and fatal). Doses for antiprotozoals commonly used to manage amphibians can be found in Table 5-3.

Levamisole has been used topically in a number of animals; however, flaccid paralysis can occur in caecilians and Surinam toads with prolonged exposure. If used topically, the drug should be rinsed off with aged water after 1 hour of contact.[61] Oronasal flushes of levamisole can be used to treat the larvae of the toadfly, which infest nasal passages, at a dose of 100 mg/L. Praziquantel can cause injection site reactions in *Typhlonectes* sp. Ivermectin can be used to eliminate nematodes, acariasis, and ticks. Some ivermectins have propylene glycol, which may irritate amphibian skin. Species-specific reactions can occur, and some animals may succumb at doses of 0.2 mg/kg. Paralysis can occur with high doses (200 mg/kg) of ivermectin, which can occur with inappropriate dilutions. Given supportive care and time, many animals recover. Ivermectin flushes of nasal passages can be performed at 10 mg/L for fly larvae. Fenbendazole is very effective against nematodes. Doses for anthelminics commonly used to manage amphibians can be found in Table 5-3.

Don't neglect to clean or treat the environment when there is a heavy parasite load. It is best to remove and replace soil and porous items.

Antifungals[39]

Immersion baths with salts, benzalkonium chloride, and dyes (malachite green) are useful for treating topical fungal infections. Anecdotal information suggests that caecilians may be sensitive to methylene blue, but this is untested.[5] Preparations of miconazole or ketoconazole cream can be applied to focal lesions. Daily, 5-minute baths in a 0.01% itraconazole solution (Sporanox, Janssen Pharmaceuticals, Beerse, Belgium; 1%

suspension diluted with 0.6% saline) for 11 days has been found to be curative for chytridiomycosis.

Documented reports of mucormycosis in amphibians have not addressed treatment options. Long-term systemic antifungal therapy may be attempted with amphotericin, which has shown good in vitro activity against *Mucor* species. Mortality from *Basidiobolus* was greatly reduced when dwarf African clawed frogs were bathed in benzalkonium chloride (2 mg/L) for 30 minutes every other day for three treatments, given a 5-day rest, and then retreated. Treatment of chromomycosis has been unsuccessful. In human cases, itraconazole is used with cryosurgery or surgical excision of lesions.

Antivirals

Reports using antivirals to treat amphibians are rare. The primary reason for this is that viral diseases are rarely diagnosed, because of a general lack of testing and because there are few affordable antiviral agents available in veterinary medicine. Veterinarians considering an antiviral for an amphibian should extrapolate the dose from the reptile literature.

Analgesics

Pain medication should be preemptive when there is an anticipation of pain (e.g., as with surgery). Opioids,[55,63] alpha-adrenergic, and nonsteroidal antiinflammatory agents can be used to provide pain relief (see Table 5-3). Pain in the amphibian can be recognized by the following signs:[63,64] immobility, lethargy, closed eyes, vocalization, color change, abnormal behavior, flick foot at affected area, aggression, lameness, and rapid respiration. Much more research is needed to fully comprehend the best methods to manage pain in amphibians.

Miscellaneous Drugs and Products

For amphibians, bandages or wraps can be difficult to apply and unrewarding. However, temporary liquid bandages or dental products can be used to provide a solid barrier against osmotic losses and a protective covering over abrasions and lacerations due to trauma. Products that are useful include Orabase (Colgate Inc., Canton, MA), Ilex (Medcon Biolab Technologies, Grafton, MA), facilitator (Idexx Corp., Elgin, IL), and Band-Aid Liquid Bandage (Johnson and Johnson Inc., Somerville, NJ), as well as other cyanoacrylate products. Regranex (Johnson and Johnson) and Carravet (Veterinary Product Laboratories, Phoenix, AZ) are additional wound care products that can be used to facilitate healing. Finally, the application of an artificial slime layer (Shield-X, Malibu, CA) before and after handling can be used to reduce the likelihood of further injuring the skin.

Emergency Treatment

When an amphibian presents for an emergency, a minimum database should be collected if the animal can tolerate it. Fluid therapy can be administered by soaking an animal in amphibian ringers (see Box 5-2), ensuring that the head stays above the water line. If the animal has fluid overload (e.g., ascites, anasarca), then use hypertonic amphibian ringers (see Box 5-3). Fluid overload might occur with hypotonic fluids, like a freshwater bath. Supplemental oxygen can also be used and administered directly or nebulized, taking care not to dry the animal out. There has been suggestion that cooling an animal[59] in the first 3 to 4 days after presentation may reduce the growth of potential pathogens and allow the medications to work. However, many bacteria are capable of regeneration at a range of environmental temperature, and lowering an ectotherm's body temperature will reduce its metabolic rate and, in turn, the distribution of various chemotherapeutics. Broad spectrum antibiotic therapy should be initiated and focused on Gram-negative and anaerobic organisms. If there is a suspicion of chytrids or *Chlamydophila,* then antifungals or doxycyclines should be given. Overall, the goals of emergency therapy are to isolate the animal, ensure appropriate temperature zones, provide oxygen, correct fluid deficits, and initiate treatment for an appropriate differential.

An entire chapter dedicated to critical care in the amphibian has been written;[62] salient points will be summarized. Hypotension in the amphibian can be recognized by pallor of the mucous membranes, collapse of the intraoral vessels (e.g., lingual plexus), and lack of definition of the ventral abdominal vein. A cut down to the abdominal vessel may be necessary for catheterization. Catheters have been placed this way experimentally, but not practically, in clinical medicine. Systemic corticosteroids may offset adrenal exhaustion and possibly increase the survivability of a patient.

The principles of the ABCs (airway, breathing, cardiac) of emergency medicine cannot be readily applied to amphibians; however, intubation and ventilation in addition to some drug therapies may prove successful (Box 5-4).

BOX 5-4	Emergency Drug Doses for Amphibians

Drug	Dose
Prednisolone sodium succinate	5-10 mg/kg IM
Epinephrine 1 : 1000	0.01-0.05 ml/100 g
Doxapram	5 mg/kg
Dexamethasone	1 mg/kg IM, IV
Calcium gluconate 10%	100 mg/kg IM, IV, ICe
Atropine	0.1 mg/kg SC, IM
Fluids 9 : 1 (0.9% saline: sterile water); use only if isotonic solutions are not available	2%-5% body weight ICe
Furosemide	5 mg/kg IM, IV

ICe, intracoelomic; IM, intramuscular; IV, intravascular; SC, subcutaneous.

NUTRITION

Assisting an animal through anorexia and illness by the provision of calories is a critical therapy to institute. The first goal of nutritional support is to feed a highly digestible product, as a sick animal may not be able to digest food at the same level as a healthy animal. The second most important goal is to make sure the food can pass through a feeding tube. This can be a problem with smaller animals and can be overcome by thoroughly grinding food or using powdered food products.

Some clinicians base caloric replacement on a calculation derived from the animal's body weight (~10% of the body weight q24h). It is more appropriate to calculate the basic requirements of the animal and give nutritional support in volumes that support the patient's digestion and comfort level (e.g., regurgitation may occur with assist feeding). The following formula can be used to calculate an amphibian's basal metabolic rate (BMR):[62]

$$BMR = 5 \times BWkg^{0.75} \text{ to } BMR = 10 \times BWkg^{0.75}$$

For diseased animals this should be increased to 1.25-2 × BMR. Additional species-specific and temperature-specific BMR formulas have been published[12,44] and may serve as a more specific tool. In general, monitoring weight is a good way to assess a feeding strategy. Observe trends and reevaluate the patient weekly. If there is weight loss in the face of caloric replacement, reconsider the quantity of calories, types of calories, and frequency of feeding, taking care not to overload the animal. Feeding a patient daily is not required to maintain condition, and it may cause unnecessary stress. Most prey items are 1 to 2 kcal/g.[44]

Nutritional products that are commercially available include Hill's A/D (Hill's, Topeka, KS), baby food that is meat based (note that these foods need supplementation to maintain Ca : P ratio), feline liquid CliniCare (Pet-Ag. Elgin, IL), Repta-Aid (Fluker Farms, Port Allen, LA), and Emeraid I or Emeraid II (Lafeber, Cornell, IL). Most of these are 0.6 to 1.4 kcal/ml. A gruel can also be made from a gel food normally offered to amphibians (Amphibian & Carnivorous Reptile, Mazuri/PMI Nutrition International, St. Louis, MO).

Whole foods can be offered, but should be prepared in advance to maximize the nutritional value. Predigesting the foods with pancreatic enzymes may be useful for amphibians with gastrointestinal disease (Prozyme, San Leandro, CA 94577-1258). Insects should have their heads removed to speed digestion. Whole rodents should be skinned to reduce digestion time. Frozen foods are easier to digest than nonfrozen foods due to cell lysis.

EUTHANASIA[15,64]

There are many different methods of euthanasia considered acceptable in amphibians. Barbiturates, MS-222, and isoflurane can all be used for euthanasia. MS-222 (overdose 200 mg/kg ICe) is rapid and does not harm organs for pathology. Phenobarbital can be used at 100 mg/kg ICe or via lymph sacs,

and death occurs within 30 minutes; intracardiac phenobarbital results in rapid death. The coelomic method may result is some histologic artifacts. Pithing an anesthetized animal into the foramen magnum is rapid, but it precludes histopathology on the brain. To ensure death, open the body cavity and remove the heart.

Hypothermia is not considered a humane method of euthanasia. Freezing an anesthetized animal has been done but only in small animals (<40 g), and the process must be rapid. A standard freezer (−20° C) is unacceptable, as it is too slow and some amphibians can tolerate short-term cold temperatures. CO_2 is considered by some to be inhumane because amphibians tolerate hypercarbia.

SURGERY[62,67]

Surgery should not be a daunting prospect to the exotic animal clinician. Amphibians heal well, tolerate blood loss, and tend to have fewer postsurgical complications than do higher vertebrates.

Preoperative Considerations

Animals should be fasted before surgery. For small amphibians, a 4-hour fast is sufficient, whereas for larger amphibians (>20 g), a 24- to 48-hour fast is more appropriate. The patient should be soaked before surgery in amphibian Ringer's solution for 60 minutes. Prophylactic antibiotics should be considered as appropriate, such as in cases of coeliotomy. Preemptive analgesia should be administered.

It is very difficult to maintain a moist patient in a sterile field. Most amphibian surgeries are considered "clean-contaminated." After soaking, the animal can be coated in ShieldX. Lubrication should not be used, as it can interfere with cutaneous respiration. Alternately, the patient can be moistened regularly with distilled or aged water during the procedure.

A 0.5% to 1% chlorhexidine solution should be used to gently disinfect the surgical site, avoiding active scrubbing. A disinfectant-soaked gauze can also be placed on the animal and allowed contact for 5 to 10 minutes. Draping is not easy in small patients, but it may be possible with larger animals. Ophthalmic instruments are preferred for amphibian surgery because they are delicate on tissues and enable the clinician to manipulate small tissues.

Postsurgical Considerations

Everting sutures should be used when closing an incision. Absorbable sutures absorb faster in a moist environment; therefore, nonabsorbable monofilament can be used instead. In most clinical cases, I observe healing before using suture absorption. Interrupted sutures should be used, as amphibians dehisce readily. Cyanoacrylate tissue adhesives can be used over sutured incisions to ensure a waterproof barrier and to prevent bacterial colonization.

Common Surgical Procedures

Common, minor surgical procedures include biopsies, identifying animals by marking or tagging, and performing cryosurgery (e.g., removal of cutaneous masses). Laparoscopy is a minimally invasive tool that is used for reproductive assessment and for internal organ biopsies. Insufflation may not be necessary, but if it is, CO_2 insufflation is appropriate as long as the animal is deflated after the procedure.

Amputation of the hindlimb can be done successfully and usually results in the return to all functions but reproductive. The entire femur should be removed; a stump should not be left, because it can become abraded and develop into an infection. Forelimb amputation can be done, but some animals need both forelimbs for posture, ambulation, and manipulation of food. Strong consideration for a species' natural behavior must be taken into account before performing amputation. Newts can regenerate missing limbs. Tail amputations can also be done in urodelans, and some species actually experience tail autonomy. Fracture repair is possible in larger specimens and should follow standard orthopedic practices.[65] In smaller animals, amputation may be more appropriate.

When performing a coeliotomy, care must be taken to avoid puncturing the lungs and gastrointestinal tract. Depending on season, the presence of large fat bodies and ovaries can make visualization of other organs difficult. A paramedian incision should be made to avoid the ventral midline blood vessel. Palpebral retractors can be used in small patients to maintain the incision and provide direct visualization into the coelomic cavity. In caecilians, surgery has not been reported, but several small paramedian incisions are recommended for exploration. I have performed a coelomic mass removal in a caecilian, but the approach was simple as the mass was well circumscribed. When performing a gastrotomy and enterotomy, the coelom should be packed with moist gauze to minimize contamination. Noninvasive methods should be attempted first. Two layer closures, as suggested in small animal medicine, would be ideal but are often not possible. A cystotomy can be performed to remove cystic calculi. Ovariectomies can be performed if care is taken to note vascularity. Many ovarian pedicles can be removed without hemostasis, but for complete ovariectomy, hemoclips may prove useful. Removing oviductal tissue is unnecessary.

Enucleation is considered a last resort and is used primarily as a pain management tool. There is a membrane between the eye and buccal cavity, which must not be damaged. Hemostasis must be foremost as exsanguination can occur, especially in small amphibians.

■ ZOONOSES[31]

Few cases of zoonotic disease transmission from amphibians have been reported; however, caution should still be exercised because many animals harbor organisms that can be pathogenic to humans. These would include *Salmonella* spp., *Leptospiral* spp., *Listeria* spp., *Edwardsiella tarda*, *Yersinia* spp., sparganosis, and *Escherichia coli*. Mycobacterial species that cause disease in amphibians can also be zoonotic and cause atypical mycobacteriosis in humans.

Acknowledgments

I would like to personally thank all of the individuals that helped to see this chapter to completion, including Hilary Corcoran, Marty Greenwell, Diedre Fontenot, Kathryn Gamble, Leigh Clayton, Michael Yuratovac, Alice Bereman, Ashley VanSimpa, Tom Meehan, Amy Shima, Ann Manharth, and Robert VanValkenburg. Many special thanks go to Kevin Wright and Brent Whitaker for their insight and their editorship of *Amphibian Medicine and Captive Husbandry,* the "encyclopedia of amphibian medicine," which I strongly suggest for the exotic animal veterinary bookshelf.

REFERENCES

1. Wright K: Taxonomy of amphibians kept in captivity. In Wright KM, Whitaker BR, editors: *Amphibian Medicine and Captive Husbandry,* Malabar, Fla, 2001, Krieger.
2. Wright K: Anatomy for the clinician. In Wright KM, Whitaker BR, editors: *Amphibian Medicine and Captive Husbandry,* Malabar, Fla, 2001 Krieger.
3. Wright K: Applied physiology. In Wright KM, Whitaker BR, editors: *Amphibian Medicine and Captive Husbandry,* Malabar, Fla, 2001, Krieger.
4. Duellman WE, Trueb L: *Biology of amphibians.* Baltimore, 1994, Johns Hopkins University Press.
5. Mylniczenko ND: Caecilians. In Fowler ME, Miller RE, editors: *Zoo and Wild Animal Medicine,* St. Louis, 2003, WB Saunders.
6. Wright K: Amphibian husbandry and housing. In Wright KM, Whitaker BR, editors: *Amphibian Medicine and Captive Husbandry,* Malabar, Fla, 2001, Krieger.
7. Vosjoli P: Designing environments for captive amphibians and reptiles, *Vet Clin North Am* 2(1):43-68, 1999.
8. Whitaker BR: Water quality. In Wright KM, Whitaker BR, editors: *Amphibian Medicine and Captive Husbandry,* Malabar, Fla, 2001, Krieger.
9. Fleming GJ, Isaza R, Spire MF et al: The use of digital thermography for environmental evaluation of reptile enclosures, *J Herpetol Med Surg* 13(1):38-42, 2003.
10. Cooper JE: Urodela. In Fowler ME, Miller RE, editors: *Zoo and Wild Animal Medicine,* St. Louis, 2003, WB Saunders.
11. Goodman G: Oral biology and conditions of amphibians, *Vet Clin North Am Exot Anim Prac* 6:467-475, 2003.
12. Wright K: Diets for captive amphibians. In Wright KM, Whitaker BR, editors: *Amphibian Medicine and Captive Husbandry,* Malabar, Fla, 2001, Krieger.
13. Wright K: Quarantine. In Wright KM, Whitaker BR, editors: *Amphibian Medicine and Captive Husbandry,* Malabar, Fla, 2001, Krieger.
14. Lewbart GA, Stoskopf MK: Amphibian medicine, selected topics, *Exot DVM* 4(pt 3):36-39, 2002.
15. Wright K: Restraint techniques and euthanasia. In Wright KM, Whitaker BR, editors: *Amphibian Medicine and Captive Husbandry,* Malabar, Fla, 2001, Krieger.
16. Stetter MD, Raphael B, Indiviglio F et al: Isoflurane anesthesia in amphibians: comparison of five application methods, *Proc AAZV*:255-257, 1996.
17. Downes H: Tricaine anesthesia in amphibia: a review, *Bull ARAV* 5(2):11-16, 1995.
18. Smith JM, Stump KC: Isoflurane anesthesia in the African clawed frog, *Cont Topics* 39(6):39-42, 2000.
19. Lafortune M, Mitchell, MA, Smith J: Evaluation of medetomidine, clove oil and propofol for anesthesia of leopard frogs, *Rana pipiens, J Herpetol Med Surg* 11(4):13-18, 2001.
20. Riggs SR, Mitchell MA, Diaz-Ferueroa O et al: Evaluating the clinical effects of clove oil and propofol on tiger salamanders (*Ambystoma tigrinum), Proc ARAV,* Minneapolis, Minn, 2003.

21. Keller CB, Shilton CM: The amphibian eye, *Vet Clin North Am Exot Anim Pract* 5(2):261-274, 2002.

22. Heatley JJ: Medication administration in amphibia, a clinical review, *J Herpetol Med Surg* 10(1):30-33, 2000.

23. Wright K: Applied hematology. In Wright KM, Whitaker BR, editors: *Amphibian Medicine and Captive Husbandry,* Malabar, Fla, 2001, Krieger.

24. Wright, K: Clinical techniques. In Wright KM, Whitaker BR, editors: *Amphibian Medicine and Captive Husbandry,* Malabar, Fla, 2001, Krieger.

25. Hoegman S: Diagnostic sampling of amphibians, *Vet Clin Exot Anim* 2:731, 1999.

26. Crawshaw GJ, Weinkle TK: Clinical and pathological aspects of the amphibian liver, *Sem Av Exot Pet Med* 9(3):165-173, 2000.

27. Wright K: Diagnostic imaging. In Wright KM, Whitaker BR, editors: *Amphibian Medicine and Captive Husbandry,* Malabar, Fla, 2001, Krieger.

28. Shildger B, Triet H: Ultrasonography in amphibians, *Sem Av Exot Pet Med* 10(4):169-173, 2001.

29. Wright K: Clinical microbiology of amphibians for the exotic practice. In Wright KM, Whitaker BR, editors: *Amphibian Medicine and Captive Husbandry,* Malabar, Fla, 2001, Krieger.

30. Wright K: Protozoa and metazoa infecting amphibians. In Wright KM, Whitaker BR, editors: *Amphibian Medicine and Captive Husbandry,* Malabar, Fla, 2001, Krieger.

31. Wright K: Bacterial diseases. In Wright KM, Whitaker BR, editors: *Amphibian Medicine and Captive Husbandry,* Malabar, Fla, 2001, Krieger.

32. Frye FL, Williams DL: *Self-Assessment Color Review of Reptiles and Amphibians.* Ames, 1995, Iowa State University Press.

33. Wright KM: Chlamydial infections of amphibians, *Bull ARAV* 6(4):8-9, 1996.

34. Green SL, Lifland BD, Bouley DM et al: Disease attributed to *Mycobacterium chelonae* in South African clawed frogs *(Xenopus laevis), Comp Med* 50(6):675-679, 2000.

35. Clayton LA, Manharth A, Pessier AP: Systemic mycobacteriosis due to *Mycobacterium avium* complex in a marine toad (Bufo *marinus), Proc ARAV,* Naples, Fla, p 148, 2004.

36. Crawshaw G: Anurans: frogs and toads. In Fowler ME, Miller RE, editors: *Zoo and Wild Animal Medicine,* St Louis, 2003, WB Saunders.

37. Reavill DR: Amphibian skin diseases, *Vet Clin Exot Anim* 4:413-440, 2000.

38. Daszak P, Berger L, Cunningham AA et al: Emerging infectious diseases and amphibian population declines, *Emerg Infect Dis* 5(6):735-748, 1999.

39. Pare JA: Fungal diseases of amphibians: an overview, *Vet Clin Exot Anim* 6:315-326, 2003.

40. Wright K: Mycoses: In Wright KM, Whitaker BR, editors: *Amphibian Medicine and Captive Husbandry,* Malabar, Fla, 2001, Krieger.

41. Pessier AP, Nichols DK, Longcore JE et al: Cutaneous chytridiomycosis in poison dart frogs (*Dendrobates* spp) and White's tree frogs *(Litoria caerula), J Vet Diagn Invest* 11:194-199, 1999.

42. Ackermann J, Miller E: Chromomycosis in an African Bullfrog, *Pyxicephalus adspersus, Bull ARAV* 2(2):8-9, 1992.

43. Wright KM, Whitaker BR: Metabolic bone disease in amphibians, *Exotic DVM* 1(pt 6):23-26, 1999.

44. Wright K: Nutritional disorders. In Wright KM, Whitaker BR, editors: *Amphibian Medicine and Captive Husbandry,* Malabar, Fla, 2001, Krieger.

45. Wright K: Cholesterol, corneal lipidosis, and xanthomatosis in amphibians, *Vet Clin Exot Anim* 6:155-167, 2003.

46. Wright K: The amphibian eye. In Wright KM, Whitaker BR, editors: *Amphibian Medicine and Captive Husbandry,* Malabar, Fla, 2001, Krieger.

47. Wright K: Clinical toxicology. In Wright KM, Whitaker BR, editors: *Amphibian Medicine and Captive Husbandry,* Malabar, Fla, 2001, Krieger.

48. Wright K: Idiopathic syndromes. In Wright KM, Whitaker BR, editors: *Amphibian Medicine and Captive Husbandry,* Malabar, Fla, 2001, Krieger.

49. Whitaker BR, Wright KM, Barnett SL: Amphibian respiratory diseases, *Vet Clin Exot Anim* 2:265-290, 1999.

50. Nichols DK: Amphibian respiratory diseases, *Vet Clin Exot Anim* 3:551-554, 2000.

51. Wright K: Trauma. In Wright KM, Whitaker BR, editors: *Amphibian Medicine and Captive Husbandry,* Malabar, Fla, 2001, Krieger.

52. Johnson D: External fixation of bilateral tibial fractures in an American bullfrog, *Exotic DVM* 5(pt 2):27-30, 2003.

53. Wright K: Spontaneous neoplasia in amphibian. In Wright KM, Whitaker BR, editors: *Amphibian Medicine and Captive Husbandry,* Malabar, Fla, 2001, Krieger.

54. Stacy BA, Parker JM: Amphibian oncology, *Vet Clin Exot Anim* 7:673-695, 2004.

55. Elkan E, Reichenbach-Klinke H: *Color Atlas of the Diseases of Fishes, Amphibians and Reptiles,* Neptune City, NJ, 1974, TFH.

56. Reichenbach-Klinke H, Elkan E: *The Principal Diseases of Lower Vertebrates: Diseases of Amphibians,* Neptune City, NJ, 1965, TFH.

57. Woodhams DC, Alford RA, Marantelli G: Emerging disease in amphibians cured by elevated body temperature, *Dis Aquat Organ* 55:65-67, 2003.

58. Wright K: Pharmacotherapeutics. In Wright KM, Whitaker BR, editors: *Amphibian Medicine and Captive Husbandry,* Malabar, Fla, 2001, Krieger.

59. Carpenter JW, Mashima TY, Rupiper D: *Exotic Animal Formulary,* ed 2, Philadelphia, 2000, WB Saunders.

60. Walker IF, Whitaker BR: Amphibian therapeutics, *Vet Clin Exot Anim* 3:239-256, 2000.

61. Crawshaw GJ: Amphibian emergency and critical care, *Vet Clin North Am Exot Anim Pract* 1:207-232, 1998.

62. Machin KL: Amphibian pain and analgesia, *J Zoo Wildl Med* 30(1):2-10, 1999.

63. Bradley T: Pain management considerations and pain associated behaviors in reptiles and amphibians, *Proc ARAV,* Reno, Nev, pp 45-50, 2001.

64. Wright K: Surgical techniques. In Wright KM, Whitaker BR, editors: *Amphibian Medicine and Captive Husbandry,* Malabar, Fla, 2001, Krieger.

Javier Nevarez

CHAPTER 6

CROCODILIANS

■ COMMON SPECIES KEPT IN CAPTIVITY

Modern-day crocodilians date back to the Mesozoic era over 65 million years ago, surviving to the present with relatively few evolutionary changes. Their biology, physiology, and anatomy are unlike those of any other reptiles. However, some species have suffered the effects of a changing environment and human encroachment; this situation has led to the formation of international programs dedicated to the preservation of threatened or near-extinct species. Of the 23 species of crocodilians, 13 can be found on the red list of endangered species.[1] Taxonomic identification varies among all species, and there is debate over the proper classification of species and subspecies (Tables 6-1 and 6-2; Box 6-1). In addition to having wild crocodilian populations, countries such as Australia, India, Mexico, Papua New Guinea, South Africa, and the United States maintain intensive production operations for various species.

In North America, the American alligator *(Alligator mississippiensis)* is the best-known crocodilian. Second to it is the American crocodile *(Crocodylus acutus),* a vulnerable species found in small numbers in Florida. The American alligator was considered a threatened species during the 1960s, but a captive rearing program in Louisiana has been successful at maintaining the estimated population at over 1 million animals.

The first type of captive rearing operations consisted of alligator farming. In farming operations, breeding pairs of alligators were kept in enclosed areas where they could mate and nest (Figure 6-1). The eggs were collected from the nests and incubated. The farming operations led to ranching operations in which eggs are harvested from the wild and incubated in private facilities (Figure 6-2). The alligators hatched on an "alligator ranch" are then raised for their hide and meat. To help maintain the wild populations, 14% of the hatched alligators are eventually returned to the wild. Louisiana is the primary producer of American alligators in the world. Captive rearing operations can also be found in Florida, Texas, Georgia, and other southern states within the United States where alligators naturally inhabit. In Louisiana the majority of the operations are ranches, whereas many farms still exist in Florida. Other crocodilian species, such as the Nile crocodile *(Crocodylus niloticus),* are primarily raised under farming operations in other countries.

In those states where alligator productions are present, there are opportunities for veterinarians to get involved with the industry. Some veterinarians, regardless of practice concentration, have alligator farmers or ranchers as part of their clientele and meet new challenges in their daily practice. A population management approach is necessary when working with these alligator production facilities. It is also advisable for veterinarians and farmers alike to be aware of the rules and regulations imposed by the local department of Wildlife and Fisheries.

In addition to being found in their natural environment, crocodilians are also found in zoos. Zoologic parks house different species of crocodilians for educational purposes, reproductive efforts, or both. As is the case with many other threatened species, zoologic institutions play a critical role in the captive reproduction of threatened species of crocodilians. Here the animals can be observed by specialists in a more controlled environment that mimics their natural habitat, although design and maintenance of the enclosures can be difficult. Disease prevention and control are other important considerations when it comes to oversight of threatened species.

TABLE 6-1	Taxonomy of the Family Alligatoridae	
Common name	**Scientific name**	**Geographic distribution**
American alligator	*Alligator mississippiensis*	Southeast United States
Chinese alligator	*Alligator sinensis*	Eastern China
Spectacled/Common caiman	*Caiman crocodilus*	Central and South America
Broad-snouted caiman	*Caiman latirostris*	South America
Jacare caiman	*Caiman yacare*	South America
Black caiman	*Melanosuchus niger*	South America
Cuvier's dwarf caiman	*Paleosuchus palpebrosus*	South America

TABLE 6-2	Taxonomy of the Family Crocodylidae	
Common name	**Scientific name**	**Geographic distribution**
American crocodile	*Crocodylus acutus*	North, Central, and South America
Slender-snouted crocodile	*Crocodylus cataphractus*	Africa
Orinoco crocodile	*Crocodylus intermedius*	South America
Fresh water crocodile/Johnston's crocodile	*Crocodylus johnstoni*	Australia
Philippine crocodile	*Crocodylus mindorensis*	Philippines
Morelet's crocodile	*Crocodylus moreletii*	Central America
Nile crocodile	*Crocodylus niloticus*	Africa and Madagascar
New Guinea crocodile	*Crocodylus novaeguineae*	Papua New Guinea and Irian Java
Mugger crocodile/Swamp crocodile	*Crocodylus palustris*	Indian subcontinent
Saltwater/Estuarine crocodile	*Crocodylus porosus*	Australia and Southeast Asia
Cuban crocodile	*Crocodylus rhombifer*	Cuba
Siamese crocodile	*Crocodylus siamensis*	Southeast Asia
African dwarf crocodile	*Osteolaemus tetraspis*	Africa
False gharial	*Tomistoma schlegelii*	Southeast Asia

BOX 6-1	Taxonomy of the Family Gavialidae	
Common Name	**Scientific Name**	**Geographic Distribution**
Indian gharial/True gharial	*Gavialis gangeticus*	Indian subcontinent

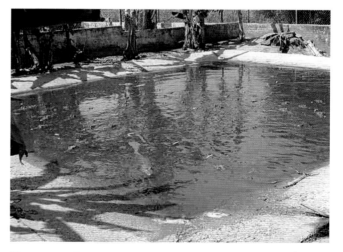

Figure 6-1 Outside enclosure at a Morelet's crocodile *(Crocodylus moreletii)* farm in Mexico.

Veterinarians may also encounter crocodilians as privately kept "pets." In the past, the spectacled caiman *(Caiman crocodilus)* and even the American alligator *(A. mississippiensis)* have been sold to the general public. There are many reasons why crocodilian species should not be maintained as pets. In addition to the physical dangers and risks associated with keeping crocodilians, there is the misfortune of inadequate husbandry, adversely affecting the reptile's health. Most crocodilians grow to be larger than other reptile species and therefore have significant space requirements. Like most animals requiring an aquatic environment, crocodilians need water that is clean and free of disease. Another husbandry issue is an incorrect diet, which can lead to metabolic abnormalities and overall poor health. Many private owners are unable or unwilling to provide these conditions for their crocodilians. In addition to these issues, most states will require special permits to own these

animals. Most people lack the proper ownership permits, and veterinarians could be liable if they treat these illegal patients. The biggest challenge that veterinarians face when treating illegally owned animals is that they are often the last chance for humane treatment for these animals. It is the duty of

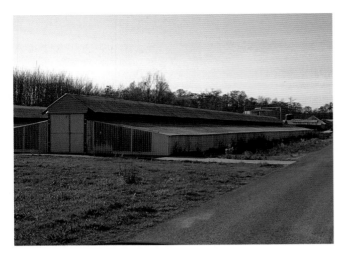

Figure 6-2 Building used in the ranching operation of American alligators *(Alligator mississippiensis)* in Louisiana.

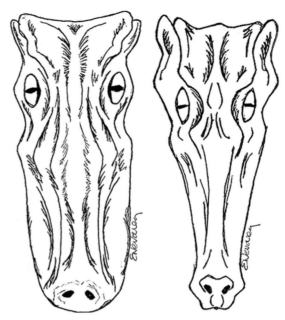

Figure 6-3 The dorsal aspect of the head of a crocodile and an alligator. Notice the V-shaped head of the crocodile vs. the more U-shaped head of an alligator.

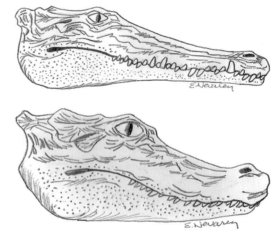

Figure 6-4 The lateral aspect of the head of a crocodile and an alligator. Notice that mandibular teeth are not visible in the alligator, whereas in the crocodile, the fourth mandibular tooth is clearly visible.

veterinarians to educate these clients and persuade them to place these animals in appropriate zoologic institutions or other accredited facilities.

Most of the material presented in this chapter specifically relates to the American alligator *(A. mississippiensis)*. Although most of the alligator information will apply to other crocodilian species, there are variations among groups that will be mentioned. The natural environment and geographic distribution of a species will often determine disease exposure. Once in captivity, all species are susceptible to the same diseases within that environment. In addition, there are some inherent differences among the three families of crocodilians—Alligatoridae, Crocodylidae, and Gavialidae—that have emerged from studying them in captivity.

BIOLOGY: ANATOMY AND PHYSIOLOGY

One of the most common questions a veterinarian may encounter regarding reptiles is "What is the difference between alligators and crocodiles?" The first difference is that they belong to two different families: the family Alligatoridae (see Table 6-1) includes the alligators and caimans, and the family Crocodylidae (see Table 6-2) includes all crocodiles. There is a third family, the Gavialidae (see Box 6-1), which contains the gharial, or gavial. Geographic location may help in the identification of some species. Alligators are thought to tolerate colder temperatures and live at higher latitudes, whereas crocodiles and caimans are less cold resistant and live in warmer areas.[2] However, there are some anatomic features that will be most useful in differentiating alligators from crocodiles. The alligators and caimans have a broad, u-shaped snout, whereas crocodiles have a more narrow, v-shaped snout. This difference can be observed by looking at the dorsal aspect of the head (Figure 6-3). A more obvious distinction can be made when looking at their mouth from the side (Figure 6-4). Alligators

and caimans have notches in the maxilla that fit the mandibular teeth. Therefore, they have no mandibular teeth visible if observed from the side with their mouth closed. On the other hand, crocodiles have the fourth mandibular tooth exposed when looking at them from the side with their mouth closed. *Integumentary sensing organs,* also known as *dome pressure receptors* (DPRs), are clear to gray pits present on the skin of crocodilians. Their function is not completely understood, but they may play a role as mechanoreceptors in prey detection or even

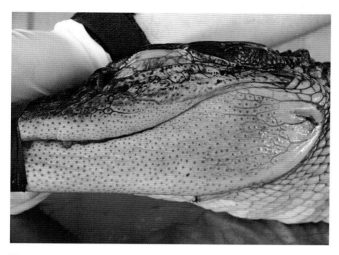

Figure 6-5 Dome pressure receptors (DPRs) on the lateral mandible of an alligator. The DPRs appear as gray dots over the skin.

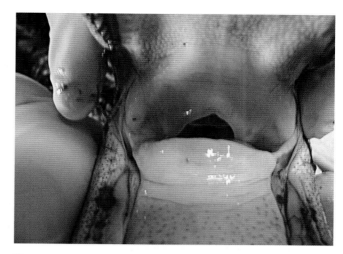

Figure 6-7 The velum palati (dorsocaudal) and gular fold (ventrocaudal) of an alligator. Together these structures comprise the palatal valve.

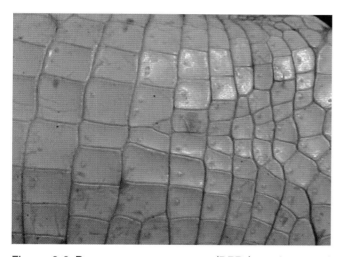

Figure 6-6 Dome pressure receptors (DPRs) on the ventral scales of a crocodile. The DPRs appear as clear to gray indentations on the scales.

as chemoreceptors aiding in detection of salinity levels.[3,4] Alligators and caimans have DPRs only on the lateral aspect of the mandible (Figure 6-5), whereas crocodiles and gharials have DPRs all over the body, most noticeably on the ventral scales (Figure 6-6). The presence of DPRs can be used to differentiate the two main groups of crocodilian skins in the leather market. An additional feature that could be used for differentiation of alligators and crocodiles is the salt glands, which are absent from the tongue of alligators and caimans but well developed in crocodiles and gharials.

An interesting anatomic feature of crocodilians is the *palatal valve,* also known as the *gular valve.* There is some discrepancy as to the name of this structure and its two components, but I will attempt to describe them based on the anatomic location.

Crocodilians have a true hard palate in the roof of the mouth that ends caudally in a soft palate. This soft palate has a ventral flap that is referred to as the *velum palati.* The velum palati is the dorsal component of the palatal valve, with its second and ventral component being the gular fold. This structure projects in a craniodorsal direction from the base of the tongue and has a cartilaginous base to it that is part of the larynx. Together, the velum palati and the gular fold form what is known as the palatal, or gular, valve (Figure 6-7). The function of this valve is to seal the pharyngeal cavity while under water to prevent aspiration. Crocodilians also have control of the nares and are able to open and close them as needed to prevent aspiration of water.

The respiratory system of crocodilians consists of well-developed lungs benefiting from a very effective inspiration aided by the intercostal muscles and the septum post hepaticum. The septum post hepaticum is a diaphragm-like muscle that creates a partial separation of the thoracic and abdominal viscera. A number of membranous connections separate the lungs and the liver, and an intricate mesentery system encompasses the gastrointestinal tract and viscera. All of these tissue structures may be necessary for allowing the changes in pressures that occur during diving.

The cardiovascular system of crocodilians also has special characteristics. Crocodilians have a four-chambered heart as opposed to the three-chambered heart found in other reptiles and amphibians. The circulation of blood through the crocodilian heart is like that in the heart of mammals, but the crocodilians possess a viable foramen of Panizza. This opening is located at the base of the heart between the left and right aortic arches and allows for venous admixture, which is essential during periods of diving to conserve oxygen.[5] During diving, there is pulmonary hypertension. This in turn creates increased pressure in the pulmonary artery and the right ventricle, which forces deoxygenated blood through the foramen of Panizza

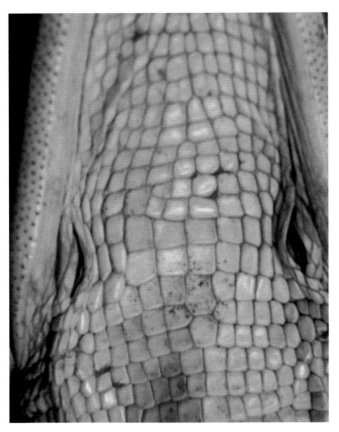

Figure 6-8 The submandibular glands of an alligator. These sometimes appear everted while an animal is being restrained.

into the left side of the heart and the aorta to be distributed through the body. This mechanism allows for conservation of oxygen and supplies oxygenated blood to those organs that require it the most, allowing some crocodilian species to stay submerged for up to 6 hours.[6] A second anastomosis may be present in other crocodilian species as a vessel connecting the two aortic arches.[2]

Submandibular (Figure 6-8) and paracloacal glands and a gall bladder are present in crocodilians. The hard dorsal scales are known as *osteoderms,* bony plates lined by skin. Crocodilians have a smaller gastric compartment distal to the stomach that is a gizzard-like structure in which rocks and other materials may be found. It does not appear as evolved as the ventriculus in birds, however. Crocodilian intestines have a thick wall and can have well-developed diffuse aggregates of lymphoid tissues like Peyer's patches. There is no urinary bladder, but the colon can hold large amounts of urine and water. Sexing can be performed by palpation of the cloaca; males have a phallus that can be palpated and extracted from the cloaca. Females have a well-developed clitoris that, depending on size, can be confused with a phallus. Internally paired gonads are found near the ventral surface of the kidneys.

Physiologic data, including body temperature, heart rate, and respiration, vary with species, age, and environmental factors (e.g., environmental temperature, season of the year).

■ HUSBANDRY
Environmental Considerations

Environmental considerations are variable depending on where a crocodilian species lives or is farmed. The aim of captive rearing operations is to produce a large number of animals in the most efficient way possible. In a zoologic or other educational institution, the goal is to exhibit the animals in an environmentally accurate artificial environment. The underlying policy of any aquatic enclosure should be clean water, appropriate diet, and enough space to accommodate the growth of the animals. As with most exotic animals, the challenge is to mimic a captive animal's natural environment.

ENCLOSURE SIZE

There are no specific references for the enclosure size of crocodilian species in captivity. The size of the enclosure will largely depend on the species of reptile and the purpose of their captivity. A general understanding of biology and natural behavior of the captive species is essential to designing appropriate enclosures. Although a zoologic institution housing the species might provide more specific advice, there are some general enclosure guidelines for the commercial production of American alligators: 1 square foot per alligator up to 24 inches in length (snout to tip of tail), 3 square feet per alligator for those between 25 and 48 inches in length, and an additional square foot of space for every 6 inches in body length beyond 48 inches.[7] These are the recommendations for the maximum stocking rate for alligators in commercial operations.

The recommendations for a zoo or educational facility are to make the exhibit as large as possible, taking into consideration the species being housed. A consideration for larger species is territoriality requiring an expanded enclosure. Male crocodilians may become more aggressive during the reproductive season, and keeping them separated should be a consideration if space is a concern. Exhibits can be outdoor, indoor, or a combination of both. Outdoor exhibits can closely mimic the natural environment but also present more challenges for maintaining water and environmental quality as well as for controlling diseases. Geographic location will also play a role in the creation of outdoor exhibits, as not all species of crocodilians can tolerate cold weather. Finally, some species can dig considerably, and measures must be taken to prevent an escape.

TEMPERATURE AND HUMIDITY

The temperature and humidity requirements for crocodilians in captivity vary with the species. Once again, an understanding of crocodilian biology and natural history is needed to try and duplicate their natural environment. An important consideration is the allowance of circadian variations in light cycle and temperatures to mimic their natural environment. This is not the case in many commercial operations, where they are maintained at a fairly constant temperature and humidity to achieve faster growth. From a health standpoint, this may allow for cross exposure of reptiles in commercial operations to infectious organisms that typically affect mammals. As the commercial reptiles are maintained at higher temperatures, new diseases commonly associated with mammals may adapt to living inside a reptile host and lead to clinical disease. In an enclosure, the temperature can be maintained via heating elements contained within the concrete slab, in line water heaters, or both. The water temperature must also be maintained during the refilling of the pen or enclosure to avoid significant temperature variations.

LIGHT

Light requirements for reptiles are still a controversial subject. In general, a source of ultraviolet B (UVB) light for herbivorous and omnivorous reptiles is recommended. Ultraviolet light is essential for the synthesis of vitamin D_3, specifically its active form 1, 25 dihydroxyvitamin D, which is essential for the metabolism of calcium and phosphorus. A lack of vitamin D_3 can lead to inappropriate calcium absorption, which in turn creates a metabolic imbalance resulting in metabolic bone disease. Metabolic bone disease, specifically secondary nutritional hyperparathyroidism, is recognized in many reptile species housed with an inappropriate source of UVB light, fed a diet deficient in calcium, or both. Carnivorous reptiles may also benefit from UVB light but are thought to obtain enough vitamin D_3 and calcium from their prey. The UVB light requirement of crocodilians is unknown, but as true carnivores they may thrive with minimal exposure to UVB light. It is a common practice on alligator ranches to raise animals in darkness with no source of UVB light or a normal light cycle. Most animals will grow well under these conditions, and some have reached adulthood without signs of metabolic diseases. However, I have also observed evidence of metabolic bone disease in a subset of captive American alligators being fed a commercial diet with no exposure to UVB light. In these cases veterinarians must also consider the possibility that the commercial diet may be deficient in calcium. Anecdotal stories from alligator ranches claim that weak, anorectic animals appear to improve after being exposed to sunlight over a period of time. Further research is needed to determine the UVB light requirements of crocodilians and the potential benefits of exposure to UVB light. Natural unfiltered sunlight is the best source of UVB light, but various artificial sources are available (e.g., fluorescent UVB light bulbs, mercury vapor light bulbs).

SUBSTRATE

The two main substrates in crocodilian exhibits are water and soil/sand. The species, age, and feeding habits must be taken into account; avoid substrates that may be ingested by accident and may lead to impactions. It is also important to prevent the public from throwing coins and trash into exhibits, as this may represent a source of toxicity and a cause of impactions. In commercial operations, a smooth covering is applied to the concrete to preserve the quality of the hide. Either an epoxy coating or plastic liners are routinely used as substrate.

◾ NUTRITION
Dietary Requirements

Crocodilians are true carnivores, as evidenced by their short gut and oral cavity. As such, they require a high protein diet, low in fiber. Their feeding habits in the wild will vary with age and food availability. Early on, their diet will consist of small invertebrates, amphibians, and reptiles. As they grow, they will eat larger prey of the type described earlier and will incorporate fish and birds into their dietary regime. With time, and depending on the species, size, and food availability, crocodilians will start eating mammals. There have been few studies investigating the nutritional requirements and feeding protocols of alligators.[8-10] Various commercial feeds are available for alligators maintained in captivity. The commercial rations consist of dry pelleted diets that try to provide full nutritional requirements. These diets can be found with a 45%, 47%, or 56% protein content, less than 11% fat, and approximately 3% fiber content.[11] Refined commercial alligator diets are widely used in production operations but may prove too expensive and/or inappropriate for the long term. A variety of whole prey feeds, such as chicken, nutria, and fish, are also recommended. If using nutria, be sure that it has not been killed using lead shot; if the lead is ingested, toxicosis can occur.[12] When feeding frozen fish to crocodilians, provide a vitamin B supplement or another meat source to prevent thiamine deficiency. To prevent dietary associated problems, purchase meat from a reputable source.

◾ PREVENTIVE MEDICINE
Quarantine

All animals should be quarantined before their introduction to a production or zoologic facility. A detailed history should be obtained from the source facility, including information regarding diseases to which the animals in question may have been exposed. One should always purchase animals from a reputable individual or institution. Little information will be known about wild-caught animals. A minimum quarantine period of 60 to 90 days is recommended in a building that is separate from the main facility. During the quarantine period, the animals can be examined for any sign of illness, and diagnostic tests (complete blood count [CBC], plasma or serum chemistry, West Nile virus antibodies, etc.) can be performed to assess their overall health status. If the alligators originated from an area where WNV is endemic, it is advisable to test for previous exposure to this virus.

Unfortunately, a true quarantine process does not often occur. Quarantine is limited by the availability of appropriate facilities, as well as by the time and production budget. Quarantine is also a challenge in commercial operations where there may be a large population of animals. Nonetheless, zoologic institutions and production facilities should try to establish an adequate quarantine program for their crocodilians.

Routine Exams

Routine physical exams of crocodilians may be incorporated into a zoologic institution's preventive health program. As animals get larger in size, performing physical exams becomes more hazardous. Chemical immobilization can be used, if needed, to perform necessary examinations, particularly on large crocodilian species. In commercial operations, the skins of a subset of the production animals will be examined at intervals before the anticipated time of slaughter. The time of hide examination presents an opportunity for veterinarians to examine the animals in more detail. Other than hide examinations, routine physical exams are not commonly performed in crocodilians from commercial operations.

Disinfection and Sanitation

Biosecurity is an essential part of disease prevention in any animal facility. The creation of a sanitation station at the entrance of each building is recommended to prevent introduction of disease organisms. These stations should contain a foot bath and a hand-washing station to decrease the opportunity of disease transfer between exhibits or buildings. A brush should be provided at each foot bath to thoroughly clean boots and shoes. The solution for the bath can be made of bleach or other commercial disinfectants, preferably with virucidal activity, and should be changed daily. Organic material will contaminate a foot bath, rendering it ineffective. The foot bath should be used before and after entering the building. A hand-washing station should consist of a water source, a sink, hand soap, and disposable hand towels. A waterless hand sanitizer product or exam gloves will suffice in lieu of a hand-washing station. In addition to the sanitation station, separate tools for working in each building are required. Separate working tools also prevent the transfer of diseases via nets, brooms, rakes, and so on. The buildings themselves must also be maintained free of pests and thoroughly cleaned whenever possible. In commercial operations, it is common practice to empty and disinfect the buildings after the slaughter period, before the introduction of new animals. Water quality is one of the main issues of concern when keeping crocodilians in captivity, and many health problems can be prevented if attention is paid to acceptable water quality.

◼ RESTRAINT

Manual restraint of crocodilians is essential for physical examination, administration of medications, administration of anesthetics, and relocations. The size and species of crocodilian will determine the best and safest restraint methods to be used. An experienced crocodilian handler must be available to help restrain the animal. Although alligators and caimans are usually thought of as being less aggressive than crocodiles, this may not always be true. All sizes and species should be handled with the safety of the people as well as the animal in mind. Crocodilians less than 1 m in length (snout to tip of tail) may be handled by one or two individuals. Those between 1 and 2 m in length should be handled by at least two or three individuals. Those longer than 2 m in length will require at least four to five individuals. Various tools (e.g., pole snares, nets, squeeze cages, traps) also can be used to restrain crocodilians. The head, tail, and limbs must be immobilized and controlled. Once the animal is under control, the mouth is secured with strong tape or a rope. Albino and leucistic animals can have increased skin sensitivity compared to the normal pigmented individual; therefore, additional care should be employed to avoid irritation of the skin. Restraint is stressful for the animal, and contact must be limited to the time it takes for the procedures being performed. (See Anesthesia for more discussion on chemical restraint.)

◼ HISTORY AND PHYSICAL EXAMINATION

Signs of illness in captive crocodilians are usually nonspecific. Anorexia, lethargy, a change in behavior, or death may be the first indication that something is wrong in a collection of animals or commercial operation. Adequate observations of the animals made by the personnel in the facility should be taken seriously. A visit to the facility is best undertaken during feeding time to avoid additional stress to the animals. At this time, the feeding and water quality policies can be evaluated. A thorough history should include information about the number of animals, source, age, most recent introduction, quarantine practices, feed, frequency of feeding, water quality parameters, clinical signs, time since first signs were observed, recent changes in management techniques, and any treatments such as salt, bleach, or antibiotics. Within a commercial operation, a subset of animals should be collected for disease diagnostics and necropsy. In addition to the obtaining of routine samples, tissues should be frozen for possible bacterial, fungal, or viral cultures. Within a zoologic institution, sacrificing live animals may not be possible, but veterinarians should obtain diagnostic samples from those with and without clinical signs. Necropsies should be performed in all dead animals. Live animals should undergo physical examination.

Once the animal is properly restrained, a physical examination can be performed. For safety purposes, veterinarians must be aware of the location of the head and tail at all times when performing the examination. A protocol should be followed for the examination process in crocodilians as in any other species. The oral examination can be performed if a speculum (e.g., PVC pipe, piece of wood) is inserted in the mouth before securing it with tape or a rope (Figures 6-9 and 6-10). Examine the eyes for evidence of discharge and assess their function (Figure 6-11). Examine the skin for any evidence of trauma or dermatitis, and then palpate the extremities, joints, musculature of neck, pelvic region, and tail. Joint swelling is often noted with infectious disease such as mycoplasmosis or trauma. Poor body condition may be reflected in atrophy of the muscles. In commercial operations, it is important to examine the skin on the animal's ventral aspect because this is the area where many disease manifestations will be noted. It is also common to find tooth marks, scratches, and lacerations on the ventral

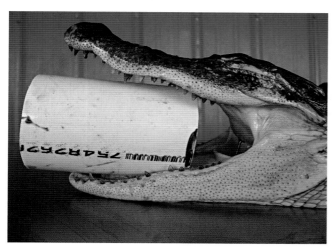

Figure 6-9 A PVC pipe used as a speculum. This allows for oral examination, endotracheal intubation, and any other procedure that requires access to the oral cavity.

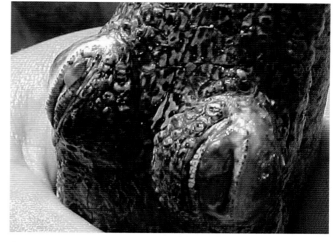

Figure 6-11 Severe conjunctivitis and periocular edema in a Morelet's crocodile *(Crocodylus moreletii)*. Chlamydiosis and mycoplasmosis should be a differential for this presentation.

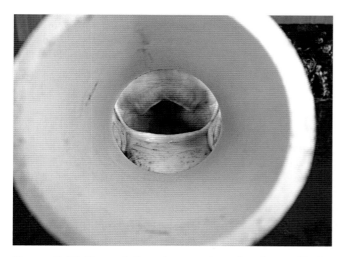

Figure 6-10 View of the pharyngeal cavity of an alligator through a PVC speculum inserted in the mouth.

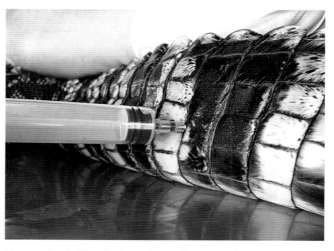

Figure 6-12 Blood draw from the ventral coccygeal vein approached from the lateral aspect of the tail in an alligator.

epithelial surface. Finally, examine the vent and cloaca for abnormalities. If working in a commercial operation, a veterinarian must examine multiple animals to determine if an observation is associated with disease. If working in a zoologic institution and any findings are suspected to be infectious in origin, other animals in the exhibit should be examined. As with any species, an examiner must know what a normal presentation is in order to recognize clinical signs of disease.

DIAGNOSTIC TESTING

Diagnostic tests used to determine crocodilian health status are no different than those used with other animal groups. CBCs, chemistry panels, and bacterial cultures can all be performed in crocodilians. However, there are limitations when it comes to the interpretation of test results because of the lack of reference ranges available for the multiple crocodilian species.

In addition, other diagnostic tests, such as those based on polymerase chain reaction (PCR) technology, enzyme-linked immunosorbent assay (ELISA), and other antibody or antigen serologic tests, are usually not validated for crocodilians. A clinician must inquire about the specifics of the tests being performed to make an accurate interpretation of the results. Published literature and the experience of other colleagues are invaluable for interpreting diagnostic test results of crocodilian species. Also there may be generally accepted diagnostic tests for diseases that have been recognized and studied in crocodilians, such as mycoplasmosis and WNV.

Venipuncture

There are various sites for venipuncture in crocodilians. The ventral coccygeal vein can be accessed from either the ventral or the lateral aspect of the tail (Figure 6-12). This vessel lies

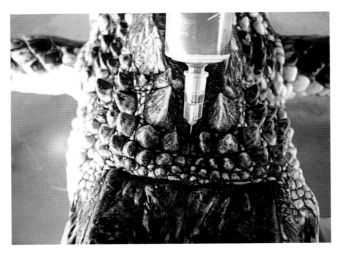

Figure 6-13 Blood draw from the supravertebral sinus in an alligator. Care must be employed to avoid inserting the needle too deep.

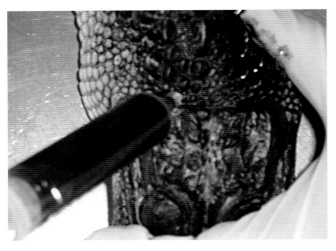

Figure 6-14 Blood draw from the lateral occipital sinus (unnamed) on the lateral aspect of the head/neck of an alligator.

ventral to the vertebral processes and on midline with the vertebrae. A second alternative is the supravertebral sinus, located on midline at the junction of the head and the neck (Figure 6-13). The examiner must be careful not to go too deep at this site, or physical damage may occur. A third site is an unnamed vessel located on both the left and right sides of the neck. This vessel can be approached from the dorsal aspect of the neck and is surrounded by muscles, decreasing the risk of coming in contact with nervous tissue (Figure 6-14).[13] A 3-ml syringe and a 22-gauge needle are recommended for collecting blood from crocodilians. Lithium heparin and EDTA tubes are used for plasma chemistry analysis and CBCs, respectively. If collecting serum, the tubes may have to sit for at least 45 to 60 minutes before centrifugation to allow proper separation of the serum from the blood cells.

Clinical Pathology

As with other species, CBCs and chemistry panels are a fundamental part of diagnostic testing of crocodilians. These tests can help assess the overall health status of the animals. A CBC can show evidence of acute or chronic inflammation that may prompt further investigation or lend direction to a definitive diagnosis. Chemistry panels can give insight into the hydration status and the health of the liver and kidneys. Also of importance are electrolyte values, which can show abnormalities related to poor diet and husbandry. A measurement of packed cell volume and total solids and/or total proteins is also an essential health indicator for crocodilian species. Fine needle aspirates, impression smears, and fluid analysis are diagnostic tools that can be useful in determining a definitive diagnosis. Urinalysis is not a practical test in crocodilians due to the absence of a urinary bladder and the fact that urine will be highly contaminated in a voided sample.

The hemocytometer with the Unopette Eosinophil Determination for Manual Methods stain (Becton Dickinson and Company, Franklin Lakes, NJ 07417-1885) is often used to obtain a CBC of crocodilian species and other reptile and avian species. A blood smear stained with Diff-Quick (Quik-dip stain, Mercedes Medical Physician and Laboratory Products, 7490 Commerce Ct., Sarasota, FL 34342) is also needed to complete the total estimated white blood cell count and obtain the cell differential count. Interpretation of CBCs from crocodilians can be challenging for veterinarians unfamiliar with the morphology of their white blood cells, which can vary from that of other reptile species. This variation found in crocodilian species is typical and more pronounced among reptiles. To become familiarized with the different cell types and their appearance, veterinarians should spend time scanning blood smears. This will often help veterinarians differentiate heterophils from eosinophils before the initiation of the differential count. Alternatively the samples can be submitted to a commercial laboratory that runs CBCs on blood collected from exotic animal species.

Imaging

Most imaging modalities (radiographs, computed tomography [CT] scan, magnetic resonance imaging [MRI], ultrasound, etc.) can be used on crocodilian species as long as there is a general understanding of their anatomy. Knowledge of normal anatomy is crucial for the interpretation of radiographs, CT scans, and MRI images. Knowledge of the anatomy will also help locate organs during ultrasound examination. Radiographs can be used to locate foreign bodies as well as diagnose fractures. Contrast studies can also be performed if the facilities and personnel are allowed to hospitalize the animal for an extended period of time. Barium sulfate (Liquid E-Z-Paque, E-Z-EM Inc., Westbury, NY 11590) and iohexol (Omnipaque, Amersham Health Inc., Princeton, NJ 08540) can be administered at 5 to 20 ml/kg PO. Iohexol can be diluted with water at a 1 : 1 to 2 : 1 ratio depending on the concentration.[14] Depending on the size of the animal and the site of interest, some imaging procedures may be performed with manual restraint or, if needed, chemical restraint. Neuromuscular blocking agents may be beneficial as chemical restraint agents if used appropriately and if the animal is monitored closely.

COMMON DISEASE PRESENTATIONS

Stress and Immunosuppression

Stress has been defined as "a physiological answer to a perceived threat that includes, but is not restricted to, increased adrenal secretion."[15] Stress can also be any event that challenges homeostasis. The response of the body to that event is complex and involves more than an adrenal response. The autonomic nervous system, the hypothalamic adrenal axis, neuropeptides, neurotransmitters, and neuroimmunologic mediators all have a role in the response of the immune system to stress.[16] Measuring stress and immunosuppression is a challenge in veterinary medicine. There are no specific tests available to provide a clinical measure of stress. Veterinarians concentrate on identifying a combination of physiologic changes that give them an idea of what is involved in a stress response. The stress response in crocodilians has been examined in relation to restraint, long-term corticosterone implants, cold shock, and stocking densities.[15,17-20] Lance et al. provides an overview of the physiology and endocrinology of stress in crocodilians.[21] Catecholamines, glucocorticoids, glucose, and lactate have been implicated in the stress response of crocodilians. Changes in the white blood cells have also been implicated with immunosuppression and the stress response.[17-19,21] There is enough evidence to suggest that stress plays an important role in the physiology of crocodilians and may indeed predispose them to illness. Overcrowding, handling, excessive noise, diet changes, temperature irregularities, and so forth, should be considered as predisposing or confounding factors of disease. All of these factors must be considered in the history of a clinical case and when determining treatment.

An example of how stress can play a role in disease susceptibility was observed in a case at a commercial alligator facility. This facility had animals with a history of chronic dermatitis. The alligators with the most severe lesions were consistently located on one end of the building, whereas those at the other end were unaffected or only mildly affected. The location of the severely affected animals was consistent in all buildings. One building had no affected animals. Based on a thorough history and observation of the operation, a possible explanation was determined for the occurrence of the dermatitis problem. All of the buildings with affected animals had PVC pipes on the inside walls that delivered water to each individual pen. A strong water stream fell from the pipes down into the water and the strength of the stream decreased from one end of the building (inflow) to the other end (outflow). The strength of the water stream was considerable near the inflow. The building with no affected animals did not have any source of falling water into the pens. Water quality, temperature, and feed were the same in affected and nonaffected buildings. The most affected animals happened to be in the pens at the inflow side of the building with the number of affected animals decreasing toward the outflow side of the building. This constant flow of water was creating a constant movement of the water surface and consequently stimulating the alligators via the DPRs. Once this watering system was changed, the cases of dermatitis decreased and no new cases were reported. Although other factors, such as water quality, may have contributed to the dermatitis, the change in the watering system decreased the progression and occurrence of the disease. This case demonstrates the importance of addressing the environment, as well as the animals, when working in commercial operations.

Bacterial Diseases

Bacterial diseases in captive crocodilians occur primarily as opportunistic infections. Poor water quality, trauma, and stress are some of the factors that contribute to bacterial infections in crocodilians. In their natural environment, crocodilians appear to have a stronger ability, compared with other species, to withstand bacterial infections. Reports of antibacterial properties in serum and tissues of crocodilians[22,23] offer a possible explanation. The possibility of increased antibacterial properties in the serum and tissues of alligators should not mislead people into thinking that crocodilians are resistant to bacterial infections. It is true that they appear to tolerate trauma and other lesions that would be fatal in many species, but crocodilians are still capable of succumbing to an array of microorganisms, including bacteria. In fact, a number of bacterial infections have been reported in crocodilians, and septicemias are thought to be a frequent finding. Septicemias can be diagnosed in postmortem examinations and are often associated with a wide number of bacteria, many of them normal gut flora. There is an abundance of information about bacteria recovered from the American alligator *(A. mississippiensis)*[24-39] (Table 6-3) and from African dwarf crocodiles *(Osteolaemus tetraspis)*.[40]

SALMONELLA INFECTION

Salmonella spp. are normal inhabitants of the gut in most reptile species and crocodilians.[41-43] The importance of *Salmonella* sp. arises more from its zoonotic potential rather than its ability to cause disease in crocodilians, but it has been reported to cause deaths in Nile crocodile *(C. niloticus)* hatchlings.[44] In most commercial operations the meat is sold as a by-product of the hide production. Various species of *Salmonella* and other bacteria have been isolated from the meat of crocodiles in commercial operations in an attempt to address the concern of zoonoses.[35,38,45-49] Zoologic institutions that have smaller crocodilians as part of a "petting" station should exercise caution, as fecal shedding of *Salmonella* sp. occurs. Although the zoonotic potential exists, there are no well-documented cases of human infections originating from crocodilians.

CHLAMYDIOSIS

Chlamydiosis has also been reported in crocodilian species.[44] There is a report of an isolate, closely associated to

TABLE 6-3	Bacteria Isolated from *A. mississippiensis* With and Without Clinical Signs of Disease		
Isolate	**Tissue**	**Clinical signs/lesions**	**Reference**
Aeromonas hydrophila	Blood	Yes	32
	Lungs, heart, liver, kidneys, intestines, oral cavity	Yes, No	24
	Lungs, blood	Yes	25
	Eye	Yes	26, 33
	Oral cavity, water	No	28
Aeromonas sp.	Lungs	Yes	34
Acitenobacter calcoaceticus	Oral cavity	No	28
Aerobacter radiobacter	Oral cavity	No	28
Bacillus sp.	Not specified	Yes	35
Bacteroides asaccharolyticus	Oral cavity	No	28
Bacteroides bivius	Oral cavity, water	No	28
Bacteroides loescheii/denticola	Oral cavity, water	No	28
Bacteroides oralis	Oral cavity	No	28
Bacteroides sordellii	Oral cavity	No	28
Bacteroides thetaiotamicron	Oral cavity	No	28
Bacteroides vulgatus	Oral cavity	No	28
Bacteroides sp.	Water	No	28
Citrobacter freundii	Blood	Yes	29
	Oral cavity	No	28
Clostridium bifermentans	Oral cavity, water	No	28
	Lungs	Yes	34
Clostridium clostriidoforme	Oral cavity	No	28
Clostridium innoculum	Water	No	28
Clostridium limosum	Oral cavity	No	28
Clostridium sordellii	Oral cavity, water	No	28
Clostridium sporogenes	Blood	Yes	34
Clostridium tetani	Oral cavity	No	28
Clostridium sp.	Blood	Yes	34
Corynebacterium sp.	Tail abscess	Yes	25
Dermatophilus sp.	Skin	Yes	36, 37
Diphtheroid sp.	Oral cavity	No	28
Edwardsiella tarda	Kidney, feces	Yes	30
	Fat body, pericardial fluid	Yes	34
Enterobacter agglomerans	Blood	Yes	29
Enterobacter cloacae	Oral cavity, water	No	28
Enterobacillus sp.	Lungs	Yes	25
Escherichia coli	Systemic	Yes	38
Fusobacterium nucleatum	Oral cavity	No	28
Fusobacterium varium	Oral cavity	No	28
Klebsiella oxytoca	Skin	Yes	29
	Oral cavity	No	28
Klebsiella sp.	Lungs	Yes	59
Micrococcus kristinae	Blood	Yes	32
Moraxella sp.	Oral cavity, water	No	28
Morganella morganii	Blood	Yes	29
	Oral cavity	No	28
	Lung	Yes	34
Mycoplasma alligatoris	Multiple tissues	Yes	32, 39
Pasteurella haemolytica	Oral cavity	No	28
Pasteurella multocida	Lungs	Yes	31
Pasteurella sp.	Oral cavity, water	No	28
Peptococcus magnus	Oral cavity	No	28
Peptococcus prevotii	Oral cavity	No	28
Proteus mirabilis	Blood	Yes	32

TABLE 6-3	Bacteria Isolated from *A. mississippiensis* With and Without Clinical Signs of Disease—cont'd		
Isolate	**Tissue**	**Clinical signs/lesions**	**Reference**
Proteus vulgaris	Oral cavity	No	28
	Oviduct	Yes	30
	Blood	Yes	32
	Lung	Yes	34
Proteus sp.	Blood	Yes	29
Pseudomonas cepacia	Oral cavity	No	28
Pseudomonas diminuta	Water	No	28
Pseudomonas fluorescens	Water	No	28
Pseudomonas pickettii	Oral cavity	No	28
Pseudomonas vesicularis	Water	No	28
Pseudomonas sp.	Lungs, pharynx	Yes	25
	Water	No	28
Salmonella typhimurium	Gastrointestinal tract	Yes	25
Salmonella braenderup, anatum	Cloaca	No	25
Serratia marcescens	Skin	Yes	29
Serratia odorifera	Oral cavity	No	28
Staphylococcus aureus	Lungs	Yes	31
Staphylococcus cohnii	Blood	Yes	32
Streptococcus sp. β-hemolytic	Lungs	Yes	34
Vibrio parahemolyticus	Blood	Yes	32

Chlamydophila psittaci, obtained from the livers of Nile crocodiles *(C. niloticus)* in Zimbabwe.[44] This infection is thought to have an acute course characterized by a hepatitis in which hatchling mortalities are observed. A chronic form of reptilian chlamydiosis characterized by conjunctivitis has also been reported and may be more common.[44] There have been reports of concurrent *Chlamydia* sp. isolates in cases of mycoplasmosis and adenoviral infections.[2]

DERMATOPHILOSIS ("BROWN SPOT DISEASE")

Dermatophilosis or "brown spot disease" is thought to be caused by *Dermatophilus* sp., with most of the cultures resembling *Dermatophilus congolensis,* and affects both crocodiles and alligators.[36,37,50-52] The characteristic brown to red lesions are located usually at the junction of the ventral abdominal scales, which may become ulcerated over time. This has occurred in both alligator and crocodile operations. This disease does not respond well to antimicrobial therapy; therefore, intensive hygiene practices are required to prevent and control outbreaks.

MYCOPLASMOSIS

Mycoplasma alligatoris is a recognized respiratory pathogen of crocodilians. It has been documented in *A. mississippiensis* and in the broad-nosed caiman *(Caiman latirostris).*[32,39,53] Other crocodilian species closely related to alligators also may be susceptible to this intracellular organism. Clinical signs are nonspecific and include lethargy, weakness, anorexia, white ocular discharge, paresis, and edema (facial, periocular, cervical, limbs).[34] Pathologic examination often reveals evidence of pneumonia, pericarditis, and polyarthritis. Helmick et al.

reported antimicrobial susceptibility for *M. alligatoris* with doxycycline, oxytetracycline, enrofloxacin, sarafloxacin, tilmicosin, and tylosin showing effectiveness against the bacteria.[54] A second mycoplasma species, *M. crocodyli,* was also described in Nile crocodiles with lesions similar to those observed with *M. alligatoris.*[55] Some studies have examined the use of an autogenous vaccine for *M. crocodyli,* but its efficacy has yet to be determined.[56,57]

MYCOBACTERIOSIS

Cases of pulmonary and enteric mycobacterial infections are mentioned by Huchzermeyer[2] and Youngprapakorn et al.[58] These reports include *Mycobacterium marinum* and *M. fortuitum* from different spectacled caimans *(C. crocodilus),* *M. avium* from an unspecified species of crocodile and from Nile crocodiles *(C. niloticus),* and *M. ulcerans* from Johnston's crocodiles *(C. johnstoni).*[2] Many other reported cases are based on gross findings and histopathology with acid-fast positive organisms identified microscopically. There are also some observed clinical cases of suspected yet unconfirmed pulmonary mycobacteriosis, based on necropsy and histopathologic evaluation.[59] Difficulties of growing *Mycobacterium* spp. make obtaining a definitive diagnosis challenging. Other diagnostic tools, such as PCR technology, may be beneficial in the identification of future mycobacteriosis cases.

Viral Diseases

Virus identification and diagnosis in reptiles has lagged compared to virus identification and diagnosis in other species. This delay has occurred primarily because of difficulties in developing diagnostic tests and lack of knowledge of viruses that affect reptiles and crocodilians. Many conditions that go undiagnosed may be caused by viruses. These may be new viruses or just viral diseases unknown to occur in reptilian or crocodilian species. There are only a few recognized viruses that have been documented in crocodilians.

Jacobson et al.[33] described an adenovirus-like infection in captive Nile crocodiles (C. niloticus) characterized by nonspecific clinical signs, lethargy, and anorexia. Conjunctivitis and blepharitis were also observed in one of two crocodiles.[2,33] Histopathologic examination revealed intranuclear inclusions, primarily in the liver but also in the intestines, pancreas, and lung. Both horizontal and vertical transmission have been postulated for this adenovirus-like infection.[2] Diagnosis is obtained through postmortem examination, and no treatment regimes have been established.

Coronavirus, influenza C virus, and paramyxovirus have been identified by transmission electron microscope in the feces of crocodilians.[2] Herpesvirus-like particles were identified by electron microscopy in the skin of a salt water crocodile (C. porosus).[60] There is a second finding of herpesvirus identified from the cloaca of an American alligator (A. mississippiensis) via PCR.[61] The clinical significance of these findings is unknown. Seroconversion to paramyxovirus and eastern equine encephalitis virus has also been reported in crocodilians.[2]

POXVIRUS

Parapoxvirus or pox-like viruses have been identified in five different crocodilian species: spectacled caiman (Caiman crocodilus fuscus),[62,63] Brazilian caiman (Caiman crocodilus acre),[64] Nile crocodile (Crocodylus niloticus),[65,66] saltwater crocodile (Crocodylus porosus),[67] and freshwater crocodile (Crocodylus johnstoni).[67] Pox lesions in caimans will be 1 to 3 mm in diameter, gray to white in color, and coalescing to macular. They may appear on the head, palpebra, maxilla, mandible, limbs, palate, tongue, and gingiva.[62-64] Palpebral and generalized edema also may be present. Resolution of clinical signs has been observed with and without changes in husbandry practices.[63,64] In crocodiles the lesions are described as 2 to 8 mm in diameter, yellow to brown, wart-like, sometimes firm, and unraised to raised nodules with occasional shallow ulcers. In crocodiles pox lesions appear on the head, palpebra, nostrils, sides of the mouth, oral cavity, limbs, ventral neck and coelom, and at the base of the tail.[65,66] Resolution of lesions was reported to occur as early as 3 to 4 weeks from the onset of clinical signs.[65] Histopathologic findings include epithelial hyperplasia, acanthosis, hyperkeratosis, and necrosis, with intracytoplasmic Borrel and Bollinger's bodies being visible in some cases.[62-66] Secondary bacterial and fungal infections may occur concurrently with the viral infection. At this time there are no specific treatment recommendations. The use of an autogenous vaccine to treat poxvirus in Nile crocodiles (C. niloticus) has had some success.[65] Mosquito control and good hygiene are essential in preventing and controlling poxvirus outbreaks.

WEST NILE VIRUS

West Nile virus (WNV) has been reported to affect various crocodilian species, including the American alligator (A. mississippiensis),[68] the Nile crocodile (C. niloticus),[69] and the Morelet's crocodile (C. moreletii).[70] Crocodilians likely become infected, as birds and mammals do, via a mosquito bite. There is also the possibility of infection after ingestion of an animal with a high viral load of WNV, as reported by Klenk et al.[71] This last scenario is more likely to occur when crocodilians are housed outdoors and not in enclosed buildings, as in most ranching operations. It has been demonstrated that alligators can serve as amplifiers of WNV.[71] Although there is a lot to be learned about WNV in crocodilians, it is believed that once infected, they can develop high viremias and shed the virus in the feces. Fecal shedding leads to horizontal transmission of the virus. There is clinical evidence for horizontal transmission to occur in commercial operations. Fecal shedding and high viremias also raise the concern of zoonosis, especially in commercial operations where animals are being slaughtered and people come in contact with blood and tissues. A strict building quarantine and hygiene strategies should be implemented to prevent the spread of WNV to other animals in the facility as well as to the personnel. In the state of Louisiana there are a number of recommendations provided to help alligator producers cope with episodes of WNV and prevent spread of the disease (Box 6-2).

BOX 6-2 **Recommendations Made to Alligator Producers in Louisiana on How to Prevent and Manage West Nile Virus**

1. Buildings with affected animals should be maintained under isolation from other buildings in the farm.
2. Feeding and cleaning of affected buildings should be performed last, after all other nonaffected buildings.
3. A foot bath (1 part water, 1 part bleach) should be placed at the entrance of the building to disinfect the shoes and boots of farm employees before and after entering the building. This foot bath should be changed on a daily basis. In addition, a set of shoes or boots may be kept only to be used inside affected buildings.
4. Hands should be washed before and after entering the building.
5. The water should be changed more frequently in affected buildings, at least once a day. This may create additional stress on the animals but should decrease the amount of feces and therefore viral organisms possibly present in the water. Any special treatment of the discharge water still remains to be determined.
6. Affected animals should not be transported to other alligator farms for processing of hides or meat.
7. Additional care should be exercised during the slaughter process to avoid direct contact with the blood and organs of animals known as exposed to, or affected with, West Nile virus.
8. Dead animals should be disposed of by burning the carcasses.
9. Aggressive mosquito control is required to help in the prevention of the disease.

Affected animals in captive operations have ranged in age from 1 month to over 12 months. In younger animals infection is usually acute and severe, with as much as 60% mortality. The pattern of deaths is peracute, usually seen as a sudden onset of mortalities followed by a peak and subsequent decline in the number of deaths. However, sporadic mortalities may also be noted, especially in older animals. Clinical signs of WNV in alligators include swimming in circles, head tilt, muscle tremors, weakness, lethargy, and anorexia.[72] Bloating and difficulties swimming have also been observed but occur less commonly.[72]

Gross findings from WNV-infected alligators are nonspecific. Light microscopy of tissues from infected animals may reveal diffuse severe heterophilic, histiocytic, and necrotizing enterocolitis; heterophilic meningoencephalitis; necrotizing and heterophilic hepatitis; heterophilic and histiocytic splenitis; generalized heterophilic and histiocytic lymphoid folliculitis; and necrotizing and heterophilic pancreatitis. Veterinarians may also observe a mild multifocal heterophilic and lymphohistiocytic interstitial nephritis, gastritis, and mild pulmonary congestion and edema. Strong immunopositivity results have been observed in the brain, liver, spleen, pancreas, kidney, and gastrointestinal tract after immunohistochemistry testing for WNV. Proliferative enteritis has been diagnosed in a group of alligators positive for WNV. The colon lesions tested positive for WNV via reverse transcriptase polymerase chain reaction (RT-PCR), culture, and immunohistochemistry[59,72] (Figure 6-15). These affected alligators were bloated and unable to submerge themselves; these symptoms may have been due to a blockage caused by the fibrinous membrane in the colon.

There is no known treatment for WNV-infected crocodilians. Mosquito control, strict quarantine, and biosecurity are essential for the prevention of WNV. Once WNV is present within an operation, it is critical to maintain infected and exposed animals in strict isolation. The ill and exposed animals must not be moved to other areas or buildings where WNV

has not been observed. Failure to maintain strict isolation may result in the spread of the virus throughout the facility. In addition, there should be strict biosecurity measures, especially in the affected areas or buildings. Tools such as nets, feeding utensils, boots, and so forth, must be left in the affected area and not introduced to other, "clean" areas or buildings. The surviving animals will continue to thrive after the WNV infection has run its course, but it is unknown for how long thereafter they can shed the virus. Antibody titers of 1 : 640 and 1 : 320 were observed in two alligators 14 months after exposure to WNV. These antibody titer results were obtained via a plaque reduction neutralization test. Definitive diagnosis of WNV infection should be based on history, clinical signs, and the results of diagnostic tests. Postmortem diagnosis can be performed via RT-PCR and/or viral culture of brain, spinal cord, or liver, with immunohistochemistry providing additional supportive evidence of WNV infection. Immunohistochemistry may prove useful as an antemortem test when applied to biopsies of the colon mucosa.

Fungal Diseases

Fungal infections also occur with some frequency in captive crocodilians. Most fungi are opportunistic invaders of the integument, respiratory system, and gastrointestinal tract. Poor water quality, trauma, stress, and extreme temperatures can contribute to the occurrence of fungal disease. It is thought that most fungal infections in crocodilians are of enteric origin and occur in other tissues secondary to an immunocompromised state.[2] It is important to remember that fungi are considered ubiquitous organisms in nature. Therefore, it is not uncommon to isolate fungi from tissues (e.g., skin, intestines) that are in contact with water and soil. The presence of fungi will vary with geographic location and management techniques that affect the different environments for their growth. There are a number of fungi that have been isolated from crocodilians[2,40,51,73-80] (Table 6-4). Some of these fungal organisms were associated with disease, whereas others were incidental findings. Diagnosis of fungal disease requires the identification of a fungal organism via culture or special stains of infected tissues. Positive identification of genus and species may be difficult. Treatment is expensive and may be affordable only when administering to a small number of animals. It also requires a long treatment period of at least 2 or 3 months. For these reasons, many fungal infections go untreated, and recommendations are made for prevention of disease.

Parasites

A number of parasites are known to affect crocodilians. Protozoa, nematodes, trematodes, and pentastomes have all been reported in crocodilians.[2] Cestode larvae have been found in some species, but no adult tapeworms are reported from crocodilians.[2] External parasites, such as leeches, flies, mosquitoes, ticks, and mites, can also affect crocodilians.[2] The presence of scales has created a misconception about the possibilities for external parasitism in crocodilians. However, there are a

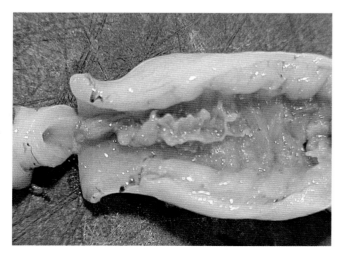

Figure 6-15 Fibrinous colitis in an alligator with West Nile virus. This animal was unable to submerge itself.

TABLE 6-4	Fungi Isolated from Crocodilians Around the World		
Fungus	**Lesions**	**Species**	**Reference**
Acremonium sp.	Intestinal contents	*Osteolaemus tetraspis*	40
Alternaria alternata	Skin	*Alligator mississippiensis*	73
Arthrinium sp.	Intestinal contents	*Osteolaemus tetraspis*	40
Aspergillus clavatus	Intestinal contents	*Osteolaemus tetraspis*	40
Aspergillus flavus	Not specified	*Crocodylus porosus*	2
	Skin	*Crocodylus porosus*	51
	Intestinal contents	*Osteolaemus tetraspis*	40
Aspergillus fumigatus	Skin	Caimans (species not specified)	2
	Lungs	*Alligator mississippiensis*	2
Aspergillus niger	Not specified	*Crocodylus porosus*	74
	Skin	*Crocodylus porosus*	51
	Intestinal contents	*Osteolaemus tetraspis*	40
	Skin	*Alligator mississippiensis*	73
Aspergillus ustus	Lungs	*Alligator mississippiensis*	2
Aspergillus versicolor	Not specified	*Crocodylus porosus*	2
Beauveria bassiana	Lungs	*Alligator mississippiensis*	75
	Lungs	*Crocodylus niloticus*	2
Beauveria sp.	Intestinal contents	*Osteolaemus tetraspis*	40
Candida albicans	Oral cavity	Caimans (species not specified)	2
Candida guillermondii	Intestinal contents	*Osteolaemus tetraspis*	40
Candida krusei	Intestinal contents	*Osteolaemus tetraspis*	40
Candida parasilosis	Skin	*Crocodylus porosus*	51
Candida sp.	Skin	*Crocodylus porosus*	51
Cephalosporium sp.	Muscle	*Caiman crocodilus*	2
	Lungs	*Caiman sclerops*	76
Chaetomium globosum	Skin	*Alligator mississippiensis*	73
Chaetomium sp.	Skin	*Alligator mississippiensis*	73
Chrysosporium sp.	Intestinal contents	*Osteolaemus tetraspis*	40
Cladosporium cladosporioides	Skin	*Alligator mississippiensis*	73
Cladosporium oxysporum	Skin	*Alligator mississippiensis*	73
Cladosporium sp.	Skin	Caimans (species not specified)	2
Cryptococcus lipolytica	Intestinal contents	*Osteolaemus tetraspis*	40
Cryptococcus luteolus	Intestinal contents	*Osteolaemus tetraspis*	40
Curvularia lunata	Skin	*Alligator mississippiensis*	73
Curvularia lunata varaeria	Skin	*Crocodylus porosus*	74
Curvularia sp.	Intestinal contents	*Osteolaemus tetraspis*	40
Epicoccum purpurascens	Skin	*Alligator mississippiensis*	73
Eurotium chevalieri	Skin	*Alligator mississippiensis*	73
Fusarium moniliforme	Lungs	*Alligator mississippiensis*	77
Fusarium solani	Internal organs	*Crocodylus porosus*	2, 74
Fusarium sp.	Not specified	*Crocodylus porosus*	2
	Gingivae	*Caiman crocodilus fuscus*	2
	Skin	*Crocodylus porosus*	51
	Intestinal contents	*Osteolaemus tetraspis*	40
Geotrichum candidum	Not specified	*Crocodylus porosus*	2
	Intestinal contents	*Osteolaemus tetraspis*	40
Geotrichum sp.	Not specified	*Crocodylus porosus*	2
Metarhizium anisopliae	Lungs	Crocodile (species not specified)	2
	Lungs	*Osteolaemus tetraspis*	2
	Lungs	*Alligator mississippiensis*	2
Monascus ruber	Skin	*Alligator mississippiensis*	73
Mucor circinelloides	Skin	Caimans (species not specified)	2
	Gastric ulcers	*Osteolaemus tetraspis*	2
	Skin	*Alligator mississippiensis*	73
Mucor sp.	Lungs	Crocodile (species not specified)	78
Nannizziopsis vriesii	Skin	*Crocodylus porosus*	79
Paecilomyces lilacinus	Liver	*Crocodylus porosus*	80

TABLE 6-4	**Fungi Isolated from Crocodilians Around the World—cont'd**		
Fungus	**Lesions**	**Species**	**Reference**
Paecilomyces farinosus	Lungs	*Alligator mississippiensis*	2
Paecilomyces variotii	Skin	*Alligator mississippiensis*	73
Paecilomyces sp.	Not specified	*Crocodylus porosus*	2
	Intestinal contents	*Osteolaemus tetraspis*	40
Penicillium citrinum	Skin	*Alligator mississippiensis*	73
Penicillium lilacinum	Lungs	Alligators and crocodiles (species not specified)	2
Penicillium oxalicum	Skin	*Crocodylus porosus*	74
Penicillium sp.	Not specified	*Crocodylus porosus*	2
	Intestinal contents	*Osteolaemus tetraspis*	40
Phoma sp.	Intestinal contents	*Osteolaemus tetraspis*	40
Syncephalastrum racemosum	Skin	*Alligator mississippiensis*	73
Syncephalastrum sp.	Skin	*Crocodylus porosus*	51
Trichoderma sp.	Skin	*Alligator mississippiensis*	2
	Intestinal contents	*Osteolaemus tetraspis*	40
Trichophyton sp.	Skin	*Alligator mississippiensis*	2
Trichosporon beigelii	Intestinal contents	*Osteolaemus tetraspis*	40
Trichosporon capitatum	Intestinal contents	*Osteolaemus tetraspis*	40
Trichosporon cutaneum	Skin	*Crocodylus porosus*	51
Trichosporon sp.	Tongue, gingivae	*Crocodylus niloticus, C. fuscus*	2

number of areas in a crocodilian's body that have soft skin and allow an external parasite to attach and/or obtain a meal. The recent cases of WNV in the American alligator (*A. mississippiensis*) are a reminder that arthropods can play an important role in disease transmission. Internal parasites are not a common problem in ranching operations where animals are maintained in concrete buildings with no organic substrate. Parasites are of major concern in wild crocodilians or those kept captive outdoors on organic substrates. External parasites are more ubiquitous, affecting both captive and wild populations. To determine the best prevention and control methods to use, veterinarians must assess the environment as well as the life cycle of the parasite.

Nutritional Diseases

With the increased knowledge of crocodilian dietary requirements, nutritional diseases are diagnosed less frequently than they were in the past. Better understanding of the biology, natural history, and physiology of the different crocodilian species has allowed implementation of better feeding schemes and diets. Over time, there has been a desire to develop commercial diets that will allow for high feed to weight gain ratios. These commercial diets are available for feeding American alligators (*A. mississippiensis*), and although the diets are not perfect, if fed appropriately, captive-hatched American alligators (*A. mississippiensis*) will grow up to 36 inches in length within a 12-month period. For zoologic institutions the goal is not rapid growth but rather normal development and a foundation for excellent health. Zoologic institutions and crocodile farms commonly provide crocodilians with fresh and/or frozen prey (e.g., poultry, swine, beef, fish, nutria,

native prey, etc.) with bones providing a source of calcium. To prevent lead toxicity in crocodilians, veterinarians must use a reputable fresh or frozen prey source that has not been killed with lead projectiles (e.g., shotgun pellets, bullets). Despite better feeding schemes and diets, veterinarians will still see crocodilians with diseases associated with nutritional deficiencies.

A common nutritional disease of reptiles is metabolic bone disease (MBD). Clinical signs of MBD include weakness, lethargy, kyphosis, scoliosis, osteodystrophy, pathologic fractures, paresis, and tooth decalcification. Various possible causes of MBD have been proposed, but it is usually associated with a calcium-phosphorus imbalance that leads to increased bone resorption. Calcium and vitamin D_3 are the two main nutritional compounds deficient in reptiles with MBD. Vitamin D_3 deficiencies are associated with a lack of exposure to UVB spectrum light, which comes naturally from the sun. Light bulbs and light tubes are commercially available to help provide adequate amounts of UVB light for reptiles. MBD is primarily observed in herbivorous or omnivorous reptiles. It appears that MBD is not commonly observed in commercial crocodilian operations, even in those were animals are raised in the dark with no source of UVB light. The carnivorous nature of crocodilians may allow them to obtain vitamin D_3 from the diet without a true requirement for UVB light. However, if an appropriate calcium source is not offered, these animals will develop MBD. Adult alligators without MBD have been observed growing in enclosed buildings with no light source while being fed a commercial diet supplemented with fresh prey meat with bones. However, anecdotal comments from various ranchers indicate that the animals appear to thrive better if exposed to sunlight. This is an area where more research is needed to determine the UVB and calcium requirements of crocodilians and their effects on growth and health.

Articular and visceral gout also have been reported in crocodilians. Some predisposing factors for gout include high protein diets, dehydration, and stress. Clinical signs associated with chronic gout in crocodilians are primarily nonspecific, but limb paresis or paralysis and joint enlargement can occur. Ariel et al. reported a case of visceral and articular gout with concurrent hypovitaminosis A in crocodile hatchlings.[81]

Deficiencies of vitamins A, B, C, or E also can lead to a variety of musculoskeletal disorders. These are thought to be less common in crocodilians fed commercial diets in addition to fresh meat products.

Respiratory Disease

Respiratory disease is one of the most common presentations of captive crocodilians in commercial operations. It is common to find lesions in the lungs associated with respiratory disease when performing postmortem examinations (Figure 6-16). Although most of the lung pathology is incidental, some animals will have a history of clinical signs associated with respiratory disease before death. Clinical signs of respiratory disease in crocodilians are nonspecific anorexia, lethargy, and weakness but may also include dyspnea, tachypnea, nasal secretion, excessive basking, respiratory stridor, and abnormal swimming (either in circles or on one side of the body). In some cases the animals may appear neurologic as they become weak and ataxic. A clear distinction must be established between respiratory disease and neurologic disease. Respiratory disease may be secondary to neurologic disease as a consequence of weakness, predisposing the animal to aspiration pneumonia. Most respiratory infections are either bacterial or fungal in origin. Upper respiratory diseases, including rhinitis and pharyngitis, also have been reported in crocodilians.[2]

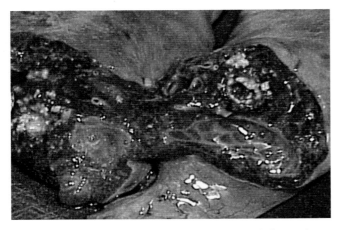

Figure 6-16 Pneumonia associated with *Klebsiella* sp. in an American alligator *(Alligator mississippiensis)*.

Neurologic Disease

Neurologic diseases are not common in crocodilians. However, the causes implicated by clinical neurologic presenting symptoms deserve special attention. The most common neurologic clinical sign is abnormal swimming behavior (e.g., swimming in circles, swimming on one side of the body, etc.). Once outside the water, these animals may show signs of lethargy, ataxia, head tilt, and muscle tremors. Anorexia may be the earliest sign observed by the facility personnel. The most recent explanation of signs of neurologic disease in crocodilian species is WNV. This virus should be in the differential diagnosis list for any crocodilian that has neurologic signs and is housed in an area where WNV is endemic. Hypoglycemia also has been reported to cause neurologic signs in alligators.[82]

Neurologic signs and deaths of alligators *(A. mississippiensis)* were identified from a commercial operation where a building was not cleaned according to the maintenance schedule. The water in the building had not been changed in a 72-hour period, and there was evidence of food debris from previous feedings. The owner found a few hundred dead alligators, and of those that remained alive, some had neurologic signs (e.g., slow reflexes, abnormal swimming patterns, ataxia, and lethargy). Necropsy and histopathologic evaluation leaned toward toxicity as the cause of death. Both dead and live animals tested negative for WNV. All other buildings were cleaned on schedule, and there was no evidence of disease in those buildings. Mortalities decreased after the building housing the sick animals was cleaned. Based on the history, clinical observations, and histopathologic findings, veterinarians believe these animals developed neurologic signs as a result of either increased ammonia level in the water, oxygen depletion in the air, or both.[59]

Musculoskeletal Disease

Musculoskeletal disease can be caused by changes in the incubation temperature or humidity; trauma from fighting, transport, or restraint; and infectious diseases (Figure 6-17). Deformities of the head, limbs, and tails are common malformations influenced by incubation rather than true genetics (Figure 6-18). Fractures and limb amputations can occur as a result of trauma and fighting, with many healing without major complications. Healed traumatic injuries are observed in captive and wild crocodilians. If the trauma is severe enough, nerve damage, muscle damage, paresis, and/or paralysis may result. The most common infectious disease known to have effects on the musculoskeletal system is mycoplasmosis. Both *M. alligatoris* and *M. crocodyli* can cause polyarthritis in affected animals.

Gastrointestinal Disease

Ingestion of foreign bodies, gastric ulcers, enteritis, and trauma to the oral cavity are gastrointestinal diseases associated with crocodilian species. Anorexia is a common sequelae to the gastrointestinal diseases listed above.

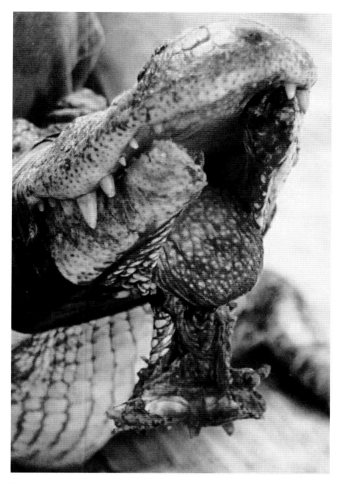

Figure 6-17 Fracture of the mandible in a wild-caught American alligator *(Alligator mississippiensis).*

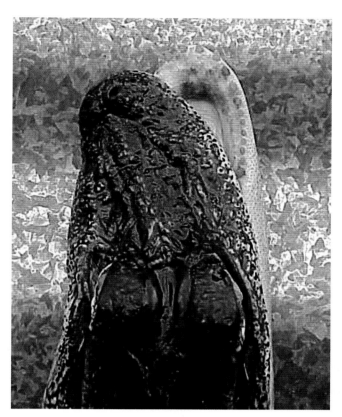

Figure 6-18 Deformity of the maxillae in a captive-reared American alligator *(Alligator mississippiensis).* These deformities are common in captivity and thought to be associated with problems during the incubation period.

Ingestion of foreign bodies occurs in both wild and captive crocodilians. Construction, malfunction of water pumps and filters, forgotten objects in the enclosure, and tossed objects by the public are some of the sources of foreign bodies for captive animals. Sharp objects such as nails may cause severe gastrointestinal problems, while other less sharp or pointed ingested material may pass without major difficulties. Infectious enteritis is usually diagnosed post mortem based on gross and histopathologic evaluation. Crocodilians appear to have an aggressive response to insult of the gastrointestinal tract. Grossly one may observe accumulation of fibrinous or fibrous material and/or necrosis of the mucosa (Figure 6-19). In some instances, this can even lead to obstruction due to accumulation of fibrinous/fibrous material. Fecal impactions and torsions are probably rare but can also occur in crocodilians, while gastric ulcerations may be associated with stress and diet. The intestinal tract of crocodilians appears to contain a significant amount of gut associated lymphoid tissue like Peyer's patches. This lymphoid tissue may allow for an aggressive inflammatory response to infectious agents in the intestinal tract.

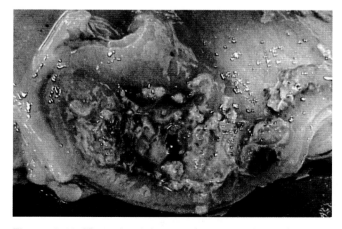

Figure 6-19 Necrosis of the gastric mucosa in an American alligator *(Alligator mississippiensis).*

Integumentary Disease

Integumentary disease is arguably the most significant disease process affecting captive crocodilians. Water quality, temperature, and stressors contribute to the occurrence of integumentary diseases. Secondary bacterial and fungal dermatitis in crocodilians can have a devastating economic impact on commercial operations. Lacerations, abscesses, and draining tracts can serve as a nidus for microorganisms. An additional predisposing factor of integumentary disease in captive operations is the accumulation of fat in the upper water column. This concentration of fat creates a slime layer on the walls and water surface, which is then transferred to the skin of the animals where it creates an ideal environment for fungal and bacterial growth. This is more of a problem when meat is the sole source of food or is provided in addition to a commercial diet. A surfactant disinfectant can be used to break down the fat accumulation in the water and on the walls of the enclosure. In most instances both bacteria and fungi will be present in the skin lesions associated with fat accumulation in the captive environment. It is important to recognize the fat accumulation problem early to institute appropriate cleaning measures and possible therapy. Mixed flora is often found in the dermal lesions, making identification of a single causal agent difficult. Antimicrobial therapy is indicated if bacterial involvement is suspected. Although the use of systemic antifungal medications is cost prohibitive in commercial operations, it can be used if only a small number of animals are affected. Improved hygiene, better water quality, stable temperatures, and decreased stress are essential for managing these dermatitis cases. In most instances those animals that are already showing clinical signs may not recover. The key to preventing and decreasing the spread of disease is improving and implementing appropriate husbandry methods.

Various alligator *(A. mississippiensis)* ranches in Louisiana have reported hatching animals with normal pigmentation that becomes "white" after a few weeks of life (Figure 6-20). Physical examination of these animals does not reveal any abnormalities other than an apparent depigmentation or hypopigmentation of the skin. The white discoloration is not unlike that described as a result of fungal or bacterial dermatitis. Upon palpation, the skin appears thinner and has

a flaky nature similar to that observed in leucistic alligators. Affected animals do not appear to grow at different rates than normally pigmented animals. The processing of the hides is not affected by the pigment deficit. A nutritional deficiency or genetics are suspected in this presentation, but there are anecdotal reports of improvement of the condition after vitamin supplementation with a multivitamin formulation.

Miscellaneous Diseases

LYMPHOHISTIOCYTIC PROLIFERATIVE SYNDROME OF ALLIGATORS ("PIX" DISEASE)

Lymphohistiocytic proliferative syndrome of alligators (LPSA), also known as PIX disease, has been recently studied in captive-reared alligators *(A. mississippiensis)* from Florida and Louisiana.[83] LPSA affects the quality of the hides in commercial operations, leading to decreased profits for alligator producers. Gross lesions of LPSA are multifocal, 1- to 2-mm, gray to red foci on the ventral mandibular and abdominal scales (Figure 6-21). They may occasionally be observed on the ventral tail scales. These lesions can be found on any section of a scale and are flush with the scale's surface; however, they may not be clearly visible in the live animal. Often, the lesions are identified during postmortem examination after close inspection of the hide using an intense backlight (Figures 6-22 and 6-23), appearing as 1- to 2-mm clearings on the scales. The lesions are circular with well-defined margins and can be confused with tooth marks and other imperfections in the skin. Therefore, antemortem identification is not very accurate at this time. Microscopic examination of the skin lesions reveals dermal nodular lymphoid proliferation with perivascular cuffing. The same changes observed in the skin

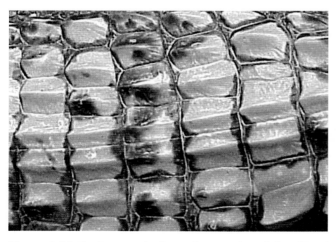

Figure 6-20 Depigmentation/hypopigmentation of the skin of an American alligator *(Alligator mississippiensis)*. A nutritional or genetic component is thought to be associated with this presenting symptom.

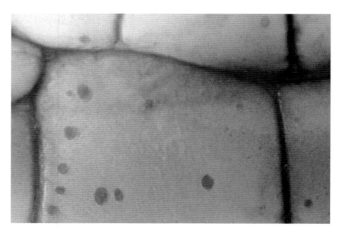

Figure 6-21 Gross lesions of lymphohistiocytic proliferative syndrome of alligators (LPSA) on the scales of an American alligator *(Alligator mississippiensis)*.

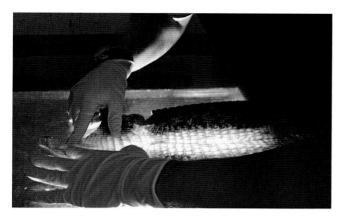

Figure 6-22 Examination of the hide of an American alligator *(Alligator mississippiensis)* using a light table to identify LPSA lesions.

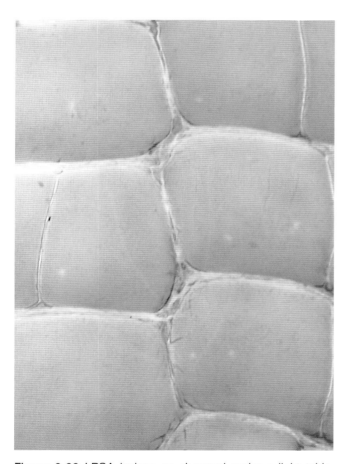

Figure 6-23 LPSA lesions as observed under a light table. Many of these lesions must be differentiated from tooth marks and other scratches. Histopathologic evaluation is used for confirmation.

have been found in the lungs, intestines, kidneys, ovaries, testicles, thyroid, gall bladder, mesentery, eyes, and nervous tissue.[84] Ongoing research has revealed a strong relationship between exposure to/infection by West Nile virus and the occurrence of PIX lesions.

TOXICITIES

Toxicities are not common in captive crocodilians. However, there have been cases of lead toxicity in alligators being fed nutria that had been killed with lead shotgun pellets.[12] Clinical signs include weakness, lethargy, anorexia, and death. Alligator ranchers and farmers are now more diligent in inquiring about the source and kill method of nutria before feeding their animals. Wild alligators, on the other hand, can be exposed to a number of toxic substances, mostly pesticides and heavy metals. Many of these substances are thought to be endocrine disrupters that affect the development and function of the reproductive organs and result in developmental defects of young crocodilians.[85-89] There is an abundance of information to support the impact of environmental contamination on crocodilians as well as other species. This reiterates the critical state of the natural habitat of many species around the world. Crocodilians have served as sentinels for anthropogenic changes that ultimately may come back to affect human health.

RUNTING

Runting is a phenomenon observed in captive crocodilian operations. It describes a general state of unthriftiness, lack of growth, and weakness. There is a visible size difference in same-age animals between the "runts" and the otherwise normally developing animals. It is not unusual to find some buildings in a commercial operation that contain the runt animals for that year. It is also in this group of animals that disease problems may be observed with higher frequency. Stress factors, including dominance by other animals, environment, and even incubation temperature, contribute to the presence of runts.[90]

■ THERAPEUTICS
Fluid Therapy

Fluid therapy of crocodilians is accomplished as in other reptile species. Veterinarians must determine hydration status, percentage of fluid deficit, and maintenance requirements to develop a plan for fluid therapy. A maintenance rate of 20 to 30 ml/kg can be administered intracoelomically (ICe), orally (PO), or intravenously (IV). In some instances, food prey items can be injected with fluid and then fed to the animal. If the animal is anorexic, manual restraint will be required for fluid administration. It is important to remember that restraint itself will be an additional stressor that may hinder the recovery of an animal. Therefore, to limit the amount of stress in the animal, treatment protocols including fluid therapy must be planned appropriately and administered quickly.

Antimicrobials

Antimicrobial therapy presents a challenge in crocodilians because of their extra label use. In commercial alligator facilities, antimicrobial treatment is complicated by the lack of drug withdrawal times for crocodilian species. Currently the U.S.

Food and Drug Administration (FDA) and the Animal and Plant Health Inspection Services (APHIS) have no recommendations on this subject. From a public health standpoint there is hope that this may change in the future. Alligator meat can be purchased from supermarkets and restaurants in the United States, primarily in the southern United States. At this time, a recommended addition of 60 to 90 days to the U.S. Department of Agriculture (USDA) food animal withdrawal time, listed for a particular drug should provide enough time for appropriate withdrawal in crocodilians, but there is no research to support this claim. If the animals are not intended for human consumption, antimicrobials can be used extra label as in other exotic species. There are few pharmacokinetic studies of antimicrobials in crocodilians. Helmick et al. examined the pharmacokinetics of both enrofloxacin and a long-acting oxytetracycline in the American alligator (*A. mississippiensis*).[91,92] Enrofloxacin was found to be effective when administered at 5 mg/kg IV every 36 hours.[91] The long-lasting oxytetracycline was found to be effective at 10 mg/kg both IV and intramuscularly (IM) every 5 days.[92] Both of these treatment regimes may be practical in a zoologic institution or a commercial operation with a small number of animals. In a large commercial operation where a higher number of animals may need treatment, it may be time, cost, and labor prohibitive to administer medications intramuscularly or intravenously to individual animals. Spectrum of coverage, method and frequency of administration, and cost should be considered when selecting an antimicrobial agent(s). Consideration should be given to those drugs that can be mixed with, or injected into, the feed. One technique of antibiotic administration is making a sausage filled with the animal's feed and placing the drug in the sausage. Manual medication by mouth or injection can be performed in smaller animals. Whenever possible, culture and sensitivity test should be obtained to identify the organism in question and determine the efficacy of the antimicrobial selected. Unless a bacterial infection is suspected, use of antibiotics is strongly discouraged. Most antimicrobial agents and their metabolites will be transported in the wastewater, potentially creating an avenue for future antimicrobial resistance.

Nutritional Support

Nutritional support of crocodilians should be approached as in other carnivorous reptiles. The main difficulties result from the handling and restraint required to force-feed an ill crocodilian. Nutritional support of an ill patient is more likely to occur at a zoologic institution than in a commercial operation. Placing an esophagostomy tube should be considered as a less stressful alternative method of feeding the critical crocodilian. Nutritional support through an esophagostomy tube will require restraint while feeding, but the stress level is reduced because the mouth does not have to be opened. Any high-protein feed (e.g., commercial feed, fresh prey) that can be blended may be used as long as it can easily pass through the tube. In larger and aggressive animals, force-feeding is a serious challenge and must be performed carefully.

■ SURGERY
Preoperative and Postoperative Considerations

Various factors should be considered before performing a surgery procedure on a crocodilian, with the initial consideration being the ultimate purpose of the animal. Is the animal part of a zoologic collection, is it from a commercial operation, or will it be released back to the wild? The next concern is the expected prognosis and time of recovery. Ultimately the animal should be able to thrive in its future environment whether it be an exhibit or in the wild. Cost of the procedure also is a major presurgical consideration. Whereas cost may not be a major decision factor in some zoologic institutions, in other programs such as conservation programs, the money needs to be carefully allocated to obtain the highest return on the investment. The available facilities, especially for postoperative management, are also an important consideration. If the procedure requires placement of sutures, the animal should be maintained in a clean environment with shallow water for a few days to prevent infection and infiltration of water into the surgical site. Depending on the species, it may be possible to spray the animal with water throughout the day instead of keeping it in water. The final consideration is the ability of the personnel to carry out the postoperative care, especially if force-feeding is required.

It would be beneficial to obtain a CBC and chemistry panel to assess the overall health status of the animal before surgery is performed. Diagnostic test results will help determine if the animal is fit for surgery and can be compared to postsurgical blood work to monitor recovery and healing, although in many instances diagnostic evaluation is an unrealistic expectation.

Anesthesia

To anesthetize crocodilian species, a basic understanding of their physiology and anatomy is needed to ensure safe delivery, induction, and maintenance of the anesthetic agent. There are various anesthetic agents, both injectable and inhalant, that can be used to anesthetize and sedate crocodilians. Procedure type, species, and size are factors that will influence the choice of anesthetic agent(s). There are no established anesthetic protocols for crocodilians, and information is often derived from field research as well as clinical experience of practitioners. Injectable anesthetic agents can be delivered in the tail muscles via a pole syringe or hand syringe or administered intravenously after immobilization or restraint.

Neuromuscular blocking agents, such as gallamine and succinylcholine, are widely used in crocodilians. When transporting large, aggressive animals, veterinarians might use these agents to prevent injury to both the handlers and the animal. However, these drugs do not have analgesic properties and should not be used alone for any surgical procedures. When using neuromuscular blocking agents, veterinarians should ensure the animal is supported with a backboard to minimize injury to the spine. Succinylcholine is a depolarizing neuromuscular blocker with primary action at the nerve end plate, and flaccid or rigid paralysis may occur depending on the dose.[5,93] There is no reversal agent for succinylcholine, so it must be used with caution and the animals monitored closely. Effects can be observed within 5 minutes of administration, and recovery takes up to 1.5 hours. Recovery will depend on the excretion of the drug in the urine and metabolism of the crocodilian. Gallamine is a nondepolarizing neuromuscular agent that competitively blocks acetylcholine at the motor end plate, resulting in flaccid paralysis. Crocodilians immobilized with gallamine will open their mouths following relaxation of the muscles; this is known as the *Flaxidil reaction.*[5] Increased respiratory rate and heart rate may be observed with gallamine immobilization.[94,95] An overdose of gallamine may lead to bradycardia, mydriasis, increased gastrointestinal motility, and paralysis of respiratory muscles.[5] Increased salivation and emesis can be prevented with presurgical use of atropine.[95] An advantage of gallamine over succinylcholine is that it can be reversed with neostigmine methylsulfate. Fatalities have been reported in American alligators *(A. mississippiensis),* Chinese alligators *(A. sinensis),* and false gharials *(Tomistoma schlegelii)* that were administered gallamine.[95] Diazepam can also be administered 20 to 30 minutes before succinylcholine or gallamine for added muscle relaxation.[96] Administration and recovery of animals with neuromuscular agents should be done far from the water to avoid drowning. Noise and light stimuli should be minimized when animals have been sedated with gallamine or any other neuromuscular agent or anesthetic. Table 6-5 shows doses for various neuromuscular agents. Following administration of a neuromuscular agent, it may be possible to intubate a crocodilian for general anesthesia with an inhalant anesthetic such as isoflurane. Remember to always provide analgesics if performing a painful procedure.

Injectable anesthestics have the added benefit of providing analgesia and decreasing the amount of inhalant anesthetics used during surgery. Dissociatives, opioids, benzodiazepines, and barbiturates have been administered to reptiles and crocodilians with various rates of success. Alpha-2 adrenergics are gaining popularity in reptile medicine and show promising results for their continued use as anesthetics in reptiles. A combination of medetomidine and ketamine works well in American alligators *(A. mississippiensis)* and has the added benefit of being able to reverse the medetomidine with atipamezole.[97] In a study involving juvenile alligators, the young animals had a higher requirement of medetomidine (220.1 ± 76.9 µg/kg IM), atipamezole (1188.5 ± 328.1 µg/kg IM), and ketamine (10.0 ± 4.9 mg/kg IM), compared to adult alligators' requirement of medetomidine (131.1 ± 19.5 µg/kg IM), atipamezole (694 ± 101 µg/kg IM), and ketamine (7.5 ± 4.2 mg/kg IM).[97] These findings are similar to those observed for other anesthetic agents used in reptiles. Metabolic differences between age classes usually require higher doses for juvenile animals.

An additional anesthetic agent that has gained popularity in reptile medicine is propofol (Abbott Laboratories, 100 Abbott Park Rd., Abbott Park, IL 60064-3500). Propofol is a lipid soluble drug with fast action and short duration of effects, which makes it an ideal anesthetic agent that allows for intubation of the animal to be followed with inhalant anesthesia. Propofol can be administered at 10 to 15 mg/kg IV[5,14] and as a constant rate infusion. The IV route of administration of propofol presents a disadvantage in cases where manual restraint is not possible or is undesired.

When choosing an anesthetic or immobilizing agent, veterinarians should take into account all the factors previously mentioned while keeping the safety of the animal and personnel in mind.

Common Surgical Procedures

Fortunately, surgeries are not routinely performed in crocodilian species. The most common surgical procedure performed in zoologic institutions is probably the removal of foreign bodies through gastroscopy. This may be performed under immobilization or general anesthesia. Enterotomies are rare but may be required if a foreign body lodges itself beyond the

TABLE 6-5	Doses of Intramuscular Administration of Neuromuscular Blocking Agents Used in Crocodilians		
Drug	**Dose (mg/kg)**	**Species**	**Reference**
Gallamine	0.4-1.25	*C. niloticus*	14
	0.6-4.0	*C. rhombifer*	94
	0.6-4.0	*C. niloticus*	5
	1.0-2.0	*C. niloticus*	5
Neostigmine	0.03-0.06	*C. niloticus*	5
	0.03-0.25	*C. niloticus*	94
	0.07-0.14	*C. niloticus*	14
Succinylcholine	0.4-1.0	*A. mississippiensis*	5, 14
	0.5-2.0	None specified	14
Succinylcholine/ Diazepam	0.14-0.37/ 0.22-0.62	*A. mississippiensis*	96

stomach, is too large to pass on its own, or both. The next most common procedure is the repair of fractures and lacerations caused by trauma. Crocodilian fracture repair can present a real challenge to the veterinarian because of an animal's large size, demeanor, and need to live in an aquatic environment. Therefore, it is preferred to perform fracture repairs with internal fixation methods, such as intramedullary pins, cerclage wire, and bone plates. Before attempting a surgical procedure, any veterinarian must realistically determine the prognosis for the animal.

REFERENCES

1. 2004 IUCN Red List of Threatened Species™, http://www.iucnredlist.org, January 2005.
2. Huchzermeyer FW: *Crocodiles: Biology, Husbandry and Diseases,* ed 1, Wallingford, UK, 2003, CABI.
3. Soares D: An ancient sensory organ in crocodilians, *Nature* 417:241-242, 2002.
4. Britton A: http://crocodilian.com, January 2005.
5. Fleming GJ: Crocodilian anesthesia, *Vet Clin North Am Exot Anim Pract* 4(1):19-145, 2001.
6. Lane TJ: Crocodilians. In Mader DR, editor: *Reptile Medicine and Surgery,* Philadelphia, 1996, WB Saunders.
7. Elsey R: Stocking rates of ranched American alligators *(Alligator mississippiensis),* (personal communication), 2004.
8. Staton MA, Edwards HM Jr, Brisbin IL Jr et al: Essential fatty acid nutrition of the American alligator *(Alligator mississippiensis), J Nutr* 120(7):674-685, 1990.
9. Coulson RA, Coulson TD, Herbert JD et al: Protein nutrition in the alligator, *Comp Biochem Physiol* 87A(2):449-459, 1987.
10. Coulson RA, Coulson TD, Herbert JD: Alligator feed evaluations, *Proc of the Louisiana Aquaculture Conf,* Baton Rouge, La, pp 48-51, 1992.
11. Burris Alligator Feeds, http://www.burrismill.com/Screens/Alligator.aspx, January 2005.
12. Camus AC, Mitchell MA, Williams JF et al: Elevated lead levels in farmed American alligators *(Alligator mississippiensis)* consuming nutria *(Myocastor coypus)* meat contaminated by lead bullets, *J World Aquaculture Society* 29:370-376, 1998.
13. Wilhite DR, Nevarez JG: Unpublished description of a new site for venipuncture in the American alligator *(Alligator mississippiensis),* 2004.
14. Carpenter JW, Mashima TY, Rupiper DJ: *Exotic Animal Formulary,* ed 2, Philadelphia, 2001, WB Saunders.
15. Rooney AA, Guillette LJJ: Biotic and abiotic factors in crocodilian stress: the challenge of a modern environment. In Grigg GC, Seebacher F, Franklin CE, editors: *Crocodilian Biology and Evolution,* p. 214, ed 1, Chipping Norton, 2001, Surrey Beatty and Sons.
16. Dohms JE, Metz A: Stress-mechanisms of immunosuppression, *Vet Immunol Immunopathol* 30:89-109, 1991.
17. Lance VA, Elsey RM: Plasma catecholamines and plasma corticosterone following restraint stress in juvenile alligators, *J Exp Zoolog* 283(6):559-565, 1999.
18. Morici LA, Elsey RM, Lance VA: Effects of long-term corticosterone implants on growth and immune function in juvenile alligators *(Alligator mississippiensis), J Exp Zoolog* 279(2):156-162, 1997.
19. Lance VA, Elsey RM: Hormonal and metabolic response of juvenile alligators to cold shock, *J Exp Zoolog* 283:566-572, 1999.
20. Elsey RM, Joanen T, McNease L et al: Growth rate and plasma corticosterone levels in juvenile alligators maintained at different stocking densities, *J Exp Zoolog* 255:30-36, 1990.
21. Lance VA, Morici LA, Elsey RM: Physiology and endocrinology of stress in crocodilians. In Grigg GC, Seebacher F, Franklin CE, editors: *Crocodilian Biology and Evolution,* ed 1, Chipping Norton, 2001, Surrey Beatty and Sons.
22. Merchant ME, Roche C, Elsey RM et al: Antibacterial properties of serum from the American alligator *(Alligator mississippiensis), Comp Biochem Physiol B Biochem Mol Biol* 136(3):505-513, 2003.
23. Shaharabany M, Gollop N, Ravin S et al: Naturally occurring antibacterial activities of avian and crocodile tissues, *J Antimicrob Chemother* 44(3):416-418, 1999.
24. Gorden RW, Hazen TC, Esch GW et al: Isolation of *Aeromonas hydrophila* from the American alligator *(Alligator mississippiensis), J Wildl Dis* 15(2):239-243, 1979.
25. Shotts EB, Gaines JL, Martin L et al: *Aeromonas*-induced deaths among fish and reptiles in an eutrophic inland lake, *J Am Vet Med Assoc* 161(6):603-607, 1972.
26. Millichamp NJ, Jacobson ER, Wolf ED: Diseases of the eye and ocular adnexae in reptiles, *J Am Vet Med Assoc* 183(11):1205-1212, 1983.
27. Jacobson ER: Immobilization, blood sampling, necropsy techniques and diseases of crocodilians: a review, *J Zoo Anim Med* 15:38-45, 1984.
28. Flandry F, Lisecki EJ, Domingue GJ et al: Initial antibiotic therapy for alligator bites: characterization of the oral flora of *Alligator mississippiensis, South Med J* 82(2):262-266, 1989.
29. Novak SS, Seigel RA: Gram-negative septicemia in American alligators *(Alligator mississippiensis), J Wildl Dis* 22(4):484-487, 1986.
30. Wallace LJ, White FH, Gore HL: Isolation of *Edwardsiella tarda* from a sea lion and two alligators, *J Am Vet Med Assoc* 149(7):881-883, 1966.
31. Mainster ME, Lynd FT, Cragg PC et al: Treatment of multiple cases of *Pasteurella multocida* and *Staphylococcal pneumonia* in *Alligator mississippiensis* on a herd basis, *Proc Am Assoc Zoo Vets,* pp 33-36, 1972.
32. Brown DR, Nogueira MF, Schoeb TR et al: Pathology of experimental mycoplasmosis in American alligators, *J Wildl Dis* 37(4):671-679, 2001.
33. Jacobson ER, Gardiner CH, Foggin CM: Adenovirus-like infection in two Nile crocodiles, *J Am Vet Med Assoc* 185(11):1421-1422, 1984.
34. Clippinger TL, Bennet RA, Johnson CM et al: Morbidity and mortality associated with a new mycoplasma species from captive American alligators *(Alligator mississippiensis), J Zoo Wildl Med* 31(3):303-314, 2000.
35. Barnett JD, Cardeilhac PT: Clinical values associated with opportunistic bacterial diseases in farm-raised alligators, *IAAAM Proc* 26:22, 1995.
36. Newton J: Brown spot disease in the Louisiana alligator industry: what we know about the disease and possible control protocols, *Proc Louisiana Aquaculture Conf,* Baton Rouge, La, pp 46-47, 1992.
37. Bounds HC, Normand RA: Brown spot disease of commercially-raised alligators: a preliminary report, Louisiana Academy of Sciences 54:62, 1991.
38. Russell WC, Herman KL: Colibacillosis in captive wild animals, *J Zoo Anim Med* 1:17-21, 1970.
39. Brown DR, Farley JM, Zacher LA et al: *Mycoplasma alligatoris sp nov,* from American alligators, *Int J Syst Evol Microbiol* 51:419-424, 2001.
40. Huchzermeyer FW, Henton MM, Riley J et al: Aerobic intestinal flora of wild-caught African dwarf crocodiles *(Osteolaemus tetraspis), Onderstepoort J Vet Res* 67(3):201-204, 2000.
41. Harvey RW, Price TH: *Salmonella* isolation from reptilian faeces: a discussion of appropriate cultural techniques, *J Hyg* 91(1):25-32, 1983.
42. Madsen M, Hangartner P, West K et al: Recovery rates, serotypes, and antimicrobial susceptibility patterns of salmonellae isolated from cloacal swabs of wild Nile crocodiles *(Crocodylus niloticus)* in Zimbabwe, *J Zoo Wildl Med* 29(1):31-34, 1998.
43. van der Walt ML, Huchzermeyer FW, Steyn HC: *Salmonella* isolated from crocodiles and other reptiles during the period 1985-1994 in South Africa, *Onderstepoort J Vet Res* 64(4):277-283, 1997.
44. Huchzermeyer FW, Gerdes GH, Foggin CM et al: Hepatitis in farmed hatchling Nile crocodiles *(Crocodylus niloticus)* due to chlamydial infection, *J S Afr Vet Assoc* 65(1):20-22, 1994.
45. Millan JM, Purdie JL, Melville LF: Public health risks of the flesh of farmed crocodiles, *Rev Sci Tech* 16(2):605-608, 1997.
46. Madsen M: Prevalence and serovar distribution of *Salmonella* in fresh and frozen meat from captive Nile crocodiles *(Crocodylus niloticus), Int J Food Microbiol* 29(1):111-118, 1996.
47. Madsen M: Microbial flora of frozen tail meat from captive Nile crocodiles *(Crocodylus niloticus), Int J Food Microbiol* 18(1):71-76, 1993.
48. Manolis SC, Webb GJ, Pinch D et al: Salmonella in captive crocodiles *(Crocodylus johnstoni* and *C porosus), Aust Vet J* 68(3):102-105, 1991.
49. Rickard MW, Thomas AD, Bradley S et al: Microbiological evaluation of dressing procedures for crocodile carcasses in Queensland, *Aust Vet J* 72(5):172-176, 1995.
50. Buenviaje GN, Hirst RG, Ladds PW et al: Isolation of *Dermatophilus sp* from skin lesions in farmed saltwater crocodiles *(Crocodylus porosus), Aust Vet J* 75(5):365-367, 1997.
51. Buenviaje GN, Ladds PW, Martin Y: Pathology of skin diseases in crocodiles. *Aust Vet J* 76(5):357-363, 1998.
52. Barnett JD, Cardeilhac PT: Brown spot disease in the American alligator *(Alligator mississippiensis), IAAAM Proc* 29:124-125, 1998.

53. Pye GW, Brown DR, Nogueira MF et al: Experimental Inoculation of broad-nosed caimans *(Caiman latirostris)* and Siamese crocodiles *(Crocodylus siamensis)* with *Mycoplasma alligatoris, J Zoo Wildl Med* 32(2):196-201, 2001.

54. Helmick KE, Brown DR, Jacobson ER et al: In vitro susceptibility pattern of *Mycoplasma alligatoris* from symptomatic American alligators *(Alligator mississippiensis), J Zoo Wildl Med* 33(2):108-111, 2002.

55. Mohan K, Foggin CM, Muvavarirwa P et al: Mycoplasma-associated polyarthritis in farmed crocodiles *(Crocodylus niloticus)* in Zimbabwe, *Onderstepoort J Vet Res* 62(1):45-49, 1995.

56. Mohan K, Foggin CM, Muvavarirwa P et al: Vaccination of farmed crocodiles *(Crocodylus niloticus)* against *Mycoplasma crocodyli* infection, *Vet Rec* 141(18):476, 1997.

57. Mohan K, Foggin CM, Dziva F et al: Vaccination to control an outbreak of *Mycoplasma crocodyli* infection, *Onderstepoort J Vet Res* 68(2):149-150, 2001.

58. Youngprapakorn P, Ousavaplangchai L, Kanchanapangka S: *A Color Atlas of Diseases of the Crocodile,* ed 1, Thailand, 1995, Style Creative House.

59. Nevarez JG: Unpublished data from clinical and research cases, LA, 2002-2003.

60. McCowan C, Shepherdley C, Slocombe RF: Herpes virus-like particles in the skin of a saltwater crocodile *(Crocodylus porosus), Aust Vet J* 82(6):375-377, 2004.

61. Johnson A: (Personal communication), March 2005.

62. Jacobson ER, Popp JA, Shields RP et al: Poxlike skin lesions in captive caimans, *J Am Vet Med Assoc* 175(9):937-940, 1979.

63. Penrith ML, Nesbit JW, Huchzermeyer FW: Pox virus infection in captive juvenile caimans *(Caiman crocodilus fuscus)* in South Africa, *J S Afr Vet Assoc* 62(3):137-139, 1991.

64. Ramos MC, Coutinho SD, Matushima ER et al: Poxvirus dermatitis outbreak in farmed Brazilian caimans *(Caiman crocodilus yacare), Aust Vet J* 80(6):371-372, 2002.

65. Horner RF: Poxvirus in farmed Nile crocodiles, *Vet Rec* 122(19):459-462, 1990.

66. Pandey GS, Inoue N, Ohshima K et al: Poxvirus infection in Nile crocodiles *(Crocodylus niloticus), Res Vet Sci* 49(2):171-176, 1990.

67. Buenviaje GN, Ladds PW, Melville L: Poxvirus infection in two crocodile, *Aust Vet J* 69(1):15-16, 1992.

68. Miller DL, Mauel MJ, Baldwin C et al: West Nile virus in farmed alligators, *Emerg Infect Dis* 9(7):794-799, 2003.

69. Steinman A, Banet-Noach C, Tal S et al: West Nile virus infection in crocodiles, *Emerg Infect Dis* 9(7):887-889, 2003.

70. Rubio A: (Personal communication), Mexico, 2003.

71. Klenk K, Snow J, Morgan K et al: Alligators as West Nile virus amplifiers. *Emerg Infect Dis* 10(12):2150-2154, 2004.

72. Nevarez JG, Mitchell MA, Kim DY et al: West Nile Virus in Alligator *(Alligator mississippiensis)* ranches from Louisiana, *J Herpetol Med and Surg* 15(3):4-9, 2005.

73. Nevarez JG: Unpublished data on fungal isolates from the skin of American alligators *(Alligator mississippiensis),* 2003.

74. Buenviaje GN, Ladds PW, Melville L et al: Disease-husbandry associations in farmed crocodiles in Queensland and the Northern Territory, *Aus Vet J* 71(6):165-173, 1994.

75. Fromtling RA, Jensen JM, Robinson BE et al: Fatal mycotic pulmonary disease of captive American alligators, *Vet Pathol* 16:428-431, 1979.

76. Trevino GS: Cephalosporiosis in three caimans, *J Wildl Dis* 8:385-388, 1972.

77. Frelier PF, Sigler L, Nelson PE: Mycotic pneumonia caused by *Fusarium moniliforme* in an alligator, *Sabouraudia* 23(6):399-402, 1985.

78. Silberman MS, Blue J, Mahaffey E: Phycomycoses resulting in death of crocodiles in a common pool, *Proc AAZV,* pp 100-101, 1977.

79. Thomas AD, Sigler L, Peucker S et al: *Chrysosporium* anamorph of *Nannizziopsis vriesii* associated with fatal cutaneous mycoses in the salt-water crocodile *(Crocodylus porosus), Med Mycol* 40(2):143-151, 2002.

80. Maslen M, Whitehead J, Forsyth WM et al: Systemic mycotic disease of captive crocodile hatchling *(Crocodylus porosus)* caused by *Paecilomyces lilacinus, J Med Vet Mycol* 26(4):219-225, 1988.

81. Ariel E, Ladds PW, Buenviaje GN: Concurrent gout and suspected hypovitaminosis A in crocodile hatchlings, *Aust Vet J* 75(4):247-249, 1997.

82. Wallach JD, Hoessle C, Bennett J: Hypoglycemic shock in captive alligators, *J Am Vet Med Assoc* 51(7):893-896, 1967.

83. Nevarez JG, Mitchell MA, Kim DY et al: Lymphohistiocytic proliferative syndrome of captive-reared American alligators *(Alligator mississippiensis)* from Louisiana, *Proc of the Assoc of Reptil and Amphib Vets,* pp 73-75, 2003.

84. Nevarez JG: Unpublished data on lymphohistiocytic proliferative syndrome of alligators (LPSA), 2004.

85. Vonier PM, Crain DA, McLachlan JA et al: Interaction of environmental chemicals with the estrogen and progesterone receptors from the oviduct of the American alligator, *Environ Health Perspect* (12):1318-1322, 1996.

86. Lind PM, Milnes MR, Lundberg R et al: Abnormal bone composition in female juvenile American alligators from a pesticide-polluted lake (Lake Apopka, Fla), *Environ Health Perspect* 112(3):359-362, 2004.

87. Stoker C, Rey F, Rodriguez H et al: Sex reversal effects on *Caiman latirostris* exposed to environmentally relevant doses of the xenoestrogen bisphenol A, *Gen Comp Endocrinol* 133(3):287-296, 2003.

88. Guillette LJ Jr, Vonier PM, McLachlan JA: Affinity of the alligator estrogen receptor for serum pesticide contaminants, *Toxicology* 181-182: 151-154, 2002.

89. Rauschenberger RH, Wiebe JJ, Buckland JE et al: Achieving environmentally relevant organochlorine pesticide concentrations in eggs through maternal exposure in *Alligator mississippiensis, Mar Environ Res* 58(2-5): 851-856, 2004.

90. Allsteadt J, Lang JW: Incubation temperature affects body size and energy reserves of hatchling American alligators *(Alligator mississippiensis), Physiol Zool* 68(1):76-97, 1995.

91. Helmick KE, Papich MG, Vliet KA et al: Pharmacokinetics of enrofloxacin after single-dose oral and intravenous administration in the American alligator *(Alligator mississippiensis), J Zoo Wildl Med* 35(3):333-340, 2004.

92. Helmick KE, Papich MG, Vliet KA et al: Pharmacokinetic disposition of a long-acting oxytetracycline formulation after single-dose intravenous and intramuscular administrations in the American alligator *(Alligator mississippiensis), J Zoo Wildl Med* 35(3):341-346, 2004.

93. Mitchell MA: Physical and chemical restraint of crocodilians, British Veterinary Zoological Society Autumn Meeting, Regents Park, London, 1999.

94. Lloyd ML, Reichard T, Odum RA: Gallamine reversal in Cuban crocodiles *(Crocodylus rhombifer)* using neostigmine alone versus neostigmine with hyaluronidase, *Proc AAZV,* pp 117-120, 1994.

95. Lloyd ML: Crocodilian anesthesia. In Fowler ME, Miller RE, editors: *Zoo and Wildlife Animal Medicine,* Philadelphia, 1999, WB Saunders.

96. Spiegel RA, Lane TJ, Larsen RE et al: Diazepam and succinylcholine chloride for restraint of the American alligator, *J Am Vet Med Assoc* 185(11):1335-1336, 1984.

97. Heaton-Jones TG, Ko JC-H, Heaton-Jones DL: Evaluation of medetomidine-ketamine anesthesia with atipamezole reversal in American alligators *(Alligator mississippiensis), J Zoo Wildl Med* 33(1):36-44, 2002.

CHAPTER 7

SNAKES

■ COMMON SPECIES KEPT IN CAPTIVITY

Snakes are listed in the class Reptilia and order Squamata. Squamata include the suborders Serpentes (snakes) and Sauria (lizards). There are over 2900 species of snakes in the world. Extant populations of snakes are generally divided into three classes: Scolecophidia, Alethinophidia, and Caenophidia.[1]

A variety of snake species are kept in captivity. The most common, by far, are the colubrids, boids, and pythons. The colubrids (1658+ species) are the largest and most diverse group of snakes and have a worldwide distribution, except for Antarctica. Both venomous and nonvenomous species are found within this family. Colubrids are found in aquatic, terrestrial, semiterrestrial, and arboreal habitats. The boas (Boidae) (40+ species) are a diverse group of snakes that can be found in fossorial, ground-dwelling, and arboreal niches from the Americas, Central Africa, South Asia, Madagascar, the West Indies, and the southwest Pacific Islands. Pythons (Pythonidae) (25+ species) were historically included in the family Boidae. However, pythons are restricted to the Old World (Africa, Asia, Australia). Pythons, like boas, may inhabit aquatic, terrestrial, and arboreal niches within their range.

The corn snakes *(Elaphe guttata)* and king snakes *(Lampropeltis* spp.) are by far the most common snakes kept in captivity. Most corn snakes and king snakes attain a total length of 1 to 2 m (3-6 feet). These animals are known for their relatively calm dispositions, although some king snakes can be aggressive. Corn snakes make good first pet reptiles. Corn snakes and king snakes have been selectively bred over the past decades for their color morphs. A wide variety of color morphs have

been developed from the common (e.g., amelanistic) to the uncommon (e.g., lavender) (Figure 7-1). The value of the snake can increase significantly based on its color. This is most evident when evaluating the other common snakes held in captivity, pythons and boids. Designer-colored ball pythons *(Python regius)* can range in price from the hundreds of dollars to tens of thousands of dollars (Figure 7-2). Pythons are popular not only for their beauty but also for their gentle disposition. There are certainly exceptions to this rule. The giant pythons, such as the Burmese *(Python molurus bivittatus)* and reticulated pythons *(Python reticulatus),* become too large for most pet owners and should not be recommended as pets (Figure 7-3). Instead, these animals should be handled only by those experienced herpetoculturists that accept the responsibility and liability that comes with giant snake ownership. Many state and local governments have established regulations banning large snakes. Veterinarians should become familiar with both state and local policies to ensure that they can make the most appropriate recommendations to their clients.

Veterinarians may be asked to work with venomous species of snakes. I recommend leaving these snakes to those with experience. Veterinarians incur a real liability, both personal and professional, when working with these animals. Unfortunately, most situations requiring a veterinarian arise after a problem has occurred rather than before an animal has been acquired. For these reasons, I limit my venomous snake medicine to those animals being housed at zoologic and educational institutions. State and local regulations regarding venomous snakes are also becoming commonplace, and veterinarians working with these animals should become familiar with these policies.

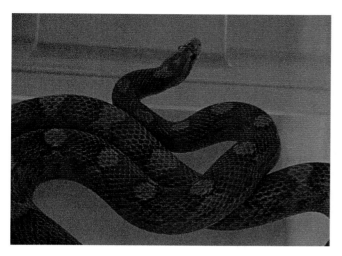

Figure 7-1 Corn snakes (*Elaphe guttata*) are members of the family colubridae. These snakes are native to North America. Corn snakes represent the first group of captive snakes bred in large numbers to promote "designer" skin patterns. Corn snakes are docile, thereby making an ideal first pet snake.

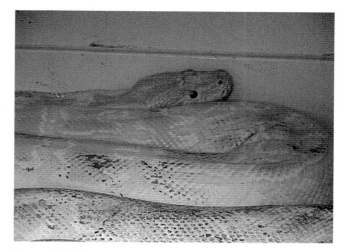

Figure 7-3 The giant species of python, such as this Burmese python (*Python molurus bivittatus*), should not be recommended as pets. These animals are best left to experienced herpetoculturists.

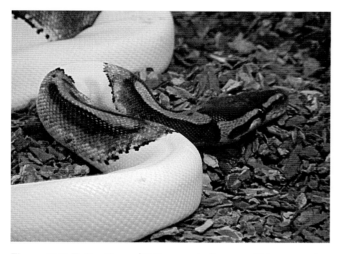

Figure 7-2 Ball pythons (*Python regius*) are an African species of python (Pythonidae) that are still routinely imported into the United States. These animals are also being captive bred in large numbers. "Designer" patterns have been developed, which can cost tens of thousands of dollars.

■ BIOLOGY: ANATOMY AND PHYSIOLOGY

The anatomy of the snake, for the most part, is consistent across species. Therefore, developing a general understanding of organ location in one species will be beneficial in working with others. When evaluating the anatomy of the snake, it may be best to separate the snake into three sections. The proximal one third of the snake generally contains the trachea, esophagus, parathyroid glands, thymus, thyroid, and the heart. The second third contains the lung(s), liver, continuation of the

esophagus, stomach, spleen, gallbladder, pancreas, proximal small bowel, and airsac. The final third contains the caudal small intestine, gonads, adrenal glands, kidneys, cecum, colon, and cloaca. This system of thirds may be useful when attempting to identify an area of interest using diagnostic imaging or when deciding on a surgical approach. In some cases, multiple images or incisions may be required to fully ascertain certain organ systems.

Snake skin is relatively inelastic, as a result of the rigid protective scales (beta-keratin). This might be considered a problem for an animal that must swallow its prey whole, but is not as a result of a thin elastic alpha-keratin region. The alpha-keratin includes the interscalar region and is most obvious in snakes during the ingestion of prey or in obese animals as their skin stretches. Snake scales originate from the epidermis. The integument of the snake is covered with two primary scale types, both originating from the epidermis. Small scales cover the dorsum and lateral surfaces of the snake, whereas larger scales cover the ventrum. It is important to make a distinction between the two scale types when considering an exploratory coeliotomy, as an incision in the ventral scales could result in significant tension on the sutures after closure and an increased likelihood of the incision becoming contaminated. I prefer to make the initial incision between the second and third rows (from the ventrum) of dorsal scales (Figure 7-4). Differences in scale shape, size, and texture can be used to differentiate snake species. For example, the presence of keeled versus nonkeeled scales is a basic taxonomic key. The snake's integument should feel dry and warm (if it is housed under appropriate environmental conditions), which is in direct contrast to the public's perception that snakes are cold and slimy. Snake skin is dry because it is relatively aglandular, although some reptiles have developed regionalized glands that are useful in attracting mates or in defending themselves against predators.

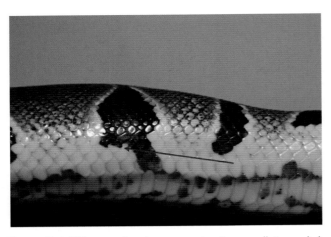

Figure 7-4 When performing an exploratory coeliotomy, it is important to make the incision between dorsal row scales. In this figure, the incision was made between the second and third rows (from the ventrum) of dorsal scales.

Ecdysis (shedding) is a naturally occurring process in the snake that is regulated by the thyroid gland. Snakes should shed their entire skin, including their spectacles, in one piece, although large snakes (>3 m) may shed their skin in pieces. Once the process of ecdysis is started, it generally takes approximately 14 days to complete. During this period it is not uncommon for a snake to become anorectic, appear listless, and avoid contact. Immediately before ecdysis, some snakes have increased respiratory sounds. This is generally associated with reduced airflow through the nares, resulting from a constriction of the shed surrounding the nares. A small-gauge hypodermic needle (25-gauge) can be used to remove any obstructive material. Excessive handling during the ecdysis period is not recommended, as it is possible to damage the newly formed underlying epidermis. Approximately 14 days before the shed, the snake will have a dull (grayish) appearance. The spectacles take on a "blue" color 7 to 10 days before the shed and then clear 2 to 3 days later. The dull color is associated with the lymphatics and enzymes that fill the space between the old and new epidermal layers. Captive snakes should be provided appropriate cage furniture (e.g., rock) to rub their rostrum against to facilitate the shedding process.

Snakes do not have eyelids. To compensate, snakes produce *spectacles* (also called *brilles*). Spectacles are a modification of the epidermis and provide protection for the exposed anterior surface of the globe. Because they originate from the epidermis, the spectacles are routinely shed during ecdysis. Retention of the spectacles has been associated with the development of corneal disease and panophthalmitis.

The skeletal system of snakes is unique among the reptiles. The skull of the snake is kinetic and does not have a mandibular symphysis, which allows it to ingest prey items larger than would be possible by a reptile with a fixed skull. The vertebral column is comprised of several hundred vertebrae that show minimal regionalization. Snakes do not have a sternum. The ventral aspect of each rib is attached by muscle to the ventral

scales. Pelvic remnants are present in all of the Scolecophidians, but hindlimb vestiges are absent. Most Alethinophidians have both pelvic remnants and hindlimb vestiges. The vestiges or spurs can be used during copulation.

Snakes do not have an external ear, tympanic membrane, or middle ear. The *stapes* (inner ear cavity) is in direct contact with the quadrate bone and transmits vibrations, enabling the snake to hear low-frequency sounds (<600 Hz).

The glottis of the snake is located on the floor of the buccal cavity. Snakes do not have vocal cords but instead make their characteristic "hissing" sound by forcing air through their glottis. The trachea of the snake has incomplete tracheal rings. Because these animals have a poorly developed mucociliary apparatus, they can have difficulty removing material from the trachea and lungs. To compensate, snakes position their head and neck in a manner that best allows unabated airflow. Snakes with respiratory disease are often found with their head and neck elevated in a 45-degree angle. Primitive snakes generally have two lungs, whereas more advanced snakes possess only one lung. The right lung is the primary lung in those species with two lungs. In general, the left lung is reduced or vestigial. Gas exchange occurs in the cranial compartment of the lung, and the caudal segment (air sac) serves to store air.

The snake heart is comprised of three chambers: two atria and one ventricle. The heart is located in the proximal one third to one fourth of the body. The heart is fairly movable in snakes, which allows for compression and displacement during the ingestion of prey. The heart is routinely used as a site of venipuncture and can be visualized by placing the animal in dorsal recumbency and looking in the approximate vicinity of the body (one third to one fourth the distance to the head) for the characteristic "beating" movement.

The digestive tract of the snake is a linear system that is modified to digest dense meals. The tongue is an important chemosensory structure. The tongue is inserted into the Jacobson organ, located in the roof of the buccal cavity, to differentiate odors. Because snakes hunt by olfaction, they can be trained to readily accept prekilled prey items. Snake teeth are homodontic, with the exception of the fangs in venomous species. The teeth of snakes have developed with the sole purpose of acquiring prey. Their general shape, being curved backward, is based on their need to apprehend and hold prey in the absence of limbs. To remove a snake that has bitten someone, it is important to consider the direction of the teeth, as pulling the animal directly from the site where it is attached will tear the skin and worsen the bite wound. Instead, the animal's head should be gently directed forward as it is being removed. Of course this is easier said than done in some cases. Snake teeth also are pleurodontic, and are therefore replaced throughout the animal's life. Of all the reptiles, snakes by far have the most teeth, with rows on the upper and lower jaws and palatine bone. Mucus excreted from the digestive glands located in the buccal cavity and esophagus lubricate prey items to facilitate ingestion. Venom glands are modified salivary glands that produce potent enzymatic compounds to assist with prey acquisition and digestion. The esophagus is a large distensible organ in the snake. The stomach is linear and produces digestive enzymes. The stomach is located approximately half the body distance from the head. The small intestine and colon are also linear structures, losing much of the coiling frequently observed in omnivores and herbivores. The cloaca is comprised of the coprodeum, urodeum, and proctodeum. The coprodeum is located in the dorsal region of the cloaca and receives fecal material from the colon. The urodeum is located ventrally and serves as the collection site for urine from the ureters. The oviducts also open into the urodeum. The proctodeum is the collecting chamber for the urodeum and coprodeum.

The snake's liver is a linear (single-lobed) organ. The liver generally begins just distal to the heart and ends at the cranial segment of the stomach. In most species the gallbladder is not directly associated with the liver. The pancreas, spleen, and gallbladder often form a triad and are located at the caudal segment of the stomach, whereas other species have a combined hepatopancreas.

Snake gonads are found cranial to the kidneys, and the right gonad is cranial to the left gonad. Male snakes do not have an epididymis. Male snakes possess paired copulatory organs called the *hemipenes*. The hemipenes are invaginated and lie in the lateral base of the tail. During copulation, a hemipenis will engorge and evaginate. All fertilization is internal. The hemipenes do not serve an excretory function.

Female snakes may be oviparous or viviparous. Snakes from the families Anomalepodae, Typhopidae, Leptotyphlopidae, Anomochilidae, Xenopeltidae, Loxocemidae, Pythonidae are oviparous; those from Uropeltidae, Cylindrophiidae, Aniliidae, and Boidae are viviparous; and snakes from the families Tropidophiidae, Acrochordidae, Viperidae, Atractaspididae, Colubridae, and Elapidae have members that are both oviparous and viviparous.

Some pythons display maternal care of their eggs. The maternal investment reduces the likelihood of predation and increases the likelihood that the eggs will hatch. The coiling also serves to regulate egg temperature.

Snakes have metanephric kidneys that are linear and lobulated. The right kidney is cranial to the left kidney. Male snakes develop sexual segments during their reproductive cycle. Snakes do not have a urinary bladder.

■ HUSBANDRY
Environmental Conditions
ENCLOSURE SIZE

The shape and size of the enclosure should be selected based on the snake's biology. For example, a fossorial species should be housed in an enclosure that is long and wide. The height of the enclosure would not be terribly important for a fossorial species. In contrast, an arboreal species should be housed in a tall enclosure to ensure that ample foliage can be placed into the enclosure. Because obesity is a common problem in large captive snakes, snakes should be provided ample area with an enclosure for physical activity. The enclosure should also be large enough to provide an appropriate environmental temperature range.

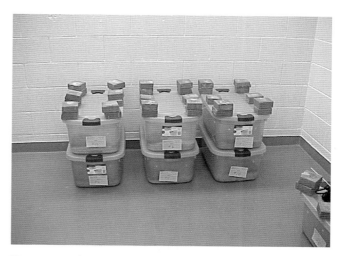

Figure 7-5 Plastic storage boxes are a common method used to store large numbers of snakes. Because of the limited size of these enclosures, developing an appropriate temperature range for the animal can be difficult. In most cases, it is easiest to set the room temperature to the desired level to accommodate the snakes.

Snake enclosures can be made from a variety of materials. The most common remains the glass fish tank. These enclosures are relatively inexpensive, are easy to clean, and provide direct visualization of the pet. Plastic storage boxes are another common commercial product used to house snakes (Figure 7-5). These enclosures are also inexpensive, easy to clean, and readily available. Many of these enclosures are not clear, so direct visualization may be limited. Commercial snake enclosures have become quite popular (Figure 7-6). These enclosures are aesthetically pleasing and easy to clean. One disadvantage of commercial enclosures is that they are more expensive than traditional enclosures.

VENOMOUS SNAKES

Venomous snakes should be housed in enclosures that have restricted access to nonessential individuals. The enclosures should have two locking mechanisms, in case one locking mechanism fails. The enclosure should be designed so that the snake can be visualized from the outside of the enclosure. There should always be at least two people involved with the handling of a venomous snake. Appropriate tongs, hooks, and collection tubes should be available for handling venomous snakes. Large, easy-to-read VENOMOUS SNAKE signs should be placed on the external walls of the enclosure. An emergency phone should be placed in the vicinity of the venomous snake enclosures with contact numbers for the local zoo, paramedics, and hospital. An antivenom protocol should be on hand at the local hospital.

TEMPERATURE

Snakes are ectotherms and depend on the environmental temperature to regulate their core body temperature. If these animals are not provided an appropriate temperature range, their metabolic rate slows. Snakes with slow metabolic rates often have a history of being anorectic, lethargic, and depressed. An inability to maintain an appropriate body temperature can also result in a reduced immune response. In my experience, many of the snakes with chronic infections are not provided exposure to an appropriate environmental temperature. To prevent these problems, snakes should be provided an environmental temperature range. The environmental temperature should mimic the animal's natural climate and should be separated into different gradients. It is important to realize that reptiles have temperature options in nature. They can bask under the sun on a rock if they wish or hide in the shade away from the heat to prevent overheating. This same system should be mimicked in captivity. I recommend that clients use variable wattage incandescent light to create a temperature gradient. Bulb wattage will depend on the size of the enclosure. A list of recommended environmental temperature zones for captive snakes can be found in Table 7-1. It is important to provide snakes a cooling period at night. For most of the temperate species, room temperature is acceptable, whereas for some tropical species, additional heat may be required. Visible light (e.g., incandescent bulbs) should not be used at night to provide heat. It is important that animals are provided a period of darkness. I generally recommend a photoperiod of 12 hours per day. This can be altered during the breeding cycle (lengthened) or aestivation period (shortened). When supplemental heat is required during periods of darkness, ceramic heat emitters or under-tank heating elements can be used.

Regardless of the heat source, snakes should not be allowed direct contact with the heating element. Animals that are allowed direct contact can develop severe thermal injuries (first to third degree). Thermal injuries should be managed aggressively. Necrotic tissue should be sharply dissected and the wound protected. I apply a hyperosmotic solution (50% dextrose) onto the wound as a microbicide. The hyperosmotic is left on the wound for 2 minutes and than rinsed away with a 0.9% saline. The fluids are always warmed (to the animal's preferred optimum) before being applied. The application of cooled or room temperature fluids can lead to a lowering of the body temperature and a reduced healing time. The hyperosmotic is applied twice daily until sufficient granulation tissue appears. The wound must be protected against desiccation. Silver sulfadiazine can be applied to the lesion to prevent desiccation and provide an antimicrobial effect. This compound is comprised of both a microbicide (silver) and an antibiotic (sulfadiazine). Bandaging these wounds can be difficult. Frye[2] has suggested using condoms, but even these can fail. I have used Tegaderm (3M, Inc., St. Paul, Minnesota) with some success. These wounds can require weeks to months to heal. Snakes with severe thermal burns should be provided fluids to replenish any losses incurred either directly as a result of the injury or after the injury until the integument heals. Systemic antibiotics also should be considered in the treatment plan.

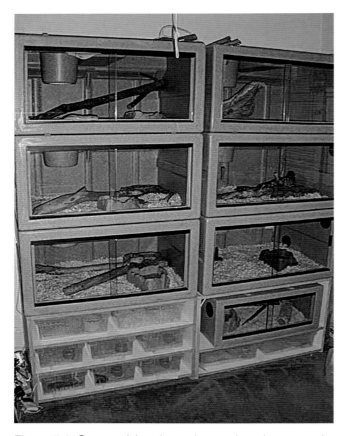

Figure 7-6 Commercial snake enclosures have become quite popular. These cages are generally easy to clean and disinfect and are aesthetically pleasing compared to plastic storage containers. (Courtesy Dr. Orlando Diaz-Figueroa.)

TABLE 7-1	Environmental Temperature Range Recommendations for Captive Snakes	
Species	Daytime temperature range	Nighttime temperature range
Corn snake	76-86° F (24-30° C)	70-75° F (21-24° C)
California kingsnake	78-88° F (25-30° C)	70-78° F (21-25° C)
Ball python	80-88° F (26-31° C)	75-80° F (24-26° C)
Boa constrictor	80-88° F (26-31° C)	75-80° F (24-26° C)
Burmese python	80-88° F (26-31° C)	75-80° F (24-26° C)
Brazilian rainbow	78-88° F (25-31° C)	75-80° F (24-26° C)
Emerald tree boa	80-88° F (26-31° C)	75-80° F (24-26° C)
Milk snake	76-86° F (24-30° C)	70-75° F (21-24° C)

HUMIDITY

Humidity is an important environmental factor to monitor for snakes. The enclosure humidity should mimic the animal's natural climate. In general, desert species tolerate humidity levels between 30% and 50%, subtropical species from 60% to 80%, and tropical species from 80% to 90%. Snakes maintained in environments with low humidity may be predisposed to dehydration and dysecdysis. Excessive humidity is frequently associated with the development of dermatitis. Humidity levels can be monitored using a hygrometer. Digital hygrometers are preferred because they can be moved around within an enclosure to determine areas that are appropriate and inappropriate. Humidity levels can be altered in an enclosure by adding a large water bowl, aerating water within a water receptacle (e.g., bowl or mason jar), adding an incubation chamber, misting the enclosure daily, or adding live plants. Large water bowls serve as a source of humidity for an enclosure as the water evaporates into the enclosure. The overall contribution of moisture to the humidity can vary based on the environmental temperature and size of the enclosure. Daily misting is a simple method for elevating the humidity, but it may provide only a temporary increase in the humidity. Incubation chambers are an excellent method for providing snakes an increased environmental humidity. I generally place moist sphagnum moss into a plastic shoe box (with ventilation holes) to create an incubation chamber. Because most snakes naturally burrow, the incubation chamber can also provide a shelter or hiding spot. Live plants can provide an improved aesthetic appearance within an enclosure, but larger snakes may damage them.

LIGHTING

Historically, lighting systems for captive snakes have not been given a great deal of attention. Many snake breeders maintain their snakes in stacks of enclosures, where the animals only receive indirect room lighting. Although many of these animals thrive and reproduce successfully, it is my belief that snakes, like other reptiles, should be provided high-quality, full-spectrum light. Full-spectrum light has many benefits, from the provision of ultraviolet radiation to rich, visible light. Recent work by my laboratory has found that certain snakes increase their 25 hydroxyvitamin D blood levels with exposure to ultraviolet B radiation (Figure 7-7). It is not known whether snakes require ultraviolet B radiation to initiate the synthesis of vitamin D. Many believe that these animals obtain their vitamin D through the ingestion of prey. Regardless, ultraviolet A and visible light remain important to snakes for regulating behavior and stimulating reproduction. I recommend providing captive snakes full-spectrum lighting to mimic the beneficial effects of sunlight. Snakes should be provided a 12-hour photoperiod. The photoperiod can be altered for the breeding season (lengthened) or brumation period (shortened). Research to elucidate the specific lighting needs of snakes should be pursued.

SUBSTRATE

Selecting an appropriate substrate for a snake is an important consideration, as these animals, especially terrestrial species,

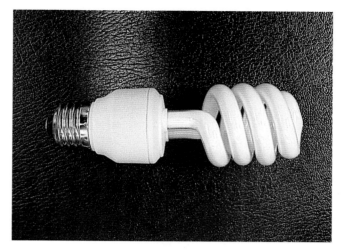

Figure 7-7 This type of coiled fluorescent bulb (Fluker Farms, Port Allen, Louisiana) has been found to increase 25-hydroxyvitamin D levels in corn snakes.

live directly on/in their substrate. When considering which substrate is best for a particular species, it is important to attempt to replicate its natural habitat. Animals that are fossorial should be provided a substrate that will allow them to burrow, while those that are arboreal need plant accessories more than a substrate. The following is a list of common substrates: newspaper, paper towels, gravel, bark chips, aspen, and sand. Snake breeders commonly use newspaper and paper towels because they are inexpensive and can be easily replaced. These substrates do not, however, allow a pet owner to regulate certain aspects of the vivarium, such as humidity. Another benefit of these substrates is that they allow a veterinarian or herpetoculturist to monitor fecal and urine output. This is especially important for recently acquired animals. Although there is an old belief that the ink found on newspaper is potentially toxic to animals, this belief is unfounded. Gravel used for aquaria can be used for snakes, but it must be large enough that it cannot be consumed. Snakes are notorious for ingesting substrate when swallowing their prey. Orchid bark chips can be used as a substrate for those species naturally found in forested areas. For burrowing species, the depth of the bark chips should be sufficient to allow the snakes to cover themselves. Natural leaf litter can also be used, but it should be thoroughly inspected for the presence of pest bugs before being placed into the vivarium. Aspen is one of the most common substrates used for captive snakes. When snakes defecate or urinate in aspen, the aspen absorbs and holds the waste, which allows the caretaker to scoop out the material using a cat litter scoop. Sand can also be used as a substrate for snakes; however, only "play sand" (e.g., the type used for children's sandboxes) should be used. Quartz-based sands used in aquaria are not recommended, as they are sharp-edged particulates and can become impacted in the skin or cause lacerations.

Accessories

A snake vivarium should mimic an animal's natural habitat. Accessories or "cage furniture" can be used to create an environment that reduces the stress an animal may otherwise encounter in captivity. It is important to always attempt to minimize stress, as it can lead to elevated corticosterone levels that affect the animal's metabolic rate and immune function. Terrestrial animals should be provided an appropriate substrate and an adequate number of hiding locations or shelters. Snakes are naturally found hiding in detritus or under rocks or fallen wood. Providing these animals a similar hiding location is highly recommended. There are a number of commercially available products that can be used to meet these needs, or a pet owner can simply find a piece of fallen wood. Again, any materials found outside should be inspected for pest bugs.

Arboreal species should be provided adequate climbing areas. Not having an opportunity to climb vertically can be just as stressful to these species as not having a hiding spot. Various materials can be used to meet these requirements. Commercially available wood branches (e.g., manzanita and driftwood) can be purchased from local pet retailers. The branches should be large enough to support the animal's weight. Branches found locally can also be used but should be free of pest bugs and insecticides.

Plants can be used to provide additional hiding areas for arboreal snakes. Plastic plants are often used because they are easy to disinfect and can withstand being climbed on. Hardy live plants can also be used. I prefer pothos *(Epipremnum aureum)* because it is inexpensive and capable of taking a great deal of neglect. Another benefit associated with live plants is that they can help to regulate or maintain the vivarium humidity. Plants also may be used for terrestrial species, but they should be well planted to avoid being destroyed.

Humidity chambers are important accessories for some snakes. These devices can be used to provide a focal area of high humidity, mimicking a burrow. In addition to their importance for providing increased humidity, they also serve as hiding spots. A plastic container (e.g., plastic shoe box) with a secure lid can be used to create a humidity chamber. Several small ventilation holes should be made in the sides of box, and a single large entrance/exit hole can be made on one end of the chamber. I generally prefer to use moistened sphagnum moss to create the humidity chamber. To moisten the moss, the material should be washed with tap water and then wrung out. The moss should be remoistened as needed. A hygrometer can be used to determine the humidity within the chamber and to determine when it should be rewashed. The moss should be replaced once it is soiled.

Snakes should be provided access to water at all times. A water bowl large enough for the animal to enter should be placed in the vivarium. Snakes routinely soak when provided access to water. Soaking is thought to increase gastrointestinal motility, assist with the removal of ectoparasites (e.g., drown mites), and serve as a stimulus to drink. The water should be changed whenever it is soiled or at least once weekly.

■ NUTRITION

Snakes are carnivorous. The dietary habits of snakes are quite diverse, and prey selection depends on their specific anatomic adaptions. Blind snakes, false blind snakes, shieldtail snakes, and thread snakes prey on soft-bodied invertebrates in fossorial habitats. Many of these snakes are specialists that feed almost exclusively on termites. Although these snakes generally remain in subterranean habitats, they will move into arboreal (tree trunk) habitats to pursue termites. Pipe snakes and false coral snakes primarily feed on other species of snakes, although false blind snakes will also prey on amphisbaenians. Sunbeam snakes, Mesoamerican pythons, boids, and pythons generally will prey on reptiles and mammals. However, Mesoamerican pythons will prey also on lizard and chelonian eggs, and arboreal species from these groups will frequently prey on avian species. Splitjaw boas and dwarf boas prey primarily on lizards. Wart snakes are adapted to aquatic systems and prey almost exclusively on fish. Vipers, pitvipers, colubrids, and elapids prey on a wide variety of vertebrates, including fish, reptiles, amphibians, birds, and mammals, depending on their range and prey availability.

Because the gastrointestinal tract of the snake is relatively short, it is important that these animals, in captivity, are provided high-quality diets. The diet for each snake should be selected based on the animal's normal feeding strategy. Arboreal snakes tend to prefer avian and mammalian prey items. Terrestrial species will consume a variety of vertebrate prey (e.g., amphibians, reptiles, birds, and mammals), although some are highly selective (e.g., ophiophagous species eat primarily other snakes). Aquatic species generally accept fish and amphibians, although they can be trained to accept mammalian prey too. Diversity in the diet is essential. Avoid feeding obese prey items. Always recommend feeding euthanized prey to snakes. Live prey items can cause life-threatening injuries if left unattended with the snake. Because snakes use olfaction to hunt, they can be readily trained to accept euthanized prey. Prey items should be humanely euthanized. Carbon dioxide or cervical dislocation may be used to effectively euthanize prey. Feeding frequency should be based on the caloric needs of the snake. I recommend waiting for the animal to defecate its previous meal before offering another meal. This will help reduce the likelihood of problems should gastrointestinal stasis occur. Based on this rule, juvenile snakes can be offered food every 2 to 7 days, whereas adult animals can be offered food every 7 to 21 days.

■ PREVENTIVE MEDICINE
Quarantine

The concept of quarantine is rather foreign to most herpetoculturists and veterinarians. Although they understand its value, it is often difficult to enforce. I recommend the following: All snakes should be quarantined for a minimum of 2 months before being introduced into a reptile collection. However, it is important to realize that even a 2-month quarantine may be insufficient time to detect certain viral, parasitic or bacterial diseases in which a snake is a latent carrier. A thorough physical examination and appropriate diagnostic screening assays should be performed before the snake is placed into quarantine and before removing the animal from quarantine. A complete blood count may be done to evaluate the animal's white blood cell status. An inflammatory leukogram may be indicative of an infectious disease. Serologic testing for snakes is limited to paramyxovirus. This is certainly a virus that a herpetoculturist would not want to introduce to a collection.

Routine Exams

Snakes should be examined by a veterinarian on at least an annual basis. Because these animals have evolved to mask their illness, a thorough examination by a veterinarian may be the only time a potential problem is identified. A complete blood count and plasma biochemistry analysis should be done at the same time to evaluate the physiologic status of the animal. When working with large snake collections, veterinarians may consider visiting a herpetoculturist at his or her own facility.

Disinfection and Sanitation

Veterinarians should develop disinfection and sanitation protocols for their clients to minimize the likelihood of disease transmission between animals or humans *(zoonoses)*. Various disinfectant compounds, including sodium hypochlorite and chlorhexidine, can be used to control pathogens in a snake habitat. For these compounds to be effective, it is important to remove all organic material from the surfaces being cleaned. Organic materials can reduce the potency and efficacy of disinfectants. I have used sodium hypochlorite (1000 ppt) as a method to eliminate *Salmonella* spp. in reptile enclosures. The compound was allowed a minimum of 15 minutes contact with the enclosure surfaces. Chlorhexidine (0.5%-1.0%) also has been found to be effective against a variety of pathogens. Again, a minimum of 15 minutes of contact time is recommended.

■ RESTRAINT
Manual Restraint

Before restraining an animal, it is important to identify its "weapons." In snakes, their primary weapon (defense) is their teeth. In some colubrids, boids, and pythons, their ability to constrict should also be considered a potential weapon. By effectively restraining the head and body of a snake, the veterinarian will remove the animal's weapons. Nonvenomous snakes can be effectively restrained by grasping the head of the animal at the level of the quadrate or mandible with one hand and supporting the snake's body with the other hand (Figure 7-8). An additional handler should be used for every 3 to 4 feet of snake to support the snake's spine. Snakes should never be draped over the neck of an individual.

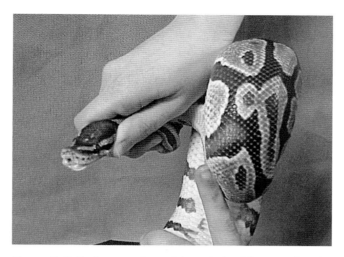

Figure 7-8 Snakes can be safely restrained by grasping the animal around the base of the mandible with the index finger and thumb. The body of the animal should be supported with the handler's free hand.

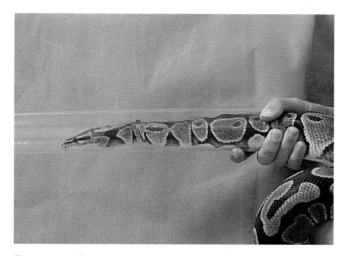

Figure 7-9 Snakes can be placed into clear plastic tubes for restraint and diagnostic sampling. This animal was placed into a tube for radiographs.

Venomous snakes should be handled only by trained professionals. Hooks and tongs should be used to remove venomous snakes from their enclosure. Once collected from an enclosure, the snake should be directed into an appropriately sized clear plastic tube. The snake should be allowed to crawl to the midpoint of the tube and then prevented from advancing (Figure 7-9). This technique allows for safe management of the snake and allows veterinarians to grossly examine the snake and collect blood from the ventral coccygeal vein. Intravenous (IV) propofol (5 mg/kg) can be administered slowly via the ventral coccygeal vein or isoflurane directed into the tube to anesthetize the snake.

Chemical Restraint

Most snakes can be safely restrained manually; however, in those cases where the snake poses a risk to the veterinarian or is too fractious for a possible procedure, chemical restraint should be considered. The dissociative agents (ketamine and tiletamine) are the preferred anesthetics for these cases. Ketamine (5-10 mg/kg intramuscular [IM]) or tiletamine (3-5 mg/kg IM) will provide sedation in most snakes. In my opinion, these doses are not appropriate for procedures that may induce pain. For more complete general anesthesia, a higher dose of these compounds may be necessary (10-20 mg/kg ketamine, 5-8 mg/kg tiletamine) or different compounds altogether (e.g., propofol or isoflurane) (see Anesthesia).

PERFORMING A PHYSICAL EXAMINATION

A snake physical examination should always be done in two parts: a hands-off exam and a hands-on exam. The hands-off exam should be done first because it can provide insight into the animal's condition. Special attention should be given to mentation, respiration, and locomotion. Abnormalities observed during a hands-off examination can be used to guide the clinician during the hands-on examination and for diagnostic testing. Abnormal mentation (e.g., a snake that does not appear aware of its surroundings), dyspnea, and/or an inability to right or move are all indicators of serious internal disease. A snake that is dyspneic should be handled cautiously during the hands-on examination or placed into an oxygen cage until it compensates. Animals that have abnormal mentation or locomotion should be restrained with care, as they may be more susceptible to injury.

The hands-on physical examination should be performed in a thorough and consistent manner. I start the examination at the head and then move caudally. The spectacles should be clear with no apparent indications of a retained spectacle or subspectacular disease. A minimal ophthalmic exam should be performed to evaluate the conjunctiva, cornea, and anterior chamber. Visual examination of the posterior chamber is difficult in snakes because of their small pupils and the fact that the iris is comprised of mixed skeletal and smooth muscle. This combination, along with the presence of a spectacle, limits the value of mydriatics in snakes. The nares should be clear and free of discharge and retained shed. The gular fold under the jaw should be examined for the presence of ectoparasites.

The oral cavity should be opened using a soft, pliable speculum. The mucous membranes should be pale to pink and free of thick ropy mucus. The tongue should be identified and evaluated. Snakes should protrude their tongue when they are in a new environment, as they use olfaction to characterize their environment. The tongue sheath should be examined closely for discharge and swelling. An abnormal tongue or tongue sheath is a significant finding and could result in anorexia in a snake. The glottis is located on the floor of the buccal cavity. Snakes have voluntary control over their glottis. The glottis should be examined closely for edema or discharge. The teeth and palate should be closely inspected for fractures or inflammation. Abscesses are a common sequela to fractured

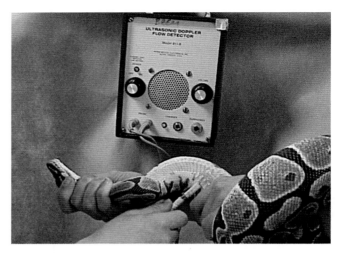

Figure 7-10 An ultrasonic Doppler can be used to obtain an audible heart beat from a snake.

teeth. Gentle expression of the surrounding soft tissue in an area with swelling may reveal a caseous discharge.

The integument should be closely inspected for ectoparasites, traumatic injuries, and inflammation (dermatitis). The spine and ribs should be palpated. The epaxial muscles should exhibit normal development. The spine will be prominent in a snake with muscle wasting. The coelomic cavity should be palpated. I generally start palpating the snake at the caudal-most aspect of the jaw and move caudally. A thumb or finger can be used to gently palpate the viscera. Any abnormal masses should be further evaluated using appropriate diagnostic tests.

It is important to assess the cardiorespiratory organs of a snake. In the past this has not always been recommended, because assessing the heart and lungs of a snake using a stethoscope can be difficult. I have found that an ultrasonic crystal Doppler can be used consistently to determine the heart rate of an animal and evaluate the snake for cardiac irregularities (Figure 7-10).

The gender of the snake should be determined as part of a routine examination. Some veterinarians charge an extra fee for determining the gender of a snake; some incorporate this into the physical examination. Knowledge of the gender of an animal is important when considering the signalment and potential differential diagnoses. Male snakes have two copulatory organs, the hemipenes. These structures are located in the base of the tail, caudal to the vent. The gender of a snake can be determined by probing for the presence or absence of these structures. Stainless steel snake probes are commercially available and highly recommended. The probe should be lubricated with a commercial lubricating jelly to facilitate passage. The probe should be inserted caudolaterally (Figure 7-11), as far as it can be directed. Once the probe cannot be inserted any further, the handler's thumb should be used to mark the position of the probe at the level of the vent. The probe should then be removed from the vent and placed on the external surface of the tail. If the probe travels farther than five scales, than the snake is (generally) a male. If the probe does not travel

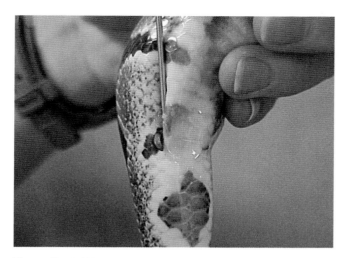

Figure 7-11 When probing a snake it is important to direct the probe caudolaterally. In most male snakes the probe can be inserted deeper than five scales.

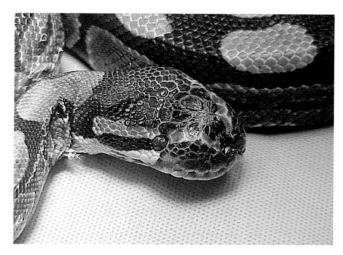

Figure 7-13 Oral abscesses are a common finding in snakes kept under inappropriate environmental temperatures. The abscesses are generally caseous in nature.

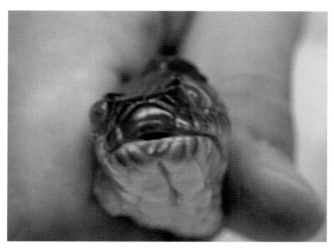

Figure 7-12 Dysecdysis is a common problem in captive snakes. Retained shed can lead to dermatitis. In this snake the spectacles were retained because of dysecdysis.

farther than five scales, then the snake is a female. Male snakes generally have longer and wider tails than do females. I will always probe the second side if the first probing suggests a female. Juvenile snakes can be sexed by gently everting a hemipenis. This technique is usually reserved for hatchlings. Holding the tail of a snake up to a bright light can also reveal the presence or absence of hemipenes.

Common Abnormalities Found on Physical Examination

Retained shed is a common finding in captive snakes suffering with dysecdysis (Figure 7-12). Animals that do not completely shed the skin from the nares may have symptoms of increased respiratory sounds, especially on exhalation. Retained spectacles also are a common problem in these cases. Rostral abra-

sions are a common finding in snakes kept in small enclosures or in "flighty" animals. Snakes can rub their rostrums to the point where they expose the frontal bones. These injuries should be treated aggressively.

Oral abscesses are a common finding in snakes with fractured teeth or injuries to the oral cavity (Figure 7-13). Affected animals often have a history of anorexia, swelling around the oral cavity, and/or oral discharge (e.g., ptyalism). A caseous discharge can often be expressed from an inflamed area.

Snakes not provided regular access to water may become dehydrated. On the physical examination these animals often show thick ropy mucus in the oral cavity, a reduced skin elasticity, and a decreased capillary refill time. In severe cases (>8% dehydration), the eyes may appear sunken as a result of the loss of fluid from the retro-orbital fat pads.

Obesity is a common finding among captive snakes, especially pythons and boids. Many of these animals are fed ad lib and not provided any exercise. Because of the calorie-rich foods that they eat (e.g., mammalian prey), these animals tend to store significant quantities of fat. Snakes store the majority of their fat within chains of intracoelomic (ICe) fat bodies. On physical examination, obese snakes often have "stretched" skin, and it is possible to observe the interscalar alpha-keratin layer.

Ectoparasites, such as mites and ticks, are a common finding on recently imported snakes. Many of these animals are maintained in less than adequate housing after capture and during transport and holding, and are rarely quarantined. Heavy burdens in young animals can lead to life-threatening anemia.

■ DIAGNOSTIC TESTING
Clinical Pathology
BLOOD COLLECTION

Blood samples can be collected from the heart, jugular, or ventral coccygeal veins of snakes. Cardiocentesis is the most frequently used venipuncture technique in snakes greater than

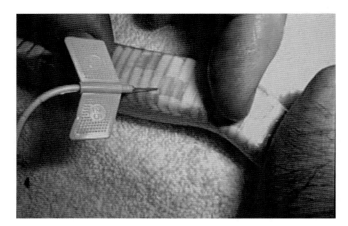

Figure 7-14 For venipuncture the heart should be isolated between an index finger and the thumb. In this corn snake, propofol is being delivered directly into the heart.

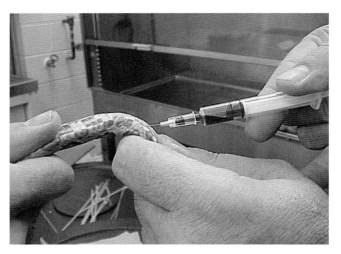

Figure 7-15 Blood can be collected from the jugular vein by inserting the needle perpendicular to the rib cage.

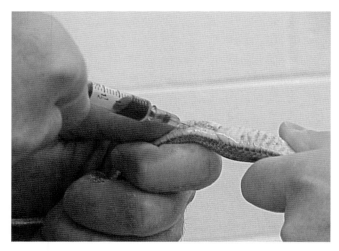

Figure 7-16 The ventral tail or coccygeal vein can be used to collect blood in larger snakes (>1 m).

200 g. The heart is located approximately one fourth to one third the distance from the snout. Placing the snake in dorsal recumbency will facilitate direct visualization of the beating heart. Venipuncture requires a minimum of two individuals: one individual to restrain the snake and a second to collect the sample. The heart should be isolated using the index finger and thumb (Figure 7-14). A 1.0- to 1.5-inch, 22- to 25-gauge needle fastened to a 3-ml syringe can be used to collect the sample. The needle should be inserted at approximately a 45-degree angle into the ventricle, and the blood will flow into the syringe with each heartbeat. If a clear fluid or diluted blood sample is obtained, the procedure should be aborted and reattempted. These samples represent lymph diluted samples and provide less than optimal results.

The jugular vein is an underutilized venipuncture site in snakes. The jugular vein of snakes is an elongate structure that is located on the medial aspect of the ribs. The heart is used as the primary landmark for locating the jugular veins. Once the heart has been identified, the location of the jugular venipuncture site(s) can be determined by counting nine ventral scales cranial to the heart. A 0.75-inch, 25-gauge needle fastened to a 3-ml syringe can be used to collect the sample. The needle can be inserted either parallel or perpendicular to the rib cage (Figure 7-15). Sample collection is based on a blind approach.

The coccygeal vein lies ventral to the caudal vertebral bodies. A 1.0- to 1.5-inch, 22- to 25-gauge needle fastened to a 3- ml syringe can be used to collect the sample. The needle should be inserted along the ventral midline at a 45-degree angle between two ventral horizontal scales approximately one third to one half the distance from the vent (Figure 7-16). Special care should be taken when collecting samples from male snakes to avoid compromising the hemipenes. The ventral coccygeal vein is most prominent in crotalids and snakes greater than 2 m.

Blood samples can be stored in ethylene diamine tetraacetic acid (EDTA) or lithium heparin microtainers (Becton Dickinson Co., Franklin Lakes, New Jersey). Complete blood counts can be performed on samples stored in either anticoagulant, although in some species the choice of anticoagulant may have an affect on the quality of the blood smear. I usually perform complete blood counts from EDTA samples and plasma biochemistry testing from lithium heparin samples. Blood smears should be made from fresh (no anticoagulant) blood samples. To reduce the likelihood of white blood cell damage during the smearing process, I premix the blood sample with 22% albumen (Gamma Biologicals, Inc., Houston, Texas). One drop of albumen to 5 drops of blood can significantly reduce the number of destroyed white blood cells in birds and reptiles (Mitchell, unpublished data). Historically, white blood cell estimates were done using the eosinophil unopette technique (Becton Dickinson Co., Franklin Lakes, New Jersey). Unfortunately, this commerical product is no longer available; however, the stain, phloxine B, can still be acquired and used to perform a white blood cell estimate.

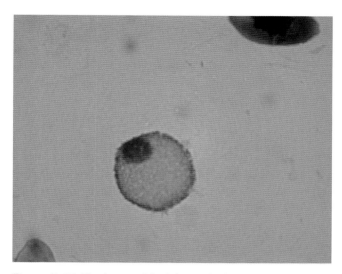

Figure 7-17 The heterophil of the snake has fusiform, eosinophilic stained granules. These cells are associated with the acute inflammatory response of snakes.

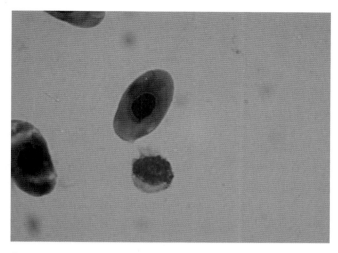

Figure 7-18 The snake lymphocyte is similar in appearance to the mammalian and avian lymphocytes. The classic lymphocyte has an acentric nucleus and high nuclear-to-cytoplasmic ratio.

Plasma biochemistries can be performed using a variety of different methods. I prefer the Abaxis VetScan (Abaxis, Inc., Union City, California), because the analyzer only requires 0.1 ml of whole blood to perform a complete biochemistry analysis. Another benefit of the system is that it does not require any time to calibrate the machine.

HEMATOLOGY

Snake erythrocytes are nucleated. Although snakes generally have fewer erythrocytes than higher vertebrates, they are longer lived (600 days).[3] Snake hematocrits tend to fall between 20% and 35%, although clinically normal snakes may have a hematocrit less than 20 or more than 35. Each individual should be evaluated on a case-by-case manner. Erythrocyte numbers can be affected by environmental conditions, reproductive status, season, and nutrition.

Heterophils are acute inflammatory cells that are frequently identified in snakes with inflammatory leukograms. Heterophils have oval to lobed nuclei and are filled with eosinophilic fusiform granules (Figure 7-17). Toxic heterophils are a common finding in chronic inflammatory responses. It is important to determine if a species depends on its lymphocytes or heterophils as the predominant cells. In species where the heterophil is the predominant cell type, the heterophil-to-lymphocyte ratio should be between 1 : 1 and 3 : 1.

Eosinophils are granulocytic cells that are often confused with heterophils. Eosinophils are filled with circular eosinophilic granules. Snakes have the largest eosinophils of all the reptiles. Although eosinophils are usually associated with allergic reactions and parasites, they likely serve other functions in an inflammatory response. Eosinophil counts may vary with stress and seasonal effects. Eosinophils are generally less than 0.5×10^3 cell/μl.

Basophils are a generally the smallest granulocytes in snakes. The nucleus of the cell is often obscured by the basophilic metachromatic granules that fill the cell. The exact function of basophils in snakes in not known; however, the cells are considered to play a role in histamine release. Basophils are generally less than 0.5×10^3 cell/μl.

Snake lymphocytes look very similar to avian and mammalian lymphocytes, with an acentric nucleus and a basophilic cytoplasm (Figure 7-18). Reptile lymphocytes function in a similar manner to lymphocytes from higher vertebrates, including moderating the immune system and producing globulins. Lymphocytes may be the predominant white blood cell in some species of snakes. Snake lymphocyte counts less than 1.5×10^3 cell/μl should be considered lymphopenic. Lymphocyte counts may vary with stress and seasonal effects.

Monocytes are the largest white blood cell encountered in snakes. The snake monocyte is similar in appearance to the monocytes described in mammals, a large nonsegmented nucleus and a blue-gray cytoplasm (Figure 7-19). Azurophils are monocyte-like but have an azure staining cytoplasm. Monocytes are primarily associated with chronic inflammatory responses and antigen processing. Absolute monocyte counts greater than 1.5×10^3 cell/μl are generally associated with a chronic inflammatory response.

Reference material for hematology in snakes is sparse. Because snake hematology can be affected by species, environmental, seasonal, and hormonal influences, interpretation of reference ranges should be made taking this information, relative to the sample population, into account. An inflammatory response in a snake may be associated with infectious agents, foreign bodies, neoplasia, traumatic injuries, and toxic exposures. In general, snakes can have an inflammatory response without an overt leukocytosis ($>15 \times 10^3$ cells/μl). In many of these cases, the leukocyte count may be within established reference ranges ($5-15 \times 10^3$ cells/μl), but the animal will have a severe monocytosis or azurophilia ($>1.5 \times 10^3$ cell/μl).

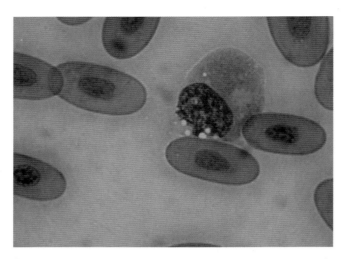

Figure 7-19 Snake monocytes are associated with the chronic inflammatory response. In some cases it can be difficult to discern a large lymphocyte from a monocyte. However, the monocyte cytoplasmic-to-nuclear ratio is higher than that of the lymphocyte.

PLASMA BIOCHEMISTRY ANALYSIS

Because ophidians have evolved to mask their illness, characterizing a disease process in a snake generally requires more than a physical examination. Plasma biochemistry analysis is an important diagnostic tool and can be used to derive important physiologic information regarding a patient. Reference material for plasma biochemistries for snakes is also sparse and variable.[4] In snakes, plasma biochemistries can be affected by environmental conditions, reproductive status, season, and nutrition.

Blood glucose is highly variable in snakes. Some species will be clinically normal with blood glucose values of 40 to 50 mg/dl. In general, blood glucose levels in snakes range from 50 to 150 mg/dl.

Calcium and phosphorus values may vary with diet and reproductive status of a female snake. In general, the calcium-to-phosphorus ratio in snakes is approximately 1.5-2 : 1. Female snakes mobilize calcium and phosphorus during the reproductive cycle and can develop significant hypercalcemias (>13 mg/dl) and hyperphosphatemias (>6 mg/dl). Snakes with renal impairment frequently have an inverse calcium-to-phosphorus ratio. Hyperphosphatemia may occur with re-feeding syndrome.

Reference ranges for the electrolytes are extremely variable. Potassium levels may vary from 2 to 6 mEq/L. Hypokalemia may occur with dietary restriction, diarrhea, and renal disease. Hyperkalemia may occur with re-feeding syndrome. Sodium levels are generally 135 to 170 mEq/L. Hypernatremia can occur with dehydration or increased salt intake. Hyponatremia is a common finding in snakes with chronic diarrhea. Chloride levels are generally between 90 and 130 mEq/L. Chloride levels, like sodium levels, increase with dehydration and dietary intake and decrease with diarrhea.

Aspartate aminotransferase (AST) is an enzyme presumed to be in all body tissues in snakes. However, an elevated AST level (>250 units/L) is generally associated with muscle or hepatic disease. Creatinine kinase (CK) is generally derived from skeletal, smooth, and cardiac muscle. An elevated CK (>300 U/L) is a strong indicator of muscle necrosis. Alanine aminotransferase (ALT) is presumed to be derived from many tissues in the body; however, unlike with AST and CK, there are no specific tissues that appear to release this enzyme in greater concentrations.

Total protein is comprised of pre-albumin, albumin, and the globulins. Protein concentrations generally increase with dehydration and inflammatory responses. Serum electrophoresis may be used to further differentiate the globulins into specific fractions. Hypoproteinemia is a frequent finding in snakes with chronic anorexia and renal disease. Hyperproteinemia is generally associated with dehydration and inflammatory disease.

Uric acid is the end product of protein catabolism in most snakes. In general, uric acid levels are <10 mg/dl in snakes. Hyperuricemia can occur as a postprandial effect in carnivores, so the time of the last meal should be considered when interpreting these results. Hyperuricemia can also occur as result of dehydration and renal tubular disease.

URINALYSIS

Urinalysis is an important diagnostic tool in mammalian veterinary medicine. The value of this diagnostic test is frequently called into question for reptiles, as these animals do not have a loop of Henle and cannot concentrate their urine. Another potential shortcoming of the urinalysis in a snake is that these animals have no urinary bladder, and urine collected from the cloaca is often contaminated with feces. However, as with any test, there is always some potential value. Urine collected directly from the ureters (via endoscopy) would likely not be contaminated and would be useful for cytology and culture. This information, in combination with other diagnostic tests, may be used to rule in or rule out disease.

Diagnostic Imaging

Diagnostic imaging is an often underutilized tool in snake medicine. Survey radiography and ultrasound can be useful tools for ruling in or ruling out specific differentials. More advanced imaging modalities, such as computed topography and magnetic resonance imaging, also can be used but are often used more sparingly because of the expense and availability to the general practitioner.

Snakes can be restrained manually, placed into a snake tube, or anesthetized for radiographs. A minimum of two images should be collected, preferably dorsoventral and lateral. The dorsoventral image can be difficult to interpret, as the spine of the snake can mask the organ systems (Figure 7-20). The lateral image provides the most insight regarding the viscera (Figure 7-21). Knowledge of normal anatomy is essential for interpreting snake radiographs. Radiographs are useful in diagnosing gastrointestinal foreign bodies, pneumonia, gastric and hepatic hypertrophy, reproductive status, and dystocia.

Ultrasound can be used to provide more specific, internal-detail, postsurvey radiographs. An ultrasound probe of 7.5 mHz or higher is recommended. I have found ultrasound invaluable in assessing snake cardiac anatomy and function, gastrointestinal motility, organ size and appearance, and reproductive status. Ultrasound also can be used to collect organ-specific fine-needle aspirates and biopsies. Both herpetoculturists

and veterinarians have found ultrasound invaluable for assessing the reproductive status of female snakes. With the value of some species topping tens of thousands of dollars, knowledge of when to combine a male and female snake to maximize the likelihood of a successful breeding event is considered priceless. Snake gonads are located in the third segment, cranial to the kidneys. I measure follicle size (>15-17 mm) and assess follicle appearance to predict ovulation (Figure 7-22). Repeated measurements should confirm that the follicle is growing in size.

Microbiology

Bacterial and fungal diseases remain significant pathogens for captive snakes. Many of the infectious agents encountered in captive snakes are directly related to inappropriate husbandry. Snakes that are not provided an appropriate thermal gradient, or are housed on a soiled substrate, may become exposed to opportunistic bacterial and fungal pathogens.

Many of the bacterial and fungal pathogens diagnosed in snakes are ubiquitous. Therefore, the techniques used to isolate these pathogens in other species (e.g., mammals) also can be used for snakes. When attempting to culture bacteria or fungi from reptiles, some advocate that the cultures should be maintained at the same environmental gradient under which the snake is housed. However, I have found that the pathogens are more likely (and more quickly) to be isolated using standard techniques (37° C). It is important to remember that many of these organisms are capable of infecting a range of hosts, including both ectotherms and endotherms.

Veterinarians interested in isolating a specific pathogen can request this of their diagnostic laboratory. Certain species, such as *Salmonella* spp., have specific requirements for growth. If these considerations are not taken into account before the sample is submitted to the laboratory, the organism may be outcompeted by more common organisms.

Parasitology

Endoparasites are a common finding in captive snakes. Although the majority of the parasites are associated with the gastrointestinal tract, there are others that can be found in the respiratory system (e.g., acanthocephalans) and integument (e.g., aberrant cestodes). When deciding which diagnostic tests should be used to confirm a diagnosis, it is best to consider the origin or location of the parasite. The presence or absence

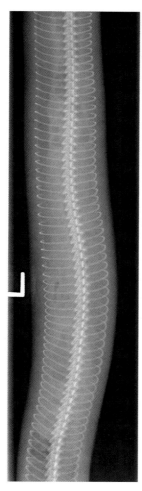

Figure 7-20 Dorsoventral radiographs in snakes may have limited value because of the prominence of the spine.

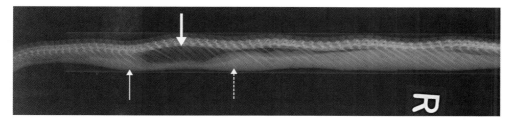

Figure 7-21 The lateral survey radiograph provides the most information regarding the viscera. In this image the heart (*thin arrow*), lung (*thick arrow*), and liver (*dashed arrow*) can be seen.

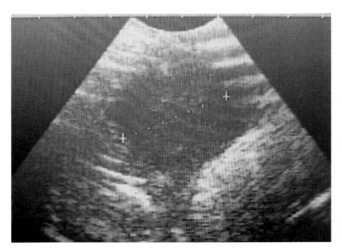

Figure 7-22 Ultrasound can be used to assess the reproductive status of a snake. Follicle size can be measured and used as a method for determining when to breed snakes.

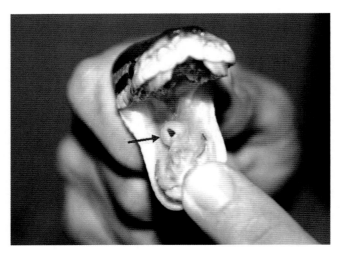

Figure 7-23 When passing a tube through the oral cavity and into the esophagus, it is important to avoid the glottis (*arrow*). The glottis is located on the floor of the oral cavity. Snakes have conscious control over the glottis.

of endoparasites was once considered useful in characterizing whether a snake was captive born or wild caught; however, this approach is often of limited value as captive-bred and imported snakes are routinely mixed in pet stores, reptile shows, and private collections.

The diagnostic tests used to confirm the presence of gastrointestinal parasites in other vertebrates are appropriate for snakes. Fecal samples should be evaluated using both a direct saline smear and a fecal flotation. The direct saline smear can be used to confirm and define bacterial and protozoal densities, whereas the fecal flotation is used to confirm the presence of trematodes, cestodes, and nematodes. Regurgitated food also can be evaluated using these techniques. If *Cryptosporidium serpentis* is suspected, then an acid-fast stain and/or Merifluor assay (Meridian Diagnostics Inc., Cincinnati, Ohio) should be considered. Any snake found to have a negative sample should be reevaluated, as all of these parasites can be transiently shed. In cases where there is no fecal output or regurgitant, a gastric lavage and/or enema can be done.

A gastric lavage can be done using a red rubber feeding tube or stainless steel gavage tube and saline. This technique requires a minimum of two individuals: one to restrain the snake and another to collect the sample. Additional assistance may be required for larger specimens. The tube should be premeasured to ensure placement into the stomach. The stomach is approximately one half the distance from the snout. The tube can be inserted into the mouth without a speculum. As the tube is being passed through the oral cavity, it is important to avoid passage into the glottis (Figure 7-23). A small quantity of lubricant can be placed on the tube to facilitate passage down the upper gastrointestinal tract. Be sure not to place excessive quantities of lubricant on the tube, as it may be aspirated into the trachea. Once the tube has been passed to the desired level, the saline solution should be instilled into the stomach. I recommend infusing no more than 5 to 10 ml/kg of saline into the stomach for this procedure. After 10 to 15 seconds, the

fluid should be aspirated back into the syringe. Once the sample has been collected, the solution should be centrifuged at 1500 rpm for 5 minutes to concentrate any pathogenic organisms. Samples should be submitted for cytologic and microbiologic testing based on the clinician's differential list.

An enema can be used to collect samples for direct visualization or as a stimulus for an animal to defecate. A red rubber feeding tube can be used for this procedure. Passing a tube into the colon of a snake is easier than it is in lizards, as snakes have no urinary bladder. The tube should be premeasured to the distance it will be passed. It is often possible to palpate feces in a colon of a snake. The tube should be lubricated to facilitate passage. I usually instill warm (snake body temperature) soapy water or 0.9% saline at a rate of 5 to 10 ml/kg. The samples should be reviewed using a direct smear and fecal flotation.

Parasites associated with the respiratory tract can generally be diagnosed via oral examination, fecal examination, or endoscopy. The eggs of lung parasites are generally passed through the trachea and into the oral cavity, where they are swallowed and passed with the feces. Sputum samples can be reviewed under light microscopy for eggs, or a direct saline smear/fecal flotation can be done to evaluate the sample for parasite eggs. A flexible endoscope can be inserted into the trachea of a snake to directly examine the lung(s) for the presence of parasites, or a rigid endoscope can be used to examine the lungs via a coelioscopy. The length of the endoscope can be a limiting factor in these cases.

Ectoparasites, including mites and ticks, are a common finding in wild-caught snakes. Adult ticks are generally easy to identify, whereas nymphs and larvae may be more difficult to visualize. Ticks are generally found around the eyes, oral cavity, and vent, although they can occur anywhere on the body. Mites are smaller in stature than ticks and thus can be more difficult to identify. Snake mites are generally found in the same areas where ticks are found, although I routinely find

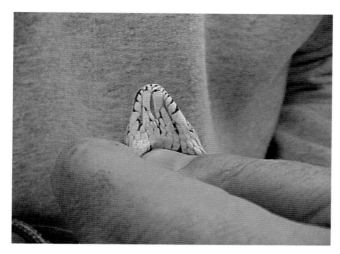

Figure 7-24 The gular fold should be inspected for ectoparasites.

them in the gular fold as well (Figure 7-24). Mites or ticks collected from a snake should be examined under a light microscope to be keyed to species.

■ COMMON DISEASE PRESENTATIONS

Infectious Diseases

BACTERIAL

Bacterial infections remain a common problem in captive snakes. The majority of the problems encountered with these animals are related to opportunistic Gram-negative bacteria, including *Escherichia coli, Pseudomonas* spp., *Aeromonas* spp., *Citrobacter freundii, C. braaki, Proteus* spp., *Serratia* spp., *Klebsiella* spp., *Enterobacter* spp., and *Salmonella* spp. Although less common, Gram-positive bacteria also have been associated with clinical disease in these animals and should be considered in a differential list. Bacterial infections can affect any system. However, most infections tend to be associated with the respiratory, gastrointestinal, and integumentary systems.

Most bacterial infections are diagnosed using standard microbiologic techniques. Because certain organisms can become injured during sample collection and transport, or are in limited numbers, an additional enrichment period may be needed. However, some organisms, such as *Chlamydophila* spp. and *Mycobacterium* spp., are difficult to isolate using standard techniques. With the advent of new molecular techniques, such as the polymerase chain reaction technique, these fastidious organisms can generally be characterized based on their 16sRNA.

Most bacterial infections in snakes are preventable. Snakes that are maintained at inappropriate environmental temperature ranges may be predisposed to opportunistic infections. Reptiles are ectotherms and rely on their environmental temperature to regulate their core body temperature. If a snake is unable to achieve an appropriate core body temperature,

then its immune function may become suppressed. Treatment should be based on antimicrobial sensitivity testing.

FUNGAL

Fungal dermatitis is a common finding in snakes maintained in moist to wet environments with poor ventilation. These conditions are frequently observed after hibernation; thus it is important to closely monitor snakes during this period. It is not uncommon to isolate multiple species of fungi from a lesion. Reptiles may harbor a large number (0-15) of different saprophytic and pathogenic fungi on their skin at any given time.[5] Cytologic examination of a skin lesion or biopsy is essential to directing the clinician's diagnostic plan. A confirmed diagnosis of a fungal disease can only be made when culture and histopathology confirm the specific pathology associated with the organism. Treatment should follow antifungal sensitivity testing. Misuse of antimicrobials may predispose snakes to fungal infections. Mycotic gastroenteritis has been reported in snakes maintained at suboptimal environmental conditions and administered inappropriate antibiotics.[6]

VIRAL

Isolating viruses from snakes is a relatively recent event. Historically, most of the infectious diseases characterized in snakes were reported to have a bacterial origin. It is possible that some of these findings were the result of limited diagnostic capabilities. With the advent of new diagnostic methods, such as enzyme-linked immunosorbent assays and the polymerase chain reaction technique, more viral diseases can be expected to be identified in the future.

Herpes virus or herpes-like viruses have been isolated from Indian cobras *(Naja naja)*, Siamese cobras *(N. naja kaouthia)*, and banded kraits *(Bungarus fasciatus)*.[7-9] The isolates from the Indian cobra and krait were incidental findings from the snake's venom.[7,8] The herpes-like virus isolated from the Siamese cobra was associated with pathologic changes in the venom gland. A herpes-like virus also has been isolated from juvenile boa constrictors *(Boa constrictor constrictor)*.[10] Intranuclear inclusions were found in the liver, pancreas, kidney, and adrenal cortex in two of the snakes.

The limited number of herpes virus infections reported in snakes might suggest that the virus is rare in ophidians; however, a lack of confirmed diagnoses may also be associated with limited diagnostic test availability or a failure of veterinarians to pursue these cases. To date, there has been no specific treatment recommendation for ophidian herpes virus infections, although acyclovir may be used to suppress infections.

Adenovirus has been isolated from a single adult boa constrictor, two rosy boas *(Lichanura trivirgata)*, and a royal python *(P. regius)*.[11-13] The histopathologic findings in the snakes were similar to those lesions described for higher vertebrates, including hepatocellular necrosis and basophilic intranuclear inclusions. The route of transmission for this virus has not been described, although minimizing contact with any secretion from an infected snake is strongly recommended.

Paramyxovirus (PMV) is one of the best-documented viral infections in snakes. The first report of this virus was from a collection of Fer-de-lance *(Bothrops atrax)* from Switzerland.[14] Since that time, PMV has been isolated from both viperid and nonviperids. All snake species should be considered susceptible to PMV. The route of transmission for this virus is likely through contact with contaminated respiratory secretions. Affected snakes may have nasal discharge and purulent hemorrhagic discharge from the glottis. Neurologic disease has also been reported to occur with PMV.[15] Diagnosis can be made using a hemagglutination inhibition assay or by viral isolation. Because the hemagglutination inhibition assay is a serologic assay, serial samples are required to confirm an active infection. In the USA, there are at least 3 laboratories performing this assay. Unfortunately, there is limited agreement between the results of these laboratories, so clinicians should use caution when interpreting the test results (M. Allender and M. Mitchell, unpublished data). Pulmonary hemorrhage and caseous debris are common postmortem findings. There is no current therapy for this virus. Trials evaluating a PMV vaccine have proven ineffective.[16] Quarantine of new acquisitions is strongly recommended. The quarantine period should be at least 3 months. A thorough examination and a minimum of two negative assays should be performed before releasing the animal from quarantine.

Inclusion body disease (IBD) can be a devastating disease in snake collections. The suspected cause of IBD is a retrovirus; however, this has yet to be confirmed. Although this disease is generally associated with boas and pythons, IBD has been reported in other species of snakes.[17] In general, boa constrictors present with a history of regurgitation and mild central nervous system dysfunction, such as a postural change (stargazing), slowed righting reflex, and impaired locomotion (Figure 7-25). Pythons generally present for more severe disturbances of the central nervous system, including a loss of the righting response, opisthotonos, and paralysis. As the disease progresses, snakes generally experience weight loss, dysecdysis, and secondary opportunistic infections, such as stomatitis, dermatitis, and pneumonia. The severe neurologic disease characterized in pythons generally limits their ability to acquire food; therefore regurgitation is rarely noted in pythons.

The route of transmission for IBD has not been determined. However, clinical disease has been identified in snakes that have direct contact with infected individuals and with snake mites *(Ophionyssus natricis)*. Diagnosis can be attempted antemortem from biopsies of the kidney, pancreas, esophagus, and liver. Eosinophilic intranuclear inclusions may be observed within the tissues when using a hematoxylin and eosin stain. Inclusion bodies may also be observed in red blood cells. However, only trained individuals should perform this procedure, as red blood cell nonviral inclusions are not uncommon findings in reptiles. Because of the low sensitivity of biopsy, false negative results are possible. One of the difficulties in characterizing IBD is that boas have been shown to harbor endogenous retroviruses. Because adenoviruses and reoviruses have also been isolated from snakes with neurologic disease, it is difficult to determine if these viruses also play a role in IBD. Postmortem examination should also include samples from the central nervous system. Encephalitis is a common pathologic finding.

There is no effective treatment for IBD. Because this disease appears to be highly contagious, affected snakes should be culled and euthanized after antemortem confirmation. Preventing the introduction of *O. natricis* into a collection and quarantining new arrivals are strongly encouraged to reduce the likelihood of introducing IBD into an ophidian collection.

Parasitic Diseases

Ticks are a common finding on wild-caught snakes. These parasites can be found anywhere on the snake but are frequently found around the eyes, oral cavity, and gular fold. Ticks can serve as vectors for disease and should be removed and disposed of properly. Special attention should be given to those tick species that are imported with reptiles from areas that harbor pathogens that could be potentially devastating to domestic livestock. The tick should be manually removed. It is important to grasp the tick at the mouthparts to prevent remnant material from causing a granuloma or abscess. The snake's enclosure should also be thoroughly cleaned to remove larval stages of the ticks.

Ophionyssus natricis is the common snake mite (Figure 7-26). This ectoparasite can be devastating in snake collections. Both larval and adult forms of the mite are parasitic. Snake mites can become reproductive within 2 to 2.5 weeks and live for 5 to 6 weeks. Chronic exposure can lead to the development of anemia. *O. natricis* also can serve as a vector for disease and can rapidly disseminate pathogens in a collection. Snake mites may play a role in the dissemination of inclusion body disease. A variety of miticides have been used to eliminate these parasites, including bathing the snake in water or applying mineral oil, topical and parenteral iver-

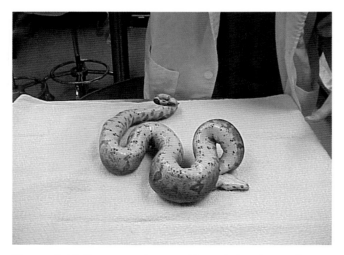

Figure 7-25 Boa constrictors with inclusion body disease often develop severe neurologic disease. This particular animal had no righting reflex.

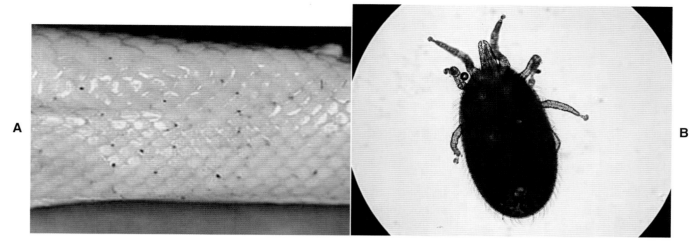

Figure 7-26 Snake mites appear as red-brown "moving specks" on snakes **(A)**. They can appear anywhere on the body. A mite infestation can be diagnosed by swabbing the red-brown moving specks with a mineral oil–coated cotton tipped applicator and reviewing the slide under a microscope **(B)**.

mectin, organophosphates, topical permethrins, and topical pyrethrins. Treatment must be twofold, including both the snake and the environment. Provent-a-mite® (Pro Products, Mahopac, New York) has been found to be both effective and safe when the directions on the label are followed.[18]

Cryptosporidium serpentis is a significant protozoal parasite in snakes. Transmission of this parasite is via the fecal-oral route. Indirect exposure via inanimate objects can also occur, as these parasites have a thick-walled oocyst that is resistant to desiccation. Snakes with cryptosporidiosis may present as asymptomatic carriers or with severe gastroenteritis. The latter may present with a history of weight loss and regurgitation. On physical examination affected snakes may be dehydrated, have obvious muscle wasting, and a mid-body swelling. Because this parasite infects the mucus-secreting cells of the stomach, it can cause severe gastric hyperplasia. Acid-fast stains of feces or the regurgitated meal may be diagnostic. The parasite can also be identified on direct smears, but this is less common (Figure 7-27). Unfortunately, because this parasite can be transiently shed, multiple samples (3-7) may be required for diagnosis. Feeding a snake may increase the reproductive cycle of the parasite and can improve the likelihood of making a diagnosis. Survey and contrast radiographs may be used to differentiate a gastric foreign body from gastric hyperplasia. A commercially available immunofluorescent antibody assay (Merifluor, Meridian Biosciences, Inc., Cincinnati, Ohio), developed for use in humans to diagnose *Giardia* and *Cryptosporidium parvum*, may be used. This assay is more sensitive than an acid-fast fecal smear and is capable of characterizing fewer organisms than is an acid-fast fecal stain.

To date, treatment of *C. serpentis* in snakes has been inconsistent. Antimicrobials have been found to reduce shedding, but they do not appear to eradicate the parasite. This organism does not appear to be zoonotic; however, strict sanitation and hygiene practices should be followed when working with infected animals. Infected animals should be culled to prevent the dissemination of the parasite into an ophidian collection.

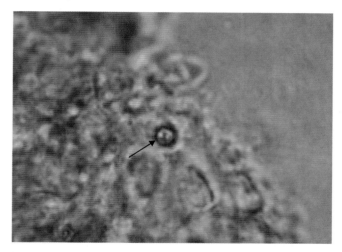

Figure 7-27 *Cryptospordium serpentis* oocyst (*arrow*) on a direct fecal smear.

Eimeria spp., *Isospora* spp., and *Caryospora* spp. are the most frequently encountered coccidian parasites in snakes. Coccidia have a direct life cycle. In higher vertebrates coccidial infections are generally self-limiting, but in snakes they generally are not. Coccidia infect primarily the intestinal and biliary epithelium, although infections of the renal epithelium also occur. Fibrosis and epithelial ulcerations are the most common histologic findings associated with coccidial infection. The clinical course of the disease and pathologic conditions is more severe in neonatal snakes. Diagnosis can be made by evaluating fecal material on a direct saline smear or fecal flotation. Treatment is generally accomplished using sulfonamides. The snake should be hydrated before it is administered sulfonamides. Most therapeutic plans recommend 5 to 7 days of treatment; however, this is generally insufficient, and treatment should continue until three negative fecal exams have been performed over a 15-day period.

Entamoeba invadens is a protozoal parasite that can cause severe, protracted disease in snakes. The life cycle is direct; thus this parasite can spread rapidly through an ophidian collection. Transmission is via the fecal-oral route. Chelonians may serve as reservoirs for this parasite. Affected snakes may develop a hemorrhagic diarrhea, severe dehydration, and muscle wasting. Mortality can approach 100%. Ulcerative gastritis and colitis are common histopathologic findings. Diagnosis can be made on a direct smear with Lugol's iodine or a fecal flotation. Metronidazole is the treatment of choice (25-50 mg/kg PO SID × 7-10 days). Supportive care, including fluid therapy, enteral support, and antibiotics for secondary bacterial infections, is also recommended.

Ciliated and flagellated protozoa are frequent findings on a microscopic examination of snake feces. Many of these organisms are commensals and likely serve an important role in the maintenance of the microecology of the gastrointestinal tract. Treatment should be considered only if the snake is demonstrating clinical disease and has pathologic symptoms associated with the protozoa. Certain flagellates, including *Giardia* spp. and *Trichomonas* spp., can be pathogenic in snakes. Affected snakes may be dehydrated and have diarrhea. Diagnosis and treatment is similar to that described for *E. invadens.*

Digenetic flukes are an infrequent finding in snakes. These flukes have an indirect life cycle, which generally includes a gastropod as the intermediate host. Styphylodoro, or renal flukes, generally parasitize the excretory system. Severe infestations can lead to significant renal pathology. Refifers, or lung flukes, may be found in the buccal cavity, pharynx, esophagus, or respiratory tract. The adult flukes generally cause mild ulcerations at their site of attachment. Because the life cycle of digenetic trematodes requires an intermediate host, the life cycle in captivity is self-limiting. Diagnosis can be made by performing a fecal or sputum flotation. Treatment can be accomplished by using praziquantel (5-8 mg/kg IM q10 days,

2-3 treatments) and manually removing flukes that are found in the buccal cavity.

Cestodes are not an uncommon finding in wild-caught snakes. The life cycle of the cestode also requires an intermediate host. *Spirometra* spp. and *Bothridium* spp. are pseudophyllideans that are found in snakes. The pleurocercoids of these cestodes are found usually in the subcutaneous (SC) tissues of the snake. On physical examination the pleurocercoids will appear as soft flocculent SC masses. Treatment can be accomplished by surgical excision of the parasite. Mesocestoides are another common cestode found in snakes. Because snakes serve as an intermediate host for this parasite, this cestode is generally found encysted in soft tissues. The snake generally serves as a definitive host for proteocephalidians. The adult cestodes are generally found in the small intestine. Identification of proglottids in fecal material or eggs from a fecal flotation is diagnostic. Treatment for those cestodes in which the reptile serves as a definitive host can be done using praziquantel (5-8 mg/kg IM q10 days, 2-3 treatments).

Nematodes are the most frequently encountered endoparasites in snakes. The life cycle of nematodes may be direct or indirect. Clinical signs may vary with the density of parasites and the location of the parasites within the host. Affected snakes may be asymptomatic or have diarrhea, intestinal obstruction and volvulus, pneumonia, renal disease, or chronic muscle wasting. Diagnosis can be made by examining a direct fecal smear or fecal flotation. There are a variety of parasiticides that can be used to treat snakes (Table 7-2).

Pentastomids are not an uncommon finding in wild-caught snakes. Affected animals may be asymptomatic or have generalized respiratory disease. Diagnosis can be made from examination of the feces (eggs) or sputum (eggs) and survey radiographs (adults). There are several recommendations for treatment, including ivermectin (0.2 mg/kg), fenbendazole (50-100 mg/kg), a combination therapy of ivermectin and fenbendazole, levamisole, and surgical/endoscopic removal of

TABLE 7-2	**Parasiticides Used to Treat Snakes**		
Parasiticide	**Dose**	**Indication**	**Comment**
Fenbendazole	25-50 mg/kg PO 25 mg/kg SID 3 days, repeat 2 weeks if necessary	Nematodes	
Ivermectin	0.2 mg/kg IM, PO q 10 days, 2-4 times	Ectoparasites, nematodes	Do not use in indigo snakes or in debilitated snakes
Levamisole	5-10 mg/kg ICe[24] once; repeat 2 weeks	Lungworms	Narrow range of safety; do not use in debilitated snakes
Metronidazole	25-50 mg/kg PO[25]	Protozoa, anaerobic bacteria	<40 mg/kg indigo snake, milk snake, tricolor kingsnake, and uracoan rattlesnake
Permethrin	0.5%	Ectoparasites	Follow label directions (Provent-a-mite, Pro Products, Mahopac, NY); apply to substrate
Praziquantel	5-8 mg/kg PO, IM[25] once; repeat 2 weeks	Cestodes	
Sulfa-dimethoxine	50 mg/kg PO, SID 7-21 days	Coccidia	Do not use in dehydrated snakes or animals with renal disease

ICe, intracoelomic; *IM,* intramuscular; *PO,* per os; *q,* every; *SID,* once a day.

the adult parasites. Because the life cycle of the pentastomids requires an intermediate host, they are self-limiting in captivity. However, treatment in captivity is often pursued because of the zoonotic potential associated with this organism.

Noninfectious Diseases
NUTRITIONAL DISEASES

Primary nutritional disease in snakes is uncommon. Most of the nutritional disorders encountered in ophidian medicine are related to the delivery, frequency, and type of food offered to the animal. Snakes that are not housed under optimal conditions may be predisposed to hypothermia, leading to anorexia or cachexia. Chronic hypothermia can also affect the immune system and reproductive status of the snake. Always reevaluate the environmental conditions for any snake with anorexia. Cachexia can also occur as a result of feeding the wrong prey type or an insufficient quantity of calories. A review of the life history and biology for a particular snake species should be done in these cases.

Obesity is one of the most common nutritional disorders observed in captive snakes. Obese reptiles may develop secondary health problems; therefore, a thorough physical examination and diagnostic work-up should be performed. Obesity can be eliminated by restricting the calories being offered to the snake and providing regular access to exercise. Obese animals should be placed on a calorie-restrictive diet and a management plan created to gradually lower the weight of the animal. Initiating a rapid weight loss program for the snake may result in secondary disease process, such as hepatic lipidosis.

Captive snakes should not be fed wild-caught prey items, as they can serve as a source of infectious diseases. Many wild prey items are exposed to pesticides or insecticides. When apex predators, such as snakes, ingest these prey items, they can bioaccumulate these hazardous toxins. Individuals responsible for the acquisition of commercially available prey items should investigate the management of the prey species to be certain they are not being treated with pesticides to manage ectoparasites.

Snakes fed commercially available soft-body insect diets may be predisposed to secondary nutritional secondary hyperparathyroidism (SNHP). Commercially available insects are frequently deficient in calcium. To reduce the likelihood of SNHP in a snake, invertebrates should be offered a high-quality, nutritionally complete diet for a minimum of 24 hours. Dusting the invertebrates with a calcium carbonate powder every other feeding also will improve the overall nutritional quality of the prey source. Snakes that are primarily offered neonatal rodents may also be predisposed to SNHP. Neonatal rodents should be removed directly from the female rodent to ensure that they are gut-loaded with calcium. Dipping the hindquarters of the neonate into a calcium carbonate powder will improve the calcium content of the prey item.

Piscivorous snakes that are offered a strict fish diet may be predisposed to thiamin and vitamin E deficiencies. Certain frozen fish produce thiaminases, which can eliminate thiamin within the tissues. Snakes fed these diets may develop neuro-logic symptoms, including a loss of the righting reflex, abnormal locomotion, muscle tremors, and blindness. Thiamin offered parenterally at 25 mg/kg once a day for 72 hours, followed by oral administration at the same dose, appears corrective. Offering live fish or fresh-killed fish is preventive. Vitamin E deficiencies may occur when piscivorous snakes are fed fish that are high in polyunsaturated fats. Steatitis is a common sequela to a vitamin E deficiency. Offering a diversity of fish prey items and restricting the quantity of obese coldwater fish species are preventive strategies.

NEOPLASIA

Neoplasia is not an uncommon finding in snakes. Many of the neoplastic tumors characterized in snakes have been previously described in domestic species, including adenoma, adenocarcinoma, carcinoma, chondrosarcoma, chromatophoromas, cystadenoma, fibroma, fibrosarcoma, granular cell tumor, hemangiosarcoma, interstitial cell tumor, leiomyosarcoma, lipoma, lymphosarcoma, melanoma, mesothelioma, myelocytic leukemia, myxosarcoma, nephroblastoma, neurofibrosarcoma, osteosarcoma, pheochromocytoma, rhabdomyosarcoma, spindle cell sarcoma, squamous cell carcinoma, thymoma, and transitional cell carcinoma.[19-21] These tumors have been found to originate from both mesenchymal and epithelial origins and affect all of the major organ systems.

Although most reports of neoplasia are derived from individual case reports, retrospective studies have been performed to estimate the prevalence of neoplasia in snake collections at zoologic institutions.[19,20,22] Zoologic institutions serve as important tumor registries for reptiles because they maintain large collections of reptiles under consistent environmental conditions and extend the lives of these animals by providing necessary nutrition and removing predators or other environmental calamities. A 20-year study at the National Zoological Park in Washington, D.C., identified neoplasia in 12.4% (36/291) of the dead snakes presented for postmortem examination during the study period.[19] A 10-year retrospective study performed at the Sacramento Zoo, California, reported a prevalence of 23.1% during the study period. These results are much different from a previously reported study, where the prevalence was less than 4%.[22] The researchers in the recent studies suggested that the higher prevalence of neoplasia may be attributed to improved husbandry and increased longevity in their collections.

The prevalence estimates for neoplasia reported from zoologic institutions may be an overestimate of the true prevalence of neoplasia for snakes. Snakes housed at these zoologic collections may be exposed to low-grade environmental toxins, including pesticide, insecticides, and heavy metals, that predispose them to the development of tumors. An increased risk of exposure to infectious disease may also occur when snakes are housed in high densities. Retroviral inclusions have been isolated from neoplasms in Burmese pythons (*P. molurus bivittatus*) and may serve a role in the development of tumors, but it is not known if a correlation exists.[23] Future studies should pursue the roles of environmental toxins and infectious dis-

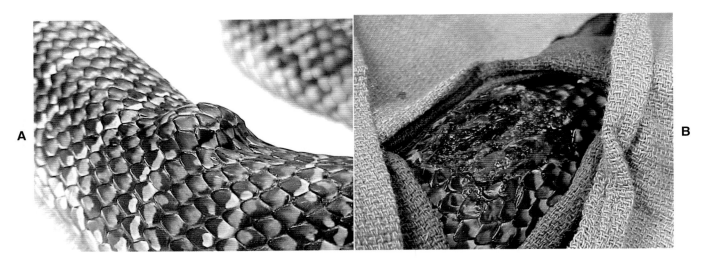

Figure 7-28 This king snake's presenting symptom was this mass **(A).** Caseous material was removed from the mass and was consistent with an abscess. Three weeks after the surgery, the problem recurred. A biopsy of the affected tissues revealed a squamous cell carcinoma **(B).**

eases in relation to tumor formation in snakes in zoologic collections.

Snakes frequently present to veterinarians for abnormal external or internal masses. The primary differentials for any mass in a snake are neoplasia, granuloma, abscess, and hematoma (Figure 7-28). The diagnostic approach for a snake case should be similar to those described for domestic species. A thorough history to define onset and progression of the disease is important. Information regarding the effect the mass has on the animal, such as limiting locomotion, prey acquisition, or eating, is also important when considering the prognosis. A thorough physical examination should be performed to assess the general health status of the snake and to develop a problem list to guide diagnostic and therapeutic plans. A complete blood count and plasma chemistry analysis are necessary to provide initial insight into the physiologic status of the snake. Certain neoplastic processes, such as lymphosarcoma, may result in gross changes to the white blood cells, including the development of obvious nucleoli and multinucleated cells. Survey and contrast radiography and ultrasonography may be used to isolate organ systems affected by neoplastic processes. Advanced diagnostic imaging, such as magnetic resonance and computed tomography imaging, can provide more specific information regarding the extent of the neoplastic process but is not routinely available to veterinarians. A fine-needle aspirate of a mass and cytologic examination of the aspirate can provide preliminary information regarding the mass. Unfortunately, the fine-needle aspirate is not a sensitive test and is susceptible to false negative results. A definitive diagnosis of a neoplastic process can be made only from biopsy and histopathologic confirmation. Histopathologic samples should be sent to a qualified veterinary pathologist. External masses can be biopsied using standard techniques. Analgesics and anesthetics should be used when performing painful procedures. Internal masses can be biopsied using endoscopic techniques or via an exploratory coeliotomy.

Treatment for neoplasia in reptiles should follow standard protocols reported in domestic animal oncology. Surgical excision of a mass is the preferred technique, especially if appropriate margins can be removed. Unfortunately, surgical excision is not possible in all cases. Chemotherapeutics have been used in reptiles with minimal success. In many cases the tumor may go into a short remission period but will return and prove fatal. Because of limited peripheral vessels to place a catheter, chemotherapeutics can be difficult to administer in snakes. However, vascular access ports have been used with success in administering chemotherapeutics long term in reptiles and may prove invaluable in these cases. Radiation therapy and photodynamic therapy have been used to treat neoplasia in snakes with some success. However, access to these therapeutic measures is currently restricted for many veterinarians.

■ THERAPEUTICS
Fluid Therapy

The cornerstone to any treatment plan should include replenishing fluids to a dehydrated animal. A failure to replenish fluids will minimize the effect of any other treatments. The first step in developing a fluid replacement plan is to determine the type of dehydration. The majority of cases are associated with isotonic dehydration, although animals not provided access to water may develop hypertonic dehydration. This information is important because it allows the veterinarian to determine which type of fluid should be used to replenish the deficit. In a perfect world, the snake's osmolarity would be determined. Unfortunately, this is rarely done. Most snakes are thought to have osmolarities between 250 and 280 mOsm;

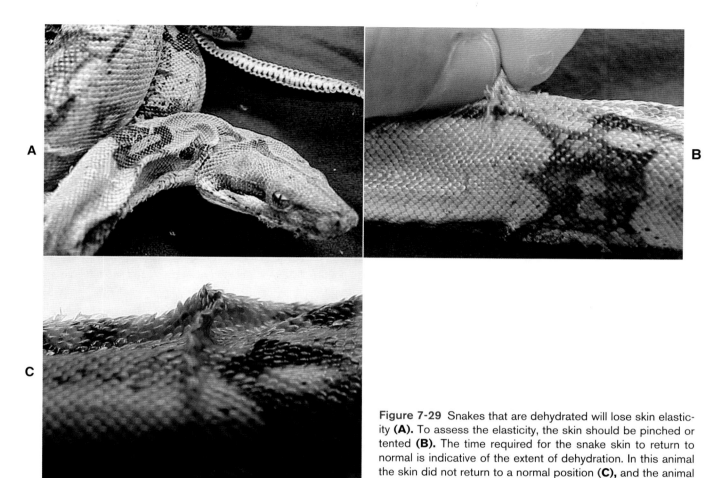

Figure 7-29 Snakes that are dehydrated will lose skin elasticity **(A).** To assess the elasticity, the skin should be pinched or tented **(B).** The time required for the snake skin to return to normal is indicative of the extent of dehydration. In this animal the skin did not return to a normal position **(C),** and the animal was estimated to be more than 15% dehydrated.

however, recent work by the author and others suggests that clinically healthy snakes can have much higher osmolarities (>2300-325 mOsm/L). Based on this, the majority of the isotonic fluids (e.g., 0.9% saline: 308 mOsmol/L; Normasol: 294 mOsmol/L) used to replenish fluid in mammals would be considered hypertonic or hypotonic depending on the individual snake's status. Calculating a snake's osmolarity using an osmometer is strongly recommended; however, when this can't be done, estimating the osmolarity using the following formula is recommended: 2(Sodium + potassium).

Assessing dehydration in snakes is more difficult than in mammals. Snake skin is not as naturally elastic as mammalian skin. To best assess the elasticity (or natural lack thereof) of snake skin, it is important to routinely examine clinically hydrated animals to develop an understanding of "normal" (Figures 7-29). The lateral body wall is the best area to assess skin elasticity in a snake. The mucous membranes of a snake should be moist. Dry, ropy mucus in the oral cavity is generally an indication of dehydration. Snake mucous membranes are typically pale pink in color, and the capillary refill time should be less than 2 seconds. An increased capillary refill time is suggestive of dehydration. The positioning of the eyes can also be used to assess snake hydration. Snakes that are severely dehydrated (>8%-10%) develop sunken eyes as a result of a loss of moisture in the retro-orbital fat pads. Blood work is often the best method for assessing the hydration status of a snake, and it is for this reason that veterinarians should recommend obtaining and testing a sample when an animal is clinically normal for comparison. A packed cell volume, sodium, chloride, total protein, and plasma osmolarity can be used to assess hydration and measure the response to treatment.

There are several routes for replenishing fluids in snakes, including per os (PO), SC, ICe, and IV. For animals that are mildly dehydrated (<5%), the PO and SC routes are appropriate. Fluids are naturally acquired via the gastrointestinal tract, so this should always be the first option. If fluids are to be replenished PO, it is essential that the gastrointestinal tract is operating normally. Any reduction in motility can lead to an osmotic diarrhea, further exacerbating the dehydration. Fluids can be administered PO via a tube. The technique is similar to the method described for gastric lavage (see Parasitology). The preferred site for SC fluids is the lateral body wall (Figure 7-30). This is the area that has, in general, the most SC space and flexibility in the skin. It may be necessary to administer

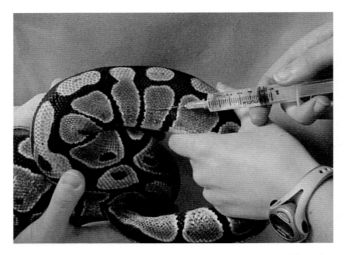

Figure 7-30 Subcutaneous fluids can be administered into the space along the lateral body wall. A maximum of 1-2 ml/100 g of fluid can be inserted into a space. However, the veterinarian or technician should use judgment when determining the volume of fluids that can be inserted into a specific injection site.

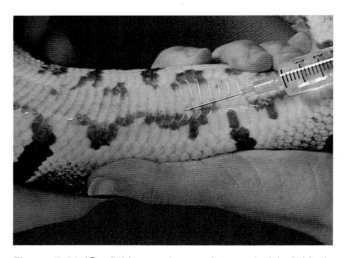

Figure 7-31 ICe fluids can be used to replenish fluids in moderately to severely dehydrated snakes. Fluids should be inserted into the ventrocaudal third of the animal to avoid the lung(s).

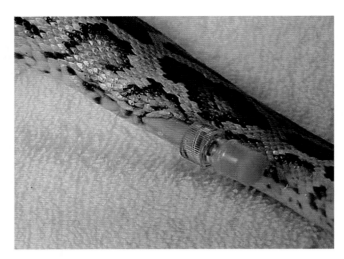

Figure 7-32 An IV catheter can be placed into the jugular vein of a snake to ensure rapid delivery of fluids and other therapeutics. The procedure requires a cut-down.

the fluids in several areas along the body wall. Snakes that are moderately to severely dehydrated (>5%) can be given fluids via the coelomic cavity or intravenously. ICe fluids should be given in the caudal third of the body. The snake should be placed in dorsal recumbency and the needle inserted between the ventral scales (Figure 7-31). Positioning the animal using this method will minimize the likelihood of introducing the fluids into the lung(s). IV catheters can be placed into a jugular vein. Jugular catheter placement generally requires a surgical cut-down. The heart is used as the primary landmark for locating the jugular veins. Place the snake in dorsal recumbency. Identify the heart. Once the heart is identified, count 9 to 10

ventral scales cranially. The surgical site should be disinfected using standard techniques. A 0.5- to 1.0-cm incision should be made between the first and second rows of the dorsal scales. Blunt dissection of the medial ridge of the ribs will reveal the jugular vein. An appropriately sized catheter should be inserted into the vein, an injection port attached, and the incision closed (Figure 7-32). Fluids can be administered via a bolus or continuous rate infusion.

Maintenance fluid rates for reptiles are much lower (10-30 ml/kg/day) than those recommended for birds (100 ml/kg/day) or mammals (80-100 ml/kg/day). When developing a fluid replenishment plan, it is important to consider both the deficit and maintenance requirements of the snake. Animals should be reassessed daily to ensure that the fluid deficit is being replaced and that the animal is not being overhydrated. Serial blood testing (e.g., packed cell volume, electrolytes, total protein, and osmolarity) can be used to assess the patient's response to therapy.

Antimicrobial Drugs

Antimicrobial drugs are likely one of the most common therapeutics administered to snakes. The dogma that all diseases are bacterial infections until proven otherwise is likely the culprit. Of course, antibiotics and antifungals do serve important purposes for captive reptiles.

When deciding whether to include an antimicrobial into a therapeutic plan for a snake, it is important to consider the pharmacology of the compound. I consider a series of questions when selecting an antimicrobial.

1. Is the drug bactericidal or bacteriostatic? Determining whether a drug is cidal or static is important because most of the bacterial pathogens isolated from snakes are Gram negative. A rapid kill of Gram-negative bacteria could lead to the release of endotoxins, resulting in the death of the host.

TABLE 7-3	Antimicrobial Drugs Used to Treat Snakes	
Drug	**Dose**	**Comments**
Amikacin	3 mg/kg IM q72h	Not to be used in dehydrated snakes or those with renal disease
Carbenicillin	400 mg/kg IM q24h[26]	
Ceftazidime	20 mg/kg IM q72h[27]	
Chlorhexidine	Topical 0.05-0.1%	Apply to external topical wounds
Ciprofloxacin	10 mg/kg PO q24-48h	
Clotrimazole	Topical	Topical application fungal dermatitis
Doxycycline	10 mg/kg PO q24h	
Enrofloxacin	5-10 mg/kg IM once, PO	
Itraconazole	5-10 mg/kg PO SID	
Ketaconazole	25 mg/kg PO SID[24]	
Silver sulfadiazine	Topical	Topical application fungal/bacterial dermatitis
Trimethoprim-sulfadimethoxine	20 mg/kg PO, IM q24h	Not to be used in dehydrated snakes or those with renal disease

IM, intramuscular; *PO,* per os; *q,* every; *SID,* once a day.

2. What is the spectrum of the antibiotic? Does it cover Gram-positive bacteria? Gram-negative? Both? Aerobes versus anaerobes?

3. Will the drug get to the desired tissues? If an infection is associated with the respiratory tract, and a selected drug does not penetrate the respiratory tissues, then it is of no value.

4. What is the mechanism of action of the antibiotic? Knowledge of how an antibiotic works is important when considering methods of resistance. Certain resistance factors occur as a result of mutations while others are plasmid generated.

5. How is the drug metabolized and excreted? If a drug must be metabolized by the liver to become active, and the snake has liver disease, the likelihood that the drug will perform as desired is decreased.

6. What are the side effects? Being able to identify the side effects associated with a drug are important, so that the compound can be discontinued before it causes irreparable harm.

7. How often does the drug have to be administered? Corticosterone is a natural hormone produced by snakes in response to stress. Elevated levels of corticosterone can lead to immune system suppression and altered metabolism. By minimizing handling time (e.g., number of treatments), veterinarians can reduce the likelihood of stimulating excessive corticosterone secretion in their snake patients.

By answering these questions veterinarians will be sure to select an antibiotic based on desired effect rather than a "best guess" approach. Table 7-3 lists antimicrobial drugs commonly used to treat snakes.

Antiparasitic Drugs

Antiparasitic drugs are commonly used to treat snakes. Many veterinarians and herpetoculturists treat animals regardless of a confirmed diagnosis. This is often done because the parasites

TABLE 7-4	Emergency Drugs Used to Treat Snakes	
Drug	**Dose**	**Indication**
Atropine	0.5 mg/kg IV, IT, IO, IM	Bradycardia, CPR, reduced secretions
Diazepam	0.5-1.0 mg/kg IM, IV	Seizures
Doxapram	20 mg/kg IV, IO, IM	CPR, respiratory stimulant
Epinephrine	0.5-1.0 mg/kg IV, (1 : 1000) IO, IT	Asystole, CPR

CPR, cardiopulmonary resuscitation; *IM,* intramuscular; *IT,* intratracheal; *IV,* intravascular.

may be shed periodically, and are thus difficult to identify, or because of a perceived problem. There are potential disadvantages to this treatment method. Regular treatment could lead to the development of resistance factors that limit the effectiveness of a drug. Antiparasitics are not without their negative side effects. Certain species of snakes may be more sensitive to certain anthelminthics. Routine treatment can lead to toxic side effects (e.g., hepatopathy, anaphylaxis, or death). I prefer to treat animals based on a confirmed diagnosis. The administration of fenbendazole to a snake with cestodes is a waste of money and may provide a false sense of security for the owner. (See Table 7-2 for a list of antiparasitics used to treat snakes.)

Emergency Drugs

Veterinarians working with snakes may find themselves in situations where they need to provide emergency drugs. Cardiac depression (bradycardia) and/or cardiorespiratory failure during an anesthetic event are the most common problems that I encounter. Table 7-4 provides a list of emergency drugs used for snakes.

Miscellaneous Drugs

In general, drugs used to manage disease processes in nonreptilian vertebrates can be used for snakes. The vast majority of the therapeutic dosages recommended for snakes are empirical or based on mammalian or avian recommendations. Veterinarians should inform their clients that the compounds used to treat their pets are being used off-label.

Nutritional Support

Nutritional support should be considered for any patient with a history of anorexia. However, defining anorexia in a snake may be easier said than done. It is not uncommon for some snakes, especially larger bodied pythons or boas, to not eat for extended periods in captivity. This may be associated with a number of factors, including that snakes are often overfed in captivity, not provided much exercise, or maintained at temperatures that lower their metabolic rate. To determine whether a period of inappetence is associated with a medical problem or is the result of a normal behavioral pattern for the snake, it would be prudent for the veterinarian to examine the body condition of the animal and perform a plasma biochemistry assay. The epaxial muscles along the spine are an excellent location for assessing body condition. A snake should have well-defined epaxial muscles. A prominent spinal column is suggestive of muscle wasting. If the spinal column cannot be easily seen or palpated, the snake should be considered obese. Ultrasound can be used on the coelomic cavity to detect the presence or absence of the linear fat bodies. Snakes that are truly anorectic may have decreased electrolyte and glucose levels.

Snakes that are judged to be in a negative energy balance should be provided supplemental calories. There are several methods that can be used for calculating the caloric requirements of a snake. Calorie replacement for snakes can be done using whole prey or a liquid enteral. Whole prey species can be used when the anorexia is short term and the gastrointestinal system is functioning normally. Mammalian and/or avian prey can be skinned before being offered to the snake to reduce the digestive load and expedite caloric uptake. Lubricating the prey with a small quantity of petroleum jelly or vegetable oil may expedite the passage of the meal. Take care not to introduce the lubricant into the glottis. Pinkie pumps are designed to macerate juvenile rodent prey items and may be used to simplify the force-feeding process. Animals with a history of long-term anorexia may benefit from a liquid enteral. Fluker Farms Carnivore Repta-Aid (Fluker Farms, Port Allen, Louisiana) is a powdered diet that can be mixed with water to provide essential replacement calories (Figure 7-33).

■ SURGERY
Preoperative and Postoperative Considerations

Surgical procedures in a snake should follow the same basic practices used for domestic mammals. A thorough physical

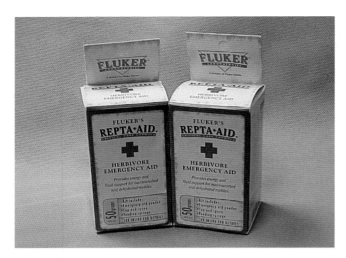

Figure 7-33 Fluker Farms Repta-Aid (Fluker Farms, Port Allen, Louisiana) can be used to replace essential calories in a snake. The product is mixed with water and can be delivered via a feeding tube.

examination and baseline data—including a packed cell volume, total solids, complete blood count, plasma biochemistries, and clotting profile—should be performed to assess the anesthetic risk and determine the suitability of the patient for the surgery. In cases where this information cannot be obtained, the client should be made aware of the added risk involved, given the lack of knowledge regarding the animal's physiologic condition.

The surgical suite should be prepared before the patient is anesthetized. A heat source should be used to maintain the animal's body temperature during the procedure. The veterinarian should attempt to maintain the animal at a temperature consistent with its optimal environmental temperature range. Convective forced air heating systems, such as the Bair hugger (Arizant Healthcare, Eden Prairie, Minnesota), recirculating water blankets, electric heating pads, and incandescent lights can be used to provide heat. It is important to monitor the animal's temperature during the procedure using an esophageal or colonic thermometer. By monitoring the animal's temperature during the procedure, it will be possible to alter the heating pattern during the procedure to maximize the efficiency of the animal's metabolism and thus the animal's ability to process the anesthetics.

The surgical site should be disinfected with 0.5% to 1.0% chlorhexidine or povidone-iodine and sterile 0.9% saline. I recommend warming the fluids for this procedure to minimize the loss of heat that may occur. Alcohol should not be used as a disinfectant, as it can also lead to the loss of body heat.

Anesthesia

Historically, clinical and surgical procedures performed on snakes were done using manual restraint or hypothermia. Fortunately, new anesthetics have become available that produce safe and effective anesthesia in snakes. Dissociative anesthetics, propofol, local anesthetics, opioids, and inhalant anesthetics are the most frequently used anesthetics in snakes. Most of the knowledge veterinarians have of these agents is based on mammalian, avian, and nonophidian reptiles, as few anesthetic research studies have been performed using snakes. When developing an anesthetic plan for an ophidian patient, veterinarians should become familiar with the physiologic needs of a particular species.

The dissociative agents, including ketamine and tiletamine, are frequently used to anesthetize snakes for clinical procedures. Although the dissociative agents are characterized as anesthetics, they do not provide sufficient visceral analgesia in mammalian species and should not be used exclusively for invasive surgical procedures in snakes. The dissociative agents are readily available, are inexpensive, and can be administered intramuscularly. One of the primary disadvantages of using dissociative anesthetics is a prolonged recovery period. Even at low doses (5 mg/kg tiletamine), snakes can require 24 to 48 hours to fully recover. Doses of ketamine as high as 80 mg/kg have been reported for the provision of surgical anesthesia; however, the dissociative anesthetics neither result in effective muscle relaxation nor provide visceral analgesia and should not be used as stand-alone anesthetics for invasive procedures. The addition of an alpha-2 anesthetic may be appropriate. However, little research has documented the effects of these drugs on snakes. I have found 10 to 20 mg/kg ketamine or 3 to 6 mg/kg Telazol (tiletamine and zolazepam) (Ft. Dodge Laboratories, Ft. Dodge, IA) sufficient to manage fractious snakes and provide anesthesia for minor surgical procedures.

Propofol (AstraZeneca, Wilmington, Delaware) is a non-barbiturate anesthetic that can be used as a sole parenteral agent to provide surgical anesthesia. The effects of propofol are not cumulative, and thus rapid recovery (30-45 minutes) occurs in most cases. To obtain a desired effect, propofol should be administered intravenously. Propofol can also be administered in the jugular vein or heart. Because of the potential cardiac and respiratory depressant effects of propofol, the snake should be intubated and ventilated during the anesthetic procedure. Propofol at 5 to 10 mg/kg administered in the ventral coccygeal vein by slow injection has been used repeatedly to anesthetize venomous snakes. In general, 5 to 15 mg/kg IV will provide general anesthesia for 30 to 45 minutes in most snake species. When longer anesthetic periods are required, additional dosing can be given to effect.

The inhalant anesthetics (e.g., isoflurane and sevoflurane) can be used to provide controlled anesthesia. The primary benefit of the inhalant anesthetics over the injectable compounds is that the veterinary surgeon has more direct control over the anesthetic. The snake should be intubated to ensure proper delivery of the anesthetic. The glottis is located on the floor of the mouth, caudal to the tongue. A noncuffed endotracheal tube should be used for the procedure. IV catheters can be used to intubate small snakes. Closely monitor the endotracheal catheter to ensure that it does not become plugged with mucus. Because snakes lack a diaphragm and can become apneic for extended periods of time, I recommend positive-pressure ventilating the snake 4 to 6 times a minute. Recovery should be done in a warmed, dark environment to reduce unnecessary external stimuli.

Local anesthetics (e.g., lidocaine, prilocaine) are often underutilized in reptile medicine. These anesthetics can be used to provide complete, local anesthesia for an animal. I generally use these compounds in combination with other anesthetics. For example, lidocaine may be used to provide anesthesia along an incision or at the base of a hemipenis for an amputation. Although there have been no studies done to determine the toxic dose for these compounds in snakes, I have found that dosing at less than 5 mg/kg is safe.

Analgesics should be used whenever an animal may feel pain. Unfortunately, knowledge of pain perception in these animals is limited. Most veterinarians accept the notion that snakes respond to noxious stimuli by moving away from a negative stimulus (e.g., injection of a drug); it is unknown, however, whether the animal feels pain during such a response. Because nothing is known about pain perception in reptiles, I err on the protective side and administer analgesics even though it is also unknown whether the analgesics have any effect. Analgesics I use in my practice are butorphanol (0.5-1.0 mg/kg IM), carprofen (2-4 mg/kg IM, PO), and meloxicam (0.5 mg/kg PO).

Surgical Procedures

The coeliotomy is routinely performed to pursue the biopsy of an abnormal mass, remove a foreign body (gastrotomy and enterotomy), or correct a dystocia. Because snake locomotion involves the direct contact of the ventral scales with a surface, surgical approaches should not be made along the ventrum through the large scales. An incision in that area may lead to excessive tension at the incision site and possible dehiscence. Approaches to the coelomic cavity of a snake should be made between the second and third rows of lateral scales to prevent contamination of the incision by the substrate. Closure of the coeliotomy should be made in two layers: the body wall and skin. The skin is considered the holding layer. An everting horizontal mattress pattern should be used to close the skin incision. An absorbable synthetic should be used to close the body wall, and nylon suture can be used to close the skin. Sutures should be removed approximately 4 to 6 weeks after surgery.

Snakes occasionally ingest foreign bodies from their environments. Affected animals may become anorectic or may regurgitate. The general location of the foreign body often can be isolated by digital palpation. Survey and contrast radiographs can be done to confirm location. Although the approach to a gastrotomy or enterotomy in a snake is similar to that used in mammals, special care should be taken when manipulating the thin walled intestine of the snake. While a two-layer closure may be used to close the bowel in mammals, this is often not possible in small snakes. Once the bowel is closed, the coelomic cavity should be irrigated with warm sterile saline. Broad-spectrum antimicrobials are indicated if the coelomic cavity becomes contaminated during the procedure.

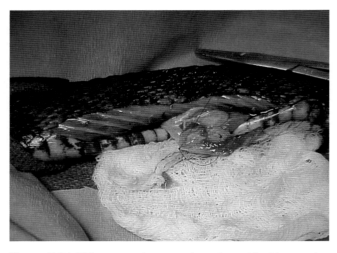

Figure 7-34 When removing eggs from the oviduct in a snake, it is important to make the incision in an avascular region. Stay sutures should be placed into the oviduct to allow the surgeon the ability to manipulate the incision and direct the eggs through the incision. The stay sutures also prevent the surgeon from losing the oviduct into the coelomic cavity.

Dystocias in snakes are generally postfollicular. Approach to the dystocia in snakes should follow standard surgical protocol. The value of the snake and the embryos or eggs should be considered before the surgery. If the snake is used exclusively for reproductive purposes, then a hysterectomy is not an option. When performing a cesarean section in a snake, the incision should be made into a relatively avascular region of the oviduct (Figure 7-34). Once the embryos or eggs are removed, the incision should be closed using a two-layer closure.

Subspectacular abscesses can develop in snakes with obstructed nasolacrimal ducts, retained spectacles, and penetrating wounds. To facilitate draining the abscess, an incision into the spectacle is needed. A ventral triangular spectaculotomy is the preferred method of treatment. By removing a ventral section of the spectacle, the veterinarian can drain the abscess, irrigate the area, unblock the nasolacrimal duct, and treat the corneal surface. Medical treatment, including topical antibiotics and artificial tears, is required until the spectacle heals.

During excitement or stress, male snakes may evaginate a hemipenis and cause damage to the structure. A damaged hemipenis should first be evaluated for tissue viability. If the tissue is viable, then it should be lavaged with copious quantities of warm sterile 0.9% saline and a mild disinfectant (0.5% chlorhexidine). Once cleaned, the structure should be replaced. If the hemipenis is edematous and cannot be replaced, a hypertonic solution (50% dextrose) may be applied topically to reduce the edema. Copious lavage with sterile saline should be done after the swelling has been reduced to remove any of the residual irritating dextrose. Two simple interrupted sutures may be placed through the anal plate and the scale caudal to the vent to prevent the hemipenis from reprolapsing. The

sutures should remain for approximately 72 hours, and the animal should be monitored closely to ensure that it can evacuate feces and urine. If the hemipenis is necrotic, it must be amputated. The hemipenes can be removed at the base of the organ using circumferential and transfixation sutures. The snake can remain in a breeding program as long as it retains one functional hemipenis.

■ZOONOSES

Snakes can serve as reservoirs for a number of potentially zoonotic diseases. *Salmonella* spp. is routinely isolated from captive snakes. The prevalence of this bacterium is high in captive snakes because of a relative lack of quarantine and minimal sanitation. Young children (<5 years old), infants, and immunocompromised individuals are the most susceptible to infection. Reptiles should not be in households with these particular risk groups, nor should they be in the households of individuals who are not willing to both clean the reptile's environment and practice appropriate hygiene methods after handling a reptile. Zoonotic cases associated with *Salmonella* spp. are almost always associated with owners' carelessness.

Snakes may harbor other Gram-negative bacteria (e.g., *Campylobacter* spp.) that can also be potentially zoonotic. To minimize the likelihood of accidental disease transmission, it is important for veterinarians to educate their clients on the importance of using appropriate disinfection and sanitation protocols. Sodium hypochlorite can be used to eliminate most bacterial agents that are zoonotic. Gloves should be worn when cleaning an animal's cage to reduce the likelihood of transmitting bacteria.

Ophionyssus natricis, the common snake mite, is known to infest people and bite them. In most cases, the mites leave humans once they realize they are not their primary host. In some cases, humans can develop dermatitis from snake mite exposure.

Humans can serve as intermediate hosts for pentastomids. These parasites are found in wild-caught reptiles. Eggs pass with sputum or feces, and humans can be exposed when cleaning the animal's environment. To minimize exposure to zoonotic pathogens, people should practice strict hygiene whenever handling snakes or cleaning the snakes' environment.

REFERENCES

1. Zug GR, Vitt LJ, Caldwell JP: *Herpetology,* ed 2, San Diego, 2001, Academic Press.
2. Frye F: Use of a condom as an occlusive bandage in snakes: a new wrinkle on an old resource, *J Small Exot An Med* 2(1):13-14, 1992.
3. Sypek J, Borysenko M: Reptiles. In Rowley AF, Ratcliffe NA, editors: *Vertebrate Blood Cells,* Cambridge, 1988, Cambridge University Press.
4. Ramsay EC, Dotson TK: Tissue and serum enzyme activities in the yellow rat snake *(Elaphe obsolete quadrivittata), Am J Vet Res* 56:423-428, 1995.
5. Pare JA, Sigler L, Rypien K et al: Cutaneous fungal microflora of healthy squamate reptiles and prevalence of the *Chrysosporium* anamorph of *Nannizziopsis vriesii, Proc ARAV,* Orlando, Fla, pp 125-127, 2001.
6. Raiti P: Mycotic gastroenteritis in a diamond python *(Morelia spilota spilota)* and two Honduran milksnakes *(Lampropeltis triangulum triangulum), Proc ARAV,* Tampa, Fla, p. 97, 1996.

7. Monroe JN, Shibley GP, Schidlovsky T: Action of snake venom on Rausher virus, *J Natl Cancer Inst* 40:135, 1968.

8. Padgett F, Levine AS: Fine structure of Rauscher leukemia virus as revealed by incubation in a snake venom, *Virology* 30:623, 1966.

9. Simpson CF, Jacobson ER, Gaskin JM: Herpesvirus-like infection of the venom gland of the Siamese cobra, *J Am Vet Med Assoc* 175:941, 1979.

10. Hauser B, Mettler F, Rubel A: Herpesvirus-like infection in two young boas, *J Comp Pathol* 93:515, 1983.

11. Jacobson ER, Gaskin JM: Adenovirus-like infection in a boa constrictor, *J Am Vet Med Assoc* 187:1226, 1985.

12. Ogawa M, Ahne W, Essbauer S: Reptilian viruses: adenovirus-like agent isolated from a royal python *(Python regius), J Vet Med* 39:732-736, 1992.

13. Schumacher J, Jacobson ER, Gaskin JM et al: Adenovirus infection in two rosy boas *(Lichanura trivirgata), J Zoo Wildl Med* 25(3):461, 1994.

14. Foelsch DW, Leloup P: Fatale endemische Infection in einem Serpentarium, *Tierrztliche Praxis* 4:527, 1976.

15. West G, Garner M, Raymond J et al: Meningioencephalitis in a Boeleni python *(Morelia boeleni)* associated with paramyxovirus infection, *J Zoo Wildl Med* 32(3):360-365, 2001.

16. Jacobson ER, Gaskin JM, Flanagan JP et al: Antibody responses of western diamondback rattlesnakes *(Crotalus atrox)* to inactivated ophidian paramyxovirus vaccines, *J Zoo Wildl Med* 22(2):184, 1991.

17. Garner M, Raymond JT, Nordhauser RW et al: Eight cases of inclusion body disease in captive palm vipers *(Bothriechis marchi), Proc AAZV,* New Orleans, La, pp 45-47, 2000.

18. Burridge MJ, Simmons LA: Control and eradication of exotic tick infestations of reptiles, *Proc ARAV,* Orlando, Fla, pp 21-23, 2001.

19. Catao-Dias JL, Nichold DK: Neoplasia in snakes at the National Zoological Park, Washington, DC (1978-1997), *J Comp Pathol* 120:89-95, 1999.

20. Ramsay EC, Munson L, Lowenstine L et al: A retrospective study of neoplasia in a collection of captive snakes, *J Zoo Wildl Med* 27(1):28-34, 1996.

21. Done LB: Neoplasia. In Mader DR, editor: *Reptile Medicine and Surgery,* Philadelphia, 1996, WB Saunders.

22. Hubbard GB, Schmidt RE, Fletcher KC: Neoplasia in zoo animals, *J Zoo Anim Med* 14:33-40, 1983.

23. Chandra AM, Jacobson ER, Munn RJ: Retroviral particles in neoplasms of Burmese pythons *(Python molurus bivittatus), Vet Pathol* 38(5):561-564, 2001.

24. Jacobson ER: Antimicrobial drug use in reptiles. In Prescott JF, Baggot JD, editors: *Antimicrobial Therapy in Veterinary Medicine,* Ames, 1993, Iowa State University Press.

25. Jacobson ER: Snakes, *Vet Clin North Am: Small Anim Pract* 23:1179-1212, 1993.

26. Lawrence K, Needham JR, Palmer GH et al: A preliminary study on the use of carbenicillin in snakes, *J Vet Pharmacol Ther* 7:119-124, 1984.

27. Lawrence K, Muggleton PW, Needham JR: Preliminary study on the use of ceftazidime, a broad spectrum cephalosporin antibiotic, in snakes, *Res Vet Sci* 36:16-20, 1984.

Javier Nevarez

CHAPTER 8

LIZARDS

■ COMMON SPECIES KEPT IN CAPTIVITY

Lizards are members of the class Reptilia, subclass Lepidosauria, order Squamata (Box 8-1). They are further classified under the suborder Sauria, which distinguishes them from the snakes, worm lizards, and Tuataras *(Sphenodon punctatus)*. There are more than 4000 known species of lizards.[1] Lizards are one of the most diverse and successful reptile groups living today and exist in a variety of habitats, including arboreal (e.g., chameleons, geckos, iguanas), aquatic (e.g., Galapagos marine iguana [*Amblyrhynchus cristatus*], crocodile lizard [*Shinisaurus crocodilurus*]), fossorial (e.g., skinks, limbless lizards, blind lizards), and terrestrial (e.g., monitors, agamids, iguanids). Most lizard species have the ability to live and survive in multiple habitats but have a preference for which environment they spend most of their time.

Of the more than 4000 extant lizard species, fewer than 30 species are routinely found in the pet trade. In an effort to protect wild populations, many species are successfully bred in captivity. The green iguana *(Iguana iguana),* inland bearded dragon *(Pogona vitticeps),* and many gecko and chameleon species are successfully propagated in captivity. Nonetheless, there are many species in which wild-caught animals are still imported for the pet trade. Whereas obtaining wild-caught specimens may be essential for some breeding programs, keeping wild-caught lizards as pets for nonreproductive purposes should be discouraged. Wild-caught animals are usually exposed to diseases not found in captive-bred animals, and their life expectancy and quality of life are much reduced when compared to captive-bred animals.

This chapter will concentrate on the husbandry and health issues of common captive lizard species. Nutritional and environmental requirements will be presented as a general guideline for maintaining herbivorous, carnivorous, insectivorous, and omnivorous lizard species in captivity. Husbandry requirements will be discussed with the natural habitats of lizards in mind. The success of maintaining healthy lizards in captivity depends on the owner's ability to achieve two main goals: provide (1) adequate nutrition and (2) proper environment. Veterinarians must be aware of the specific requirements for the lizard species they are treating before making any assessment or recommendation. There is an abundance of misinformation about the captive care of lizard species. This misinformation may start with the breeder or seller of the animal, the pet store clerk, friends, or others, who, out of ignorance, disseminate incorrect pet care information. There are also many companies that manufacture products specifically for use with lizards and other reptiles. Some of these companies are responsible and manufacture products with input from knowledgeable veterinarians or herpetologists, whereas others manufacture products that may adversely affect the animals' health.

The majority of diseases observed in captive reptiles are directly associated with improper husbandry. Discussion regarding specific lizard species will be excluded purposefully, despite their presence in the pet trade, as they are either not well suited for life in a captive environment or limited to the care of expert hobbyists or herpetologists. In addition to presenting husbandry information, I will discuss the veterinary care of lizards. The veterinary information will focus on treatment protocols that range from basic to advanced veterinary skills that are needed to properly care for these reptile patients.

BOX 8-1	**Taxonomy of Lizards**

Class Reptilia
Subclass Lepidosauria
Order Squamata
Suborder Sauria (Lacertilia)
Infraorder Iguania
Family Agamidae (Agamas)
Family Chamaeleonidae (Chameleons)
Family Iguanidae (Iguanas)
Subfamily Corytophaninae (Casquehead lizards)
Subfamily Crotaphytinae (Collared and Leopard lizards)
Subfamily Hoplocercinae (Wood lizards and Clubtails)
Subfamily Iguaninae (Iguanas and Spinytail iguanas)
Subfamily Leiocephalinae
Subfamily Leiosaurinae
Subfamily Liolaeminae
Subfamily Oplurinae (Madagascar iguanids)
Subfamily Phrynosomatinae (Earless, spiny, tree,
    side-blotched, and horned lizards)
Subfamily Polychrotinae (Anoles)
Subfamily Tropidurinae (Neotropical ground lizards)
Infraorder Gekkota
Family Gekkonidae (Geckos)
Family Pygopodidae (Legless lizards)
Family Dibamidae (Blind lizards)
Infraorder Scincomorpha
Family Cordylidae (Spinytail lizards)
Family Gerrhosauridae (Plated lizards)
Family Gymnophthalmidae (Spectacled lizards)
Family Teiidae (Whiptails and tegus)
Family Lacertidae (Lacertids, wall lizards)
Family Scincidae (Skinks)
Family Xantusiidae (Nightl)
Infraorder Diploglossa
Family Anguidae (Glass lizards and alligator lizards)
Family Anniellidae (American legless lizards)
Family Xenosauridae (Knob-scaled lizards)
Infraorder Platynota (Varanoidea)
Family Helodermatidae (Gila monsters)
Family Lanthanotidae (Earless monitor lizards)
Family Varanidae (Monitors)

■ANATOMY

Integumentary System

Like other reptiles, most lizards have thick skin with varying degrees of scaling. Lizards have ectodermal scales that can be smooth or keeled depending on the species.[2,3] Those species with keeled scales have a rough or spiny appearance. Some lizards may incorporate osteoderms, especially around the head region as is the case with gila monsters and beaded lizards (*Heloderma* spp.). Unlike snakes, which have a continuous shed, lizards shed their skin in patches. Appropriate humidity for the particular species is essential for proper shedding or ecdysis. Some species, such as chameleons (*Chamaeleo* spp.), are known for their ability to blend into their environment

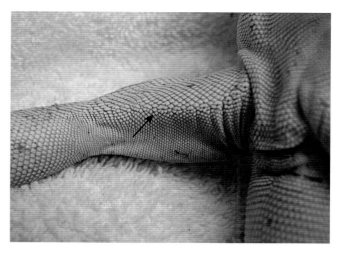

Figure 8-1 Small femoral pores *(arrow)* in a female green iguana.

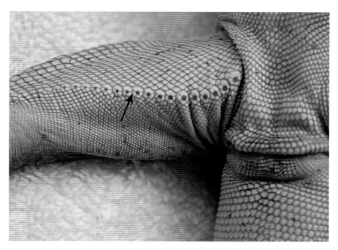

Figure 8-2 Large femoral pores *(arrow)* in a male green iguana.

because their skin contains chromatophores that allow changes in color. The mechanism of these changes is not fully understood, but they appear to involve a complex group of reactions based on their environment. Chameleons also have the ability to change colors based on their moods and perhaps even as a way to communicate with others chameleons and fend off potential predators. Another way in which lizards have evolved and adapted to their environments is via ornamentation in the form of coloration as well as skin extensions expressed as dewlaps, spines, crests, and skin folds.[2] These features may help veterinarians differentiate males from females, whereas others are designed for protection against predators. Lizard skin is largely aglandular, although some species have femoral pores/glands on the ventral aspect of the thigh. In these species, the males have pores of considerable size whereas they are barely visible in the females (Figures 8-1 and 8-2). Others have both femoral and precloacal pores. This is one form of sexual dimorphism in lizards. The subcutaneous space of lizards varies with the species and should be a consideration

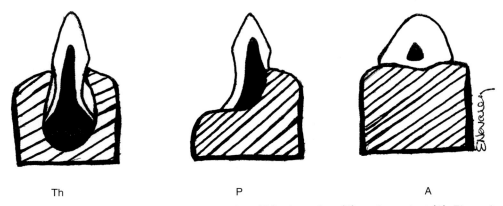

Th   P   A

Figure 8-3 Different types of dentition. Thecodont (Th), pleurodont (P), and acrodont (A). Pleurodont and acrodont are the two types found in lizards.

at the time of fluid administration. Finally, some species have well-developed claws that can inflict damage on handlers. Therefore, regular trimming is recommended for those lizards in captivity.

Gastrointestinal System

TEETH

Lizard teeth are classified as pleurodont or acrodont. Pleurodont teeth have longer roots with weak attachments to the mandible and no socket (Figure 8-3). They rest on the lingual side of the mandible; the buccal side has a prominent ridge of bone. Pleurodont teeth can be replaced throughout the life of the lizard.[2] Acrodont teeth have shorter roots with a firmer attachment, lack sockets (see Figure 8-3), and are fused with the bone itself. Acrodont teeth are not replaced in adulthood.[2] These considerations should be taken into account when performing oral examinations so as to avoid damage to the teeth, especially those with acrodont dentition. The teeth of lizards have varied functions depending on the species. In some lizards, they aid in the grinding of coarse food material before passing to the stomach. Other lizards rely on their teeth to tear or break larger pieces of food into smaller pieces that are then swallowed whole. Teeth also play a role in defense from predators and during mating. Some males latch on to the females during copulation by biting them on the neck or head. Nonetheless, the teeth of most lizards probably do not play as important a role as they do in other groups of animals. The size of lizards' teeth is small compared with the size of their heads and bodies.

TONGUE

There are distinct variations of tongues among lizard species. For example, bearded dragons have a yellowish coloration of their mucous membranes and tongue. Green iguanas have a red coloration on the tip of their tongues. Chameleons have a complex structure that houses their long tongues at the base of the oral cavity. The tongue of lizards can be fleshy or snake-like, as in monitor lizards. Veterinarians must be familiar with these normal variations as part of the physical exam process.

With the exception of chameleons, few species of reptiles have presenting problems related to the tongue.

STOMACH AND INTESTINES

Lizards have a relatively simple stomach with no compartmentalization. The stomach empties into the small intestine and then, in some species, into a well-developed cecum. From there it follows its course into the colon, which also may be well developed and include multiple sacculations. This type of colon is usually present in herbivorous reptiles that require a high degree of hindgut fermentation. Carnivorous lizards have a less developed cecum and colon and an overall shorter gastrointestinal tract. The colon then empties into the coprodeum section of the cloaca. Gastrointestinal disease occurs with some frequency in lizards as a result of foreign bodies or infectious organisms.

CLOACA

The cloaca is a common space that collects the waste and opens into the outside of the body. The outer opening is commonly referred to as the *vent*. The cloaca is divided into three main sections: the coprodeum, the urodeum, and the proctodeum. The *coprodeum* collects the fecal matter from the colon. The *urodeum* is the area that collects urine directly from the ureters or bladder. The reproductive tract also connects with the urodeum. The urodeum and coprodeum then empty into the *proctodeum* before being excreted outside of the body. It is in the proctodeum that the urine and fecal matter mix. The cloacal mucosa is usually moist and can be examined to help determine the hydration status of the animal. It can be very difficult to identify the three main areas in a live animal.

Cardiovascular System

Lizards have a three-chambered heart comprised of two atria and a single ventricle. An anatomic-physiologic body function of lizards and other reptiles, which has raised some controversy in the veterinary literature, is the renal portal system (RPS). Under certain physiologic conditions, the RPS allows blood from the caudal aspect of the body to circulate through the kidneys and/or liver before reaching the systemic circulation. This renal portal blood flow has been perceived as a problem for drug administration. Some drugs may be nephrotoxic and lead to adverse effects if carried directly into the kidneys. The metabolism of drugs also may be affected if they pass through the kidneys before generalized tissue distribution, resulting in the drugs being excreted before reaching the target tissues. Studies have investigated the RPS in red-eared sliders (*Trachemys scripta elegans*)[4] and green iguanas.[5] Both investigations concluded that blood flowing from the hind limbs is directed primarily at the liver, bypassing the kidneys. In red-eared sliders, blood flowing from the tail region was shown to flow into the kidneys or bypass the kidneys and go straight into the liver.[4] In green iguanas, blood flowing from the tail was shown to flow into the kidneys.[5] Benson and Forrest stated that "the renal portal vasculature joins the primary renal circulation at the level of the efferent arterioles."[5] This would imply that drugs excreted by glomerular filtration would be spared by the RPS, whereas those excreted by tubular secretion would be adversely affected.[5] This idea is further supported by findings of a study in red-eared sliders that evaluated the effects of the RPS on the pharmacokinetics of gentamicin and carbenicillin.[6] In mammals, gentamicin is excreted via glomerular filtration and carbenicillin through tubular secretion. After comparison of cranial and caudal injections of these drugs, it was concluded that gentamicin pharmacokinetics was not affected by site of administration.[6] However, carbenicillin was observed to have a perceived reduction in bioavailability after injection in the caudal limbs as opposed to the cranial limbs.[6] This reduction in bioavailability was determined not to have clinical relevance. A first-time passage through the renal tubules for a drug excreted at the tubules would explain the perceived decrease in bioavailability. Despite these findings, there is not enough evidence to support a clinically relevant decrease in the effectiveness of drugs administered in the caudal musculature of reptiles. Conversely, these studies are limited and do not take into consideration multiple variables that may affect the RPS. A valve system was proposed as a part of the control of the RPS but was not proven in all species.[4,5] Factors affecting the metabolism of the reptile, such as temperature, nutrition, time of the year, and health status, may influence the physiologic mechanisms of the RPS and regulate when it will or will not direct blood flow into the kidneys and/or liver. Further studies are needed to evaluate the RPS under various conditions in lizards and other reptile species.

From a clinical veterinarian's standpoint the conflicting information is confusing, with current research showing little evidence of concern for drug administration in the caudal aspect of the body. Clinicians should have precise knowledge of the metabolism and excretion of drugs to determine the best site of administration, being especially critical for antibiotic injections. Even with the RPS, the drugs still may reach adequate plasma levels despite a first passage through the kidneys. Until further pharmacokinetic studies are performed, I recommend the continued administration, when feasible, of therapeutic agents in the musculature of the cranial limbs. One

limitation of the cranial musculature, in some species, is that the muscle mass may be less than that found in the caudal limbs. Injecting large volumes of therapeutic agents over a long period of time may lead to nerve and muscle damage or tissue necrosis. Lack of a limb, due to amputation, trauma, or focal dermatitis, is another presenting condition that may preclude administration of drugs in the cranial limbs. In instances where a veterinarian cannot administer medications in the cranial limbs, the best alternative would be the caudal limbs or epaxial musculature. Ultimately, this decision is based on the clinician's experience, knowledge, and case situation. There is enough evidence to support the presence of an RPS but not enough evidence to explain all of its functions.

Renal System

Lizards, like most reptiles, are uricotelic. The end product of protein catabolism is the production of uric acid by the liver, which is then transferred over to a metanephric kidney. The kidney goes through three main stages of development: pronephric, mesonephric, and metanephric. In higher vertebrates, the mesonephric kidney dominates into adulthood and is comprised of an elaborate arrangement of nephrons with a well-developed renal pelvis and a loop of Henle that allows efficient urine concentration. The reptilian kidney, on the other hand, is dominated by the metanephric arrangement in which there are far fewer nephrons and a poorly developed renal pelvis. The reptilian kidney lacks a loop of Henle and therefore is not able to concentrate urine as a mesonephric kidney would. Uric acid is filtered by the glomeruli and secreted by the proximal tubules.[7] Because of this, lizards are not able to concentrate urine beyond the osmolarity of their plasma.[7] The urine follows a path through the mesonephric duct into the urodeum. Most lizard species have a urinary bladder, which receives urine from the urodeum. Together with the liquid urine, there is excretion of urates, which are the insoluble salts that aid in the conservation of water.

The posterior segment of some lizard kidneys express sexual dimorphism during the reproductive period, increasing in size to produce seminal fluid in males.[2] The uricotelic nature of reptiles allows them to conserve fluids in a way different from other animal groups. Reptiles, in general, excrete urates and retain as much fluid as possible. This adaptation is essential for those animals living in desert environments. However, this adaptation also contributes to the difficulties of managing renal disease in reptiles.

Reproductive System

Sex determination may not be easily accomplished in some reptile species. Others have sexual dimorphism that allows differentiation of males and females based on external characteristics. In the green iguanas, males tend to have large heads with big dewlaps, operculum scales, and dorsal spines, all considered to be male-associated characteristics. Females have smaller heads and smaller dewlaps. Other lizard species may also have increased ornamentation in the males in the form of

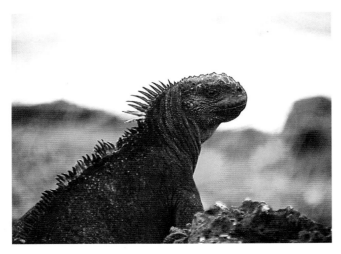

Figure 8-4 Compared with male marine iguanas, female marine iguanas have smaller heads and darker coloration.

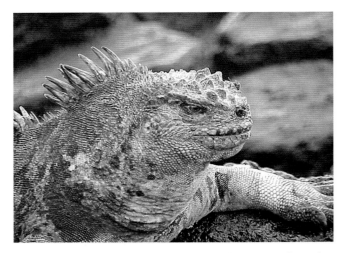

Figure 8-5 Compared with female marine iguanas, male marine iguanas are more robust, with a larger head and neck, and are more colorful, with varying shades of red, green, brown, and black.

colors, crests, spines, casques, and other exaggerated external features as compared with the females (Figures 8-4 and 8-5). This distinction in masculine versus feminine characteristics is not evident in all lizard species. Instead, veterinarians must rely on more precise ways to differentiate the sexes. Large femoral pores can easily be observed in the adult male of many species (see Figure 8-2). Females have smaller femoral pores as compared to the males (see Figure 8-1). Another distinction comes from the presence of the male copulatory organs, the *hemipenes,* which are located on the ventral aspect of the base of the tail caudal to the location of the vent. A hemipenal bulge can be observed on adult males of some species. The hemipenes are a purely copulatory organ with no association with the urinary system. Therefore, the copulatory organs can be amputated in cases of trauma or unresolved paraphimosis. This occurs with lizards and other reptiles.

Reproduction in lizards is stimulated by environmental effects, such as temperature, humidity, and photoperiod. The presence of natural substrates, such as soil, may stimulate reproduction in females. Before folliculogenesis, the females may decrease food consumption and become anorectic. Anorexia is often the first sign that a female is reproductively active. Males have paired internal testes that will increase in size during the reproductive season, and females have paired ovaries with follicles that grow to considerable size during the reproductive season. Females also can produce and lay infertile eggs in the absence of a male. Egg retention/binding is a common presenting symptom in some female iguanas. Frequently, egg retention is associated with inappropriate husbandry and diet, and an ovariohysterectomy is the treatment of choice in these patients. Aggressive behavior may be observed in intact adult lizards, especially during the reproductive season. Early sterilization may prevent hormonally induced behavior in adulthood, but the owner must understand the treatment may not be effective.

The birthing and reproductive methods of lizards are quite varied. Lizards can be oviparous, ovoviparous, or parthenogenic. *Oviparous* species lay eggs that require incubation until the hatching of the young. Many species dig nests in the ground where they lay the eggs. *Ovoviparous* species give birth to live animals without the need for laying an egg. *Parthenogenic* species do not require mating to produce young (e.g., whiptail lizards *[Cnemidophorus tigris]*). Instead, the females are able to reproduce by themselves. Green iguanas and bearded dragons are oviparous species. Blue-tongued skinks *(Tiliqua spp.)* are ovoviviparous. Chameleons can be oviparous or ovoviparous.

Nervous System

The nervous system of reptiles is poorly understood. This presents a challenge in the recognition, diagnosis, and treatment of neurologic diseases of reptiles. The lack of knowledge regarding the reptile nervous system also makes it difficult for clinical veterinarians to differentiate pain responses from reflex responses. A primitive system that has evolved little over the years may be more adapted to reflex stimulation than conscious pain perception. In some species there is considerable movement of the body after death, most commonly observed in crocodilian species. The response of these species after death may indicate stimuli of peripheral innervations without a conscious perception of pain. Because there is no current information to substantiate this possible physiologic pathway in reptiles, veterinarians must assume that all reptiles have conscious pain perception and take appropriate measures to provide analgesia. Selection of appropriate anesthetic and analgesic agents is also limited because of a lack of understanding about the type of receptors present in the many reptile species as compared with mammals.

To treat a reptile with neurologic signs, it is important to be knowledgeable of the animal's normal behavior, both in the wild and in its captive environment. This will help determine if the clinical signs, as described by the owner, are abnormal. Although muscle tremors may be diagnosed as a neurologic problem, a veterinarian must consider primary underlying causes such as a dietary calcium deficiency. Head tilt, abnormal posture and ambulation, slow righting reflex, and lack of awareness of their environment are some of the more obvious neurologic signs that may be observed in affected reptiles. Others signs, such as decreased proprioception, pupillary light reflexes, and strength, may be more difficult to assess. A thorough history is needed when trying to assess exposure to toxins and trauma. Reptile patients with metabolic disorders may also present with neurologic signs (e.g., secondary nutritional hyperparathyroidism). Diagnosis of primary neurologic disease is rare in reptile species maintained as pets and often is determined after ruling out other disease processes.

Musculoskeletal System

The musculoskeletal system of lizards is very similar across species lines. Most lizards have well-developed extremities and tails, with limbs being used for locomotion (e.g., running, climbing). Some species are capable of bipedal locomotion for short periods of time (e.g., basilisk [*Basiliscus plumifrons*]). The tails of some lizards can undergo autotomy, an adaptation by which the tail will break off at a predetermined place to facilitate escape from predators. The tail will then regenerate but not to the original size, shape, or color. For this reason it is important to avoid restraining lizards by the tail, especially iguanids. Other species do not undergo tail autotomy but may have prehensile tails (e.g., chameleons). Most lizards have a rib attached to every vertebra except on the sacral vertebrae, which can be palpated during the physical examination and noted when viewing radiographic images. Trauma to the extremities and tail are common clinical presenting signs. Although the objective of a tail or extremity surgery is to save the affected appendage most species tolerate amputation if necessary. Arboreal species may have a more difficult time adjusting after amputations because of their need to use a limb for climbing.

Respiratory System

Nostrils are clearly visible in most lizards. Nasal salt glands also are present in some lizard species (e.g., green iguanas). A prime example of nasal salt glands can be found in the Galapagos marine iguanas, which have extensions from their nostrils to aid in the expulsion of salt away from the body (Figure 8-6). Lizards have a single tracheal opening (glottis) located at the base of the tongue. With the mouth closed, the glottis is in close apposition to the internal opening of the nares, similar to the arrangement of the choana in birds. The lungs of lizards have evolved over time whereby the lung structure can be air sac–like and lined with a minimal number of falveoli, or a more elaborate, reticulated tissue with a higher number of falveoli. In either case the lung structure is less elaborate than in mammals. The lungs usually comprise a significant volume of the coelomic cavity and can extend caudally into the lumbar region of some lizard species during inspiration. Lizards also use their lungs as air reserves to inflate their bodies and remain wedged between rocks to defend against a predator attack; they may display this behavior during a physical examination. Because they lack a diaphragm, lizards rely on the mechanical action of the ribs during inspiration and expiration for respiration to occur. Care must be taken to avoid a tight grip around the body of lizards, as this may interfere with respiration. Auscultation of normal lungs should reveal minimal respiratory noise. Increased respiratory noises may be due to normal vocalization (e.g., hissing) or a true anomaly (e.g., pneumonia). Diagnostics such as radiographs and blood work may be used to investigate a suspected anomaly.

Auditory System

Most lizards have external ear openings, and in many species an external tympanic membrane may be observed (Figure 8-7).

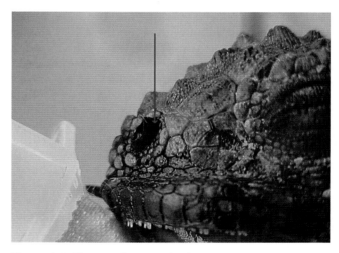

Figure 8-6 The nostrils of marine iguanas have a slight extension of tissue to aid in the excretion of salts away from the head and eyes *(arrow).*

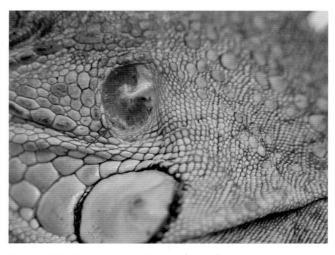

Figure 8-7 Tympanic membrane *(arrow)* of a green iguana.

This membrane is usually translucent and may be covered by skin. The posterior side of the membrane should appear dry with no indication of fluid accumulation. Behind the tympanic membrane lies the middle ear cavity and structures of the inner ear with their vestibular function. These structures are as varied as the species of lizards in which they are found. Ultimately, the hearing of lizards may be limited to detecting vibrations from their environment, with little acuity for noise. There is little vocalization among the many lizard species, but some may communicate in frequencies outside of the range of human hearing. From a clinical standpoint few diseases of the ear are recognized in lizards. Aural abscesses are a common clinical finding in certain tortoise species but are rarely noted in lizards.

Ocular System

The anatomy of the lizard eye is quite varied and interesting. Some species have eyelids, whereas others rely mostly on spectacles for protection of the cornea. Lizards with eyelids may also have a nictitating membrane. Species without eyelids (e.g., gecko) may use their tongues to keep the spectacle/cornea clean and moist. Some species also possess scleral ossicles, similar to those present in many bird species, which maintain the shape of the globe. The cornea lacks a Descemet's membrane, and the iris is controlled primarily by striated muscle (similar to avian species), precluding the diagnostic return of pupillary light reflexes.[2] The shape of the pupil varies with the species. Diurnal species usually have larger round pupils, whereas nocturnal species usually have vertical pupils that are able to constrict to a very small size. Most species have avascular retinas and a *conus papillaris*.[2] A pineal eye, not a visual structure is present in some species (Figure 8-8) and is responsible for detecting variations in light cycles and may aid with thermoregulation through determining optimum basking periods. Some lizards have very special adaptations to their eye structure. For example, chameleons have the ability to move each eye independently, whereas the horned lizard *(Phrynosoma spp.)*, can squirt blood from its periocular tissue to fend off predators. Overall veterinarians must be aware that ocular diseases occur with some frequency in reptiles.

■ HUSBANDRY
Environmental Considerations
CREATING A VIVARIUM

An enclosure for a lizard should be designed to accommodate that species and its natural habitat. Ideally, a vivarium is created to provide the same conditions found in nature by that particular species; however, this is often not practical. Nonetheless, some people are able to provide elaborate enclosures for their lizards. I concentrate here on explaining the minimum environmental requirements for the common lizard species maintained in captivity. The requirements can be broken down into five categories: enclosure type and size, temperature and humidity, lighting, substrate, and accessories. Regardless of the species, these five elements must be considered before obtaining a lizard.

ENCLOSURE TYPE AND SIZE

The rule of thumb for enclosure size is the bigger the better, with an underlying consideration to plan for an appropriate enclosure size for the adult lizard. Often an appropriate enclosure size is provided for juvenile lizards, but they quickly outgrow this space. The main orientation of the enclosure depends on the species. Arboreal lizards benefit from enclosures with a vertical orientation (Figure 8-9), whereas terrestrial and fossorial lizards require enclosures with a horizontal orientation (Figure 8-10). In addition to the size of the enclosure, construction materials must be appropriate. Synthetic nonporous materials are preferred, as they are easier to clean and lighter in weight. However, cages made of these materials can be expensive and need to be purchased from a manufacturing company. Wood is still a popular material for the construction of reptile enclosures. Wood is readily available and inexpensive, and most people can build a lizard's enclosure. The main disadvantages of wood are its weight and its ability to retain water and organic matter. Pressure treated wood that contains chemical compounds to prevent decay must be avoided because of potential toxin exposure. Wood used in reptile enclosures must be properly sealed against water damage by using stains and polyurethane. It is also advisable to seal the seams and corners with a silicon caulking material for ease of cleaning. The wood stains, polyurethane, and caulking must be allowed to cure for several days to avoid any toxicity. It is important to inspect the enclosure on a regular basis to ensure that the wood is completely sealed and intact. A more durable, safe but expensive option is the use of synthetic decking material that is now available. Plexiglas® is a lightweight material that may be used in combination with wood to create enclosures for lizards. Glass tanks can make adequate enclosures for juvenile lizards and those species that mature to a smaller size (e.g., anoles).

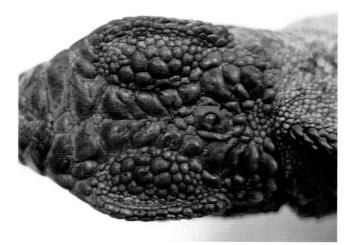

Figure 8-8 Pineal eye *(arrow)* of a green iguana.

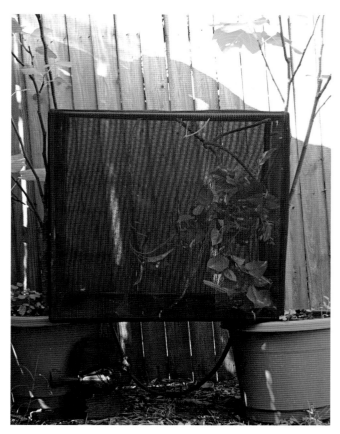

Figure 8-9 Vertical enclosure ideal for arboreal lizards such as chameleons.

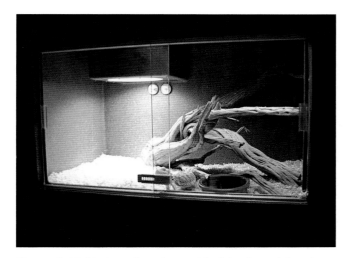

Figure 8-10 Horizontal enclosure ideal for fossorial and terrestrial lizards, such as skinks and bearded dragons.

Glass tanks must have screen tops to provide proper ventilation. One material that should be avoided when building an enclosure is uncoated metal wire mesh. This material will lead to skin abrasions when the animals rub against or climb on it. Also, galvanized wire has the potential of causing zinc toxicity in lizards if they chew on the wire and accumulate toxic levels

of the metal over time. A plastic coated wire mesh is available and appropriate for use in enclosures. The size of the wire mesh should be such that it does not cause injuries from escape attempts and does not allow other animals to enter the enclosure (e.g., domestic dogs or cats, wild raccoons). As a general rule, the size of the mesh opening should be smaller than the size of the head of the animal. One major advantage of using mesh is than the enclosure is well ventilated. In addition, wire mesh is lightweight and relatively inexpensive.

The size of an enclosure will depend on the adult size of the animal as well as its natural habits. Some species are more sedentary and do not travel a long distance in nature in search of food or territory and therefore do not require much space for their captive environment. Green iguanas are arguably the most popular pet lizard species and also require one of the largest enclosure sizes for any pet lizard. Green iguanas can grow up to 6 feet in length. Unfortunately, many owners do not realize this when they obtain a green iguana. The minimum enclosure size for a single adult green iguana should be approximately $4' \times 3' \times 6'$ (length × width × height). Some chameleon species (e.g., veiled chameleon [*Chamaeleo calyptratus*]) can grow up to 24 inches in length and require a vertically oriented enclosure with minimum dimensions of $3' \times 3' \times 4'$. Other species (e.g., bearded dragons) will benefit from a longer and wider enclosure, with the basic dimensions for housing a single animal being $3' \times 3' \times 2'$. The size of the lizard enclosures usually is not considered by the novice lizard owner. Unfortunately, many pet lizards end up confined to inappropriate enclosures for most of their lives because of inadequate owner education.

TEMPERATURE AND HUMIDITY

Reptiles rely primarily on the environmental temperature to regulate their internal body temperature. In a natural environment there are normal variations in body temperature during a 24-hour period. Many reptile species take advantage of the early morning and mid-day sun to bask and warm their bodies. As the day progresses, the reptile's internal body temperature begins to decrease as the environmental temperature decreases. I have observed greater than 20° F variations in the cloacal temperature of green iguanas over a 12-hour period. This apparently wide temperature gradient is part of the normal biology of many lizard species. Reptiles and lizards strive to achieve an optimal body temperature during the day, which is essential for the physiologic processes of digestion, immune function, acid-base balance and reproduction.[8] Ultimately, the animal must maintain an adequate metabolic rate to sustain homeostasis. The temperature at which a lizard has an adequate metabolic rate sustaining homeostasis has been referred to as the *preferred optimal temperature zone* or the *thermal neutral zone*.[8] Regardless of which term is used, reptiles have an optimal temperature, a single temperature, at which physiologic function is at its peak. In an ideal situation this temperature would be achieved for a certain period of time every day, but in reality most reptiles thrive within a range of acceptable temperatures that allow them to maintain appropriate physiologic function. Ultimately, achieving an acceptable temperature range is the goal of temperature regulation for captive lizards, allowing for diurnal variations in temperature and a reduction in the nocturnal temperature. Although actual requirements vary among lizard species, some generalizations can be made about the most common species maintained in captivity. A recommended diurnal temperature range for tropical and desert lizard species is 85° F to 95° F, with a basking light provided to allow for a concentrated area of heat (reaching a maximum of 100° F to 105° F) in the area directly underneath it. To avoid thermal burns on the animal, it is essential to monitor the temperature under the basking light. There should always be a barrier between the light and the animal, with enough room to allow basking as desired. The nocturnal temperature range for most species should be between 72° F and 78° F. Ceramic heat emitters (Figure 8-11) and basking lights (Figure 8-12) are good sources of radiant heat. Various types of heating pads are available for use under the reptile enclosures, with most having an adhesive that attaches them to the underside of the enclosure. The most important consideration regarding the heating pads is to ensure that they are calibrated to achieve a maximum safe temperature or that a rheostat is used to control the heat output. A layer of substrate is recommended between the heated area and the animal for added protection against thermal burns. Most veterinarians suggest leaving the heating pad on at all times and utilizing the basking lights or ceramic heaters to increase the diurnal temperature. The room temperature also can be regulated to provide an adequate environment. If the room is maintained at a warmer temperature, it will be easier to achieve the desired temperature within the enclosure. Various types of thermometers are available to monitor temperature inside reptile enclosures. Some thermometers record temperatures at different intervals or provide maximum and minimum temperatures, giving the owner a daily temperature gradient within the enclosure.

A second factor closely associated to temperature is humidity. Humidity has a direct impact on the heat index, so two enclosures with the same temperature may have a different physiologic impact based on the humidity level. Higher humidity increases the heat effect on a lizard by increasing the heat index within the enclosure. With higher heat indexes and increased moisture, proper ventilation is essential for temperature regulation and reduction of microorganism growth. The recommended humidity for tropical species is 80% to 90%, with desert species requiring a lower humidity (30%-50%). There are various ways to increase humidity in an enclosure, including adding large water bowls, moist sphagnum moss, or water mister systems. The main idea is to increase the presence of water in the enclosure to increase the relative humidity. A humidifier may be used in the room containing the enclosure, especially during the winter months when the calefaction results in decreased humidity. Humidity is measured with a hygrometer, and appropriate humidity for the species in question is essential to maintain hydration, allow shedding, and prevent disease.

LIGHTING

Lighting requirements of reptiles vary with the nutritional requirements of the species in question. It is generally thought that herbivorous, insectivorous, and most omnivorous reptiles have an absolute requirement for ultraviolet (UV) radiation, specifically in the UVB spectrum. Light in the UVB spectrum is essential for the synthesis of vitamin D_3 and consequently the absorption and metabolism of calcium. Nonetheless, there are no specific requirements for these species to indicate how much exposure they really need. Carnivorous species are

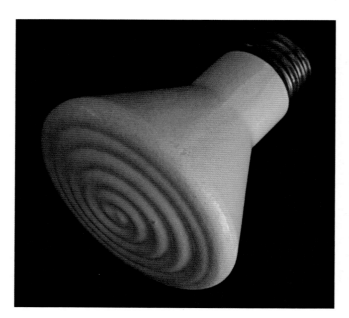

Figure 8-11 Ceramic heat emitters used to provide radiant heat without light.

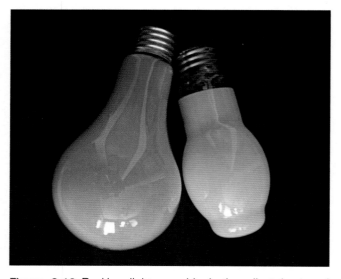

Figure 8-12 Basking lights provide both radiant heat and visible light, but most have no ultraviolet B radiation output.

thought to have the ability to obtain enough vitamin D_3 from their prey; however, studies have shown that carnivorous species may still benefit from exposure to UVB.[9] The best source of UVB is direct, unfiltered sunlight. Owners must remember that glass and other materials filter beneficial UVB rays. Lizards in captivity maintained indoors should be exposed to natural sunlight 2 to 3 times a week, especially in the summer, in addition to artificial UVB. During the winter an owner may need to rely only on artificial sources of UVB. Many sources of artificial UVB lights are available in the market. Although many of these bulbs are referred to as full spectrum, owners must make sure that the one purchased has an appropriate output in the UVB spectrum. There are two main types of bulbs that provide UVB: fluorescent bulbs and mercury vapor bulbs. Fluorescent bulbs come in a variety of UVA and UVB percentage outputs. The main output of consideration should be the UVB, which should be at least 5%. Fluorescent bulbs are available as long tubes or strip lights and as a coiled bulb version that can be used with regular incandescent light fixtures (Figure 8-13). The type for use with incandescent light fixtures shows promise of providing a more effective UVB output.[10] The average price of a fluorescent bulb

with UVB spectrum is approximately US$25 to $35. One disadvantage of fluorescent bulbs is their effective working distance. Most bulbs will provide adequate UVB within 12 inches from the bulb, but the UVB output decreases exponentially beyond 12 inches from the bulb. This dramatic reduction in UVB radiation is an important consideration when designing the enclosure. In enclosures taller than 12 inches, a climbing surface must be provided to allow the lizard to get within 12 inches of the bulb. Placing a basking light nearby will ensure that the animal effectively uses the area under the light. These bulbs usually have an effective life span of 6 months, at which point they must be replaced by a new bulb, whether or not they still provide light.

Mercury vapor bulbs are generally self ballasted and can be used with a regular incandescent light fixture with an appropriate wattage rating. Non-ballasted mercury vapor lamps require the purchase of an external ballast. Good quality mercury vapor bulbs start at approximately US$40 to $50 and are available as spotlights, which provide light in a concentrated area, or as flood lights, which cover a widespread surface area. These bulbs have the advantage of providing heat in addition to the UVB light, and providing effective UVB output at distances greater than 12 inches. The mercury vapor lights must be set up at a distance recommended by the manufacturer to prevent overheating and provide adequate exposure to UVB. The major disadvantages associated with these bulbs are that they are fragile, suffer early burnout, and are expensive. Their effective UVB output is also approximately 6 months and therefore should be replaced twice a year. These bulbs provide a very strong UVB output that may be damaging to humans if not used properly. Most manufacturers recommend turning off the bulb while working within the enclosure. Owners must be made aware of both the possible consequences of using this light source and the precautions required.

SUBSTRATE

The choice of substrates for reptile enclosures is a main subject of discussion among veterinarians and owners. The primary substrate consideration should be a nontoxic, easily digestible product that is absorbable and easy to clean. Unfortunately, most commercially available products do not meet these requirements. In my opinion, the best substrates are newspaper, other nontoxic paper, or artificial turf (also known as indoor/outdoor carpeting). Newspaper is inexpensive, nontoxic, easy to clean, and, if ingested, easily digestible. Unfortunately many owners do not find newspaper to be very esthetic. Newspaper as a substrate also does not meet the goal of creating a natural vivarium. Artificial turf is readily available in green and brown colors, thereby being more aesthetically pleasing while meeting the necessary criteria for a substrate. The artificial turf must be of good quality and not the type that will lose strands of material easily, as these pieces may be ingested and result in intestinal blockage. Other commercially available products that may be recommended include recycled paper products, ornamental bark chips (not cedar or pine), aspen bedding, and cypress mulch. All substrate products have

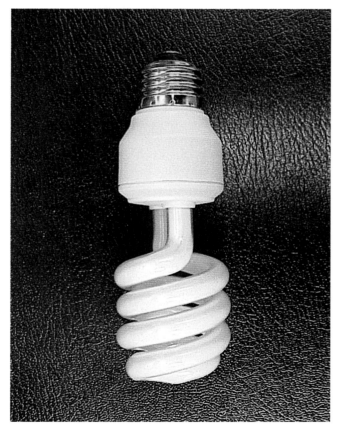

Figure 8-13 Compact fluorescent bulb used as a source of UVB light for reptiles. These bulbs are designed to provide UVB output for reptiles; not all fluorescent lights produce adequate UVB.

the potential of being ingested by the animal and causing an obstructions. Some substrates hold more moisture and are more difficult to clean. One consideration in choosing a substrate is that the individual substrate particle should be too large for the lizard to swallow. Accidental ingestion usually occurs while feeding the lizards; therefore, an appropriate feeding bowl or container should be provided that is deep enough to prevent spillage of the food within it. Alternatively, owners can try to feed the lizard in a separate container with no substrate in it; although well-acclimated lizards may tolerate this, for most lizards it would be a stressful situation. There are some products that should not be used as substrate in reptile enclosures, including cedar chips, cat litter, corn cob, and other products sold as a digestible reptile substrate, such as calcium carbonate sand. The so-called digestible sands sold in many pet stores are not as digestible as advertised and may cause severe impactions when ingested. They are also advertised as a source of calcium for reptiles, but this is misleading. (Proper sources of calcium are discussed in Nutrition.) Many veterinarians have treated cases of gastrointestinal impaction in lizards that ingested sand substrate. For experienced breeders or hobbyists that have the time and knowledge to monitor their collection very closely and desire a sand substrate, one alternative is the use of play sand that has been sifted very carefully to remove the larger particles. Sand substrate should be reserved for adult specimens only, because young lizards are more curious and may be more prone to accidental ingestion. In addition, newborn and juvenile animals have a smaller diameter to their intestinal tract, and even a small amount of sand can cause gastrointestinal obstruction. Novice hobbyists should avoid the use of all sand products. Although many people have successfully used sand and other particulate substrates over the years, these materials continue to be a cause of intestinal impaction for many lizards maintained as pets.

ACCESSORIES

Accessories, or *cage furniture,* refers to items that not only enhance the aesthetics of the enclosure but also serve a functional purpose as a psychologic stimulus for the lizard. Accessories include water and food bowls, branches for climbing, plants, and hiding places. Water and food bowls should be of appropriate size to allow easy access for the animal while minimizing food spillage. Artificial branches or rock formations can be used to promote exercise and create basking areas under the light. Natural branches and rocks may be used, but extra care is required to disinfect these materials both before placing them in the enclosure and after contact with organic material such as feces. Appropriate nontoxic, natural or artificial plants may be provided depending on the species of lizard. Natural plants (e.g., pothos, ficus) may be consumed by certain lizard species and require frequent replacement. Lizards should also be provided with accessories to promote hiding and a sense of security where they can sleep at night undisturbed. An array of items ranging from cardboard to PVC and other synthetic and natural products can be used for this purpose. The most important thing to remember when selecting accessories is to be sure that they are nontoxic and easily disinfected.

◼ NUTRITION
Dietary Requirements

This section will concentrate on the four main dietary schemes of lizards: herbivorous, carnivorous, omnivorous, and insectivorous. Which scheme a species falls under determines its recommended dietary requirement. As with other groups of animals, some lizard species (e.g., bearded dragons) vary in their dietary scheme according to age and even season. It is also important to remember that in nature, lizards may deviate slightly from their normal dietary scheme on occasions. Dietary deviations may be prompted by seasonal changes, physiologic need, or scarcity of food.

Herbivores

Herbivorous reptiles have a primary dietary requirement of plant material, including grasses, leaves, and fruits. Most herbivorous reptiles have a colon that aids in the fermentation of feedstuffs and require a diet with moderate to high fiber content and moderate to low fat and protein content. Not all herbivorous lizards have the same nutritional requirements, and it is incumbent on the owner to become knowledgeable about the particular requirements of the species being maintained in captivity. Even with green iguanas there are many variations with respect to dietary recommendations. Therefore, a general recommendation for feeding herbivorous lizards will be presented. Specifics for each species of lizards can be located in other published sources. A common mistake is feeding the captive herbivorous lizard too many carbohydrates in the form of fruits and/or diets too high in protein (e.g., dog or cat food). The key management point is to introduce a balanced diet that not only provides fiber, protein, and fat but also other nutritional elements, such as vitamins and minerals. The source of the protein is also an important consideration, because for herbivorous reptiles, the protein source should be of primary plant origin. Allen and Oftedal's recommendations for the dietary requirements of green iguanas consist of 22% to 26% protein level on a dry matter basis for juvenile iguanas and 15% to 17% protein on a dry matter basis for adult, nonreproductive iguanas.[11] This is accompanied by recommendations of 6% to 10% crude fiber or 10% to 18% acid detergent fiber.[11] At first this may seem contraintuitive to what herbivores should require, but these recommendations are based on a primary diet of plant matter. The protein content of plants is smaller when compared to animal sources and it is also not as digestible. This explains why, on a dry matter basis, the protein requirement is larger than fiber requirements and why the protein requirement would be smaller if the source of the protein was more easily digestible. Baer et al. found that diets with 12% crude fiber or 20% acid detergent fiber led to decreased weight gain and energy retention in juvenile green iguanas.[12] A proposed explanation for this observation is that the iguana's digestive system is not as specialized as that of ruminants and may not be able to efficiently process dietary fiber. An additional observation is that little grinding of the plant material occurs before ingestion; therefore, the material reaches the intestinal tract with a large particulate size that is harder to digest.[11] Perhaps offering finely chopped plant material would help the digestibility of the fiber in the intestinal tract of herbivorous lizards. The nutrition of green iguanas has been studied more than that of most lizard species. The same principles may or may not apply to other herbivorous lizards, depending on their natural habitat, available feedstuffs, and efficiency of their digestive tract. A critical aspect of the nutrition of herbivorous reptiles is the ability to maintain an overall balance of calcium and phosphorus at a ratio of 1.5 : 1 to 2 : 1, which is essential for optimum calcium availability and metabolism.

Even with different views of what and how to feed herbivorous lizards, the primary recommendation is to offer as varied a diet as possible. Some commercial diets are available for different lizard species, but many are limited in their nutritional composition. Also the nutritional analysis of these commercial diets is not regulated and is often inaccurate.[11] Commercial diets should not be used as the sole source of feed for any lizard species. Some companies have the input of properly trained nutritionists and herpetologists to assist in the manufacture of their commercial feed products, whereas others do not. Some diets are readily available to the public, whereas others may only be purchased by zoologic institutions or sold in bulk quantities. The alternative to commercial diets is feeding what is known as the "salad-based diet." The salad-based diet consists of different greens and vegetables from the local grocery store or produce stand. The variety of vegetables offered varies according to season and geographic location. A list of some greens and vegetables that are recommended for feeding herbivorous reptiles is provided in Box 8-2. A controversial item in this table is the feeding of lettuce (red or romaine). It is argued that red and romaine lettuce have little nutritional value and therefore should not be fed to reptiles. Although the concern about lettuce has its merits, these items should be offered as part of a mixed, varied diet and not as a sole source of plant matter. Red and romaine lettuces are both readily available and represent a dietary source of fiber that can be used as part of a balanced diet. The more diversity that can be offered, the more balanced a diet is likely to be. In addition to

items that may be purchased at the grocery store, the local garden store will sell some plants with leaves and flowers or fruits that may be used to feed reptiles. Both the flowers and leaves of the hibiscus plant can be offered to herbivores and are part of the natural diet of some tropical lizards. Dandelions are a favorite of most reptiles and can be offered as part of a varied diet. All plants offered to reptiles must be free of pesticides and fertilizers to avoid potential toxicities. A controversial dietary recommendation is what source of protein should be made available to herbivorous reptiles? If iguanas are considered to be true herbivores, then the protein should come from a plant source. Alfalfa has been advocated as an ideal source of protein for reptiles. Alfalfa can be found as the fresh plant (not the sprouts), pellets formulated for mammals, and even tablets for humans. Although alfalfa is likely the best source of plant protein, it should not constitute the majority of any reptile's diet. Like other food items, alfalfa should be used as a component of the dietary plan.

Although there is a general consensus on what not to offer nutritionally, few are in agreement on what to feed herbivorous lizards. High-protein dog and cat foods should not be offered to herbivorous lizards. Some expert hobbyists and herpetologists have included dog or cat foods as part of the dietary plan for certain lizards, which is done under a closely observed nutritional plan that takes into consideration the amount, frequency, and nutritional value of all items fed. For the average pet lizard owner, this nutritional oversight can be an overwhelming task and many times leads to excessive feeding of a high-protein diet, which, in turn, may lead to renal disease. Some leafy greens and nonleafy vegetables are rich in oxalic acid. If ingested in excessive amounts, oxalic acid can bind calcium and reduce the absorption of this important mineral. Food items with high oxalic acid (OA) content should be limited (e.g., parsley (1.7 g OA/100 g), spinach (.97 g OA/100 g), and chives (1.48 g OA/100 g)).[13] Alfalfa also is known to have increased levels of oxalic acid and therefore should be fed in moderation. Other greens and vegetables may contain high amounts of glucosinolates. These are goitrogenic glycosides present in some plants that have been associated with toxicity.[14] Plants with high levels of glucosinolates are being studied for potential benefits in treating cancer (e.g., cabbage, Brussels sprouts, broccoli, cauliflower, kale, kohlrabi, Swiss chard, radish, pak choy, and watercress).[14] Plants with high glucosinolates should also be used sporadically and not as a main ingredient in the diet.

Feeding herbivorous reptiles is complex and full of contradictions, depending on the reference sources. No plant material by itself is nutritionally balanced, and some may cause additional problems if fed frequently and/or in large amounts. The best and most simple approach to feeding herbivorous reptiles is to provide a combination of fresh dark leafy greens, vegetables, plants (e.g., leaves, flowers, and fruits), alfalfa, commercial diet, and vitamin/mineral supplementation. Plant material should constitute 50% to 80% of the diet. The rest of the diet should be a commercial formula deemed appropriate for the species being fed. Alfalfa can also be added to the diet but should not be used in conjunction with food items

---

BOX 8-2	**Recommended Greens and Vegetables for Feeding Herbivorous Lizards**

Bell peppers	Mustard greens
Bok choy	Okra
Carrots	Parsnip
Collard greens	Red leaf lettuce
Dandelion	Romaine lettuce
Eggplant	Squash (variety)
Endive	Sweet potatoes
Faba beans	Turnip greens
Green beans	

containing high levels of oxalic acid. Vitamin and mineral supplements designed for reptiles can be sprinkled over the food with the amount limited to that of the allowed dose of vitamin A in reptiles (56 international units/kg body weight).[11] Vitamin and mineral supplements should be used with caution when feeding a commercial diet to prevent nutritional toxicity or imbalance. All greens and vegetables should be thoroughly washed before being offered to remove organic debris and prevent contamination with bacteria and other organisms.

Carnivores

Carnivorous reptiles have a primary dietary requirement for prey items such as small mammals, birds, and even other reptiles. These animals rarely deviate from animal prey items as their primary food source. Carnivorous reptiles require high-protein diets with moderate fat and low fiber. In captivity, mice and rats have served as a primary source of nutrition for these reptiles and should be offered prekilled to avoid trauma to the captive reptile. Mice and rats can also be purchased frozen and then thawed before being offered. If offering immature rodents, it is advisable to coat them with a calcium supplement to increase the calcium intake. The calcium supplement should contain calcium only or have an appropriate calcium-to-phosphorus ratio (2 : 1).

Insectivores

Insectivorous reptiles have a true requirement for insects as their primary food source. Unfortunately, many believe that all lizards and most reptiles are insectivores. This misconception has led to years of inappropriate nutrition for many lizard species, including the green iguana. Insects such as crickets, mealworms, and waxworms are readily available through pet stores, breeders, and Internet retailers. Insects and their larvae do not provide enough nutrition by themselves and must be gut loaded before being offered to the reptile. In nature, these insects feed on decaying matter and naturally load their guts with nutrients from their feedings. Veterinarians and responsible reptile owners try to mimic the insects' natural nutritional supplementation by what is commonly known as gut loading. This consists of feeding the insects a diet rich in nutrients for 1 or 2 days before offering them to the reptile, thereby increasing the nutritional value of the insect. Mealworms have a lot of natural body fat, and excess feeding of mealworms is a common cause of obesity in lizards. In addition to crickets, mealworms, and waxworms, earthworms may be readily accepted by insectivores. Insects are available in various sizes depending on the species. All prey items fed to insectivorous lizards should be of appropriate size. As a general rule the prey should be smaller than the lizard's head and able to fit easily in the lizard's mouth. Feeding too large of a prey can lead to intestinal impaction and delayed gastric emptying. There are few truly insectivorous reptile species. Although bearded dragons are primarily insectivores early in life, they later develop an interest in plant material and become more omnivorous.

Omnivores

Omnivorous reptiles are indiscriminate in what they eat and are thought to be true scavengers ingesting plant material as well as prey items. Seasonality may influence their choice of foods, and some species have a predilection for certain food items such as insects. Omnivorous lizards require a well-balanced, varied diet with moderate amounts of protein, fat, and fiber. They can tolerate higher levels of protein than can herbivores but should not be maintained on an exclusive carnivore diet. Omnivores can be maintained on a diet that combines the recommendations for herbivores, carnivores, and insectivores.

■ PREVENTIVE MEDICINE
Quarantine

Any new lizard being introduced into a household or collection of animals where there are other reptiles or lizards present should be quarantined a minimum of 60 to 90 days. The quarantine procedure should be performed in a separate building or room from the one in which the other reptiles are housed. The new specimen should be fed and handled last after all other animals in the collection have been attended to. The enclosure, substrate, bowls, and accessories should be disinfected daily and separately from the others in the collection. During this quarantine period it is also advisable to have the new lizard examined by a veterinarian. Once the quarantine process has begun, no new animals should be introduced until the ongoing quarantine is finished.

Routine Exams

Routine veterinary care for pet lizards is recommended as with any other species of exotic pet. A thorough annual examination by a qualified veterinarian provides a forum for addressing husbandry issues and monitoring the growth and development of the patient. A complete blood count (CBC) and/or chemistry panel can provide a reference of the patient's values and overall health status. If the animal develops an illness, then the established CBC/chemistry panel reference ranges may be used as a baseline. Establishing a baseline is important for many lizard patients because of the paucity of information regarding normal, species-specific reference values for blood parameters. Seasonality may influence the results of the CBC and chemistry panel; therefore, these samples must be obtained at approximately the same time each year. The seasonal variations may become even more prominent in female lizards during the reproductive season. Together, the blood work and physical exam allow veterinarians to retain a yearly record of the health of the patient, which will be invaluable in case of illness. These recommendations also should be carried out with any new animal to determine its health status before implementing a quarantine period or before transferring the lizard to an established collection.

Disinfection and Sanitation

Hygiene is an essential part of maintaining healthy animals, and with lizards, feces, urine, and food are the main sources of organic waste. The type of cage and substrate will influence the ease of cleaning the waste material. Most lizards defecate/urinate a few times per week, depending on the diet and frequency of feeding. Organic waste should be removed from the enclosure immediately. Any surface that comes into contact with the organic waste must also be cleaned and disinfected. A complete cleaning and disinfection of the enclosure, including removal of substrate and accessories, should be performed every 3 to 6 months. A mild soap solution or an organic nontoxic cleaner is recommended for cleaning and disinfecting the interior surfaces, accessories, and cage furniture. Chemical cleaners and disinfectants may prove toxic to the animal and therefore should not be used. There are some products sold for use in reptile enclosures, but the ingredients of these products must be examined carefully before their use. The most common disinfectant used is a 1 : 10 solution of bleach and water, applied after removal of all organic material. The bleach solution should be rinsed off and the enclosure ventilated thoroughly before placing the lizard back in the enclosure. Other acceptable disinfectants include quaternary ammonium compounds, chlorhexidine, and iodophores.[15] Disinfectants must be used in a dilute solution and rinsed thoroughly after use in a reptile habitat. Finally, it is important to take appropriate measures to prevent cross-contamination of household items and surfaces bacterial contaminants (e.g., *Salmonella* spp.). Individuals must thoroughly wash their hands after coming in contact with a reptile and their environment. Avoid hand washing in the kitchen sink; use a bathroom sink instead, and if possible, wash the cage and accessories outside of the house. If no outdoor facility is available, thoroughly disinfect sinks and/or bathtubs after the accessories and cage are cleaned. An antibacterial disinfectant should be used on household surfaces that come in contact with reptiles and the contents of their enclosures. Children, the elderly, and immune-compromised individuals should consider additional measures if handling reptiles and their enclosures. These recommendations are aimed at preventing the transfer of zoonotic diseases from reptiles to humans.

■ RESTRAINT
Manual Restraint

Most lizard species can be restrained manually by a single individual. Larger species such as monitors and iguanas may require multiple individuals. Because a lizard may bite, its head should be restrained. Placing an index finger and thumb around the base of the mandible will secure the head. The handler's free hand should be used to restrain the rear legs and the tail (Figure 8-14). Lizards should not be grabbed by their tail, as some species have the ability to lose the distal part of the tail as a defense mechanism; this is known as *tail autotomy*. Extra care must be taken when restraining species with auto-

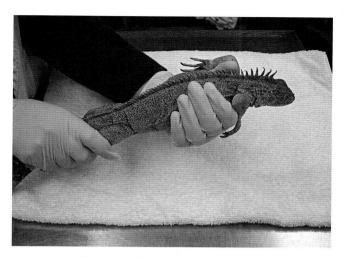

Figure 8-14 Restraint of a green iguana. This animal remained calm with support of the thorax and rear legs, but some may require additional restraint of the front legs, head, or both.

tomy (e.g., green iguanas). Some lizards will be accustomed to handling and may be placed with their ventrum resting on your forearm, but the handler must remain vigilant to avoid being bitten. A technique that may calm some species of lizards is to cover both eyes with cotton balls or gauze and wrap their heads with bandaging material. This will create vagal stimulation and lead to a calming effect that may be beneficial when obtaining radiographs or performing a physical examination.

Chemical Restraint

Chemical restraint of pet lizards is rarely warranted for routine physical examination and diagnostic testing. Using therapeutic measures to restrain lizards is usually reserved for painful procedures and surgery. (Anesthesia and analgesia are discussed in depth under Surgery.)

■ PERFORMING A PHYSICAL EXAMINATION

The physical exam provides the initial health assessment of any animal, including the lizard. Veterinarians must be familiar with the normal anatomy of the lizard species being examined to differentiate between normal and abnormal findings. Experience and other resources will help veterinarians become familiar with individual differences between species. Once the animal is properly restrained, the physical examination should begin. The eyes are examined for any evidence of dryness, blepharospasm (in those species with eyelids), and asymmetry. Looking at the dorsal aspect of the head is useful in determining symmetry of the eyes. Sunken eyes are indicative of dehydration. The function of the third eyelid, if present, should be assessed. Some species will have external ear openings or tympanic membranes. Oral examination can be performed with the help of a speculum (e.g., tongue depressors, rubber spatulas, wood applicators). One must exercise caution when opening the mouth to avoid breaking the teeth. The appearance of the oral cavity is quite varied depending on the species. Look for evidence of asymmetry, which may be related to root tooth abscesses, ocular disease, trauma, or all of these things. It is common in most species to have accumulation of saliva in the caudal aspect of the pharyngeal cavity. This saliva can be slightly viscous at times and should not be confused with a sign of dehydration, as in mammalian species. The mucous membranes normally appear as pale pink, pink, or even pigmented depending on the species. Blood vessels in the oral cavity can be used to help assess hydration and perform a capillary refill–like test similar to that used with mammals. Although it may not be as accurate as in mammals, a slow refill of the vessel (greater than 3-5 seconds) should prompt further assessment of the hydration status. Cotton tip applicators may be used to press against the vessels and determine a capillary refill time.

After examination of the oral cavity, the extremities should be palpated for any evidence of swelling, fractures, or decreased range of motion. The palmar and plantar surfaces of the feet are examined for evidence of pododermatitis. The tip of the digits and tail are examined for any evidence of dysecdysis that may be causing constriction and necrosis. The spine and tail are examined for any signs of kyphosis or lordosis. Although it may be difficult to elicit and interpret pain in reptiles, any motion that appears to cause a reaction and can be duplicated may indicate a problem in that region and should be investigated further.

Coelomic palpation can be challenging in lizards, as they have the ability to hold air within their lungs and stay inflated for extended periods of time. However, firm but gentle and steady pressure of the coelomic cavity will enable the examiner to palpate the animal. The examiner's familiarity with the lizard's anatomy will play an important role in the interpretation of the results. Herbivorous lizards may have a prominent colon during palpation. Bearded dragons have large, prominent fat pads on the caudal coelomic cavity that may impede palpation of other organs. The main goal of coelomic palpation is to ensure there is no large, firm or hard mass that may associated with disease. In green iguanas with renomegaly, the cranial poles of the kidneys may be palpated at the point of the pelvic inlet, prompting further testing. Chameleons are laterally compressed and present an additional challenge for coelomic palpation. Nonetheless, an understanding of the patient's normal anatomy should facilitate identification of abnormalities. After coelomic palpation, the vent and cloaca are examined. The cloaca can be everted to look for any evidence of sand or foreign material, which is commonly observed in animals that present with an impaction. The color and moisture level of the mucosa are additional ways to assess the hydration of the patient.

The examiner should assess the condition of the skin. Scales should be flat against the skin with a uniform overall appearance. Areas of abnormal pigmentation with raised skin or scales

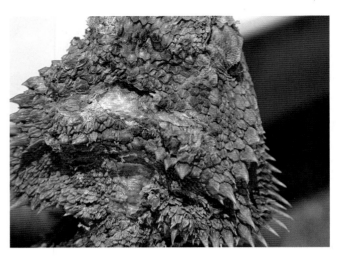

Figure 8-15 Dermatitis on the head of a bearded dragon. This animal was housed outdoors in a subtropical environment.

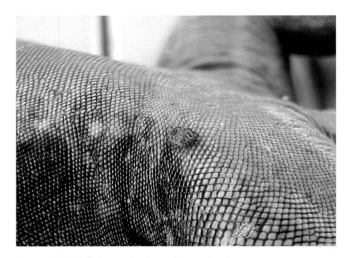

Figure 8-16 Tick on the leg of a marine iguana.

and a sharp line of demarcation may be indicative of fungal or bacterial dermatitis (Figure 8-15). These areas should not be confused with normal shedding, which, in lizards, occurs in a nonuniform pattern over time. The examiner also must look for evidence of external parasites such as ticks and mites (Figure 8-16). Ectoparasites are commonly found between the scales/skin under the mandible, axillary and inguinal regions, and at the base of the tail.

■ DIAGNOSTIC TESTING
Clinical Pathology

Clinical pathology of lizards is used on an everyday basis to help diagnose diseases and monitor response to therapy. CBCs and chemistry panels (plasma or serum) are two common tests that are highly recommended to determine a lizard's baseline

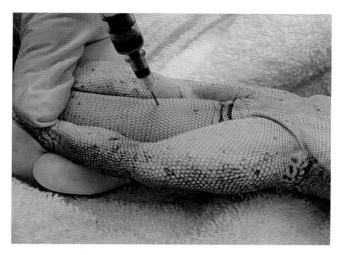

Figure 8-17 Venipuncture of the ventral coccygeal vein in a green iguana. In males, the entry site should be distal to the hemipenes to avoid trauma to these structures.

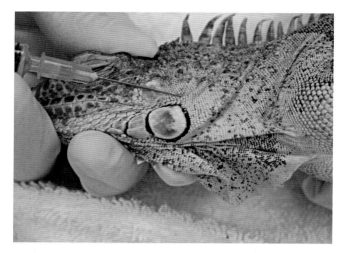

Figure 8-18 The landmarks for the jugular vein in a green iguana are the tympanic membrane and the point of the shoulder. In this case the needle was inserted from a craniocaudal direction entering caudal to the tympanum.

health status. In addition, clinical pathology involves the examination of cytologic specimens and urine samples as well as other tests like protein electrophoresis. Veterinarians must explain to the clients the importance of performing these tests and how they will help monitor the patient's health. The veterinarian should also be aware of the factors that may influence the results of these tests (e.g., species, age, sex, reproductive status, and season of the year).

Venipuncture

Venipuncture can be accomplished with a 1- to 3-ml syringe and a 22- to 26-gauge needle depending on the size of the animal and the collection site. There are three main sites used to collect blood from lizards. Site selection depends on personal experience, size of the animal, species, and health of the animal. The ventral coccygeal vein can be accessed from either the ventral or lateral aspect of the tail (Figure 8-17). This vessel lies along the ventral midline of the coccygeal vertebrae. Hypothermia and hypovolemia may increase the difficulty of a blood draw from the ventral coccygeal vein because of peripheral vasoconstriction. The jugular vein is located on the lateral aspect of the neck from a point near the caudal mandible to the point of the shoulder (Figures 8-18 and 8-19). In lizard species with an external ear opening, the opening or tympanic membrane can be used as the cranial landmark. Jugular venipuncture in lizards is usually a blind procedure with the needle being inserted at a location based on the anatomic landmarks described earlier. The third site for blood collection in lizards is the ventral abdominal/coelomic vein, which is located on the ventral midline. This vessel bifurcates at the umbilicus; therefore, venipuncture must be attempted cranial to the umbilicus (Figure 8-20). Cardiac puncture is not recommended in lizards.

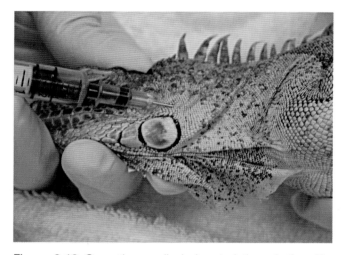

Figure 8-19 Once the needle is inserted through the skin, aspirate gently until a flash of blood is obtained. Steady the syringe and obtain the blood sample.

Veterinarians also must be mindful of the maximum amount of blood that can be drawn safely from the reptile patient. As a general rule, obtaining a maximum blood volume equal to 0.5% of the total body weight is recommended. This is equivalent to 0.5 ml of blood per 100 g of body weight. In large healthy animals a slightly larger volume (1 ml/100 g) can be obtained. If the maximum amount of blood is obtained in one draw, one must wait 5 to 10 days before collecting another blood sample. The amount of blood drawn and period between sample collections are dependent on the size and health status of the patient.

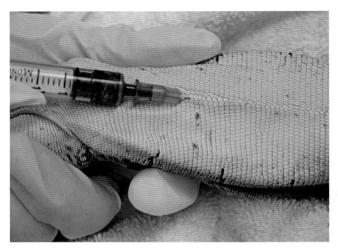

Figure 8-20 Venipuncture of the ventral abdominal vein in a green iguana. This site may be more challenging than the ventral coccygeal and jugular veins.

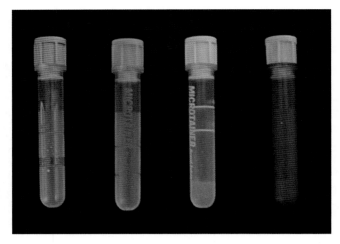

Figure 8-21 Small blood tubes with a 0.25- to 0.5-ml capacity can be used to store small volumes of blood from lizards. These are available with sodium EDTA *(purple)*, lithium heparin *(dark green)*, lithium heparin with plasma separator *(light green)*, and non-anticoagulant tubes with serum separator *(yellow)*.

Blood Handling

The sample must be handled carefully to avoid hemolysis, which will affect the results of the CBC and chemistry panel. Hemolysis can damage the integrity of the cells and lead to difficult interpretation of the differential count and artificial decreases in the total white blood cell (WBC) count. Hemolysis was shown to affect plasma levels of phosphorus, potassium, total protein, and aspartate aminotransferase in 10 green iguanas.[16] The blood cells of many exotic species are fragile and have a tendency to clot quickly. To obtain a better sample, one should remove the needle from the syringe before transferring the blood into the tube. The blood must be transferred immediately after collection and mixed well with the anticoagulant to avoid clotting. Because the blood volume that can be collected safely from lizards tends to be very small compared to that from mammalian species, the use of Microtainer® blood tubes (BD Vacutainer Systems, Becton Dickinson and Company, Franklin Lakes, NJ) (Figure 8-21) is recommended. These tubes require a minimum of 0.25 ml and a maximum of 0.5 ml of blood for an appropriate ratio of blood to anticoagulant. For the majority of reptiles (except chelonians), a sodium ethylenediaminetetraacetic acid (EDTA) tube (purple top) will be appropriate. EDTA has been shown to provide better results than lithium heparin in samples obtained from 32 green iguanas.[17] Lithium heparin (green top) can also be used if EDTA tubes are not available, but the cells will be more susceptible to degradation. Lithium heparin tubes come in two varieties. One has a gel that will separate the plasma after centrifugation (see Figure 8-21) and is ideal for samples destined for plasma chemistry panels that may sit overnight because the separation of plasma from red blood cells (RBCs) will prevent hemolysis and artifacts. The other lithium heparin tube has no separator gel and can be used for both CBCs and chemistry panels. In addition, there are plain tubes with no anticoagulant, which are used for collection of serum

for chemistry panels or serologic testing. The plain tubes also are available with a gel to separate the serum. To obtain optimum results, veterinarians should consult with technicians at the diagnostic laboratory to ensure that the samples are properly collected and processed. Poor quality samples will yield nonreliable results.

Complete Blood Count

There are three main interpretations of a CBC: normal leukogram, leukocytosis (elevated total white cell count), or leukopenia (decreased total white cell count). In addition, a stress leukogram (heterophilia with possible monocytosis and lymphopenia) may be commonly observed in reptile patients. A complete blood count will provide the veterinarian with information regarding a possible inflammatory process. A finding of leukocytosis does not directly correlate to an infectious process, but it may provide information that, together with the history and presentation, is consistent with an infectious disease (e.g., bacteria, fungi, viruses, parasites). Other tests are required (e.g., cultures, biopsies, serology) to aid in the identification of a potential infectious agent. Other differential diagnoses, such as stress, neoplasia, immune-mediated disorders, trauma, metabolic imbalances, and endocrine disorders may contribute to the physiologic response of a leukocytosis. The other possible abnormality observed in a CBC is a leukopenia, or decreased WBCs. Possible differential diagnoses associated with a leukopenia include neoplasia, viral infection, septicemia, toxicity, immune-mediated disease, bone marrow disease, drug-induced toxicity, and white blood cell sequestration in the tissues. In addition to determining the total white cell count, the veterinarian must also be familiar with the morphology of WBCs in lizards. A major challenge is the varied morphology that occurs between different lizard species.

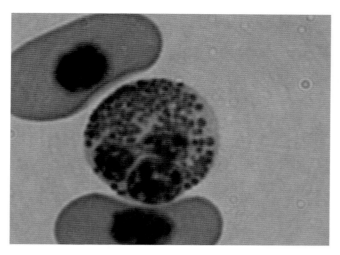

Figure 8-22 Heterophil of a green iguana. These cells may be easily confused with mammalian eosinophils because of the rounded granules and brighter red-pink color. (Modified Wright-Giemsa stain; ×1000.)

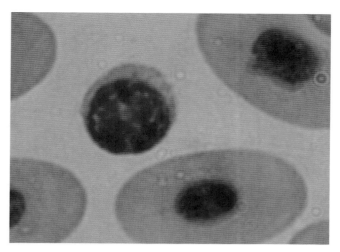

Figure 8-23 Lymphocyte of a green iguana. Notice the scan basophilic cytoplasm. (Modified Wright-Giemsa stain; ×1000.)

In reptiles the heterophil is the equivalent to the neutrophil in mammals (Figure 8-22; also see Figure 8-24). The difference comes as a result of different staining characteristics and the enzymatic content of the cells. Heterophils lack many of the peroxidases and other enzymes present in mammals. This leads to the formation of more caseous abscesses as opposed to a liquified abscess. In most species of lizards, the heterophil is the most abundant WBC and phagocytizes foreign organisms during the early part of an inflammatory event. The second most abundant cell is the lymphocyte, although some reptile species may normally have more lymphocytes than heterophils (Figure 8-23). The function of lymphocytes lies mainly with the production of antibodies (B cells) and moderation of the immune function (T cells). Monocytes are the largest WBCs and are in charge of antigenic processing and granuloma formation (Figure 8-24). Monocytes are often called upon after heterophils have initiated the process of phagocytosis. Eosinophils are another WBC that is normally activated during parasite infections and allergic reactions (Figures 8-25 and 8-26). The role of eosinophils in reptiles may be more complex then currently recognized, possibly having a more active involvement in the inflammatory process. Finally, the basophil is a small cell that may occur with some frequency in certain species of lizards and may be negligible in others (Figure 8-27). Basophils carry histamines, surface immunoglobulins, and enzymes. The function of basophils in the reptile inflammatory response is not completely understood at this point in time. Thrombocytes should not be confused with lymphocytes, with the main difference being the clear, almost invisible cytoplasm of thrombocytes (Figure 8-28).

Unfortunately, arriving at a conclusion as to whether a CBC is normal or abnormal is not an easy task in many reptile species, including lizards. This is due primarily to a lack of normal reference values for most species. It is important to remember that a true normal reference range for any species

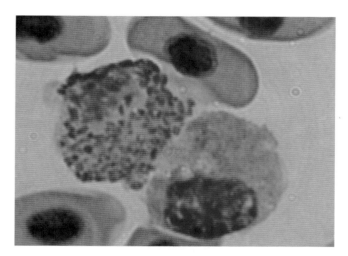

Figure 8-24 Monocyte and heterophil of a green iguana. Notice the abundant basophilic cytoplasm of the monocyte. (Modified Wright-Giemsa stain; ×1000.)

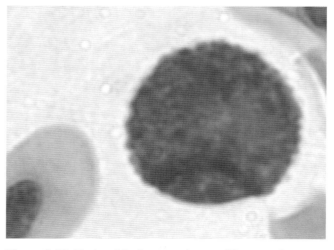

Figure 8-25 Eosinophil of a green iguana. They are characterized by a large amount of granules that protrude from the cytoplasm. (Modified Wright-Giemsa stain; ×1000.)

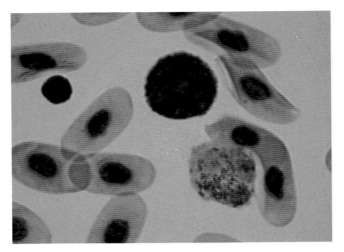

Figure 8-26 Eosinophil (top) and heterophil (bottom) of a green iguana. (Modified Wright-Giemsa stain; ×1000.)

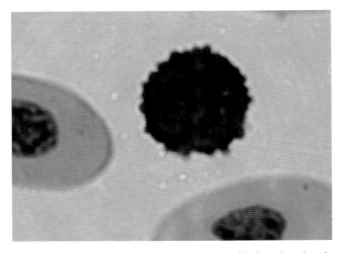

Figure 8-27 Basophil of a green iguana. Notice the deeply basophilic granules. (Modified Wright-Giemsa stain; ×1000.)

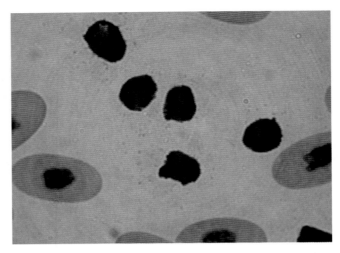

Figure 8-28 Thrombocytes of a green iguana. Notice the clear cytoplasm, which is barely visible as compared to that of lymphocytes. Thrombocytes also tend to be found in aggregates. (Modified Wright-Giemsa stain; ×1000.)

BOX 8-3	General Reference for Interpretation of Complete Blood Count

Total WBCs	$5.0\text{-}18.0 \times 10^3$
Heterophils:	
Lymphocytes	1 : 1 to 3 : 1 (may be inversed in some species)
Monocytes	$<1.0 \times 10^3$
Eosinophils	$<0.5 \times 10^3$
Basophils	$<0.5 \times 10^3$

of animal should not include values from diseased animals. Unfortunately, these values are sometimes included in the so-called normal ranges. Another limitation is the sample size of many reference values. It is not accurate to interpret blood values for all lizards in a group based on a limited sample size. A final limitation is the report of the WBC differential on a percentage basis without consideration of the absolute numbers. Interpretation of a leukogram based on percentages of the cells alone can be misleading. To illustrate, let's assume that the normal reference range for green iguana heterophils has been reported to be 45% to 55%. Taking two green iguanas (Ig1; Ig2) with different total WBC count numbers (Ig1 WBC = 8,000; Ig2 WBC = 36,000) but the same percentage of heterophils (50%): Ig1 has a WBC count within acceptable limits, whereas Ig2 has an elevated WBC, or a leukocytosis. If one looks at the percentage alone, both of these iguanas appear to have normal heterophil counts. However, if one looks at the absolute numbers of heterophils (Hets) (Ig1 Hets = 8,000 × 0.5 = 4,000; Ig2 Hets = 36,000 × 0.5 = 18,000), it becomes obvious that Ig2 has a heterophilia that is contributing to the leukocytosis. If a veterinarian had not analyzed the leukogram as a whole and had concentrated on the percentages alone, he or she would have determined erroneously that the heterophils were normal for this animal. This is a common mistake if the absolute differential count is not determined or is ignored. Veterinarians must rely on their clinical experience in combination with the limited resources available to interpret the CBC of reptiles and many exotic species. A general rule for interpretation of the CBC is described in Box 8-3. The values in Box 8-3 are derived from the experience of veterinarians that work with reptiles and are a general starting point to help clinicians differentiate normal leukograms, stress leukograms, leukocytosis, and leukopenias. These values should not be interpreted as scientifically or statistically accurate for all reptile species. Veterinarians also can refer to studies that have examined CBC values for certain lizard species.[7,9,18-20]

Because of a lower metabolism, lizards have a lower packed cell volume (PCV) when compared to mammals and birds. Reptiles can have PCVs in the range of 20% to 35%. Some values may be higher or lower depending on season, sex, and species. This variation reemphasizes the importance of obtaining annual blood parameters to establish normal patterns for each patient in a practice. When faced with a suspected anemia in a lizard, veterinarians should always approach the case as with any other species. A thorough history and physical examination will help determine if the animal appears to be clinically anemic in correlation with the PCV. Once the PCV has been established and anemia diagnosed, a determination of whether the anemia is regenerative or nonregenerative is in order. Unfortunately, veterinarians rely primarily on polychromasia as evidence of regeneration of the RBCs. Other useful values, such as reticulocyte percent, mean corpuscular volume, mean corpuscular hemoglobin, and hemoglobin, are not readily available for the reptile patient. Four possible causes for anemia are blood loss, hemolysis, lack of RBC production, and anemia of chronic disease. Blood loss anemia may be associated with external or internal RBC loss, possibly caused by trauma or infectious disease. In mammals, acute blood loss usually appears as a nonregenerative anemia during the acute stage, but evidence of regeneration will appear within 48 to 96 hours.[21] Differentials leading to hemolysis are not common in reptiles, but infectious disease, autoimmune disease, and toxicity may be implicated in this process. Anemias linked to hemolysis are usually regenerative in nature. A lack of production of RBCs usually presents as a nonregenerative anemia and can be caused by bone marrow disease, endocrine disease, iron deficiency, or disease of hematopoietic organs (e.g., kidney and spleen). Anemia of chronic disease (e.g., inflammation, infection, neoplasia) is nonregenerative in nature and is likely a common cause of anemia in reptiles.[21]

Hemacytometer

The presence of nucleated RBCs in reptiles requires a manual estimate of CBCs. Manual CBCs are commonly estimated using a hemacytometer (Figure 8-29) with the Unopette® Eosinophil Determination for Manual Methods stain (Becton Dickinson and Company, Franklin Lakes, NJ). A stained blood smear is also needed to complete the total estimated WBC count (TEWBC) and obtain the differential cell count. Alternatively a blood smear alone can be used to calculate both an estimated WBC count and differential cell count. However, the blood smear method is less reliable than the hemacytometer method.

The instructions provided with the Unopette system for mixing the blood with the stain are easy to follow. After mixing the blood with the stain, let the mixture sit for approximately five minutes before placing it into the hemacytometer chambers. After filling both chambers, the hemacytometer should sit for five to ten minutes in order for the cells to settle; if one waits too long, the RBCs will pick up the stain increasing the chance of a false elevation in the final count. The hemacytom-

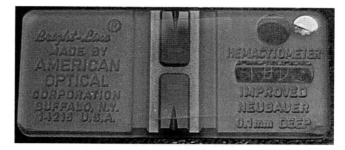

Figure 8-29 Hemacytometer used to perform complete blood counts in reptiles.

eter chambers can be examined under the microscope using the 10X objective. All nine squares of each chamber of the hemacytometer should be counted. Once the hemacytometer reading and the differential count have been performed, one can calculate the TEWBC:

$$\frac{\text{Number of stained cells in both sides of chamber} \times 1.1 \times 16}{\%\ \text{heterophils} + \%\ \text{eosinophils}} = \text{TEWBC}$$

Example:

The hemacytometer count is 110 cells on side 1 and 100 cells on side 2.

The differential is as follows:
Heterophils 65%
Lymphocytes 25%
Monocytes 6%
Basophils 1%
Eosinophils 3%

$$\frac{(110 + 100) \times 1.1 \times 16}{0.65 + 0.03} = 5435\,\text{WBC}$$

Then obtain absolute values for the differential WBC by multiplying the WBC by the percentage of each cell type. Notice that numbers are rounded to the nearest decimal point):

Total WBC = 5435
Heterophils (5435 × .65) = 3533
Lymphocytes (5435 × .25) = 1359
Monocytes (5435 × .06) = 326
Basophils (5435 × .01) = 54
Eosinophils (5435 × .03) = 163

Smear Preparation

The first step in preparing the blood smears is to remember the fragile nature of reptilian cells. One technique used to help preserve the integrity of the cells involves the use of 22% bovine albumin (Gamma Biologicals, Inc., Houston, TX) (Figure 8-30). In a separate clean vial, mix one drop of 22% bovine albumin with five drops of blood. This mixture is gently mixed, and the smears are prepared. Experienced technicians

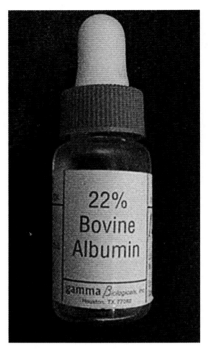

Figure 8-30 Bovine albumin (22%) used for blood smear preparation. Five drops of blood mixed with one drop of albumin help preserve the integrity of the cells.

who are adept at making blood smears may have good results without the use of the bovine albumin. Blood smears are then prepared in a routine manner using the slide method. To perform the slide method, place a small drop of the blood on the slide surface and the using the edge of a second slide at approximately 45 degrees, smear the blood. This technique provides better cell preservation and distribution in the monolayer as opposed to the coverslip technique or the slide-to-slide technique.[22] The smears can then be air dried and stained with a modified Wright's stain or Wright-Giemsa stain. If using bovine albumin, allow the smears to dry for 30 to 45 minutes for better stain retention.

Once the slides are stained, a differential WBC count is determined to identify the percentage of each white cell present in the blood. Using the 10X and 40X objectives, locate a section of the blood smear with an even distribution of RBCs and WBCs. This area is usually near the feathered edge and is described as an area where there is no clumping or grouping of cells. Excessive cell clumping will lead to differential WBC counts that are not representative of the patient's condition. Once an area with good cell distribution is identified, proceed to engage the 100X objective with oil immersion. At 100X a technician will be able to identify and differentiate the five types of WBCs. The next step is to count and differentiate the first 100 white cells observed using a manual counter that records multiple cell types. When counting, move in a constant direction (e.g., zigzag pattern) without going over the same area twice. Continue moving into a new field to count and differentiate the white cells in that field, and so on. Stop count-

ing once 100 cells have been identified. The total number of each cell type can be expressed as a percentage:

Heterophils 65 = 65%
Lymphocytes 25 = 25%
Monocytes 6 = 6%
Basophils 1 = 1%
Eosinophils 3 = 3%
Total 100 = 100%

These values are used in the formula to determine the WBC count as well as to determine the absolute values for the differential cell count. A list of equipment needed to perform CBCs in reptiles is presented in Box 8-4.

Biochemistries

Biochemical values can be obtained from either plasma or serum samples. There is no clear evidence of one sample being better than the other for reptilian biochemical evaluations. Which sample is submitted will depend on the laboratory and/or equipment being utilized. Regardless of which sample is used, consistency in sampling and interpretation is important. Avoid comparing plasma chemistry results to serum chemistry results, as these vary even if submitted concomitantly from the same animal. To obtain reliable results, contact the diagnostic laboratory to inquire about desired sample handling, packaging, and submission. Hemolysis and delayed separation of the plasma or serum are two main factors contributing to degradation of the chemistry samples. The same techniques of venipuncture described previously can be used to obtain samples for biochemistries. The sample is placed in a lithium heparin tube for plasma biochemistries or in a tube with no anticoagulant for serum chemistries. Always remove the needle before transferring the blood sample to the Microtainer® tube to avoid additional hemolysis. Centrifuge and separate the serum or plasma as soon as possible and place the sample in a separate container. If using a tube with a gel separator, the sample can be left in the original tube after centrifugation. Once the plasma or serum is separated, the sample is ready for analysis or submission to a diagnostic laboratory. If there is a delay in analyzing the sample (e.g., overnight shipping), refrigerate or freeze the sample immediately after separation of the plasma or serum.

Interpretation of biochemistries in lizards is limited by the lack of references available for the different species. Nonetheless, there are a few studies that have examined the chemistry values in Komodo dragons *(Varanus komodoensis)*[9] and green iguanas.[7,18-20,23] Interpretation of biochemistries is also limited to fewer values than in mammals because of the low activity of many enzymes in reptilian tissues. Plasma and tissue (e.g., liver, kidney, epaxial muscle, heart, lung, spleen, small intestine, pancreas) activities of alkaline phosphatase (ALP), aspartate transaminase (AST), alanine transaminase (ALT), lactate dehydrogenase (LDH), gamma-glutamyltransferase (GGT), creatine kinase (CK), glutamate dehydrogenase (GMD), and amylase (AMS) were evaluated in six juvenile green iguanas by Wagner and Wetzel.[24] CK was the only enzyme with high tissue activity (epaxial muscles and heart).[24] LDH and AST had moderate activities in all tissues while GGT, GMD, ALT, and ALP had low activities in tissues.[24] It was also reported that low tissue activities were consistent with low plasma activities.[24] Although the number of iguanas in this study was limited, the results are consistent with similar studies in reptiles and birds.[25,26] There appears to be a distinct lack of enzymatic activity in most reptilian tissues, leaving the values of CK, AST, and LDH as clues of abnormalities in the chemistry panels. Even then, a definitive association may not be established between these values and clinical diseases. In addition to CK, AST, and LDH, the chemistry panel will provide information about levels of proteins (albumin, globulin), electrolytes, minerals, and other metabolites such as uric acid. Blood urea nitrogen (BUN) and creatinine are not values considered to be clinically relevant in reptile medicine because of the differences in metabolism of protein/nitrogen. Instead, uric acid is a more clinically relevant protein/nitrogen metabolite. Uric acid is the main end product of nitrogen catabolism in lizards and is excreted via the kidneys. Although many believe that elevations in uric acid (>11-12 mg/dL) are indicative of renal disease, this is not usually the case. The two most common reasons for elevations in uric acid are dehydration and postprandial sampling. If renal disease is a concern, examine the calcium-to-phosphorus ratio (Ca : P), which is a more accurate indicator of renal disease. Normal reptiles will have a Ca : P ratio of 1.5-to-1 or greater. With renal disease an inverse ratio is seen because the calcium is not reabsorbed at the kidney, and phosphorus is not actively excreted.

A measurement that is not usually provided in routine biochemistries is ionized calcium. Ionized calcium is the biologically active form of calcium. This value is important in determining the true calcium deficiencies in animals with suspected metabolic disease and during folliculogenesis. It is common in reptile species to observe a hypercalcemia and possibly a hyperphosphatemia associated with reproduction in females. In these animals an increase in the total calcium is observed, but it is impossible to distinguish the bound from the unbound calcium. Obtaining a level of ionized calcium would facilitate determination of whether or not the reptile has enough biologically active calcium to support reproductive demands. Plasma levels of ionized calcium have been examined in green iguanas.[23,27] These values vary with age, sex, and reproductive status. Further work is needed to determine the fluctuations of ionized calcium in relation to the reproductive cycle of reptiles. In addition, ionized calcium levels may be decreased under alkalosis and increased under acidosis.[27]

Diagnostic Imaging

Radiography, contrast radiography, ultrasonography, fluoroscopy, magnetic resonance imaging (MRI), and computed tomography (CT) have been applied to reptiles in clinical and research cases. Diagnostic imaging techniques have been used to evaluate the RPS in green iguanas,[28] the mechanism of the chameleon's tongue,[29] and the relationship between metabolic bone disease and bone density in green iguanas.[30] Smith et al. evaluated the use of 25% suspension of barium at 25 ml/kg administered by stomach tube for performing gastrointestinal contrast studies in five green iguanas maintained between 27° C and 29° C.[31] The investigators determined a median time for gastric emptying of 8 hours with a 4-hour small intestine transit time and a 16-hour small intestine emptying time.[31] Median colon transit time was 15 hours, and the emptying time was 66 hours.[31] Barium should not be used if a gastric rupture is suspected or if there is risk of aspiration. If gastric rupture or aspiration is a concern, a dilute iodine contrast agent (e.g., iohexol) should be substituted for barium. These are just a few examples of advanced diagnostic imaging techniques that have been used to evaluate lizards.

EQUIPMENT

Most standard diagnostic imaging equipment can be used to perform procedures for lizard cases. The small size of many lizard species necessitates the ability to obtain high-detail radiographs for an appropriate diagnostic evaluation. The radiograph machine should have a capacity of at least 300 milliampere (mA) at 1/60 seconds or faster exposure time.[32,33] The machine should have a kilovolt peak (kVp) range of at least 40 to 100 kVp with the ability to change the exposure in 2-kVp increments.[32,33] The machine also should have the ability to rotate the tube 90 degrees to the table surface to allow for exposure with a horizontal beam, a technique widely used with exotic animals such as lizards and tortoises. The type and quality of the film and screens are also important factors in obtaining high-detail images. Rare-earth, high-detail films and screens are recommended.[32-34] Alternatively, single-emulsion slow speed films (e.g., mammography films) are also used for enhanced detail.[33,34] Double-emulsion films provide the least detailed images for lizard patients.[33,34] There are new technologies being applied to films and screens that may also satisfy the needs for exotic animal radiography. In addition there are two newer modalities: computed radiography (CR) and digital radiography (DR). CR replaces the regular film with a special erasable film that can be used for multiple exposures. Some CR units require specific screens and cassettes, whereas others can be used with the existing screens and cassettes. Radiographs are obtained with CR in the same way, using existing equipment. The processing of the film using a CR unit requires a special developer that reads the film and provides a digital image that can be stored in a computer loaded with special software. The film can be erased and used again once the image has been digitally stored. The ease of use and equipment required vary with the manufacturing company, but in essence any radiographic machine can be used to expose an image on a special film that is developed with a special processor. The CR technology provides a high-quality digital image and is less expensive than DR. Main disadvantages of CR are that it does not save much time in the developing process, and it may take some time to adjust the exposures to obtain optimum results. The second technology, DR, relies on a completely digital system. With DR there is a specialized digital plate that replaces the conventional cassette. Digital radiography also can be used with an existing radiograph machine. The image is processed straight from the digital plate into a computer for viewing. This technology provides instant high-quality images without the need for developing films. One major disadvantage of early DR systems was the inability to perform horizontal beam radiography because the cassettes were attached to the table. However, there are more mobile DR systems that provide horizontal beam imaging. The major disadvantage of DR is that it is more expensive than CR. There is much debate regarding which of the two technologies provides a better quality image (CR or DR). Most believe that DR will be the modality of the future and CR will be phased out. For exotic animal medicine the major advantage of CR and DR is the ability to manipulate images digitally and magnify areas that would otherwise be difficult to assess using nondigital systems. Digital manipulation of radiographs is extremely helpful in small patients where detail of small structures is minimal. As the cost of these technologies decreases, their use in exotic animal practices will increase.

POSITIONING

A minimum of two radiographic views should be obtained for all species, including lizards. A ventrodorsal (VD) or dorsoventral (DV) view and an orthogonal lateral view are recommended. The DV view may be more easily obtained in animals that are awake or fractious. In laterally compressed species such as chameleons, a DV/VD view is more difficult to obtain and interpret. An attempt should be made to obtain these view(s) regardless of a patient's disposition or anatomic makeup. Placing bandage material over the eyes (e.g., blinders) will calm most animals sufficiently to collect the radiographs, reducing the radiographs, reducing the need for chemical restraint. After the animal has calmed down, the lizard can be positioned and secured (e.g., taped) to the cassette. Some lizards may resist restraint but will stand still for exposure. The lateral view is more easily obtained if the x-ray machine is capable of a 90-degree tube (e.g., horizontal beam) to the table. This

90-degree tube rotation yields a lateral view with the animal standing on a flat surface, with the cassette behind the animal. Another alternative is to have a technician hold the animal during the procedure. This may be possible in larger lizards but impractical for small species. Always remember to practice appropriate safety and to not expose body parts of the personnel to the x-rays. If manual restraint does not allow proper radiographic positioning, the animal may require sedation. Other alternatives for restraint and positioning include providing branches or radiolucent climbing surfaces for the lizards to hold onto while obtaining the radiographs. The animal may also be placed inside a radiolucent container such as an acrylic chamber. These radiographic positioning methods are useful for certain examinations but do not allow for straight positioning of the animal. It is important to label the cassettes properly. In some instances additional markers may be needed, and these can be placed directly on the animal to mark areas of interest. Additional markers are particularly useful if examining the vertebral column. Small markers can be taped at different intervals on the lizard's skin, allowing for ease of interpretation on both views.

INTERPRETATION

One of the main challenges associated with of lizard radiography comes from the anatomic differences between species. Veterinarians must become familiar with the anatomy of each lizard species to accurately interpret the radiographic images. There is little published information about the radiology of lizard species. However, this should not prevent extrapolation of techniques from other species and applying them to the lizard patients if it provides useful information. Some of the applications of diagnostic imaging in lizards include the diagnosis of fractures, metabolic bone disease, osteophytes,[35] arteriosclerosis,[36] foreign bodies, intestinal impactions, enteritis, dystocia, reproductive disorders,[37] ascites, neoplasia, uroliths, cystic calculi, fecoliths, pneumonia, and others.[33,34,38] An understanding of the anatomy as well as the expected disease process facilitates better interpretation of the radiographs.

▪ COMMON DISEASE PRESENTATIONS

Infectious

VIRUSES

Viruses have been identified in lizard species; however, the pathogenicity associated with some of these infectious agents has not been established. Whereas the ability to recognize and diagnose viruses in reptiles is improving, the ability to effectively treat viral infections is still lacking. Supportive therapy remains the mainstay of management for these cases, as the use of antiviral drugs is not widespread in reptile medicine. The primary reasons these drugs are not routinely used in lizard patients are lack of pharmacokinetics information and expense. Nonetheless, continued research in this area is needed to better characterize and understand the epidemiology of these organisms. The results of this research will lead to improved prevention, control, and treatment strategies. An understanding of the viruses affecting lizards is also essential for conservation efforts of wild species. Histopathologic examination and electron microscopy are available diagnostic techniques that can be used to help identify viruses in suspect animals.

Adenoviruses

Adenoviruses or adeno-like viruses have been identified in a mountain chameleon (*Chamaeleo montium*),[39,40] Jackson's chameleon (*Chamaeleo jacksoni*),[41] bearded dragons,[39,42-44] fat-tailed geckos (*Hemitheconyx caudicinctus*),[39,44] Tokay gecko (*Gekko gecko*),[44] leopard gecko (*Eublepharis macularius*),[44] blue-tongued skink (*Tiliqua scincoides intermedia*),[44] Gila monster (*Heloderma suspectum*),[44] Savannah monitor (*Varanus exanthematicus*),[45] and Rankin's dragon lizards (*Pogona henrylawsoni*).[46] Identification of the mentioned adenoviruses was carried out by PCR or electron microscopy. Clinical signs associated with adenovirus infection are nonspecific and vary from neurologic signs (head tilt, circling) to poor body condition and death.[39,40,42] Two reports found coinfection of adenovirus and dependovirus in bearded dragons.[42,43] Lesions of this dual infection were found mostly in the liver and intestines. In one report the animals also had a coccidial (*Isospora sp.*) infection in the small intestine.[42] In the mountain chameleon the viral particles were also detected in the small intestine, and the animal had a concurrent enteric nematodiasis.[40] Enteritis was also reported in fat-tailed geckos with chronic weight loss in which adenovirus was identified via PCR.[39] Transmission of this virus is thought to occur via the fecal-oral route. No treatment is currently available, although some animals do respond to supportive care for lizards other than supportive therapy. The disease is usually fatal, especially in juvenile animals, and diagnosed on postmortem examination.

Paramyxovirus and reovirus

Paramyxovirus has been described in the caiman lizard (*Draecena guianensis*).[47] Combined paramyxovirus and reovirus infections/exposures have also been described in Mexican lizards (*Xenosaurus* and *Abronia* spp.),[48] spiny-tailed iguanas (*Ctenosaura* spp.),[49] and iguanas (*Iguana iguana rhinolopha*).[49] The caiman lizards had histologic evidence of a proliferative pneumonia.[47] Paramyxovirus was identified based on electron microscopy, immunoperoxidase staining, viral culture, and hemagglutination inhibition assay.[47] In the Mexican lizards, viral isolation was performed from a cloacal swab of a *Xenosaurus platyceps*.[48] Antibodies were also detected for *Xenosaurus* sp. and *Abronia* sp.[48] In addition, this study found antibodies against a reovirus from three *X. grandis*.[48] Antibodies against paramyxovirus and a reovirus were also detected in spiny-tailed iguanas (*Ctenosaura* spp.) and iguanas (*Iguana iguana rhinolopha*) from the Honduran islands via virus neutralization test (reovirus and paramyxovirus) and hemagglutination inhibi-tion (paramyxovirus).[49] Maxwell cites a report of a reovirus isolated from a green iguana,[50] and Drury et al. reported the isolation of a reovirus from a spiny-tailed lizard (*Uromastyx hardwickii*).[51]

Iridoviruses

The family Iridoviridae is comprised of four genera: *Iridovirus, Chloriridovirus, Lymphocystivirus,* and *Ranavirus*. An invertebrate iridescent virus was isolated from two bearded dragons, a four-horned chameleon (*Chamaeleo quadricornis*), and a frill-necked lizard (*Chamydosaurus kingii*).[52] Marschang et al. isolated irido-like viruses of two different genera, *Iridovirus* and *Ranavirus*, from a four-horned chameleon, a green iguana, and a leaf-tailed gecko (*Uroplatus fimbriatus*).[53] The genus *Iridovirus* had been described in insects but not reptiles, which suggests the possibility of transmission of iridoviruses from insects to reptiles.[53] Lizard erythrocytic viruses (LEVs) have been described under the family Iridoviridae[54] and their pathogenicity (e.g., LEVs) is poorly understood. Alves de Matos et al. performed an experimental infection of two lizard species (*Lacerta monticola* and *Lacerta schreiberi*) and demonstrated that the infection was mostly restricted to erythrocytes.[55] However, in some instances the virus infected leukocytes and killed the infected animals.[55] Other reports of LEVs include nine flap-necked chameleons (*Chamaeleo dilepis*),[54] one Fischer's chameleon (*Bradypodion fischeri*),[54] two four-horned chameleons,[56] and a high-casqued chameleon (*Chamaeleo hoehnelli*).[56]

Herpesviruses

Herpesviruses are one of the more widespread viruses in nature. It is not surprising that they have been identified in various lizard species. There are three main subfamilies of herpesviruses: Alphaherpesvirinae, Betaherpesvirinae, and Gammaherpesvirinae. The literature suggests that this classification is restrictive and that herpesviruses found in non-mammalian species should be classified under new subfamilies.[57] Based on the available information, the currently recognized herpesviruses in reptiles have been classified under the subfamily Alphaherpesvirinae.[57] One of the earliest reports was from green iguana cell cultures.[58] A viral agent was observed in the cell cultures and determined to be cytopathic in *Terrapene* spp. and *Iguana* spp.[58] Suspicion of it being a herpes-type virus was supported by electron microscopy.[59] A later report comes from electron microscopy examination of papillomatous growths on the skin of a green lizard (*Lacerta viridis*).[60] More recently herpesviruses have been implicated with stomatitis in three green tree monitors (*Varanus prasinus*),[61] a Sudan plated lizard (*Gerrhosaurus major*),[62] and a black-lined plated lizard (*Gerrhosaurus nigrolineatus*).[62] Wellehan et al. also described a case of hepatic necrosis in a San Esteban chuckwalla (*Sauromalus varius*) in which a herpesvirus was identified.[57] This chuckwalla died without apparent signs of illness.[57] Herpesvirus infection has also been reported in red-headed agamas (*Agama agama*) with evidence of disease in the liver, lung, and spleen.[63]

West Nile virus

West Nile virus (WNV) has recently been identified as a disease in crocodilians.[64-67] These cases have enlightened veterinarians about the possibility of other reptile species becoming infected with WNV and serving as amplification hosts. Experimental and natural infections of WNV have been proposed for Mediterranean house geckos (*Hemidactylus turcicus*).[68] Low viral loads of WNV were detected in green iguanas after experimental infection.[69] Further studies will determine if lizard species can play a role in the cycle of WNV in North America.

Miscellaneous viruses

Besides those already mentioned, other viruses have been described in lizards. A concurrent chlamydial and poxvirus infection was reported in a flap-necked chameleon (*Chamaeleo dilepis*),[70] and three rhabdoviruses were isolated from lizards by Monath et al.[71] Experimental infection with Japanese encephalitis virus (JEV) was demonstrated in the Japanese grass lizard (*Takydromus tachydromoides*), Japanese five-lined skink (*Eumeces latiscutatus*), Barbour's five-lined skink (*Eumeces barbouri*), and Ryukyu five-lined skink (*Eumeces marginatus*).[72] They were also able to show transmission of JEV from infected mosquitoes to uninfected lizards (*Takydromus tachydromoides* and *Eumeces latiscutatus*).[73] In the same study they were also able to infect mice via infected mosquitoes that had fed on the infected lizards.[73] Overwintering of JEV was demonstrated in captive (experimental) and wild lizards.[73]

FUNGI

Fungal infections have been reported as affecting various tissues in a variety of reptile species. Fungal infections are a diagnostic challenge because the identification of a fungus on cytology and culture does not necessarily implicate that it is responsible for the disease. Classification of the fungi may also be difficult and require analysis by an outside laboratory. This is due to the large number of saprophytic organisms that live in the soil, decaying matter, and in the environment. Saprophytic fungi are often opportunistic disease organisms and not necessarily primary infectious agents. Most fungal infections are opportunistic and occur secondary to an underlying disease process. It is important to analyze carefully the presentation, clinical signs, and diagnostics to determine if a fungal infection is truly present. A biopsy of the affected tissue showing fungal elements and changes consistent with a fungal infection can provide convincing evidence of disease. Treatment of fungal infections can be expensive and side effects of systemic therapy can be encountered. In addition, the treatment should be performed for a minimum of 4 to 8 weeks to ensure resolution of the disease. Many infections occur on the skin and allow for use of topical antifungal medications. Dilute iodine and chlorhexidine can also be used as an aid in the treatment of superficial skin mycoses. Systemic drugs are required for the treatment of systemic mycoses and deep skin mycoses. Itraconazole, ketoconazole, and amphotericin B are some of the therapeutic choices for systemic therapy. Newer generation drugs are becoming available and may have a place in reptile medicine in the future. Resistance to antifungal drugs does occur, and there is the option of performing a sensitivity test for fungal cultures, but this can be expensive and unreliable. Morphology of the organism in cytologic examination and growth media are used for identification. Rate of growth, type of culture media and temperature of incubation may also be used to help identify a fungus. Successful antifungal therapy may depend on appropriate identification of the organism. If a fungal infection is diagnosed in a lizard, be sure to explore the literature and learn from the experience of others. Fungal infections can be devastating to the infected lizard and frustrating for the clinician to treat.

Aspergillus spp.

Aspergillosis was diagnosed in a black-pointed teguexin (*Tupinambis nigropunctatus*) with generalized mycosis,[74] and *Aspergillus terreus* was diagnosed in two San Esteban chuckwallas.[75] These animals had a necrotizing dermatitis, and fungal hyphae were identified on biopsy. Both animals died, despite treatment, and necropsy revealed systemic involvement, with one of the animals having evidence of fungal disease in the heart, lungs, spleen, and brain.[75]

Candida spp.

Jacobson et al. cited reports of *Candida albicans* from the necrotic liver of a two-banded chameleon (*Chamaeleo bitaeniatus*) and the necrotic esophagus of a crocodile tegu (*Crocodilurus lacertinus*).[74] Schumacher cited reports of *Candida guilliermondii* in Fischer's (*Chamaeleo fischeri*) and Jackson's chameleons.[76]

Cryptococcus spp.

Hough reported a case of *Cryptococcus neoformans* in an eastern water skink (*Eulamprus quoyii*). This organism was isolated from a subcutaneous lesion near the spine.[77]

Chrysosporium spp.

The *Chrysosporium* anamorph of *Nannizziopsis vriesii* (CANV) has been reported in various cases of skin mycoses in lizards. Affected species include Parson's chameleon (*Chamaeleo parsonii*),[78] Jackson's chameleon,[78] jewel chameleon, (*Chamaeleo lateralis*),[78] veiled chameleon, and a day gecko (*Phelsuma sp.*).[79] Experimental infection was also accomplished in veiled chameleons via cutaneous contact.[80] An attempt to culture CANV from the skin of healthy squamates was only successful in an African rock python (*Python sebae*).[79] A report of fungal dermatitis in bearded dragons provided a diagnosis of *Trichophyton terrestre* for the condition known as "yellow fungus disease."[81] However, it may be possible that the lesions were actually caused by the CANV, which is easily misidentified as a *Trycophyton* sp.[81] Another species of *Chrysosporium*, *C. keratinophilum*, is cited by Jacobson et al. as being found in lung and stomach lesions of two green iguanas.[74]

Miscellaneous mycoses

A case of unspecified phycomycosis was reported in a Jackson's chameleon that presented with a rectal prolapse.[82] Despite attempts to correct the problem, the animal's condition deteriorated and it was euthanized.[82] Histopathology revealed mycotic enteritis with organisms identified morphologically as belonging to the class Phycomycetes.[82] Reavil et al. reported histopathologic findings of mycotic infections in various lizard cases; however, none of the organisms were identified.[83] Nonetheless, it is worth noting the sites of infection: skin, liver, lung, digestive tract, bone, and one case of ocular mycoses.[83] Some of the lizard species implicated included the bearded dragon, panther chameleon *(Furcifer pardalis),* New Caledonia giant gecko *(Rhacodactylus leachianus),* Standing's gecko *(Phelsuma standingi),* fat-tailed gecko, leaf gecko *(Phyllodactylus sp.),* and green iguana.[83]

BACTERIA

Bacterial infections are probably the most common infectious disease observed in reptiles. Rather than review the abundant literature on this topic, I should emphasize the basic approach to bacterial infections in reptiles. Bacterial infections can occur in a variety of lizard tissues. Some are primary pathogens, whereas others may occur secondarily to trauma, as an underlying disease, or when an animal is in an immunocompromised state. Gram-negative bacteria are most often associated with infections in lizards, although Gram-positive bacteria can also cause serious disease. Carnivorous reptiles have a predominance of Gram-negative bacteria as part of their normal oral and gastrointestinal flora. Knowledge of a lizard's normal flora should be considered when interpreting diagnostic tests. Improper husbandry may contribute to bacterial dermatitis, which is seen in lizards with some frequency, presenting as areas of discoloration with a dark brown to black color change. Fungal dermatitis may present in a similar fashion or occur concurrently with bacterial dermatitis. The first step in diagnosing a bacterial infection is determining if there are gross lesions that may harbor the bacteria or whether a particular tissue or organ may be affected. This will determine what samples to obtain and how to collect them. Cytology can help clinicians identify if bacteria are present in the tissue in question. A Gram stain will identify bacteria as Gram positive or Gram negative. A wet mount may help identify the bacteria as motile or nonmotile. A bacterial culture is the second and most important diagnostic tool for the identification of bacterial pathogens. Often aerobic cultures are performed, but some cases may require anaerobic culture depending on clinical signs and tissues affected. Anaerobic cultures should be pursued for aggressive infections or those that do not respond to standard therapy. After a positive culture and identification of a suspected pathogen, an antibiotic sensitivity panel is needed to help select the most appropriate drug or ensure that current therapies are effective in treating the illness. Cultures have some disadvantages. The main disadvantage of diagnostic cultures is that a negative result does not rule out the absence of bacteria or disease. A negative culture may simply be the effect of the culture medium and/or growth conditions on the bacterial population. Second, the bacterium isolated on culture may not be the primary pathogen; therefore, culture results must be interpreted in conjunction with clinical presentation. New developments in biomedical sciences may also provide molecular tests, such as those using PCR technology for identification of certain bacteria.

Obtaining a culture sample is best performed using a sterile swab or after biopsy. If a biopsy sample is obtained, it should also be submitted for histopathologic examination. Histopathologic examination may provide additional information to help characterize the lesion(s). Additional sampling techniques may require a special medium, such as that used for blood or anaerobic cultures. The specialized media can usually be obtained from the laboratory performing the tests. Veterinarians must resist the temptation to indiscriminately use antimicrobials without attempting to determine the cause of the disease. In some cases, this may be difficult because of monetary constraints or limited resources. Nonetheless, bacterial diagnostic techniques, when indicated, should be provided as part of the diagnostic workup to the reptile owner.

Parasites

Lizards are also susceptible to parasitic infections. Parasitism is more common in wild-caught animals and those maintained outdoors, but it also may occur in groups of lizards maintained indoors. Ticks and mites can attach to a lizard's skin, and in an unsanitary environment, infestations can be severe. Although they can attach anywhere in the body, ectoparasites are usually found on the inguinal or axillary region, near the vent, on the ventral aspect of the mandible, and around the head. To break the life cycle of parasites, both the animal and its living environment must be treated. Ivermectin (0.2 mg/kg PO, SC q2wk × 3) has been used safely in reptiles, except for chelonians in which it is toxic. I have observed toxicity in a group of snakes after they were administered Ivomec® Plus (Merial Ltd, 3239 Satellite Blvd., Duluth, GA), an ivermectin and clorsulon combination. This formulation should not be used in reptiles. Fipronil (Frontline®) (Merial Ltd, 3239 Satellite Blvd., Duluth, GA) and imidacloprid (Advantage®) (Bayer Health Care LLC, Animal Health Division, Shawnee Mission, KS) have been used safely in reptiles, but toxicities may be observed if used in large amounts. It is generally recommended to apply a small amount of the medication to gauze and then rub the skin of the reptile with the gauze. Avoid getting these compounds close to the eyes and mucous membranes. An alternative to pharmaceuticals is to rub mineral oil over the body of the reptile, theoretically drowning the external parasites. Treatments can be repeated on a weekly basis as needed. The enclosure must be cleaned and disinfected daily to aid in breaking the life cycle of the parasites. The substrate can be changed to newspaper for ease of cleaning.

Internal parasitism is diagnosed via fecal floats and wet mounts as with other species. A cloacal flush can be performed if no feces are available. Tracheal washes are also used to diagnose lung parasites. Trematodes and cestodes can be treated with praziquantel at 5 to 10 mg/kg PO every 14 days.[84] Nematodes can be treated with ivermectin (0.2 mg/kg PO, SC q2wk × 3) or fenbendazole (50-100 mg/kg PO q2wk × 2-3).[84] If a high parasite load is present, it may be advisable to start treatment with fenbendazole first to avoid the rapid kill caused by ivermectin. This rapid kill could lead to toxicity associated with microthrombi or obstructions of the intestinal tract.

Oxyurids are commonly observed in low numbers in bearded dragons and other species without clinical signs of parasitism. These are thought to be commensal or even mutualistic in some species. Treatment should be considered in cases in which clinical disease (e.g., diarrhea) is associated with the presence of the parasites.

Protozoan parasites can be normal inhabitants of the gastrointestinal tract of lizards, but some can cause severe disease (e.g., *Entamoeba invadens*). Metronidazole (100 mg/kg PO once, repeat in 2 wk) or dimetridazole (100 mg/kg PO once, repeat in 2 wk) may be used for the treatment of most flagellated and ciliated protozoa.[85] *Cryptosporidium* spp., however, a coccidian protozoa, will not respond to therapy, and the infections are fatal. *Cryptosporidium serpentis* and *C. saurophilum* have been described in snakes and lizards, respectively.[86] Diagnosis of *Cryptosporidium* spp. may be attempted from feces, cloacal wash, stomach wash, and regurgitated material by use of a modified acid fast stain. Molecular techniques are becoming available but have the limitation of being unable to differentiate between *Cryptosporidium* species. Euthanasia should be considered for animals with clinical signs consistent with cryptosporidiosis and positive identification of the organism. Presence of the organism, however, may not always indicate disease, but the animal may be capable of shedding. Other coccidian parasites also occur in lizards and may respond to treatment with sulfa drugs or potentiated sulfa drugs.

Hemoparasites may be observed in reptiles and appear to be nonpathogenic; thus, no treatment is required. Rarely some patients will have clinical signs of anemia in conjunction with a high hemoparasite load. Those patients suffering from hemoparasite-caused anemia may be treated with iron-dextran and quinidine.[50] Success with this therapy is largely unknown because of the infrequent need to treat hemoparasites in lizard patients.

Nutritional

Nutritional secondary hyperparathyroidism (NSH) is a common disease process of reptiles. Although the terms *NSH* and *metabolic bone disease (MBD)* are often used interchangeably, MBD encompasses NSH, renal secondary hyperparathyroidism (RSH), primary hyperparathyroidism, and other metabolic diseases affecting bone health. Clinical signs may be the same for all diseases leading to MBD, but the history of each case will vary. NSH is primarily associated with a deficiency in dietary calcium, excessive dietary phosphorus, a vitamin D_3 deficiency, or a combination of these factors. A lack of calcium in the body eventually leads to hyperparathyroidism in an effort to maintain adequate calcium levels. Increased parathyroid hormone leads to increased osteoclastic and consequently osteoblastic activity. This increased activity over time is the cause of the clinical signs observed in NSH. Calcium deficiencies occur as a result of inappropriate levels in the diet, often associated with with an inverse Ca : P ratio. This is commonly observed in herbivorous lizards, but carnivores and omnivores also may be affected. A lack of UVB light exposure either directly from the sun or via artificial bulbs leads to decreased synthesis of vitamin D_3, which is essential for calcium absorption and metabolism. An animal that is fed an appropriate diet but has no source of UVB light can develop the same clinical signs as one with an improper diet. In some animals NSH develops as a consequence of both inadequate diet and UVB exposure. Clinical signs of NSH include weakness, lethargy, decreased growth or stunting, abnormal posture, decreased appetite, weight loss, muscle fasciculations, paresis, pathologic fractures, and fibrous osteodystrophy of the long bones and mandible ("rubber jaw"). The severity of clinical signs varies with the age of the animal and the chronicity of the disease. Some young animals show signs of NSH early in life, but in most cases it is a chronic disease. Some animals with NSH may appear to be juveniles but in reality are several years old and have stunted growth caused by an inadequate calcium and general malnutrition. It appears that NSH is not as commonly observed in carnivorous reptiles. One explanation is that carnivorous reptiles can obtain enough vitamin D_3 from the diet without a true requirement for UVB. However, if an appropriate calcium source is not offered, these animals will likely develop NSH. Carnivorous lizard species may still benefit from UVB exposure; therefore, a UVB source in their environment is recommended.[9]

Diagnosis of NSH can be achieved using various methods. A history of an inadequate diet and/or lack of exposure to UVB, together with clinical signs, are strong indicators that the patient is suffering from NSH. However, diagnostic tests are essential to characterize the severity of the disease. Radiographs may be obtained to evaluate the patient for the presence of pathologic fractures and to characterize the overall bone density. If present, fractures may be recent and require external coaptation for stability. A decrease in bone density may be observed as a diffuse decrease in the opacity of the bony cortices. In some areas there may be little contrast between bone and soft tissue. Chemistry panels are the best diagnostic test to help a veterinarian determine the severity of disease. In the early stages of NSH the calcium levels may be normal or even slightly elevated as the body is actively reabsorbing bone to keep up with the calcium demand. Phosphorus levels may also be normal during the early phase of NSH. As the disease progresses without therapy, the continued resorption of the bones will lead to a depletion of calcium and an appreciable decrease in the calcium levels in the blood. At the same time, phosphorus levels will remain normal or slightly elevated, leading to an inverse calcium-to-phosphorus ratio. It is important to evaluate other parameters in the chemistry panel such as AST, CK, uric acid, proteins, and electrolytes. It may be difficult to differentiate NSH from RSH, as they may occur concurrently and both may have an inverse Ca : P ratio. RSH should be considered in reptiles that are maintained on an appropriate diet and UVB source but show signs consistent with MBD.

The first step in the treatment of NSH is correction of the dietary and/or UVB deficiencies. Therapy includes administration of calcium supplements in either oral or injectable form. Calcium glubionate can be given orally at 10 mg/kg every 12 hours.[84] Alternatively, 10% calcium gluconate can be administered IM at 10 to 50 mg/kg.[84] Other treatment alternatives include Tums® (Glaxo Smith Kline, Moon Twp, PA) tablets or other calcium carbonate sources. These calcium carbonate products can be sprinkled over the food or made into a suspension with water. No specific doses are available, but I recommend $\frac{1}{4}$ to $\frac{1}{2}$ of a tablet once a day as needed. Many lizards will find the fruit flavors more palatable and readily eat the food with the crushed tablets. Oral supplementation is preferred when possible. Parenteral vitamin D treatment is also recommended until the environmental deficiencies are corrected (e.g., addition of UVB light). The rest of the NSH therapy consists of cage rest and supportive therapy, including fluids and force-feeding as needed. Phosphate binders are another recommended adjunct therapy and work at the level of the gut, reducing phosphorus absorption; however, they do not directly reduce phosphorus levels in the blood. If the animal is fed a proper diet with an adequate Ca : P ratio, the use of phosphate binders is not necessary.

Another nutritional disease that may be observed in reptiles is hypovitaminosis A. This disease is common in tortoises but does not appear as common in lizard species. Chameleons appear to be most commonly affected. Most chameleon species are insectivores, and if the insects are not gut loaded properly, they will not provide adequate nutrition. Clinical signs of hypovitaminosis A may include anorexia, stunted growth, periocular edema, squamous metaplasia, dermatologic disease, and overall unthriftiness.[87] Determining blood levels of vitamin A may help diagnose the disease, but normal values are not recognized for all species and the assay may not be readily available to most clinicians. A combination of history and clinical signs may provide enough evidence for suspicion of vitamin A deficiency. Treatment of hypovitaminosis A should be performed judiciously to avoid hypervitaminosis A, which can have serious physiologic effects. Some products include vitamin D and E as part of an injectable formulation and are available in high concentrations, making it difficult to provide appropriate doses for smaller animals. An alternative formulation is Aquasol A® (Astra USA, Inc., Westborough, MA), which is a water-miscible formulation that can be administered PO, SC, or IM at 1000 to 2000 international units/kg. Most reptiles will require this dose for treatment of hypovitaminosis A administered once every 7 to 14 days for a total of two or three treatments. Some chameleon species may require regular vitamin A supplementation[87]; however, certain chameleons, such as the Jackson's, mountain, Johnston's, and panther chameleons, may be more susceptible to oversupplementation, and the dose should be decreased by half.[87] The true requirements of vitamin A for lizard species are largely unknown, and the information available is based primarily on clinical experience.

Other nutritional deficiencies probably occur but go unrecognized or present concurrently with NSH and hypovitaminosis A. The key to prevention of nutritional disease is a well-balanced diet with appropriate husbandry for the lizard species being maintained in captivity.

Renal Disease

Chronic renal disease (CRD) appears to be a common presentation in adult green iguanas, whereas acute renal disease occurs with less frequency. Green iguanas form a large percentage of the lizards maintained as pets, and perhaps CRD is overrepresented in this species, but it can also occur in other lizard species. The term *CRD* encompasses a number of diseases that can affect the kidney. Some of these include interstitial nephritis, gloemrulonephritis, pyelonephritis, tubulonephrosis, amyloidosis, gout, bacterial nephritis, neoplasia, and an assortment of sclerotic diseases.[7] Predisposition to renal disease may come from the metanephric nature of reptile kidneys, which have an inherent inability to concentrate urine because of the absence of the loop of Henle and a small number of nephrons. The specific etiology or pathophysiology of renal disease in lizards is not completely understood, but there are some proposed predisposing factors, including poor nutrition, dehydration, neoplasia, infectious diseases, nephrotoxic drugs, gout, and metastatic mineralization.[50] Gout could either contribute to, or be caused by, renal disease. Metastatic mineralization, as explained by Maxwell, is commonly seen in conjunction with CRD.[50] The etiology of metastatic mineralization is relatively unknown, but it is believed to be associated with calcium and vitamin D_3 imbalances. The signs of metastatic mineralization usually accompany those of CRD and include soft tissue mineralization and renomegaly.[50]

History, clinical signs, a chemistry panel, radiographs, and biopsy can aid in the diagnosis of CRF. Clinical signs are nonspecific but include anorexia, lethargy, dehydration, and in some cases, obstipation if renomegaly is present. Polydipsia and polyuria may be observed in some cases. These animals may also have a less than adequate husbandry without enough access to water. One of the most rewarding diagnostic parameters is the presence of an inverse Ca : P ratio. Although a slight inverse Ca : P ratio may be found with advanced stages of NSH, a severely inversed ratio is frequently seen with CRD. Significant elevation in uric acid may be noted with CRD but is often associated only with dehydration. Other parameters, such as CK and AST, may also be elevated but are nonspecific for the diagnosis of CRD. Radiographs may be of value in the effort to differentiate CRD from NSH or determine if the two diseases are present together. Soft tissue (metastatic) mineralization may be observed with CRD. Evidence of renomegaly is helpful in differentiating CRD from NSH, with the enlarged kidneys being palpated cranial to the pelvic inlet and/or seen on radiographs. Renal biopsy is the only definitive way to diagnose renal disease, and there are various biopsy techniques that can be used in lizard species. Biopsy samples may be obtained by laparoscopy, coeliotomy, ultrasound-guided technique, or cut-down technique.[7] The cut-down technique is one of the most common methods and works well in green iguanas. The cut-down procedure can be performed under general or local anesthesia with analgesia. The approach is between the caudal aspect of the femur at its most proximal aspect and the lateral aspect of the tail. A horizontal incision is made on the lateral aspect of the tail on midline below the lateral processes of the coccygeal vertebrae.[7] The kidney is visualized after minimal dissection through the musculature. Renal biopsies are sometimes not procured because some owners are unwilling to provide consent for the procedure or the veterinarian is unable to perform this procedure. In some instances the lizard may be too critical to withstand the stress of anesthesia. Even without a renal biopsy, veterinarians can often gather enough evidence to implicate renal disease as the primary cause of disease.

Treatment of renal disease consists primarily of fluid therapy, being mindful to avoid overhydration. Placement of an IV or IO catheter, if possible, is strongly recommended. Daily PCV percentages and regular biochemistries will help monitor hydration and levels of calcium and phosphorus. Calcium supplementation can also be implemented to help counteract the deficiency of this important nutritional element. Phosphate binders are recommended to decrease the absorption of phosphorus at the level of the intestine. Nutritional support is also essential to maintain the health of the animal. Products selected should be appropriate for the species being treated and have low protein levels, even in carnivorous lizards.

Gout

Gout can occur as visceral, articular, or periarticular forms. Uric acid can be present in the blood as free uric acid or as urate salts.[88] Elevations in any of these forms of uric acid in the blood lead to hyperuricemia. Sustained hyperuricemia of greater than 25 mg/dl exceeds the solubility of uric acid.[50] Temporary elevations beyond the solubility of uric acid may be observed with dehydration and will not lead to gout. Therefore, uric acid levels are not always a consistent indicator of gout. The presence of hyperuricemia and a decreased ability to clear uric acid through their kidneys lead to precipitation of insoluble uric acid crystals in the tissues. The presence of these crystals in the body/organ tissues is considered gout. Controversy still exists about the predisposing factors of gout, but dehydration, chronic disease, renal disease, and excessive protein intake may all contribute to gout. Diagnosis of gout is determined based on history and physical examination with blood work and radiographs providing additional supportive evidence. Diseased animals may be lethargic, weak, dehydrated, and in poor body condition. Articular and periarticular gout are very painful to the lizard patient. Subcutaneous nodules may be observed near the joints, and radiographically it may be possible to visualize bone lysis in the affected joint as well as evidence of crystals in the tissues. In some cases white nodules may also be observed in the mucosa of the oral cavity. Definitive diagnosis of gout requires microscopic examination of crystals or tophi from the joint or soft tissues. Treatment of gout is based on what is known from human medicine, but its effectiveness in the reptile patient is largely unknown. Fluid therapy and correction of nutritional imbalances are significant components of the therapeutic approach. Allopurinol and probenecid are used in human medicine to help reduce the synthesis and increase the excretion of uric acid, but their value in reptiles is unknown. Probenecid is contraindicated in dehydrated patients and with concomitant use of some antimicrobials. Antiinflammatory drugs may be warranted for those patients with severe pain. Surgical removal of the tophi from the joints should be pursued if possible.

However, once the crystal deposits are dispersed throughout the body, the prognosis is grave. Proper hydration, nutrition, and husbandry are essential for the prevention of gout, with preventive measures preferred over treatment.

Urinary Calculi

Cystic calculi can occur in lizard species, whereas renal calculi are rarely encountered. Cystic calculi occur with some frequency in iguanas and other species with a urinary bladder. Food with high amounts of calcium oxalates may be a predisposing factor for calculi formation. High protein diets, especially when fed to herbivorous lizards, have also been proposed as a potential cause of cystic calculi. Cystic calculi may also be secondary to renal disease and gout. Dehydration and inadequate humidity levels likely play a role in disease development. Animals may present with nonspecific signs of lethargy, weakness, and anorexia. Others will have no clinical signs, and diagnosis is incidental. In some patients the owners may report an increased amount of urates visible on urination. At times the urates may appear coarse, dry, and gritty. Radiographs may help diagnose calculi if the material is radioopaque. Otherwise, endoscopy or exploratory surgery may be required to obtain a definitive diagnosis. Treatment consists of surgical removal of the cystic calculi and all of the sludge present in the bladder. In addition, the animal must be hydrated and nutritional deficiencies corrected. If the husbandry is improved and there are no underlying diseases, most patients will have a good prognosis with little chance of reoccurrence.

Neoplastic Disease

Neoplastic disease is being diagnosed with increased frequency in lizards. It is unclear whether there is an increased incidence of neoplasms or veterinarians are becoming more skilled at diagnosing them. An increase in the number of owners who seek veterinary care for their lizards may also contribute to the perceived increase in neoplasia cases. Neoplastic disease should be a differential diagnosis whenever a mass is detected either radiographically or during physical examination. Neoplasia should also be considered in cases that present with nonspecific clinical signs. Physical exam, radiographs, and blood parameters may help diagnose neoplasia and any secondary disease process. Cytologic examination may be helpful in diagnosing a tumor type but may be misleading on occasion. Bone marrow aspirates may be beneficial for staging some tumors or for the diagnosis of leukemia. A surgical biopsy with histopathologic examination remains the best way to definitively diagnose a neoplastic condition. The tissues must be submitted to a pathologist who is familiar with exotic animal species or is willing to consult out of the laboratory. Once a diagnosis is made, a treatment scheme can be decided. Unfortunately, the treatment for neoplasia in reptiles is lagging behind the advances made in small animal medicine. The expense associated with certain treatments, such as radiation or chemotherapy, may be prohibitive for some reptile owners. In addition, little is known about the effectiveness of cancer therapy in reptiles. Even if an owner decides to treat his or her pet lizard, little information is available about treatment planning and expected outcome of therapy. For these reasons, surgical removal, whenever possible, remains the treatment of choice in most cases. A major limitation is the small physical size of most lizards, which reduces the ability of veterinarians to remove large margins of tissue around the tumor, often leading to recurrence of disease. In some cases, surgical removal may actually result in resolution of disease. The type of tumor, location, size, and duration are factors that may influence the outcome of cancer therapy.

Veterinarians must inform the owners about the limitations associated with cancer treatment of lizard species but also point out the benefits of learning from each case. Independent of treatment response, the knowledge gained through each case provides experience when developing therapeutic protocols and assessing prognosis for future patients.

Some of the neoplasias reported in lizard species include, but are not limited to, visceral hemangiosarcoma in a green iguana,[89] peripheral benign nerve sheath tumor in a Savannah monitor[90] and bearded dragons,[91] malignant nerve sheath tumor in bearded dragons,[92] malignant chromatophores in veiled chameleons,[93] lymphoid neoplasia in Egyptian spiny-tailed lizards (Uromastyx aegyptius),[94] disseminated lymphoma in two Savannah monitors and a green iguana,[95] monocytic leukemia in a bearded dragon,[96] ovarian papillary cystadenocarcinoma with metastasis in a green iguana,[97] thyroid adenoma with hyperthyroidism in a green iguana,[98] and renal adenocarcinoma in desert iguanas (Dipsosaurus dorsalis).[99]

There is also a report of radiation treatment for lymphoblastic leukemia in a sungazer lizard (Cordylus giganteus).[100] The lizard was originally treated with prednisone (0.2 mg q72hr for 6 months), but the treatment was discontinued due to a lack of treatment response. Whole body radiation therapy was then initiated, and the lizard responded favorably but died 11 months later as a consequence of a recurrent femoral pore abscess. At necropsy there was evidence of squamous metaplasia and fibrosis of some tissues, which were attributed to postradiation side effects.[100]

■ THERAPEUTICS
Fluid Therapy

Replacement fluid therapy for reptiles should be based on the animal's hydration status and condition and available products. A physical exam and thorough history are essential before developing a fluid replacement plan. The physical exam will help determine clinical evidence of dehydration as evidenced by sunken eyes, decreased capillary or venous refill, and pale, possibly dry, and tacky mucous membranes. A number of lizard species may have a relatively dry oral cavity, whereas others have a considerable amount of mucus. This may complicate the assessment of the animal's hydration status. The color of the mucous membranes may be lighter than that in mammals or difficult to assess due to the presence of pigment. The palatine vessel is located on the roof of the mouth and may be used to

assess venous refill similar to a capillary refill test. The skin may lose its elasticity and become wrinkled and dry with overt fluid loss, but this observation is also subjective and may not be noted until the animal's condition is more severe. An increase in the PCV and total protein/solids is also helpful when determining the hydration status of a lizard patient. In addition, evidence of hypernatremia and hyperchloremia may be observed in acutely dehydrated patients. Uric acid is an important biochemical parameter that is frequently elevated when the animal has had a fluid deficit for a prolonged period of time. Dehydration may be initiated and sustained by a number of conditions (e.g., blood loss, diarrhea, trauma, hypovolemic shock), but chronic disease and anorexia are often the primary causes in captive lizards. Dehydration is usually determined subjectively by establishing a percentage rating. This method is not very accurate and only utilizes the information obtained from the physical exam and/or CBC/chemistry panel.

When developing a fluid replacement plan for a patient, it is important to account for ongoing fluid losses. In addition to correcting fluid deficits, it is also important to provide the patient maintenance fluids during its convalescence to replace the fluids it doesn't take in while it is anorexic or not drinking. Maintenance fluid requirements are an objective measurement to be given daily in the same amount regardless of hydration status. Recommendations for maintenance fluid rates in reptiles vary from 10 to 30 ml/kg every 24 hours. A fluid volume accounting for the percentage of dehydration and ongoing fluid losses should be added to the maintenance requirements to determine the total fluid volume a patient will require. Some authors suggest that the total volume of fluids given to lizards in a 24-hour period should not exceed 1% to 2% of the animal's total body weight in grams (10-20 ml/1000 g body weight),[101,102] which is close to the recommended maintenance requirements. With many cases it is not possible to administer the total amount of fluids calculated when taking into account maintenance, percent dehydration, and losses. The decision of volume and frequency of fluid administration will depend on the severity of dehydration and size of the animal. Patients that are severely dehydrated require larger volumes of fluid, and replacement therapy should be more aggressive. However, this aggressive therapy is also dependent on the lizard's ability to properly absorb and distribute the fluid volume. Larger lizards generally handle a higher percentage of fluids on a body weight basis. When administering fluids, veterinarians must consider the distribution of fluids in the body. Unfortunately, the knowledge about the extracellular fluid (ECF) distribution and the intracellular fluid (ICF) distribution in reptiles is lacking compared to what is known about mammals. As the name implies, the ICF is present within the cells and comprises the main fluid compartment in reptiles. The ECF is subdivided into interstitial, plasma, lymph, and transcellular fluid. Transcellular fluid encompasses cerebrospinal, synovial, pericardial, intraocular, and peritoneal fluid.[103] In humans the total fluid volume varies with age, sex, and fat content. Younger, leaner individuals have a higher percentage of total body water as compared to older or more obese individuals. On average, humans have a total body water content of 60% in relation to their body weight.[103] Of this amount, 40% is in the ICF and 20% in the ECF. Despite the difference in percentages, both the ICF and ECF remain in constant homeostasis. Blood contains both ICF and ECF components and is thought by some to be a separate fluid compartment of its own within the circulatory system.[103] Homeostasis is achieved by maintaining a close osmolarity between the ICF, interstitial fluid, and plasma. Uncorrected values of osmolarity for these fluids in humans are 301.2 mOsm/L, 300.8 mOsm/L, and 301.8 mOsm/L, respectively.[103] Plasma has a slightly higher osmolarity because of the proteins within it. Maxwell and Helmick provide one of the most comprehensive discussions about the distribution of fluids in reptiles, but no recent studies have added to this body of knowledge.[102] Their investigations show that iguanas have a total body water content of approximately 71% of their body weight, with 54% distributed in the ICF and 17% in the ECF.[102] Therefore, the water composition of iguanas is similar to that of mammals with the exception of a higher total body water content and ICF.[102] Maxwell and Helmick also provide a value of approximately 330 mOsm/L for the plasma of green iguanas, 300 mOsm/l for the plasma of desert iguanas, and a range of 300 mOsm/L to 400 mOsm/L for other reptiles.[102] A plasma osmolarity of approximately 250 mOsm/L has been reported in chelonians.[104] A wider range in osmolarity may be due to differences among desert and tropical species, age, sex, and body fat content. Much controversy still exists regarding the plasma osmolarity in reptiles, and further research in this area is needed.

All of the previously mentioned information can be applied clinically for the selection of fluid products and route of administration in lizards. Until further research findings are published, veterinarians must consider the wide range of osmolarities found in reptiles and plan their fluid therapy regimens accordingly. Box 8-5 shows the osmolarity of commonly used fluids used in veterinary medicine. The best fluid for a particular case should be determined based on the animal's osmolarity. In most cases with acute fluid loss, an isotonic fluid should be used.

BOX 8-5   **Various Fluid Types Available for Use in Reptiles and Their Respective Osmolarities**

Fluid Type	Osmolarity (mOsm/L)
2.5% Dextrose	126
5% Dextrose	253
Lactated Ringer's	272
2.5% Dextrose in 0.45% saline	280
Normosol-R	294
0.9% Sodium chloride	308
Ringer's	309
5% Dextrose in lactated Ringer's	525

Various routes for fluid administration are available for lizards, including oral (PO), intravenous (IV), subcutaneous (SC), intracoelomic (ICe), and intraosseous (IO) routes. Hypotonic fluids are preferred for SC administration to facilitate absorption. The goal is to administer fluid therapy via a route that will achieve rapid replacement of the fluid deficit without compromising homeostasis. Ultimately, treatment is based on replacement of the intravascular space with eventual redistribution into the ICF and ECF. Therefore, direct IV administration via a catheter is the most efficient fluid administration route, but it is also invasive and may be difficult in some species. The IO route also provides efficient fluid absorption, but it is invasive and requires placement of a needle or IO catheter into a bone. Intraosseous catheters require increased maintenance to remain patent. The oral route is minimally invasive but requires an active gastrointestinal tract for proper absorption, and even under the best circumstances is not as effective as the IV route. With some patients it may be beneficial to provide PO fluids concurrently with IV administration to stimulate gut movement and maintain hydration of the gastrointestinal tissue. SC fluid administration can be performed in some lizards but the fluid absorption is limited at this site, dependent on the health of the underlying capillary bed. Peripheral vasoconstriction will also slow down the rate of absorption of SC fluids. If too much fluid is injected at one SC site, absorption may also decrease because of capillary collapse. The ICe route remains one of the most popular routes for replenishing fluids in reptiles. Absorption is not as efficient as the IV or IO routes but is better than SC and PO. At the time of fluid administration, avoid using fluid products that have a higher osmolarity than normally found in the fluid compartment of the animal. Administering a fluid product via the ICe or SC route to a green iguana with a higher osmolarity than the plasma osmolarity of the patient (300 mOsm/L) will stimulate additional shifts of fluid from the intravascular space/plasma and the interstitial space into the coelomic cavity or SC space. The best approach is to give slightly hypotonic fluids that will then be drawn to areas with higher osmolarity, such as vascular and interstitial spaces. When giving fluids IV or IO, the best choice is an isotonic fluid that will help maintain homeostasis. If volume expansion is desired, a slightly hypertonic solution can be administered IV until the animal's hydration status improves; an isotonic solution should be selected for maintenance. Once fluid therapy is initiated, the animal must be monitored on a daily basis and hydration reassessed to adjust the treatment plan.

Antimicrobials

Antimicrobial therapy is commonly used to treat animals diagnosed with infectious diseases. In reptile medicine there are additional challenges associated with the lack of pharmacokinetic studies for most drugs, extra label use, small patient size, cost, ease of administration, frequency of administration, and safety. Use and selection of antimicrobial agents must be done judiciously, taking into account a number of clinical considerations. First, select drugs that have been used safely in the lizard species being treated and that will cause no harm to the animal. Second, choose an appropriate drug based on the spectrum of coverage, tissue distribution, and results of culture and sensitivity testing. The best antimicrobial agents will be effective against a number of organisms and are classified as broad-spectrum antibiotics. Broad-spectrum antibiotics may show effectiveness against Gram-positive and Gram-negative organisms as well as aerobes and anaerobes. Not all drugs are considered broad spectrum, and a combination of drugs may be needed to cover all four treatment areas. In addition to the four areas just listed, also consider if the drug is cidal or static. Cidal drugs will kill the organism, whereas static drugs will inhibit or slow its growth. The method of action of the antimicrobial product must also be considered especially when choosing penicillin. Table 8-1 shows some of the major drug groups available, with examples of specific drugs, coverage spectrum, and method of action.

Other limitations associated with the use of antimicrobial agents in lizards are related to the ease and frequency of administration. In fractious animals, it may be more challenging to give a drug by mouth, especially when multiple treatments are required over a 24-hour period. Therefore, try to select a product that has a low frequency of administration and one that the patient will tolerate. A final point about antimicrobial therapy and prevention of antimicrobial resistance involves the dosing and length of treatment. Always select and calculate appropriate dosages for the patient. This may require finding multiple references for comparison of recommended doses. Once a dosage is calculated, it must be administered for the correct period of time and not discontinued before the end of the treatment period. Some people follow the practice of giving one injection of an antimicrobial agent and discharging the patient with no additional treatments. Not only will this promote antimicrobial resistance, but it will not effectively treat the patient's condition. Antimicrobial treatment should only be discontinued 7 to 10 days after resolution of clinical signs.

It is the responsibility of the veterinarian to choose the appropriate drugs to avoid the perpetuation of antimicrobial resistance. Unfortunately, many veterinary practitioners have formulated the habit of using a single antibiotic (e.g., enrofloxacin) as a sole source of therapy for all infectious diseases, even in cases in which a bacterial infection is questionable. Although fluoroquinolones are very good broad-spectrum antimicrobials with good tissue distribution, other antimicrobials may be equally effective. This is one reason why culture and antibiotic sensitivity testing is important. The same principles also apply to the use of topical antimicrobials. The indiscriminate use of topical antimicrobial products can also lead to antimicrobial resistance. When appropriate, bacterial cultures and sensitivity testing should always be offered as part of the diagnostic plan of lizards. It is imperative that the veterinarian inform the pet owner of the benefits of appropriate antimicrobial selection and the prevention of drug resistance.

Nutritional Support

Nutritional support is an essential aspect of the supportive care of lizard patients. Various physiologic parameters can be used to determine when to initiate nutritional support. In most species an acute 10% body weight loss or a chronic 20% body weight loss indicates a need for nutritional support. The ability to determine a percentage body weight loss assumes the normal weight of the patient is on file. Because of the slower metabolism of lizards, it may take a longer period of time to lose 10% or 20% of their body weight when compared to mammals and birds. Therefore, the weight guidelines used to determine the need for nutritional support in lizards may be misleading on their own, and other factors should be considered. Other concurrent factors to consider include the status of the animal upon presentation, body condition, and date of the last meal. An animal with signs of weakness, anorexia, and poor body condition will benefit from nutritional support even if considerable weight loss has not occurred. Having information regarding the last date the animal ate is also an important consideration. While some lizards will become anorexic at certain times (e.g., reproduction, winter), prolonged periods (>7-10 days) of anorexia outside of that normally observed in the past is an indication for examination by a veterinarian. As one would suspect, nutritional support may be a consideration in these cases. In addition to history and physical examination, a CBC, chemistry panel, and radiographs may provide additional information regarding the treatment of the patient. An intestinal tract impaction or blockage by either a foreign body or a mass must be ruled out before starting nutritional support. If an impaction or obstruction is found, this condition must be resolved before beginning nutritional support. If the intestinal obstruction is not resolved, continued supportive feeding can develop into gut stasis and distension of the intestinal tract, which may lead to rupture. If additional food is placed in a gut with little to no peristaltic activity, there is a risk of the material breaking down without effective digestion, creating additional complications. Nutritional support and fluid therapy are interrelated, with the amount of fluids used in feeding being subtracted from the total amount of the fluid therapy to avoid over hydration.

There are a limited number of products that are specifically designed for the nutritional support of lizards. Most of these products are in a powder formulation that is reconstituted with water for gavage feeding. Gavage feeding is achieved using ball-tipped gavage needles or red rubber catheters. Feeding via tube may be stressful for the lizard patient, especially those with long-term needs; therefore, an esophagostomy tube may be indicated. Some of the commercial nutritional products are manufactured specifically for herbivores, carnivores, and insectivores to meet the different nutritional needs of each group. Another nutritional option for herbivorous lizards is crushed alfalfa pellets mixed with water. Slurries of crushed alfalfa pellets can be processed into a consistency that will allow passage through a gavage tube. The same technique can be used with vegetables after grinding them into a fine consistency

TABLE 8-1   **Antimicrobial Properties**

Type	Method of action	Static or cidal	Gram-positive (+) or Gram-negative (−)	Aerobes (AB) or anaerobes (AN)	Examples and doses	Side effects
Cephalosporins 1st generation	Inhibit cell wall synthesis	Cidal	+ and −	AB	Cefazolin (20 mg/kg SC, IM q24h), cephalexin (20 mg/kg PO q12h)	Anaphylaxis
2nd generation			+ and −	AB and AN	Cefoxitin (20 mg/kg IM q24h)	
3rd generation			+ and −	AB and AN	Ceftazidime (20 mg/kg IM q72h), ceftiofur (2-4 mg/kg IM q24h)	
Aminoglycosides	Inhibit protein synthesis (50sR)	Cidal	−		Amikacin (3-5 mg/kg IM q24-48h), gentamicin (3 mg/kg IM q72h)	Nephrotoxicity, ototoxicity
Tetracyclines	Inhibit protein synthesis (30sR)	Static	+ and − (*Mycoplasma, Chlamydophila, Rickettsia*)	AB	Doxycycline (5-10 mg/kg PO q24h)	Nephrotoxicity, cholestasis, pyrexicity, discolored teeth
Macrolides	Inhibit protein synthesis (50sR)	Static	+	AB and AN	Erythromycin, clindamycin (5 mg/kg PO q24h)	GI toxicity
Fluoroquinolones	Inhibit bacterial DNA synthesis	Cidal	+ and −	AB	Enrofloxacin (5-10 mg/kg PO, IM q24h), ciprofloxacin (10 mg/kg PO q24h)	Cartilage erosion in young
Metronidazole	Not well understood; damages DNA	Cidal	−	AB	(25-50 mg/kg PO q24-48h) Also antiprotozoal	CNS toxicity
Potentiated sulfas	Function as competitive PABA antagonists	Cidal	+ and −	AB (*Pasteurella, Staphylococcus, Streptococcus*)	Trimethoprim-sulfas (30 mg/kg PO q24h)	KCS, crystalluria, arthropathy, thrombocytopenia
Chloramphenicol	Inhibits protein synthesis	Static	+ and −	AB and AN	Chloramphenicol (50 mg/kg PO, SC q12-24h)	Bone marrow aplastic anemia (humans)
Penicillins	Inhibit cell wall synthesis	Cidal				GI sensitivity, anaphylaxis
Natural penicillin			+	AB and AN	Procaine G (10,000 IU/kg SC, IM q12-24h)	
Aminopenicillins Antipseudomonal			+ and −		Amoxicillin (20 mg/kg PO q12-24h), ampicillin (5 mg/kg PO, SC, IM q12-24h)	
			− best (beta-lactamase sensitive)		Ticarcillin (200 mg/kg IM q24h), carbenicillin (200 mg/kg IM q24h), piperacillin (200 mg/kg IM q24h)	
Clavulanic acid	Inhibits beta-lactamase				Clavamox (20 mg/kg PO q24h)	

CNS, central nervous system; *GI*, gastrointestinal; *KCS*, keratoconjunctivitis sicca; *PABA*, *p*-aminobenzoic acid.

with a food processor. Human baby foods are a readily available alternative for nutritional support. Human baby foods are available in vegetable- and meat-based formulas. Careful evaluation of the nutritional composition of human baby food is necessary because of significant variations in protein and vitamin A content. Baby food products with a small percentage of vitamin A based on the daily requirements for humans are recommended for lizards to reduce the possibility of developing hypervitaminosis A. There are certain nutritional products designed for mammals (e.g., rabbits, rodents, ferrets) that may be used to feed the critically ill lizard. When using mammal products to feed the lizard patient, regulation of protein intake may be needed, especially in those patients requiring protein restriction (e.g., renal disease). How much and how often to feed will depend on the basal metabolic rate (BMR), also known as *standard metabolic rate (SMR)*, and maintenance energy requirement (MER) of the individual animal. To use the feeding formulas, knowledge of the animal's body weight and the kcal/ml or kcal/g of the formula being used is necessary. Some feeding formulas provide a table in which the MER has already been calculated. When using products without published kcal/ml or kcal/g (e.g., human baby food), feeding intervals and volume should be based on body weight of the patient.

The following formulas can be used to calculate the nutritional support needs for a lizard:

Basal Metabolic Rate of Reptiles (BMR)[105]

$BMR = 32W^{0.77} = kcal/day$, where W = body weight in kg

$MER = n \times BMR = kcal/day$, where *n* ranges from 1.1 to 2.5 depending on the animal's condition.

Amount to feed = MER (kcal/day) $\div A$ = ml/day or g/day, where *A* = kcal/ml or kcal/g of the food being used.

Once the BMR is calculated, adjust for the physical condition of the animal at the time that support is needed. The MER is usually considered the amount of kcal required for maintenance; however, MER can be adjusted based on the status of the animal at the time by multiplying BMR by a constant *n*. A value of *n* = 1.5 is considered adequate for maintenance. Values below 1.5 will allow nutritional support without additional stress on the intestinal tract. Values above 1.5 will allow additional support to those with an active intestinal tract that have a negative energy balance and will benefit from increased calories to recover from injury or disease. Higher values of *n* can also be used for animals that have been on long-term nutritional support and have improved enough to process additional nutritional supplementation. In critical cases it is extremely important to start feeding with small amounts, slowly and with longer intervals between feedings. In many critical cases the intestinal tract will have reduced peristaltic action and needs time to recover. To account for reduced peristaltic activity, begin feeding at 50% to 80% of the MER and slowly build up to the calculated MER over 1 to 2 weeks. The frequency of feeding will depend not only on the MER but also on the capacity of the stomach for the lizard species being supplemented. As a general rule, estimate 2% to 5% of body weight (g) as the capacity in milliliters that can be fed at once (i.e., a 1-kg lizard has the stomach capacity to hold 20-50 ml of food in its stomach.) Larger lizards can generally tolerate a larger feeding volume, approaching 5% of the body weight. The recommended approach is not to feed the maximum amount at once but to divide the amount into several feedings a day so as to avoid overloading the digestive capability of the stomach. Once the MER and the amount of food required for supplementation has been determined, one can calculate the maximum amount to be fed at one time. Even if it is possible to provide the MER in one feeding, it is advisable to split the amount over two or three feedings. One of the main thoughts behind splitting the MER is to prevent refeeding syndrome. Refeeding syndrome is characterized by an electrolyte imbalance as a consequence of reintroduction of energy and amino acids after prolonged anorexia. The main effect of the electrolyte imbalance is a shift of potassium and phosphorus from the extracellular to the intracellular space following glucose movement, leading to a peracute hypokalemia and hypophosphatemia. Clinical signs of refeeding syndrome in humans include muscle weakness, tetany, seizures, myocardial dysfunction, hemolytic anemia, water retention, and death.[106] Although little is known about the occurrence of refeeding syndrome in reptiles, it is suspected that similar changes to those noted in humans could occur. Finally, it is important to remember that the diets used for nutritional support are intended for short-term use only and should not be used for the long-term feeding of the patient. Despite all products and information currently available, these supplements may not be nutritionally complete and therefore are aimed at providing calories and energy in an easily digestible form. A conservative approach should be used initially until the response from the animal is observed. If any regurgitation is noted after feeding, decrease the amount and/or frequency of feeding and then increase the amount slowly until the animal is able to compensate. Defecation is an important sign indicating food movement and a functional intestinal tract. These general guidelines provide a starting point for the nutritional support of lizards. Each patient should be evaluated on a daily basis and therapy adjusted according to treatment response.

■SURGERY
Preoperative and Postoperative Considerations

Species, age, sex, overall health status, procedure to be performed, and available equipment should all be considered when evaluating the status of a lizard for a surgical procedure. In addition, the surgeon should have an understanding of the anatomy and physiology of the lizard species being treated and the procedure to be performed. In some instances it may be the surgeon's first surgery on a particular species. Although performing a procedure for the first time on a particular species should not be a deterrent, it would be helpful to consult available literature or colleagues about any peculiarities of the species that may relate to the specific procedure. Examples of differences among lizard species include the presence or absence

BOX 8-6 **Physical Status Classification for Patients Undergoing Anesthesia**

Status	Description
1	Healthy patient with no abnormalities observed on physical exam
2	Patient with evidence of mild systemic disease
3	Patient with evidence of severe systemic disease
4	Patient with severe systemic disease that is a constant threat to life
5	Moribund patient that is not expected to survive without intervention requiring anesthesia

Adapted from the guidelines of the American Society of Anesthesiologists.

of a urinary bladder, normal pigmentation of the internal coelomic wall and mesentery, and abundant fat reserves within the coelomic cavity. Being informed may save surgical time and decrease potential anesthetic complications.

Surgical procedures may be divided into two categories: elective surgeries and surgeries that are required for diagnosis and/or treatment of a disease process. Animals undergoing elective surgeries must be in good health with no evidence of disease. Health abnormalities identified in a patient scheduled for elective surgery must be corrected before the procedure is performed. Those requiring nonelective surgery should be stabilized before the procedure, with the appropriate supportive therapy being maintained intraoperatively and during recovery. Establishing IV access for fluid therapy and possible emergency drug administration is recommended but not always possible. If the patient requires long-term nutritional support, an esophagostomy tube may be placed at the time of surgery. The same categories of physical status adopted by the American Society of Anesthesiologists can be applied to reptiles (Box 8-6). These guidelines will help the veterinarian determine the risks involved, based on the patient's condition, and decide the best time for surgical intervention. The surgeon must determine if a patient can physically withstand an anesthetic and surgical procedure with minimal risk of fatality. Evaluation of all treatment options is important for all concerned, to verify that surgery is the most appropriate and effective route of therapy. The anesthetic plan is also an important preoperative consideration. Anesthetic drugs, monitoring equipment, and anesthetist experience are factors associated with the success of anesthesia and surgery, especially in critical lizard patients.

Postoperative management of a case should be planned prior to the procedure to limit the likelihood of complications. All lizard patients should be provided a warm, clean environment (e.g., critical care incubator unit), appropriate fluid therapy products, and analgesics and other essential therapeutics during their recovery period. The animal's movement may need to be restricted to prevent incision dehiscence, internal trauma, and pain. Restraint and movement of the animal must be done carefully to avoid inflicting pain or damaging the incision site. A quiet place to recover is recommended, along with an available nurse observer to monitor the patient after extubation.

ANESTHESIA

Adequate anesthesia requires planning that takes into consideration the health status of the animal, procedure to be performed, and expected complications. Critical animals must be adequately supported before, during, and after the procedure. Adequate patient support may require placement of an IV catheter for administration of fluids, antibiotic therapy, and nutritional support. Thermoregulation is critical to maintain metabolic activity in reptile species. Invasive procedures, especially those involving a coeliotomy, carry a higher risk of hypothermia. It is important to monitor the reptile patient aggressively during and after administering the anesthetic. Sedation may be used with fractious animals that may pose a danger to the handlers or to perform minor procedures. General anesthesia should be used for any major surgical procedure. As part of the anesthetic plan, also consider the use of systemic and local analgesic agents. Even though little information is available concerning the pharmacokinetics of opioids and nonsteroidal antiinflammatory drugs (NSAIDs) in reptile species, these therapeutic agents should be considered for the reptile patient. Ideal anesthesia will combine preemptive analgesia with injectable premedication for induction followed by maintenance with gas.

Analgesic agents used in lizards include opioids (e.g., butorphanol, buprenorphine, and morphine) and NSAIDs (e.g., carprofen and meloxicam). Dosages for most of the analgesic agents are empirical and lack pharmacokinetic data. Nonetheless, clinical experience and ongoing studies provide promising evidence that analgesics may be of benefit in the reptile patient. The ideal use of analgesic agents requires preemptive administration at least 1 hour before the scheduled procedure. Preemptive analgesia and premedication initiate the analgesic benefits in the patient and may actually reduce the dose of general anesthetic agents required to maintain a surgical plane of anesthesia. Unless new scientific studies provide evidence of disadvantages to using analgesic agents, it is recommended to incorporate analgesics as part of the pain management program of lizards.

Injectable anesthetic agents are used for premedication/induction of anesthesia. There are various published protocols for injectable anesthetics that can be used in lizards (Table 8-2). Propofol, a white solution that must be injected IV or IO, has gained popularity in recent years. In small or hypovolemic animals, IV or IO access may be difficult, and a different anesthetic must be chosen. The use of propofol has been evaluated in green iguanas via IO administration,[107] and it has been used with success in marine iguanas[108] and other lizard species. The most common side effects of propofol are apnea and cardiovascular depression, both of which are dependent on dose and rate of administration. A high dose and/or fast rate of injection increases the chance of side effects occurring. The

TABLE 8-2	Injectable Anesthetics Used in Lizards	
Drug(s)	**Dosage (mg/kg)**	**Comments**
Ketamine	5-10	As preanesthetic followed by inhalant anesthesia
Ketamine with medetomidine	5-10 (K) with 0.1-0.2 (M)	Start with low dose of ketamine; medetomidine is reversible with atipamezole
Atipamezole	0.5-1.0	Reversal for medetomidine; can split amount SC and IM or IV
Propofol	10-15	Give IV at a slow rate to avoid apnea; allows enough relaxation for endotracheal intubation; provides 20-30 min anesthesia
Tiletamine/zolazepam	5-10	Severe respiratory depression possible; good for muscle relaxation before intubation
Butorphanol	0.05-1.5	Used in combination with other protocols for analgesia

dose of propofol for lizards ranges from 10 to 15 mg/kg IV or IO. Although extravasation injection decreases the effectiveness of the drug, it does not cause damage to the tissues. Propofol is somewhat expensive and once a bottle is opened, the contents must be refrigerated and used within 24 hours. In small patients, the cost-benefit ratios must be discussed with the patient's owner. Other injectable anesthetics commonly used in lizards include ketamine, tiletamine-zolazepam, and medetomidine (see Table 8-2). These last anesthetic agents have a longer shelf life and are more cost effective than propofol.

Inhalant anesthetics (e.g., isoflurane and sevoflurane) are routinely used in exotic animal practice and are preferred over older inhalant agents (e.g., halothane). Gas anesthesia, using isoflurane or sevoflurane, provides fast, smooth induction with a rapid recovery. One major limitation of the use of gas anesthetic agents in lizards is the requirement of the gas to be actively inhaled for full benefit of anesthesia. Some lizard species hold their breath upon the initial exposure to the gas, prolonging the induction period. Although chamber induction may work with certain patients, it is not reliable, and a considerable amount of waste gas is produced. A better alternative to chamber induction is to induce the lizards with an injectable anesthetic agent, allowing adequate relaxation for endotracheal intubation. Once the animal is intubated, gas anesthesia can be initiated. Mosley et al. have determined the minimal alveolar concentration (MAC) of isoflurane in green iguanas and the effects that butorphanol may have on the MAC.[109] Results indicated a MAC of 2.1% with no significant effects from butorphanol.[109] Another study looked at the cardiovascular dose response of isoflurane alone and in combination with butorphanol.[110] The results revealed that a dose-dependent cardiovascular depression resulted from isoflurane alone but that the combination of isoflurane and butorphanol produced no detrimental effects on the cardiovascular function.[110] A third study evaluated the cardiac anesthetic index of isoflurane in green iguanas.[111] Results of these studies suggest that isoflurane by itself or in conjunction with butorphanol is a safe anesthetic in green iguanas. In a separate study, Hernandez-Divers et al. compared isoflurane and sevoflurane anesthesia after premedication with butorphanol in green iguanas.[112] This study showed sevoflurane was superior to isoflurane in quality, speed of induction, and recovery of anesthesia. Many clinical

veterinarians, however, do not believe there is a significant enough clinical difference between isoflurane and sevoflurane to warrant the additional expense of sevoflurane.

MONITORING
Reflexes
The most basic method of monitoring an anesthetized patient is by assessing body system reflexes. The loss of the righting reflex is an initial assessment used to determine if a reptile is becoming sedated or anesthetized. Palpebral reflexes are usually not accurate in reptiles; instead, the corneal reflex gives a more adequate indication of anesthetic depth. A cotton swab moistened with ophthalmologic lubricant can be used to assess the corneal reflex. Tongue withdrawal is also a very useful parameter to monitor anesthetic depth in reptiles, especially in lizards and snakes. A positive tongue withdrawal is usually observed in a light plane of anesthesia or during recovery. The toe pinch reflex can be used to assess deep pain in reptiles. To elicit a toe pinch response, hemostats are used with the tips covered with rubber tubing to avoid skin trauma. Despite controversy regarding pain perception in reptiles, a positive withdrawal following a toe pinch should not occur in a properly anesthetized reptile. Information from reflexes, together with heart rate and respiration rate, can be used to monitor the induction, maintenance, and recovery of anesthesia in lizards.

Thermoregulation
Hypothermia is a major inciting factor associated with anesthesia-related complications during reptile surgical procedures. Body heat loss occurs by convection, radiation, conduction, and evaporation.[113] Convective heat loss occurs as a result of air exchange at the body surface: As warm air is exchanged with colder air, heat loss occurs. Patient convective heat loss is an important concern in rooms that are maintained cold and have a rapid air exchange. Radiation heat loss is a result of the difference in temperature between the animal and the surrounding surfaces and environment. Conduction heat loss occurs from contact with cold surfaces (e.g., stainless steel tables). Most veterinary personnel are aware of conductive heat loss but often disregard convection and radiation heat loss. Evaporative loss occurs at the lung and skin and through procedures that open the coelomic cavity.

Lizards must have thermoregulatory support during and immediately after an anesthetic procedure. Failure to maintain proper body temperature leads to prolonged recoveries and death. There are a number of tools and techniques available to maintain the body temperature of an anesthetized patient, but none is perfect on its own. Instead attempts should be made to provide a combination of methods to address all four forms of heat loss (e.g., convection, radiation, conduction, and evaporation), thus reducing the occurrence of hypothermia in lizard patients.

Forced Air Warmers

Forced-air warmer systems have gained popularity in both human and veterinary medicine. These systems consist of a main unit that blows warm air into a blanket. Forced-air warmers address mainly convective heat loss but may also prevent conductive heat loss depending on the type of blanket used. An advantage of the forced-air warmer system is that heat is generated instantly without the delays experienced with heating pads. The heat output from the forced-air warmer can also be adjusted, and they are less prone to causing thermal injuries when used properly. The blankets can be fitted to surround the patient, and once a drape or towel is placed over the blanket, they create a warm environment that is very effective at thermoregulation.

Heating Pads

Heating pads are usually placed between the patient and the surgical table. The main function of heating pads is to prevent heat loss due to conduction. Recirculating water blankets are an excellent choice for providing even heat distribution and minimizing the risk of thermal burns to the patient. A major disadvantage of recirculating water blankets is they are easily punctured. Alternatively, an electric heating pad can be used, but these have the major disadvantage of causing thermal burns and are difficult to regulate. Electric heating pads must be used at a low setting and with a barrier, such as a towel, between the pad and the patient. In addition, electric heating pads may present a fire hazard and should not be left unattended for extended periods of time. Heating pads help maintain the patient's body temperature and decrease conductive heat loss.

Other Heat Sources

In addition to heating pads and forced-air warmers, heat lamps and ceramic heat emitters can be used to thermoregulate the anesthetized lizard. A low-cost way to provide direct contact heat is by using stockings filled with dry beans or rice. These can be placed in the microwave for a few minutes to warm them up. A disadvantage of the bean or rice bags is that heat is not evenly distributed; therefore, they must be tested by touch before placing them against the animal. They only provide heat for a short period of time but are a good heat source to be used outside of a clinic or when additional thermal support is needed. Warm fluid bags can be used for the same purpose as the bean or rice bags. Water baths can be made by filling a plastic container with warm water and then placing the container inside a trash bag. To reduce the incidence of thermal burns, the water should not be too hot and a towel should be placed between the animal and the plastic bag. To prevent further heat loss, the top of the container can be covered with towels.

Thermometers

Thermometers are essential for monitoring the core body temperature of the patient during anesthesia. Placement of the thermometer is critical to getting an accurate reading of the core body temperature. Flexible temperature probes are essential for accurate temperature readings because they can be inserted in the esophagus up to the point of the heart. The esophageal location is thought to provide the most accurate reading of core body temperatures. Flexible temperature probes can be found as accessories for some pulse oximeters as well as electrocardiogram (ECG) machines. Alternatively, there are digital thermometers equipped with flexible probes. A major disadvantage of these temperature probes is that they are delicate and tend to malfunction with time if not properly handled. In addition, some models can be expensive, and the size of the probe can be a limitation for use in smaller lizards.

CARDIOVASCULAR MONITORING

Cardiovascular monitoring is essential when monitoring lizards under general anesthesia. Cardiovascular monitoring includes gathering information about the heart rate and rhythm as well as the blood pressure. Other tools and parameters, such as pulse oximetry and blood gases, are closely linked to cardiovascular physiology. Unfortunately, cardiovascular monitoring is an area in which there is a lack of both information and appropriate equipment for lizard patients. A disparity in the size of instruments (e.g., blood pressure cuffs) and size of the patients is the main limiting factor. In addition, there is a lack of information about normal parameters (e.g., blood pressure, oxygen saturation). The continued use of these monitoring tools despite these challenges will continue to stimulate research as well as expand veterinarians' understanding of their clinical application in exotic species.

The most basic method to monitor the cardiovascular system is via the heart rate. Heart rate monitoring can be done externally with a stethoscope placed against the cranial lateral coelomic body wall (e.g., thoracic region). In some lizards, placement of a stethoscope on the body surface does not provide an easily audible heart sound. Therefore, an esophageal stethoscope or Doppler transducer is required to obtain audible heart sounds. Besides heart rate, other cardiovascular parameters (e.g., blood pressure, heart rhythm) require specialized equipment.

Doppler

A Doppler unit may be the most reliable method to monitor heart rate. A Doppler unit can also be used to obtain indirect blood pressure readings with the aid of a cuff. The units are moderately expensive and the transducer probes fragile, but with proper care, Doppler units are reliable and require little maintenance. Placement of the transducer probe varies with the species. For lizards the probe can be placed on the thoracic cavity or in the axillary region. Conduction gel must be used to obtain a good signal. Once the signal is audible, it is essential to secure the probe firmly in position to avoid displacement during the procedure. The level of pressure placed on the probe may also influence the signal reading and is often the reason for unreliable function. To keep the transducer in place once the signal is found, gauze, cotton balls, or tongue depressors can be secured with tape over the probe. After the transducer has been secured, it is also helpful to tape the cord of the probe in place to prevent turning of the probe.

Electrocardiography

Electrocardiograms (ECG) have a long history of use as a diagnostic tool and for monitoring the anesthetized patient in human and veterinary medicine. The ECG provides heart rate and rhythm information that may influence the anesthetic management of a patient. Heart rates can be obtained from the rhythm strip and are an accurate measure of true heart rate, second only to auscultation or Doppler. There are various models of ECG machines in the market that range from portable ECG units to elaborate monitoring stations that include ECG as well as capnography, pulse oximetry, and temperature probes.

For the lizard patient the recommendation for lead placement is to insert a needle through the skin at the point of placement and attach the alligator clips to the needle. In larger lizards the alligator clips may be used without the needle, but care must be taken to avoid skin trauma. Alcohol is required for proper signal conduction through the leads.

Blood Pressure

Blood pressure can be obtained via direct or indirect methods. Direct blood pressure monitoring involves the placement of an arterial catheter connected to a pressure transducer. The direct blood pressure technique is difficult to set up in lizards, and the equipment may not be readily available in practice. Indirect blood pressure monitoring can be performed by using a Doppler or via the oscillometric method. The Doppler method is thought to be more accurate than the oscillometric method when compared with the direct blood pressure technique.[114] The Doppler technique involves the use of a pressure cuff with a sphygmomanometer placed on an extremity. The cuff width should be 30% to 50% of the limb circumference.[114] The Doppler probe should be placed distal to the cuff, which is then inflated to a point where the Doppler signal is cut off. Then the cuff is allowed to deflate slowly while the manometer is observed and the systolic blood pressure is recorded as that coinciding with the first audible signal of the Doppler.[114] It is recommended to obtain an average of multiple measurements for accuracy. The size and placement of the cuff, instrumentation, and personal experience may influence the results. Unfortunately, this tool is rarely used in reptile medicine because of the lack of both proper equipment and scientific information relating to interpretation of monitoring data.

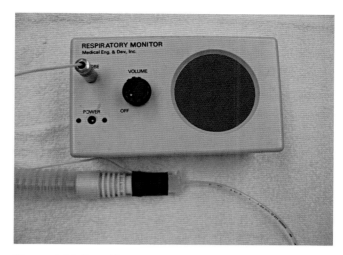

Figure 8-31 Breathing monitor used with exotic patients such as lizards. The sensor is placed in line with the anesthetic circuit.

RESPIRATION

The respiration of the anesthetized animal is often under control of the anesthetist via a mechanical ventilator. When a mechanical ventilator is not used, it is important to monitor the spontaneous ventilation of the patient. Apnea is frequently the first indication that a problem is occurring with the anesthetized patient. Apnea may be a result of the level of anesthesia or a more complicated physiologic response that can lead to death.

Breathing Monitors

There are breathing/apnea monitors that can be used with small exotic patients (Medical Engineering & Development Inc., 3334 Vrooman Rd., Jackson, MI) that have an audible signal during exhalation (Figure 8-31). An absence of that signal may indicate apnea in the anesthetized patient. Breathing monitors are useful in patients that remain on spontaneous ventilation and provide a way for the anesthetist to count breaths. Different sensors are available depending on the size of the animal. Choosing the appropriate sensor for the size of the animal is critical to the proper functioning of the monitor. Breathing monitors are very useful, especially when the patient is covered with drapes and thoracic excursions are not visible.

Pulse Oximetry

Pulse oximeters are used to detect arterial hemoglobin oxygen saturation (SaO_2). Pulse oximeter probes have an infrared light that is transmitted through the blood and then picked up by the other side of the probe. The difference in the absorption of the light determines the readout of oxygen saturation. Most pulse oximeters also provide a heart rate reading but are not considered a reliable measure of heart rate. Pulse oximetry is an excellent way to monitor for hypoxemia and provides data that help the veterinarian determine changes in the ventilation rate. Pulse oximeters can be used with small mammals, reptiles, and birds, but their placement in these patients is more problematic than in dogs and cats. Probes must be placed in an area with adequate blood perfusion. There are various types of probes available, with the anal reflectance probe being most useful for reptiles. These probes can be placed in the cloaca or esophagus, after which a cotton ball or gauze sponge can be used to help keep them in place. Tissue perfusion, tissue thickness, and pigmentation can all influence the reading of a pulse oximeter. The use of pulse oximetry is controversial in lizards because of the many factors that can adversely influence accurate readings. Time and experience will increase the ease of use of pulse oximetry. As a general rule, SaO_2 readings greater than 95% indicate adequate perfusion, whereas values between 90% and 95% indicate mild hypoxemia. Values below 90% are indicative of severe hypoxemia. The trend of the SaO_2 readings in a lizard patient over the course of a procedure is more important than individual readings at a single point in time.

Capnography/Capnometry

Capnography is a useful tool for monitoring the ventilation and acid-based status of the anesthetized patient. Capnographs monitor the end tidal CO_2 ($ETCO_2$) and are available as mainstream or sidestream monitors, depending on their location in the circuit. Mainstream capnographs have the monitor directly between the endotracheal tube and the ventilator circuit. Sidestream capnographs retrieve expired gas through a tube that sends it to a separate unit outside the circuit. Although $ETCO_2$ values have not been established for lizards, veterinarians are more interested in changes in trend than individual values. Type of capnograph, breathing frequency, gas mixture, and foreign material in the sensors (e.g., saliva, condensation) may affect the reliability of the reading.

Blood Gases

Blood gases are an integral part of anesthetic monitoring for large and small animal patients. In exotic pet medicine, blood gases are seldom used in the practical clinical setting. For lizard patients, difficulties that limit the application of this technique begin with obtaining arterial blood samples, limited blood volumes, and the requirement for specialized equipment. To monitor blood gases during anesthesia, veterinarians must have an understanding of the physiology involved in creating changes in the values. Both metabolic and respiratory disturbances can be diagnosed with the aid of blood gas analysis. As with other monitoring parameters, there are no normal blood gas values for lizard species. Some reptile species may be able to tolerate physiologic changes that are classified as lethal in mammals.

The recovery phase of anesthesia is also critical for the reptile patient. Much of the stimulus for respiration comes from decreased oxygen levels. If a reptile is maintained on 100% oxygen after anesthesia, it is likely to remain apneic for extended periods of time. For lizard patients, discontinue 100% oxygen 5 to 10 minutes after the end of the procedure and continue to ventilate the animal with an ambu bag at a rate of 1 to 4 breaths per minute. The mechanical ventilation will provide room air with a lower oxygen concentration, leading to a faster recovery. If the animal appears cyanotic, 100% oxygen should be maintained for a longer period of time. Once spontaneous respiration begins, the endotracheal tube should remain in place until the animal appears to be strong and is able to maintain respiration without the aid of the tube. The endotracheal tube can become clogged with mucoid secretions and must be cleaned and reinserted if the animal is not ready to be extubated. Atropine and glycopyrrolate do not appear effective in decreasing oral secretions in lizards. The experience of the anesthetist with the species at hand will influence anesthetic choice, monitoring techniques, and the approach to recovery. If problems are encountered during the anesthesia, the same resuscitation drugs (atropine, doxapram, and epinephrine) used in other species can be used in lizards. The success of cardiopulmonary resuscitation is low in reptiles, and many lizard patients die within 24 hours after a resuscitation event.

Instrumentation

There are a variety of instruments that have been designed or adapted for small exotic patient use (e.g., lizards). Small surgical instruments (ophthalmic instruments) are preferred when working with small patients. Normal-sized instruments may work well in larger patients. Magnification loops or operating microscopes enhance the visualization of the surgical field (Figure 8-32). Radiosurgery and CO_2 laser units are useful for many lizard surgical procedures because of the need for hemostasis and decreased tissue trauma. If a radiosurgery unit is not available, small fine-tip hemostats can be used to occlude bleeding vessels. Epinephrine applied topically will initiate vasoconstriction and control bleeding. Gel Foam® (Upjohn, Kalamazoo, MI) is a product that can be used to control hemorrhage and promote clotting. Hemoclips can be used to ligate larger vessels and may be used to control hemorrhage as well as obtain biopsies. Monofilament, absorbable suture that

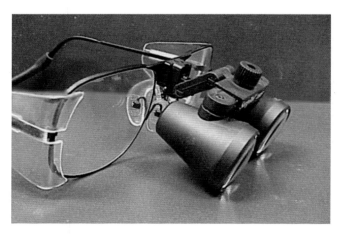

Figure 8-32 Magnifying glasses used for microsurgeries in exotic pets such as lizards. They allow better visualization of small structures such as blood vessels.

Title: The veterinary clinics of North America. Exotic animal practice.Additional Info: None available Subject(s): <u>Veterinary medicine --Periodicals.</u> <u>Exotic animals --Periodicals.</u> <u>Veterinary Medicine --Periodicals.</u> <u>Animal Diseases --Periodicals.</u> Peer reviewed / refereed Publisher: Philadelphia : W.B. Saunders Co., c1998-

Location: King Periodicals, one week loan Call Number: <u>Shelved by title</u> Number of Items: 20 Status: Available Library has: 2002 to present. Catalogued individually by subject/title until May 2002; then as periodical Recent Issues: v. 12, no. 1 (2009 Jan.) Cardiology
v. 11, no. 3 (2008 Sept.) Hematology and Related Disorders
v. 11, no. 2 (2008 May) Toxicology
v. 11, no. 1 (2008 Jan.) Endocrinology
v. 10, no. 3 (2007 Sept.) Neuroanatomy and Neurodiagnostics

Title: BSAVA manual of exotic pets / editors: Anna Meredith, Sharon Redrobe.Additional Info: <u>Check for more information on this title.</u> Subject(s): <u>Veterinary medicine.</u> <u>Exotic animals --Diseases.</u> Publisher: Quedgeley, Gloucester, UK : British Small Animal Veterinary Association, c2002.

Location: King Reference, in library use only Call Number: <u>REF SF981.B72 2002</u>

Main Author: <u>Girling, Simon.</u> Title: Veterinary nursing of exotic pets / Simon Girling.Additional Info: <u>Check for more information on this title.</u> Subject(s): <u>Exotic animals --Diseases.</u> <u>Wildlife diseases.</u> <u>Pet medicine.</u> <u>Veterinary nursing.</u> <u>Animal Diseases --therapy</u> <u>Animal Technicians</u> <u>Veterinary Medicine</u> Publisher: Malden, MA : Blackwell Pub., 2003.

Location: King General Collection Call Number: <u>SF997.5.E95 G57 2003</u> Number of Items: 1 Status: Available

Main Author: <u>Tully, Thomas N.</u> Title: A technician's guide to exotic animal care / Thomas N. Tully, Jr., Mark A. Mitchell.Additional Info: <u>Check for more information on this title.</u> Subject(s): <u>Exotic animals --Diseases.</u> <u>Wildlife diseases.</u> <u>Pet medicine.</u> <u>Veterinary nursing.</u> Publisher: Lakewood, Colo. : AAHA Press, c2001.

Location: King General Collection Call Number: <u>SF997.5.E95 T85 2001</u> Number of Items: 1 Status: Available

Title: Laboratory medicine : avian and exotic pets / edited by Alan M. Fudge.Additional Info: <u>Check for more information on this title.</u> Subject(s): <u>Avian medicine.</u> <u>Pet medicine.</u> <u>Cage birds --Diseases.</u> <u>Exotic animals --Diseases.</u> <u>Wildlife diseases.</u> Publisher: Philadelphia : Saunders, c2000.

Location: King General Collection Call Number: <u>SF994 .L33 2000</u> Number of Items: 1 Status: Available

degrades by hydrolysis is preferred for use in reptiles. Skin staples are used by some as an additional layer of closure but are not needed in most instances.

TECHNIQUE

Surgical technique and skills vary according to the experience and training of the veterinarian. Skin incisions should be made between the scales. The ventral abdominal vein must be avoided; thus, for a ventral approach into the coelomic cavity, a paramedian incision is required to avoid the vessel. Veterinary surgeons should exercise care when cutting through the skin to avoid puncturing the large colon. The tissues within the coelomic cavity should be handled in a delicate manner, as they may be more fragile than in mammals, especially in patients with intestinal disease. Closure of the coelomic cavity can be done in two or three layers depending on the species and size of the animal. The skin will form a strong barrier, and an everting pattern must be used for proper healing of the lizard's skin. Horizontal or vertical mattress patterns are used commonly for lizard skin closure. Surgical glue may also be used to provide additional strength as well as a hydrophobic barrier. The surgeon must remember that blood loss and hypothermia are two critical factors to consider when performing surgeries on lizards.

When repairing a skin wound, take caution not to undermine too much tissue because it can result in the loss of the vascular supply to the affected epithelium, thereby affecting the healing process. Avascular epithelial lesions will benefit from multiple procedures to slowly advance the skin flaps. The bone cortices of lizards can be very thin compared with those of mammalian species. Placement of intramedullary pins and other hardware fixation methods should be done carefully when performing orthopedic procedures on lizard patients to avoid iatrogenic fractures. Continued innovation is critical for improving the surgical options available for lizards and reptiles in general.

COMMON SURGICAL PROCEDURES

The two most common elective procedures performed in lizards are orchidectomy and ovariectomy with salpingectomy. Orchidectomies should be performed in younger males to reduce the likelihood of sexual aggression. Ovariectomy and salpingectomy procedures are often performed after females present for chronic egg laying or dystocia. The follicles are easily visualized during the reproductive season. Other common nonelective procedures include tail and extremity amputations, removal of cystic calculi, exploratory coeliotomy, renal biopsies, removal of foreign bodies, repair of wound lacerations, and orthopedic procedures. Surgical procedures are not as common as medical procedures in most practices that treat lizard species.

■ZOONOSES

Salmonella spp. are normal inhabitants of the gut flora of reptiles and are shed intermittently in the feces. The shedding of *Salmonella* spp. organisms may be exacerbated by stress and poor husbandry. The reptile industry has focused on eliminating *Salmonella* spp. in pet reptile species. Unfortunately, there are, as yet, no successful methods for eliminating the shedding of this zoonotic bacterium. Small children and immune-compromised individuals have a higher risk of infection through exposure than does the average person. The recommended practice to prevent the transmission of *Salmonella* spp. from reptile to human is to maintain good hygiene techniques (e.g., washing hands with soap immediately after handling the reptile). It is also recommended is to wash hands in an area other then the kitchen to prevent contamination of the kitchen sink. The enclosure of the reptile must be cleaned regularly, and feces must be removed shortly after the reptile defecates. The water and food bowls should be cleaned and disinfected thoroughly in a sink other than the kitchen sink. The task of cleaning the enclosure and feeding the pet lizard should be left to an adult and not a child until the child is old enough to understand the risks and take appropriate precautions. It is the responsibility of the adults in the household to understand the risks associated with salmonellosis and the measures that should be followed to reduce exposure. Individuals have maintained pet reptiles for many years without any adverse effects to their health by following recommended hygiene practices. In most instances where reptile-associated salmonellosis occurs, inadequate hygiene is the cause.

In addition to *Salmonella* spp., there are a number of other zoonotic agents that can be transmitted from reptiles to humans. Whereas some organisms are very species specific, others are found in many species. Under the right conditions, many bacteria, fungi, or viruses presenting in animals can also affect humans. Unfortunately, the practice of collecting wild lizards in their natural environment and selling them in the pet trade continues to be a common practice. Collecting lizards from their natural environment not only affects the wild populations and their environments but also presents a risk of introducing new diseases to both captive animals and humans. Captive-bred reptiles generally are in better health than wild-caught reptiles and therefore represent less of a risk for disease transmission. Once again, young children, the elderly, and immune-compromised individuals are more susceptible to becoming ill from exposure to a disease organism that may be present in pet lizards. Although it is the veterinarian's responsibility to educate the pet owner about the risks involved with salmonellosis and other zoonoses, it is ultimately the individual's responsibility to take appropriate measures to prevent exposure to disease organisms.

REFERENCES

1. http://www.embl-heidelberg.de/~uetz/LivingReptiles.html
2. Barten SL: Lizards. In Mader DR, editor: *Reptile Medicine and Surgery,* Philadelphia, 1996, WB Saunders.
3. Sprackland RG: *All About Lizards,* New Jersey, 1977, TFH.

4. Holz P, Barker IK, Crawshaw GJ et al: The anatomy and perfusion of the renal portal system in the red-eared slider *(Trachemys scripta elegans)*, *J Zoo Wildl Med* 28(4):378-385, 1997.

5. Benson KG, Forrest L: Characterization of the renal portal system of the common green iguana *(Iguana iguana)* by digital subtraction imaging, *J Zoo Wildl Med* 30(2):235-241, 1999.

6. Holz P, Barker IK, Burger JP et al: The effects of the renal portal system on pharmacokinetic parameters in the red-eared slider *(Trachemys scripta elegans)*, *J Zoo Wildl Med* 28(4):386-393, 1997.

7. Hernandez-Divers SJ: Green iguana nephrology: a review of diagnostic techniques, *Vet Clin North Am Exot Anim Pract* 6(1):233-250, 2003.

8. DeNardo DF: Reptile thermal biology: a veterinary perspective, *Proc ARAV*, pp 157-163, 2002.

9. Gillespie D, Frye FL, Stockham SL et al: Blood values in wild and captive Komodo dragons *(Varanus komodoensis)*, *Zoo Biol* 19(6):495-509, 2000.

10. Mitchell MA: (Personal communication), 2005.

11. Allen ME, Oftedal OT: Nutrition in captivity. In Jacobson ER, editor: *Biology, Husbandry, and Medicine of the Green Iguana*, Melbourne, Fla, 2003, Krieger.

12. Baer DJ, Oftedal OT, Rumpler WV et al: Dietary fiber influences nutrient utilization, growth and dry matter intake of green iguanas *(Iguana iguana)*, *J Nutrit* 127:1501-1507, 1997.

13. USDA Nutrient Data Laboratory: Oxalic acid content of selected vegetables, http://www.nal.usda.gov/fnic/foodcomp/Data/Other/oxalic.html, April 2005.

14. Cornell University Poisonous Plants Informational Database: Toxic agents in plants, glucosinolates, http://www.ansci.cornell.edu/plants/toxicagents/glucosin.html, April 2005.

15. Divers SJ: Clinical evaluation of reptiles, *Vet Clin North Am Exot Anim Pract* 2(2):291-331, 1999.

16. Benson KG, Paul-Murphy J, MacWilliams P: Effects of hemolysis on plasma electrolytes and chemistry values in the common green iguana *(Iguana iguana)* *J Zoo Wildl Med* 30(3):413-415, 1999.

17. Hanley CS, Hernandez-Divers SJ, Bush S et al: Comparison of the effect of dipotassium ethylenediaminetetraacetic acid and lithium heparin on hematologic values in the green iguana *(Iguana iguana)*, *J Zoo Wildl Med* 35(3):328-332, 2004.

18. Harr KE, Alleman AR, Dennis PM et al: Morphologic and cytochemical characteristic of blood cells and hematologic and plasma biochemical reference ranges in green iguanas, *JAVMA* 218(6):915-921, 2001.

19. Divers SJ, Redmayne G, Aves EK: Haematological and biochemical values of 10 green iguanas *(Iguana iguana)*, *Vet Rec* 138(9):203-205, 1996.

20. Jacobson ER: Clinical evaluation and diagnostic techniques. In Jacobson ER, editor: *Biology, Husbandry, and Medicine of the Green Iguana*, Melbourne, Fla, 2003, Krieger.

21. Couto CG: Anemia. In Nelson RW, Couto CG, editors: *Small Animal Internal Medicine*, St Louis, 1998, Mosby.

22. Perpinan D, Hernandez-Divers SJ, Hernandez-Divers SM et al: Comparison of three different techniques to perform blood smears in the green iguana *(Iguana iguana)*, *Proc ARAV*, p 108, 2004.

23. Nevarez JG, Mitchell MA, Le Blanc C et al: Determination of plasma biochemistries, ionized calcium, vitamin D3, and hematocrit values in captive green iguanas *(Iguana iguana)* from El Salvador, *Proc ARAV*, pp 87-93, 2002.

24. Wagner RA, Wetzel R: Tissue and plasma enzyme activities in juvenile green iguanas, *Am J Vet Res* 60(2):201-203, 1999.

25. Ramsay EC, Dotson TK: Tissue and serum enzyme activities in the yellow rat snake *(Elaphe obsoleta quadrivitatta)*, *Am J Vet Res* 56(4):423-428, 1995.

26. Franson JC, Murray HC, Bunck C: Enzyme activities in plasma, kidney, liver, and muscle of five avian species, *J Wildl Dis* 21(1):33-39, 1985.

27. Dennis PM, Bennett RA, Harr KE et al: Plasma concentrations of ionized calcium in healthy iguanas, *J Am Vet Med Assoc* 219(3):326-328, 2001.

28. Benson KG, Forrest L: Characterization of the renal portal system of the common green iguana *(Iguana iguana)* by digital subtraction imaging, *J Zoo Wildl Med* 30(2):235-241, 1999.

29. de Groot JH, van Leeuwen JL: Evidence for an elastic projection mechanism in the chameleon tongue, *Proc Biol Sci* 271(1540):761-770, 2004.

30. Zotti A, Selleri P, Carnier P et al: Relationship between metabolic bone disease and bone mineral density measured by dual-energy X-ray

absorptiometry in the green iguana *(Iguana iguana)*, *Vet Radiol Ultrasound* 454(1):10-16, 2004.

31. Smith D, Dobson H, Spence E: Gastrointestinal studies in the green iguana: technique and reference values, *Vet Radiol Ultrasound* 42(6):515-520, 2001.

32. Silverman S, Janssen DL: Diagnostic imaging. In Mader DR, editor: *Reptile Medicine and Surgery*, Philadelphia, 1996, WB Saunders.

33. Mitchell MA: Diagnosis and management of reptile orthopedic injuries, *Vet Clin North Am Exot Anim Pract* 5(1):97-114, 2002.

34. DeShaw B, Schoenfeld A, Cook RA et al: Imaging of reptiles: a comparison study of various radiographic techniques, *J Zoo Wildl Med* 27:364-370, 1996.

35. Chiodini RJ, Nielsen SW: Vertebral osteophytes in an iguanid lizard, *Vet Pathol* 20:372-375, 1983.

36. Schuchman SM, Taylor DO: Arteriosclerosis in an iguana *(Iguana iguana)*, *JAVMA* 157(5):614-616, 1970.

37. Mehler SJ, Rosenstein DS, Patterson JS: Imaging diagnosis-follicular torsion in a green iguana *(Iguana iguana)* with involvement of the left adrenal gland *Vet Radiol Ultrasound* 43(4):343-345, 2002.

38. Schildger BJ, Hafeli W: The radiologic differential diagnosis in girth increases of the gastric cavity and the body of lizards *(Squamata: Sauria)*, *Tierarztl Prax Oct* 20(5):531-543, 1992 (abstract).

39. Wellehan JFX, Johnson AJ, Jacobson ER et al: Nested PCR amplification and sequencing of reptile adenoviruses, including a novel gecko adenovirus associated with enteritis, *Proc ARAV*, p 14, 2003.

40. Kinsel MJ, Barbiers RB, Manharth A et al: Small intestinal adeno-like virus in a mountain chameleon *(Chamaeleo montium)*, *J Zoo Wildl Med* 28(4):498-500, 1997.

41. Jacobson ER, Gardnier CH: Adeno-like virus in esophageal and tracheal mucosa of a Jackson's chameleon *(Chamaeleo jacksoni)*, *Vet Pathol* 27(3):210-212, 1990.

42. Kim DY, Mitchell MA, Bauer RW et al: An outbreak of adenoviral infection in inland bearded dragons *(Pogona vitticeps)* coinfected with dependovirus and coccidial protozoa *(Isospora sp)*, *J Vet Diagn Invest* 14(4):332-334, 2002.

43. Jacobson ER, Kopit W, Kennedy FA et al: Coinfection of a bearded dragon *(Pogona vitticeps)* with adenovirus- and dependovirus-like viruses, *Vet Pathol* 33(3):343-346, 1996.

44. Wellehan JF, Johnson AJ, Harrach B et al: Detection and analysis of six lizard adenoviruses by consensus primer PCR provides further evidence of a reptilian origin for the atadenoviruses, *J Virol* 78(23):13366-13369, 2004.

45. Jacobson ER, Kollias GV: Adenovirus-like infection in a savannah monitor, *J Zoo Anim Med* 17:149, 1986.

46. Frye FL, Munn RJ, Gardner M et al: Adenovirus-like hepatitis in a group of related Rankin's dragon lizards *(Pogona henrylawsoni)*, *J Zoo Wildl Med* 25(1):167, 1994.

47. Jacobson ER, Origgi F, Pessier AP et al: Paramyxovirus infection in caiman lizards *(Draecenea guianensis)*, *J Vet Diagn Invest* 13(2):143-151, 2001.

48. Marschang RE, Donahoe S, Manvell R et al: Paramyxovirus and reovirus infections in wild-caught Mexican lizards *(Xenosaurus and Abronia spp)*, *J Zoo Wildl Med* 33(4):317-321, 2002.

49. Gravendyck M, Ammermann P, Marschang RE et al: Parmyxoviral and reoviral infections of iguanas on Honduran islands, *J Wildl Dis* 34(1):33-38, 1998.

50. Maxwell LK: Infectious and noninfectious diseases. In Jacobson ER, editor: *Biology, Husbandry, and Medicine of the Green Iguana*, Fla, 2003, Krieger.

51. Drury SE, Gough RE, Welchman Dde B: Isolation and identification of a reovirus from a lizard, *Uromastyx hardwickii*, in the United Kingdom, *Vet Rec* 151:637-638, 2002.

52. Just F, Essbauer S, Ahne W et al: Occurrence of an invertebrate iridescent-like virus *(Iridoviridae)* in reptiles, *J Vet Med B Infect Dis Vet Public Health* 48(9):685-694, 2001.

53. Marschang RE, Becher P, Braun S: Isolation of iridoviruses from three different lizard species, *Proc 9th ARAV Conf*, pp 99-100, 2002.

54. Telford SR, Jacobson ER: Lizard erythrocytic virus in East African chameleons, *J Wildl Dis* 29(1):57-63, 1993.

55. Alves de Matos AP, Paperna I, Crespo E: Experimental infection of lacertids with lizard erythrocytic viruses, *Intervirology* 45(3):150-159, 2002.

56. Drury SEN, Gough RE, Calvert I: Detection and isolation of an iridovirus from chameleons *(Chamaeleo quadricornis and Chamaeleo hoehnelli)* in the United Kingdom, *Vet Rec* 150(14):451-452, 2002.

57. Wellehan JFX, Jarchow JL, Reggiardo C et al: A novel herpesvirus associated with hepatic necrosis in a San Esteban chuckwalla, *Sauromalus varius, J Herpetol Med and Surg* 13(3):15-19, 2003.

58. Clark HF, Karzon DT: Iguana virus, a herpes-like virus isolated from cultured cells of a lizard, *Iguana iguana, Infect Immun* 5(4):559-569, 1972.

59. Zeigel RF, Clark HF: Electron microscopy observations on a new herpes-type virus isolated from *Iguana iguana* and propagated in reptilian cells in vitro, *Infect Immun* 5(4):570-582, 1972.

60. Raynaud A, Adrian M: Cutaneous lesions with papillomatous structure associated with viruses in the green lizard (*Lacerta viridis), C R Acad Sci Hebd Seances Acad Sci D* 283(7):845-847, 1976.

61. Wellehan JFX, Johnson AJ, Latimer KS et al: Varanid herpesvirus 1: a novel herpesvirus associated with proliferative stomatitis in green tree monitors (*Varanus prasinus), Vet Microbiol* 105(2):83-92, 2005.

62. Wellehan JF, Nichols DK, Li LL et al: Three novel herpesviruses associated with stomatitis in Sudan plated lizards (*Gerrhosaurus major*) and a black-lined plated lizard (*Gerrhosaurus nigrolineatus), J Zoo Wildl Med* 35(1):50-54, 2004.

63. Watson GL: Herpesvirus in red-headed (common) agamas (*Agama agama), J Vet Diagn Invest* 5:444-445, 1993.

64. Nevarez JG, Mitchell MA, Kim DY et al: West Nile Virus in alligator (*Alligator mississippiensis*) ranches from Louisiana, *J Herpetol Med and Surg* 15(3):4-9, 2005.

65. Miller DL, Mauel MJ, Baldwin C et al: West Nile virus in farmed alligators. *Emerg Infect Dis* 9(7):794-799, 2003.

66. Steinman A, Banet-Noach C, Tal S et al: West Nile virus infection in crocodiles. *Emerg Infect Dis* 9(7):887-889, 2003.

67. Klenk K, Snow J, Morgan K et al: Alligators as West Nile virus amplifiers, *Emerg Infect Dis* 10(12):2150-2154, 2004.

68. Gruszynski K, Nehlig R, Mitchell MA et al: Evaluating the role of the Mediterranean house gecko (*Hemidactylus turcicus*) in the epidemiology of West Nile virus: part 1, experimental infection, *11th ARAV Conf*, pp 133-134, 2004.

69. Klenk K, Komar N: Poor replication of West Nile virus (New York 1999 strain) in three reptilian and one amphibian species, *Am J Trop Med Hyg* 69(3):260-262, 2003.

70. Jacobson ER, Telford SR: Chlamydial and poxvirus infections of circulating monocytes of a flap-necked chameleon (*Chamaeleo dilepis), J Wildl Dis* 26(4):572-577, 1990.

71. Monath TP, Cropp CB, Frazier CL et al: Viruses isolated from reptiles: identification of three new members of the family *Rhabdoviridae, Arch Virol* 60(1):1-12, 1979.

72. Oya A, Doi R, Shirasaka A et al: Studies on Japanese encephalitis virus infection of reptiles: I. experimental infection of snakes and lizards, *Jpn J Exp Med* 53(2):117-123, 1983 (abstract).

73. Doi R, Oya A, Shirasaka A et al: Studies on Japanese encephalitis virus infection of reptiles: II. Role of lizards on hibernation of Japanese encephalitis virus, *Jpn J Exp Med* 53(2):125-134, 1983 (abstract).

74. Jacobson ER, Cheatwood JL, Maxwell LK: Mycotic diseases of reptiles, *Sem Av Exot Pet Med* 9(2):94-101, 2000.

75. Tappe JP, Chandler FW, Liu S et al: Aspergillosis in two San Esteban chuckwallas, *JAVMA* 185(11):1425-1428, 1984.

76. Schumacher J: Fungal diseases of reptiles, *Vet Clin Exot Anim* 6(2):327-335, 2003.

77. Hough I: Cryptococcosis in an eastern water skink, *Aust Vet J* 76(7):471-472, 1998.

78. Pare JA, Sigler DB, Hunter RC et al: Cutaneous mycoses in chameleons caused by the *Chrysosporium* anamorph of *Nannizziopsis vriesii (Apinis)* Currah, *J Zoo Wildl Med* 28:443-453, 1997.

79. Pare JA, Sigler L, Rypien KL et al: Cutaneous mycobiota of captive squamate reptiles with notes on the scarcity of *Chrysosporium* anamorph of *Nannizziopsis vriesii, J Herpetol Med and Surg* 13(4):10-15, 2003.

80. Pare JA Coyle KA, Sigler L et al: Pathogenicity of the *Chrysosporium* anamorph of *Nannizziopsis vriesii* for veiled chameleons (*Chamaeleo calyptratus), Proc ARAV*, pp 9-10, 2004.

81. Johnson DH: An emerging dermatomycosis and systemic mycosis syndrome in bearded dragons (*Pogona vitticeps*): two case reports of "yellow fungus disease," *Proc ARAV*, pp 26-28, 2004.

82. Shalev M, Murphy JC, Fox JG: Mycotic enteritis in a chameleon and brief review of phycomycoses of animals, *JAVMA* 171(9):872-875, 1977.

83. Reavill DR, Melloy M, Schmidt RE: Reptile mycotic infections from the literature and 55 cases, *Proc ARAV*, pp 62-71, 2004.

84. Carpenter JW: *Exotic Animal Formulary*, St Louis, 2005, WB Saunders.

85. Jacobson ER: Reptiles, *Vet Clin North Am Small Anim Pract* 17(5):1203-1225, 1987.

86. Klaphake E: Cryptosporidiosis: an update for reptile veterinarians, *Proc ARAV*, pp 84-89, 2003.

87. Klaphake E. (moderator): Chameleons and vitamin A: roundtable discussion, *J Herpetol Med and Surg* 13(2):23-31, 2003.

88. Mader DR: Gout. In Mader DR, editor: *Reptile Medicine and Surgery*, Philadelphia, 1996, WB Saunders.

89. Levine BS: Visceral hemangiosarcoma and egg yolk peritonitis in a common green iguana, *Iguana iguana, Proc ARAV*, pp 69-71, 2002.

90. Diaz-Figueroa O, Toomey J, Mitchell MA et al: Peripheral nerve sheath tumor in the coelomic cavity of a Savannah monitor (*Varanus exanthematicus), Proc ARAV*, pp 135-137, 2004.

91. Lemberger KY, Manharth A, Pessier AP: Multicentric peripheral nerve sheath tumors in two related bearded dragons (*Pogona vitticeps), Proc ARAV*, pp 55-56, 2003.

92. Mikaelian I, Levine SG, Harshbarger JC et al: Malignant peripheral nerve sheath tumor in a bearded dragon, *Pogona vitticeps, J Herpetol Med and Surg* 11(1):9-12, 2001.

93. Reavill DR, Schmidt RE, Stevenson R: Malignant chromatophoromas in three veiled chameleons (*Chamaeleo calyptratus), Proc ARAV*, pp 131-133, 2004.

94. Gyimesi ZS, Garner MM, Burns RB et al: High incidence of lymphoid neoplasia in a colony of Egyptian spiny-tailed lizards (*Uromastyx aegyptius), Proc ARAV*, p 7, 2003.

95. Hernandez-Divers SM, Orcutt CJ, Stahl SJ et al: Lymphoma in lizards: three case reports, *J Herpetol Med and Surg* 13(1):14-22, 2003.

96. Gregory CR, Latimer KS, Fontenot DK et al: Chronic monocytic leukemia in an inland bearded dragon, *Pogona vitticeps, J Herpetol Med and Surg* 14(2):12-16, 2004.

97. Stacy BA, Vidal JD, Osofsky A et al: Ovarian papillary cystadenocarcinoma in a green iguana (*Iguana iguana), J Comp Pathol* 130(2-3):223-228, 2004.

98. Hernandez-Divers SJ, Knott CD, MacDonald J: Diagnosis and surgical treatment of thyroid adenoma-induced hyperthyroidism in a green iguana (*Iguana iguana), J Zoo Wildl Med* 32(4):465-475, 2001.

99. Burt DG, Chrisp CE, Gillett CS et al: Two cases of renal neoplasia in a colony of desert iguanas, *J Am Vet Med Assoc* 185(11):1423-1425, 1984.

100. Martin JC, Moore AS, Ruslander D et al: Successful radiation treatment of leukemia in a sungazer lizard (*Cordylus giganteus), ProcARAV*, p 8, 2003.

101. Klingerberg RJ: Therapeutics. In Mader DR, editor: *Reptile Medicine and Surgery*, Philadelphia, 1996, WB Saunders.

102. Maxwell LK, Helmick KE: Drug dosages and chemotherapeutics. In Jacobson ER editor: *Biology, Husbandry, and Medicine of the Green Iguana*, Fla, 2003, Krieger.

103. Guyton AC, Hall JE: The body fluids compartments: extracellular and intracellular fluids; interstitial fluid and edema. In Guyton AC, Hall JE, editors: *Textbook of Medical Physiology*, Philadelphia, 1996, WB Saunders.

104. Wilkinson R: Therapeutics. In McArthur S, Wilkinson R, Meyer J, editors: *Medicine and Surgery of Tortoises and Turtles*, Oxford, 2004, Blackwell.

105. Stahl S, Donoghue S: Feeding reptiles. In Hand MS, Thatcher CD, Remillard RL et al, editors: *Small Animal Clinical Nutrition*, Topeka, Kan, 2000, Mark Morris Institute.

106. Remillard RL, Armstrong PJ, Davenport DJ: Assisted feeding in hospitalized patients: enteral and parenteral nutrition. In Hand MS, Thatcher CD, Remillard RL et al, editors: *Small Animal Clinical Nutrition*, ed 4, Topeka, Kan, 2000, Mark Morris Institute.

107. Bennett RA, Schumacher J, Hedjazi-Haring K et al: Cardiopulmonary and anesthetic effects of propofol administered intraosseously to green iguanas, *J Am Vet Med Assoc* 212(1):93-98, 1998.

108. Nevarez JG, Mitchell MA, Wilkelski M: Evaluating the clinical effects of propofol on marine iguanas (*Amblyrhynchus cristatus), Proc ARAV*, pp 48-49, 2003.

109. Mosley CA, Dyson D, Smith DA: Minimum alveolar concentration of isoflurane in green iguanas and the effect of butorphanol on minimum alveolar concentration, *J Am Vet Med Assoc* 222(11):1559-1564, 2003.

110. Mosley CA, Dyson D, Smith DA: The cardiovascular dose-response effects of isoflurane alone and combined with butorphanol in the green iguana *(Iguana iguana), Vet Anaesth Analg* 31(1):64-72, 2004.

111. Mosley CA, Dyson D, Smith DA: The cardiac anesthetic index of isoflurane in green iguanas, *J Am Vet Med Assoc* 222(11):1565-1568, 2003.

112. Hernandez-Divers SM, Schumacher J, Read M et al: Comparison of isoflurane and sevoflurane anesthesia following premedication with butorphanol in the green iguana *(Iguana iguana), Proc ARAV,* pp 1-2, 2003.

113. Rembert MS, Smith JA, Hosgood G et al: Comparison of traditional thermal support devices with forced-air warmer system in anesthetized Hispaniolan Amazon parrots *(Amazona ventralis), J Avian Med Surg* 15(3):187-193, 2001.

114. Haberman ChE, Morgan JD, Kang ChW et al: Evaluation of Doppler ultrasonic and oscillometric methods of indirect blood pressure measurement in cats, *Intern J Appl Res Vet Med* 2(4):279-289, 2004.

Megan Kirchgessner
Mark A. Mitchell

CHAPTER 9

CHELONIANS

COMMON SPECIES KEPT IN CAPTIVITY

There are over 285 different species of chelonians in the world.[1] Chelonians represent one of the most unique and recognizable groups of animals in the world. Characterized by their bony shell, no other tetrapod has both its pectoral and pelvic girdles encased in bone.[1] The chelonians are the longest lived of the reptiles, with some animals living over 100 years. Over the years, chelonians have been classified using a number of different taxonomic classifications, including morphologic and molecular features. However, for the purpose of this text, we will classify them based on habitat selection. For the captive chelonian, this is a preferred method because it is useful for defining the captive needs of the chelonian. The two primary classifications based on this system are the turtle and the tortoise. Turtles include species that are aquatic. These animals generally leave the water only to move to another body of water or to lay their eggs. Examples of this group can be found in Box 9-1 and Figures 9-1 and 9-2. For this group it is important to determine what type of aquatic system the animals originate from. There are three different types of aquatic systems: freshwater, brackish, and marine systems. The provision of the most appropriate system is critical to the long-term care of these animals in captivity. The tortoises include animals that are completely terrestrial. These animals are generally considered poor swimmers, and if provided a deep body of water in captivity, could drown. Common examples of these animals can be found in Box 9-1 and Figures 9-3 and 9-4.

BIOLOGY
Integumentary System

The epidermis is composed of an outer keratinized layer (stratum corneum) and an inner actively dividing layer (stratum germinivatum). The dermis represents the vascular region of the integument and supplies nutrition to the epidermis. The dermis is also the location of the osteoderms. There are limited glandular structures within the integument of chelonians. Ecdysis tends to be random and uncoordinated and results in fragmentary shedding, which continues throughout the life of the chelonian.[2]

The majority of the chelonian shell is comprised of membranous bone (osteoderms). The membranous bone is covered by horny scutes, which form the outer, visible part of the shell. The scutes are formed from the epidermis and are equivalent to the scales of reptilian skin (Figure 9-5). Growth of the scutes occurs by the addition of new keratinized layers to the base of each scute.[3] The shell is a vascular structure. In the past, recommendations were made to subtract the weight of the shell when determining drug doses; however, this is not recommended, as the shell is a living tissue and should be included when calculating a therapeutic plan.

Cardiovascular System

The chelonian heart lies in a pericardial cavity and is located slightly caudal to the pectoral girdle and cranial to the lungs.[3] Externally, the heart is generally located where the humeral and

Common Species of Chelonians Kept in Captivity (Pet and Institutional)

Turtles

Alligator snapping turtles	*Macroclemys temminickii*
Snapping turtles	*Chelydra serpentina*
Red-eared slider	*Trachemys scripta elegans*
Diamond-backed terrapins	*Malaclemys terrapin*
Soft-shelled turtles	*Apalone* spp.
Mata mata	*Chelus fimbriatus*

Tortoises

Sulcata tortoise	*Geochelone sulcata*
Russian tortoise	*Testudo horsfieldii*
Red-footed tortoise	*Geochelone carbonaria*
Box turtle (tortoise)	*Terrapene* spp.
Leopard tortoise	*Geochelone pardalis*

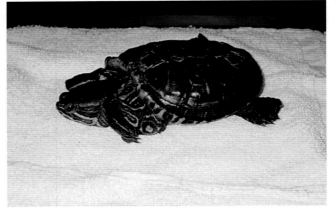

Figure 9-2 Red-eared slider turtles *(Trachemys scripta elegans)* are native to the United States and are the most commonly bred turtle in captivity. This particular animal has metabolic bone disease.

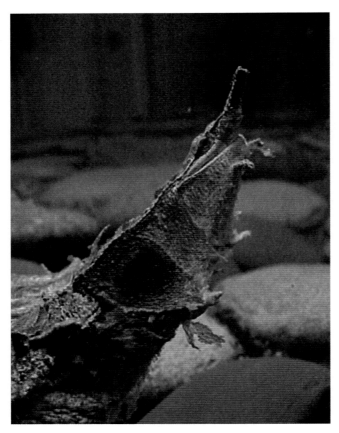

Figure 9-1 Mata mata turtles *(Chelus fimbriatus)* are an extreme example of an aquatic turtle.

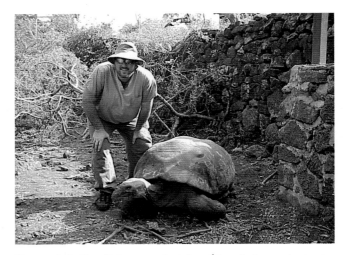

Figure 9-3 The Galapagos tortoise *(Geochelone elephantopus)* is the largest of the tortoises.

thoracic plastron scutes meet. The heart is three chambered, with two separate atria and an incomplete ventricular septum. The right atrium receives deoxygenated blood from the left and right precaval veins, postcaval vein, left hepatic vein, and other, smaller vessels. The left atrium receives blood from the left and right pulmonary veins. Numerous muscular folds in the walls of the ventricle shunt oxygenated and deoxygenated blood into the appropriate arterial pathways.[2] The left aorta gives rise to the celiac, left gastric, and cranial mesenteric arteries before converging with the right aorta.[3]

Renal Portal System

Venous return from the pelvic limbs drains into the kidneys to form the renal portal system in reptiles.[3] The primary function of the renal portal vein is to maintain adequate blood flow to the renal tubules when the glomerular blood flow is low. This large vessel arises near the junction of the epigastric and external iliac veins and enters the kidney centrally.[2] The chelonian renal portal vein contains valves that effectively shunt blood drained from the caudal half of the body directly into either the kidney or the liver and central venous reserve.[4-6]

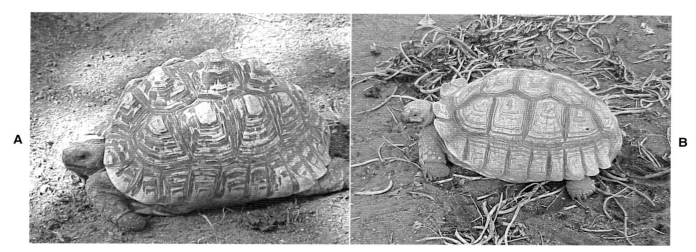

Figure 9-4 The leopard tortoise *(Geochelone pardalis)* **(A)** is commonly bred in captivity. These tortoises have a good disposition and do not get as large as other common captive species (e.g., *Geochelone sulcata)* **(B)**.

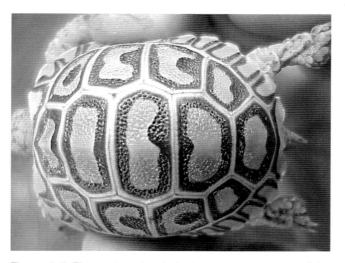

Figure 9-5 The scutes of a chelonian are a component of the chelonian integument. They play an important role in preventing desiccation and protecting the outer surface of the shell.

Although avoidance of the hindlimbs for intramuscular and intravenous injections of drugs has traditionally been advocated, research has demonstrated that this may be an unsubstantiated theory. Results of research conducted by Holtz et al. demonstrated that it is unlikely that the injection site has any influence over the activity of a drug and that the caudal half of the reptile body is suitable for drug administration.[5] Both Beck et al. and Holtz et al. found no significant difference in drug metabolism when gentamicin (excreted by glomerular filtration) was administered into the hindlimb, as opposed to the forelimb.[5,7] Studies conducted by Malley revealed that adrenaline released during caudal intramuscular injections may reduce perfusion of the renal portal system, thereby increasing hepatic circulation.[8] It is important to consider that these studies were conducted on a limited number of species. Addi-

tional research is required to further elucidate if there is an effect based on species or an animal's physiologic status.

The Dive Reflex

It has been suggested that the pathway of blood flow from the heart into the pulmonary vessels is under some degree of physiologic control. The dive reflex in anesthetized turtles *(Trachemys scripta)* has been studied intensely, and it was consequently discovered that hypoxia resulted in an increase in the resistance of pulmonary blood vessels. Because this effect persisted in the face of atropine administration and cervical vagotomy, locally mediated resistance was suggested. Considering the fact that chelonians have only one ventricle, thereby limiting the separation of oxygenated and deoxygenated blood, alterations in vascular resistance may have a significant effect on the perfusion of organs, including the lungs. Consequently, the rates of elimination of inhalation agents by the lungs may be reduced in those situations where the dive reflex is observed.[9]

Respiratory System
UPPER RESPIRATORY TRACT

Chelonians are obligate nasal breathers.[3] The nares open into a keratinized vestibule, which is divided cranially by a cartilaginous septum into right and left nasal chambers. The nasal chambers do not contain either turbinates or sinuses and extend caudally until converging into a single passageway dorsal to the hard palate. The passageway terminates at the choana. A soft palate is not present in chelonians.[10,11]

LOWER RESPIRATORY TRACT

The chelonian glottis is easily identified at the back of the tongue. The tracheal rings are complete[3] and the trachea, bronchi, and lungs are all covered by a ciliated glandular epithelium that is ineffective at eliminating particulate foreign material and excessive respiratory secretions.[10] The trachea divides into paired bronchi relatively cranially in most chelonians.[12] Because of this, it is important to resist passing an endotracheal tube far into the lower respiratory tract. Doing so may result in intubating a single lung and lead to inconsistent anesthesia.

Chelonian lungs occupy a large volume in the dorsal half of the coelomic cavity. The borders of the lungs include the periosteum of the carapace dorsally, the pectoral girdle cranially, and the pelvic girdle caudally.[3] The lungs are multicameral, with a single intrapulmonary bronchus that divides into a complicated network of bronchioles and faveoli.[13] Chelonian faveoli differ from mammalian alveoli in that they are compartmentalized, and oxygen exchange occurs on the reticulated surface of these compartments.[2] The lungs are separated from the other coelomic viscera by a thin, nonmuscular, postpulmonary septum or pleuroperitoneal membrane (also called the septum horizonatale or the pseudodiaphragm).[2,13,14] Chelonians do not have a true diaphragm and are therefore not dependent on negative pressure for breathing. The volume of the lungs is reduced to one fifth when the head and limbs are retracted.[15]

VENTILATION

To compensate for the absence of an expandable chest, chelonians have developed strong trunk muscles that help to expand and contract the lungs with active inspiration and expiration.[15-17] It is the movement of the septum horizontale, powered by the movements of the trunk muscles, the viscera, and the limb girdles, that alters the intrapulmonary pressure and effectively draws air in and out of the lungs.[2,3] When the septum horizontale is pulled taut and downward by the trunk muscles (e.g., limb movement), the area occupied by the lungs increases. This increase in lung volume thereby facilitates inspiration.[2] For terrestrial chelonians, inspiration is passive and expiration is active, but this scenario is reversed for aquatic chelonians due to the effect of hydrostatic pressure on visceral volume.[18,19]

SUPPLEMENTAL RESPIRATORY ORGANS AND METHODS

Selected semiaquatic freshwater turtles possess the ability to absorb oxygen via the presence of well-vascularized cloacal bursae. This mechanism of oxygen absorption is utilized principally during periods of underwater hibernation. Some soft-shelled turtles can remain submerged for hours in the mud, utilizing oxygen in the water via exchange through the plastron and carapace, the villiform oral papilla, and the pharyngeal mucosa.[3,20] Frye suggests that chelonians possess methods of glycolytic respirations, based upon the discovery that these animals can survive up to 8 hours in pure atmospheric nitrogen.[12]

Gastrointestinal System
UPPER DIGESTIVE TRACT

The chelonian oral cavity does not contain any teeth. Rather, chelonians use a sharp horny beak, or tomia, to grasp and tear food. The salivary glands of chelonians do not secrete digestive enzymes, but the stomach, small intestine, pancreas, liver, and gall bladder produce these proteolytic substances. The esophagus travels down the left side of the neck and terminates in the stomach, which is embedded in the left lobe of the liver.[3]

LOWER DIGESTIVE TRACT

The simple chelonian stomach is the proximal boundary of the lower digestive tract. The small intestine of chelonians is not well divided into a duodenum, jejunum, or ileum, and the tract is located in the caudal coelomic cavity.[21] The mucosa of the small intestine is composed of single columnar epithelium,[2] and regeneration of the intestinal epithelium takes an estimated 8 weeks in *Chrysemys picta* at a temperature of 20° C to 24° C (68° F to 75° F).[22]

The large intestine begins with the cecum, which is not a distinct organ but is rather a widening of the distal colonic wall.[23,24] The cecum is located in the right caudal quadrant of the coelomic cavity. The large intestine is typically divided into ascending, transverse, and descending portions. The mucosal epithelium is comprised of a large number of glandular cells.[2] Passage of food through the chelonian digestive tract is quite slow when compared to mammalian transit times (up to 2-4 weeks), but this allows for maximal nutritional absorption.[25]

The distal boundary of both the lower digestive tract and the urogenital tract is the cloaca. The cloaca is subdivided into three sections: the coprodeum, urodeum, and proctodeum. Of all the reptiles, subdivision of the cloaca is the least prominent in chelonians. The colon terminates at the coprodeum, and the coprodeum is separated from the more cranial urodeum by a distinct fold of tissue. The proctodeum is the most caudal aspect of the cloaca.[2]

LIVER

The chelonian liver is separated into indistinct lobes, and a small gall bladder is located at the caudal border of the right side. The liver functions basically in the same manner as the liver of other vertebrates, participating in lipid, glycogen, and protein metabolism. It is believed that the chelonian liver plays a pivotal role in the activation of calcitriol (vitamin D). It is important to note that the functionality and appearance of the chelonian liver is affected by both hibernation—when large amounts of fat may be deposited in the liver and decreased synthesis, storage, and release of liver products occur—and, in females, by reproduction—when vitellogenesis and increased protein synthesis occur. Primary hepatic pathology must therefore be differentiated from normal reproductive and seasonal hepatic variation.[2]

PANCREAS

As in other vertebrates, the chelonian pancreas is located adjacent to the proximal segment of the duodenum. The exocrine and endocrine physiologic functions of the chelonian pancreas are similar to that of higher vertebrates. Pancreatic secretions include a variety of different digestive enzymes, including amylase, trypsin, chymotrypsin, carboxypeptidase, elastase, lipase, ribonuclease, and chitinase. The other major pancreatic product is an alkaline secretion that neutralizes the acidic gut contents and creates a more suitable environment for the digestive enzymes.[2]

DIGESTIVE PHYSIOLOGY

Chelonian digestion is dependent on environmental temperature. More specifically, the amount and activity of secreted enzymes[26,27] and the absorptive capability of the intestinal mucosa are directly related to temperature.[21] Maximum digestion occurs within the animal's appropriate temperature range (ATR), and the degree of digestion decreases when either above or below the ATR.[2] At high temperatures, gastric hydrochloric acid production is reduced, thereby altering the pH of the stomach. Consequently, pepsinogen activity is reduced and digestion is slowed.[2] Cell membrane permeability of the gut mucosa is also altered at different temperatures, thereby changing the absorptive processes of glucose and amino acids and the substrate affinity to trypsin.[21] Seasonal fluctuations in digestive rates of chelonians also exist, with rates in summer being higher than those in spring.[27]

It has been determined that extremely slow digestion occurs between 10° C and 15° C (50° F to 59° F) and absolutely no digestion occurs below 7° C (45° F).[21] When temperatures are below this critical level, putrefaction of the ingesta occurs. This occurs often in captive, hibernating chelonians and in captive, imported chelonians that rely on supplemental heat to maintain normal physiologic activities. The absorption of toxic putrefaction products may affect the normal functioning of the nervous or other body systems.[2] Chelonian gastrointestinal contractions have been found to be temperature dependent as well.[2] Chelonian gut contractions are not continuous but rather occur in a series.[28,29] Gastric contractions begin at the cardia, run down the gastric wall in intervals of 21 to 31 seconds, and then terminate at the pylorus. These gastrointestinal contractions are controlled via vagal impulses, and the process is temperature dependent.[30] Contractions of the small intestine occur at intervals of approximately 45 seconds.[31] The first type of large intestinal peristalsis begins at the cecum and ends at the coprodeum. The speed of this type of contraction ranges from 0.15 to 0.5 mm/sec and typically results in defecation. The second type of contraction is an antiperistalsis, which starts at the coprodeum and pushes ingesta cranially for 2 to 3 cm. This type of antiperistalsis occurs at intervals of 18 to 25 seconds and allows urine to be shunted into the caudal parts of the colon where water and ions can be reabsorbed.[21] Gastrointestinal transit time appears to be shortest in omnivorous species and longest in herbivorous species.[21] The large intestines of herbivorous species tend to have a greater volume than those of omnivorous species.[31]

Renal System

Chelonians have two large, flat, lobulated kidneys that are located in the retrocoleomic cavity, ventral to the caudal lung fields and cranial to the pelvic girdle. The chelonian kidney lacks both a loop of Henle and a renal pelvis.[2] The renal nephron is comprised of a glomerulus, a proximal tubule, an intermediate segment, and a distal tubule.[32] The chelonian kidney produces urine that is hypotonic to isotonic to blood and actively excretes uric acid. Bilateral ureters enter the urodeum of the cloaca at approximately the 10 and 2 o'clock positions. As stated previously, antiperistalsis of the urodeum allows urine to be transported caudally into the coprodeum and colon to maximize water and ion absorption. Urine may also travel cranially from the urodeum to the bladder for water reabsorption. The bladder wall is lined with ciliated cells and secretes mucus. The urethra is relatively short in chelonians and enters the bladder through the midventral floor of the urodeum.[2]

RENAL PHYSIOLOGY

The chelonian kidney serves many important functions, including osmoregulation, fluid balance regulation, excretion of metabolic waste products, and the production of various hormones and vitamin D metabolites.[31,33-36] Research has shown that the urine in the renal tubules and ureters of *Gopherus agassizii* is always hypo-osmotic to blood until passage through the urinary bladder, where it becomes isosmotic via presumptive electrolyte and fluid exchange.[34]

Urinary nitrogen is excreted in chelonians as a balance of ammonia, urea, uric acid, amino acids, allantoin, guanine, xanthine, and creatinine.[32-34,37] There are four described chelonian excretion patterns, each largely reflecting the environment in which an animal lives. Uricotelic and ureo-uricotelic chelonians tend to live in arid or desert environments, where water must be conserved. Uricotelic chelonians excrete predominately uric acid and urates, whereas ureo-uricotelic chelonians produce uric acid and urea as their major urinary excretory products. These chelonians are able to conserve water because uric acid is poorly soluble and can be excreted with minimal associated water.[2] In uricotelic chelonians, hypo-osmotic tubular and ureteral urine is thought to decrease urate precipitation within the renal tubules during periods of dehydration.[35] With uricotelism, urates precipitate out of solution in the bladder and do not need to be actively reabsorbed. Ureotelic and amino-ureotelic chelonians live in environments where water is plentiful. Ureotelism occurs when the major urinary excretory product is urea, whereas amino-ureotelism occurs when the major urinary excretory products are both ammonia and urea. Urea is highly water soluble and difficult to concentrate; therefore, it must be excreted with significant amounts of water.[2]

Ureteral urine has three possible pathways to follow once exiting the ureters, and the pathway decided upon is influenced by hydration status, fluid intake, and other biochemical factors. Urine may be directed into the coprodeum/proctodeum upon exiting the ureters. Some fluid reabsorption may occur in the colon or proctodeum, and the urine ultimately mixes with fecal material and is voided simultaneously. Urine may also be directed into the bladder, where electrolyte and fluid exchange occurs and isotonicity, regarding osmolarity and electrolyte composition, results. The bladder of uricotelic and amino-ureotelic species plays a significant role in fluid and electrolyte homeostatic regulation. Uric acid is precipitated out of solution, mainly as potassium urate, within the bladder and is consequently voided at urination. Finally, some ureteral urine may be excreted with no alterations to the fluid or electrolyte composition. It has been suggested that tortoise urination strongly coincides with drinking and bathing, and this is suggestive of an evolutionary mechanism that was developed to ensure the conservation of water in arid environments.[2]

Reproductive System
REPRODUCTIVE ANATOMY

The male chelonian has a single penis (phallus), which protrudes from the floor of the proctodeum. Unlike the mammalian penis, the chelonian phallus is not involved in urination. Paired oval-shaped testes lie within the dorsal coelomic cavity, just cranioventral to the retrocoelomic kidneys. The testes generally fluctuate in size seasonally. The ductus deferens travels alongside the ureters. In the female, two ovaries are present in the coelomic cavity and are suspended from the dorsal coelomic membrane. At ovulation, ova are released into the paired oviducts and are eventually deposited at the urodeum of the cloaca. All chelonians are oviparous.

GENDER IDENTIFICATION

The majority of chelonians are sexually dimorphic, though differences are often not apparent in sexually immature juveniles. There are a number of ways to identify the gender of a chelonian. Male chelonians have a large, fleshy penis that is often heavily pigmented. The chelonian penis also has a median groove to assist in directing sperm during copulation. It must be remembered that clitoral hyperplasia, which may resemble a penis, has also been documented in chelonians. This typically occurs in females treated with oxytocin during dystocia and in debilitated, hypocalcemic, or edematous females. Males typically have longer, broader tails than females, and the distance from the caudal edge of the plastron to the cloacal opening is also generally longer in males than females (Figure 9-6).[2]

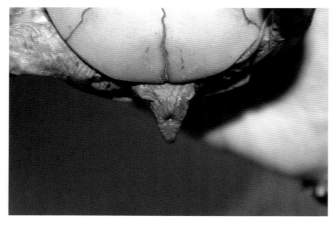

Figure 9-6 The vent of the adult male chelonian opens caudal to the carapace.

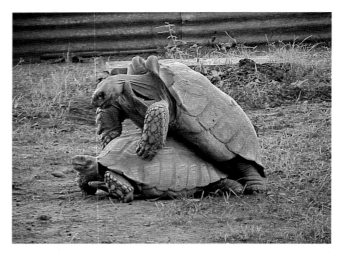

Figure 9-7 The plastron of male tortoises is generally concave. This allows them to mount the females during copulation.

The male plastron of some terrestrial species is concave or indented compared to a female's (Figure 9-7). This is thought to be an adaptation to assist with mounting. Adult males are frequently smaller than females of the same age. Male gopher tortoises *(Gopher polyphemus)* develop large mental glands in their mandibles. Red-eared sliders *(Trachemys scripta elegans)* develop long claws on their front legs and use them to visually stimulate the female turtle. Male box turtles *(Terrapene carolina)* develop red-colored irises, whereas females have yellow-colored irises. The gender determination of hatchling sea turtles has been described using testosterone levels of residual egg fluid.[38] Environmentally sex determined species can potentially be sexed by monitoring the temperature of incubation.[2] Oxygen concentration during incubation is also believed to affect the sex ratio of a clutch.[39] Endoscopy is a useful, yet more invasive, technique to determine the gender of a chelonian.

MATING

In most terrestrial species of chelonians, the male mounts the female from above and behind, and the engorged penis is inserted into the female cloaca. Aquatic species mate underwater. Male courtship behavior, which oftentimes precedes mating, frequently includes characteristic vocalizations and aggression. Males of some chelonian species repeatedly ram females with their gular scutes or bite the head and limbs of trapped females. This behavior is considered necessary to induce females to be submissive for mating. The aggressive behavior, along with pheromones and mating itself, may also induce ovulation in receptive females. Not all ovulation is induced by mating, as evidenced by the fact that some female chelonians may store sperm for up to 4 to 6 years.[2]

REPRODUCTIVE PHYSIOLOGY

Females of most chelonian species exhibit annual reproductive cycles, but some species breed only every 3 to 4 years.[40] Temperate chelonians tend to breed seasonally, whereas tropical species continuously breed.[41] Reproductive physiology is influenced by many different environmental factors, including rainfall, humidity, food availability, presence of a suitable mate, and photoperiod.[2]

Two classes of chelonian vitellogenesis have been described. In the first type, vitellogenesis and follicular growth typically begin in late summer or autumn and are completed just before the winter hibernation. In the second class, which occurs in nonhibernating tropical chelonians, slow follicular growth occurs continuously but is not completed until just before ovulation. Ovulation typically occurs in the spring, and follicular development occurs directly before ovulation. The second type of vitellogenesis occurs less commonly.[42] Some species of chelonians can exhibit both types of vitellogenesis, depending on the environmental conditions. Research in the area of reproduction suggests that some chelonian species may be induced ovulators.[43] Ovulation may be influenced by pheromones, male courtship behavior (e.g., butting, biting, vocalizations), or the act of mating itself.

In chelonians, a distinct corpus luteum is formed following ovulation, and evidence suggests that both the corpus luteum and the chelonian ovary secrete progesterone.[44,45] Progesterone has been shown to inhibit ovulation completely and to reduce oviduct and follicle size in *Chrysemys picta*.[46] Estrogen stimulates vitellogenesis, the production of lipophosphoproteins by the liver, and their incorporation into the egg.[41,45,47,48] It is thought that both estrogens and progesterone influence the hypothalamic release of gonadotropins.[44]

As stated previously, females of some species are capable of storing sperm for 4 to 6 years. Consequently, eggs from females obtained from the wild within this time frame should be considered possibly viable and worthy of incubation.[12,49] Stored sperm is thought to reside in the narrow tubules of the albumin-secreting region of the oviducts,[50] and internal fertilization is thought to occur within the oviduct, postovulation.[12] Fertilized ova continue down the paired oviducts, and the cranial and middle portions of this structure function to produce both yolk and egg components. Calcification of the egg occurs in the caudal portion of the oviduct.[12]

Nesting behavior in chelonians includes a reduction in food ingestion, increased territorial behavior, climbing, and perimeter walking or pacing.[39] Dystocias in captive chelonians can often be attributed to failure to provide a suitable nesting site with an adequate substrate at an appropriate temperature.[51] During oviposition, most chelonians build a nest site via excavation with their hindlimbs. Clutch size varies depending on the species of chelonians, and multiple clutches are possible within one breeding season.

As stated previously, incubation temperature can play a significant role in gender determination in some chelonian species. Research in the area of reproduction of the leatherback turtle *(Dermochelys coriacea)* has revealed a proposed mechanism behind environmental sex determination. It is hypothesized that when eggs are incubated at higher temperatures, the enzyme aromatase is activated and this activation converts available androgen steroid substrate to estrogens. Without the activation of aromatase, no estrogen will be produced and the embryo will remain male.[52,53]

EGG DEVELOPMENT AND ANATOMY

Chelonian eggs are generally deposited in a protected environment and left to develop and incubate in the absence of maternal care. The shell of the egg is comprised of an external mineral layer and an internal fibrous layer. Soon after oviposition, the embryo begins to rise to the dorsal portion of the egg and the yolk settles to the ventral aspect.[54] The first extraembryonic membrane to form is the vitelline or yolk sac membrane. This membrane eventually becomes vascularized and provides the early nutritional and respiratory needs of the embryo. Later in development, the amnion, chorion, and allantois form. The innermost membrane, the amnion, surrounds the embryo and provides fluid support. The allantois acts as a nitrogenous waste container and eventually fuses with the outermost membrane, the chorion. The chorion serves as the major gas exchange organ for the embryo.[2] The development of an air space is variable among chelonian species, along with its location. The importance of this structure is unknown at this time but may play a role in gas exchange before pipping.[55]

The full-term embryo uses the egg tooth, or caruncle, to "pip" its way out of the egg. The extraembryonic membranes are eventually absorbed by the embryo, and after a variable amount of time, the hatchling leaves the egg.[2]

Nervous System

Chelonians have 12 cranial nerves.[56,57] The brain is comprised of approximately 1% of the body mass and contains fairly well-developed optic lobes. The spinal cord travels to the tail tip and no cauda equina is present.[57] A true arachnoid space is not present, and the area between the leptomeninges and the dura mater is known as the subdural space.[3]

Musculoskeletal System

The chelonian beak consists of an upper keratinized horny beak, known as the rhamphotheca, which overlies the maxilla. The horny beak attaches to the mandibular ramus at the dentary and contains no dentition.[2] Unlike in mammals, the chelonian skull is devoid of articulations, except at the jaw.[58] The skull also lacks true temporal openings. On either side of the bony skull, chelonians have large supratemporal fossae. The retractor muscles extend from the fossae and the supraoccipital crest and attach to the base of the skull, thereby allowing chelonians to retract their heads into their shells. The adductor muscles of the chelonian jaw run through a trochlear pulley system, which increases the length of the muscle fibers and provides extra strength. The pulley is formed by a process on the pterygoid bones in Pleurodira and by the quadrate bone in Cryptodira. The pulley system redirects the adductor muscle fibers in a vertical manner for maximum force, thereby allowing the skull of chelonians to remain small yet retain a strong bite.[17,25] Chelonians open their beaks by lowering the mandible.[3]

The thoracic and lumbar ribs are integrated into the shell, and no sternum is present.[2] There are 8 cervical and 10 trunk vertebrae, and the 10 ribs attach to the trunk vertebrae. Whereas the trunk vertebrae are fused together, the cervical vertebrae remain independent of one another, allowing for the bending of the neck sideways (Pleurodira) or retraction into the shell (Cryptodira).[3] Modified thoracic and pelvic limb girdles are present inside the ribs and are fused to the carapace in Pleurodira but not in Cryptodira.[3] The pectoral girdle consists of the epiplastron (clavicle), the entoplastron (interclavicle), the scapula, the acromion process, and the coracoid bone. The pelvic girdle is comprised of the ilium, ischium, and pubic bones, all of which are paired and meet at the acetabula. The ilium is attached dorsally to the sacral ribs.[3] Chelonians generally have pentadactyl limbs that extend more laterally than mammalian limbs. The humerus and femur are short in length, and the carpus and tarsus are both fused. Chelonians have five claws on each foot, with the exception of tortoises—which have short stubby toes and only four claws on the hind feet—and three-toed box turtles (Terrapene carolina).[3]

Sensory System
SIGHT

Vision is highly developed in chelonians.[3] Chelonian eyes are located within orbits in the bony skull and are separated medially by bony structures. In some species, the septum is partially fibrous. A nictitans membrane is present in the majority of chelonian species. The muscles controlling eye movements are the same as those in mammals and consist of the superior and inferior obliques, anterior and posterior retractor bulbi, levator bulbi, and superior and inferior optic rectus muscles. The Harderian gland produces an aqueous secretion and lies in the nasal area. The gland opens into the ventral conjunctival sac, and the ducts of the Harderian gland drain into the craniomedial angle of the eye between the membrane nictitans and the conjunctiva bulbi. The lacrimal gland also produces an aqueous secretion and opens into the conjunctival sac. It is located in the temporal region of the orbit.[2] Due to the lack of nasolacrimal ducts, tears are removed via simple overflow, evaporation, and absorption by the conjunctival mucosa.[59] Evaluation of tear production via the Schirmer tear test is not useful in chelonians.

The cornea of chelonians lacks a Bowman's layer, which is present in the cornea of higher vertebrates. The epithelium of the cornea is very thick and is lined by a thin Descemet's membrane. The iridocorneal angle is less developed than in mammals, and the shape of the anterior chamber is maintained via the production of aqueous humor. Research conducted by Selmi et al. determined that the right and left intraocular pressures of red-footed tortoises (Geochelone carbonaria) were 14.5 ± 8.2 and 15.7 ± 9.3 mmHg, respectively. No change in intraocular pressure was noted as the animals aged.[60] As in birds, the iris sphincter of chelonians is under voluntary control.

The chelonian retina is avascular. Nutrition is provided by choroidal vessels and a vascular projection into the vitreous from the optic nerve head, the conus papillaris, as in the avian pectin. The retina also contains more cones than rods, allowing

chelonians to discern color differences. Many North American box turtle (Terrapene) species are attracted to red and orange,[61] whereas Testudo species prefer red and/or yellow.[2] Herbivorous species appear to recognize the color green. Species that have evolved in low light intensity environments typically have larger globes relative to the overall head size. This grants these species a greater ability to see in low light intensity areas.[2]

OLFACTION

Chelonians have a well-developed olfactory system, and extensive and highly refined chemosensory cells are located within the nasal epithelium.[2] The Jacobson's organ is an accessory olfaction organ that all reptiles possess. It is a paired organ that is located on the rostral roof of the oral cavity over the vomer bones. The Jacobson's organ is simply a localized area of sensory epithelium that is innervated by the vomeronasal nerve (a branch of the olfactory nerve) and is less developed in chelonians than other reptiles.[3] Gular movements in semiaquatic species, which occur when water is pumped through the nasal chamber by pharyngeal contractions, are believed to be related to the olfactory system rather than the respiratory system. Taste buds are also located throughout the oral epithelium, and both taste and smell appear to play a role in appetite stimulation and normal feeding.[2]

HEARING

Chelonians do not have a well-developed sense of hearing. Chelonians do not have external ears but rather exhibit the tympanic membrane (a layer of simple undifferentiated skin). The tympanic membrane lies caudal to the eye, at the level of the commissure of the beak. The function of the tympanic membrane is to protect the middle ear cavity. The tympanic cavity is separated by a process of the quadrate bone into a lateral tympanic cavity and a medial recessus cavi tympani. The inner ear is protected by this bony process. Sound is transferred from the tympanic membrane to the underlying extracolumella, a cartilaginous disc that is connected to an ossicular process, known as the columella. The columella is made up of a thin osseous shaft that penetrates through a small hole in the bony ventral process of the quadrate bone to contact the inner ear. The inner ear then ends in a funnel-shaped plate. Rotational movement is also transferred to the inner ear in the same manner, and it is believed that chelonian ears may be more important for balance than for hearing. It is thought that chelonians are only capable of hearing low tones, which may be due more to vibrations than to auditory signals.[2]

▆ HUSBANDRY
Environmental Conditions
ENCLOSURE SIZE

The shape and size of the enclosure should be selected based on the chelonian's habitat preference. Aquatic species should be provided deep, leak-proof enclosures, whereas tortoises can be provided shallow containers. All chelonians should be provided the largest enclosure possible. Some recommendations call for the enclosure to be at least four times the size of the turtle's carapace; however, we feel this is too small. Instead, we prefer that the enclosure be at least 10 times the carapace diameter. Maximizing the surface area of the enclosure is important for ensuring ample area for exercise and an appropriate thermal gradient. Providing a large enclosure is also important because of the feeding habits of the chelonians. Tortoises are grazers and can generally consume large quantities of grass hay in their enclosure. If the enclosure is too small, the animals will overconsume their substrate. For aquatic animals it is important because these animal consume their food in the water. For those species that require live food, a larger enclosure ensures that the animal must exercise, providing enrichment, to capture its prey. A larger enclosure also helps to ensure better water quality, as small enclosures can become fouled relatively quickly.

Chelonian enclosures can be made from a variety of materials. The most common enclosure for aquatic species remains the glass fish tank. These enclosures are relatively inexpensive, easy to clean, and provide direct visualization of the pet. These are not considered as ideal for tortoises because they are poorly ventilated; however, limited ventilation can also be a problem for aquatic species. Plastic storage boxes are another common commercial product used to house chelonians. These enclosures are also inexpensive, easy to clean, and readily available. Many of these enclosures are not clear, so direct visualization may be limited; however, with chelonians the risk of escape is minimal so lids are not generally necessary unless they are being used to prevent unauthorized contact with children or domestic pets. Tortoises do not generally fare well in wire-based cages, as they may develop rostral or limb abrasions while trying to pass through the cage. We have found that tortoises can be kept outdoors in pens created from wood or tin (Figure 9-8). Any tortoises or turtles kept in outdoor pens should be protected from both domestic pets (e.g., dogs) and wildlife predators.

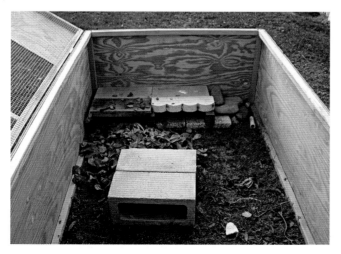

Figure 9-8 Tortoises can be housed outdoors in a variety of enclosures. This is an example of a simple wooden pen.

TEMPERATURE

Chelonians are ectotherms and depend on the environmental temperature to regulate their core body temperature. If these animals are not provided an appropriate temperature range, their metabolic rate slows. Chelonians with reduced metabolic rates often present with a history of being anorectic, lethargic, and depressed. An inability to maintain an appropriate body temperature can also result in a reduced immune response. In our experience, many of the chelonians that presented with chronic infections are not provided exposure to an appropriate environmental temperature. To prevent these problems, chelonians should be provided an environmental temperature range. The environmental temperature should mimic the animal's natural climate and should be separated into different gradients. It is important to realize that reptiles have temperature options in nature. They can bask under the sun on a rock if they wish or hide in the shade away from the heat to prevent overheating. This same system should be mimicked in captivity. Chelonians generally bask during the early morning and late afternoon and recover to shelter during the middle of the day when the heat is the highest. We recommend that clients use variable wattage incandescent light to create a temperature gradient. Bulb wattage will depend on the size of the enclosure. The following temperature gradients are appropriate for chelonians: temperate species (75° F to 85° F; 23.9° C to 29.4° C), tropical species (80° F to 88° F; 26.7° C to 31.1° C), and desert species (85° F to 95° F; 29.4° C to 35.0° C). It is important to provide chelonians a cooling period at night (5° F to 10° F). Water temperatures for aquatic species should range between 75° F and 80° F (26.6° C to 31.1° C). Visible light (e.g., incandescent bulbs) should not be used at night to provide heat. It is important that animals are provided a period of darkness. We generally recommend a photoperiod of 12 hours per day. This can be altered during the breeding cycle (lengthened) or aestivation period (shortened). When supplemental heat is required during periods of darkness, ceramic heat emitters or under-tank heating elements can be used. Regardless of the heat source, chelonians should not be allowed direct contact with the heating element. Animals that are allowed direct contact can develop severe thermal injuries (first to third degree). For thermal injury treatment options, please refer to the snake chapter.

HUMIDITY

Humidity is an important environmental factor to consider for tortoises, but it is less important for aquatic species because they live in a moist environment. In general, desert tortoise species tolerate humidity levels between 30% and 50%, subtropical species from 60% to 80%, and tropical species 80% to 90%. Chelonians maintained in environments with low humidity may become anorectic and dehydrated and develop reduced gastrointestinal transit times. Excessive humidity is frequently associated with the development of dermatitis and respiratory disease. Humidity levels can be monitored using a hygrometer. Digital hygrometers are preferred because they can be moved around within an enclosure to determine areas that are appropriate and inappropriate. Humidity levels can be altered in an enclosure by adding a large water bowl, aerating water within a water receptacle (e.g., bowl or mason jar), adding an incubation chamber, misting the enclosure daily, or adding live plants. Large water bowls serve as a source of humidity for an enclosure, as the water evaporates into the enclosure. The overall contribution of moisture to the humidity can vary based on the environmental temperature and size of the enclosure. Daily misting is a simple method for elevating the humidity but may provide only a temporary increase to the humidity.

LIGHTING

Historically, lighting systems for captive chelonians have not been given a great deal of attention. Herpetoculturists who maintain their animals indoors often provide only ambient light. Animals maintained outdoors derive the most benefit from routine exposure to direct or indirect sunlight. A recent study in red-eared sliders (*Trachemys scripta elegans*) found that animals provided exposure to full-spectrum fluorescent lighting were significantly more likely than controls to have higher 25-hydroxyvitamin D plasma levels.[62] Full-spectrum lighting has many benefits, from the provision of ultraviolet radiation to rich, visible light. Although the benefits of full-spectrum lighting have not been evaluated in other species of chelonians, we recommend providing captive chelonians full-spectrum lighting to mimic the beneficial effects of sunlight. Chelonians should be provided a 12-hour photoperiod. The photoperiod can be altered for the breeding season (lengthened) or brumation period (shortened).

SUBSTRATE

Substrate selection for chelonians is an important consideration, as many of these animal are geophagic and can develop foreign bodies if provided an inappropriate substrate. Aquatic species should be provided a gravel substrate. Larger pieces of gravel that are not edible are preferred. Sand may be used but is generally more difficult to manage, is easily stirred, and may increase the water turbidity. Aquatic species not provided a substrate may develop pressure sores, especially if maintained in plastic enclosures. Terrestrial species may be housed on a variety of different substrates. When considering which substrate is best for a particular species, it is important to attempt to replicate its natural habitat. Most of these animals are naturally found on grass, detritus, or rock-based substrates. Maintaining tortoises in outdoor facilities, when weather permits, provides the most realistic substrate. This type of substrate also provides a regular food source. The provision of a grass substrate is more difficult for captive, indoor tortoises. The following is a list of common substrates used for tortoises held indoors: newspaper, paper towels, alfalfa pellets (Figure 9-9), large gravel, orchid bark chips, grass hay, and straw. Newspaper and paper towels are commonly used for juvenile animals and recently acquired animals because they are inexpensive, can be easily replaced, and allow a veterinarian or herpetoculturist to monitor fecal and urine output. There is a wives' tale that the ink found on newspaper is potentially toxic to animals, but this belief is unfounded. Gravel can be used but should be

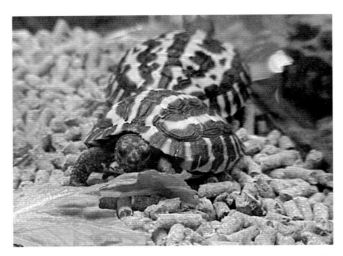

Figure 9-9 Chelonians can be housed on a variety of substrates. These spider tortoises *(Pyxis arachnoides)* are being housed on rabbit pellets.

sufficiently large enough to prevent ingestion. Orchid bark chips can be used as a substrate for those species naturally found in forested areas. Natural leaf litter can also be used but should be thoroughly inspected for the presence of pest bugs before being placed into the vivarium. Alfalfa pellets and grass hay are commonly used because they can serve as both a substrate and source of nutrition. However, these substrates are easily soiled and can serve as a source of infection (e.g., bacterial or fungal) to these animals. In any case, the type of substrate to be used should be selected based on the specific needs of a particular animal. If one substrate does not appear to be of value, another should be evaluated.

WATER QUALITY

Aquatic species must be provided access to a clean water source. The best method for ensuring that the animal's aquatic environment is clean is to use filtration. Many of the filtration methods used to maintain aquatic systems for ornamental fish can be used for turtles, although turtles can produce significantly more biologic waste than ornamental fish. The primary filtration units used for aquatic systems are mechanical, chemical, and biologic. Mechanical filtration consists primarily of material that traps organic material. Many of the new power or canister filters use sponge-like materials and floss as mechanical filters. Chemical filtration is generally done using the addition of specific chemicals (e.g., those that chelate ammonia) or charcoal. Charcoal binds to noxious chemicals, rendering them nontoxic. Ultraviolet radiation can also be used as a chemical filter to kill potential pathogens. Biologic filters are based on the premise that living bacteria naturally degrade potential toxins (e.g., ammonia and nitrite) to less toxic compounds (e.g., nitrate). These filters work by providing surface area within the enclosure for the bacteria (e.g., *Nitrosomonas* spp. and *Nitrobacter* spp.) to colonize. All three of these filtration methods can be used in aquatic turtle systems. It is important to recognize that because turtles produce significant quantities of organic waste, mechanical filters must be changed more regularly than in ornamental fish systems.

ACCESSORIES

A chelonian vivarium should mimic an animal's natural habitat. Accessories or "cage furniture" can be used to create an environment that reduces the stress an animal may otherwise encounter in captivity. It is important to always attempt to minimize stress, as it can lead to elevated corticosterone levels that affect the animal's metabolic rate and immune function. Terrestrial animals should be provided an appropriate substrate (see Substrate) and an adequate number of hiding locations or shelters. Shelters can be made from cardboard boxes, plastic potting containers, or any material that can shelter the animal. For fossorial species, a packed substrate should be used to allow the animal to burrow. Chelonians should be provided access to water at all times. A water bowl should be placed in the vivarium that is large enough for the animal to enter. Chelonians routinely soak when provided access to water. Soaking is thought to increase gastrointestinal motility and serve as a stimulus to drink. The water should be changed daily or as it is soiled.

◼ NUTRITION
Dietary Requirements

Chelonians may be herbivorous, omnivorous, or carnivorous, depending on the species. An ideal diet for captive chelonians mimics their natural diet as closely as possible and provides a diversified selection of food. Some herbivorous species will often readily eat an omnivorous diet,[63] but eventually these animals will reveal signs of nutritional deficiencies.[64] Therefore, it is important to remember that food preferences do not always correlate with appropriate nutrition.

Herbivorous Chelonians

Herbivorous tortoises and marine turtles are classified as hindgut fermenters,[65,66] with microbial fermentation occurring in the large intestine. Consequently, the bulk of the diet of herbivorous tortoises should be vegetable fiber. The vegetable fiber offered to tortoises should be rich in vitamins A and D_3 and should have more available calcium than phosphorous.[39] An ideal Ca : P ratio of at least 1.5 : 1 to 2 : 1 should be present.[67] The diet should also be low in fats, oils, proteins, thiocyanates, and oxalates.[39] In captivity, tortoises are typically fed weeds, flowers, and grasses on a daily basis. Tortoises will forage for themselves if provided an appropriately planted enclosure, but additional food is usually required. It is important to periodically peruse the yard and rule out the presence of any poisonous plants, such as rhubarb,[63] daffodils, potatoes, buttercup, and yew. A variety of foods should be offered and can be mixed with calcium, iodine, vitamin D_3, and vitamin A supplementation. It is important to remember that grocery greens are generally higher in protein and lower in fiber and

may have an inverse calcium-to-phosphorus ratio to natural forage.[68] Spinach, cabbage, and beet greens should not be fed in excess due to their high oxalate content. The majority of foods designed for dogs, cats, humans, and other mammals should not be fed to tortoises. Debilitated tortoises requiring force-feeding or tube-feedings should be fed a critical care diet designed for herbivorous reptiles.

Omnivorous Chelonians

It has been suggested that omnivorous chelonians do best when offered plant and animal matter in proportions that range from 75:25 to 90:10.[69] Dietary requirements in these species tend to change with age, with most juveniles requiring a diet comprised of a higher proportion of animal matter. As the juveniles mature, their dietary requirements shift to a more herbivorous diet.[68]

Free-ranging omnivorous chelonians will ingest earthworms, slugs, snails, millipedes, pupae, and maggots. It is essential to monitor the diets of captive invertebrates to avoid nutritional deficiencies in the chelonians that are ingesting them. The insects, worms, and pupae should be offered a diet rich in minerals and vitamins to ensure that the prey is "gut-loaded" and will meet the nutritional needs of the predator species. The invertebrate prey should also be dusted with calcium powder before feeding to ensure that the proper calcium-to-phosphorus ratio is maintained.[63] Chelonians appear to prefer "slightly rotten" fruits and vegetables, and their diets may be occasionally supplemented in very small amounts with meat, fish, or low-fat dog or cat food.[68] However, it is important to consider that "slightly rotten" foods may have more microbes associated with them and may predispose the chelonian to food poisoning. In addition, mammalian diets should generally be avoided long term as they may be too potent (e.g., excess protein and vitamins) for a chelonian. Liver and yellow or dark orange colored vegetables (squash, carrots, sweet potatoes) are excellent sources of vitamin A,[70] and Swiss chard, kale, beet greens, escarole, parsley, watercress, and green beans all have a positive Ca : P ratio.

Most semiaquatic chelonians are omnivorous. There are many commercial pelleted diets available (e.g., Aquatic Turtle Diet, Fluker Farms, Port Allen, LA) that suit the nutritional needs of these particular chelonians (Figure 9-10). Some species, such as the Chinese three-striped box turtle *(Cuora trifasciata)* and the Malayan box turtle *(Cuora amboinesis)*, prefer to be fed in the water. Abnormal shell and bone growth may occur if the diet being offered is too high in animal protein. These diets are often also high in phosphorus, which disrupts the normal calcium-to-phosphorus ratio. Fruits and vegetables should be dusted with calcium and vitamin powder just before being offered. Obesity can be avoided by feeding adults three to four times per week.[68]

Asian box turtles *(Cuora* spp.) are a commonplace captive semiaquatic chelonian. Hatchlings feed almost entirely on animal prey, whereas adult turtles require vegetable and fruit supplementation. It has been suggested that one third to one half of the diet offered to adults should be plant based, and

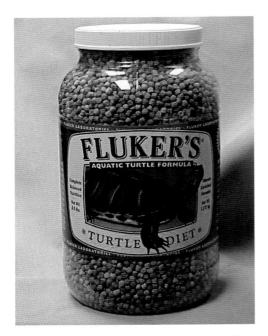

Figure 9-10 Commercial turtle chows can be used in combination with natural food items to diversify an animal's diet.

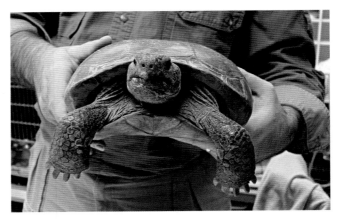

Figure 9-11 For nonaggressive chelonians, the animal can be restrained by grasping the sides of the shell.

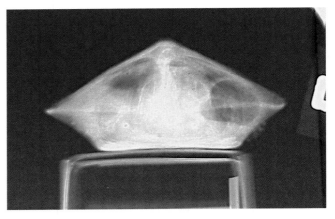

Figure 9-12 Chelonians can be placed onto a roll of tape or other support to minimize movement during a radiograph.

the remaining one half to two thirds should be animal matter. The plant portion of the diet should be made up of 70% to 80% vegetable matter and 20% to 30% fruit matter.[70] Plant matter offered should include collard and mustard greens, kale, bok choy, dandelions, apples, grapes, strawberries, bananas, and pears. Animal matter suitable for ingestion includes whole, skinned, chopped mice; pinkies; trout chow; earthworms; crickets; slugs; maggots; and sardines.[68]

The red-eared slider *(T. scripta elegans)* also feeds on a variety of animal and vegetable matter and almost exclusively feeds in the water. Greens, fruit, commercial turtle chow, pond fish pellets, raw whole fish, liver, and insects are commonly offered.[68] The adult red-eared slider is primarily herbivorous.[68]

Carnivorous Chelonians

There are a number of aquatic chelonians that are considered true carnivores. One species, the snapping turtle *(C. serpentina)*, has also been found to have vegetation mixed with its stomach contents and is presumed by some to have omnivorous tendencies, although others suggest this finding is more directly related to their feeding strategy. When snapping turtles pursue their food, they strike and grab everything they can at once, which may include the surrounding vegetation. Most carnivorous species (e.g., mata mata turtle; *C. fimbriatus)* are piscivorous. It is important to provide these animals a prey species that mimics their natural diets. Goldfish *(Carassius auratus)* are generally offered because of availability but are a very fatty fish and can provide a potential hepatic toxin. When offering wild fish, it is important to consider that they may serve as reservoirs for infectious diseases and parasites. Pretreating with a salt bath (5-10 ppt) may help to reduce some (but

not all) of the burden. If frozen fish are offered, then the turtle should be supplemented with thiamine, as frozen-thawed fish can produce thiaminases.

■ RESTRAINT
Manual Restraint

The chelonian patient rarely requires significant or forceful restraint; however, large freshwater snapping turtles and marine turtles may pose exceptions to this. Small chelonians can easily be handled with a hand on either side of the carapace (Figure 9-11). Larger chelonians may be restrained with the placement of one hand around the cranial carapace, dorsal to the neck, with the other hand around the caudal carapace, dorsal to the tail. The beak should always be directed away from the handler. To passively restrain a chelonian patient for radiographs or some other procedure, the patient may be placed on a raised object, such as a roll of tape or a circular feeding dish, which is positioned in the center of the plastron (Figure 9-12). With nothing for their limbs to make contact with, the patient is effectively immobilized. It is very important to note that hypothermia is an inappropriate method of restraint. The chelonian head can be restrained by grasping the base of the skull at the point of the mandibular rami with the index finger and thumb. Gentle traction should be used to extend the head and neck. Never use excessive pressure, as this can lead to cervical spinal injury.

Chemical Restraint

Most chelonians can be restrained manually; however, in those cases where it is necessary to immobilize the patient, chemical restraint may be necessary. Of all of the reptiles, chelonians, in our opinion, require the highest dosing levels. Appropriate chemical immobilization drugs and dosages can be found in the Anesthesia section of this chapter.

■ PERFORMING A PHYSICAL EXAMINATION

The physical examination of the chelonian patient should be performed in a systematic manner to ensure that all organ systems are examined.

Head and Associated Structures

The cornea and lens of the chelonian eye should both be transparent. Suspicious areas of the cornea may be stained with fluorescein to assess for corneal ulceration. The eyes, conjunctiva, and eyelids should be examined for evidence of swelling, discharge, conjunctivitis, or conjunctival hyperplasia, which may be consistent with vitamin A deficiency. The pupillary and menace ocular reflexes should be assessed. It is important to realize that, depending on the species, some chelonians will blink in response to the menace reflex, whereas others will retract their heads into their shells.

The position of the eyes in the sockets should also be closely examined. The eyes may appear bilaterally enophthalmic in cases of severe dehydration, whereas bilateral exophthalmia may be observed concurrently with generalized edema. Unilateral enophthalmia is suggestive of injury or trauma, and unilateral exophthalmia is consistent with either trauma or the presence of a retrobulbar abscess or tumor.[71]

The nares should be inspected for the presence of discharge. Cutaneous erosion, softness, and depigmentation are often associated with chronic upper respiratory tract disease. The jaw and beak should both be palpated and closely assessed. A soft and flexible jaw may be discovered in juveniles suffering from fibrous osteodystrophy secondary to nutritional hyperparathyroidism. Instability of the jaw may result from trauma or pathologic fractures. An overgrown beak is oftentimes associated with a nutritional disease, such as vitamin A deficiency; however, we have found most of these cases to have acceptable nutrition. Instead, we have found that overgrown beaks are associated with limited diets that do not provide much wear on the beak.

The oral cavity should be assessed with the help of an oral speculum or other nontraumatic instrument. The oral mucous membranes should be examined for pallor, cyanosis, or conges-

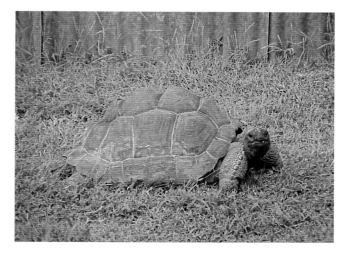

Figure 9-13 Shell pyramiding has been associated with high protein diets and limited exposure to water. It is likely that this issue is multicausal.

tion. Stomatitis may appear as erythema, hemorrhage, pallor, or yellow diphtheroid membrane formation. Ulceration of the mucous membranes, petechiation, and caseation are also consistent with stomatitis. The glottis should be examined for erythema, edema, or discharge. The glottis is located at the base of the tongue and can be visualized by gently pushing on the intermandibular (gular) space. The tympanic membranes should be assessed for the presence of swelling, which may be consistent with abscessation or hypovitaminosis A.

Shell

The shell should be examined for scute quality. Pyramiding of the scutes has been associated with excessive dietary protein ingestion and limited access to water (Figure 9-13). Abnormal keratinization, ulceration of the shell, discharges, swelling, soft areas, and malodorousness should be recorded. Poor calcification of the shell is often associated with secondary nutritional hyperparathyroidism, and a reddish hue of the plastron may be suggestive of septicemia (e.g., vasculitis). Ulcerative shell disease is most consistent with the presence of shell ulceration and discharge.

Appendages

All limbs should be thoroughly palpated and the range of motion of each joint assessed. Each limb should be compared to the opposite appendage to detect any asymmetric abnormalities, such as fractured bones or joint abnormalities (e.g., infection or articular gout). The musculature overlying the radius and ulna and tibia is indicative of the body condition. A well-fleshed lower limb is indicative of a positive energy state, whereas the palpation of musculature that closely follows the contour of the bones is supportive of a negative energy balance or emaciation. The distal limbs should be examined for the presence of nail abnormalities, which may be consistent with lameness or inappropriate husbandry conditions. Frost damage may appear as edema of the lower limbs.

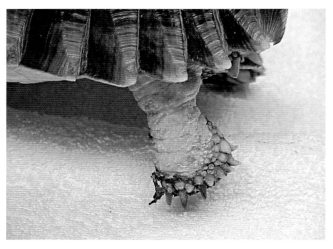

Figure 9-14 Iatrogenic hypervitaminosis A can occur as a result of oversupplementing vitamin A. In this sulcata tortoise case, the animal sloughed its skin.

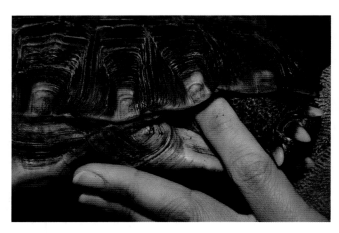

Figure 9-15 During a routine examination, it is important to palpate the coelomic cavity. This can be done by inserting a finger into the prefemoral area. This is generally not possible in larger specimens.

Skin

The skin should be examined for abnormal shedding, sloughing, edema, ulceration, abscessation, or discharge. Decreased skin elasticity is often consistent with dehydration. Excessive administration of vitamin A may result in blistering and sloughing of the skin on the limbs (Figure 9-14). The exudate is often clear. The skin should also be examined for parasitic infestation. This is most commonly observed in chelonians recently captured from the wild.

Coelom

The coelom may be palpated via insertion of one to two fingers just in front of the caudal limbs in the prefemoral fossae (Figure 9-15). The presence of ascites, visceral enlargement, a space-occupying mass, or a calcified egg can be assessed via digital palpation. Calcified eggs can also sometimes be found inside the coprodeum via gentle palpation on either side of the tail.

Cloaca

The cloaca should be examined for the presence of erythema, edema, trauma, or discharge. Cloacal digital examination may be necessary in cases of suspected dystocia, cystic calculi, or space-occupying lesions or to check choanal and cloacal tone.

Auscultation

It is generally considered difficult to auscultate the heart and lungs of a chelonian using a standard stethoscope. We have found that a crystal ultrasound Doppler is the best method for assessing the heart. The Doppler probe should be placed between the head and forelimb (either side) and directed cau-

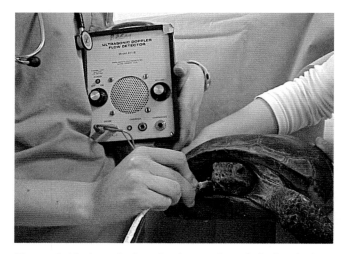

Figure 9-16 Auscultating the heart of a chelonian is best achieved using a Doppler. The probe should be inserted in the distal cervical area and directed caudally toward the heart.

dally toward the heart (Figure 9-16). The same technique can be used to assess the heart during anesthesia.

■ DIAGNOSTIC TESTING
Hematology

Blood can be extracted from the chelonian patient using a variety of techniques and venipuncture sites. A maximum of 5 to 8 ml/kg body weight of blood may be collected, but typically 1 to 1.5 ml/kg is sufficient. The jugular vein yields blood samples that are least likely to be lymph diluted and is the vessel of choice in patients weighing less than 4 kg. The head and neck may be extended and restrained via placement of a finger and thumb behind the occiput. The chelonian can then be placed in lateral recumbency, and the jugular vein can oftentimes be visualized as it extends caudally from the angle of the mandible. The vessel should be entered in a caudal-pointing direction (Figure 9-17). The dorsal venous sinus, or the dorsal coccygeal vein, may be utilized in some species of chelonians and is typically found in the dorsal midline of the tail. It must be mentioned that lymph dilution may occur in this site and potential damage to the central nervous system may ensue if the subarachnoid space is entered and cerebral spinal fluid is sampled without proper disinfection of the sampling site.

The subcarapacial venous sinus can also be utilized for blood sampling or intravenous drug administration. A 22- or 25-gauge, 1- to 1.5-inch hypodermic needle is inserted dorsal to the cervical neck directly on midline just ventral to the carapace at an approximately 60-degree angle (Figure 9-18). The turtle's neck may be flexed or extended. If a cervical ver-

tebra is contacted with the tip of the needle, the needle is slightly withdrawn and redirected cranially or caudally. Other venipuncture sites can also be utilized but are also subject to lymph contamination. These sites include the brachial venous plexus, femoral venous plexus, and the femoral vein.

Once the blood is collected, a packed cell volume may be determined using a microhematocrit tube. Calcium-ethylenediaminetetraacetic acid has been reported to cause hemolysis in chelonian blood samples[71]; however, more recent research suggests this may not be consistent across all species. Blood smears should be prepared with fresh, nonclotted, whole blood, as lithium heparin can cause leukocyte and thrombocyte clumping. The coverslip technique has been recommended over the conventional, second slide technique to decrease cell lysis.[73] We have found that mixing five drops of reptile blood with one drop of bovine albumin (22%, Gamma Biologics, Houston, TX) minimizes white blood cell lysis on the slide and allows for a more accurate white blood cell estimate. The blood smears, regardless of the method of creation, should be stained with Diff-Quick, Wright-Giemsa, or another rapid stain. An automated total white blood cell counting system is not currently available for the reptilian patient; therefore, this task must be manually performed via the eosinophil Unopette system or Natt and Herrick's or Rees and Ecker's staining solutions. There is currently no recommended, accurate method to determine thrombocyte counts. Examples for white blood cell types in chelonians can be found in Figures 9-19 through 9-22 and Table 9-1.

Biochemical Analysis

Biochemical analysis of blood can be run on either serum or plasma. Reference ranges for biochemistry analysis for various chelonian species are found in Table 9-2. It must be remembered that the validity of "normal" values depends upon the knowledge of the circumstances of their source (species, sex, age, season, sample size, nutrition, and general husbandry).

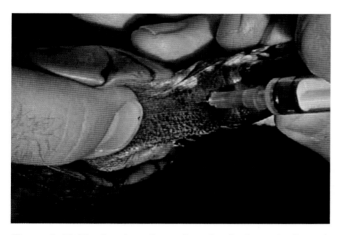

Figure 9-17 The jugular vein tends to be the best site for collecting lymph-free blood samples. This vessel can be located on the lateral surface of the neck. The tympanum is an excellent landmark for locating the vessel.

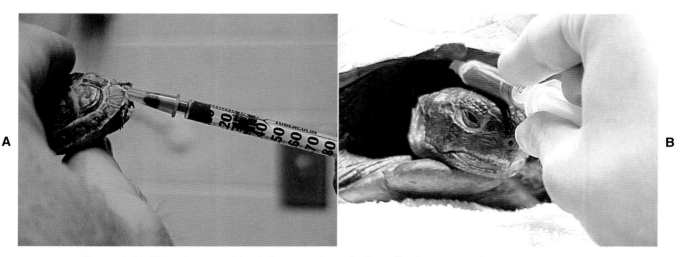

Figure 9-18 The subcarapacial vein is an excellent site for collecting samples in fractious chelonians or animals where the neck cannot be withdrawn (**A** and **B**).

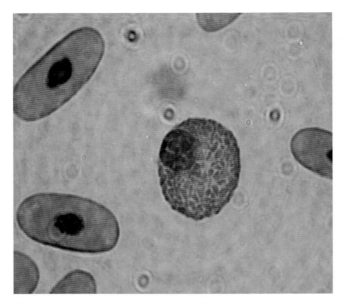

Figure 9-19 A gopher tortoise *(Gopherus polyphemus)* heterophil.

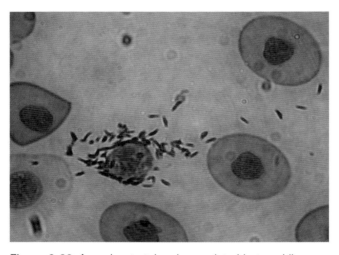

Figure 9-20 A gopher tortoise degranulated heterophil.

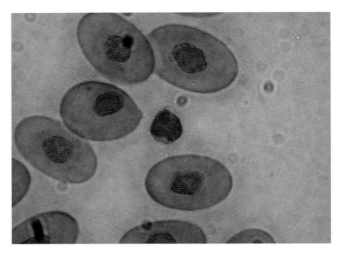

Figure 9-21 A gopher tortoise lymphocyte.

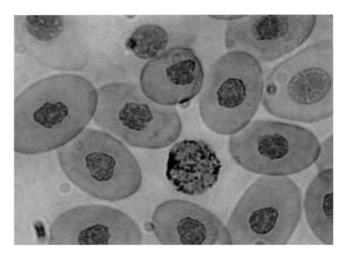

Figure 9-22 A gopher tortoise basophil.

Urinalysis

Chelonians frequently urinate during stressful handling or stimulatory procedures, such as venipuncture. Although a urine culture should not be performed on a free-catch sample, urinalysis values can still be accurately interpreted. Culturing urine is generally not recommended in chelonian patients, regardless of the method of collection, because the urodeum is continuous with the coprodeum and feces may retrograde back into the bladder and cause contamination. Although cystocentesis is easily preformed via insertion of a needle and syringe in the prefemoral fossa, the bladder wall is very thin and there is significant risk of consequent urine leakage. Urethral catheterization of the chelonian patient, an alternative to cystocen-

tesis, typically requires anesthesia or sedation and the use of a rigid endoscope.

Although urine examination has proven to be useful in the diagnosis of several pathologic conditions, not all values commonly utilized in the mammalian urinalysis have been validated in chelonian medicine. Urine samples from a variety of grossly normal terrestrial herbivorous chelonians maintained in captivity revealed urine-specific gravity values ranging from 1.003 to 1.012.[86] The urine-specific gravity of desert tortoises *(Gopherus agassizii)* was assessed at peak rainfall, and values of 1.005 to 1.009 were obtained. At other times of the year, the urine-specific gravity of *Gopherus agassizii* was determined to be 1.005 to 1.029. It is important to keep in mind both that the chelonian kidney is designed to produce hypo- to isosmotic urine and that the urine-specific gravity is furthered modified by water and electrolyte exchange across the bladder wall.[34] Conclusions about renal function can therefore not be drawn based upon urine-specific gravity values alone.

| TABLE 9-1 | Hematologic Reference Ranges for Various Chelonian Species |

Parameter	Radiated tortoise (*Geochelone radiata*)[74]	*Testudo marginata;* dorsal coccygeal vein[75]	*Testudo marginata;* brachial vein[75]
Erythrocyte count (10^6/µl)	0.53-0.67	0.2-0.49	0.43-0.77
Hematocrit (%)	19.0-45.0	19-58	52-73
Hemoglobin (g/dl)	4.5-8.6		
Leukocytes (10^3/µl)	2.5-5.9	0.70-4.20	2.70-7.80
Lymphocytes (10^3/µl)	0.40-3.4	0.31-2.90	1.12-5.54
Monocytes (10^3/µl)	0.025-0.47	0.00-0.08	0.00-0.31
Eosinophils (10^3/µl)	0.025-0.53	0.00-0.76	0.00-0.86
Basophils (10^3/µl)	0.10-0.94		
Heterophils (10^3/µl)	0.68-3.4	0.37-1.85	0.57-3.9

Parameter	Aldabra tortoise *Geochelone giganteus*[76]	Gopher tortoise *Gopherus polyphemus*[77]
PCV (%)	17 (11-27)	23 (15-30)
RBC (10^6/µl)	0.4 (0.3-0.7)	0.54 (0.24-0.91)
Hb (g/dl)	5.4 (3.2-8.0)	6.4 (4.2-8.6)
MCV (pg)	452 (375-537)	
MCH (g/dl)	146 (118-185)	
MCHC (g/dl)	33 (28-40)	
WBC (10^3/µl)	3.4 (1.0-8.3)	15.7 (10-22)
Heterophils (%)	71 (32-79)	30 (10-57)
Lymphocytes (%)	22 (2-40)	57 (32-79)
Monocytes (%)	2 (0-8)	7 (3-13)
Eosinophils (%)	0.5 (0-7)	
Basophils (%)	2 (0-4)	6 (2-11)

Parameter	Red-eared slider *Trachemys scripta*[78]
PCV (%)	29 (25-33)
RBC (10^6/µl)	0.3-0.8
Hb (g/dl)	8.0
MCV (pg)	
MCH (g/dl)	
MCHC (g/dl)	
WBC (10^3/µl)	13 (3.5-25.5)
Heterophils (%)	
Lymphocytes (%)	
Monocytes (%)	
Azurophils (%)	
Eosinophils (%)	
Basophils (%)	

Parameter	Common box turtles *Terrapene carolina*[79,80,81]
PCV (%)	22 (7-35)
RBC (10^6/µl)	0.5 (0.09-1)
Hb (g/dl)	5.1
MCV (pg)	420 (229-1000)
MCH (g/dl)	102
MCHC (g/dl)	28 (26-29)
WBC (10^3/µl)	7 (1.7-16)
Heterophils (%)	11
Lymphocytes (%)	56
Monocytes (%)	9.4
Azurophils (%)	
Eosinophils (%)	
Basophils (%)	9

TABLE 9-2 Biochemistry Analyte Reference Ranges for Various Chelonian Species

Parameter	Radiated tortoise Geochelone radiata[74]	Testudo marginata; coccygeal vein[75]	Testudo marginata; brachial vein[75]	Desert tortoise Gopherus agassizii[82]
Albumin (g/dl)	0.8-1.3			
Alkaline phosphatase (ALP) (IU/L)	72-120	53-164	180-295	
Calcium (mg/dl)	10.8-14.4			9-17
Cholesterol (mg/dl)	60.2-153.5			
Glucose (mg/dl)	46.2-92.8			30-150
Aspartate aminotransferase (IU/L)	42.0-134.0	25-83	47-98	
Lactate dehydrogenase (IU/L)	213.4-591.5	31-431	182-882	25-250
Phosphorous (mg/dl)	2.6-4.3			
Total protein (g/dl)	3.2-5.0	8.0-32.0	32.0-39.0	2.2-5.0
Uric acid (mg/dl)	0.0-0.6			2.2-9.2
Sodium (mEq/L)	121.0-132.0			130-157
Potassium (mEq/L)	5.1-5.8			2.2-4.5
Chloride (mEq/L)	92.0-99.0			
Carbon dioxide (mEq/L)	24.0-29.0			

Parameter	Aldabra tortoise Geochelone giganteus[76]	Gopher tortoise Gopherus polyphemus[77]
Alkaline phosphatase (IU/L)	111 (29-182)	39 (11-71)
Alanine aminotransferase (IU/L)	7 (0-26)	15 (2-57)
Aspertate aminotransferase (IU/L)	57 (5-138)	136 (57-392)
Bilirubin, total (mg/dl)	0.2 (0-0.3)	0.02 (0-0.1)
Urea (mg/dl)	33 (21-57)	30 (1-130)
Calcium (mg/dl)	12 (6-20)	12 (10-14)
Chloride (mEq/L)	93 (87-107)	102 (35-128)
Cholesterol (mg/dl)	275 +/− 135	76 (19-150)
Creatinine kinase (IU/L)	303 +/− 635	160 (32-628)
Creatinine (mg/dl)	0.1 (0.1-0.2)	0.3 (0.1-0.4)
Glucose (mg/dl)	50 +/− 16	75 (55-128)
Lactate dehydrogenase (IU/L)	532 +/− 430	273 (18-909)
Magnesium (mEq/L)	5.1 +/− 0.3	4.1 (3.3-4.8)
Phosphorus (mg/dl)	4.3 (1.6-12.1)	2.1 (1.0-3.1)
Potassium (mEq/L)	4.7 (3.2-6.1)	5.0 (2.9-7.0)
Protein, total (g/dl)	4.1 (0.6-6.2)	3.1 (1.3-4.6)
Albumin (g/dl)	1.5 (0.3-2.6)	1.5 (0.5-2.6)
Globulins (g/dl)	2.6 (0.3-3.6)	
Sodium (mEq/L)	133 (129-136)	138 (127-148)
Uric acid (mg/dl)	1.6 (0-4.9)	3.5 (0.9-8.5)

Parameter	Red-eared slider Trachemys scripta[78]	Mediterranean tortoise Testudo hermanni[83]
Alkaline phosphatase (IU/L)	212 (81-343)	196-425
Alanine aminotransferase (IU/L)	16 +/− 22	
Aspertate aminotransferase (IU/L)	202 (0-419)	19-103
Bilirubin, total (mg/dl)	0.3 +/− 0.3	
Urea (mg/dl)	22	
Calcium (mg/dl)	14 (14-15)	10.8-14.0
Chloride (mEq/L)	102 (97-107)	96-115
Cholesterol (mg/dl)	167 +/− 43	
Creatinine kinase (IU/L)	1288 (1093-1483)	
Creatinine (mg/dl)	0.3 +/− 0.1	<0.3
Glucose (mg/dl)	67 (20-113)	
Lactate dehydrogenase (IU/L)	3625 (2389-4861)	161-473
Magnesium (mEq/L)	2.2	
Phosphorus (mg/dl)	4.0 (3.7-4.3)	5.1-9.9

TABLE 9-2	Biochemistry Analyte Reference Ranges for Various Chelonian Species—cont'd	
Parameter	Red-eared slider Trachemys scripta[78]	Mediterranean tortoise Testudo hermanni[83]
Potassium (mEq/L)	6.3 (4.3-8.3)	4.5-5.0
Protein, total (g/dl)	4.5 +/−1.1	3.1-5.4
Albumin (g/dl)	1.8 +/− 0.5	
Globulins (g/dl)	2.6 +/− 0.9	
Sodium (mEq/L)	137 (133-140)	130-144
Uric acid (mg/dl)	1.2 +/− 0.7	2.1-9.8
Parameter	Leopard tortoise Geochelone pardalis[84]	Pancake tortoise Kinixys erosa[85]
Alkaline phosphatase (IU/L)	3.2-5.0	
Alanine aminotransferase (IU/L)		
Aspertate aminotransferase (IU/L)		
Bilirubin, total (mg/dl)		
Urea (mg/dl)		
Calcium (mg/dl)	9.4-14.0	9.6-18.4
Chloride (mEq/L)		83-116
Cholesterol (mg/dl)		26-231
Creatinine kinase (IU/L)		
Creatinine (mg/dl)	0.9-2.5	0.1-0.3
Glucose (mg/dl)		
Lactate dehydrogenase (IU/L)		
Phosphorus (mg/dl)	2.1-4.0	2.1-4.2
Potassium (mEq/L)	3.8-5.1	4.2-6.1
Protein, total (g/dl)	3.2-4.9	2.4-4.1
Albumin (g/dl)	1.2-2.2	1.2-2.1
Globulins (g/dl)		
Sodium (mEq/L)	128-145	111-146
Uric acid (mg/dl)	1.2-1.6	0.9-9.2
Parameter	Common box turtles Terrapene carolina[79,80,81]	
Alkaline phosphatase (IU/L)	62 (29-102)	
Alanine aminotransferase (IU/L)	7 (2-14)	
Aspertate aminotransferase (IU/L)	124 (2-620)	
Bilirubin, total (mg/dl)	0.5 (0.1-1)	
Urea (mg/dl)	49 (20-102)	
Calcium (mg/dl)	13.6 (6.5-26.4)	
Chloride (mEq/L)	106 (101-112)	
Cholesterol (mg/dl)	240 (65-496)	
Creatinine kinase (IU/L)	463 (37-898)	
Creatinine (mg/dl)	0.4	
Glucose (mg/dl)	84 (33-155)	
Lactate dehydrogenase (IU/L)	206 (111-313)	
Phosphorus (mg/dl)	4 (1.6-8.2)	
Potassium (mEq/L)	5.6 (3-9.7)	
Protein, total (g/dl)	5.6 (2.7-7.5)	
Albumin (g/dl)	2.2 (1.2-3.2)	
Globulins (g/dl)	3.4 (2.5-4.7)	
Sodium (mEq/L)	144 (138-149)	
Uric acid (mg/dl)	1.6 (0.5-3.1)	

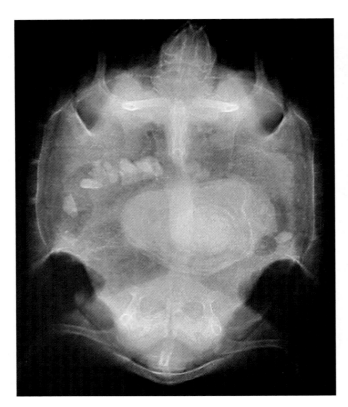

Figure 9-23 Radiographs confirming the presence of cystic calculi in a desert tortoise *(Gopherus agassizii)*.

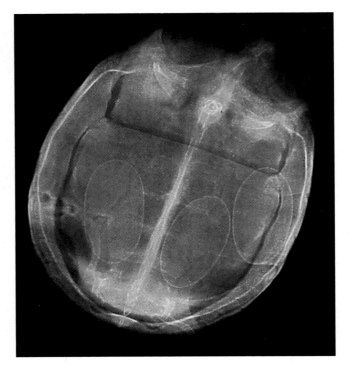

Figure 9-24 A dorsoventral radiograph of a box turtle *(Terrapene carolina)*. Generally, these images are difficult to interpret because they are "shell on shell" or "bone on bone." In some cases, such as this image showing a gravid female, it is possible to diagnose abnormalities or confirm the reproductive state of the animal.

The urine pH of apparently healthy herbivorous terrestrial chelonians has been documented to range from 8.0 to 8.5.[86] The urine pH of posthibernation patients ranged from 5.0 to 6.0 but was noted to rise to 8.0 to 8.5 within 1 month of normal feeding.[86] Protein levels of up to 30 mg/dl have been recorded by Innis in apparently healthy *Testudo graeca*.[86] Cystic calculi are commonly seen in chelonians fed diets of inappropriate mineral content. Uric acid crystals,[87] ammonium oxalate,[88] calcium phosphorus, and struvite crystals[89] have all been reported in chelonian urine sediments.

Diagnostic Imaging

Diagnostic imaging can play a vital role in reaching a diagnosis in the chelonian patient. Radiology is frequently employed to assess for the presence of cystic calculi (Figure 9-23), visualize the contents of the female reproductive tract, check for the presence of joint disease or fractures, and monitor for radiographic evidence of pneumonia. Typically, little information will be gained concerning the liver, kidneys, heart, thyroid, pancreas, gastrointestinal tract, or spleen unless the organs are mineralized or grossly enlarged. A survey radiographic assessment should ideally include the dorsoventral (Figure 9-24), craniocaudal (Figure 9-25), and lateral (Figure 9-26) views to allow for proper radiographic examination. Barium sulfate (0.3%) or water-soluble iodine compounds are helpful in assessing gastrointestinal function. The following recommendations have been developed to assist with the production of

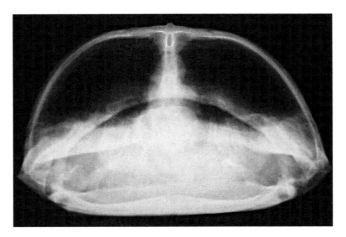

Figure 9-25 A craniocaudal (or anterior-posterior) radiograph of a box turtle *(Terrapene carolina)*. These images provide distinct views into each lung.

a useful image: 40 to 60 kVp for small to medium chelonians (<2 kg), 60 to 80 kVp for medium-sized chelonians (2-8 kg), and 80 to 100 kVp for large chelonians (>8 kg).[90]

Ultrasound is typically not utilized as frequently as radiographs in the chelonian patient, but its use is becoming more frequently reported in the literature. The two acoustic windows utilized in the chelonian patient include the prefemoral acous-

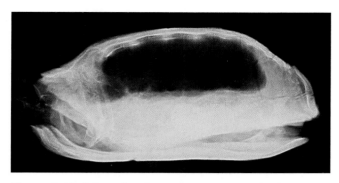

Figure 9-26 A lateral radiograph of a box turtle *(Terrapene carolina)*. These images provide the best view of the viscera. Note that on lateral radiographic images of chelonians, the viscera and lung field generally account for the ventral 50% and dorsal 50% of the coelomic cavity, respectively. Any changes to this percentage may be an indication of an abnormality.

tic window and the cervicobrachial window. Visualization of the female reproductive tract, liver, gastrointestinal tract, urinary bladder, and kidney is possible via the prefemoral window, whereas visualization of the heart, liver, thyroid, and great vessels can be achieved through the cervicobrachial window.[90] A 3.5- or 5-MHZ curvilinear probe is recommended for use in sea turtles.[91] Frequencies of 5 to 10 MHz have been recommended to provide appropriate examination of chelonians weighing less than 4 kg.[90]

Both rigid and flexible endoscopes can be utilized to examine chelonians. Entrance to the coelomic cavity through the prefemoral fossa permits visualization of the reproductive organs, the liver, and the digestive tract and allows proper access to the kidneys for biopsy. The upper digestive and respiratory tracts may be examined via insertion of an endoscope or bronchoscope though the oral cavity; and the lower digestive, urinary, and reproductive tracts can be examined via insertion of an endoscope through the cloaca. Appropriate biopsies may be obtained in this manner as well. Both magnetic resonance imaging and computed tomography have yielded excellent diagnostic potential in the chelonian patient.[90]

Microbiology

When submitting a sample for bacterial culture, it is advantageous to request antibiotic sensitivities as well. Anaerobes are commonly isolated from chelonian samples along with opportunistic pathogens (*Pseudomonas* spp., *Proteus* spp., *Klebsiella* spp.); therefore, both anaerobic and aerobic cultures should be requested. Due to the common microorganisms isolated from chelonians, sensitivities to fluoroquinolones, ceftazidime, amikacin, and ticarcillin should be specifically requested. It is also important to review the appropriate culture media and storage requirements for both aerobic and anaerobic cultures. If specific bacteria that are difficult to culture are suspected, such as *Mycoplasma* spp., special transport media may be necessary. If

a mycobacterial infection is suspected, tissue biopsies should be divided into three parts. One part should be submitted for histopathology with a request to examine for acid-fast organisms, the second sample should be submitted for aerobic and anaerobic culture and sensitivity in an appropriate growth medium, and the third sample should be placed in a sterile container with sterile saline and submitted for specific mycobacterial culture.[92]

Parasitology

A fecal sample should be obtained from any thin, anorectic, or otherwise debilitated patient, regardless of the consistency of the feces. A wet fecal smear is constructed by mixing a small amount of sample with a few drops of saline on a slide. A coverslip is applied and the sample is examined under 10 to 40 times magnification. Fecal sedimentation should be utilized to concentrate protozoans or trematodes, and the visualization of protozoans is enhanced via phase-contrast microscopy. Fecal flotation is used to concentrate parasites, but it must be remembered that trematode and cestode eggs may not float. Dried fecal smears may be stained with acid-fast stain to examine for the presence of *Cryptosporidium* spp. Because parasites can be shed transiently, serial samples may be required to determine the true status of the chelonian. For recently acquired animals, it is also important to consider that each parasite has a prepatent period. Fecal samples should be tested over a period of time that considers the prepatent period.

Miscellaneous Diagnostics

Novel diagnostic modalities, such as polymerase chain reaction (PCR), virus isolation, and serology (enzyme-linked immunosorbent assay [ELISA], immunohistochemistry), are becoming increasingly more available. Compared to PCR, virus isolation is a more specific diagnostic test, whereas PCR is more sensitive. Heavy bacterial contamination may denature viral particles, resulting in a false negative result. Virus isolation is generally utilized when cytology or histopathology reveals results consistent with a viral infection.[91] Samples appropriate for viral isolation include excreted material, body fluid, tissue biopsies inoculated into appropriate viral transport medium, or fresh or rapidly frozen samples. Once collected, the samples should be placed in sterile containers and stored at low temperatures (approximately 5° C [41° F]). Specific transport recommendations should be sought from the virology laboratory.

PCR can be applied to any of the same samples that are utilized for viral isolation, and PCR is less affected than virus isolation by inappropriate temperatures during transport. A PCR assay has been developed for the detection of herpesvirus stomatitis in tortoises[93] and chelonian *Mycoplasma* infections.[94] Serology may be utilized for specific infectious agents, such as herpesvirus infections, and the receiving laboratory should always be consulted regarding current submission requirements.

■ COMMON DISEASE PRESENTATIONS

Chelonians are susceptible to a range of different pathogens, including viruses, bacteria, fungi, and parasites. It is important to note that much of the knowledge we have today regarding these disease agents is based on recent research over the past 2 to 3 decades. Our overall understanding of the epidemiology of these diseases remains limited.

Viral Diseases

HERPESVIRUS

Herpesvirus infection is often diagnosed in animals that have been exposed to other chelonians presumed to be carriers of the disease. It is believed that an asymptomatic carrier state exists, and husbandry conditions are often inappropriate. Herpesvirus infection is frequently observed in chelonians that have recently experienced a stressful event and consequent immunosuppression and recrudescence of infection, such as inappropriate hibernation, a sudden change in temperature, nutritional deficiencies, metabolic disease, or the onset of breeding season.[95]

All chelonian species should be considered susceptible to herpesvirus infection. Depending on the infected species, herpesvirus infection is also called "gray-patch disease" *(Chelonia mydas)*, "necrotic stomatitis" *(Chersina angulata)*, "lung, eye, trachea disease" *(Chelonia mydas)*, and "lymphoproliferative disease" *(Testudo hermanni, Geochelone pardalis)*.[95]

Herpesvirus may be isolated from fresh or rapidly frozen tissue samples or from tissue swabs. Research suggests that it may be easier to isolate the virus from oropharyngeal swabs than from conjunctival or cloacal samples.[96] Research also suggests that the virus may be shed only transiently in oral secretions, either during primary infection or recrudescence.[97] Virus particles may be detected in the blood of viremic animals[96] along with herpesvirus antibodies. Viral particles may also be detected via electron microscopy.

Histopathology, impression smears, and skin scrapes may demonstrate the presence of eosinophilic intranuclear inclusion bodies. A PCR assay is currently available for the detection of chelonian herpesvirus infection,[98] and the development of both an ELISA and immunoperoxidase-based serologic test for the detection of herpesvirus antigen in tissue samples is currently underway.[99,100] It is important to state that even though a viral agent may be isolated from a diseased individual, this does not necessarily mean that the cause of the disease has been determined.

The most frequent complaint associated with herpesvirus infection is the stomatitis/rhinitis/conjunctivitis complex (Figure 9-27). Edema of the ventral neck, dehydration, depression, neurologic signs, hypersalivation, dysphagia, dyspnea, and yellow diphtheritic membrane formation on the tongue, oropharynx, and nasopharynx are also commonly described. Nasal discharge and exfoliation of the skin of the head and neck have occasionally been noted.[95] Because this virus travels along nerves, it can affect many different organ systems.

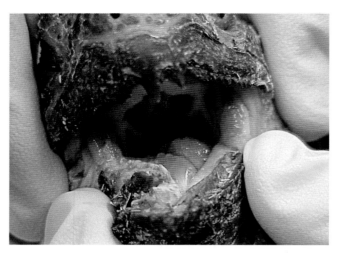

Figure 9-27 Stomatitis is a common finding in chelonians with herpes virus. This desert tortoise *(Gopherus agassizii)* had a diphtheritic membrane associated with the mucous membranes and tongue.

Mycoplasmosis, iridovirus infection, immunosuppression, metabolic disease, the hibernation of recently fed animals, penetrating injuries from food items, local irritation, and chemical intoxication should all be considered in patients displaying clinical signs of stomatitis.[95]

Herpesvirus infections are thought to lie dormant in the central nervous system and other tissues following primary infection. Recrudescence occurs during periods of physiologic stress, which causes immunosuppression and the consequent production of viral particles and active shedding of the virus.[95]

At this time, it is not possible to eliminate herpesvirus from an infected individual. Treatment is therefore mostly directed at supportive care and attempts to eliminate stresses until the body's natural defenses are able to induce a reprieve from the recrudescence state. The placement of an intraosseous or intravenous catheter, continuous fluid administration, appropriate antibiotic selection to prevent secondary bacterial infections, and analgesic administration should be considered on an individual basis. Nutritional support is mandatory in anorexic, debilitated patients, and the placement of a esophagostomy tube is often appropriate. The oral cavity should be rinsed and cleansed with dilute chlorhexidine (0.5%) or povidone-iodine (0.5%) and a cotton-tipped applicator once per day. This procedure typically requires anesthesia or analgesic administration. Infected animals should be isolated and placed into quarantine. Anecdotally, acyclovir (80 mg/kg) three times per day via a stomach or esophagostomy tube has been utilized with variable results. The drug is typically administered until resolution of clinical signs is observed, and it appears to be most effective when treating initial infections and/or when treatment is initiated early in the course of disease.[95] Clients should be informed that these animals still pose a risk to other chelonians.

Quarantine for newly acquired chelonians is generally recommended for 12 to 18 months. Captive chelonians should also be subdivided into small, isolated groups to limit the spread of infectious disease. Diseased or ill chelonians should be removed from a collection immediately.[95]

IRIDOVIRUS

Research suggests that chelonian infection with iridovirus may follow exposure to amphibians carrying the disease.[101] The history of infected chelonians may therefore include inhabitance of an outdoor pond that is shared with frogs or other amphibians.

Iridovirus induces many of the same clinical signs as herpesvirus infection, including the appearance of the stomatitis/rhinitis/conjunctivitis complex. Edema of the ventral neck, dehydration, depression, hypersalivation, dysphagia, dyspnea, and yellow diphtheritic membrane formation on the tongue, oropharynx, and nasopharynx have also been described. Reports of herpesvirus-associated stomatitis vastly outweigh reports of iridovirus-associated stomatitis.[95]

Herpesvirus infection, mycoplasmosis, immunosuppression, metabolic disease, the hibernation of recently fed animals, penetrating injuries from food items, local irritation, and chemical intoxication should all be considered in patients displaying clinical signs of stomatitis.[95]

Basophilic cytoplasmic inclusion bodies are compatible with iridovirus infection and can be viewed via impression smears, histopathology, or skin scrapes. Virus-like particles may also be viewed via electron microscopy within biopsy samples, skin scrapes, or urine, feces, or sputum samples. Virus isolation may also be pursued, but proper transport media, transport conditions, and sample collection procedures must be followed. As stated previously, even though a viral agent may be isolated from a diseased individual, this does not necessarily mean that the cause of the disease has been determined.[95]

Treatment is directed mostly at nursing care and the management of secondary bacterial infections. The placement of an intraosseous catheter and continuous fluid administration, appropriate antibiotic selection to treat secondary bacterial infections, and analgesic administration should all be considered on an individual basis. Nutritional support is imperative in anorexic, debilitated patients, and the placement of a pharyngostomy tube is often appropriate. If severe diphtheritic membrane formation is present, the oral cavity should be rinsed and cleansed with dilute chlorhexidine (0.5%) or povidone-iodine (0.5%) and a cotton-tipped applicator once per day. This procedure typically requires anesthesia or analgesic administration. Infected animals should be isolated and treated following an appropriate quarantine protocol.[95]

Quarantine for 12 to 18 months for newly acquired chelonians is generally recommended. Captive chelonians should also be subdivided into small, isolated groups to limit the spread of infectious disease. Diseased or ill chelonians should be removed from a collection immediately.[95]

MISCELLANEOUS VIRAL DISEASES

Although herpesvirus is the most commonly described virus affecting chelonians, other viruses can be found sporadically in the literature. Viral particles consistent with adenovirus have been observed via electron microscopy in *Testudo graeca* afflicted

with necrotic stomatitis.[102] Paramyxovirus-like inclusions were observed in one chelonian involved in an outbreak of disease characterized by necrotic stomatitis, respiratory disease, and high mortality.[103] Papilloma virus, poxvirus, and flavivirus have also been suspected in other outbreaks of disease.

Chelonians appear to act as intermediate hosts for some viral agents. Toga viruses (eastern and western equine encephalitis virus), rhabdoviruses (vesicular stomatitis virus group), and bunyaviruses (Bunyamwera virus and Crimean Congo hemorrhagic fever virus) have been documented in various chelonian species, but no clinical disease has been associated with the infections.

Bacterial Diseases

GRAM-POSITIVE ORGANISMS

The majority of Gram-positive bacteria are not considered pathogenic in chelonians. However, Gram-positive organisms are capable of causing disease in immunocompromised or debilitated patients, and treatment should be considered when no Gram-negative bacteria are cultured or no response to therapy is noted for a Gram-negative infection. There are some examples of Gram-positive bacterial infections in chelonians, but most are probably unreported because they are not considered significant enough for publication. *Corynebacterium* spp. was reported to be the cause of a liver abscess in a desert tortoise *(Gopherus agassizii)*,[104] and coagulase positive *Staphylococcus* spp. are generally considered pathogenic.

GRAM-NEGATIVE ORGANISMS

Yersinia spp., *Mycobacterium* spp., *Pasturella* spp., and *Pseudomonas* spp. are considered to be important Gram-negative opportunistic pathogens of chelonians.[95] *Pseudomonas* sp. is considered part of the indigenous florae of the chelonian oral cavity and intestinal tract; however, it is frequently isolated from lesions associated with ulcerative stomatitis, dermatitis, septicemia, and pneumonia.[105] *Yersinia* spp. and *Mycobacterium* spp. are potential Gram-negative zoonotic agents of reptiles, along with *Vibrio* spp., *Salmonella* spp., *Aeromonas* spp., and *Campylobacter* spp.[95] *Pasturella* spp. infections are typically treated with fluoroquinolones. *Aeromonas* sp. infection is frequently associated with pneumonia, septicemia, and lesions of the oral cavity and skin.[105] *Chlamydia* (*Chlamydophila* spp.), another Gram-negative pathogenic organism, has been reported in chelonian species and should be considered in the differential list for any granulomatous lesions.[105] *Salmonella* spp., due to its zoonotic potential, and *Mycoplasma* spp., one of the most commonly diagnosed Gram-negative microorganisms, will be discussed in further detail.

MYCOPLASMOSIS (*MYCOPLASMA AGASSIZII*)

Mycoplama sp. infection is frequently diagnosed in animals that have been exposed to other chelonians presumed to be carriers of the disease. It is also often observed in chelonians in the immediate posthibernation period when the patient may be immunosuppressed. Husbandry conditions are often inappropriate.[95]

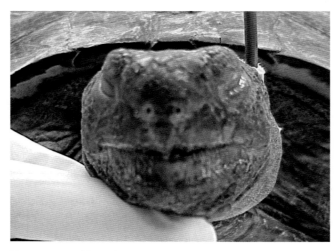

Figure 9-28 Mycoplasmosis is becoming a problem in both wild and captive tortoises. This gopher tortoise presented with clinical signs associated with the upper respiratory tract, including conjunctivitis and rhinitis.

Mycoplasma agassizii has been isolated from the airways of desert tortoises *(Gopherus agassizii)*, Horsfield's tortoises *(Testudo horsfieldi)*, and leopard tortoises *(Geochelone pardalis)*.[106-108] It has also been "identified" in gopher tortoises *(Gopherus polyphemus)*, Indian star tortoises *(Geochelone radiata)*, Asian tortoises *(Indotestudo* spp.), spur-thighed tortoises *(Testudo* spp.), and box turtles *(Terrapene carolina bauri)*.[99] All species should be considered susceptible.[95]

Mycoplasma spp. infections are frequently characterized by serous, serosanguineous, and purulent nasal discharge (Figure 9-28). Inactivity, anorexia, lethargy, ocular and oral discharge, and/or abnormal or increased respiratory sounds often accompany the nasal discharge.[95]

A complete blood count, biochemistry panel, and radiographs should be performed in patients with upper respiratory tract disease. In chelonians suspected to be infected with *Mycoplasma agassizii*, *Mycoplasma* PCR and *Mycoplasma* isolation from ocular and nasal swabs should be pursued. It has been suggested that ocular swabs may result in less secondary bacterial contamination. *Mycoplasma* isolation requires specific harvest techniques, transport media, storage requirements, and transport conditions to reduce the chance of a false negative result. *Mycoplasma* culture requirements are extensive and it may take 3 or more weeks before colonies are apparent. *Mycoplasma* serology has also been utilized to detect anti-*Mycoplasma* antibodies (via ELISA testing). Although ELISA testing is sensitive, it does not distinguish past exposure from current infections, and cross-reactivity with antibodies to similar bacterial antigens may result in a false positive result.[95]

There are a number of oral and parenteral antimycoplasmid therapies, including enrofloxacin, tylosin, doxycycline, or clarithromycin. Flushing the nasal cavity with these medications (with the exception of tylosin) has also been effective in alleviating clinical signs associated with *Mycoplasma* infection. None of these medications has been proven to be completely effective for treating *Mycoplasma* infections, and patients with confirmed

Mycoplasma infections should consequently be isolated and given a guarded prognosis for complete recovery.[95] Research suggests the possibility of an asymptomatic carrier state.[109]

SALMONELLA SPP.

It has been suggested that most, if not all, reptiles have *Salmonella* spp.; however, a review of the literature suggests that the presence of *Salmonella* sp. is more dependent on the environment than anything else. The prevalence of *Salmonella* sp. can approach 100% in captive chelonians, whereas it has been found to be 0% in some wild populations.[110] Research one of us has done (MAM) has found that the prevalence of *Salmonella* sp. in captive-raised red-eared sliders can range from 0% to 38% (Mitchell, unpublished data). In most cases, only a single egg in a clutch is positive (Mitchell, unpublished data). Other animals likely become exposed when they are in close quarters with their shedding sibling.

The isolation of *Salmonella* sp. from chelonians is typically not associated with the presence of disease. It may, however, be reflective of husbandry conditions, with omnivorous species a more likely potential source of the bacteria than herbivorous species. *Salmonella* sp. can occasionally cause disease in chelonians. Confirmation of infection should be based on a combination of culture and pathology.

Salmonella sp. can be diagnosed antemortem via culture, ELISA, and PCR. Culture and PCR are the two most common diagnostics used. *Salmonella* sp. can be shed transiently, so it is important to submit several samples to confirm an animal's true status. Clients will often ask their veterinarian to determine the *Salmonella* sp. disease status of their pets. This is fine, but a positive culture should not result in treatment. Instead, clients should be made to recognize the importance of practicing strict hygiene practices. The Centers for Disease Control and Prevention (CDC) published the following guidelines for preventing turtle-associated salmonellosis:

1. Pregnant women, children under 5 years of age, and people with impaired immune systems should not handle reptiles. Reptiles should not be housed in facilities where pregnant women, young children, and immunosuppressed individuals live.
2. All handlers should wash their hands with soap immediately after any contact with either a reptile or a reptile cage.
3. Reptiles should be housed away from areas of food preparation.
4. Kitchen sinks should not be utilized to wash reptilian food or water bowls or to soak reptiles. Any sink that is used for these purposes should be appropriately disinfected.[111]

Fungal Diseases

High humidity, malnutrition, overcrowding, and inadequate environmental hygiene may predispose an individual to the development of a fungal infection.[112] The use of antibiotics may also contribute to the development of fungal overgrowth. Discussions of gastrointestinal fungal infections are not common in the literature, but a *Penicillium* sp. infection has been reported in *Chelonidis nigra, Basidobolus ranarum* has been isolated from the mouth of *Chelonidis gigantea,* and *Paecilomyces* sp. has been documented in the mouth and stomach of *Chelonidis gigantean.*[112] A yeast infection of the gastrointestinal tract of an anorexic *Testudo graeca* that was successfully treated with nystatin has also been reported.[113] Although nystatin is appropriate to treat gastrointestinal fungal overgrowth, systemic fungal infections must be treated with ketoconazole, fluconazole, or itraconazole. Shell fungal infections have been documented as a result of the placement of fiberglass patches on shell fractures, and these infections should be treated with topical medications and possibly a systemic antifungal medication.

Parasitic Diseases

CESTODES

Cestode infections appear to be uncommon in chelonians. *Ophiotaenia* sp. has been reported in freshwater chelonians,[114] along with *Glossocercus* sp. and *Bancroftiella* sp.[115] No pathogenic effects of any of these cestode species have been reported. Cestode eggs are easiest to detect via fecal flotation with zinc-sulfate solution. Treatment of cestode infections in debilitated or immunocompromised individuals consists of oral or systemic praziquantel,[116] dichlorophen, niclosamide, or bunamidine. Some species of cestodes are also susceptible to benzimidazoles.

TREMATODES

These metazoan parasites are all parasitic flatworms.[117] Monogenetic (direct life cycle) trematodes inhabit the nasopharynx or urinary bladder of aquatic chelonians and are believed to be nonpathogenic. Digenetic trematodes, which require an intermediate host, have been reported to reside in different internal organs. These parasites are generally thought to be nonpathogenic in terrestrial and freshwater chelonians. Eggs of both mono- and digenetic trematodes are common in chelonian feces, and they are typically not associated with clinical signs of pathology.[117] They are most easily detected via fecal flotation with zinc-sulfate solution. Trematode eggs can also be visualized with the help of centrifugation of feces and examination of the resulting sediment. Treatment of excessive numbers of trematode eggs in debilitated or ill chelonians typically consists of oral or systemic praziquantel.[95] For the digenetic flukes, the parasite does not usually persist in the absence of intermediate hosts or final hosts.

CILIATED PROTOZOA

Nyctotherus sp. and *Balantidium* sp. cysts and trophozoites are commonly identified in fecal examinations. Treatment for ciliates is often not indicated unless large numbers are present or the patient is already debilitated or ill. Metronidazole is the treatment of choice for severe ciliate infections.[95]

FLAGELLATES

The presence of flagellates is generally considered normal in chelonians. However, in stressed or debilitated chelonians, high numbers of flagellates may be noted on fecal wet mounts. An excessive flagellate load has been associated with anorexia, weight loss, and unthriftiness over time.[118] Flagellate overgrowths are generally treated with dimetridazole (40 mg/kg PO for 5 days)[119] or metronidazole (50-100 mg/kg as a single dose; the same dose may be repeated in 2 weeks if warranted by fecal examination or clinical signs).[119,120] Alternatively, metronidazole may be administered at 20 mg/kg every 48 hours until eradication of the parasite.[121,122]

HEXAMITA

Hexamita is described as a slowly progressing disease causing no specific clinical signs. Nephromegaly, anorexia, weight loss, and gradual onset of renal failure have been described in cases of advanced disease.[123] Renal biopsy and histopathology are necessary to determine if the clinical signs are caused by the presence of *Hexamita*-like organisms. The presence of flagellates in urine is potentially normal. Dimetridazole, administered at a dose of 40 mg/kg PO for 5 days, has been used in cases of *Hexamita* infection.[119] Metronidazole has also been used as a single dose of 125 to 275 mg/kg. This dose is often repeated in 2 weeks if fecal examination is not negative or if the clinical signs are still present.[119,120]

PROTOZOANS

Amoebiasis (Entamoeba spp.)

Amoeboid organisms are commonly detected in chelonian feces. Oftentimes they are considered nonpathogenic, but cases of pathology in chelonians have been reported. More important, chelonians may serve as a source of infection for other, more susceptible species, in which pathogenicity of the organism is much greater. In snakes and lizards, for example, the organism is considered highly pathogenic, and separate housing facilities for chelonians, snakes, and lizards is consequently advised.[120]

All chelonian species are considered susceptible to infection. Giant species of chelonians are thought to be particularly susceptible.[124] As stated previously, amoeboid organisms do not commonly cause clinical disease in chelonians. In particularly pathogenic infections, anorexia, listlessness, and watery diarrhea may be observed. Death can occur with severe infestations.

Fecal examination is the most widely employed method of diagnosis, with cysts and trophozoites being indicators of infection.[120] Culture techniques and repeated sampling may be necessary to identify intermittent shedders and carriers.[125] ELISA testing can also be utilized to diagnose amoeba infection.

Metronidazole is effective against amoebic trophozoites and is considered an effective extraintestinal amoebicide. Pharmacokinetic studies in the green iguana and yellow rat snake have shown that a dose of 20 mg/kg every 48 hours is appropriate.[121,122] Treatment should continue for at least 2 weeks although longer treatment is often required. Combination therapy may be required to completely clear an infection, as metronidazole is only partially effective against amoebic cysts.[126]

Chloroquine, a medication commonly used to prevent and treat malaria in humans, is also labeled for treatment of extraintestinal amoebiasis and is effective against trophozoites.[127] It is available in both oral and intramuscular formulations. Combination therapy is recommended due to the ineffectiveness of chloroquine in treating amoebic cysts.

Paromomycin is an aminoglycoside that is not well absorbed from the gastrointestinal tract. It is generally used in humans as a luminal amoebicide to eradicate amoebic cysts. It has been used to eliminate a *Cryptosporidium* sp. infection in Gila monsters at a dose of 300 to 360 mg/kg every 48 hours for 14 days[128] and in snakes at a dose of 25 to 100 mg/kg daily for 4 weeks to eliminate amoebiasis.[118] Systemic absorption across a compromised intestinal mucosa may result in acute renal failure and death.

In addition to amoebicidal drugs, patients often require fluid administration (via intraosseous catheter or intracoelomically), nutritional support, and antibiotics.

Repeated negative fecal examinations over a 3-month-long quarantine procedure are required to ensure resolution of infection.

Coccidians

Over 30 species of *Eimeria* and *Cryptosporidium* have been reported to infect both terrestrial and semiaquatic chelonians.[129] Both *Eimeria* and *Cryptosporidium* species are rarely associated with disease in chelonians, but infection may contribute to debility in sick animals.[112,130] It is generally believed that *Cryptosporidium* uneventfully inhabits the chelonian upper digestive tract.

Eimeria oocysts are shed in the feces and are generally described as 10 to 15 μm × 25 to 37 μm. Each oocyst contains four spherical sporocysts.[130] Fecal shedding is not always present and, consequently, histopathology may be required to look for intranuclear coccidiosis. Electron microscopy may be utilized to identify trophozoites, merozoites, microgametes, and macrogametes.

Cryptosporidium oocysts are approximately 5 μm in diameter and most easily detected using phase-contrast microscopy after fecal flotation. The oocysts are also readily identified with acid-fast stains on wet fecal smears. Gastric and cloacal wash fluids may be evaluated via immunofluorescent assays.

Sulfonamides are effective against *Eimeria*. Sulfadimethoxine can be used at a dosage of 50 mg/kg PO every 24 hours for 5 to 7 days and then every other day as needed. Unfortunately, chelonian *Cryptosporidium* sp. infections are not so easily treated. Virtually all anticoccidial agents have failed to resolve reptilian cryptosporidiosis. Research has shown that resolution may be possible in Gila monsters treated with paromomycin[128] and in monitor lizards treated with hyperimmune bovine colostrum.[131] Unfortunately, hyperimmune bovine colostrum is not commercially available at this time, and paromomycin is no longer produced. Because of the risk of contagion, affected animals should be culled, sent to a place where they cannot infect others, or euthanized.

Nematodes

Nematodes are tubular worms that are commonly known as round worms. Adult nematodes reside in the gastrointestinal

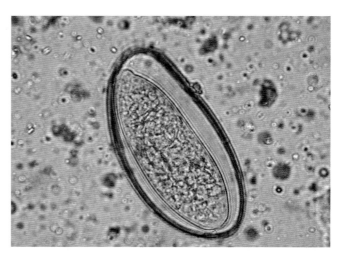

Figure 9-29 Nematodes, such as this oxyurid, are a common funding in chelonian feces. These organisms are generally considered to serve as commensals; however, many veterinarians treat them as parasites.

tract, lungs, or nasopharynx and exist free in the coelomic cavity of their host.[132] Pinworms (order Oxyurida) have a direct life cycle. These nematodes typically reside in the lower gastrointestinal tract, and affected animals are usually asymptomatic. Adult organisms are visible to the naked eye, and oxyurid eggs have variable morphology. The eggs are commonly asymmetric and do not contain a thick wall or scalloped surface (Figure 9-29). Excessive numbers of these organisms in debilitated chelonians or in chelonians that reside in inappropriate environmental conditions may require medical treatment. Oxyurid infestation is typically treated with mebendazole (20-25 mg/kg, repeat in 2-3 weeks), thiabendazole (50 mg/kg, repeat in 2-3 weeks), fenbendazole (50-100 mg/kg, repeat in 2-3 weeks), or oxfenbendazole (66 mg/kg, repeat in 2-3 weeks). Fenbendazole, oxfenbendazole, and thiabendazole may be administered either intracloacally or orally. Treatment with ivermectin or piperazine is not advised.

Ascarids

Sulcascaris spp. and *Angusticaecum* spp. are commonly observed in chelonian feces. Ascarids may reach 10 cm in length and typically inhabit the gastrointestinal tract. Eggs may be visualized via examination of stomach washes and fecal floats. The eggs are typically thick walled and measure 80 to 100 μm × 60 to 80 μm. Pathology may result from visceral larval migrans or via damage to the gastrointestinal mucosa from embedding adults. Clinical signs may be a result of intestinal perforation or visceral migration and disseminated bacterial infections.[63] Multiple anthelminthics have been utilized in reptiles for ascarid infections, including mebendazole (20-25 mg/kg, repeat in 2-3 weeks), thiabendazole (50 mg/kg, repeat in 2-3 weeks), fenbendazole (50-100 mg/kg, repeat in 2-3 weeks), or oxfendazole (66 mg/kg, repeat in 2-3 weeks). Piperizine and ivermectin are not recommended.[95]

Nutritional Disorders

Nutritional disorders in chelonians commonly present as a chronic problem, and the diet is oftentimes centered on chelonian food preference or human convenience. In most cases, deficient diets are comprised of limited numbers of food items and/or are not supplemented with calcium and vitamin powders.[68]

HYPOVITAMINOSIS A

Vitamin A is a critical component in the production and maintenance of epithelial cells and is also intimately associated with several structures related to vision. Hypovitaminosis A is a common clinical entity in chelonian medicine, especially in chelonians fed predominately low vitamin A foods, such as iceberg lettuce and cucumbers, or a limited number of meat products. Dark leafy greens—such as bok choy, spinach, dandelions, turnip and mustard greens, broccoli—and yellow/orange fruits and vegetables—such as squash, peppers, and carrots—are rich in B-carotene, the precursor to vitamin A.[132] The yolk sac, which is not totally resorbed until approximately 6 months of age, is able to satisfy the vitamin A requirements of hatchlings until resorption.[133]

The most obvious clinical abnormality associated with hypovitaminosis A is squamous metaplasia, which results in the degeneration of epithelial surfaces (e.g., conjunctiva, gingiva, pancreatic ducts, renal tubules, skin, and lung faveoli)[134,135] (Figure 9-30). Due to the multiple epithelial surfaces of the body, squamous metaplasia can manifest itself in several different ways. Blepharospasm, conjunctivitis, blepharedema, blindness, rhinitis, blepharitis, lower respiratory tract

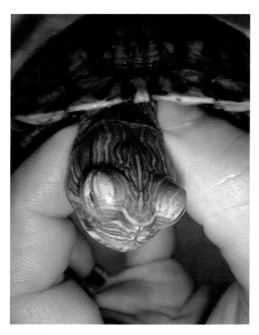

Figure 9-30 Hypovitaminosis A can result in squamous metaplasia of various tissues in a chelonian. In this box turtle, the animal presented with blepharedema. (Courtesy Dr. David Sanchez-Migallon Guzman.)

disease (nasal discharge, depression, dyspnea, open-mouth breathing), and/or cutaneous abnormalities may be observed. Middle ear infections and aural abscesses have also been linked with hypovitaminosis A,[132] along with hepatic lipidosis.[134] Acute deficiency in semiaquatic chelonians generally presents as ocular changes, whereas chronic deficiency in terrestrial chelonians is typically associated with respiratory, hepatic, renal, and/or pancreatic epithelial abnormalities.[68]

The diagnosis of hypovitaminosis A can be met via dietary history, clinical signs, measuring vitamin A levels, or histopathology of tissue samples (squamous metaplasia of the epithelial surfaces). Supportive treatment should be utilized when there are clinical manifestations of vitamin A deficiency, and appropriate husbandry and dietary changes should be instituted. Vitamin A deficiency can be corrected by oral supplementation with vitamin A products or by offering small amounts of liver once per week. Injectable vitamin A should be used very cautiously, as hypervitaminosis A can occur with a single injection (see Figure 9-14). Oral dosing with natural sources of B-carotene, or preformed vitamin A, is safer and the preferred method of supplementation.[68] Studies suggest that hepatic uptake of vitamin A following parenteral administration was much higher when water-miscible products, as opposed to oil-based products, were used.[136] It can therefore be surmised that if injectable supplementation must be used, an oil-based product should be selected. We have found that 1500 to 2000 IU vitamin A is a safe parenteral dose for treating deficient animals. A single parenteral injection followed by dietary correction and oral supplementation is recommended. It is, however, important to recognize that other diseases can present with similar clinical signs (e.g., herpesvirus, mycoplasmosis) and that not every animal that presents has hypovitaminosis A. This persistent misconception, similar to the idea that every rabbit abscess is associated with *Pasteurella multocida,* needs to be corrected.

METABOLIC BONE DISEASE/SECONDARY NUTRITIONAL HYPERPARATHYROIDISM

Metabolic bone disease (MBD) is defined as any metabolic defect that alters the morphology and functioning of bones. MBD is usually related to low levels of calcium or excessive levels of phosphorus, which consequently bind to calcium and render it physiologically unavailable. Decreased calcium availability results in increased parathyroid activity and mobilization of stored calcium from the shell and bone cortices. Factors predisposing chelonians to the development of MBD include dietary deficiency of calcium and/or suitable vitamin D_3, inappropriate calcium-to-phosphorus ratio in the diet, lack of exposure to ultraviolet light (ultraviolet B radiation increases activation of vitamin D precursors and facilitates gastrointestinal resorption of calcium), dietary excess of protein during rapid growth periods, anorexia, or abnormal vitamin D_3 metabolism secondary to renal, hepatic, intestinal, or parathyroid disease. Renal disease alters phosphate excretion and calcium absorption and may induce MBD, while diseases of the small intestine may interfere with gastrointestinal absorption of calcium. The absence of bile salts may also reduce calcium absorption. MBD may be observed in chelonians that are offered excessive amounts of beet greens, kale, and spinach, as these vegetables store a large percentage of their calcium as calcium oxalate, thereby rendering the calcium as physiologically unavailable.[95]

MBD is commonly observed in rapidly growing juveniles, presumably secondary to the demands of shell growth.[137] MBD may manifest itself as pyramiding of the scutes, which occurs when the central scute grows at a differential rate to the outer scutes. Excessive protein supplementation in early life and inadequate humidity may also cause pyramiding.[95]

Clinical signs consistent with MBD vary depending on the age and species of the patient. The most common clinical finding in the semiaquatic turtle is "soft-shell." Semiaquatic turtles may also exhibit extensive secondary erosive infections of the plastron and carapace. Juvenile chelonians present with pyramiding and/or distortion of the rhamphotheca.[132] This commonly occurs as a result of fibrous osteodystrophy, which is observed when osteoclastic resorption of osteoid is replaced by highly cellular connective tissue. Juveniles may also exhibit splayed hindlimbs, secondary to flattening of the pelvis, and an abnormal gait. Adult chelonians have large calcium reserves in the bones of the carapace, plastron, and limbs; therefore, they typically exhibit nonspecific signs of illness. These clinical signs include dystocia, anorexia, cloacal prolapse, abnormal fecal character, muscular weakness, collapse of the femoral head, renal compromise, hepatic lipidosis, and/or constipation.[95]

A thorough history is required before a diagnosis of MBD can be met. An appropriate diet should include the following: Ca : P ratio of 1.5 : 1 to 2 : 1, suitable amounts of calcium and phosphorus (Ca: 0.6%-1% dry matter, P: 0.5%-0.8% dry matter), and appropriate mineral and vitamin supplementation. Calcium-binding foods should not be present in large amounts, and animal matter should not be included in an herbivore's diet. The details concerning ultraviolet light exposure should also be discussed with the handler. The type and brand of light source (290-310 wavelength), the position of the bulb (8-12 inches from the animal), the replacement period (6-12 months), and the photoperiod (reflective of the natural photoperiod) should be discussed.

Radiography may reveal osteomalacia (adult failure of bone calcification), which manifests itself as loss of bone density, thinning of the cortices, coarsened trabecular pattern, mottled radiolucent areas, folding fractures, and bowed bones.[138] Radiography may also be suggestive of osteoporosis (resorption of osteoid exceeds formation), which appears as thinning of the cortices and an increased medullary cavity.[138] Soft tissue swelling of the neck and forelimbs may also be observed on radiographs, along with pathologic fractures of the long bones.

Low blood calcium levels are highly suggestive of MBD, but calcium blood levels are frequently not low in cases of MBD because of hyperparathyroid activity. It must be remembered that blood levels of calcium are not reflective of physiologically available levels of calcium. Ionized levels of calcium are more indicative of the availability of calcium, but, unfortunately, published reference levels are difficult to find in the literature. Significantly low available calcium levels manifest as muscle weakness and may be correlated with cloacal prolapse, dystocia, and generalized weakness. Hyperparathyroidism also occurs as a result of hyperphosphatemia, as parathyroid hormone causes decreased phosphate absorption from the gastrointestinal tract and increased phosphate excretion at the level of the kidney.[95]

Treatment of MBD is dependent upon the correction of inappropriate husbandry. An unsuitable calcium-to-phosphorus ratio of the diet should be corrected, the proper provision of ultraviolet light should be instituted, and oral supplementation of calcium and vitamin D_3 should be initiated. Romaine lettuce, Swiss chard, kale, beet greens, escarole, parsley, watercress, and green beans all have a positive Ca : P ratio and should be added into the recommended diet.

GOUT

Gout is defined as the deposition of uric acid and urate salts within visceral tissues and on articular surfaces. Gout occurs as a result of hyperuricemia, which arises secondary to increased production or decreased excretion of uric acid. Increased production of uric acid may occur secondary to the ingestion of excessive amounts of protein (e.g., an herbivorous chelonian that is regularly offered animal protein). Decreased excretion of uric acid may occur secondary to reduced perfusion of renal tissues, which may be a result of dehydration, hemoconcentration, water deprivation, or renal disease. Reduced glomerular filtration eventually leads to a decrease in the overall excretion of urate salts, which results in hyperuricemia. Hyperuricemia, in turn, leads to the precipitation of urate complex microcrystals within tissues. These deposits are known as "gout tophi." Considering the fact that the urinary bladder in chelonians participates in electrolyte and fluid exchange, gout may also occur as a result of saturation of the bladder contents with urate toxins during dehydration.[95]

Common sites of deposition of uric acid include articular joints (Figure 9-31), the pericardial sac, the liver, the renal cortex, and the spleen. Clinical signs associated with gout include joint swelling and pain, depression (associated with tophi deposition in the central nervous system), and dehydration. Affected animals are also commonly anorectic and lethargic.[95] The diagnosis of gout can be met via the use of several different diagnostic modalities. Radiography may reveal the presence of radiopaque mineralized urate crystals, and ultrasonography may demonstrate echodense areas of crystallization within the heart or kidneys. Cytology of aspirated material from tissue affected by gout will usually reveal inflammatory cells and urate crystals.[139,140] Unfortunately, blood uric acid levels are not reliable indicators for the presence of gout because levels have often normalized by the time the patient presents.

Once gout tophi have been deposited, they are rarely reabsorbed. Therapy is therefore directed at the prevention of further deposition of gout tophi. The mainstay of therapy is rehydration to correct the hyperuricemia and the correction of any dietary imbalances or other predisposing causes of gout. In acute conditions, intraosseous or intravenous fluids should be utilized. In chronic cases, the oral, cloacal, and coelomic

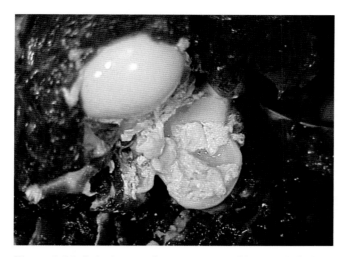

Figure 9-31 Articular gout is a common problem in chelonians not provided regular access to water. A pet retailer told this client that African sulcata tortoises do not require water, as they derive it exclusively from their diet. The provision of high water content greens and grasses, in addition to water, can prevent this problem from occurring.

routes of fluid administration can be utilized. Diets restricted in purines should be recommended. In cases of anorexic animals, placement of an esophagostomy tube should be considered. Critical care formulas for carnivorous and herbivorous reptiles are available and can be administered through the tube. Allopurinol (50 mg/kg PO SID[141]), a urease inhibitor, is commonly used in hyperuricemic animals to reduce uric acid production. It must be mentioned that studies concerning the efficacy of this drug and the possible long-term effects of the drug in chelonians have not been conducted. Probenecid (250 mg/animal PO BID[142]), which increases the renal excretion of uric acid, should not be used until the glomerular filtration rate is considered acceptable. Any concurrent infections in affected joints or organs that occur secondary to gout deposition should be treated appropriately. Surgery is occasionally indicated when uric acid deposits are compromising joints.[95]

HEPATIC LIPIDOSIS

Hepatic lipidosis appears to be a normal physiologic occurrence that is observed during hibernation and vitellogenesis. It therefore must be interpreted in light of the season, reproductive status, and species of the patient. Lipidosis can also be considered a pathologic process, for example when it occurs in obese, anorectic chelonians. Chronic hyperparathyroidism has also been linked to derangement in lipid metabolism.[64] Hepatic lipidosis rarely occurs without a preceding clinical condition. Predisposing causes of deranged lipid metabolism include chronic hyperestrogenism, abnormal thyroid metabolism, diabetes mellitus, a chronic nutrient-deficient diet, starvation, excessive levels of dietary fat, excessively long hibernation periods, inappropriate hibernation temperatures, anorexia, secondary nutritional hyperparathyroidism, or inappropriate photoperiod.[95]

Clinical signs related to hepatic lipidosis are generally non-specific and include obesity, lethargy, reduced fertility, weight loss, abnormal fecal character, and anorexia. Biochemical analysis and complete blood counts are usually reflective of chronic disease. Currently, there is no liver function test that has been validated for use in chelonians and no enzymes have been determined to exhibit a high liver specificity. Ultrasonography may reveal the presence of a hyperechoic liver,[144,145] and ultrasound-guided liver aspirates or biopsies may be obtained. Gross examination of the liver, via prefemoral coeloscopy or an exploratory coeliotomy, often reveals the liver to be friable, pale, yellow, and abnormally textured. Biopsies may be obtained in this manner as well.[95]

Treatment of hepatic lipidosis is dependent upon treating the underlying cause. Inappropriate husbandry issues must be addressed as well. Treatment is oftentimes quite prolonged and may required extensive nursing care. Rehydration can be achieved via intravenous or intraosseous administration methods or via intracoleomic, intracloacal, or oral administration. Affected chelonians are frequently anorectic, and placement of an esophagostomy tube alleviates the stress of force-feeding. Critical care formulas for carnivorous and herbivorous reptiles are available for administration through the feeding tube.[146]

OVERFEEDING

Obesity is frequently observed in chelonians that are offered excessive amounts of food and in individuals that are not encouraged to exercise. In cases where exercise is restricted, both the amount and frequency of feedings should be reduced. Dry matter intake can be reduced in 10% increments over a period of several weeks. In large exhibits, food can be scattered around to encourage exercise.[68]

EARLY MATURITY AND ACCELERATED GROWTH

Accelerated growth rates can be obtained in juvenile and hatchling chelonians fed high protein diets,[147-149] such as beans or meats. The excessive growth rate of juveniles has been associated with high mortality, renal disease, and irreversible deformities of the skeletal system. It appears as though "pyramiding" of the scutes can be correlated with ingestion of large amounts of protein early in life (Figure 9-32).[150] The shell may also appear a bit small in size when compared to the size of the head and limbs. The absence of a hibernation period, the provision of high-quality foods, and an extended winter photoperiod have also been suggested as potential causes for accelerated growth and pyramiding of the scutes.[68]

Alternate day feedings and timed daily feedings can be used to stem accelerated growth. Hibernating juveniles for short, closely monitored periods and varying temperature, humidity, and photoperiod to mimic natural conditions may prevent continuous annual growth.[68]

INTESTINAL DYBIOSIS

Indigenous intestinal flora can be depleted or altered after a course of oral antibiotic therapy. Affected animals will

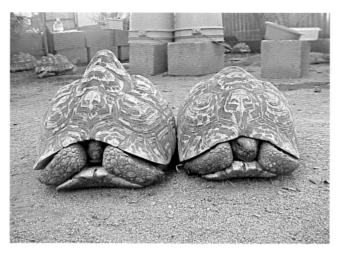

Figure 9-32 These two leopard tortoises were provided similar diets. The tortoise on the left has obvious carapacial pyramiding.

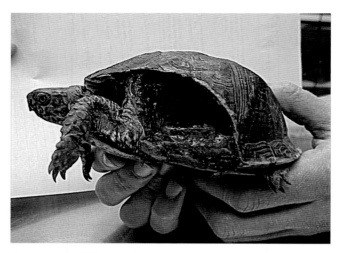

Figure 9-33 Wild chelonians can sustain severe traumatic shell injuries. The shell deficit seen in this animal healed over a 6-month period by developing a bridge of connective tissue. Eventually it remineralized.

commonly become anorexic and may act lethargic or exhibit diarrhea. To repopulate the gastrointestinal tract, an appropriate reptilian probiotic may be administered. Feces, passed before the commencement of the antibiotic, or feces from another individual from the same species may be administered via a stomach tube after the discontinuation of the antibiotics. Pathogenic *Candida* overgrowth may also occur and can be treated with oral nystatin.[68] Foods from untreated areas can also be offered to refaunate the animal's intestine.

Neoplasia

Neoplasia is defined simply as "abnormal tissue growth." The growth of a tumor can act as a space-occupying lesion, invade surrounding tissues and organs, secrete noxious substances, and/or negatively impact the host's immune system.[151] With the increased availability of diagnostic modalities and the rising interest in chelonian medicine, neoplasias of various types have been documented in turtles and tortoises, some with more frequency than others. It is believed that this recent unveiling of chelonian neoplasias is a reflection of underdiagnosis of neoplasia in the past rather than the start of a new trend in the incidence of neoplasia in chelonians.

One of the best-known and better characterized neoplasms of chelonians is fibropapillomatosis in marine turtles. A herpesvirus is the confirmed causal agent,[112,152-155] and the tumors are typically solitary or multicentric cutaneous growths. The tumors are typically characterized histologically as papilliform epidermal hyperplasia, but unlike in conventional papillomas, a prominent stromal component is observed as well. A number of affected turtles have concurrent and often multicentric visceral fibromas, frequently involving the kidneys.[156]

Renal adenocarcinoma has been documented in chelonians as well. These tumors are typically large, solitary, and unilateral in nature and typically have a tubular pattern with little anaplasia, a low mitotic index, and frequent capsular invasion and

scirrhous response. The development of urate tophi within neoplastic tubules and in the adjacent scirrhous stroma is commonly reported in affected chelonians. Metastases of this tumor are uncommonly observed, and nephrectomy is a recommended treatment option in many of the cases.[156,157] Acinar cell adenocarcinoma has also been observed in a small number of chelonians,[156] along with thyroid carcinomas.[156-158] Gastric adenocarcinoma has been detected in chelonians, both with[159] and without metastases.[160] These tumors are typically invasive and are associated with a marked scirrhous response, resulting in thickening of the gastric wall.[156] Cutaneous squamous cell carcinoma tumors have also been reported in chelonians.[156,160,161] It has been documented both on the limbs and in the intermandibular skin. In all cases, although the tumors were locally invasive, no vascular invasion or evidence of metastasis was noted.[156]

Although each of the neoplasias listed above have been documented in at least three patients, some neoplasias have been reported in only isolated individual chelonians. Oros et al. documented the first case of multicentric lymphoblastic lymphoma in a juvenile female loggerhead sea turtle (*Caretta caretta*). Metastases were noted in the plastron, thyroid gland, heart, aorta, left lung, spleen, liver, kidneys, stomach, and small intestine.[162] Although ovarian neoplasia is considered rare in chelonians, a single case of a malignant ovarian teratoma in a 7-year-old red-eared slider has been documented.[163]

Miscellaneous Conditions

Wild chelonian patients are frequently presented to the veterinary hospital for traumatic shell injuries. Although the majority of these injuries are the result of negative encounters with a car (Figure 9-33), domestic (Figure 9-34) and wild animal bites, lawn mowers, and gun shots have also been associated with shell trauma. Shell fractures can involve the plastron,

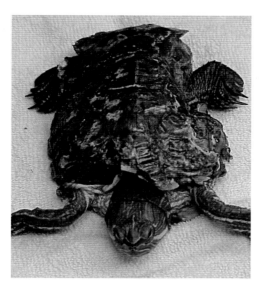

Figure 9-34 This captive red-eared slider turtle was mauled by the family pet. Domestic pets should not be provided direct contact with these animals.

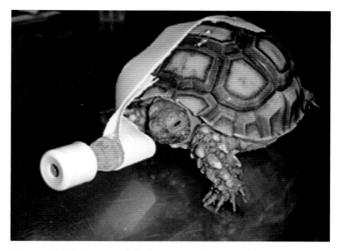

Figure 9-35 The cranial plastron (gular scutes) can be used as a site for intraosseous catheter placement in juvenile tortoises.

carapace, bridge, or all three and may be simple or comminuted. There are various methods to repair turtle shell fractures. The use of orthopedic plates, wires, and screws requires drilling into the shell, which runs the risk of further fragmentation of the shell or damage to the underlying viscera. Fiberglass patches can also be placed across the fracture site and epoxied on either side of the fracture. Some veterinarians believe that fiberglass patches should not be used on chelonians that physiologically shed scutes or peel portions of the keratin of the carapace with growth. This is due to the belief that the fiberglass patches predispose the patient to the development of shell rot or infection.[164] Many of the epoxies used for shell repair are exothermic. If this material enters the coelomic cavity, it can cause severe thermal burns, and for this reason should be avoided. The application of a fiberglass patch is not ideal for managing open wounds that require extensive treatment.

The use of metal bridges should be considered in cases involving open wounds, as this technique allows access to the fracture site and permits continued cleansing and monitoring of the wound. The bridges may be made of aluminum, brass, stainless steel, or plastic zip ties. Most bridges are 0.5 cm wide and 3.0 cm long. The bridges may be used to create appropriate stabilization of the plastron, carapace, or bridge by straddling the fracture and attaching to the uninjured shell and to the unstable fragment via the use of epoxy. Certain portions of the fracture can be left open for cleaning, and the metal bridges can easily be removed for further wound treatment without damage to the underlying shell. Stabilization of the fracture site should be pursued to prevent additional damage to the fragments, contamination by bacterial and parasitic microorganisms, and pain associated with fragment instability. Fracture stabilization is also required to promote normal granulation tissue and callus formation between shell fragments.[165] One of the primary reasons for failure when treating a shell

fracture is closing the wound before it is completely decontaminated. Shell fractures should be managed as open wounds, unless found and treated within less than 6 hours, and closed only after they are considered decontaminated.

■ THERAPEUTICS
Fluid Therapy

There are a number of different methods that can be used for replenishing fluids in a chelonian, including intravenous, intraosseous, epicoelomic, intracoelomic, oral, or intracloacal administration. Intravenous catheters can be placed within the jugular vein and may require a jugular cut down before placement. The intravenous route is preferable for severely dehydrated animals (>8%). Intraosseous fluids can be delivered into the bridge or gular scute. The approach through the gular scute is especially useful for juvenile chelonians (Figure 9-35). A standard hypodermic needle can be inserted into the osteoderms and a continuous rate infusion delivered. In adult animals, the placement of the catheter requires the veterinarian to predrill an insertion site for the catheter. Intracoelomic fluids are administered via the prefemoral fossa, and the space is able to safely handle a maximum of 20 to 30 ml/kg/day of fluids (Figure 9-36). Intracoelomic fluids are generally considered to be rapidly absorbed by the coelomic membrane and visceral serosa. Epicoelomic fluid administration occurs by injection through the cranial inlet of the shell, laterodorsal to the head and neck, just dorsal to the plastron, and slightly below/into the pectoral muscles. In this area, 10 to 20 ml/kg/day of fluids can safely be administered. If the fluids are being given orally via a stomach tube, it is important to extend the neck to facilitate passage of the tube. Attempts to force the tube may otherwise result in perforating the esophagus.

Mammalian fluid preparations (Normosol, 0.9% sodium chloride; Abbott Laboratories, North Chicago, IL) are suitable for fluid administration in chelonians.[146] It has been suggested

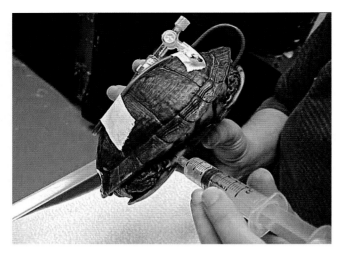

Figure 9-36 Chelonians can be rehydrated using a variety of different methods. In this picture, the box turtle is being given fluids via the intracoelomic route.

that fluids containing lactate should be avoided in reptiles because lactic acidosis is a common problem in debilitated chelonians,[166] but this view is controversial. The calculation of serum osmolarity can be helpful in deciding the fluid type to administer, and the following equation is used in this assessment:

$$\text{osmolarity} = 2\,(Na + K) + \text{glucose} + \text{urea (all measured in mmol/L)}$$

The blood osmolarity appears to vary depending on the species, and research has revealed that the blood osmolarity values of *Gopherus agassizii* range from approximately 250 to 350.[167,168] Hypertonic dehydration is typically treated with 0.45% saline, whereas isotonic or hypotonic dehydration is usually treated with 0.9% saline ± 5% dextrose. Hyperkalemic patients should be administered 5% dextrose. Ongoing losses (diarrhea, regurgitation) should be counteracted with administration of a balanced electrolyte solution (e.g., Normosol).

Maintenance fluid requirements for chelonians are estimated to be approximately 10 to 30 ml/kg/day, depending on the species. This amount can be divided into two to three boluses administered several hours apart, or it can be administered as a continuous rate infusion via an intraosseous or intravenous catheter. Fluid deficits should be slowly corrected over 3 days. Once the deficit has been corrected, the fluid administration rate can be decreased to account for maintenance requirements only.

Antimicrobial Drugs

It is important for veterinarians to consider the implications of antibiotic usage for their patients to decrease the risk of creating an antibiotic-resistant bacterial superinfection. Ideally, bacterial culture and sensitivity should always be pursued to ensure appropriate therapeutic selection. When this is not possible, antibiotics should be selected based upon careful consideration of the most likely organism present. The most common bacteria isolated from chelonians are Gram-negative opportu-

nists, such as *Pseudomonas* sp., *Proteus* sp., *Aeromonas* sp., *Providencia* sp., *Salmonella* sp., and *Klebsiella* sp. It must be remembered that these same bacteria are oftentimes cultured from healthy individuals, and the isolation of these microorganisms does not necessarily implicate them in a disease process. Anaerobic bacteria are commonly isolated as well. Table 9-3 contains recommendations for antibiotics that are commonly used in the chelonian patient. It must be remembered that many of the doses favored by clinicians were derived anecdotally, rather than by pharmacologic studies.

Miscellaneous Drugs

Table 9-4 contains a list of miscellaneous compounds commonly used to manage chelonian patients.

Emergency Drugs

Table 9-5 contains a list of emergency drugs commonly used to manage chelonian patients.

Nutritional Support

Nutritional support is an often ignored, yet extremely important, aspect of care for debilitated chelonians. The chelonian patient can be force-fed, syringe-fed, tube-fed via gavage or fed through the use of an esophagostomy tube. An esophagostomy tube permits administration of oral medications, fluids, a critical care diet, and greatly reduces stress in the patient. The tube is usually placed with sedation. First, the red rubber feeding tube should be premeasured to the junction of the pectoral and abdominal scutes. A small amount of lubricant placed on the tube will assist with passing the tube. The head of the patient should be extracted from the shell and, while holding the neck in extension, long-handled crocodile forceps inserted through the mouth and into the esophagus. The forceps should be pushed laterally to protrude in the mid to distal esophageal wall and skin. Visualize the carotid artery and jugular veins, if possible. The carotid is generally in the ventral neck and the jugular in the lateral neck. Cut down horizontally over the protruding forceps with a scalpel blade, and push the tips through the incision. Grasp the end of the red rubber feeding tube in the forceps and draw it though the skin, into the esophagus, and out the mouth by withdrawing the instrument. Reverse the grip on the end of the tube and gently feed the tube down the esophagus into the stomach. The tube can be sutured into place via a purse string suture or a horizontal mattress suture and a Chinese finger trap pattern. The tube should always be capped and can be taped to the carapace to prevent self-removal (Figure 9-37). Radiographs or endoscopy can be performed to confirm proper tube placement.

The tube should always be flushed with water after use to prevent clogging. Feeding tubes are often well tolerated for up to 6 weeks in very debilitated chelonian patients and can remain in place for 3 months or more. Most animals are able to eat normally while the tube is in place; therefore, a fresh diet should always be made available. There are many different critical care diets available for use in chelonians, and it is very

TABLE 9-3	Common Antibiotics Used to Treat Chelonians			
Drug	**Species**	**Dose**	**Route**	**Frequency**
Ampicillin	*Testudo hermanni*	50 mg/kg[169]	IM	BID
Amikacin	*Gopherus polyphemus*	5 mg/kg[170]	IM	q48h
Gentamicin	*Chrysemys picta*	10 mg/kg [171]	IM	q48 h
	Chrysemys scripta elegans	6 mg/kg[172]	IM	q2-5d
Neomycin	Terrapins	200-400 mg per 5 gallons of tank water[173]		
Chloramphenicol	Snakes	50 mg/kg[174]	SC	q12-72h
Doxycycline		50 mg/kg	IM, PO	
Enrofloxacin	*Testudo hermanni*	10 mg/kg[169]	IM	SID
	Gopherus polyphemus	5 mg/kg[175]	IM	q24-48h
	Geochelone elegans	10 mg/kg[176]	IM	BID for *Pseudomonas* and *Citrobacter*
Clindamycin	*Caretta caretta*	5 mg/kg[177]	IM	SID
Trimethoprim/sulfadiazine	*Testudo hermanni*	30 mg/kg[169]	PO	SID for first two doses then q48h
Metronidazole	Reptiles (antibacterial)	50 mg/kg[178]	PO	SID
	Reptiles (antiprotozoan)	260 mg/kg[64]	PO	Once
	Reptiles (antiprotozoan)	160 mg/kg[179]	PO	SID
	Reptiles (antiprotozoan)	100 mg/kg[179]	PO	Days 1 and 14
Ceftazidime	Reptiles	20 mg/kg[180]	IM, IV	q72h
Clarithromycin	*Gopherus agassizii*	15 mg/kg[181]	PO	q48-72h
Tylosin	Reptiles	25 mg/kg[182]	IM, PO	SID
	Reptiles	5 mg/kg[183]	IM	SID

BID, Twice a day; *IM*, intramuscular; *IV*, intravenous; *PO*, per os; *SC*, subcutaneous; *SID*, once a day.

important to select the appropriate diet based on the dietary requirements of the patient. Instructions pertaining to the amount to be fed can usually be found in the package insert. It is very important to avoid refeeding syndrome in patients that have not eaten for extended periods of time. No more than 50% of the calculated metabolic energy requirement (MER) should be fed for the first 2 to 4 days, and gradually this can be increased to 100%. If the patient suddenly reverts to extreme lethargy or weakness once feedings have been initiated, recheck the electrolyte and mineral values (e.g., potassium and phosphorous) and initiate appropriate treatment.

■SURGERY

Anesthesia

Chelonian anesthesia is oftentimes described as a "challenging endeavor." This is primarily a reflection of the need to be proficient with chelonian anatomy, physiology, health, and disease. Knowledge of anesthetic drugs and equipment is vital as well. Nevertheless, if all aspects of preparation are accounted for and potential emergency precautions are taken, chelonian anesthesia can also be extremely satisfying.

PREANESTHETIC PRECAUTIONS

All potential anesthetic candidates require a thorough physical examination before anesthesia. Baseline diagnostics should be recommended before anesthesia, including determining a packed cell volume, total protein, and blood glucose. As with higher vertebrates, all potential candidates should be stabilized before the induction of anesthesia to reduce the potential for anesthetic complications. Once stabilized, chelonian patients should ideally be anesthetized in the morning to allow for recovery under direct supervision throughout the remainder of the day. The anesthetic candidate should be maintained within its preferred optimal temperature during the preanesthetic period. Whereas Heard[196] recommends preoperative fasting because of impaired digestion following the procedure, Bennett[197] does not recommend fasting, because it takes several days to decrease the intestinal volume of hindgut fermenters, and aspiration with an intubated glottis is highly unlikely.

PREMEDICATION AND LOCAL ANESTHESIA

Local anesthesia is a feasible option when procedures are scheduled for superficial sites. The pharmacokinetics of lidocaine in chelonians has not been thoroughly studied, but it should be remembered that the mammalian toxic dose ranges from 5 to 20 mg/kg. Opioids should be utilized preoperatively in patients when a painful procedure is anticipated. Butorphanol is generally administered at a dose of 0.5 to 1 mg/kg intramuscularly. Our understanding of anesthesia in chelonians is limited, but it is generally considered more important to do no harm, and thus why we recommend analgesics. Nonsteroidal antiinflammatories (e.g., meloxicam 0.2-0.5 mg/kg, PO SID; carprofen

TABLE 9-4	Common Miscellaneous Drugs Used to Treat Chelonians				
Drug	**Species**	**Dose**	**Frequency**	**Route**	**Use**
Acyclovir	*Gopherus agassizii*	80 mg/kg[178]	SID	PO	Herpesvirus outbreak
Allopurinol	*Testudo graeca*	20 mg/kg[142]	SID	PO	
	Reptiles	20 mg/kg[178]	SID	PO	
	Chelonians	50 mg/kg[141]	SID	PO	
Calcitonin	Chelonians	1.5 IU/kg[39]	Once	IM	
Calcium-EDTA	*Chelydra serpentina*	2 mg/kg[184]	q10d	IM	Lead toxicity
Calcium glubionate	Reptiles	10 mg/kg[185]	SID–BID	PO	
Calcium gluconate	Chelonians	100 mg/kg[188]	SID	IM	
Fenbendazole	Reptiles	30-50 mg/kg for nematodes[180]	Once or repeat in 3 weeks	PO	Anthelmintic
		50-100 mg/kg for spirurids[116]			
Furosemide	Chelonians	5 mg/kg[186]	SID–BID	IM	Diuretic
Itraconazole	*Chamaeleo* spp.	10 mg/kg[187]	SID for 21 days	PO	Antifungal
Ketoconazole	*Gopherus polyphemus*	15-30 mg/kg[188]	q24h	PO	Antifungal
Levamisole	Tortoises	50 mg/kg[189]	Once	PO	Anthelmintic
	Tortoises	300 mg/kg[190]	Once	PO	
Metoclopromide	*Gopherus agassizii*	1 mg/kg[191]	SID	PO	Antiemetic Gastric motility modifier
Nystatin	Chelonians	100,000 IU/kg[192]	SID	PO	Antifungal
Oxytocin	Chelonians	2-10 IU/kg[39]	Once, repeat in 4-8 h if necessary	IM	Stimulates smooth muscles contraction
Praziquantel	Chelonians	5-8 mg/kg[39]	Once	PO	Anthelmintic
	Reptiles	5-30 mg/kg[116]	Once	PO or IM	
Probenecid		250 mg/animal[142]	BID	PO	
Vitamin A		1500-3000 IU/kg	IM once every 14d PO daily	IM, PO	Caution recommended with parenteral administration due to risk of overdose
Vitamin B1 (thiamine)	Reptiles	25 mg/kg[186]	SID	PO or SQ	
		50-100 mg[193]	PRN	IM	
Vitamin B12		0.05 mg/kg[193]		IM, SQ	
Vitamin B (complex)		25 mg/kg[194]	SID	PO	
Vitamin C		100-250 mg/kg[195]	PRN	IM	
		10-20 mg/kg[195]	PRN	IM	
Vitamin D	Reptiles	100 IU/kg[137]	Days 0 and 7	IM	
	Chelonians	10-40 IU/kg[39]	SID	PO	
Vitamin E		100 IU/kg[195]	Repeat in 7 days	IM	

2 mg/kg, PO IM) are also routinely given as analgesics; however, their efficacy is unknown.

VASCULAR ACCESS

Vascular access can be achieved in chelonians via intravenous, supracarapacial sinus, and intraosseous catheterization. The jugular vein is visualized in the chelonian patient on the dorsolateral surface of the neck at the level of the auricular scale. Some patients must be anesthetized to allow extension of the neck and placement of the catheter (18-24–gauge catheter). A 19- or 24-gauge butterfly catheter facilitates drug administration in the jugular vein in the awake patient. The dorsal cervical sinus is another potential drug administration site in the awake chelonian, along with the dorsal coccygeal vein. In smaller chelonians, intraosseous catheterization of the plastron has been described. If vascular access is achieved, intravascular fluid administration during anesthesia, at a dose of 5 to 10 ml/kg/h, is recommended.[198,199]

TABLE 9-5	Common Emergency Drugs Used to Treat Chelonians		
Drug	**Dose**	**Frequency**	**Route**
Atropine	0.1-0.2 mg/kg[194]	PRN	SC
Dexamethasone sodium phosphate	0.1-0.25 mg/kg[192]	PRN	IV
Furosemide	5 mg/kg[194]	q12-24h	IM
Iron dextran	12 mg/kg[195]	Weekly	IM
Sodium bicarbonate	0.5-1 mg/kg[195]	PRN	IV

SC, Subcutaneous; *IM,* intramuscular; *IV,* intravenous; *PRN,* as needed; *SC,* subcutaneous.

TABLE 9-6	Anesthetic Agents Commonly Used to Anesthetize Chelonians		
Drug	**Dosage**	**Route**	**Comments**
Ketamine	10-20 mg/kg	IM	Mild sedation
Ketamine	20-40 mg/kg	IM	Moderate sedation
Tiletamine	5-10 mg/kg	IM	Mild sedation
Propofol	10-15 mg/kg	IV	General anesthesia
Ketamine + Medetomidine	5-10 mg/kg (K) 0.075-0.1 mg/kg (M)	IM	Mild sedation
Ketamine + Medetomidine	10-15 mg/kg (K) 0.1-0.15 mg/kg (M)	IM	Moderate sedation
Isofluorane	5% / 1 L oxygen	Inhalant	Induction
Isofluorane	3% / 1 L oxygen	Inhalant	Maintenance

IM, Intramuscular; *IV,* intravenous.

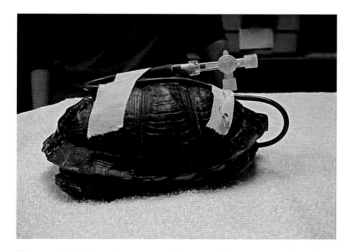

Figure 9-37 The placement of an esophagostomy tube is an excellent idea for any anorectic turtle.

INDUCTION

Gaseous induction via an anesthetic chamber or facemask is generally inappropriate for chelonians due to their ability to breath hold for long periods of time or convert to anaerobic respiration. Injectable anesthetics are frequently employed to obtain an acceptable plane of anesthesia for intubation. Due to the lack of available resources for pharmacokinetic studies on anesthetic agents in reptiles, it is very important to remember that many of the drug dosages used by clinicians have been developed anecdotally. Considering the prolonged drug clearance in chelonians, drugs with reversible, antagonistic agents should be used as frequently as possible. A list of anesthetic agents commonly used in chelonians is found in Table 9-6.

INTUBATION AND VENTILATION

Intubation and assisted ventilation is recommended in all chelonian anesthetic procedures. The chelonian glottis is located at the caudal aspect of the fleshy tongue and is easy to visualize with gentle finger pressure in the intermandibular space. The trachea is comprised of complete cartilaginous rings, and the choana is located in the cranial one third of the cervical area. It is therefore quite easy to inadvertently intubate a single bronchus. Intravenous catheters, uncuffed endotracheal tubes, or shortened urethral catheters can all be used to intubate a chelonian. Topical lidocaine can be applied conservatively to the glottis via a cotton-tipped applicator to decrease the incidence of laryngospasms. Muscular, respiratory, and cardiac depression have been observed in cases of excessive topical anesthetic application.[200]

Chelonians utilize movements of the pelvic and axillary limbs and muscles to alter the size of the coelomic cavity and generate negative pressure in the lungs. This is essential for effective ventilation to occur. Once anesthetized, these movements are obviously hindered, and positive pressure ventilation should be administered throughout the entire procedure. Four to six breaths per minute is generally recommended, depending on the size of the anesthetized patient. Dorsal recumbency also hinders ventilatory movements due to reduced lung volume, unaided tidal volume, and decreased blood perfusion. Large chelonians should not be maintained in dorsal recumbency for prolonged periods of time.[200]

PATIENT MONITORING

It can be quite difficult to assess the depth of anesthesia in the chelonian patient, but it is imperative that this be closely monitored. Neither the tail or limb withdrawal reflexes nor the head withdrawal reflex are present during a surgical plane of anesthesia.[199] The loss of the palpebral reflex generally occurs at a light plane of anesthesia, whereas the loss of the corneal blink reflex and the vent reflex are both indicative of a dangerously deep level of anesthesia.[199]

MONITORING EQUIPMENT

A pulse oximeter is a two-wavelength spectrophotometer that detects the color of pulsating blood and equates this color with oxygen saturation.[200] Pulse oximetry has not been adequately validated for use in chelonians, but a lingual clip or esophageal or cloacal probe[8,201] may be used to monitor trends in oxygenation saturation[202] and to monitor the peripheral pulse. An ultrasonic Doppler flow detector can also be used to monitor heart rate by placing it over the carotid artery or directing it caudally toward the heart. The use of an 8-MHz Doppler probe detects blood flow in small to medium-sized vessels. The probe is usually attached to a loudspeaker, which translates the blood flow into an audible signal and allows easy, consistent heart rate monitoring. Alterations to the heart rate or rhythm are easily and rapidly detected. The three-chambered reptilian heart renders electrocardiograph interpretation difficult, and, considering the fact that the reptilian heart continues to beat for some time after removal from the body, it appears as though electrocardiogram monitoring is of little value in assessment of anesthetic plane. Maintaining the patient's temperature at the upper range of its preferred optimum will minimize the risk of hypoxia by increasing oxygen consumption and will decrease recovery time. Core temperature may be monitored via esophageal or cloacal probes.[203]

Surgery

Chelonians may present for a number of different surgical needs. The following will be a description of the most common surgical procedures performed in our practice, although it is important to recognize that any procedure that can be done in a domestic species can be pursued in chelonians.

AURAL ABSCESSES

Aural abscesses are a common problem in captive chelonians, especially red-eared sliders and box turtles. Many of these animals present with a history of unilateral or bilateral swelling at the site of the tympanic membrane. The diagnosis associated with these lesions is generally straightforward, although identifying a specific etiology may not be as simple. These lesions are generally associated with opportunistic infections, although exposure to organochlorines may also be associated with the development of disease. Opportunistic infections are generally considered to originate in the oral cavity and ascend the eustachian tube. Most aural abscesses are associated with the middle ear. When examining an affected animal, it is important to evaluate the oral cavity, pharynx, and eustachian tube for obvious signs of inflammation. Treating these abscesses requires both a medical and surgical approach. Medicinal treatment should be based on bacterial culture and sensitivity. Before receiving the results, a potent broad-spectrum antibiotic, such as a fluoroquinolone, is recommended. Analgesics and antiinflammatories should also be provided in these cases. Although our understanding of analgesia in chelonians is limited, we generally rely on opioids (Butorphanol, 0.5-1.0 mg/kg twice daily) or nonsteroidal antiinflammatories (meloxicam, 0.2-0.5 mg/kg once daily) to provide comfort for our patients.

The chelonian patient should be anesthetized for this procedure, as it requires extensive exploration and flushing in the aural canal and oral cavity. A general anesthesia is preferred, and the animal should be intubated to minimize the likelihood of aspiration. The external surface of the tympanic membrane should be disinfected using standard techniques. A large "X" should be made over the tympanic membrane. With gentle expression, a liquid and caseous material will be expressed from the middle ear. This material should be completely removed, and the site irrigated with warmed, dilute chlorhexidine/Betadine and 0.9% saline. The tympanum should be left open to allow for continued irrigation. The incision should be allowed to heal by secondary intention healing. Antibiotics and analgesics should be continued until the wound is healed. Reoccurrence is possible, so it is important to identify any deficiencies in the animal's husbandry and correct them.

INTEGUMENTARY ABSCESSES

Chelonians, like other reptiles, generally respond to infectious agents by producing large inflammatory responses. These inflammatory responses generally result in the development of a caseous abscess and can occur anywhere on the body. To successfully manage these abscesses, it is essential that the veterinary surgeon remove the caseous material (or nidus of infection). Attempts to treat chelonian abscesses using antimicrobial therapy only are often met with limited/poor results. Surgical removal of these abscesses is similar to that described for the aural abscesses. The integument should be disinfected before being incised. The incision should be made over or just off to the side of the abscess. All attempts should be made to remove the cyst wall. Once the abscess is opened, the caseous material should be removed and the site irrigated with an appropriate disinfectant. These lesions should be left open and managed as open contaminated wounds. Delayed primary closures

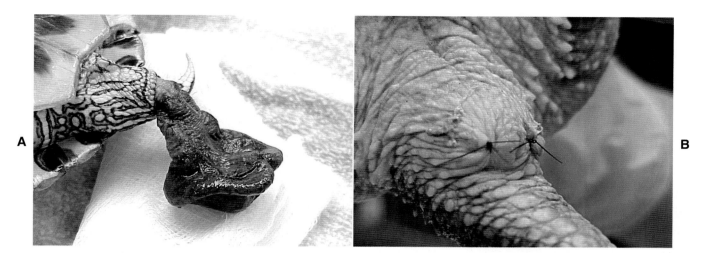

Figure 9-38 The phallus of this red-eared slider is prolapsed **(A)**. It is important to clean and disinfect the organ before replacing it. Two simple interrupted stay sutures may be placed through the vent to prevent the phallus from reprolapsing **(B)**.

may be attempted once the site is no longer considered contaminated.

CLOACAL/RECTAL/ OVIDUCTAL PROLAPSE

When a chelonian presents for a prolapse from the vent, it is important to determine which organs are involved. Generally, the prolapse is associated with the cloaca, rectum, or phallus. Phallus prolapses are the easiest to diagnose, as these structures have a stalk attached to the cranial floor of the cloaca (see Phallus Prolapse). When tubular structures are prolapsed, it can be more difficult to determine exactly which structure is affected. In the simplest case, the cloaca will be prolapsed. The cloaca is comprised of three chambers: the proctodeum, coprodeum, and urodeum. Openings to the urodeum will often have urates being expelled, the coprodeum will have feces, and the proctodeum may have both materials mixed. If the cloacal tissues are viable, they can be irrigated with saline and 50% dextrose (for reduction) and then reduced. We prefer to perform these procedures under anesthesia or at least mild sedation. If the tissues are not viable, an endoscope should be inserted into the cloaca to assess tissue viability. Necrotic tissues should be removed surgically. If the prolapsed structure appears to be associated with the intestine or reproductive tract, radiographs, ultrasound, or coelioscopy may be necessary to assess the extent of the damage. For chronic cloacal or rectal prolapses, the rectum may need to be surgically tacked to the rib cage via a plastron osteotomy. In cases where there is generalized necrosis to the cloaca or rectum, the prognosis is guarded.

For chronic oviductal prolapse cases, an ovariohysterectomy is recommended.

PHALLUS PROLAPSE

Male chelonians have a single phallus. This structure, like the hemipenes of lizards and snakes, serves a single function as a copulatory organ. In captivity, and occasionally in wild specimens, it is not uncommon for chelonians to present with a prolapsed phallus (Figure 9-38). There are a number of different suspected etiologies for this presentation (e.g., arousal, hypocalcemia, trauma, foreign body obstruction, and cystic calculi), although most cases go undiagnosed. Once prolapsed, the organ can become desiccated and necrotic if it is not reduced. In cases where an animal presents with a prolapsed phallus, attempts should be made to assess the status of the organ, determine its viability, and consider whether the organ should be reduced or amputated. In cases where the tissue is still considered viable, the organ should be reduced. Before being reduced, the phallus should be cleaned with dilute chlorhexidine (0.5%) and saline. To reduce the size of the phallus for replacement, we generally liberally irrigate the phallus with 50% dextrose. Once the organ is reduced to a size that will allow it to be reduced, it should be rinsed, removing the dextrose, and replaced to the floor of the cranial base of the tail. To reduce the likelihood of the phallus reprolapsing, two simple interrupted nonabsorbable sutures can be placed through the vent. It is important to place the sutures at a distance that prevents reprolapse of the phallus without affecting the animal's ability to defecate or urinate. In cases where the phallus is determined to be necrotic, it should be removed. Phallus amputation can be achieved by placing sutures around the base of the phallus. We generally use transfixation sutures for this procedure. It is important to remove all of the necrotic tissues to prevent the dissemination of necrotic thromboemboli. Once removed, the base of the phallus can be replaced into the cranial base of the tail.

PLASTRON OSTEOTOMY

The chelonian shell can pose a real problem for the veterinary surgeon. Many of the surgical procedures that need to be performed on these animals require significant exposure to the coelomic cavity. A plastron osteotomy will provide the most

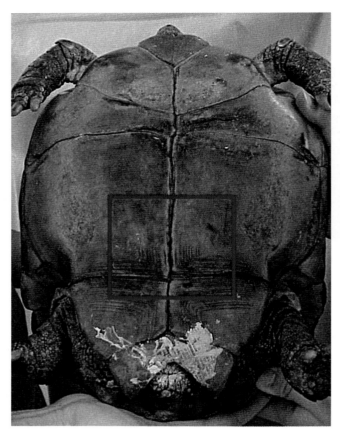

Figure 9-39 The approach to a plastron osteotomy should be through the abdominal and cranial femoral scutes. Care should be taken to avoid cutting into the pelvis.

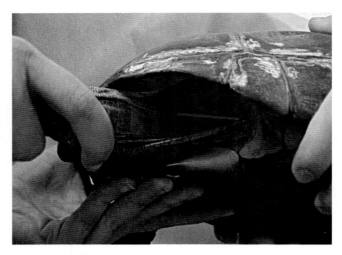

Figure 9-40 We prefer to approach coelomic surgery through the prefemoral fossae whenever possible, as it is less invasive then a plastron osteotomy.

appropriate exposure for most procedures. A plastron osteotomy should be attempted only with the animal under general anesthesia. The surgical approach should go through the abdominal and femoral scutes (Figure 9-39). Care should be taken to avoid the middle to caudal femoral scutes, as the pelvis lies under these sections of the scutes. The surgical site should be disinfected using standard techniques. A high-speed saw should be used to make the incision through the osteoderms. It is important to cool the tissues (e.g., spraying sterile 0.9% saline) while cutting them to minimize the collateral thermal damage associated with the saw. The blade should be angled to create a beveled edge on the osteoderm. This will ensure that the excised osteoderm will fit nicely back into place after surgery. The excised osteoderm should be stored in warm sterile 0.9% saline during the procedure to minimize autolysis. Once the excised osteoderm section is removed, the first tissues generally encountered are the ventral abdominal veins and coelomic membrane. The vessels can be ligated if they limit exposure to the coelomic membrane. A standard exploratory should be done, taking time to evaluate all tissues that can be visualized or palpated. Once the planned procedure is completed, the coelomic membrane can be closed using a simple continuous suture pattern. In some species, the membrane is too friable to close. The excised section of osteoderms should

be replaced and held in place with dental acrylic. We always place dental acrylic first because it is not exothermic. A rapid drying epoxy can be placed over the dental acrylic to waterproof the incision.

PREFEMORAL FOSSAE APPROACH

The prefemoral fossae approach can be attempted for those procedures that can be done in the caudal coelomic cavity. The most common procedures attempted using this approach are enterotomy, cystotomy, liver and renal biopsy (endoscopic preferred), and egg removal. This approach is preferred over the plastron osteotomy because it induces less tissue damage and the healing times for soft tissues are much more rapid than for bone. Unfortunately, this approach is limited in many species because of the small size of the fossae, which limits any real access to the coelomic cavity.

This approach can be attempted by placing the chelonian in lateral recumbency and distracting the rear leg caudally (Figure 9-40). The surgical site should be disinfected using standard techniques. The incision into the coelomic cavity should be made carefully, as the skin, subcutaneous tissues, and muscle layers are thin and it is easy to penetrate the coelomic cavity and accidentally damage underlying tissues (e.g., urinary bladder, intestine). A spay hook may be required to access tissues. Closure for this approach is routine, with simple interrupted sutures being used to close the body wall and horizontal mattress sutures used to close the skin.

GASTROTOMY/ENTEROTOMY

Foreign bodies are a common finding in captive tortoises housed on gravel-based substrates. Because many of these species are geophagic, it is natural for them to consume mineral-based materials. Unfortunately, the substrate often becomes impacted in the small intestine. On occasion the large intestine becomes impacted, but it is generally a large enough organ that it does not become completely impacted. Gravel in the large intestine of some species may play a role in mechanical digestion of plant material. Aquatic species offered large quantities of molluscs or gastropods occasionally become impacted with the shells of these invertebrates. Survey radiographs or contrast surveys are generally sufficient to diagnose an obstruction.

Foreign materials entrapped in the stomach can either be removed by endoscopic removal or via a gastrotomy. Because of the location of the stomach in the chelonian, gastrotomies are best approached via a plastron osteotomy. Intestinal foreign bodies may also be approached via a plastron osteotomy or through an incision through the prefemoral fossae. The approach to a gastrotomy or enterotomy in a chelonian is similar to that described for domestic species. One exception, however, is due to the fragility of the tissue. The intestinal tissues of chelonians are more friable than in mammals. Because of this, it is important to handle the tissues carefully during a procedure, especially if there is concern about the viability of the tissues. Necrotic or hypoperfused tissues are more likely to tear during manipulation or dehisce at the incision. Coeliotomy sponges should be inserted into the coelomic cavity before incising the intestine to limit the likelihood of intestinal spillage and a coelomitis. Stay sutures should be used to facilitate handling of the intestine. The initial incision for an enterotomy should be made on the dorsal surface of the intestine in an avascular area. The foreign material should be removed, the site lavaged with sterile saline, and the incision closed using a simple interrupted suture pattern. A double layer closure (e.g., Lembert-Cushing) may be used to close a gastrotomy incision.

CYSTOTOMY

Cystic calculi are a common finding in captive chelonians that are not provided routine access to water and/or are fed high protein diets. Cystic calculi are also occasionally observed in wild tortoises. Cystic calculi can become rather large in chelonians and should be removed to minimize traumatizing the urinary bladder. In addition to the surgery, any underlying deficiencies in husbandry should be accounted for. A cystotomy can either be approached through a plastron osteotomy or prefemoral fossae approach. It is important to consider the size of the cystic calculi when deciding the approach to ensure that the stone can be removed. In some cases, the stone may have to be broken into pieces to facilitate removal. The urinary bladder of chelonians is thin and friable. Coeliotomy pads should be inserted around the bladder to minimize spillage into the coelomic cavity. Removing excess urine from the bladder may reduce spillage, although it can be difficult to aspirate urine from the bladder if there are considerable urate salts in the urine. The bladder can be expressed digitally during the procedure, but care should be taken to avoid contaminating the surgical field. Stay sutures should be placed in the bladder to maintain control of the incision. The incision should be made in an avascular area. The cystic calculi should be removed and the bladder flushed. Closure can be accomplished using a simple interrupted pattern.

OVARIOIHYSTERECTOMY

Reproductive surgeries in chelonians are generally associated with dystocias. It is always important to ask a client the importance of the reproductive status of a particular animal before attempting a surgery. For some clients their chelonian is a pet, whereas for others they are considered a breeder animal. In cases where a dystocia or chronic reproductive problem occurs in a pet-only animal, an ovariohysterectomy can be done. In breeder animals, eggs are generally removed via a salpingotomy, and the reproductive tract spared. The most common approach to an ovariohysterectomy in a chelonian is through a plastron osteotomy. Endoscopic approaches are becoming more common, but the general practitioner is unlikely, at the time of this writing, to pursue this approach. Salpingotomies can be approached either through the plastron osteotomy or prefemoral fossae.

An ovariectomy in a chelonian is similar to that described for other species. We prefer to use hemoclips over suture to remove the gonads, as placement of the hemoclips is more rapid and easier to do. Gentle traction on the ovary will reveal the ovarian vessels in the mesovarium. A sufficient number of hemoclips should be placed over the vessels to achieve hemostasis. It is important to remove the entire follicular ovary. This procedure is generally easier to perform during the breeding season, as the mesovarium has more play and can be manipulated to apply the hemoclips. The oviducts or shell glands can be removed by ligating the base of the structures at the level of the cloaca and gently dissecting any mesometrium. In cases where the reproductive tract is to remain (e.g., breeder animal), a salpingotomy can be performed following the same techniques used for an enterotomy.

■ZOONOSES

Many of the zoonotic agents that can be transmitted by the chelonian patient have been discussed previously. The most commonly encountered microorganisms include *Salmonella* spp., *Mycobacterium* spp., *Campylobacter* spp., *Chlamydia* spp., *Yersinia* spp., *Vibrio* spp., *Aeromonas* spp., and *Escherichia coli*. Various intestinal parasites may also be transmitted from the chelonian patient. Considering the potential for transmission of infectious agents, all chelonians, healthy and sick, should be treated as contaminated individuals. Ideally, gloves should be worn during handling, and hands should always be washed after handling. Turtles and tortoises should not be housed near food preparation areas, and any sinks or tubs that are used for soaks or baths should be appropriately disinfected. Clients should be advised of the importance of hand washing each time they handle their pets.

REFERENCES

1. Zug GR, Vitt LJ, Caldwell JP, editors: *Herpetology*, San Diego, Calif, 2001, Academic Press.
2. McArthur S, Meyer J, Innis C: Anatomy and physiology. In McArthur S, Wilkinson R, Meyer J, editors: *Medicine and Surgery of Tortoises and Turtles*, Ames, Iowa, 2004, Blackwell.

3. O'Malley B: *Clinical Anatomy and Physiology of Exotic Species*, Edinburgh, 2005, WB Saunders.

4. Holz PH, Barker IK, Crawshaw G et al: The anatomy and perfusion of the renal portal system in the red-eared slider, *J Zoo Wildl Med* 28(4):378-385, 1994.

5. Holz PH, Conlon PD, Crawshaw GJ et al: The reptilian renal portal system and its effect on drug kinetics, *Proc Ann Meeting ARAV/AAZV*, Pittsburgh, Pa, pp 95-96, 1994.

6. Holz PH: The reptilian portal system: influence on therapy. In Fowler ME, Miller ER, editors: *Zoo and Wild Animal Medicine, Current Therapy, vol 4*, Philadelphia, 1999, WB Saunders.

7. Beck K, Loomis M, Lewbart G et al: Preliminary comparison of gentamicin injected into the cranial and caudal limb musculature of the eastern box turtle *Terrapene carolina carolina*, *J Zoo Wildl Med* 26(3):265-268, 1995.

8. Malley AD: Reptiles. In Seymour C, Gleed R, editors: *BSAVA Manual of Small Animal Anaesthesia and Analgesia*. Ames, Iowa, 1999, Blackwell.

9. Crossley D, Altmiras J, Want T: Hypoxia elicits an increase in pulmonary vasculature resistance in anesthetized turtles, *J Exp Biol* 201(24):3367-3375, 1998.

10. Fowler ME: Comparison of respiratory infection and hypovitaminosis A in desert tortoises. In Montali RJ, Migaki G, editors: *Comparative Pathology of Zoo Animals*, Washington DC, 1980, Smithsonian Institution Press.

11. Jacobson ER: Diseases of the respiratory tract of chelonians, *Verh Ber Erkrg Zootiere* 38:1-5, 1997.

12. Frye FL: *Biomedical and Surgical Aspects of Captive Reptile Husbandry*, ed 2, Melbourne, Fla, 1991, Krieger.

13. Perry SF: Structure and function of the reptilian respiratory system. In Wood SC, editor: *Comparative Pulmonary Physiology: Current Concepts*, New York, 1989, Dekker.

14. Murray MJ: Pneumonia and respiratory function. In Mader DR, editor: *Reptile Medicine and Surgery*, Philadelphia, 1996, WB Saunders.

15. Gans C, Hughes GM: The mechanism of lung ventilation in the tortoise (*Testudo graeca*), *J Exp Biol* 47(1):1-20, 1967.

16. McCutcheon FH: The respiratory mechanism of turtles, *Physiol Zool* 16:255, 1943.

17. Pough FH, Andrew RM, Cadle JE et al: *Herpetology*, Englewood Cliffs, NJ, 1998, Prentice Hall.

18. Jackson DC: Mechanical basis for lung volume variability in the turtle *Pseudemys scripta elegans*, *Am J Physiol* 220(3):754-758, 1971.

19. Wood SC, Lenfant CJ: Respiration. In Gans C, editor: *Biology of the Reptilia, vol 5*, London, 1976, Academic Press.

20. Girgis S: Aquatic respiration in the common Nile turtle (*Trionyx triumgis*), *Comp Biochem Physiol* 3:206, 1961.

21. Guard CL: Comparative gut physiology and diets for reptiles, *Proc AAZV*, Washington, DC, pp 32-34, 1980.

22. Wurth SM, Musacchia XJ: Renewal of the intestinal epithelium in the freshwater turtle *Chrysemys picta*, *Anat Rec* 148:427-439.

23. Ashley LM: *Laboratory Anatomy of the Turtle*, ed 1, Dubuque, Iowa, 1962, WMC Brown.

24. Guibe J: L'appareil digestif. In Grassé PP, editor: *Traité de Zoologie, Tome XIV*, Paris, Masson, 1970.

25. King G: Turtles and tortoises. In *Reptiles and Herbivory*, London, 1996, Chapman & Hall.

26. Wright RD, Florey HW, Sanders AG: Observations on the gastric mucosa of *Reptilia*, *Quart J Exp Physiol* 48:1-14, 1957.

27. Riddle O: The rate of digestion in cold-blooded vertebrates: the influence of season and temperature, *Am J Physiol* 24:447-458, 1909.

28. Patterson T: Comparative physiology of the gastric hunger mechanism, *Ann NY Acad Sci* 34, 1933.

29. Hukhara T, Naito T, Kameyama H: Observations on the gastrointestinal movements of the tortoise *Geoclemys reevesii* by the means of the abdominal-window technique, *Nippon Heikatsukin Gakkai Zasshi* 11(2):39-46, 1975.

30. Wright RD, Florey HW, Sander AG: Observations on the gastric mucosa of *Reptilia*, *Quart J Exp Physiol* 48:1-14, 1957.

31. Skoczylas R: Physiology of the digestive tract. In Gans C, editor: *Biology of the Reptilia, vol 8*, London, 1978, Academic Press.

32. Dantzler WH: Renal function (with special emphasis on nitrogen excretion). In Gans C, editor: *Biology of the Reptilia, vol 5*, London, 1978, Academic Press.

33. Moyle V: Nitrogenous excretion in chelonian reptiles, *Biochem J* 44:581-584, 1949.

34. Dantzler WH, Schmidt-Nielson B: Excretion in the fresh-water turtle (*Pseudemus scripta*) and desert tortoise (*Gopherus agassizii*), *Am J Physiol* 210:198-210, 1966.

35. Minnich JE: The use of water. In Gans C, Harvey Pough F, editors: *Biology of the Reptilia, vol 12*, London, 1982, Academic Press.

36. Mader DR: Reptilian urogenital system and renal disease, *Proc 21st Ann Waltham/OSU Symp for the Treatment of Small Anim Dis Exot*, Columbus, Ohio, pp 71-74, 1997.

37. Khalil F, Haggag G: Ureotelism and uricotelism in tortoises, *J Exp Zool* 130:423-432, 1955.

38. Owens DW: Hormones in the life history of sea turtles. In Lutz P, Musick JA, editors: *Biology of the Sea Turtles*, London, 1996, CRC Press.

39. Highfield AC: *Practical Encyclopedia of Keeping and Breeding Tortoises and Freshwater Turtles*, London, 1996, Carapace Press.

40. Carr AF, Carr MH: Modulated reproductive periodicity in *Chelonia*, *Ecology* 51:335-337, 1970.

41. Duval D, Guillette LJ Jr, Jones RE: Environmental control of reptilian reproductive cycles. In Gans C, Pough FH, editors: *The Biology of the Reptilia, vol 13*, New York, 1982, John Wiley & Sons.

42. Licht P: Reproductive cycles of vertebrates: Reptiles. In Lamming GE, editor: *Marshall's Physiology of Reproduction, vol 1*, Melbourne, 1984, Churchill Livingstone.

43. Kuchling G, Razandrimamilafiniarivo OC: The use of ultrasound scanning to study the relationship of vitellogenesis, mating, egg production and follicular atresia in captive ploughshare tortoises *Geochelone yniphora*, *Dodo* 35:109-115, 1999.

44. Bentley PJ: *Comparative Vertebrate Endocrinology*, ed 3, Cambridge, UK, 1998, Cambridge University Press.

45. Kuchling G: Hormones and reproduction. In: *The Reproductive Biology of the Chelonian*, Berlin, 1999, Springer-Verlag.

46. Klicka J, Mahmoud IY: The role of hormones in the reproductive physiology of the painted turtle (*Chrysemys picta*), *Gen Comp Endocrinol* 31:407-413, 1977.

47. Callard IP, Doolittle J, Banks WI et al: Hypothalamic regulation of endocrine function: recent studies on the control of the reptilian ovarian cycle, *Gen Comp Endocrinol, Supplement* 3:65-75, 1972.

48. Licht P: Reproductive endocrinology of reptiles and amphibians: gonadotrophins, *Ann Rev Physiol* 41:337-351, 1979.

49. Frye FL: *Biomedical and Surgical Aspects of Captive Reptile Husbandry*, ed 1, Edwardsville, Kans, 1981, Veterinary Medicine Publishing.

50. Galbraith DA: Multiple paternity and sperm storage in turtles, *J Herpetol* 117-123, 1993.

51. Lloyd ML: Reptilian dystocias review: causes, prevention, management and comments on the synthetic hormone Vasotocin, *AAZV Ann Meeting*, pp 290-294, 1990.

52. Desvages G, Girondot M, Pieau C: Sensitive stages for the effects of temperature on gonadal activity in embryos of the marine turtle *Dermochelys coriacea*, *Gen Comp Endocrinol* 92(1):54-61, 1993.

53. Gross T, Crain D, Bjorndal K et al: Identification of sex in hatchling loggerhead turtles *Caretta caretta* by analysis of steroid concentrations in chorioallantoic/amniotic fluid, *Gen Comp Endo* 99:204, 1995.

54. Ewert M: Embryology of turtles. In Harless M, Morlock H, editors: *Turtle Perspectives and Research*, New York, 1985, John Wiley & Sons.

55. Ferguson M: Reproductive biology and embryology of the crocodilians. In Gans C, editor: *Biology of the Reptilia*, New York, 1985, John Wiley & Sons.

56. Barten: Shell damage. In Mader DR, editor: *Reptile Medicine and Surgery*, Philadelphia, 1996, WB Saunders.

57. Bennet RA: Fracture management. In Mader DR, editor: *Reptile Medicine and Surgery*, Philadelphia, 1996, WB Saunders.

58. Bellairs A, Kamal AM: The chondrocranium and the development of the skull. In Gans C, Parson TS, editors: *Biology of the Reptilia*, London, 1981, Academic Press.

59. Millichamp NJ, Jacobsen ER, Wolf ED: Diseases of the eye and ocular adnexae in reptiles, *JAVMA* 183(11):1205-1212, 1983.

60. Selmi AL, Mendes GM, McManus C et al: Intraocular pressure determination in clinically normal red-footed tortoise (*Geochelone carbonaria*), *J Zoo Wildl Med* 33(1):58-61, 2002.

61. Dodd CK: *North American Box Turtle: A Natural History*, Norman, Okla, 2001, University of Oklahoma Press.

62. Acierno M, Mitchell MA, Zachariah T et al: Evaluating the effects of ultraviolet B radiation on plasma 25-hydroxyvitamin D levels in red-ear slider turtles (*Trachemys scripta elegans*), *Am J Vet Res*, article in press.

63. Frye FL: *A Practical Guide for Feeding Captive Reptiles*, Malabar, Fla, 1991, Kreiger.

64. Bone RD: Gastrointestinal system. In Beynon PH, Cooper ME, Lawton MP, editors: *Manual of Reptiles*, Cheltenham, UK, 1992, British Small Animal Veterinary Association.

65. Edwards MS: Dietary husbandry of large herbivorous reptiles, *Proc ARAV*, pp 139-143, 1991.

66. Fenchel TM, McRoy CP, Ogden JC et al: Symbiotic cellulose degradation in green turtles, *Appl Environ Microbiol* 37(2):348-350, 1979.

67. Scott PW: Nutritional diseases in reptile medicine and surgery, *Proc BVZS*, London, 1996.

68. McArthur S, Barrows M: Nutrition. In McArthur S, Wilkinson R, Meyer J, editors: *Medicine and Surgery of Tortoises and Turtles*, Ames, Iowa, 2004, Blackwell.

69. Donoghue S: Nutrition of the tortoise, *Proc ARAV*, pp 21-30, 1996.

70. Boyer TH: Box turtle care, *Bull ARAV* 2(1):9-14, 1992.

71. Jacobson ER, Greiner E, Terrell S et al: Intranuclear coccidiosis of tortoises, *Proc ARAV*, pp 85-86, 1999.

72. Muro J, Cuenca R, Pastor J et al: Effects of lithium heparin and tripotassium EDTA on haematologic study of Hermann's tortoises *(Testudo hermanni)*, *J Zoo Wildl Med* 29(1):40-44, 1998.

73. Raskin RE: Reptilian complete blood count. In Fudge AM, editor: *Laboratory Medicine: Avian and Exotic Pets*, Philadelphia, 2000, WB Saunders.

74. Marks SK, Citino SB: Hematology and serum chemistry of the radiated tortoise *(Testudo radiata)*, *J Zoo Wildl Med* 21(3):342-344, 1990.

75. Lopez-Olvera JR, Montane J, Marco I et al: Effect of venipuncture site on hematologic and serum biochemical parameters in marginated tortoise *(Testudo marginata)*, *J Wildl Dis* 39(4):830-836, 2003.

76. Samour JH, Hawkey CM, Pugsley S et al: Clinical and pathological findings related to malnutrition and husbandry in captive giant tortoises *(Geochelone* species), *Vet Rec* 15:299-302, 1986.

77. Taylor RW Jr, Jacobson ER: Hematology and serum chemistry of the Gopher tortoise, *(Gopherus polyphemus)*, *Comp Biochem Physiol* 72A:425-428, 1982.

78. Crawshaw G J: Comparison of plasma biochemical values in blood and blood-lymph mixtures from red-eared sliders, *Trachemys scripta elegans*, *Bull ARAV* 6:7-9, 1996.

79. Frye FL: Reptile Clinician's Handbook, Malabar, Fla, 1994, Krieger.

80. Mitruka BM, Rawnsley HM: *Clinical, Biochemical, and Hematological Reference Values in Normal Experimental Animals and Normal Humans*, ed 2, New York, 1981, Masson.

81. Stein G: Hematologic and blood chemistry values in reptiles. In Mader DR, editor: *Reptile Medicine and Surgery*, Philadelphia, 1996, WB Saunders.

82. Rosskopf WJ: Normal hemogram and blood chemistry values for California desert tortoises, *Small Anim Clin* Jan:85-87, 1982.

83. Gobel T, Sporle H: Blutentnahmetechnik und Serumnormalwerte wichtige Parameter bei der griechischen Landschilkroete *(Testudo hermanni hermanni)*, *Tieraertzliche Praxis* 20:231-234, 1992.

84. Raiti P, Haramati N: Problems of reptiles: magnetic resonance imaging and computerized tomography of a gravid leopard tortoise *(Geochelone pardalis pardalis)* with metabolic bone disease, *J Zoo Wildl Med* 28(2):189-197, 1997.

85. Oyewale JO, Ebute CP, Ogunsanmi AO et al: Weights and blood profiles of the west African hinge-backed tortoise, *Kiniyxys erosa* and the desert tortoise, *Gopherus agassizii*, *Zentralbl Veterinarmed A* 45(10):599-605, 1998.

86. Innis CJ: Observation on urinalyses of clinically normal captive tortoises, *Proc ARAV*, pp 109-112, 1997.

87. Mader DR, Ling GV: Cystic calculi in the Californian desert tortoise *Gopherus agassizii*: evaluation of 100 cases, *Proc ARAV*, pp 81-82, 1999.

88. Wilkinson R: Clinical pathology. In McArthur S, Wilkinson R, Meyer J, editors: *Medicine and Surgery of Tortoises and Turtles*, Ames, Iowa, 2004, Blackwell.

89. McKown RD: A cystic calculus from a wild western spiny softshell turtle *Apalone (Trionyx) spiniferus hartwegi*, *J Zoo Wildl Med* 2(93):347, 1998.

90. Wilkinson R, Hernandez-Divers S, Lafortune M et al: Diagnostic imaging techniques. In McArthur S, Wilkinson R, Meyer J, editors: *Medicine and Surgery of Tortoises and Turtles*, Ames, Iowa, 2004, Blackwell.

91. Whitaker BR, Krum H: Medical management of sea turtles in aquaria. In Fowler ME, Fowler RE, editors: *Zoo and Wild Animal Medicine, vol 4*, Philadelphia, 1999, WB Saunders.

92. Wilkinson R: Clinical Pathology. In McArthur S, Wilkinson R, Meyer J, editors: *Medicine and Surgery of Tortoises and Turtles*, Ames, Iowa, 2004, Blackwell.

93. Une Y, Uemura K, Nakano Y et al: Herpesvirus infection in tortoises *(Malacochersus tornieri* and *Testudo horsfieldi)*, *Vet Pathol* 36:624-627, 1999.

94. McLaughlin GS, Jacobson ER, Brown DR et al: Upper respiratory tract disease in gopher tortoises: pathologic investigation of naturally occurring disease in Florida, *J Wildl Dis* 36:272-283, 2000.

95. McArthur S: Problem-solving approach to common diseases of terrestrial and semi-aquatic *chelonians*. In McArthur S, Wilkinson R, Meyer J, editors: *Medicine and Surgery of Tortoises and Turtles*, Ames, Iowa, 2004, Blackwell.

96. Marschange RE, Gravendyck M, Kaleta EF: Herpesviruses in tortoises: investigations into virus isolation and the treatment of viral stomatitis in *Testudo hermanni* and *T graeca*, *J Vet Med B* 44:385-394, 1997.

97. Origgi R: Tortoise herpesvirus and stomatitis-rhinitis in tortoises, *Proc ARAV*, Orlando, Fla, pp 101-102, 2001.

98. Marschange R, Milde K, Bellavista M: Virus isolation and vaccination of tortoises against a *chelonid* herpesvirus in a chronically infected population in Italy, *Dtsch Tierartzlich Waschr* 108:376-379, 2001.

99. Origgi FC: Development of an ELISA and an immunoperoxidase-based test for a herpesvirus exposure detection in tortoises, *Proc ARAV*, Columbus, Ohio, pp 65-57, 1999.

100. Origgi FC, Klein PA, Mathes K et al: An enzyme linked immunosorbent assay (ELISA) for detecting herpesvirus exposure in Mediterranean tortoises [spurthighed tortoise *(Testudo graeca)* and Hermann's tortoise *(Testude hermanni)*], *J Clin Microbiol* 39:3156-3163, 2001.

101. Cunningham AA: Emerging infectious diseases and amphibian declines, *Proc BVZS*, pp 35-37, 2000.

102. Cooper JE, Gschmeissner S, Bone RD: Herpesvirus-like particles in necrotic stomatitis of tortoises, *Vet Rec* 123(21):544, 1988.

103. Jacobson ER, Gaskin JM, Brown MB et al: Chronic upper respiratory disease of free-ranging desert tortoises *(Xerobates agassizii)*, *J Wildl Dis* 27:296-316, 1991.

104. Berschauer R, Mader D: Hepatic abscess due to *Corynebacterium* sp. in desert tortoise, *Gopherus agassizii*, *Bull ARAV* 8:13-15, 1998.

105. Pare JA, Sigler L, Rosenthal KL et al: Microbiology: fungal and bacterial diseases of reptiles. In Mader DR, editor: *Reptile Medicine and Surgery*, ed 2, St Louis, 2006, WB Saunders.

106. Brown MB, Schumacher IM, Klein PA: *Mycoplasma agassizii* causes upper respiratory disease in the desert tortoise *(Gopherus asassizii)*, *Infect Immunol* 62:4580-4586, 1994.

107. Lederle PE, Rautenstrauch KR, Rakestraw DL et al: Upper respiratory disease and mycoplasmosis in desert tortoises from Nevada, *J Wildl Dis* 33(4):759-765, 1997.

108. McArthur SD, Wilkinson RJ, Barrows MG: Tortoises and turtles. In Redrobe S, Meredith MA, editors: *BSAVA Manual of Exotic Pets*, Cheltenham, UK, 2002, British Small Animal Veterinary Association.

109. McArthur SD, Windsor HM, Bradbury JM et al: Isolation of *Mycoplasma agassizii* from United Kingdom captive chelonians *(Testudo horsfieldi* and *Geochelone pardalis)* with upper respiratory tract disease, poster display, *Ann Conf ARAV*, Reno, Nev, 2002.

110. Saelinger CA, Lewbart GA, Christian LS et al: Prevalence of *Salmonella* spp. in cloacal, fecal, and gastrointestinal mucosal samples from wild North American turtles, *J Am Vet Med Assoc* 229(2):266–268, 2006.

111. Angulo F: Here we go again? Reptile-associated salmonellosis in humans, *Proc ARAV*, Houston, Texas, pp 65-66, 1997.

112. Jacobson ER, Schumacher J, Telford SR et al: Intranuclear coccidiosis in radiated tortoises *(Geochelone radiata)*, *J Zoo Wildl Med* 25:95-122, 1994.

113. Zwart P, Buitelaar M: *Candida tropicalis* enteric infections and their treatment in chelonians, *Ann Proc AAZV*, pp 58-59, 1980.

114. Frank W: Endoparasites. In Cooper JE, Jackson OF, editors: *Diseases of the Reptilia, vol 1*, London, 1981, Academic Press.

115. Pichelin S, Cribb TH, Bona FV: *Glossocercus chelodinae* (MacCallum 1921) n comb (Cestoda: Dilepididae) from freshwater turtles in Australia and a redefinition of the genus *Bancroftiella johnston*, *Syst Parasitol* 39:165-181, 1998.

116. Frank W, Reichel K: Erfahrungen bei der Bekaempfung von Nematoden und Cestoden bei Reptilien und Amphibien. In *Erkankungen der Zootiere, Verh Ber XIX Int Symp Erk De Zootiere, Poznan*, Berlin, 1977, Akademik Verlag.

117. Greiner EC, Mader DR: Parasitology. In Mader DR, editor: *Reptile Medicine and Surgery*, St Louis, 2006, WB Saunders.

118. Lane TJ, Mader DR: Parasitology. In Mader DR, editor: *Reptile Medicine and Surgery*, Philadelphia, 1996, WB Saunders.

119. Jacobson ER: Parasitic diseases of reptiles. In Kirk RW, editor: *Current Veterinary Therapy VIII, Small Animal Practice*, Philadelphia, 1986, WB Saunders.

120. Jacobson ER, Clubb S, Gaskin JM et al: Herpesvirus-like infection in Argentine tortoises, *JAVMA* 187:1227-1229, 1983.

121. Kolmstetter CM, Frazier D, Cox S et al: Metronidazole pharacokinetics in yellow rat snakes *(Elaphe obsolete quadrivittata)*, *Proc AAZV*, Houston, Tex, p 26, 1997.

122. Kolmstetter CM, Frazier D et al: Pharmacokinetics of metronidazole in the green iguana *(Iguana iguana)*, *Bull ARAV*, 8(3):4-7, 1998.

123. Zwart P, Truyens EH: Hexamitiasis in tortoises, *Vet Parasitol* 1:175-183, 1975.

124. Klingenberg RJ: *Understanding Reptile Parasites: A Basic Manual for Herpetoculturalists and Veterinarians*, Lakeside, Calif, 1993, Advanced Vivarium Systems.

125. Denver M, Cranfield M, Graczyk T et al: A review of reptilian amoebiasis and current research on the diagnosis and treatment of amoebiasis at the Baltimore Zoo, *Proc AAZV*, pp 11-15, 1999.

126. Plumb D: *Veterinary Drug Handbook*, White Bear Lake, Minn, 1999, Pharma Vet.

127. *Physicians' Desk Reference,* ed 51, London, 1997, Random House.

128. Paré JA, Crawshaw GJ, Baren JR: Treatment of cryptosporidiosis in Gila monsters *(Heloderma suspectum)* with paromomycin, *Proc ARAV*:23-24, 1997.

129. McAlister CT, Upton SJ: The coccidians of testudines, with descriptions of three new species, *Can J Zoo* 67:2459-2467, 1989.

130. Barnard SM: Color atlas of reptilian parasites, part II: flatworms and roundworms. *Compend Contin Educ Pract Vet* 8:259, 1986.

131. Cranfield M, Graczyk T: New approaches for diagnosis of *Entamoeba* infections in captive reptiles, *Proc ARAV*, pp 17-18, 1999.

132. Boyer TH: Differential diagnosis by symptom: turtles, tortoises, terrapins. In Mader DR, editor: *Reptile Medicine and Surgery*, Philadelphia, 1996, WB Saunders.

133. Frye FL: Vitamin A sources, hypovitaminosis A and iatrogenic hypervitaminosis A in captive *chelonians*. In Kirk RW, Bonagura JD: *Current Veterinary Therapy X*, Philadelphia, 1989, WB Saunders.

134. Elkan E, Zwart P: The ocular disease of young terrapins caused by deficiency of vitamin A, *Pathol Vet* 4:201-222, 1967.

135. Fowler ME: Comparison of respiratory infection and hypovitaminosis A in desert tortoises. In Montali RJ, Migaki G, editors: *Comparative Pathology of Zoo Animals*, Washington, DC, 1980, Smithsonian Institution Press.

136. Palmer DG, Rubel A, Mettler F et al: [Experimentally induced skin changes in tortoises by high parenteral doses of Vitamin A] [Article in German], *Zentra Veterinarmed A* 31:625-633, 1984.

137. Donoghue S, Langenberg J: Nutrition. In Mader DR, editor: *Reptile Medicine and Surgery*, Philadelphia, 1996, WB Saunders.

138. Fowler ME: Metabolic bone disease. In Fowler ME, editor: *Zoo and Wild Animal Medicine,* ed 2, Philadelphia, 1986, WB Saunders.

139. Mautino M, Page DC: Biology and medicine of turtles and tortoises, *Vet Clin North Am* 23(6), 2001.

140. Speer BL: Disease of the urogenital system. In Altman RB, Clubb SL, Dorrestein GM et al, editors: *Avian Medicine and Surgery*, Philadelphia, 1997, WB Saunders.

141. Kolle P: Efficacy of allopurinol in European tortoises, part 2, *Proc ARAV*, Orlando, Fla, pp 185-186, 2001.

142. Martinez-Silvestre A: Treatment with Allopurinol and Probenecid for visceral gout in a greek tortoise *(Testudo graeca)*, *Bull ARAV* 7(4):4-5, 1997.

143. Center SA, Crawford MA, Guida L et al: A retrospective study of 77 cats with severe hepatic lipidosis 1975-1990, *J Vet Intern Med* 31(1):1-7, 1993.

144. Redrobe S: An introduction to *chelonian* radiography and ultrasonagraphy, *Proc BVZS*, pp 1-7, 1996.

145. Divers SJ, Cooper JE: Reptile hepatic lididosis, *Semin Av Exot Pet Med* 9(3):153-164, 1999.

146. McArthur S: Feeding techniques and fluids. In McArthur S, Wilkinson R, Meyer J, editors: *Medicine and Surgery of Tortoises and Turtles*, Ames, Iowa, 2004, Blackwell.

147. Jackson CG, Trotter JA, Trotter TH et al: Accelerated growth and early maturity in *Gopherus agassizii*, *Herpetol* 32:139, 1976.

148. Lambert MR: On the growth of the captive-bred Mediterranean *Testudo* sp. in Northern Europe. In Rocek Z, editor: *Studies in Herpetology*, Prague, 1986, Charles University.

149. Reid D: Notes on the dietary regimes of juvenile spur-thighed tortoises *(Testudo graeca)* and a comparison of their growth over 12 months, *J Assoc Study Rep Amph* 1(3):2, 1986.

150. Innis C: Considerations in formulating captive tortoise diets, *Bull ARAV* 4(1):8-12, 1994.

151. Hernandez-Divers S, Garner M: Neoplasia of reptiles with an emphasis on lizards. *Vet Clin Exot Anim* 6:251-272, 2003.

152. Herbst LH, Jacobson ER, Klein PA et al: Comparative pathology and pathogenesis of spontaneous and experimentally induced fibropapillomas of green turtles *(Chelonia mydas)*, *Vet Pathol* 36(6):551-564, 1999.

153. Lackovich JK, Brown DR, Homer BL et al: Association of herpesvirus with fibropapillomatosis of the green turtle *Chelonia mydas*, and the loggerhead turtle, *Caretta caretta* in Florida, *Dis Aquat Organ* 37(2):89-97, 1999.

154. Quackenbush SL, Work TM, Balazas GH et al: Three closely related herpesviruses are associated with fibropapillomatosis in marine turtles, *Virology* 246(2):392-399, 1998.

155. Norton TM, Jacobson ER, Sundberg FP: Cutaneous fibropapillomatosis and renal myxofibroma in a green turtle *Chelonia mydas*, *J Wildl Dis* 26(2):265-270, 1990.

156. Garner MM, Hernandez-Divers SM, Raymond JT: Reptile neoplasia: a retrospective study of case submission to a specialty diagnostic service, *Vet Clin Exot Anim* 7:653-671, 2004.

157. Machotka SV: Neoplasia in reptiles. In Hoff GL, Frye FL, Jacobson ER, editors: *Diseases of Amphibians and Reptiles*, New York, 1984, Plenum Press.

158. Frye FL, Carney FD: Parathyroid adenoma in a tortoise, *Vet Med Small Anim Clin* 70(5):582-584, 1975.

159. Frye FL: Diagnosis and surgical treatment of reptilian neoplasms with a compilation of cases 1966-1993, *In Vivo* 8(5):885-892, 1994.

160. Cowan DF: Diseases of captive reptiles, *JAVMA* 153(7):848-859, 1968.

161. Billips LH, Harshbarger JC: Neoplasia: reptiles. In Melby EC, Altman NH, editors: *Handbook of Laboratory Science, vol 3*, Cleveland, 1976, CRC Press.

162. Oros J, Torrent A, Espinosa de los Monteros A et al: Multicentric lymphoblastic lymphoma in a loggerhead sea turtle *(Caretta caretta)*, *Vet Pathol* 38(4):464-467, 2001.

163. Newman SJ, Brown CJ, Patnaik AK: Malignant ovarian teratoma in a red-eared slider *(Trachemys scripta elegans)*, *J Vet Diagn Invest* 15(1):77-81, 2003.

164. Bonner BB: *Chelonian* therapeutics, *Vet Clin North Am* 3(1):257-289, 2001.

165. Richards J: Metal bridges: a new technique of turtle shell repair, *J Herpetol Med and Surg* 11(4):31-34, 2001.

166. Prezant RM, Jarchow JL: Lactated fluid use in reptiles: is there a better solution? *Proc ARAV*, pp 83-87, 1997.

167. Minnich JE: Comparison of field water budgets in the tortoises *Gopherus agassizii and G polyphemus*, *Am Zoo* 16:219, 1976.

168. Christopher MM, Brigmon R, Jacobson E: Seasonal alterations in plasma beta hydroxyl-butyrate and related biochemical parameters in the desert tortoise *Gopherus agassizii*, *Comp Biochem Physiol* 108A:303-310, 1994.

169. Spörle H, Göbel T, Schildger B: Blood levels of some anti-infectives in the Hermann's tortoise *(Testudo hermanni)*. In *4th Int Colloq Pathol Med Reptiles Amphibians*, Germany, 1991.

170. Caligiuri RL, Kollias GV, Jacobson ER et al: The effects of ambient temperature on amikacin pharmacokinetics in gopher tortoises, *J Vet Pharm Ther* 13:287, 1990.

171. Bush M, Custer RS, Smeller JM et al: Preliminary study of gentamicin in turtles, *Proc AAZV*, p 50, 1970.

172. Raphael B, Clark CH, Hudson R: Plasma concentrations of gentamicin in turtles, *J Zoo Anim Med* 16:136,1985.

173. Thorsen TE: Salmonellosis in pet turtles, *Mod Vet Pract* 55(1):31-32, 1974.

174. Clark CH, Rogers ED, Milton SL: Plasma concentrations of chloramphenicol in snakes, *Am J Vet Res* 46:2654, 1985.

175. Prezant RM, Isaza I, Jacobson ER: Plasma concentrations and disposition kinetics of enrofloxacin in gopher tortoises, *Gopherus polyphemus*, *J Zoo Wildl Med* 25:82-87, 1994.

176. Raphael B, Papich M, Cook RA: Pharmacokinetics of enrofloxacin after a single intramuscular injection in Indian Star tortoises, *J Zoo Wildl Med* 25:88-94, 1994.

177. Nutter FB, Lee DD, Stamper MA et al: Hemiovariosalpingectomy in a loggerhead sea turtle *(Caretta caretta)*, *Vet Rec* 146:78-80, 2000.

178. Klingenberg RJ: Therapeutics. In Mader DR, editor: *Reptile Medicine and Surgery*, Philadelphia, 1996, WB Saunders.

179. Jackson OF. In Cowie AF, editor: A manual of the care and treatment of children's and exotic pets, pp. 19-37, Cheltenham, UK, 1976, British Small Animal Veterinary Association.

180. McArthur S, Wilkinson R, Meyer J, editors: *Medicine and Surgery of Tortoises and Turtles*, Ames, Iowa, 2004, Blackwell.

181. Wimsatt J, Johnson J, Mangone BA et al: Claithromycin pharmacokinetics in the desert tortoise *(Gopherus agassizii)*, *J Zoo Wildl Med* 30(1):36-43, 1999.

182. Murphy JB: The use of the macrolide antibiotic tylosin in the treatment of reptilian respiratory infections, *Brit J Herpetol* 4:317-322, 1973.

183. Jacobson ER, Behler JL, Jarchow JL: Health assessment of *chelonians* and release into the wild. In Fowler ME, Miller RE, editors: *Zoo and Wild Animal Medicine, vol 4*, Philadelphia, 1999, WB Saunders.

184. Borkowski R: Lead poisoning and intestinal perforations in a snapping turtle *(Chelydra serpentina)* due to fishing-gear ingestion, *J Zoo Wildl Med* 28(1):109-113, 1997.

185. Allen DG, Pringle JK, Smith D: *Handbook of Veterinary Drugs*, Philadelphia, 1993, JB Lippincott.

186. Frye FL: *Biomedical and Surgical Aspects of Captive Reptile Husbandry*, ed 2, Melbourne, Fla, 1991, Krieger.

187. Pare JA, Sigler L, Hunter DB et al: Cutaneous mycoses in chamaeleons caused by the *Chrysosporium* anamorph of *Nanniziosis vriesii (Apinis) currah*, *J Zoo Wildl Med* 28(3):443-453, 1997.

188. Page CD, Mautino M, Derendorf H et al: Multiple dose pharmacokinetics of ketoconazole administered to gopher tortoises, *Gopherus polyphemus*, *J Zoo Wildl Med* 22:191-198, 1991.

189. Zwart P, Ham van B. *Tijdschrift diergeneesk* 97:1285-1286, 1972.

190. Frank W. In Klos HG, Lang EM, editors: *Zootierkrankheiten*, Berlin, 1974, Paul Parey.

191. Tothill A, Johnson JD, Wimsatt J et al: Effects of cisapride, metoclopromide and erythromycin on the prokinetic passage of ingested markers in the desert tortoise *Gopherus agassizii, Proc ARAV*, pp 143-144, 1999.

192. Jacobson ER: Necrotising mycotic dermatitis in snakes: clinical and pathological features, *J Am Vet Med Assoc* 177:1169-1175, 1980.

193. Benson KG, Tell LA, Young LA et al: Pharmacokinetics of ceftiofur sodium after intramuscular or subcutaneous administration in green iguanas *(Iguana iguana)*, *Am J Vet Res* 212:1278-1282, 2003.

194. Bennet RA: Reptile anesthesia, *Semin Av Exot Pet Med* 7:30-40, 1998.

195. Dennis PM: Plasma concentration of ionized calcium in healthy iguanas, *JAVMA* 219:326-328, 2001.

196. Heard DJ: Principles and techniques of anaesthesia and analgesia for exotic practice, *Vet Clin North Am Small Anim Pract* 23(6):1301-1327,1993.

197. Bennet RA: Reptile anesthesia. In *Kirk's Current Veterinary Therapy XII*, Philadelphia, 1995, WB Saunders.

198. Johnson JH: Anaesthesia, analgesia and euthanasia of reptiles and amphibians, *Proc AAZV*, Calgary, Alberta, Canada, pp 132-138, 1991.

199. Bennet RA: Anaethesia and analgesia. In Cornick-Seahorn J, editor: *Semin Av Exot Med* 7(1):30-40, 1998.

200. McArthur S: Anaesthesia, analgesia and euthanasia. In McArthur S, Wilkinson R, Meyer J, editors: *Medicine and Surgery of Tortoises and Turtles,* Ames, Iowa, 2004, Blackwell.

201. Mader DR: Critical care and anesthesia workshop, *ARAV*, Columbus, Ohio, 1999.

202. Allen JL: Use of pulse oximetry in monitoring anaesthesia. In Fowler ME, Miller RE, editors: *Zoo and Wild Animal Medicine: Current Therapy 4,* Philadelphia, 1999, WB Saunders.

203. Bailey JE, Pablo LS: Anaesthetic monitoring and monitoring equipment in small exotic pet practice. *Semin Av Exot Med* 7(1):53-60, 1998.

Thomas N. Tully, Jr.

CHAPTER 10

BIRDS

■ COMMON SPECIES KEPT IN CAPTIVITY

Avian species are commonly maintained in captivity for the enjoyment and pleasure of the owner. The companion bird is generally classified as an interactive animal that recognizes the owner, and a human-animal bond develops. The aviary or cage bird may recognize the owner, but its purposes are to propagate the species and/or provide companionship and enjoyment. Of avian species that are maintained in zoologic parks, some species are endangered and others are displayed to educate the patrons. Many of the species kept in zoologic parks are difficult to keep in captivity and have little, if any, companionship qualities. This chapter will focus on the common avian species that present most often to veterinary clinics.

Passerine Species

Passerine species usually are cage birds, purchased for their beauty, singing ability, or both.

CANARY

The canary is one of the most popular cage birds because of its singing ability (Figure 10-1). Male canaries sing to attract mates and establish territory. The light cycle has a direct effect on a canary's singing quality. The canary molts feathers during the longer days of summer and has full plumage for finding a mate and breeding during the shorter days of fall and winter. It is during the shorter days that the male canary sings to find and keep a mate. During the longer summer days it is not unusual for the male canary to stop singing as new feathers are developing.

Numerous types of canaries exist, including both common (e.g., Fife, Border, Gloster) and rare (e.g., Lizard, Yorkshire, Norwich, frilled) examples. Canary types known to be excel-

lent singing birds include the waterslager, German roller, and American Singer. Showing canaries during the fall is a popular pastime among canary owners. Some of the canaries that are shown are called red canaries. The red factor canary is a cross between the red siskin and the border fancy canary. To enhance the red coloring in a red factor canary's feathers, the bird may be fed a commercial produce supplement or a diet high in similar compounds (e.g., carrots, broccoli). The commercially manufactured pigment can be placed either in the food or in the drinking water during the molting process. The color supplement will only work through the uptake of pigment in developing feathers. Once the feathers are mature, the color additive will no longer be effective. This is one reason why most of the canary shows are in the later months of the year, when the feathers are mature and the bird is ready to select a mate. For the red canary the feathers are fully developed and colored during the winter months.

There are two different physical characteristics of canary feathers with each type; straight-feathered birds and the birds with a disk-shaped crest of feathers on their head. Different feather characteristics are part of the genetic makeup of the birds, which contributes to the development of breeding programs. The crest is a dominant mutation, and crested birds should never be mated with crested birds. Only birds that have the crested gene should be bred to normal birds for the possibility of producing both crested and noncrested offspring. Canaries are extremely susceptible to avian pox and genetic disorders (e.g., congenital cataracts). Care must be taken when breeding canaries to prevent exposure to mosquitos that will expose the birds to the avian poxvirus, and care must be taken in selection of adults to reduce the incidence of genetic disorders.

GOULDIAN FINCH

The Gouldian or lady Gouldian, an Australian finch, is one of the most beautiful caged birds. The normal coloration is a red face, olive green wings, purple breast, and yellow belly

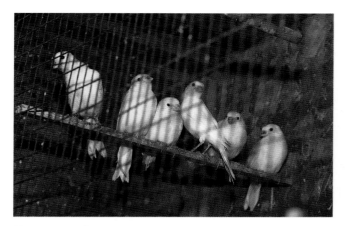

Figure 10-1 Canaries are popular caged birds that are revered for their beauty and singing qualities.

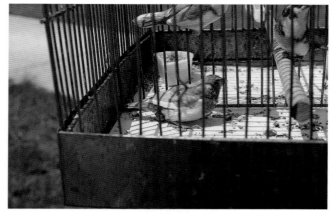

Figure 10-3 Society finches are commonly used as surrogate parents for other finch species, such as the Gouldian finch.

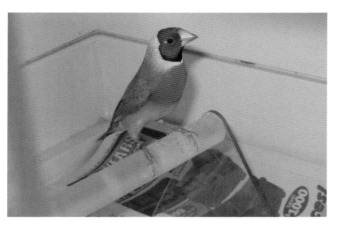

Figure 10-2 Gouldian finches are very colorful and are bred for different color mutations.

(Figure 10-2). The male bird has more vivid coloration than the female, and the hen's beak has a color change from white to gray during the breeding season. This bird is popular with aviculturists trying to develop new color mutations. Accepted color mutations are white-breasted green, lilac-breasted green, pastel green, white-breasted pastel green, lilac-breasted pastel green, blue, white-breasted blue, lilac-breasted blue, and combinations of these colors. There are nonaccepted color mutations, such as cinnamon, sea green, and dilute, but they have not been approved by the Gouldian finch societies at this time. These colorful birds need to have the proper caging and diet to reduce the stress they often exhibit in captivity. High stress levels contribute to poor reproductive results and chronic illness. To increase reproductive success, Bengalese (aka society) finches are used as foster parents. The use of Bengalese finches as foster parents also promotes the exposure of air sac mites, *Syngamus trachea,* to the Gouldian finch offspring. Air sac mites are one of the most common disease conditions associated with the Gouldian finch and are difficult to clear from an affected animal because of the constant immunocompromised

state of the patient in captivity. Strict oversight of appropriate husbandry and dietary issues will aid in maintaining a healthy pet finch or a productive aviary of these attractive birds.

BENGALESE FINCH (SOCIETY FINCH)

The true name of this bird is the Bengalese finch, but it is commonly called the society finch (Figure 10-3). This bird is not found in nature but was developed through the crossbreeding of the sharp-tailed munia *(Lonchura acuticauda)* and the striata munia *(Lonchura striata).* This genetic variant has a variety of color patterns of white, brown, and tan. The society finch is best known as an excellent foster parent for Gouldian finch babies, but it also makes an excellent caged bird on its own. These birds are easy to breed and are entertaining to watch when housed together in a group. Although the Bengalese finch is known for its breeding and foster-parenting ability, caution must be used when these birds are sitting eggs or raising babies. Success in producing finch or other avian species offspring is obtained through minimal contact with the parents. It is not uncommon for birds to abandon their nest, eat their eggs, or kill their babies if too much interference is generated by the owner incessantly checking the nest or nest box.

ZEBRA FINCH

This colorful interactive bird is a popular caged bird. With its red bill and black-and-white tail, the Zebra finch not only is attractive but also appears adaptable to a captive environment (Figure 10-4). Excellent reproductive success, particularly in an outdoor aviary, is one of the positive aspects of owning these birds. As with the society finch, the zebra finch is so prolific that clutch numbers should be regulated to 3 or 4 per season to maintain the health of the adults. There are commercially available nests manufactured for zebra finches, constructed of small rattan slats or grass fiber. These nests usually are oblong in shape and have an opening near the top (Figure 10-5). To discourage egg laying, all nesting material should be removed from the enclosure and/or the nest box taken out. As with the

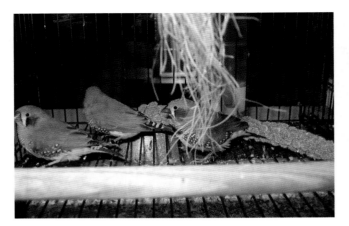

Figure 10-4 Zebra finches have a pleasant chirping sound and are very popular caged birds that are easy to maintain.

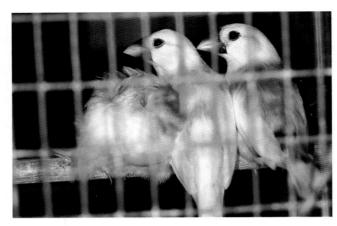

Figure 10-6 Java rice birds are a common caged bird in many parts of the United States. In certain states and countries this bird may be illegal to own because of potential agricultural damage if released.

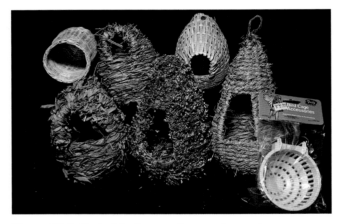

Figure 10-5 Typical finch nests that may be used to encourage reproductive activity between a pair of birds.

Gouldian finch, color mutations are common with zebra finches. Having a number of birds in a cage or aviary setting will generate lively entertainment along with a pleasant chirping vocalization within the group.

STRAWBERRY FINCH AND CORDON BLEU FINCH

The strawberry finch is a brownish red bird covered with white spots over the body. One of the desired qualities of this bird is its beautiful song, stronger and clearer in the male than in the female. The strawberry finch is more difficult than the previously mentioned finches to propagate successfully in captivity; most success is attained in naturalized aviary settings. Live food (e.g., mealworms) should be provided all year round.

The cordon bleu finch, although found in aviary and cage settings, is relatively expensive compared with the other described finches. This finch has a light blue face and chest area with the rest of the body being whitish tan. The male cordon bleu finch has a red ear patch that is lacking on the female. Attention to detail and especially naturalized aviary settings generate the best reproductive results with this finch. As with the strawberry finch, the cordon bleu finch requires live food throughout the year.

JAVA RICE BIRD

The Java rice bird is small, has a large pink beak (Figure 10-6), and is a very popular, inexpensive cage and aviary bird. There are many different color mutations (e.g., white, pied), in part because of their ability to reproduce in captivity. As with other passerine species that breed readily in captivity, it is recommended to limit the clutch size of this bird. Before purchase, one should check with the local wildlife regulations regarding ownership status of this bird. There is a concern in some regions of the country that if released, the Java rice bird will be a future threat to the destruction of grain fields; thus, the ownership of this bird is prohibited in those areas.

OTHER PASSERINE SPECIES

There are a variety of passerine species maintained in caged and aviary settings. The list includes weavers, whydahs, manikins, waxbills, cardinals, and a variety of other finches. Before purchasing a bird to maintain in captivity, prospective owners must research the husbandry and dietary requirements of that bird species. This research will educate the owners not only on the commitment necessary for the particular bird of interest but also on whether they have the resources to provide the care required to maintain the health of that animal. Many of the uncommon passerine species are difficult to propagate in captivity; therefore, the majority of birds enter the market through importation. Imported birds that are uncommon are often expensive, making the initial investment for this type of bird less appealing for a new owner.

Small passerines require oversight and care, especially in outdoor aviaries. The birds will denude foliage for nesting purposes and have territorial disputes within and outside of species groups. Maintenance of the aviary is required, for keeping the plants healthy, keeping unwanted predators out, and keeping the birds inside. Rats often invade outdoor aviaries and will capture psittacine species when they are roosting at night. Rodents are attracted to aviaries because of the food provided the birds and eventually the birds and eggs themselves. Making an aviary rodent proof will protect birds and eggs and will reduce the stress on breeding pairs that may not mate or may abandon the nest as a response to the presence of vermin.

Food must be provided at all times, with appropriate variety to meet the species' requirements. For live food, small mealworms, insect larvae, pupae, aphids, and spiders are commonly fed. Millet, rape, sesame, hemp, niger, canary, thistle, and poppy seed are the seed varieties most often used for passerine diets. Egg food diets are recommended for hand-rearing young birds and for providing adult females increased nutrition during the reproductive process. The perishable nature of egg food contributes to quick spoilage, which may adversely affect the health of the birds. A time-tested egg food diet should be used for the passerine species being fed. The egg food diet should be fed in the proper amount at the proper time and removed before it is spoiled. The husbandry oversight intensifies when egg food is being offered to reproductively active birds. Passerine species must always have water available; they have little ability to survive once the water container is empty. (A more detailed passerine nutritional overview will be provided in Nutrition.)

Psittacine Species

Psittacine species are birds usually purchased for their beauty and companionship.

BUDGERIGAR (COMMON PARAKEET)

The budgerigar (budgie) is commonly called a *parakeet* in North America (Figure 10-7). Unfortunately, there are many different species of parakeets, so it is in the public's best interest to differentiate between the species when identifying a bird. To identify this bird within this chapter and for future use, one should become familiar with using the term *budgerigar*. The normal budgie color is a green body with a yellow head and wings speckled with black over the face. As with the passerine species, there are many color mutations ranging from lutino to blue. A generalized dimorphic characteristic for "normal" green budgies is that the female has a pink/brown cere, whereas the male has a blue cere. One may use the cere color to determine gender in a green color budgie, but this method is not helpful with the various color mutations. A blue budgie with a blue cere may be female. Palpating the distance between the pubic bones with the right index finger may give some indication of gender, females having a wider pubic distance than males.

Budgerigars may be an individual's first and only bird purchased as a pet. The single budgie can be easily tamed or can

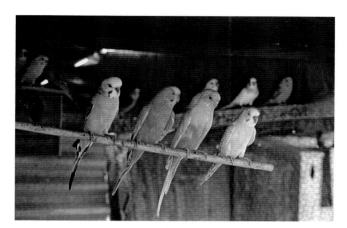

Figure 10-7 The budgerigar (budgie) is one of the most popular companion avian species in the United States and is most commonly called the parakeet.

be obtained as a hand-raised young bird. As companion animals, these birds are easy to train to "talk." In most cases, when the action of speaking is applied to psittacine species, it refers to the ability to mimic the voice and sounds of humans or inanimate objects (e.g., telephone ring tones, microwave beeping, doors squeaking). Budgerigars have been known to have a vocabulary of up to 500 words. The owner should understand that the voice of a bird is produced at the *syrinx*, otherwise known as the avian voice box. This anatomic structure is located at the tracheal bifurcation, deep in the cranial coelomic cavity. The diminutive budgerigar has a soft, high-pitched voice that requires a good ear for one to understand the sounds the bird is making. These birds can be housed as a single pet or in a larger cage with multiple inhabitants. Budgerigars, when housed as a group of birds, are beautiful to watch, especially if a number of different color mutations are present within the cage. The playful chirps and noises the birds commonly make when interacting with one another also are pleasant on the ear and livens up a house. The budgerigar is an easy avian species to set up for reproductive purposes. A wooden nest box in the cage will provide an adequate place for egg laying and bird raising.

COCKATIEL

The cockatiel is a small gray bird with a yellow face and orange cheek patch that is recommended for the novice bird owner. Hand-raised cockatiels have many qualities that allow first-time bird owners to interact with their pet and become comfortable with an animal with which they have little or no experience. Cockatiels are small, with an average weight of about 90 grams. Being birds with companionship qualities, they rarely bite, even if there is little interaction over a period of time. Many psittacine species (e.g., lovebirds, parrotlets) often bite their owners and are distrustful unless handled on a daily basis. For the owner that has little time for daily handling, the cockatiel is the pet bird of choice. Cockatiels can be reproductively active, with female birds laying eggs on a regular

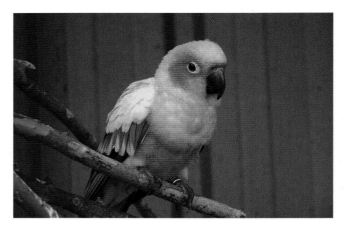

Figure 10-8 The sun conure is small and beautiful. Like most conure species, they are inexpensive, but can have a persistent irritating vocalization. (Courtesy Dr. Steve Wilson.)

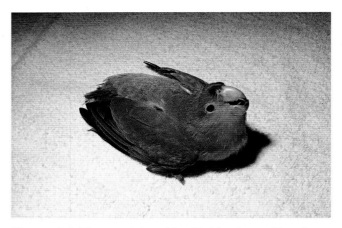

Figure 10-9 The peach-faced lovebird is often sold and promoted as a Valentine's Day gift. These birds can make excellent pets if there is daily interaction between the bird and the owner. Lovebirds that make the best companion animals are housed alone.

basis if comfortable with their environment and diet. There are many different color mutations for cockatiels, with gray being the normal color. Male gray cockatiels are darker gray, have a brighter yellow head and a bright orange cheek patch. Female gray cockatiels have more muted colors than males, and the ventral aspect of their primary and secondary flight feathers have transverse white bars. In general the birds with color mutations have fewer gender-differentiating characteristics. As with any bird, if there is no male in the enclosure, all eggs laid by the female are infertile. For the pair of birds that lay fertile eggs, a wooden nest box will be adequate for the hen to deposit eggs and raise the young. Clutch numbers should be regulated to 4 or 5 a year because a cockatiel pair will lay all year. A calcium source (e.g., cuttlebone) is required for adequate nutrition, and as with all psittacine species, a base diet consisting of extruded pellets is recommended. Seed treats (e.g., Nutriberries, Lafeber Company, Ordell, IL), along with vegetables and fruit, will provide a diverse diet that increases nutritional offerings and are psychological stimuli for the bird. Normal gray cockatiels have an average life expectancy of 16 years, with the more inbred color-mutated birds having shorter average life spans.

CONURE

Conures may be considered small parrots (Figure 10-8). This group of birds can be divided into pyrrhua (e.g., maroon-bellied, white-eared) and aratinga (e.g., red-masked, jendaya, sun, blue-crowned). In general, the pyrrhua are less noisy and make better companion animals, with the exception of the aratinga blue-crowned conure. Conures are popular companion avian species because they are beautiful, have "talking" capabilities, are a relatively small group of psittacine birds, and are relatively inexpensive. Unfortunately, because of their relatively low price, many novice bird owners purchase conures without performing the proper research on their new pet. Most conure species have beaks that are large enough to inflict a serious bite injury to the owner. These birds are independent,

even when hand-raised, and may bite without any provocation. The arantinga group can be beautiful (e.g., sun conure, jendaya) but are often so vocal that they present a significant distraction and disturbance to their owners. The exception, again, to the vocal aratinga group is the blue-crowned conure. A blue-crowned conure was used as the bird actor for the movie *Paulie*. Many conure species successfully reproduce in captivity and are readily available for the pet trade. Conures are small parrots and need adequate cage space and appropriate toys for their powerful beaks. Most conures have an average life span of 20 to 25 years.

LOVEBIRD

Lovebirds are native to central and southern Africa and Indian Ocean islands and weigh approximately 50 grams. There are a number of species of lovebirds, but the peach-faced and black-masked are the most common (Figure 10-9). Even though both the peach-faced and black-masked are lovebirds, they build their nests using very different methods. The peach-faced lovebird places nest material in its rump feathers and then flies back to the nest box and makes a concave nesting cavity with the material. The black-masked lovebird carries nest material in its beak and then builds a nest by filling the cavity with material and tunneling through to the nesting chamber. Lovebirds are aggressive and have to be handled on a daily basis to retain their companionship qualities. Only hand-raised lovebirds that are maintained as single birds are recommended as companion animals. These birds are often promoted as Valentine's Day gifts, to be purchased as a pair. It is often stated by the salesperson that it is best to purchase a pair of birds for their well-being and health. Lovebirds do not need to be purchased in pairs nor maintained as a pair of birds. Lovebirds that are purchased as a pair will make very poor interactive pets for the new owner. Most psittacine species should be maintained as either a companion animal or breed-

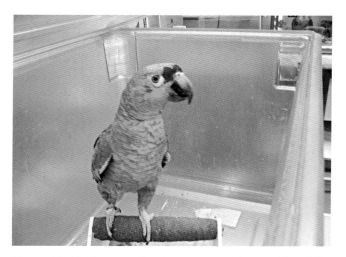

Figure 10-10 To many, the Amazon parrot is considered the typical companion avian species.

ing animal. Rarely does a breeding animal make a quality companion animal. Of course, the single companion bird will not provide fertile eggs or lay eggs at all if a male. Birds will trust and interact with their own species much better than with the human owner if given a choice. The single, hand-raised lovebird that is handled daily makes a very good companion animal. Lovebirds have an average life span of 15 years.

SOUTH AMERICAN PARROT

Typically when one thinks of a pet bird, the vision of a pirate comes to mind with a large green parrot on his shoulder. Large parrot species exist from the southwestern United States (e.g., thick-billed parrot) to Argentina (e.g., Quaker). The most common South American parrots sold for companion animals are the yellow-headed parrot species and Central American parrot species. The green-cheeked, yellow-cheeked, and lilac-crowned Amazon parrots are common Central American species, whereas the yellow-nape, double-yellow-head, and blue-front Amazon parrots may be considered common South American parrots maintained in captivity (Figure 10-10). Although many of these species have overlapping territories, these birds are found from Mexico into South America. South American parrots are relatively difficult to reproduce in captivity, but experienced aviculturists have been able to keep up with the demand for domestic, hand-raised babies since the cessation of wild bird imports into the United States in the early 1990s. In general South American parrots can make excellent companion animals but are extremely vocal during the early morning and early evening hours. These birds can mimic human voices and interact with their owners. With their large beaks, if frightened, these birds can seriously injure their owners. Amazon parrots are seasonal breeders, with reproductive activity at its height during the spring months. Male parrots are very temperamental during this time; mild-mannered birds may become aggressive and are prone to unprovoked attacks on the owner. This activity has led to

owners searching for behavior modification options to prevent this hormonally induced aggressive behavior. The popularity of Amazon parrots as pets has produced an active illegal smuggling operation on the U.S. border with Mexico. To enhance a bird's value in the eyes of an uneducated buyer, the bird smugglers will bleach a green parrot's head feathers yellow. This bleaching process will not affect a parrot's underlying skin in most cases, but it can cause a severe dermatitis if the bleach is not applied properly or with a great deal of care. Small conures and parrots that have had have their heads bleached as adults have been offered for sale as baby yellow-head Amazon parrots. A program sponsored by the United States Fish and Wildlife Service (USFWS) and the United States Department of Agriculture (USDA) takes confiscated birds and puts the birds through the required quarantine procedure. After the birds have been successfully quarantined for exotic Newcastle disease and are disease free, they are auctioned off at sanctioned events with proceeds supporting the efforts of the USFWS and USDA. A common disease presentation noted in the captive Amazon parrot is obesity. A regulated diet and exercise, if possible, are highly recommended to maintain a companion animal with a healthy body condition. The average life span of South American parrots is 35 to 40 years.

COCKATOO

Cockatoos are native to Australia and the surrounding south Pacific Islands. As a group of birds, cockatoos are classified as black (e.g., palm, gang gang) and white (e.g., umbrella, salmon crested, sulfur crested). As companion animals the black cockatoos are extremely expensive and rare, whereas the white cockatoos are considered a common large pet bird. White cockatoos are easily reproduced in captivity and have the ability to mimic the human voice and inanimate objects. The characteristic that makes cockatoos a desirable pet is also the source of owner disappointment: the intense companionship quality of the single pet bird. It has been said that a cockatoo's main goal in life is to become physically attached to its owner. If an owner's time interacting with the bird satisfies the animal's apparent need for companionship, then there are relatively few behavioral problems that will develop with the bird. If the bird desires more time with the owner than can be provided, behavioral problems will be common among white cockatoo species, including screaming and neurotic feather picking. Screaming occurs when the bird wants attention but the owner is unwilling or unable to meet the bird's demands. Cockatoos are large birds with loud vocal abilities, and the screaming produced is very disruptive to the household. Psychological feather picking is a physical response to stress within the bird's environment. There are many conditions that can increase the stress level of cockatoos, one being the inability to meet the bird's demand for companionship interaction. As mentioned previously, it is imperative that potential owners educate themselves regarding the characteristics of the birds they are considering for companion animals and how the birds will adjust to their lifestyle. Through prepurchase education, the result of the ultimate decision will not only satisfy the new owner but their avian

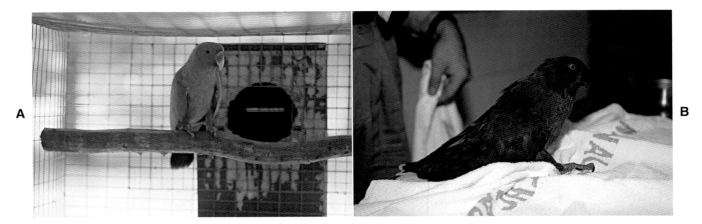

Figure 10-11 Eclectus parrots have dimorphic coloration with the male being green **(A)** and the female being red **(B).**

companion as well. The average life span of a cockatoo is 30 to 45 years.

AFRICAN GREY PARROT

There are a number of large parrot species found on the continent of Africa, including the African grey parrot. The African grey parrot may be the most popular large companion bird because it mimics inanimate objects and the human voice (in the tone and range of the person) and is an elegant, slate-gray color with a bright red tail. There are three species of African grey parrot: Congo, Timneh, and Ghanan. The most common and most desired by pet bird owners is the Congo African grey. These species of African grey parrots are easy to reproduce in captivity and are stimulated to breed by moving the birds to a different cage or location. Once hatched and hand-raised, the bird should be introduced to as many people as possible when the bird is still young. As the African grey parrot ages, it becomes less trusting of people and objects that are set up in its cage. New objects and people must be introduced slowly to prevent increased stress, which manifests itself in a vocalized growling by the bird. Also if an African Grey parrot is started on a diverse diet when weaned from hand-feeding formula, it will continue to accept an assorted diet throughout its life. Because these birds are generally mistrusting, there is a problem of psychological feather picking, similar to that described in cockatoos. A number of husbandry issues need to be addressed to determine the cause(s) of the feather picking condition. It is not uncommon for the feather picking African grey to stop the abusive behavior and just as suddenly, some time later, reinitiate the painful process. The average life span for Congo African grey parrots is 30 to 40 years.

ECLECTUS PARROT

This beautiful bird is found on the South Pacific islands and in Australia. The unusual characteristic of the eclectus parrot is the dimorphic color characteristics of the male and female.

The male is bright green, and the female is red (Figure 10-11). When the eclectus parrot was first discovered, aviculturists believed the male and female were two different species. The eclectus parrot, in general, is a very good choice for a companion animal. Aggressive behavior, minimal mimicking ability, and a propensity for psychological feather picking are traits that potential owners should consider before owning these beautiful birds. It is the beauty of the eclectus parrot that draws the interest of potential owners. The birds commonly reproduce in captivity and are hand-raised for the pet market. The availability of the birds makes them easy to obtain. Aviculturists who successfully reproduce eclectus parrots are also aware that the female will abuse, and sometimes kill, unwilling or nonaggressive male birds. Great care must be followed when setting up breeding pairs of eclectus parrots to prevent cage mate mortality.

MACAW

Macaws are new world species, and within this group, the largest of the pet birds are found. The hyacinth macaw is the largest of the macaw species, weighing well over a kilogram, whereas the Hahn's macaw weighs between 150 and 200 grams, on average. The diversity of size with the macaw species also provides a diversity of companionship characteristics with this group of birds. The hyacinth macaw is a very interactive bird, is known as "the gentle giant," and is very expensive. The smaller macaw species are relatively inexpensive but can be very vocal and not as interactive as some of the species previously mentioned. The beauty of the macaw species and their size make these animals desirable. A large macaw demands adequate room for its enclosure and the understanding from the owner that they have a loud vocalization. Macaws do not mimic clearly and usually do not have a large vocabulary of imitated words or sounds. Macaws can be affectionate, but researching the companionship qualities of each species is recommended before purchase. The average life span of the large macaw species is 45 to 50 years.

OTHER PSITTACINE SPECIES

There are a number of smaller psittacine species that are maintained either as companion or aviary birds. South American species include the Quaker parrot, parrotlet, pionus, and caiques. The Meyer's and Sengel parrots, common birds within the pet trade, are native to Africa, whereas rosella's and Bourke's parakeets, moustache parrotkeets, hanging parrots, and lories, are indigenous to Asia, the South Pacific islands, and Australia. Many of these species are maintained as smaller parrots with similar cage and nutritional requirements. The lory species has a specialized tongue: when extended, the tongue reveals papilla on the dorsal surface that allows the copious ingestion of nectar and pollen. Captive lories are fed a special lory diet that is either powdered or dissolved in water. This sweet liquid diet results in soft, thin fecal material. Many potential owners would view the specialized diet and diarrhea-like stool as a disadvantage of owning a lory. The Quaker parrot is a temperate zone bird found in the central areas of Argentina. The Quaker is the only psittacine that builds a nest and is a very adaptable species outside of its native habitat. In areas of the United States, feral Quaker parrots have reproduced in the wild. This has led to the formation of laws making the ownership of Quaker parrots illegal in certain jurisdictions within the United States. With the popularity of bird ownership and widespread interstate transport of companion avian species, potential owners should be aware of laws regulating the possession of specific avian species within their city, state, or both. As with all birds mentioned in this chapter, each species has its positive and negative qualities as a companion animal. There are many venues in which one can review these characteristics to determine which bird would fit their lifestyle and ultimately their ability to properly care for that particular animal.

■ BIOLOGY

Beak

Birds have a number of anatomic and physiologic parameters that separate them from mammalian species. The most obvious is the bill and feathers. The bill, or beak, is a complex anatomic structure. The upper beak is attached to the frontal bone with the craniofacial hinge, whereas the lower mandible is attached through the articulation of the articular and quadrate bones.[1] Passerine and psittacine beak anatomy is a complex system of support and germinal epithelium. Bone is the foundation of the beak and is covered by a vascular layer and the germinal epithelium, which is covered by the keratinized epidermis called the *rhamphotheca*.[1] The rhamphotheca is subdivided into the *rhinotheca* of the upper beak and the *gnatotheca* of the lower beak. The complex structure of the beak poses a problem to medical personnel trying to correct beak injuries or loss. The beak will not regrow if a substantial section of the beak has been traumatically removed or if the beak sloughs because of a disease process (Figure 10-12). The beak will heal at the interface of the damage and viable tissue, but it will not regen-

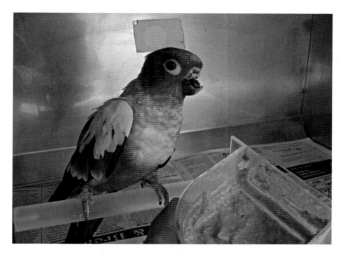

Figure 10-12 The upper beak of a conure that has healed after being traumatically removed by the hen when the animal was a nestling. The beak will not regrow if the underlying tissue has been damaged.

erate to its original size and shape. The pressure applied by the animal when climbing or eating adversely affects the ability of a beak prostheses to stay attached for any period of time. Many companion avian species will be able to adapt to dietary modifications if they are unable to eat a normal diet as a result of a severe beak injury. Working with an affected patient to adapt to its challenged condition should be the first priority of veterinarians and owners, not euthanasia.

Feathers

The feathers of a bird are analogous to the hair on mammals. Feathers protect the animal from the elements and also provide a significant means to maintain normothermia. For passerine and psittacine species the normal body temperature is between 102° F and 104° F. An elevated body temperature has advantages of restricting the incidence of bacterial infections but also is problematic when trying to maintain or dissipate heat. Birds are much more sensitive to elevated than reduced temperatures. When acclimatized, pet birds generate an increased down feather coat to compensate for lower environmental temperatures, but they have relatively few options to disperse heat even if placed outdoors before the onset of the hot summer months. Birds that are suffering from hyperthermia will pant and breath with mouths open to reduce body temperature. If the environmental temperature is too warm, the birds will not survive for long without significant temperature modifications (e.g., air movement, placing the animal in an air conditioned environment). If the bird is hypothermic, one of the first body reactions detected by the owner is fluffed feathers. Fluffed feathers are a bird's reaction to cold temperatures externally or an internal inability to maintain normothermia. The fluffed feathers allow a bird to trap air between the outer feathers and the body, creating an insulating barrier. The condition of erecting the feathers to create an insulating barrier requires a significant amount of energy; therefore, the cause of this protective process should be identified and eliminated.

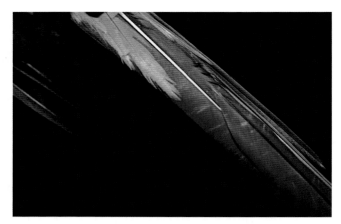

Figure 10-13 Transverse lines in a feather that were created by an endogenous corticosteroid released during the feather growth phase.

All birds go through a process of growing what are called *blood feathers*. The emergent feather shaft is filled with blood, which brings nourishment to the developing feather. The most obvious blood feathers are the large primary and secondary wing feathers, *remiges,* and major tail feathers, *retricies.* During the growth phase, the feathers are innervated and will be painful to the bird if cut or traumatized. Once developed, the bird will not experience pain when feathers are cut, only if forcefully pulled from the follicle. If there is generalized stress to the animal during the feather growth phase, feather growth will be adversely affected. This adverse affect will be noted in the mature feather as transverse lines (Figure 10-13). These transverse lines are disruptions in the barb and barbule architecture due to the increase in the endogenous corticosteroid production caused by stress.

Bird feathers consist of the calamus, base of the feather within the follicle, main shaft, barbs extending off the main shaft, and barbules that hold the barbs together. The incessant preening observed in birds is, in part, a process to make sure the barbules are interlocked between the barbs, making the outer feathers smooth. Bird owners, especially concerned novice bird owners, should be made aware that preening is normal and feather loss in preening is a natural occurrence. The highly publicized disease condition of psychologic feather picking leads many owners to believe that any feather loss in the act of preening is abnormal. Molting will occur at least once a year and often twice a year. Birds will molt in temperate climates in the spring and fall in relation to the environmental temperature shifts. It is very easy to distinguish an indoor bird from one that has been acclimatized to cooler weather and lives in an outdoor aviary in the winter. The outside bird will have significantly more down feathers than the one kept inside.

Respiratory System

The upper respiratory system in the bird begins with the nares, and within the nares is the visible operculum or keratinized flap. Avian species have only one sinus, the infraorbital sinus,

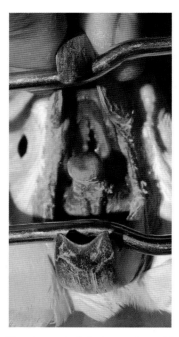

Figure 10-14 The choanal slit is the oral-nasal interface on the dorsal surface of the oral cavity.

with many diverticula within the head. The infraorbital sinus is extensive once the upper airway passes the nares and conchae. The terminus of the upper respiratory system is the choana leading to the choanal slit. The choanal slit is the interface between the upper airway and oral cavity. The choanal slit is a V-shaped structure in the dorsal surface of the oral cavity, with the base of the V being most rostral (Figure 10-14). Lining the choanal slit are epithelial projections that are easily eroded during an infectious disease process and/or when irritated.

The lower respiratory system begins with the glottis, which leads to the trachea. There is direct air flow from the choana into the trachea when the beak is closed. There is no epiglottis; this absence of an epiglottis predisposes avian species to aspiration of ingested material, especially when under the stress of struggle or an agonal event. It is recommended, when treating or tube feeding an avian patient, to administer oral medications or food before putting a bird into its cage to prevent aspiration. A bird will be able to control the glottis in order to prevent aspiration of regurgitated material when there is not a struggle against restraint. The trachea of avian species has closed signet-shaped rings.

When intubating a bird, a decision must be made to determine which style of tracheal tube should be used. If an endotracheal tube is used with an inflatable cuff, the anesthetist can be assured of a proper fit. The inflatable cuffed endotracheal tube is a concern when used on animals with closed tracheal rings because of the possibility of pressure necrosis occurring at the site of the cuff. It is recommended to use noncuffed endotracheal tubes on avian patients to prevent the occurrence of pressure necrosis (Figure 10-15). If noncuffed endotracheal tubes are used, it is imperative that the veterinary surgeon

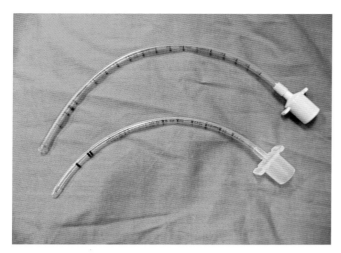

Figure 10-15 A noncuffed endotracheal tube is recommended for use with avian patients.

selects the proper size to ensure a tight fit. The proper sized noncuffed endotracheal tube will allow the use of a ventilator and a respiratory monitor and will prevent the aspiration of blood or ingested food.

At the terminus of the trachea as it bifurcates, there are specialized tracheal rings that form the syrinx. The *syrinx* is the "voice box" of a bird. The more developed an avian species' vocal abilities are, the more developed is its syrinx. The tracheal bifurcation is deep within the cranial coelomic cavity, making surgical access very difficult. In certain species (e.g., peafowl), veterinarians are often asked to perform devocalization procedures. Devocalization surgery is not recommended on avian species because of the difficulty in gaining surgical access to the structure and the thin margin of performing a successful devocalization surgery.

Birds take two cycles of respiration to move one volume of air through their respiratory system. Once the bird inhales, the volume of air goes through the trachea, bypassing the lungs, and is held in the caudal air sacs. When the animal exhales, that volume of air goes into the lungs through the air capillaries, and there in the lungs, gas exchange takes place. When the bird inhales for the second time, the air from the lungs enters the cranial air sacs and then leaves the body on the second exhalation. The air sac system usually contains four paired (cervical, cranial thoracic, caudal thoracic, abdominal) air sacs and one unpaired (clavicular) air sac. These air sacs are uniformly avascular and allow for large volumes of air to pass through the lungs for gas exchange in a relatively small animal. The air sac system in birds allows for excellent endoscopic viewing of the coelomic cavity and the internal organs without having to insufflate the patient. The flow through air capillaries within the lungs is a much more efficient gas exchange mechanism than the dead end alveoli found in mammalian lungs. The efficiency and sensitivity of the avian respiratory system have led to birds being used as air quality monitors in coal mines and in wars where toxic gas may be used as a weapon.

Birds also have an extension of air sacs into the bones. These bones are pneumatic bones and are lined with air sac epithelium. Bones that are classified as pneumatic bones in avian species include the humerus, keel, and vertebra. Interosseous catheters for fluid administration should not be placed in a pneumatic bone.

Digestive System

The oral cavity is the beginning of the avian digestive system. Most birds have a dry oral cavity due to the lack of salivary glands. Birds do have salivary glands, but they are few in number, do not produce a significant amount of mucus, and are not an active location for digestion to occur. At the base of the tongue lies the glottis, and over the glottis is the beginning of the cervical esophagus. The cervical esophagus dilates into the ingluvies or crop at the level of the thoracic inlet. In caged and companion birds the crop is well developed. The crop is often the location of thermal burns that occur after feeding young birds formula that is too hot. Thermal burns of the crop take place on the gravity-dependent side or ventral surface. The patient may present with an edematous hyperemic area of skin at the thoracic inlet. The crop injury must be allowed to mature in order to delineate the affected tissue from the nonaffected tissue. Once a determination of the viable from nonviable tissue is made, surgery should be initiated to remove the affected tissue and appose the viable tissue margins. If the surgery does not take place, the necrotic plug will slough, leaving a fistula from the crop to the external body surface. It is not unusual for owners of fully feathered birds to first notice food at the thoracic inlet in fistulated birds.

The cervical esophagus extends from the crop into the proventriculus, or true stomach, which produces hydrochloric acid and pepsin. Major digestive processes occur within the proventriculus. Ingesta leaving the proventriculus enters the ventriculus, where it is mechanically broken down. In most instances companion avian species do not need grit to break down the ingested food. If a toxic foreign body (e.g., lead, zinc) enters the ventriculus, it is difficult to remove. Between the proventriculus and ventriculus is the intermediate zone, a transitional section of the gastric anatomy that is lined with interfacing proventricular and ventricular mucosa. This section of the stomach is most often cited as the primary location of gastric tumors.[2] The ventriculus in avian species is more developed in birds that use it as a grinding organ (e.g., chickens, pea fowl, pigeons). To grind the food, a bird ingests grit. *Grit* can be defined as a nondigestive tool that is ingested and used to break down food. Companion avian species and common cage birds do not need grit to digest their food. This is truer today because of the availability of processed avian diets. The ventriculus is lined with a hard kolin layer consisting of a hardened carbohydrate protein matrix. The kolin layer hardens when exposed to the hydrochloric acid from the proventriculus and obtains its color from the retrograde movement of small intestinal biliverdin.[2] The grinding process of the ventriculus is aided by rotating the food in this muscular organ. There are four quadrants of muscle that comprise the ventriculus. The muscle thickness rotates between quadrants, switching from thick (cranioventral, caudodorsal) to thin (craniodorsal, caudoventral). The different muscle thicknesses aid in the digestive process of birds but make it difficult to remove ingested foreign bodies.

The small intestine begins after the ventriculus. The pancreas is located within the descending loop of the duodenum. Both pancreatic and bile ducts open into the duodenum.[2] There may be two or three pancreatic ducts, depending on the species.[2] Bile ducts enter the intestine from the gall bladder (cysticoenteric) in some birds; in birds with no gall bladder (e.g., Amazon parrot, ostrich), bile ducts enter the intestine from the liver (hepatoenteric duct).[2]

The vitelline or Meckel's diverticulum is the remnant of the yolk sac and may be located at the jejunum-ileum interface. The vitelline diverticulum is a small epithelial projection from the intestinal wall. The avian digestive system continues with the ileum, which terminates at the rectum. Where the ileum intersects with the rectum is also the location of the caeca. Not all birds have caeca. When present, the caeca are the most developed in species in which a large percentage of the diet consists of fibrous plant material. The rectum empties into the coprodeum, a chamber of the cloaca. The other chambers of the cloaca are the urodeum, terminus of the reproductive and urinary tracts, and the proctodeum. The proctodeum is the collecting chamber of the coprodeum and urodeum before the material is evacuated through the vent. Lymphatic tissue, most developed in young birds, is called the cloacal bursa and is located on the dorsal surface of the cloaca. If visible, the male phallus is located on the ventral floor of the cloaca.

Reproductive System

The reproductive organs of birds (testis and ovary) are located at the cranial pole of the kidney, caudal to the adrenal gland. In companion and cage birds the female has one ovary, located on the cranial ventral aspect of the left kidney. The ovary is connected to the urodeum by the oviduct. The oviduct is divided into five sections: infundibulum, magnum, isthmus, uterus, and vagina. The developing egg remains in the uterus longer than in any other section of the oviduct, and it is in the uterus where the egg shell is formed. The male bird has two testes, and they are connected to the urodeum by the ductus deferens. Companion and cage birds have a nonintromittent or nonprotruding phallus.[2]

Renal System

Birds are uricotelic, the end product of nitrogen metabolism is uric acid.[1,3] The three-lobed avian kidney is located within an area of the dorsomedial coelomic cavity. The kidney lobes are situated within and against the ventral aspect of the cranial rib and vertebral surface. Birds do not have a bladder or urethra; instead, urine enters the urodeum through the ureters. A renal portal valve is found within the lumen of the common iliac vein, and when the valve is open, blood flows into the caudal vena cava, away from the kidney tissue.[1,3] There are two types of nephrons within the avian kidney: cortical (reptilian) and medullary (mammalian).[1,3] The cortical nephron, which is found in the greatest number of bird species, lacks a loop of Henle, whereas the medullary nephron has a loop of Henle.

Avian Skeleton

Bird bones are lightweight and strong. For the bones to be both light and strong, the cortices have a high density of calcium and are very thin. Bones with a high tensile strength are appropriate for flight, but when fractured, they have a tendency to shatter. As mentioned earlier, some bones are extensions of the air sac system (e.g., humerus). In flighted birds the sternum is modified for attachment of the large pectoral muscles. The pelvic bones are fused into the synsacrum to withstand the pressures of perching, landing after flight, and capturing prey.

Eye

The avian globe is large and has similar anatomy as that of the mammalian eye. Differences between the avian and the mammalian eye include voluntary control of the iris tissue, a scleral ring of bone, and the *pecten oculi*. The scleral ring of bone gives the eye structure and form. On the surface of the retina over the optic nerve lies the pecten oculi. The pecten oculi extends into the posterior chamber and is able to inject fluid into the globe for organ pressure and environmental stabilization within the anterior chamber.

■ HUSBANDRY
Environmental Considerations

One of the most important owner influences on a bird's health is its environment. An environment that promotes psychological well-being leads to a happy, healthy, reproductively active bird. For small cage birds, a large cage or aviary will allow for flight and space needed to reduce territorial stress that is often associated with common species maintained in captivity. Overcrowding will lead to injury and stress. Aviary design is often based on an individual's imagination and monetary investment. Aviaries can be small areas within a house or large outdoor flights (Figure 10-16). Large free flight aviaries require plants for hiding, perception of safety, and building of nests. Maintenance is often required with the free-flighted aviaries because small birds have a habit of pulling the leaves off the plants and trees within the enclosure. As with all aviaries, rodent and vermin control is important. Rodents and insects are drawn to the food debris produced by pet birds. Bird food not stored properly is also a magnet for rodents and insects. In the southeastern United States, fire ants, drawn to an aviary by spilled food, are potential deadly pests to young chicks. Roaches, found in many aviaries and houses, are the intermediate host for *Sarcocystis falcatula*. Food debris will draw pests, and the nutritional composition of bird food degrades when exposed to the environment, especially heat. Storage of bird

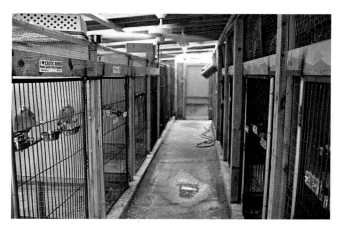

Figure 10-16 A large outdoor aviary that was developed to enhance breeding of psittacine species.

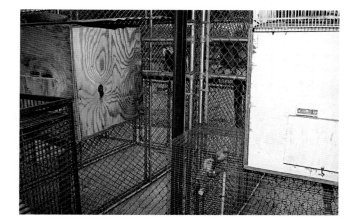

Figure 10-17 Observation doors on nest boxes allow the owner to view the interior without causing too much stress to the breeding pair.

BOX 10-1	Minimum Recommended Sizes for Nest Boxes in a Psittacine Flight

Birds	Nest Box Size in Inches (Height × Width × Depth)
Large macaws	48 × 16 × 16
Large cockatoos, medium macaws	36 × 12 × 12
Large parrots, Amazon parrots, African grey parrots	24 × 12 × 12
Pionus, small macaws	24 × 12 × 12
Conures, caiques	18 × 12 × 12
Small conures, cockatiels	16 × 10 × 10
Lovebirds, parrotlets, budgerigars	8 × 8 × 24

From Clubb SL, Flammer K: The avian flock. In Ritchie BW, Harrison GJ, Harrison LR, editors: *Avian medicine: Principles and Application,* Lake Worth, Fla, 1994, Wingers.

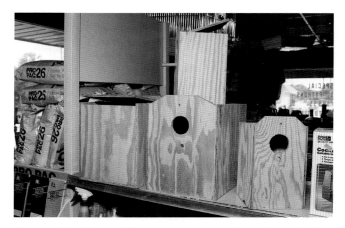

Figure 10-18 Two different nest box designs for psittacine birds.

food is important to maintain nutritional integrity and prevent the introduction of pests. People that establish large outdoor aviaries may desire individual flights that are occupied by a single pair of birds. The paired flight cages are set up in most cases for breeding purposes. Food and environment have an effect on the success of breeding pairs producing offspring. Knowledge by the bird owner is essential on what is needed to give the pair the best opportunity for successful reproductive activity by that particular species. Information on nest box size is important, as is the material from which the nest box is made (Box 10-1).

All nest boxes should have an observation door so that owners can view the interior with minimal disturbance to the bird (Figure 10-17). It is important for bird owners to view the inside of the nest box for laying activity and egg production. Once the eggs hatch, proper development of the babies should be monitored and the babies pulled if treatment is needed or if hand-feeding is required. Some birds like a wooden

nest box in an elongated shape with the hole near the top (Figure 10-18). Some species, such as macaws and cockatoos, will "modify" their nest boxes by chewing wood; this activity may stimulate reproductive activity. If the breeding pair is too destructive to the nest box, material such as sheet metal can be used to build the structure. It is important to make sure that smooth slick surfaces on nest box bottoms are lined with wood chips to ensure proper positioning of legs during the rapid skeletal growth of young birds. Slick nest box bottoms lead to splay-legged birds and other developmental abnormalities that affect the joints and long bones of the legs. Hardwood chips are recommended for lining the bottom of the breeding box because they do not produce the volatile oils associated with softwoods (e.g., cedar, pine). The volatile compounds cause irritation to the respiratory system and exposed dermis of both parents and baby birds. For species in which there may be cagemate trauma or death (e.g., cockatoos, rosellas, eclectus), two-holed T nest boxes allow for the mate to escape if being attacked. Other recommendations to prevent cagemate trauma include trimming the aggressive mate's wings so that

BOX 10-2 Recommended Cage Bar Spacing for Psittacine Species Maintained as Companion Animals

Bird	Cage Bar Spacing (in Inches)
Large macaws and cockatoos	$\frac{3}{4}$-$1\frac{1}{2}$
Large parrots, Amazon parrots, African grey parrots	$\frac{3}{4}$-1
Cockatiels and small conures	$\frac{1}{2}$-$\frac{3}{4}$
Budgies and lovebirds	$\frac{3}{8}$

From Gallerstein GA: *The Complete Pet Bird Owner's Handbook,* Minneapolis, 2003, Avian.

BOX 10-3 Recommended Perch Diameters for Cage and Aviary Birds

Bird Weight	Perch Diameter in Inches
<25 g	$\frac{3}{8}$
25-70 g	$\frac{1}{2}$
70-150 g	$\frac{5}{8}$
150-300 g	$\frac{3}{4}$
300-650 g	1
650 g-2 kg	2

From Gallerstein GA: *The Complete Pet Bird Owner's Handbook,* Minneapolis, 2003, Avian.

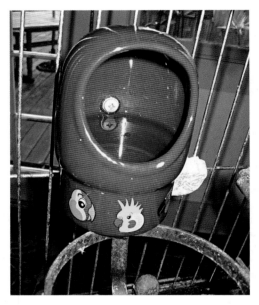

Figure 10-19 An example of a protected water source. The overhead protection reduces exposure to fecal and food contamination.

the bird being attacked has better flight capabilities. Custom-made, outdoor flights for aviaries should be made out of wire produced especially for that purpose. Custom-made indoor cages can be painted with nontoxic paint, but owners should be aware that over time the bird will probably pick at the paint, affecting the overall look of the enclosure. The most common cage material for outside cages is galvanized caging wire that is produced in sheets and cut to form the appropriate cage size for the bird(s) to be housed. The cut wire sections are then held together using binders called "J" clips. This galvanized cage wire may lead to zinc toxicosis through birds scraping the wire with their beak and ingesting the galvanized pieces. The galvanized protective coating can also be leached into water droplets that form on the wire and are then licked off by the birds. To reduce the amount of excess galvanized coating on new wire, washing with vinegar and abrading the cleaned material with a wire brush are recommended. There are many different types of cages available commercially for the bird that is to be housed inside, with the main options being metallic bars and acrylic. Stainless steel cages are of the highest quality cage material that can be used for companion bird enclosures. Stainless steel is usually not painted and does not rust. The most common cage material used for indoor psittacine enclosures is powder-coated steel. These powder-coated cages are available in many colors and sizes. Smaller cages may be nickel or brass-plated wire that can become dull after the clear coat finish ages or is disturbed by the birds. It is imperative that all bird cages have appropriate space between the cage bars to prevent the animals from getting their head stuck between the bars (Box 10-2).

There are many specialty cages using a variety of material for cage bars. Research is required to make sure the size and material are suitable for the bird being housed. This also applies to cage furniture, perches, and bowls (e.g., food, water). Cages and aviaries that contain small birds must be easy to clean and must be easy for the owner to change the food and water. Perches can be made out of hardwood or formed plastic. Appropriate perch material is recommended to prevent ingestion of foreign bodies leading to gastrointestinal disease. A natural hardwood (e.g., oak, hickory, maple) perch offers various diameters for birds to grasp, exercise their feet, and chew; also, they are inexpensive and can be readily replaced (Box 10-3).

Any wood that is gathered from a tree for perch material should be cleaned and disinfected before it is placed in the cage. Toys and cage furniture are usually marketed for specifically sized birds. Under no circumstances should one place toys manufactured for smaller birds in a cage with larger species (e.g., budgie toys should not be placed in an Amazon parrot's cage). The large bird will break the toy and may ingest the parts, initiating gastrointestinal disease. Always purchase toys and cage furniture that are size appropriate and manufactured as such for that specific pet bird.

For water, a bottle with a stainless steel sipper tube is best for birds. This type of watering system allows for easy access for refilling and cleaning and also prevents the bird from defecating in its water supply. If a water bottle with a sipper tube is not used, there are ceramic water receptacles that attach to the side of a cage with a hole in the side. This design also reduces defecation into the water receptacle (Figure 10-19). Food dishes containing pelleted food, seed, fruit, and vegetables should be easy to remove, difficult for the bird to turn over, and easy to clean and disinfect. Stainless steel is the material of choice for food dishes, but thick ceramic bowls are also acceptable. Heavy plastic is appropriate for small bird bowls and is the food and water receptacle material of choice for passerine species. Food and water should be changed daily, and depending on the bird, the cage should be cleaned every 2 to 3 days. There are many different cage substrates used to line the bottom of pet bird cages. The cage substrate of choice is newspaper because it allows the owner to see the bird's stool for evaluation, and it is inexpensive and readily available. Newspaper also becomes dirty, which is apparent to the owner, indicating a need to clean the cage. If other cage substrates are used (e.g., crushed corn cob, ground walnut shell, and shredded paper), it is difficult to determine how dirty a cage may be; these substrates can hide the extent of fecal and urine buildup, often prolonging the perception of a clean cage. The best disinfectant for cleaning bowls, toys, and cage furniture is dilute sodium hypochlorite, or household bleach. It should always be remembered that dirt cannot be disinfected. To properly disinfect a cage or material within a cage, organic material first must be removed from all surfaces. After the organic material has been removed, the action of the disinfectant can be effective in cleaning the surface to which it has been applied.

Lighting is important for canaries, because their molting and breeding is directly correlated to the length of daylight to which they are exposed. During the summer (long daylight hours), canaries molt and will stop singing. When the daylight hours wane (autumn, winter), the feathers are in place and the bird sings to attract a mate. Shortening a cockatiel's exposure to daylight has been recommended for cessation of egg laying. Indoor birds should be exposed to artificial, full-spectrum light (UV-A and UV-B) to enhance breeding activity and vitamin D metabolism and subsequent calcium absorption from the gastrointestinal tract.[6] The bulbs should be placed within 12 inches of the animals, turned on for at least 1 hour every 24 hours, and replaced every 6 months.[6] Birds prefer to go to sleep at sundown and awake at sunrise. If a bird's cage is in a room in which a family watches television and is light well into the night, a cage cover is recommended. A cage cover is not required for pet birds, but if used, it should be part of the nightly routine and removed early in the morning. One should remember that birds are much more susceptible to heat than cool weather or "drafts" within a house. If birds are allowed to acclimatize during the temperate autumnal season, down feathers will grow in under the cover feathers, increasing the animal's ability to withstand cool weather. Birds will play in the snow or stay outside of a nest box when temperatures are below freezing if they are properly acclimatized. Birds have a normal body temperature of approximately 103° F and have little ability to dissipate environmental heat. External heat generated within a bird's environment is considered dangerous, and the animal should be removed as soon as possible. An acrylic cage with very little ventilation generates elevated temperatures within that space when placed in direct sunlight (Figure 10-20). If acrylic cages are used, they must be placed away from direct sunlight. Cages should never be placed in a kitchen or in an area that will disturb the bird when it is sleeping. Kitchens are the area in which vapors generated from

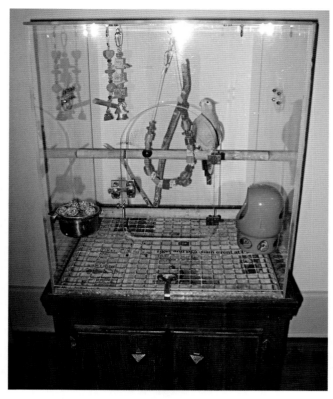

Figure 10-20 An acrylic cage keeps debris from falling on the floor but must be kept away from direct sunlight and requires regular cleaning of the panels.

cooking are emitted, and many are toxic to a bird's sensitive respiratory system.

Identification

There are currently two specific methods for identifying birds: leg bands and microchips. It is required by law that birds be identified, and either leg banding or microchips within the pectoral muscle are acceptable. Leg bands are the most common method for bird identification. Closed or open bands can be purchased by the breeder and placed on a young bird's leg shortly after hatch. It is easy to place a band on a bird's leg when the bird is young because the bones are pliable and the foot joints have more laxity early in life. Oversized closed leg bands or open bands can be placed on an older bird. Information on leg bands includes the year, owner's initials, and a statement that the animal was hatched. The benefits of identification are somewhat diminished because leg bands pose a health risk due to the possibility of the bird getting the band entangled in cage wire or toys. Even if the bird is able to free itself from entrapment, the result of the injury can lead to swelling and vascular impingement, resulting in foot necrosis distal to the band. If at all possible, leg bands should be removed to prevent injury or possible death to the bird. Placing a microchip in the pectoral muscle is the recommended identification method for companion avian species. The microchip (Figure 10-21) most commonly used to identify pet birds is the AVID

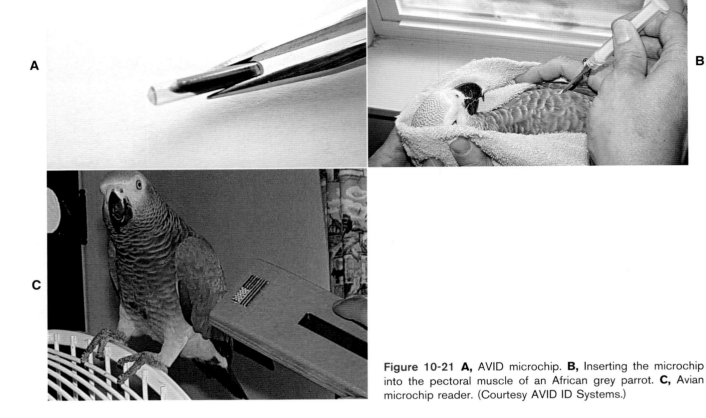

A

B

C

Figure 10-21 **A,** AVID microchip. **B,** Inserting the microchip into the pectoral muscle of an African grey parrot. **C,** Avian microchip reader. (Courtesy AVID ID Systems.)

microchip system (AVID Microchip ID Systems, Folsom, LA). Microchips can be placed successfully in birds weighing more than 150 grams. For birds that weigh less than 150 grams, leg bands are the identification method of choice.

■ NUTRITION

A bird's diet is one of the most important factors affecting its health. Health is directly correlated to quality of life and life span of that animal. There are many different species of birds that can be classified as companion animals and cage birds. Each avian species has its own nutritional requirement, and owners are encouraged to research the proper diet for their bird(s). For companion avian species and caged birds, a base pelleted or seed diet is recommended and should be fed ad lib. Pelleted diets are manufactured using two processes: bound and extruded. With bound pellets the food material is finely ground and mixed with a substance that under pressure and pressed will form a pellet. In most cases with bound pellets, the food material is not cooked. Extruded pellets start with a very finely mixed batter of food ingredients that is cooked and pressed through a processing machine into shapes. Bound pellets retain much of the food ingredients' color and smell after they are made, whereas extruded pellets come in different shapes and colors and may have a sweet odor (Figure 10-22).

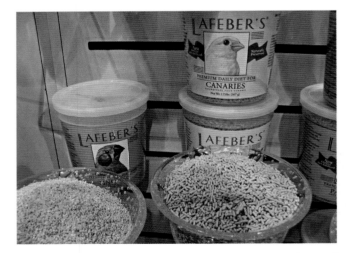

Figure 10-22 An example of pellets that are manufactured specifically for passerine species.

Pelleted diets come in a variety of sizes and should be selected based on the size of bird being fed. One disadvantage for feeding multicolored pellets is the bird may select certain colored pellets and not eat others. Selection of specific colors or shapes is expensive and leads to waste. By offering multicolored pellets that have different shapes, a bird is psychologically stimulated by the offering. A proper diverse diet is not only psychologically stimulating, which leads to a high quality of life, but is speculated to improve reproductive activity within an aviary.

Seed-based diets have been the staple of cage bird nutrition for many years. The advent of pelleted diets has improved owners' ability to provide a better balanced diet to their bird without having to offer vitamin and mineral supplementation. Not every bird will eat pelleted diets, although there are bound pellets with large pieces of exposed food bits that may be considered a formulated dietary offering. Some avian species, including many canary and finch species, require seed as their base diet. Providing the seed diet not only is natural to the bird but also delivers the nutrients that its body requires. For many psittacine species, seeds are considered a treat to be offered in small quantities. Most seed diets are high in fat content and have low quantities of other essential elements. Seed-based diets for canaries contain millet, rape, niger, sesame, hemp, and linseed, among other seed varieties. Many of the psittacine diets, including those developed for cockatiels, parrots, and macaws, have a high percentage of sunflower seeds, safflower seeds, or both. For the larger birds, including macaws, nuts (e.g., peanuts, hazelnuts, almonds) are added to the commercial diets. Some pet stores offer individual seeds that can be mixed into a homemade diet. To check for freshness of the seed, a sample of the product can be placed on a wet towel to observe for sprouting. Most birds, even the small caged birds (e.g., canaries, finches), will shell the seed before ingesting the kernel. To prevent seed waste, sifting the uneaten seed from the hulls will save money and reduce the amount of food discarded. Seed will degrade in nutritional quality over time, especially if exposed to heat and sunlight. Keeping seed cool will extend its shelf life. Insects, especially seed moths, can infiltrate storage containers. Keeping the seed in insect-proof containers in a refrigerator is a recommended method for reducing seed moth infestations. For psittacine species in which a seed diet is not the diet of choice, a pelleted product is recommended as the base diet. Introducing an older bird to a pelleted diet is often difficult when a seed diet has been their regular diet. Even older birds that are over 30 years old will convert to a pelleted diet. It is important to observe birds converting to a pelleted diet for ingestion of the food and not just crushing the pellet looking for an interior kernel. Two signs that indicate if a bird is eating pellets are the production of fecal material and a color change of the fecal material that correlates to the color of the pellets being ingested. Birds will produce "pellet dust" even when the food is being eaten. There are formed seed products, for example, Nutriberries® (Lafeber Co., Cornell, IL), that aid in the transition from seed to pellets (Figure 10-23). These formed products introduce birds to a bound product that the bird must pick off the seed to eat. Another way to transition birds from seed to pellets is by slowly introducing more pellets in the seed mixture over time. With the slow introduction of pellets, within 1 or 2 weeks, the diet is 100% pellets. When a bird is hospitalized, it is preferable not to change the diet until the animal is at home and free of

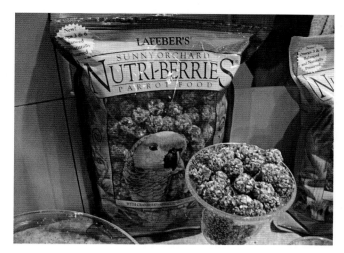

Figure 10-23 Processed food items, such as Nutriberries®, can be used to transition birds from an all-seed diet to an all-pellet diet.

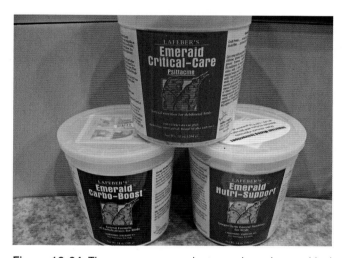

Figure 10-24 There are many products, such as these critical care products, that are fed to the bird via a crop feeding tube.

disease. The main goal for dietary measures within the hospital setting is for the animal to eat. Adding significant stress of a dietary change during hospitalization does not benefit the patient. If the animal does not eat and needs nutritional supplementation, there are commercial products available that provide the necessary dietary requirements. These products are easily reconstituted from a powder form and may be given via a crop feeding tube (Figure 10-24). Tube feeding a bird or giving an oral therapeutic agent via a crop tube should be performed last before putting the bird into its cage. Because avian species do not have an epiglottis, they readily aspirate material that is regurgitated from the crop when struggling. If the bird has just had materials placed in its crop and is not struggling but standing in the enclosure, it will be able to control the closure of the glottis and prevent aspiration of the food or drug.

Water is a very important component of avian nutrition. Fresh clean water should always be made available in a bird's enclosure. For small caged birds the container can have an attached plastic lid forming a hole in which the bird can place its head to drink. For psittacine species, a water bottle attached to the outside of the cage with a stainless tube inserted through the cage bars is the water container of choice. The outside water bottle is easy to fill without disturbing the bird and prevents "poop soup" (i.e., the result of a bird defecating and urinating in its water container). Water should be changed on a daily basis and is an especially important maintenance objective for the owner to follow. Birds are able to tolerate the quality of municipal tap water, but well water should be boiled before being given to birds. Although well water may be clean coming out of the ground, it can be contaminated easily by bacteria colonizing the pipes leading to the faucet. Many automatic watering systems use small rubber tubes and stainless steel nibs placed in the cage and thus are difficult to clean. Often the rubber diaphragm behind the stainless steel nib is a site for bacterial colonization. If possible, automatic watering systems should not be used in an aviary setting.

Calcium is an important dietary element for companion and caged birds. Many birds on a seed diet and reproductively active hens need calcium supplementation. In general all birds should have calcium supplementation in their cage. Calcium supplementation can be provided in the form of a cuttlebone, mineral block (Figure 10-25), crushed oyster shell, or baked crushed eggshell. Most cage and companion birds do not need grit. *Grit* can be defined as a nondigestible, nonnutritional dietary aid to crush food material in the ventriculus (e.g., quartz). As mentioned previously, most companion and cage birds shell their seeds before ingestion. Many of the psittacine species actually crush the kernel or pellet before eating. These birds do not need grit. Crushed oyster shell will deliver calcium to the body if ingested and will possibly stay in the ventriculus to aid in crushing up food. Because crushed oyster shell has a nutritional value in that it is providing a source of calcium, it is not considered grit. Birds will eat the calcium if provided and when needed to meet physiologic demands. Cuttlebones should be placed in the cage with the soft side facing the bird. Cuttlebones are strictly a calcium source and are not beak sharpening devices. If vitamin or mineral supplementation is added to the water, the water must be changed on a daily basis. Vitamin and mineral supplements degrade starting at the time of placement into the water source. Adding vitamin and mineral supplements provides an excellent medium for bacterial growth. To reduce growth and subsequent exposure to bacteria, the water should be changed daily and the water receptacle disinfected.

The ability of the adults to feed their young without the danger of thermal burns is not the only advantage of having parent birds raise their offspring. As adult birds feed their young through regurgitation, they inoculate their young with their crops' autochthonous bacterial flora. This autochthonous flora (beneficial bacteria) usually is comprised of *Bacillus* spp.,

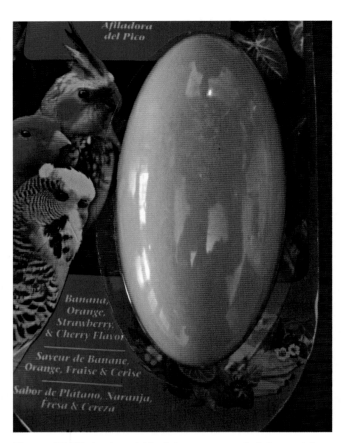

Figure 10-25 A mineral block is a source of dietary calcium, not a beak-sharpening device.

Corynebacterium spp., *Streptomyces* spp., and *Lactobacillus* spp.[7] The regurgitated food containing this soup of microorganisms normally proliferates within the gastrointestinal tract of the neonate, promoting digestion and providing immune support against gastrointestinal infections caused by bacteria that contribute to sour crop and diarrhea.[8,9] It is common practice for aviculturists to give probiotic supplements to birds that are being hand-fed, that are showing signs of crop stasis, and/or have been taking antibiotic medication. The autochthonous flora usually colonize the crop, stomach, and intestinal tract in the first 3 to 4 weeks after hatching.[9] These beneficial bacteria aid in digestion by promoting optimal environmental conditions for the breakdown of the food for utilization by the intestinal tract.[1] Also, the autochthonous flora protect the bird by occupying attachment sites on the intestinal mucosa; secreting metabolic products that inhibit growth, function, and reproduction of disease-causing bacteria; and maintaining an environment with a low pH.[7] There have been studies using readily available cow- and goat-processed probiotic supplements for hand-fed psittacine species, and no significant improvements in survival or growth were demonstrated.[10,11] Again, this would help support the belief that nonspecies specific, in particular mammalian, obtained probiotic organisms may have minimal beneficial effects on the avian digestive system. Studies have shown that the mammalian *Lactobacillus* sp. reduces intestinal pH if administered daily over a period of

2 to 4 weeks, which may help with the digestive process if no other beneficial organisms are being supplemented by the hand-feeder or the parent birds.[7] If the birds are supplemented an avian-specific or species-specific bacterial supplement, the beneficial bacteria will start to protect the intestinal tract at 4 to 6 weeks of age.[12] At 4 to 6 weeks of age, the birds are often in a highly immunocompromised condition and remain so until they are eating food on their own. Any protection or support that an owner can give the bird at this time will be beneficial for the bird's overall health and condition.

Fruits and vegetables are also dietary supplements that are presented as part of a bird's diet. Fruits should be used sparingly in most bird diets because they are composed of mainly sugars and water. Some psittacine species (e.g., eclectus, lories) require a significant amount of fruit in their diet, but these are exceptions. Fruit should be offered only a couple of times a week. To reduce the cost of providing fresh fruits and vegetables, a large discount can be obtained from fruit and vegetable markets on produce that is old or unappealing to customers. As with most food products, the younger birds are when exposed to different foods, the more readily they accept diversity in their diet. Vegetables offer more of a nutritional benefit than do fruits. Fresh or cooked dark green, red, and orange vegetables should be offered on a daily basis if possible. A separate container should be in the enclosure to add any food material other than the base diet. Because of the likelihood of microorganism growth, it has been recommended that fresh fruit and vegetables or cooked food should only be left in the cage for 30 minutes.[5] Vitamin and mineral supplements can be added to food as well as water. It is best to add the supplements to food in which it will adhere. Powder is likely to fall through the seed and end up in the bottom of the container. Coating the seed first with food oil (e.g., sesame) will give the supplement an attachment surface. The supplements can also be sprinkled on fresh fruit and/or vegetables or cooked foods.

Some foods are toxic to birds. Avocados and chocolate are the most commonly known foods that are toxic to birds. Comfry, a green leaf herb that is popular with canary breeders as a fresh food for their birds, may lead to liver damage. Any food that is high in sugar or salt content is not recommended for captive avian species. Zinc-coated water containers should also be avoided because of the possibility of leaching chemicals from the plated surface.

Special bird diets have been formulated for certain species and for young growing birds. Lories, birds native to Australia and the South Pacific islands, eat fruit, nectar, and pollen as the main part of their diet. Powdered and liquid Lory diets are commercially available and should be provided to this species as its primary food source (Figure 10-26). Myna birds and toucans are susceptible to hemochromatosis, or iron storage disease of the liver. The iron content of many diets has resulted in special myna and toucan diets that have low iron composition. Grapes are high in iron and should not be fed to toucans, mynah birds or those avian species predisposed to iron storage disease. Tea has been advocated as a supplement that binds iron and may be used to reduce dietary iron intake in birds

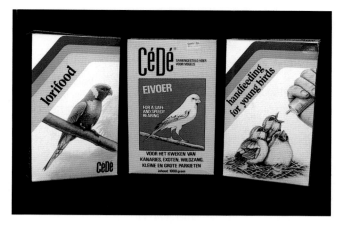

Figure 10-26 The lory diet is an example of special formulation avian products that meet the nutritional demand of specific species.

susceptible to hemochromatosis. Hand-raised baby birds need a liquid diet. The advent of commercially available hand-feeding formula has revolutionized the ability of bird owners to adequately feed baby parrot species. These commercially available hand-feeding diets are easy to reconstitute using warm water, and they provide the nutrition needed for proper growth and development. For most situations in which psittacine species are being hand-raised, a commercial product is preferable to homemade formulas. The use of warm water to reconstitute the powder has decreased the incidence of burned crops caused by overheated baby bird formulas that needed to be cooked before administration. If heating a baby bird formula for feeding, it must be remembered that a bird's body temperature is approximately 103° F; therefore, the formula should be fed 2 to 3 degrees cooler than the body temperature. If the food is warmed in a microwave oven, it should be thoroughly mixed to prevent hot spots from forming within the food. Owners have the ability to control a bird's diet, thereby having a significant effect on its overall health and quality of life. Educating the owner on recommended diets is one of the most important aspects of the postpurchase physical examination.

▪ PREVENTIVE MEDICINE

Birds that are imported into the United States have to be quarantined in USDA facilities for 30 days. During this 30-day quarantine period, the birds are monitored for any signs of illness and may be treated with a tetracycline-impregnated food. The quarantine regulation for birds was established to prevent the introduction of velogenic viscerotropic Newcastle disease into the United States. Since the passage of the Wild Bird Conservation Act in 1992, there has been a significant reduction of parrot species importation into the United States. With the majority of companion avian species being captive bred, the widespread exposure to infectious diseases observed during the importation period appears to be reduced. At the same time there has been a significant advancement in avian medicine and surgery and general knowledge relating to husbandry, nutrition, and management.

For birds entering homes in which there are other cage or companion avian species, the new arrival should be quarantined for at least 30 days. This 30-day quarantine period should take place in a building with a separate air space, away from the established avian presence. Unfortunately, not everyone has the ability to quarantine a new bird in a separate building. In cases where the recommended quarantine protocol cannot be followed, one should try to separate the new bird as far as possible from its housemates. Once the bird has acclimatized for a few days to its new environment, an examination should be performed by a veterinarian with an interest in, and knowledge of, avian medicine. The most important part of the examination, aside from determining the health status of the animal, is educating and informing the owner of husbandry and nutritional requirements of the patient. Also included in the education process is a review of clinical signs associated with illness. When a bird becomes ill, there are signs that an owner should look for, and if this knowledge is lacking then it may be too late to help the patient once the abnormalities are recognized and is presented to the veterinarian. Most avian owners have never owned a bird and therefore lack the general knowledge that is obtained through previous ownership. The general physical examination of the bird and educating the owner will take a significant amount of time if correctly performed. An owner must be reminded that the bird should not be treated with any medication during the quarantine period unless it is for a specific disease problem. Prophylactic treatment will often mask diseases and inadequately treat those diseases, resulting in the placement of the bird in the house or aviary with subclinical illness. If the bird is harboring a disease organism, it is best for the disease process to become evident during quarantine so it can be treated. Young birds should be vaccinated against polyoma virus infection. The first vaccine is given subcutaneously at 6 weeks of age and the second injection 3 weeks later. A certificate is given to the owner, signed by the veterinarian, validating the vaccination process. After the bird is examined, a routine physical evaluation is recommended every year. This yearly physical will track the bird's growth and health over time and is especially useful to use as a benchmark if it becomes ill. Often birds will present more often for grooming procedures that include wing feather trimming, nail trimming, and beak smoothing.

For any disinfectant to be effective, all organic debris must be removed from the surface to be treated. Dirt or organic material cannot be disinfected through traditional methods used in aviaries with the compounds employed. A dilute sodium hypochlorite solution is the most cost-effective and efficient disinfectant one can use. Phenol-based disinfectants are more expensive than sodium hypochlorite and will effectively kill mycobacterial organisms. If newspaper or a disposable sheet paper product is placed on the bottom of cages and within baby bird containers, much of the fecal material is removed when the cage or aviary is cleaned. Outside flight cages should be elevated (Figure 10-27), which allows for raking and debris removal from the area. All birds should be

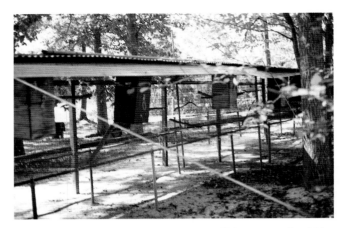

Figure 10-27 When possible, outdoor flight cages should be elevated to prevent bird exposure to the ground, reduce predator attacks, and ease cleaning.

removed from their cages if a volatile chemical compound is being used to disinfect the flights, cages, or enclosures. Once the smell has dissipated, the birds will be able to safely return to the area without fear of respiratory damage due to the irritating chemical compounds within the environment. The avian respiratory tract is much more sensitive to irritating environmental toxins than is the mammalian lung. The amount of volatile compound a human can withstand is significantly greater than that of a bird. It is also recommended to rinse a cage and cage bowls and toys thoroughly before placing the bird back into its enclosure. All disinfecting should take place in a well-ventilated area and strictly follow the manufacturer's instructions regarding usage and dilutions. If wooden cage furniture or perches cannot be cleaned or disinfected, they should be discarded and new toys and/or perches procured.

■ PHYSICAL EXAMINATION AND RESTRAINT

To the uninitiated, the avian physical examination can be an imposing task. There are many aspects of the avian examination that pose problems and concern to the veterinarian and veterinary technician. The examination of birds is basically the same as examination of other animals, but it should be performed in steps to gain a full appreciation of the owner's concern, patient's clinical condition, and evaluation of the patient's physical status.

Veterinarians must never underestimate the value of questioning the owner when obtaining the history of the case. With all species of animals there are basic questions veterinarians should ask when formulating a historical perspective on the case, and there are species-specific questions that pertain only to the animal being examined. Figure 10-28 is a guide that may be used for questioning the owners of these feathered companions.

It does help to understand some of the basic nutrition and husbandry issues that are recommended for the care of

Avian History Form	Date:	
RDVM info	Admitting Clinician	
	Appt. Time:	

Name of Bird: _____	Species: _____	Age: _____	Pet Bird/Breeder

Background Information:
Length of time owned:_____   Where acquird? Breeder ☐ Pet Store ☐ Other_____
Vaccination History _____   When was last molt?_____   Character of feces _____
How often is bird handled? Daily ☐   Occasionally ☐   Never ☐   Is bird ever taken outside? Y/N

Husbandry:
Housed Indoors/Outdoors? _____   Where is cage located? _____
Type of Caging:_____   Size of Caging_____   Galvanized? Yes ☐ No ☐
Cage Substrate?_____   How often is cage cleaned? _____
What type of disinfectant is used when ckeaning cage?_____
Types of toys/perches offered? _____

Nutrition:
Type of food offered:
--Pellets? No ☐ Yes☐   If yes. what brand?_____   Amount fed/frequency _____

--Seed?   No ☐ Yes☐   If yes. what type?_____   Amount fed/frequency _____

--Fruits?   No ☐ Yes☐   If yes. what type?_____   Amount fed/frequency _____

--Vegetables? No ☐ Yes☐ If yes. what type?_____ Amount fed/frequency_____

Type of Supplements/Treats offered?_____

Water Source:_____   How often is water changed?_____

Any other pets?:No ☐ Yes☐   If yes, specify:_____

Any other pets?: No ☐ Yes☐   Specify: _____

Birds are housed together or singly?_____   If not housed together, where are other birds located?_____
Any new additions to the bird population? No☐ Yes☐   If yes, specify _____
      −Were the new additions properly quarantined separate from rest of bird population? _____

Past Medical History/Problems :

Current Presenting Problem:

Duration of Problem:

Figure 10-28 Sample avian history form.

companion avian species. First, it is important to learn the owner's general knowledge regarding pet bird care. If the owner is experienced, how much of this knowledge has been transferred into the overall environment and nutritional offerings of the animal being examined? Important issues regarding the bird's age, where it was purchased, exposure to other birds, and past medical history will help determine possible exposure to infectious disease. Cage location, other animals within the house, and household environment will aid the examiner in determining possible stress-induced illness or provide information that will lead to helpful recommendations that will improve the patient's quality of life and possibly health. All information that can be gathered relating to the presenting condition before an examination will help the veterinarian to develop a plan for examination and diagnostic testing used to establish a definitive diagnosis and treatment plan.

Once the history has been taken, the examining veterinarian should observe the bird from a distance, preferably out of sight of the patient. This observation can be accomplished through a one-way mirror or small window in the exam room door. If a patient is extremely ill or moribund, emergency care must be initiated as soon as possible. For the routine, postpurchase, or annual physical examination or a noncritical presentation, the "external" physical examination is useful. In cases where the bird is with the owner, thereby providing a sense of protection and comfort, the veterinarian has an opportunity to witness clinical signs that otherwise may be lost if the patient is excited. The external examination consists of observing the patient's respiration, perching/walking ability, posture, feather condition, and any abnormality mentioned by the owner. The external examination will also give the veterinarian and/or veterinary technician a good indication if the bird is in a condition that will allow for a thorough "hands-on" physical evaluation. Conditions that preclude a hands-on physical examination of an avian patient include severe dyspnea or respiratory distress in the form of open beak breathing, wings out and tail bobbing, or standing or sitting, depressed with its feathers fluffed on the bottom of the cage.

If it is determined that the bird is able to withstand a thorough hands-on physical examination, then the animal must be captured and restrained. The capture and restraint of birds is one of the most traumatic events for veterinarians, owners, and birds during the physical examination process. The smooth and uneventful capture of a pet bird for physical examination goes a long way in developing confidence of the owner in the veterinarian. When restraining a bird, the less stress there is, the better the examination will be. First, the bird should be quickly and confidently captured. For small caged birds (e.g., finches, canaries), the cage should be placed on the examination table. With one person at the light switch and the other with their hand in the cage, the bird is observed for capture when the light is turned off. Within seconds of the light being turned off, the bird should be grabbed before it has time to accommodate to the darkness of the room. Once the bird is captured, the light is turned on and the bird's head is placed between the middle and index fingers in a dorsal recumbent position (Figure 10-29). The thumb and little

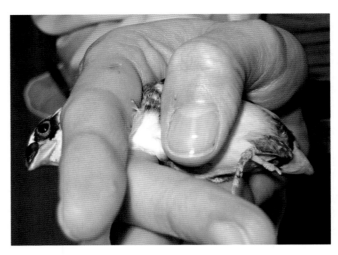

Figure 10-29 Proper way to restrain a small bird.

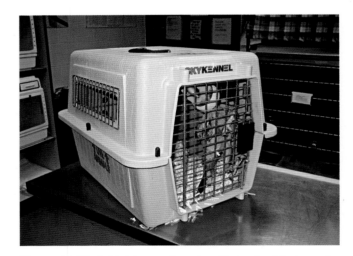

Figure 10-30 A bird in a pet carrier. Birds should always be transported to the veterinarian in a pet carrier or cage.

finger hold the body without restricting breathing. This technique works wonders in reducing the stress of chasing the bird around the cage and is very impressive to owners. The dark room technique may work for smaller psittacine species (e.g., budgerigars, lovebirds) but has little effect on parrot species.

Birds should always arrive to the veterinary clinic or hospital in cages or pet carriers (Figure 10-30). For smaller cage birds, the owner may bring the bird to the clinic in its normal living environment. Plastic pet carriers can be modified into transport carriers for birds by inserting a wooden dowel perch across the bottom half of the carrier and lining the carrier with newspaper substrate. The dowel gives the patient a place to perch out of its feces, while the newspaper can be changed after the fecal sample has been gathered. There are few if any circumstances when the bird should come to a veterinarian's

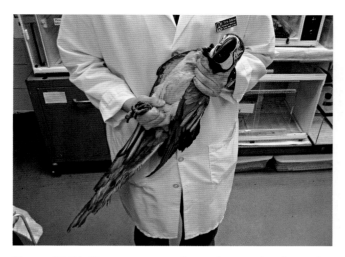

Figure 10-31 The proper way of securing a psittacine, using an Elizabethan grip.

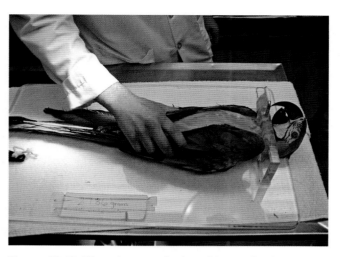

Figure 10-32 The avian restraint board is an effective method of restraining a pet bird.

office outside of a cage or a pet carrier. There are too many opportunities for the bird to get injured in an unfamiliar environment, often surrounded by dogs, cats and curious humans. After the physical examination the avian patient is often stressed and upset and may bite an owner that is only too willing to love the bird when trying to "settle it down." If the owner can remove the bird from the examination table or hand the bird to the veterinarian, this is the first step toward restraint. The bird is then placed in a position for capture with a towel. Most birds respond favorably to slow acceptance of the towel, observing the restraint as one moves the toweled hand from in front to behind the bird. If the bird is reluctant to be restrained, then a toweled hand can go into the carrier and grab the bird from behind the head when the bird bites on the side of the container. A bird cannot bite two objects at one time. If it is biting the side of the carrier to get away or stabilize its position, it cannot bite the veterinarian. Patients reluctant to be captured must be grabbed quickly, without hesitation on the part of the handler. Hesitation is an invitation to be injured from a bird bite.

Once in place, the thumb and index finger form an Elizabethan grip under the mandible. The opposite hand comes over the top of the legs and holds the bird in place while the last three digits of the hand hold the neck, securing the outside wing while the inside wing is pressed against the body (Figure 10-31). If the bird cannot be held because of the patient's intransigence or the technician's inability, an avian restraint board may be used (Figure 10-32). The little finger on the head hand can tuck the outside wing in as the inside wing is held in place against the body. A towel around the body makes it difficult to complete the physical examination, and it, the towel, gets in the way of many examination procedures. Once the bird is captured, it can be placed on an avian restraint board or held by an experienced technician.

If one is to collect samples for diagnostic testing, this should be done first. All materials used for diagnostic sample collec-

tion should be in place before capture. Blood samples should be collected before the physical examination process. The vein of choice for blood collection in pet avian species is the right jugular vein. Other diagnostic sample collection should occur on an as-needed basis, if desired by the owner or as part of a routine screening protocol.

Avian physical examinations are no different than other animal examinations once the bird is restrained. The physical examination begins at the head and ends at the vent and/or uropygial gland. The beak and head are examined straight on for symmetry and normal beak occlusion. The nares are examined for symmetry and nasal discharge. Because most birds have feathers around the nares, it is easy to determine if there is nasal discharge because there will be matted feathers. The eyes should be examined for lens opacity, anterior chamber condition, corneal health, and conjunctival inflammation. Again, if ocular discharge is present, the feathers along the cranial ventral lid margin will be matted. Eyes can be examined to determine hydration status, with sunken globes and dry corneas being indicators of a patient needing fluid therapy. Although there are few cases in which the avian ear is diseased, the ears should be examined. The ears are located caudal and ventral to the lateral canthus of the eyelids. By lifting the modified feathers covering the external ear canal, this structure can be examined for abscesses or discharge. The oral cavity and choanal slit (dorsal surface of the oral cavity) can be examined by opening the beak with a specialized avian speculum (Figure 10-33). The veterinarian must be careful to place the speculum in the leading edge of the upper and lower beak to prevent iatrogenic trauma to the lateral beak walls of the rhinotheca and rhamphotheca. The avian oral cavity should be dry and smooth. The choanal slit is lined with epithelial projections extending from the thin edge toward the center of the opening. If there is an inflammatory process occurring within the upper respiratory system, the choanal slit may be inflamed or edema-

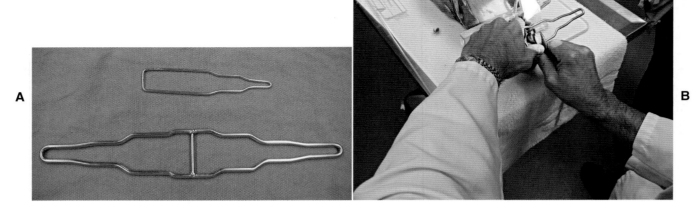

Figure 10-33 A, Two psittacine beak specula of different sizes. **B,** Examining the avian oral cavity using the oral speculum.

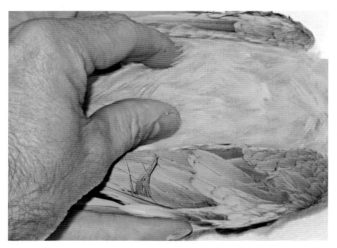

Figure 10-34 Palpation of the pectoral muscles is an excellent way to determine body condition of the companion avian patient.

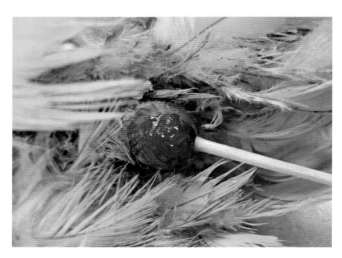

Figure 10-35 The vent area of parrots should be examined for the evidence of papillomas as shown in this figure.

tous, and the papillary projections may be eroded from the edge of the slit.

The thoracic inlet can be palpated for crop stasis, an ingested foreign object, or thermal crop trauma. The pectoral muscle of parrot species is the best site for determining body condition of the avian patient (Figure 10-34). A body score of 1 would be assigned to a patient that is extremely emaciated, whereas a body score of 5 is considered overweight. The pectoral muscles should round up to the keel without extending higher than that skeletal structure. The feathers over the body can be examined for coloration and normal architecture. Both the legs and wings should be flexed and extended to examine joint function and the patient observed for proper positioning of all limbs. The toes should be uniform in size and have a reticulated pattern on the plantar surface. There should be concern if the reticulated skin surface has been rubbed off; the smoothness can indicate hyperemic areas, especially in the weight-bearing

parts of the toes. The cause of epithelial sloughing on the plantar surface of the feet may be associated with vitamin A deficiency or improper perch material (e.g., sandpaper, cement). Swollen toes may be an indication of a foreign body stricture or, in certain large psittacine species such as macaws, a condition called constricted toe syndrome. Under the dorsal surface of the wing in the propatageal area, a black nondescript tattoo may be present indicating a bird that has been surgically sexed. Birds with the tattoos on the right wing are sexed males, whereas birds with tattoos on the left wing are sexed females. It is always recommended that anyone purchasing a bird for reproductive purposes have the animal sexed again endoscopically to examine gonads and the coelomic cavity to confirm the gender of that particular bird. It is difficult to palpate internal organs because of the extension of the keel caudally over the coelomic cavity. In palpating the caudal coelomic cavity, it is possible to feel eggs within the oviduct, the ventriculus, an enlarged liver, and the nonfused pubic bones. The nonfused pubic bones in the caudal coelomic cavity are the landmarks aviculturists use to determine the sex of certain avian species, commonly called *pelvic sexing*. The vent is examined for proper appearance and the feathers around the vent examined for fecal material. The feathers around a normal vent should be clean, without fecal soiling. In many parrot species, in particular larger birds, the vent should be everted so that the veterinarian can examine the mucocutaneous junction for evidence of papillomas. Papillomas may appear as a roughened surface on the mucocutaneous junction to proliferative tissue protruding from the vent (Figure 10-35). If there is doubt concerning the validity of a diagnosis of papillomatous tissue involving the vent, then vinegar can be used to moisten the mucocutaneous area in question. If the surface epithelium is disrupted, the vinegar will turn the unhealthy tissue white. The uropygial gland is located on the extreme caudal dorsal surface of the bird, proximal to the *pygostyle* (the last vertebra of birds). The uropygial gland or preen gland should be examined for symmetry and overall appearance. To assess heart health and respiratory condition, the bird should be ausculted. The heart is best evaluated with a pediatric stethoscope over the lateral body wall, whereas respiratory condition is best determined by listening over the craniodorsal body wall. Before the bird is returned to the carrier, it should be weighed on a digital gram scale. The digital gram scale should have a maximum weight of 6 kilograms and weigh patients in 1-gram increments. Newspaper substrate should be placed in the cage or carrier before returning the patient to the owner and all blood on the feathers or skin cleaned with hydrogen peroxide. Birds with a full crop or food in the crop should be handled carefully, and they should have the food removed or have minimal restraint until the food passes. It is very easy for an avian patient to regurgitate food in the crop and aspirate the contents into the respiratory system. Because birds' major lymph organs are the thymus and the cloacal bursa, there are no lymph nodes to palpate during an avian physical examination. The avian physical examination requires a general protocol that should be followed from the history to the hands-on health evaluation. Only through a thorough physical examination can a veterinarian develop a diagnostic plan in order to work toward a definitive diagnosis.

Chemical Restraint and General Anesthesia/Analgesia

Chemical restraint of avian patients can be classified as injectable sedation and anesthesia and inhalation anesthesia. Situations that call for chemical restraint are birds with seizures or neurologic signs, or the need to take radiographs or perform minor and major surgical procedures. Rarely, if ever, should a bird be sedated to perform a routine physical examination or to collect samples for diagnostic testing. With the advent of endoscopic gender determination, it was a common practice to use injectable anesthetic agents to sedate the patient for the procedure. The disadvantages of injectable anesthetic agents are an inability to quickly modify the drug's effect on the patient and often very traumatic induction and recovery periods. The induction period may be 5 minutes, whereas the recovery phase may last 30 minutes to 1 hour, depending on the agents being used. It is currently acceptable to use drugs for sedative purposes (Table 10-1), but injectable anesthetics are discouraged when safe, controllable gas products (e.g., isoflurane, sevoflurane) are readily available.[13]

TABLE 10-1	Common Injectable Sedation and Anesthetic Agents	
Agent	**Dose**	**Comments**
Atipamezole (Antisedan, Pfizer)	0.25-0.38 mg/kg IM	Psittacine species
Diazepam (Valium, Roche)	0.5-0.6 mg/kg IM	Most species/sedation
	or 2.5-4.5 mg/kg PO	Most species/sedation
Ketamine HCl (Ketaset, Fort Dodge)	20-50 mg/kg SC, IM, IV	Psittacine species; smaller species may require higher dose
Ketamine (K)/Diazepam (D)	(K) 5-30 mg/kg IM +	
	(D) 0.5-2.0 mg/kg IM, IV	Psittacine species
Ketamine (K)/Medetomidine (M)	(K) 2.5-7.0 mg/kg IM	
	(M) 75-150 µg/kg IM	Large psittacine species
Ketamine (K)/Midazolam (Md)	(K) 10-40 mg/kg SC, IM	Psittacine species
	(Md) 0.2-2.0 mg/kg SC, IM	
Ketamine (K)/Xylazine (X)	(K) 20-50 mg/kg IM	Psittacine species <250 g require dose at higher end of range
	(X) 1-10 mg/kg IM	
Medetomidine (Domitor, Pfizer)	60-85 µg/kg IM	Psittacine species
Midazolam (Versed, Roche)	2-3 mg/kg IM	Amazon parrots
Propofol (Rapinovet, Mallinckrodt)	133 mg/kg IV	Psittacine species
Tiletamine/zolazepam (Telazol/Fort Dodge)	4-25 mg/kg IM	Most species

From Carpenter JW: *Exotic Animal Formulary*, ed 3, St Louis, 2005, WB Saunders.
IM, intramuscular; IV, intravenous; PO, per os; SC, subcutaneous.

One of the most difficult situations that avian veterinarians face is the prospect of placing their patients under general anesthesia. There is a saying that I fully agree with that states, "There is no minor surgery when a patient is placed under general anesthesia." This statement is true, and all avian and exotic animal veterinarians should adhere to its premise. To begin with, all clients must be made aware of the consequences of placing an avian patient under general anesthesia and the possible adverse clinical situations that can and do occur when an avian patient is induced or maintained under general anesthesia. Once an owner has been properly notified of the potential side effects and risks of general anesthesia, a focus on the veterinary team must take place. An anesthetist should be assigned to the case for every procedure that requires general anesthesia. By assigning a specific anesthetist to the case, the veterinarian can concentrate on the diagnostic testing, treatment, and recovery of the patient. The assigned anesthetist should be confident and familiar with the anesthesia machine to manipulate and monitor the machine during procedures in which general anesthesia is required (e.g., radiology and ultrasound diagnostics).

The avian patient must be assessed for its ability to withstand general anesthesia and the procedures that will take place under this form of anesthesia. If it appears that the patient is too ill to cope with the rigors of general anesthesia, then that patient should be monitored for any adverse conditions and treated before going under general anesthesia.

First and foremost, the clinician treating the animal must assess its condition and the ability of that bird to withstand the risk of the anesthetic protocol. If the animal is not able to withstand the anesthetic protocol, then it must be monitored, treated, and stabilized.

A "crash kit" should be assembled to manage emergency situations. The crash kit should contain endotracheal tubes, tape, intravenous (IV) catheters, 22-gauge 1½-inch spinal needles, therapeutic agents that stimulate the heart to beat faster (e.g., epinephrine, atropine), and an agent that stimulates respiratory action (e.g., dopram). Once the crash kit has been assembled, it should be taken to every general anesthetic procedure.

If the bird appears healthy, any diagnostic procedure can take place as long as the owner has been educated on the adverse side effects of general anesthesia. In most cases the birds are not administered a preanesthetic agent. The avian patient will be examined for its ability to withstand the rigors of general anesthesia. Anesthesia procedures that are scheduled for avian patients should take place in the morning, allowing for postprocedure observation. The avian gastrointestinal system moves material through at a rapid rate. In my own observations of contrast material moving through the gastrointestinal system of a macaw, I saw barium being transferred from the crop to the distal intestinal tract in 45 minutes. Even with the rapid flow of food material, it is recommended to fast the animal for 1.5 to 3 hours before general anesthesia. Of course the fasting time should be evaluated on a case-by-case basis. If the patient is dehydrated or if there is a concern regarding hypoglycemia during the procedure, IV or intraosseous (IO) fluid therapy should be administered. The recommended sites for IV and IO catheter placement are the medial tarsometatarsal vein and the distal ulna or proximal tibiotarsal bone, respectively.

Once it has been determined that the patient is in good enough condition for the procedure, induction takes place. In most cases of avian general anesthesia, isoflurane gas is used. There has been an increased usage of sevoflurane and desflurane with avian species, but the higher price of these agents and small difference in their overall advantages to isoflurane continue to keep their usage at a low level.

A mask or induction chamber may be used for induction and preparation of the patient for intubation. An appropriate-sized plastic face mask is recommended for pet bird anesthesia induction. A problem that often occurs when placing the face mask on the patient is the bird biting the rubber diaphragm of the mask. If the rubber diaphragms have too large an opening for that size bird, some material (e.g., 4 × 4 gauze sponges, towel) must be placed in the space between the diaphragm and head to prevent gas leakage. If the bird patient bites the diaphragm and it needs to be replaced, Vet-Wrap™ (3M Inc., Minneapolis, MN) or some other self-adhesive material can be used to make a smaller, more durable diaphragm that can be removed between bird usages. For gas induction it is generally recommended to provide a 5% flow of isoflurane with a 2-liter flow of oxygen. As mentioned previously, it is extremely important to have an anesthetist specifically monitoring the patient's response to the anesthetic and the machine. At a 5% flow of isoflurane, most patients will undergo rapid induction and are ready for intubation in less than a minute. Careful attention must be given to the patient's condition for intubation.

For intubation, all materials should be prepared and ready for use before induction. Materials needed for intubation include the tracheal tube (noncuffed, 2.5-4.0 interior diameter for most companion avian species), tape, and hemostats. A noncuffed tube is used to prevent pressure necrosis from developing on the mucosal surface of the trachea. The hemostats are needed to grasp the tongue and extend it for exposure of the glottis. Once the animal is induced, the mask is removed from the bird's face, the beak opened, tongue grasped and extended, the tube placed into the trachea through the glottis, and the machine disconnected from the face mask and attached to the tracheal tube. The tracheal tube should be taped into place by attaching a strip of white cloth adhesive tape to the tracheal tube and wrapping it around the back of the bird's head and retaping it to the tube.

Monitoring devices that can be used to collect baseline data include a Doppler unit to monitor heart rate and strength of the heart beat, a respiratory monitor, an esophageal thermometer, and an ECG, if available.[14] There are other monitoring units that provide additional vital information, but the basic monitoring items mentioned at the beginning of this paragraph are essential in most, if not all, cases. Perivascular access should be achieved using the IV route (e.g., tarsometatarsal vein, jugular vein, or basilic vein) or IO route (e.g., distal ulna or proximal tibiotarsal bone). Atropine has been used with

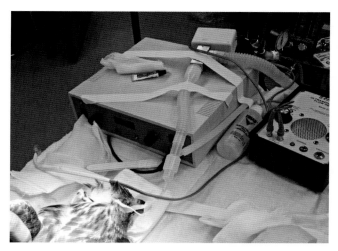

Figure 10-36 An intermittent positive pressure ventilator can be used for many avian surgeries, but a tight seal of the endotracheal tube is required for proper function.

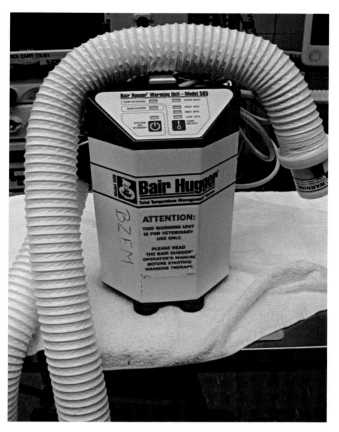

Figure 10-37 Convective thermal heating devices are highly recommended to maintain normothermia in the avian patient.

success in cases of bradycardia at a dose of 0.02-0.08 mg/kg IM or 0.01-0.02 mg/kg IM.[13]

Controlled mechanical ventilators (Figure 10-36) are being used more often in avian surgeries to maintain consistency of oxygen and anesthetic uptake by the patient. Mechanical ventilators work best when the body cavity is not entered.

It is important to maintain normothermia during general anesthesia, which is very difficult to do for the avian patient whose body temperature ranges from 101° F to 104° F. Although not commonly used, an esophageal thermometer can monitor body temperature while the bird is under general anesthesia. A cloacal probe may be used, but the patient often voids feces or urine during the surgical procedure, and there is peristaltic action of the distal gastrointestinal tract pushing the probe out of the vent. All of these conditions can adversely affect the ability of the veterinarian to properly monitor an avian patient's body temperature when using the cloacal orifice for probe placement. Historically, conductive heat, in the form of a water blanket, or radiant heat, in the form of a heat lamp placed close to the patient, has been used to maintain body temperature while the patient is under general anesthesia. In recent years the convective air blanket (e.g., Bair Hugger®) (Figure 10-37) has been more effective in maintaining normothermia for avian patients under general anesthesia than the water blanket and is less obtrusive than the heat lamp.

Analgesia

Pain management has become an integral part of patient care within veterinary medicine. This also applies to avian patients and possibly has a significant impact on the successful conclusion to many surgical cases. Box 10-4 lists dosages for nonsteroidal antiinflammatory drugs for avian species.[15]

BOX 10-4 **Nonsteroidal Antiinflammatory Drugs for Avian Species**

1. Phenylbutazone
   20 mg/kg, q8h, PO (raptors)
   3.5-7.0 mg/kg, q8h (psittacine species)
2. Acetylsalicylic acid
   5.0 mg/kg, q8h, PO
   In 250 ml drinking water, add 325 mg and change water TID
3. Flunixin meglumine
   1.0 mg/kg, q24h, IM, hydration essential
4. Ibuprofen
   5-10 mg/kg, q8h–q12h, PO use pediatric suspension for small birds
5. Ketoprofen
   2.0 mg/kg, q8h–q24h, IM or SC
6. Carprofen
   2.0-4.0 mg/kg, q8h–q12h, PO
7. Piroxicam
   0.5 mg/kg, q12h, PO
8. Meloxicam
   0.1-0.4 mg/kg, q24h, PO

From Paul-Murphy J, Ludders JW: Avian analgesia, *Vet Clin North Am Exot Anim Pract* 4:35-46, 2001.
IM, intramuscular; PO, per os (oral); SC, subcutaneous; TID, three times a day.

◼ DIAGNOSTIC TESTING

For a veterinarian treating an avian or exotic animal patient, diagnostic testing is an essential tool in formulating a definitive diagnosis, prognosis, and treatment plan. Avian patients do not allow any guesswork for the attending clinician and will quickly succumb to a disease process if not properly treated. The diagnostic test results will give the veterinarian a snapshot window to "look" inside the patient at that particular point in time. By developing a baseline of values, the practitioner can follow the progress of a disease process through a treatment period. If the patient responds to the treatment, it is continued; if the patient does not respond, a treatment alternative is considered. Veterinarians must always remember to collect the samples that will be affected by stress at the beginning of an examination and follow with those that are least affected by the physical and emotional stress. In most cases, blood is collected for a complete blood count (CBC) and plasma chemistry panel first because stress is likely to adversely affect the white blood cell count. This presentation will review the proper techniques used to collect samples from avian patients that are subsequently submitted for diagnostic testing. All patients should be properly restrained to prevent injury to the veterinarian, technician, and, most importantly, the patient.

Blood Collection

The amount of blood that can be safely collected from relatively healthy avian patients is 1 ml/100 g body weight. With this amount of blood, the basic diagnostic tests, a CBC and plasma chemistry panel, can be ordered, even on small patients. Veterinarians should always discuss submission requirements for a blood sample with their diagnostic laboratory to reduce errors that may be caused by improper shipment. If enough blood cannot be drawn from a small patient to run all tests, a practitioner has to decide which test(s) will give the most useful information.

Common sites for blood collection include the right jugular vein, basilic vein, and median tarsometatarsal vein.

The right jugular vein is the vein of choice for blood collection in most companion bird species. The jugular vein can be found in a featherless tract (apterium) on the ventrolateral aspect of the cervical region. When collecting blood from birds, the procedure should be performed when the vein is visual. One aspect of birds that makes it easy to collect blood is that their skin is thin and veins highly visible. Aspects that make blood collection difficult are that birds have mobile veins under the skin and the vessel walls are extremely elastic, making needle punctures difficult. When visualizing the vein, it should be held off with the thumb, allowing the syringe barrel to rest on the finger for stability while drawing the sample. For most avian species, a 3-ml syringe with a 26-gauge needle is adequate for collection (Figure 10-38).

The basilic vein, located on the ventral surface of the wing coursing over the proximal radius and ulna, is another choice for avian blood collection. The disadvantages to collecting blood from the basilic vein are that the vein is superficial with

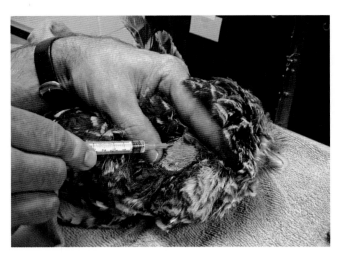

Figure 10-38 A 3-ml syringe should be used to collect blood in avian patients weighing more than 50 grams.

little support tissue to disperse a hematoma, and in most bird species it is small, precipitating collapse. Often if the basilic vein is used, the person collecting the sample must "milk" the syringe to reduce pressure on the vessel. The location of this vein is optimum for IV injections because the veterinarian can see the needle in the vessel lumen and the therapeutic agent being injected into the vein. If this vessel is used for IV injection or blood collection, the owner must be aware of the resulting hematoma because of the lack of feathers covering the proximal radius/ulna on the ventral surface of the wing.

In some avian species the medial tarsometatarsal vein can be used for blood collection or the placement of an indwelling IV catheter. This vein can be located in a groove that extends down the medial surface of the tarsometatarsal bone. The larger the bird is, the more developed and usable this vein is for blood collection or catheter placement.

Although three veins have been described for blood collection in avian patients, these locations should not limit the veterinarian in the selection process for a suitable site. Any large vessel that is readily available for blood collection should be used (e.g., humeral vein, lateral tarsometatarsal vein).

Fecal Gram Stains

Fecal Gram staining as part of a companion avian physical examination is a controversial subject. Often birds are able to mask illness, or it is difficult for the veterinarian to determine underlying conditions as the bird adapts to a new environment. Overtly the animal may appear normal but there could be pathogenic organisms within the gastrointestinal tract that are waiting for an opportunity to cause disease when the bird's immunologic system is compromised.

In a bird that is exhibiting no external clinical disease signs, Gram-negative organisms (e.g., *Pseudomonas* spp., *Klebsiella* spp.) are considered potential pathogens. Gram-positive organisms that may be problematic include the alpha- and beta-hemolytic *Streptococcus* spp. and more than three candida organisms per oil immersion field. The normal microflorae of most parrot species are primarily Gram-positive rods.

Microbiologic Cultures

When obtaining culture samples from avian patients, the veterinarian must again contact the diagnostic laboratory to make sure that proper protocol is followed for transport and maintenance of the sample to optimize organism recovery. If the veterinarian is seeking an aerobic or anaerobic organism, this must also be discussed with the laboratory to ensure the proper collection and transport medium are used for survival of the bacteria or fungal organisms. When collecting microbiologic cultures, veterinarians and technicians have a tendency to use the smallest culturette possible, commonly called the Mini-tip culturette (Becton Dickinson Microbiology Systems, Cockeysville, MD), most likely to avoid injuring the small patient. It is a known fact that the larger the surface area is on the Culturette, the better the chances are that the laboratory can isolate the organism. Veterinarians should use a regular-sized culturette when possible to increase their chances of isolating an organism.

Common sites for culture include the choana, crop, cloaca, and skin. When determining if an area needs to be cultured, a specific protocol needs to be followed. This protocol should start with evidence of clinical disease. If the choanal papillae (small epithelial projections that protrude toward the center of the opening in the dorsal respiratory/oral interface) are blunted or missing, this may indicate a condition of upper respiratory inflammation or irritation. Swelling and hyperemia along the choanal slit may be signs of a more chronic disease condition. Often these clinical signs are found in conjunction with other disease problems (e.g., sneezing, nasal and/or ocular discharge, dyspnea). A culture of the choana is recommended if disease signs are observed during the physical exam, or if the owner mentions abnormalities. To reduce the chance of culturing transitory organisms, the choana should be cultured in a specific manner. In most companion bird species the choana is a triangular opening on the dorsal surface of the oral cavity. The base of the triangular structure is missing as the skin of the choanal opening transitions into the oral cavity. The apex of the triangle points in the direction of the beak. The culturette should be directed toward the apex of the triangle and the cotton tip of the culturette buried into the underlying choana into the nasal septum. Fluid can be flushed into the nares to "push" nasal material—possibly containing the organisms desired—onto the culturette once it is in position within the choana. Another option for obtaining culture samples of the upper respiratory system is an infraorbital sinus lavage of the area between the medial canthus and nares *(lores)*. The collection site can be identified in the medial aspect of the lores area as a depression. If the area described for infraorbital sinus lavage is swollen and contains fluid, a sample of this material can be aspirated and submitted for culture.

Culturing the crop is indicated when birds are exhibiting signs of crop stasis or regurgitation. When working with hand-fed birds, in most cases it is easy to culture the crop because

they readily accept material being placed in their mouth. The baby bird should be positioned as if being hand-fed. Shown the culturette, most baby birds will open their mouth and quickly swallow the cotton-tipped swab. Once in the crop, located at the thoracic inlet, the culturette can be palpated and should be vigorously rubbed against the crop mucosa. As with all cultures, it should be emphasized to owners how important it is to identify the potential disease-causing organisms to determine the correct antimicrobials to treat the infection(s). It is not unusual to find that many complex, highly regarded new antimicrobial agents are ineffective in treating avian isolates. What is surprising is that these same organisms are sensitive to simple, commonly used antibiotics. This again emphasizes the need for culture and sensitivity for avian cases that are showing clinical disease signs.

Culturing the cloaca will often provide information on possible infections affecting the reproductive, urinary, or intestinal tract. The confluence of the three body systems at the cloaca, in particular the intestinal tract, makes it clear that organisms will be identified. The important factor for veterinarians treating avian species is to recognize what the normal intestinal flora is for that particular bird. For most parrots, Gram-positive organisms are uniformly the organisms most commonly found within the gastrointestinal tract. There may be nonpathogenic Gram-negative bacteria (e.g., *Escherichia coli* or *Enterobacter* spp.) in small numbers in many cases. Large numbers of Gram-negative bacteria are not normal florae for many parrot species, and Gram-positive bacteria, in particular *Streptococcus* spp., can cause disease. When culturing the cloaca, the cotton-tipped swab should be "buried" into the cloaca and rubbed against the cloacal lining. Upon slow removal of the swab, the cloacal mucocutaneous interface with the vent can be everted to examine for papilloma lesions. An important clinical result of the cloacal culture that should be shared with the owner is that for a short time after the examination, the bird may have a blood-tinged stool due to the irritation of the cloacal lining.

Fine Needle Aspirates

The first line of diagnostic testing for an avian patient with a tissue mass is a fine needle aspirate. Advantages of collecting and submitting a fine needle aspirate include minimal trauma to the site being sampled and the ability to obtain the sample without putting the bird under general anesthesia. Unfortunately, the results of fine needle aspirate samples are often nondiagnostic. Although most of these samples will not be helpful in determining a diagnosis, the advantages of no general anesthesia and the atraumatic nature of the sample collection make fine needle aspiration a recommended primary diagnostic technique.

Tissue Biopsies

Because most fine needle aspirate samples are nondiagnostic, full thickness biopsies are the next step in determining the cause of masses or tissue pathology. Biopsy samples that will be forwarded for histopathologic evaluation can be collected

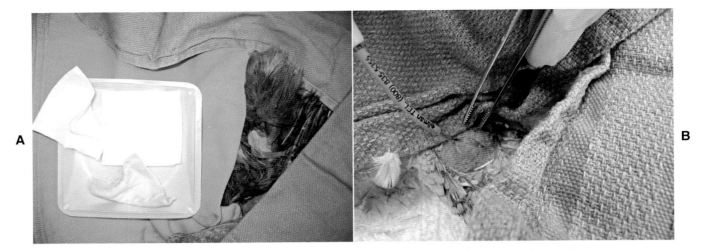

Figure 10-39 Preparation of an avian skin biopsy site is similar to that of other animals **(A)**. Because of the fragile nature of avian skin, care should be taken when collecting the sample **(B)**.

as partial sections or as the result of a total excision or resection of the affected tissue. The samples should be placed in 10% formalin solution for sample preservation.

Skin Biopsies

Avian patients are prepared for skin biopsies in a manner similar to that for other companion animals (Figure 10-39). The biopsy sample should contain a representative area of pathology to give the diagnostic laboratory the best chance of diagnosing the disease problem. Application of tape over the biopsy site and the use of a punch biopsy to take the skin sample through the tape allows the skin sample to maintain shape. The skin sample attached to the tape also aids a pathologist to easily identify the surface epithelial layers. By placing the sample in plastic cassettes within a 10% formalin solution, preservation of the sample is guaranteed for histopathologic examination. Suturing the surgical site with an absorbable suture material using a simple continuous pattern will allow for proper healing and minimal trauma from the patient. An Elizabethan collar can be used on many different species if self-trauma does occur.

Current Disease Testing

Psittacine circovirus 1 and 2 can be tested on avian patients using whole blood and environmental swabs, examining for circovirus DNA. Avian polyoma virus testing involves submission of whole blood and choanal/cloacal swabs. Pacheco's disease evaluation calls for whole blood and a combined choanal/cloacal swab. The recommended *Chlamydophila psittaci* panel includes serum, whole blood, and a combined choanal/cloacal swab. Antibody titers can also be used to determine the presence of Pacheco's disease, West Nile virus, and avian polyoma virus. Veterinarians should always maintain communication and submit samples to a single diagnostic laboratory. This will not only result in consistent results but also allow the veterinarian to develop a professional relationship with the personnel at that particular laboratory when there are questions regarding cases, test results, and/or new testing methods.

CHLAMYDOPHILA PSITTACI TESTING

Using currently available polymerase chain reaction (PCR) diagnostic tests, there is no way of determining whether the *C. psittaci* DNA sequences are coming from viable organisms infecting the bird, environmental contamination, or segments of the organism passing through the gastrointestinal tract or being immunologically neutralized by the immune system. Two new tests have been developed to detect the rRNA operon and /or the *ompA* gene for the family Chlamydiaceae: the TaqMan and multiplex tests.[16] By detecting the rRNA operon this new technology will be able to determine, if in fact, a viable organism is present in the patient. The rRNA operon will only be reproducible in replicating *C. psittaci* organisms. These tests may be available to the veterinarians in the future, and they show the bright promise of this advanced technology in clinical veterinary situations.

Serologic testing for *C. psittaci* in pet avian species has been available for a number of years.[17] These tests have often worked best when the patient was showing clinical signs associated with avian chlamydiosis. The serologic tests that are currently available to the veterinary practitioner in North America are direct complement-fixation, elementary-body agglutination, and ELISA. Serologic testing may continue to be helpful in confirming an overt clinical case of avian chlamydiosis or in determining the efficacy of antibiotic treatment. A multiparametric diagnostic approach, in which serology is part, is considered by some clinicians to be the best avenue to achieve a *C. psittaci* diagnosis. The gold standard for the definitive diagnosis of *C. psittaci* in an avian patient has been culture and isolation of the organism.[18] The problems have also been published on the difficulties of culturing this organism because of its obligate intracellular nature.[18] Using the new technology and acknowledging the previous gold standard, an updated recommendation for definitive diagnosis has been made, especially for live avian patients. The updated recommendation is the isolation of the organism on buffalo green monkey cells in combination with nested PCR or PCR followed by hybridization of the amplicon to a labeled internal probe and serology using ELISA based on antibody detection against recombinant or synthetic *C. psittaci*–specific antigens.[19] At this time, most avian diagnostic laboratories do not offer these state-of-the-art tests. To have the best opportunity for *C. psittaci* culture and isolation on a live patient, serial fecal samples or combined choana/cloaca cultures should be collected for 3 to 5 consecutive days and pooled in transport media supplied by the diagnostic laboratory.[20] For isolating the intracellular bacterium in necropsied patients, liver and spleen samples are preferred. When submitting samples for avian chlamydiosis diagnostic testing, veterinary clinics should follow all laboratory requirements so as to increase the chance for isolation in truly positive cases.

Current published information lists the time between exposure to the *C. psittaci* organism to the onset of illness from 3 days to several weeks, in most cases, but it may appear years after exposure.[21] There are three case definitions as established by the National Association of State Health Veterinarians (NASPHV) and the Centers for Disease Control and Prevention (CDC) in *Compendium of Measures to Control* C. psittaci *Infection among Humans and Pet Birds,* 2006.[21]

Case Definitions of Avian Chlamydiosis[21]

1. **Confirmed case** is defined on the basis of at least one of the following laboratory results: (a) isolation of *C. psittaci* from a clinical specimen, (b) identification of chlamydial antigen by immunofluorescence (fluorescent antibody [FA]) of the bird's tissues, (c) a greater than fourfold change in serologic titer in two specimens from the bird obtained at least 2 weeks apart and assayed simultaneously at the same laboratory, or (d) identification of *C. psittaci* within macrophages in smears stained with Gimenez or Macchiavello stain or sections of the bird's tissues.

2. **Probable case** is defined as compatible illness and at least one of the following laboratory results: (a) a single high serologic titer in one or more specimens obtained after the onset of signs or (b) the presence of *C. psittaci* antigen (identified by ELISA, PCR, or FA) in feces, a cloacal swab, or respiratory or ocular exudates.

3. **Suspected case** is defined as (a) compatible illness that is epidemiologically linked to another case in a human or bird but that is not laboratory confirmed, (b) a subclinical infection with a single high serologic titer or detection of chlamydial antigen, (c) compatible illness with positive results from a nonstandardized test or a new investigational test, or (d) compatible illness that is responsive to appropriate therapy.

These case definitions should help the clinician interpret the diagnostic test results as they relate to a patient that may have signs consistent with avian chlamydiosis or subclinical cases. To aid in diagnosis, a complete history should be taken from the owner, an external physical examination of the patient should be performed, and basic diagnostic tests, including a CBC, should be submitted to a laboratory.[22] If avian chlamydiosis is suspected, treatment should be initiated until the diagnosis is confirmed, a clinical response is achieved, or another diagnosis is determined.

WEST NILE VIRUS TESTING

The recommended diagnostic test to determine if an animal has WNV infection is the IgM capture ELISA.[23] Because WNV-induced antibodies will cross-react with other flaviviruses, including the St. Louis encephalitis virus, there is a need to specify the infectious agent if the IgM capture ELISA is positive. To definitively confirm WNV, a plaque-reduction neutralization test is recommended.[23]

Parasites

It is a rare occurrence, but ectoparasites and/or endoparasites have been diagnosed in companion avian patients that have been hand-raised from "closed aviaries." Direct fecal smears, fecal flotation parasite examinations, and necropsy examinations of the digestive system are all methods by which parasites are diagnosed.[24] Advising owners that only specific antiparasitic drugs are effective against specific parasites will promote owner compliance when using these medications. Reviewing a parasite's life cycle with owners will help prevent recurrence or transmission to unaffected birds in the aviary.

It is very unusual for companion avian species to be diagnosed with parasites. Bird owners often believe their bird has external parasites because of the animal's fastidious grooming habits and normal feather loss. This thought may be perpetuated because the only previous avian parasite exposure bird owners may have had is finding an orphaned songbird on the ground covered with lice. Caged birds are seldom exposed to environments where they would contact the parasites that live on the skin or feathers.[24] Outdoor aviaries or cages may expose their occupants to the rogue wild bird that would transmit mites or, more likely, lice. Raptors, waterfowl, and other gallinaceous birds will commonly present with ectoparasites, at which time the owner should initiate treatment of the bird and environment.

There are two common ectoparasites that infest caged birds: *Sternostoma tracheacolum* and *Knemidokoptes* spp.[25] *Sternostoma tracheacolum* is also known as the tracheal/air sac mite, and it affects mainly canaries and finches. Birds that are diagnosed with the tracheal mite, usually by clinical signs and transtracheal illumination, show signs of respiratory distress and have an audible clicking sound when breathing. Ivermectin (Ivomec, Merck AgVet Division, Rahway, NJ), 0.2 mg/kg PO or SC for 2 to 3 treatments 7 days apart and/or a 5% carbaryl powder lightly dusted on the dorsal feather surface will treat *Sternostoma tracheacolum* infestations in caged birds.[25] Tracheal/air sac mites are often transmitted to young birds from parents during the rearing process. Under stressful conditions the mites overwhelm the patient and clinical signs develop.

Scaly face/scaly leg mites (*Knemidokoptes* spp.) live in the featherless areas around the face and legs. The common names of this mite are derived from the irritation of the surface epithelium that causes a hyperkeratosis of the affected skin and beak. Budgerigars and canaries (tasselfoot) are the most common pet bird species to be diagnosed with scaly face mites.[25] Ivermectin is the treatment of choice for *Knemidokoptes* spp.

Chewing lice of the order Mallophaga and domestic poultry mites *Dermanyssus gallinae* and *Orithonyssus* spp. may infest parrot species that live outdoors in breeding flights.[25] Environmental cleaning is very important in preventing reinfestation of the lice and mites. A 5% carbaryl powder may be used in conjunction with ivermectin therapy to treat infested birds.[25] In raptors and waterfowl, I have been successful in treating feather lice and hippoboscid flies with fipronil (Frontline, Rhone Merieux)—1 pump of spray in axillary area and rub over feathers.[13]

As with external parasites, internal parasites are uncommon in companion and caged birds. All birds should have direct fecal smears and fecal flotation examinations as part of a complete health check. The two most common protozoan parasites diagnosed in avian species are *Giardia* spp. and *Trichomonas gallinae*. Giardiasis is associated with intestinal tract disease, whereas trichomoniasis presents as white plaques or necrotic masses in the mouth and esophagus.[25] The treatment of choice for both *Giardia* spp. and *T. gallinae* is metronidazole (Flagyl, G.D. Searle Co., Chicago, IL) 50 mg/kg q24h PO, 5-10 days.

Atoxoplasma spp., a coccidian parasite, affects primarily canaries, finches, and myna birds. The diagnosis is usually determined during a pathology examination of a dead juvenile bird that dies shortly after appearing depressed.[24] The juvenile birds are exposed by their parents shedding the infective oocysts in the feces. Treatment is difficult; therefore, it is recommended that disease-free birds be used for breeding. Trimethoprim/sulfadiazine (Roche Pharmaceuticals, Nutley, NJ) 100 mg/kg PO twice daily is the recommended treatment for avian coccidian parasitic diseases. As it may be difficult to treat a large group of caged birds individually, ¼ to ½ tsp sulfachlorpyridazine (Vetasulid, Solvay) per liter of drinking water for 5 to 10 days may be used.

Sarcocystis falcatula is the other coccidian parasite commonly diagnosed in companion avian species.[25] This parasite usually is found in aviary birds housed outdoors in breeding flights. The life cycle of *S. falcatula* involves the opossum (*Didelphis virginiana*) as the definitive host of the organism and cockroaches to transfer infectious sporulated oocysts or sporocysts to psittacine species (intermediate host).[25] As with *Atoxoplasma* spp., *S. falcatula* is usually diagnosed during a pathologic examination of a dead bird.[25] The extensive life cycle requirements of the parasite make environmental management extremely important if the owner wants to prevent exposure and infections within an aviary.[25]

Hemoproteus spp., *Plasmodium* spp., and *Leukocytozoon* spp. are parasites that may be found in the red blood cells of wild-caught psittacine species, raptors, doves, and pigeons.[25] These parasites are transmitted through the bite of infected arthropods. Unless there is an overwhelming infestation of these parasites, treatment is not recommended.

Nematodes, as with most of the parasites that affect avian species, commonly infect birds that live in outdoor environments. Ascarids have a direct life cycle, in which simply ingesting eggs can infect a bird, whereas *Capillaria* spp. and *Syngamus trachea* need an intermediate host.[25] Ascarids and *Capillaria* spp. live in the intestinal tract, whereas *S. trachea* is found in the oral cavity and esophagus.[25] Birds infested with intestinal parasites will be depressed and emaciated. In most cases nematode eggs are shed in the feces and can be observed in a fecal flotation exam. It is important to treat the bird and, if possible, the environment.

Although parasites are not commonly diagnosed in companion avian species, veterinarians that treat birds need to be familiar with diagnosis and treatment. Aviary birds are exposed through vermin, insects, and wild birds. Birds that live in pens outside are naturally exposed through direct contact and intermediate hosts. Successful resolution of a case includes not only treating the individual bird but also reducing future exposure to the parasite, parasite eggs, or intermediate host.

Diagnostic Imaging

Veterinary medicine has made advances in diagnostic imaging capabilities that parallel human medicine. Imaging techniques available to veterinarians include radiography, contrast radiography, ultrasonography, endoscopy, computed tomography, and magnetic resonance imaging. All of these techniques have and can be used on psittacine species. For the safety of the avian patient and veterinary staff and quality of images, isoflurane or sevoflurane general anesthesia is recommended.

A critical assessment of the patient should be made before the animal is placed under general anesthesia for radiographic evaluation. Even if the bird appears to be an excellent candidate for general anesthesia, the owner(s) must be informed on the dangers of general anesthesia and the rare but real chance the patient may die. Precautions for emergency therapy are necessary for any avian hospital administering general anesthesia. The first step in emergency preparations is putting together a "crash kit." Recommended items to include in a crash kit are therapeutic agents to revive a patient that is not breathing or has a slow or nonexistent heart beat, syringes, needles, tracheal tubes, tape, and an ambu bag (bag valve mask). If the bird presents in a condition that is not conducive for general anesthesia, it may be amenable for quick images that may be diagnostic (e.g., heavy metal objects or a foreign body within the gastrointestinal system). All birds should be intubated when placed under general anesthesia for radiographs. Birds are induced via a facemask and then intubated and maintained on isoflurane or sevoflurane anesthesia. If images of the skull are desired, an air sac tube may be placed in the caudal thoracic air sac after the patient is induced. To maintain an avian patient in the proper plane of anesthesia with administration of the anesthetic agent through an air sac tube, oxygen flow and percent of anesthetic agent should be higher than used in routine tracheal intubation.

To obtain the best radiographic images, high-definition screen film combinations are recommended.[26] Rare-earth screens have a higher intensifying capacity without the loss of detail found in calcium tungstate screens. The higher intensifying capacity is generally needed given the short exposure times used on pet bird species. The best combination of screen and film for avian practice at this time is a rare-earth screen and film emulsified on one side.[26] Rare-earth screens with greater intensifying capabilities (sensitivity of 200) are needed for marginal quality machines. The small size of avian patients require short exposure times (0.015-0.05 seconds) using at least a 200-300 mA machine.[26] To obtain the highest degree of contrast, 10 to 20 kV is optimal.[26] Inflating the air sacs during radiographic exposure will result in increased contrast of internal organs. For smaller avian patients, less than 100 grams, and for specific focal areas of interest in larger birds (e.g., toes), dental radiographic units using high-detail dental film will provide greater detail, in most cases, than will larger radiographic views.

As mentioned previously, general anesthesia is recommended for most avian patients being radiographed or undergoing a diagnostic imaging examination. Before induction, the radiographic team needs to designate an anesthetist, have the endotracheal tube and tape prepped for placement, have the positioning board ready and the emergency crash kit available. The anesthetist must understand his or her position, be able to focus on the job, and be able to relay vital information to the radiographic team.

For positioning the patient, a Plexiglas® restraint board is recommended. The restraint board allows for consistent positioning between patients and when taking serial radiographs of the same patient. The head/neck restraint allows the patient to be stretched for better positioning. The standard avian radiographic views are ventrodorsal and lateral. The legs are stretched down and the wings stretched out, with all extremities taped to the board on the ventral dorsal view. When the bird is positioned in lateral recumbency, the wings are placed over the dorsum and taped, the bottom leg is stretched cranially, and the top leg is stretched caudally and taped to the board. Other positions can be achieved depending on the case. For radiographic gastrointestinal contrast studies, iohexol is the contrast material of choice although barium sulfate has been used successfully in the past. The main benefit of iohexol over barium sulfate is that iohexol has been proven to cause less tissue damage to the lungs if aspirated.[27] Iodine-based agents have been used when IV contrast material has been needed for urography or computed tomography studies.

Ultrasonography is a relatively recent advance in avian diagnostic imaging techniques. The recommended transducer for avian patients is a sector scanner with a frequency of 7.5 MHz.[26] General anesthesia is not as important for patients undergoing a sonographic examination, but for sensitive heart examinations it may be beneficial when viewing those images. Avian patients should be fasted for at least 3 hours, and birds of prey for 1 or 2 days, before undergoing a sonographic examination.[26] Because of the avian air sac system, there are only a few windows into the body that are effective in obtaining diagnos-

tic ultrasound image results. Caudal to the keel, with the bird in dorsal recumbency, the transducer can be directed in a cranial dorsal direction to obtain images of the liver and heart. Directing the transducer dorsally in the mid to caudal coelomic cavity will highlight the intestinal and urogenital tracts.

One of the more common imaging techniques used on avian patients is endoscopy. Rigid endoscopes having a diameter of 1.9 to 2.7 mm are commonly used for minimally invasive coelomic, respiratory, and cloacal imaging. As with any imaging technique, there is a learning curve, and endoscopy is no exception. Knowledge of the avian anatomy is imperative when viewing images of the coelomic cavity through the endoscope or on a video monitor. Required instrumentation for endoscopic imaging includes the scope, biopsy port cannula, blunt-tipped trocar, biopsy forceps, and scissors. To perform this procedure, it is extremely useful to have aspiration capabilities and an endoscopic camera with a video monitor. Common sites of entry into the coelomic cavity with an endoscope are the caudal air sac, choanal slit, upper infraorbital sinus, trachea, and cloaca. Other areas of the bird may be accessed, but the aforementioned sites are the most commonly viewed. By accessing the caudal thoracic air sac, the entire coelomic cavity may be viewed. Through this portal, the lungs, heart, liver, kidney, proventriculus, spleen, kidneys, gonads, urogenital tract, and intestinal tract can be assessed. If any suspicious pathologic condition is encountered, a biopsy sample may be taken of that organ or tissue. Through the choanal slit, viewing the nasal bifurcation, granulomas may be observed. When viewing the choana with the endoscope, aspiration capabilities are warranted. Often there is a buildup of mucoid nasal discharge in and around the infraorbital sinus and extending down through the choanal slit. This nasal discharge should be removed to obtain an unobstructed view of the anatomy in question. An air sac breathing tube is required for the endoscopic examination of the trachea. The most common disease condition identified through examination of the trachea is granuloma formation caused by aspergillosis. Aspiration and culture of the granuloma will often provide a definitive diagnosis of the disease for the veterinarian. To view the cloacal mucosa, sterile saline is needed to fill this anatomic structure during the examination. Nonspecific cloacal prolapses are a common reason cloacoscopy is done in an avian patient. Biopsies of the cloaca mucosa may provide an answer for the cloacal prolapse presentation. To view the upper infraorbital sinus, an incision is made in the depression found between the medial canthus and nare. The endoscope is then placed through this incision and the cranial aspect of the infraorbital sinus is viewed. Granulomas and tissue masses may be seen from this location and biopsy samples taken of lesions observed.

Computed tomography (CT) was first introduced in 1972. Computed tomography images are radiography-based thin cross-sectional scans that remove the complications of superimposed structures. Transverse and longitudinal scans can be performed on a patient in 1- to 5-mm slice thickness or a distance recommended by the clinician. With the updated computer programs, three-dimensional models can be generated from most CT studies. One advantage of CT is that it can produce images of individual anatomic structures within a serial study. A complete transverse scan of an avian patient can take place within 15 minutes. Birds should be under general anesthesia for CT scans, and plans for table movement during the scan must be made before the scan is initiated. To highlight tissue masses, IV iodine-based contrast material is often used as a comparison to a survey scan. One of the major disadvantages of CT technology is cost. A complete avian scan may cost between $350 and $500.

Another expensive but very useful image technology is magnetic resonance imaging (MRI). This technique uses a superconducting magnet as part of its imaging technology. MRI is more complicated to use for avian patients because of the superconducting magnet. No metal that would be affected by magnetic forces can be in the room during the scan. Unless nonconductive material is used in the construction of the anesthesia machine, injectable general anesthetic agents are required. Any monitoring equipment must also be compatible with the super conducting magnet, thereby making nonmagnetic equipment extremely expensive to purchase. As with CT scans, MRI scans are relatively expensive when compared to the other available diagnostic techniques currently available.

■ COMMON DISEASE PRESENTATIONS

Respiratory conditions are the most common disease presentations of companion avian species treated at veterinary hospitals. There are many reasons for this repeated finding, but the most likely reason is that avian species possess an efficient and complex respiratory system. African grey parrots are one of the most common companion avian species diagnosed with *Aspergillus* spp. respiratory infections. For a veterinarian to properly assess, diagnose, and treat avian respiratory disease, he or she must understand the basic upper and lower respiratory anatomy of birds.

Upper Respiratory Anatomy

The nares are located within the cere, either surrounded or covered by feathers. There are opercular bones within the nasal opening, which is a normal anatomic structure. The nares should be clear and symmetric. The right and left infraorbital sinuses of parrot species allow air exchange, whereas the infraorbital sinuses of passerine species are separated by the nasal septum. Nasal conchae project from the lateral wall of the nasal cavity. There are eight diverticula originating from the single infraorbital sinus, which extends from the beak to the distal cervical area, culminating in the cervicocephalic air sac. There is no connection between the infraorbital sinus and lower respiratory air sac system. The upper respiratory system terminates at the paired choanae, with the air exiting the choanal slit. Normal appearance of the choanal slit includes epithelial projections (papillae) pointing toward the center of the opening.

Lower Respiratory Anatomy

When the beak is closed, the rima glottis fits against the choanal opening, allowing conditioned air to flow into the lower respiratory system. The rima glottis is not covered by epiglottic cartilage and can be visualized easily by pulling the tongue cranially and observing the tracheal opening at the base of the tongue. The trachea, which includes the syrinx (voice box), is made up of complete, signet-shaped rings. The syrinx, located at the tracheal bifurcation, is composed of modified tracheal cartilage. The trachea bifurcates into the paired primary bronchi leading to the lungs. Avian lungs have a dorsal position in the thoracic cavity and are fixed and firmly attached to the vertebral column and ribs. Lung structures include primary, secondary, and tertiary bronchi that lead to the atria and infundibula of the air capillaries where gas exchange occurs. The air sacs are connected to the lungs and incorporate most of the coelomic cavity not occupied by major internal organs. The air sac space allows for increased air capacity within the bird and extends into the pneumatized bones.

Respiratory Physical Exam

Taking a good history will often aid in developing a differential diagnosis list for the respiratory condition affecting the avian patient. Environment, diet, past and current abnormal clinical signs the owner may have noticed, and review of the body systems are important considerations when examining a bird with a respiratory condition.

An external physical examination has its limitations. The nares, infraorbital sinus, and oral-respiratory interface, can be quickly assessed, over and above the bird's external appearance and demeanor. A minimum database should include weight (on a digital gram scale), Gram stain/cytology, culture, and CBC. Other tests, if needed, to definitively diagnose a respiratory disease include plasma chemistry panel, bacterial/fungal/viral testing, radiographs, ultrasound scan, endoscopic examination, and ECG.

Specific Respiratory Diagnostic Techniques

Radiographs should be taken when the bird is under general anesthesia. Two views are required to properly assess the patient's condition. An avian restraint board will allow for reproducible positioning of the patient for ventrodorsal and lateral views.

Sinus aspiration, of the right and left infraorbital sinus, and tracheal lavage are needed to obtain samples for cytology and/or culture when clinical signs dictate the use of these testing methods.

Common Disease Presentations of Aspergillosis in African Grey Parrots

Upper respiratory aspergillosis usually presents as nasal granulomas that grow to deform the nasal anatomy. These fungal granulomas must be debrided and the underlying tissue cultured in order to obtain a definitive diagnosis.

Lower respiratory aspergillosis is seen more often than upper respiratory fungal granulomas. Unfortunately, lower respiratory aspergillosis is more difficult to diagnose than the overt nasal granuloma. The bird infected with aspergillosis involving the lungs and air sacs may be depressed and present with mild dyspnea. A CBC, plasma chemistry panel, and radiographs are the basic diagnostic protocol for African Grey parrots presenting with the clinical signs described above. Many times the CBC will show a severe, chronic inflammatory leukogram. The heterophil count can range as high as 70,000 to 80,000 cells/ml. Radiographic evidence can range from cloudy air sacs and obvious radiopaque granulomas to no abnormalities, even in the most severe cases. At this time the best way to definitely diagnose aspergillosis in an African grey parrot is via coelomic endoscopy. Serologic antigen and antibody testing has not been perfected to the point of offering reliable results for antemortem diagnosis.

TREATMENT

Once the diagnosis is confirmed or a differential diagnosis list is formulated, treatment can begin. The proper treatment may be aided by specific methods that are effective in treating the avian respiratory system.

SYSTEMIC THERAPY

Itraconazole 5-10 mg/kg. Comment: Caution should be used when contemplating the use of this drug in African grey parrots, as they are extremely sensitive to itraconazole and may become anorexic and depressed when treated with this drug. Alternative treatments should be considered.

Terbinafine 5-15 mg/kg. Comment: This is the systemic antifungal drug of choice for African grey parrots.

SINUS FLUSH

3.5 mg neomycin, 124.5 mg trypsin, 10 mg amphotericin B—all added to 30 ml of a water-soluble base. Comment: Add 0.1-0.4 ml of the base solution to 10-20 ml of saline for direct flushing through the nares once daily. Flush until there is an easy uniform flow out of the choana from both sides and with equal resistance.

NEBULIZATION

Equipment: nebulizer compressor (Sportneb, model 3050, Medical Industries America, Adel, IA), infant nebulizer, nebulizing chamber.

Nebulize for about 15 minutes twice daily, antimicrobial agent, saline, and 3-5 drops acetylcysteine (Mucomyst).

Amphotericin B: 7 mg/ml saline

Clotrimazole: 1% × 30-60 min

Chlamydophila psittaci

Chlamydophila psittaci, the name veterinarians commonly call the parrot fever organism, is one of the most common bacterial diseases that infect pet birds. This intracellular bacterium has been the subject of much research regarding avian species as well as humans and other animal groups. The purpose of this research is not only to improve diagnostic capabilities and animal health, but also to protect humans from becoming infected. *C. psittaci* is a zoonotic disease that can cause death in humans who are infected. The advent of antibiotics and development of modern diagnostic techniques have lessened the pathogenic impact of *C. psittaci* but have not removed much of the mystery surrounding its diagnosis and treatment in animals, especially avian species. Molecular biology has enabled scientists to unravel some of the mysteries, with many of these findings annually contributing to the scientific knowledge base. Recent scientific studies have led to new findings on classification and diagnostic testing of the *C. psittaci* organism. A protocol to control *C. psittaci* infection among humans and pet birds has recently been published by the Centers for Disease Control and Prevention.[21]

The name change of a diagnostic test parameter, organism, or disease is often wrought with initial disdain and a reluctance of usage. With this preface, *Chlamydia psittaci* has been reclassified as *Chlamydophila psittaci.*[28] The family Chlamydiaceae has been divided into two genera: *Chlamydia* (*Chlamydia trachomatis, Chlamydia muridarum,* and *Chlamydia suis*) and *Chlamydophila* (*Chlamydophila pneumoniae, Chlamydophila pecorum,* and *Chlamydophila psittaci*).[28] The type species for the *Chlamydia* genus is *Chlamydia trachomatis,* whereas *Chlamydophila psittaci* is the type species for the *Chlamydophila* genus.[28]

The new classification of *C. psittaci* allows for better differentiation from other, similar organisms. The *Chlamydophila* spp. are identified through ribosomal signature sequences; they do not produce detectable quantities of glycogen; they are slightly larger than the *Chlamydia* genome and contain a single ribosomal operon; and they have varying morphology and a varying resistance to sulfadiazine.[28,29] To the veterinary clinician treating a bird infected with avian chlamydiosis, the new classification may seem esoteric. But it is these new discoveries leading to this reclassification that will allow for a better understanding of *Chlamydia* spp. and *Chlamydophila* spp. Specifically, and most importantly for veterinary practitioners, *C. psittaci* diagnostic tests, treatments, and vaccines will be developed from the material generated from the studies used to further identify these organisms.

The molecular discoveries that have led to reclassification of the *C. psittaci* organism have also led to the development of new diagnostic tests. There have been a number of *C. psittaci* diagnostic tests advertised that utilize DNA amplification techniques, but unfortunately, the new tests have not given the veterinary community one highly sensitive and specific product. Polymerase chain reaction (PCR) molecular diagnostic techniques are based on the detection of target DNA sequences, specifically of the pathogen in question.[30] It must be remembered that with current commercially available diagnostic techniques, the target DNA sequences cannot determine if the material is from a viable organism.[30] Moreover, because of the sensitivity and specificity of molecular testing, false positives from environmental contamination, contamination by sample-to-sample DNA carryover, or contamination by DNA carryover from previous amplifications of the same target may occur.[21]

Even with the disadvantages listed above, detection of *C. psittaci* genes by amplified and nonamplified nucleic acid–based detection methods is still a viable method for screening for this disease. Newer, better molecular testing methods are being discovered yearly, thereby aiding the practicing veterinarian. PCR sample collections are easy and noninvasive and have simple transport and storage requirements.[19] Other listed advantages of PCR testing include the minimal sampling, ease of testing large bird populations, rapid results, and high sensitivity and specifity.[19] Current technology allows for further identification of PCR testing either to specifically identify the species or to confirm a positive test. A nested PCR test, which is a second, more specific PCR test on a smaller gene base taken from the original material, is one way of improving molecular diagnostic test results. The other method to help improve routine PCR test results is hybridization of the amplicon to a labeled internal probe specific for the *C. psittaci* organism.

Medicated protocols that have been used successfully in treating avian chlamydiosis depend on a number of factors, including owner administration of the antibiotic for 45 days and owner compliance with bringing the bird in for weekly injections, giving full dosage of the medication, and reducing the amount of calcium chelation of doxycycline by restricting calcium supplementation at the time of treatment.[20] Owner compliance is often enhanced by the knowledge that avian chlamydiosis is a zoonotic disease. Whether the owner is treating the bird at home with medicated pellets or giving weekly Vibravenous injections, the treatment should be under the direction of, and supervised before, during, and after treatment by, a veterinarian.

There are recommendations of dosing 400 mg doxycycline hyclate (50 and 100 mg capsules, Pfizer Inc., New York, NY) per liter of drinking water for cockatiels and 400 to 600 mg doxycycline hyclate per liter of drinking water for parrots and macaws.[21] There have been limited pharmacologic studies investigating doxycycline hyclate–impregnated water therapy, but drug toxicity can occur in birds on this treatment program. Clinical conditions associated with toxicity include depression, inactivity, anorexia, biliverdin-stained urine, and altered liver enzymes.[21] It is essential that veterinarians monitor birds placed on this treatment regimen for possible toxic side effects. If any signs of toxicity occur, treatment should be discontinued immediately and another treatment protocol initiated.

Medicated pellets containing 1% chlortetracycline are commercially available and are one of the easiest, least stressful ways to medicate one or more birds (Box 10-5). The pellets come in different sizes to correspond to species size variations. It is

---

BOX 10-5   Sources of Medicated Pellets

1. Avi-Sci Inc., 4477 South Williams Rd., St. Johns, MI 48879; 800-942-3438; Fax 989-224-9227.
2. Pretty Bird International, Inc., 5810 Stacy Trail, P.O. Box 177, Stacy, MN 55079; 800-356-5020.
3. Rolf C. Hagen (Tropican®), P.O. Box 9107, Mansfield, MA 02048; 800-225-2700; 888-BY-HAGEN.
4. Roudybush, P.O. Box 908, Templeton, CA 93456; 800-326-1726.
5. Ziegler Brothers, Inc., P.O. Box 95, Gardners, PA 17324-0095; 800-841-6800.

---

advantageous for birds to eat pellets before treatment because there is usually no transition between the regular food and the medicated diet. Unfortunately, birds unfamiliar with a pelleted diet may not make the transition and may have to be treated orally (PO) or with intramuscular (IM) injections. As with any treatment protocol, birds on a medicated pellet diet need to be weighed on a weekly basis to determine if they are eating; treatment progress also should be monitored.

Oral doxycycline treatment is advantageous because a known amount of the antibiotic is applied directly into the body. The disadvantages are potential gastrointestinal upset and direct calcium chelation of the antibiotic by ingested foodstuffs. Administering the oral doxycycline before the bird eats may help reduce regurgitation and chelation of the antibiotic. If a bird is treated with oral doxycycline and the crop is full of food, this scenario results in reduced efficacy of the drug and a loss of available dietary calcium. The loss of dietary calcium through chelation is extremely problematic in young, fast-growing birds. Dosage recommendations for doxycycline monohydrate or doxycycline calcium syrup (Pfizer Inc., New York, NY) are listed in Table 10-2.[21]

Intramuscular and IV injections offer treatment options for the critically ill patient and birds that cannot be treated by the previously described methods. The IV doxycycline hyclate product (Pfizer Inc., New York, NY), 25-50 mg/kg, should be administered only once or twice during the initial critical presentation, after which the patient should be switched to the PO or IM formulation.[18] The long-acting parenteral doxycycline formulation (Vibravenos®, Pfizer Laboratories, London, UK) dosage recommendation is 75 to 100 mg/kg given IM every 5 to 7 days for the first 4 weeks, then every 5 days for the remainder of the 45-day treatment period.[13]

Feather Loss

Feather loss through self-induced trauma is one of the most difficult diagnoses to make. There are many factors that have been identified as causing birds to pluck feathers that may eventually lead to skin mutilation. The list of possible causes of pathologic feather plucking includes, parasitism (internal/external), hypersensitivity, external neoplasia, internal pain/granuloma, feather folliculitis, bacterial/fungal dermatitis, and environmental irritants (e.g., cigarette smoke, zinc toxicosis).

TABLE 10-2	Psittacine Doxycycline Dosage Recommendations	
Bird	**Frequency**	**Dose**
Cockatiels, Senegal parrots, blue-fronted and orange-winged Amazon parrots	SID	40-50 mg/kg
African Grey parrots, Goffin's cockatoos, blue and gold macaws, and green-winged macaws	SID	25 mg/kg
Cockatoos and macaws	SID	25-30 mg/kg (starting dose)
Other psittacines	SID	25-50 mg/kg

From Compendium of measures to control *Chlamydophila psittaci* infection among humans (psittacosis) and pet birds (avian chlamydiosis), 2006, http://www.nasphv.org/Documents/Psittacosis.pdf, July 12, 2006.
SID, once a day.

NORMAL PREENING, MOLTING

The first condition a veterinarian must consider when a case presents for abnormal feather loss is whether the feather loss is normal. Not only must a veterinarian consider if the feather loss is normal but also if the bird is exhibiting normal preening behavior. Birds are fastidious with their grooming habits. The body is covered with feathers, and the feather architecture requires normal preening by the birds to align the feather barbs for normal positioning on the body. During the process of preening, molting feathers are naturally removed, often giving the owners the impression that the bird is pulling out the feathers. This is a normal process and one that takes place on an almost daily basis. Molting usually takes place over weeks or months in order to maintain a full feather coat and the ability to fly. Some avian species (e.g., waterfowl) that migrate south for the winter will molt their flight feathers all at once, rendering them flightless for a short period. Pet avian species do not molt all of their flight feathers at one time. They will molt many of their feathers before the winter months as they acclimatize to the cooler weather and then again in the spring as the days grow warmer. Owners need to be aware of this periodic molting because there will be more feathers in and around the cage during the fall and spring months. Parrots will also molt their primary and secondary flight feathers in a symmetric pattern. If one notes developing feathers on one wing when performing a feather trim, then there probably will be a similar pattern of new development on the contralateral wing. Normal molting does not equate to pathologic feather picking or evidence of an external parasite problem. Normal molting does not leave the bird with featherless areas on the body. When there is an above-average amount of feather loss that is normal, there will be evidence of new feather growth in the form of "pin" feathers. Pin feathers are developing feathers that have not opened to display the barbs; they appear as small pointed shafts interspersed within the feather coat. Owners need to be educated on the normal preening behavior of their pet bird and normal feather loss and development.

Arguably the most difficult avian cases to diagnose are those that involve pathologic feather picking. With a long list of differential diagnoses, it is very important to determine the health status of the presenting patient. If the feather plucking condition is determined to be a treatable disease, then a specific therapeutic regime should be prescribed. A recommended workup for this presentation includes a complete history (Figure 10-40) and external physical examination, CBC, plasma chemistry panel, fecal examination, parasite examination (flotation and direct), cloaca and choana cultures, radiographs, and biopsies (where indicated). Veterinarians must understand that cases where feather loss is involved take an inordinate amount of time when compared to other presenting complaints. Because there will be more time involved with the initial visit, veterinarians must consider charging more for this workup than for a routine complaint. One of the most important considerations during the primary workup is the patient history. There are a number of differential diagnoses for generalized feather loss, and a standardized patient history form will allow veterinarians to take a complete history in a methodic manner, so as not to miss evidence that may lead to a diagnosis.

Veterinarians can make a quick determination if the feather loss is generalized or self-induced. If the feather loss is self-induced, feather loss will occur at body areas where the bird can reach. Feather loss to areas such as the head usually denotes a generalized disease process or cagemate trauma. Differential diagnoses for generalized feather loss include nutritional, infectious, and hormonal diseases.

Specific disease conditions that are diagnosed can be treated by therapeutic or surgical means to reduce the trauma a bird inflicts upon itself by pulling out feathers or traumatizing the underlying epithelium. Trying to find a disease cause of feather picking is almost as difficult as identifying a behavioral source. The difficulty in determining a definitive disease diagnosis for feather plucking reinforces the need to follow a history protocol, as defined earlier, and a routine diagnostic plan for a feather loss presentation.

Focal areas of feather loss are often associated with an underlying tissue mass or granuloma. The underlying mass can usually be detected through palpation of the exposed skin surface. Inspissated abscesses, granulomas, lipomas, xanthomas and squamous cell carcinomas are common diagnoses of focal feather loss in pet avian species. To diagnose the cause of the mass, a fine needle aspirate is recommended as the first step in identification, followed by an excisional biopsy if necessary. In most cases once the underlying irritant is removed, the patient stops feather picking.

PARASITES

Parasite-induced feather picking is a more complex diagnosis than most veterinary textbooks claim. The underlying basis for internal parasite-induced feather picking is that pain, stress, and general condition of the bird result in the coping mechanism of feather picking. Internal parasites that have been implicated as possible causes of self-induced feather loss include tapeworms, giardiasis, and roundworms. If any of these para-

Avian Dermatologic Patient History Form

1. Where and when did you get your bird?
2. How old is your bird now?
3. How was the bird housed before you acquired it?
4. How is the bird housed now?
   a. Isolated?
   b. In a group?
   c. In a breeding situation?
   d. Household?
   e. Aviary?
5. Describe the bird's cage/enclosure.
6. How often do you handle your bird?
7. What do you feed your bird?
8. Any treats or table scraps offered?
9. Any vitamins or minerals offered?
10. How often do you provide fresh water for your bird?
11. How often do you clean and disinfect the cage?
    a. Food/water dishes?
12. What products do you use ?
13. Have you owned or kept birds before?
14. Do you have any other birds now?
15. Do you have any other pets?
16. In what room in the house do you keep your bird?
17. Has the bird been kept in the same area or moved around?
18. Does your bird have exposure to the outdoors?
19. Has the bird been exposed to other birds?
    a. Wild birds?
    b. Neighbor's birds?
    c. Birds at shows/fairs?
20. When did your bird last molt?
21. What is the sex of your bird and how was it determined?
22. Has your bird ever exhibited breeding behavior?
23. Does your bird fly around the house or in a flight cage?
24. Has your bird ever been in a breeding situation?
    a. What was the result?
25. When does your bird vocalize the most?
26. When did you first notice your bird picking its feathers?
27. What part of the body was first affected?
28. How often does the bird pick?
    a. Do you ever see the bird pick its feathers?
29. Has the pattern of picking changed over time?
30. Has the severity of picking changed over time?
31. Has your bird been seen by another veterinarian for this problem?
32. When does the bird pick the most?
    a. The least?
33. Have any changes occurred in your life resulting in a change in your bird's routine?
    a. Have you recently moved?
    b. Have the number of people in the household changed?
    c. Have your work hours changed?
    d. Have you changed the amount of time you spend with your bird?
34. Do you or any household members smoke?

Figure 10-40 Avian Dermatologic History Form. (Adapted from Lightfoot T: Feather plucking: causes and cures, *Proc Annu Mardi Gras Avicul Conf* 11:3-8, 2000.)

sites are identified during a physical examination, the patient should be treated. It is debatable if the parasite infestation is in fact the cause of the feather picking or some other measure that is modified during the visit. If nothing else, the bird will be in better health once treated properly for the identified internal parasites. External parasites can cause feather destruction, feather loss, and/or excessive preening. *Knemidokoptes* spp., also known as the scaly leg and face mite, is commonly found in budgerigars. Feather loss around the beak and eyes is evident when birds present with this parasite. Hyperkeratosis of the facial skin, beak, and legs is a result of the dermal irritation to the mite infestation. *Dermanyssid* and *Macronyssid* mites are extremely irritating and are often observed as red or black dots moving over the feathers and skin of an agitated avian patient. *Dermanyssid* and *Macronyssid* mites are rarely found on pet bird patients.

CHRONIC HEAVY METAL TOXICOSIS

Zinc toxicity has been implicated as a cause of pathogenic feather plucking in pet birds. There is little scientific support of this assertion, but treatment of birds diagnosed with elevated zinc levels has appeared to stop the feather plucking problem. Many pet avian species are maintained in galvanized wire caging, which contains high quantities of zinc. Also, birds may chew and swallow toy parts and electronic parts or come in contact with a number of other products that contain zinc. Although zinc is a micronutrient with physiologic benefits, too much of this element can cause disease problems; whether feather picking is one of the disease conditions of zinc toxicosis still has to be scientifically determined. If identified, zinc toxicosis should be treated; once treated, the bird may stop the feather trauma.

ALLERGIES

Most animal species have been found to have allergic reactions to environmental or ingested substances. Pathologic evidence suggests that birds suffer from similar conditions. Although the immune system is slightly different in avian species than in mammals, initial skin testing studies also suggest that negative and positive controls for evaluating skin testing are possible. Unfortunately, the ability to read these tests is not practical for the veterinarian. If biopsy sample results suggest a hypersensitivity cause to the feather/skin trauma, then a review of the environment, diet, and treatment should be initiated.

FOLLICULITIS/DERMATITIS

Many fungal and bacterial organisms or a combination of both can cause underlying feather follicle and skin irritation. The results of this irritation can lead to feather picking. Culture and slide cytologic evaluation of abnormal skin and biopsies will help establish a definitive diagnosis for treatment.

ENDOCRINE SYSTEM

There has been an underlying movement to place hypothyroidism in the category of generalized feather loss. Unfortunately, until recently routine testing measures have been unavailable to the veterinarian or a lack of interpretive information for results received. Research has advanced to the point of a better understanding of avian thyroid levels and interpretation of test results, which in turn helps the veterinarian establish a viable treatment program for feather-picking birds suspected of endocrine abnormalities.

LIVER DISEASE

Hepatic disease that may result in circulating toxins has been identified as a cause of feather plucking.[32] Liver enzyme levels, liver function tests (e.g., bile acids), biopsies, and radiographs may help determine the health of a patient's liver. Evaluation for evidence of hepatic disease may help identify the cause of feather picking.

PSYCHOLOGIC

Self-induced feather loss may be initiated by a medical disease problem and be resolved when that primary cause is removed or treated. Unfortunately, many times even after the initiating cause of feather picking has been removed, the bird will continue to pull out feathers. It is the behavioral habit of pulling the feathers out that is the most difficult condition to stop once a diagnosis has been made. As with any behavior modification, self-induced feather picking/trauma is very difficult to treat, and the owner must continue to stay the course. Diet, surrounding environment, cage position, other birds surrounding the cage, and new family members are reasons for initiation or aggravating feather picking problems. There are components that can be manipulated by the owner for possible reduction or resolution of the condition. New therapeutic regimes and behavior modification techniques are being described or advanced as treatments for this multifactorial disease presentation. If the cause of the feather picking problems is determined to be psychologic in origin, many avian behaviorists believe that self-induced feather loss is misplaced behavior and a response to stress.[33]

TREATMENTS FOR THE FEATHER PICKING BIRD

A rapid effective treatment is the Elizabethan (E) collar. The use of an E collar is not recommended unless the bird is traumatizing the skin or there are epithelial injuries. The E-collar is a temporary treatment that, when removed, often does not result in modification of the problem. Box 10-6 lists several recommended behavioral modification medications.

■ REPRODUCTIVE DISORDERS

Most avian owners are separated into one of two types: companion bird owners with no interest in reproducing parrot species and owners breeding psittacine species for money or as a hobby. Bird reproduction issues and problems will affect both types of bird owners. It is important for veterinarians to understand some of the basic factors involved in companion bird reproductive disorders that may have psychologic and/or physical manifestations. Not laying eggs or laying infertile eggs is considered a reproductive disorder. The seeming inability of

---

BOX 10-6   Behavioral Modification Medication

1. Nortriptyline (Pamelor, Sandoz)
   2 mg/120 ml drinking water
2. Amitriptyline (Elavil, Stuart)
   1-2 mg/kg PO q12-24h
3. Paroxetine (Paxil, SmithKline Beecham)
   1-2 mg/kg q24h
4. Haloperidol (Haldol, McNeil)
   Antipsychotic medication, numerous adverse side
   effects, toxic to hyacinth macaws and cockatoos
   0.15-0.20 mg/kg PO q12h—Amazon parrots, other
   psittacine species <1 kg
   0.10-0.15 mg/kg PO q12h—Amazon parrots, other
   psittacine species >1 kg
   0.4 mg/kg PO q24h—psittacine species/self-mutilation,
   feather picking
   6.4 mg/L drinking water × 7 months—African grey
   parrots/feather picking
   1.2 mg/kg IM every 21 days—most psittacine species/
   feather picking

Adapted from Carpenter JW: *Exotic Animal Formulary,* ed 3, St Louis, 2005, WB Saunders; Speer B: Clinical reproductive avian medicine, *in* Foundations in Avian Medicine, *Proc Annu Conf Assoc Avian Vet,* pp 23-33, 1995.

---

many parrots to produce fertile eggs may be caused by nutritional, management, or physical disease problems. A veterinarian is most useful in reproductive cases when all aspects of the management are addressed.

Good management procedures start with owners knowing their birds through meticulous record keeping. Only through production records do owners know for sure how many eggs have been laid and hatched by a particular pair of birds. It has been my experience that there is more time between clutches than most owners realize. Following a good flock health program and an all in/all out aviary traffic flow will reduce disease introduction into an aviary, thereby protecting an investment. Production managers can use records to evaluate breeding pairs and to meet short-term goals. If a bird is not performing, it can be sold or moved into a flight cage with another mate. It must be remembered that most owners arrange the marriages of pet birds and that arranged marriages do not always result in offspring. There are testimonial accounts of a bird escaping from one flight and going three enclosures away, kicking out the bird of that gender, and having eggs in a few weeks, when for years there were no eggs between the split pairs. Birds, for the most part, will not breed if they do not feel that there is enough food to raise the babies. The hens need enough calcium and nutrients to withstand the stresses of ovulation and egg production. Birds that are not reproducing need to be replaced.

Treating disease problems affecting the avian reproductive tract is often much easier than investigating management or compatibility issues. Egg binding, or *dystocia*, is arguably the most common reproductive disease process seen by veterinarians.[34] Dystocia is the mechanical obstruction of an egg in the caudal reproductive tract, caudal oviduct/uterus, vagina, or vaginal-cloacal junction.[35] Causes of dystocia are hypocalcemia

and nutritional deficiencies; oviduct, uterus, or vaginal muscle dysfunction; excessive egg production; large, misshapen, or soft-shelled egg(s); age of hen; obesity; oviduct tumor or infection; lack of exercise; hyperthermia or hypothermia; and genetics.[34] When a patient has been diagnosed with dystocia, it is imperative to stabilize the bird as soon as possible. That would include fluid therapy, IM calcium injection, vitamin A and D_3, nutritional supplementation if needed, and placement into a heated, humidified intensive care unit. Once the patient is stabilized, removal of the egg should be contemplated; this can be accomplished by either helping the bird expel it herself or manually removing it through direct veterinary intervention. Prostaglandin E_2 (PGE_2) relaxes the uterovaginal sphincter and increases uterine contractions.[36] The application of 0.1 ml/100 g body weight of PGE_2 gel (Prepidil; Pharmacia and Upjohn, Kalamazoo, MI) directly into the dorsal area of the cloaca contacting the uterovaginal sphincter may help promote egg delivery. In optimal circumstances, Prepidil will initiate uterine contractions that expel the egg within 15 minutes of application.[36] If Prepidil is used, extreme caution is warranted regarding the exposure of human skin. The avian patient should be treated with Prepidil only at the veterinary hospital, where it should be applied with cotton-tipped applicator by a veterinarian wearing latex exam gloves. Oxytocin targets the uterus but does not relax the uterovaginal sphincter and is inferior to PGE_2.[36] Ovocentesis, or aspiration of the egg contents, can safely be performed on eggs visible in the caudal one third of the oviduct; surgical removal is recommended only in life-threatening situations. To prevent egg binding from reoccurring, it is recommended to give leuprolide acetate (0.375 mg IM in cockatiels), a mammalian LHRH (GnRH) that reduces serum gonadotropin levels by reducing the number of LHRH receptors in the pituitary.[34] Leuprolide acetate has been effective in delaying egg laying from 19 to 28 days.

Prolapsed oviduct out of the cloaca commonly occurs when there is difficulty passing the egg through the terminal part of the reproductive tract. The exposed reproductive tract becomes desiccated, adhering to the egg. Many of these cases can be resolved by hydrating the exposed reproductive tract and slowly manipulating the egg through the uterovaginal sphincter. Replacement of the oviduct, once the egg is removed and a topical medication has been applied, is often sufficient in remedying the problem. Reoccurrence of prolapsed oviduct is rare in my practice.

Egg yolk peritonitis occurs when ovulation takes place outside of the oviduct into the coelomic cavity. Ectopic ovulation is often noted secondary to reverse peristalsis, salpingitis, metritis, neoplasia, cystic hyperplasia, ruptured oviducts, and stress or physical restraint of the egg-laying hen. Treatment requires patient stabilization and diagnosis confirmation. Confirmation of egg yolk peritonitis can be made through cytologic evaluation of cellular debris from a coelomic aspirate, radiology, and CBC. The patient usually is depressed and has an enlarged caudal ventral coelomic cavity. Many patients are diagnosed with concurrent adhesions involving the intestinal tract and other major organs. Surgery, including a salpingohysterectomy is difficult when trying to address the significant pathology associated with peritonitis. Chronic egg yolk peritonitis is considered the most common fatal reproductive condition in avian species.[34]

Chronic egg laying, commonly occurring in cockatiel hens, is a life-threatening problem. Behavioral and dietary modification should be tried before therapeutic measures are used. If behavioral and dietary modifications are not successful, then leuprolide acetate (0.375 mg IM in cockatiels) (Lupron; TAP Pharmaceuticals, Deerfield, IL) is the therapeutic drug of choice.[34] Cockatiels should be injected every 18 days and budgerigars every 12 to 14 days.

Bacterial infections affecting the ovary, oviduct, and cloaca can cause reproductive abnormalities. Results of CBC, culture, and sensitivity testing of a reproductive tract or a cloacal culture will aid in the diagnosis of a reproductive tract infection. Reproductive tract infections may be secondary to neoplasias of the ovary or oviduct. Ovarian neoplasia has been diagnosed in budgerigars but is not often seen in other parrot species. There is currently no treatment for ovarian or reproductive tract tumors.

Reproductive disorders are presented to teaching hospitals on a regular basis. By performing the proper work-ups, the reproductive disorders can be diagnosed and treated, hopefully perpetuating the species for future generations to enjoy.

■ MANAGING AVIAN CASES
Critical Care Considerations

It is a clinical challenge when veterinarians have to administer therapeutic procedures to pet avian patients. The thoughtful use of therapeutic procedures on a debilitated patient is often correlated to the success or failure of treating a patient.

When a technician enters the exam room ready to question the owner regarding their beloved companion bird, care and expertise are expected. It is important not only to get a good history and understand the techniques needed to provide a professional service but also to inform and educate the owner, who may have little expertise or knowledge of husbandry and health. It is important for technicians to gain continuing educational support to add specific avian medical information to the technician's basic veterinary knowledge already learned through professional training and expertise. When veterinarians are establishing or expanding a species group within a practice, veterinary and referral support is important when faced with "in house" questions about a patient's condition or care. When treating and collecting diagnostic samples from avian patients, proper equipment must be used. This is a small but important investment for a practice to make in order to provide the quality of service that clients have come to expect. A basic history following an avian line of questioning not only provides information focused on the presenting problem but also allows the veterinarian to review deficiencies of husbandry or nutritional care. Any problems noted with owner care or nutritional offerings should be discussed with the owner in an educational manner. As mentioned previously it is not unusual for new avian animal owners to be totally unaware of the proper measures to care for and feed their feathered friends.

Continuing education opportunities exist, on both local and national levels, for the veterinary technician to gain experience about avian medicine. New texts and periodicals also provide essential information on avian medicine. The Association of Avian Veterinarians, Boca Raton, FL, www.aav.org is another excellent source for cutting-edge avian information published in journal and newsletter format.

Husbandry issues are a common source of illness and trauma to companion avian species. Questions should be asked about the cage location, substrate, size of cage, cage material, cleaning and disinfecting methods, and perches and toys. As questions are asked during the interview, a more detailed explanation may be needed if it is determined that there is a potential problem area. The other major component of questioning centers on the nutrition provided and ingested by the bird. Type of food being offered and the daily amount being offered are the first questions asked. A more important question for the owner is not what the bird is being fed, but what it is eating. (Information about water source, water container, and how often water is changed is detailed in Nutrition.)

Finally, quarantine procedures and new bird acquisitions should be covered during the case review. These questions will coincide with a review of the bird population at the owner's house and if the patient was housed alone or in a group. After questioning, the owner needs to review any past medical problems and give the veterinarian a specific historic description of the current medical problem(s).

After the history is taken and before the patient is examined, the owner may consult the veterinarian about specific concerns. For the examination the bird should be observed without the stress of holding and then, if possible, be given a complete hands-on physical examination. To properly examine the avian patient and collect diagnostic samples for testing, a few avian specific equipment items are recommended. One advantage of expanding into pet avian practice is the minimal investment needed to treat most of the disease problems associated with these animals. Grooming, which includes nail trims, beak care, and wing feather trims, can be a large part of an avian practice. A handheld motorized grinding tool is used on larger birds for nail trims and beak grooms (Dremel, Inc., Racine, WI). I use a battery-operated hot-wire cautery unit to trim small (i.e., <150 g) birds' nails (MDS, Inc., Brandon, FL) (Figure 10-41). The cautery unit appears less stressful on the smaller birds than the motorized grinding tool.

Special avian surgical equipment includes small noncuffed endotracheal tubes (Bivona, Inc., Gary, IN), radiosurgical equipment (Ellman International, Inc., Hewlett, NY) (Figure 10-42), and respiratory monitors (Medical Engineering & Development, Inc., Jackson, MI). Small ophthalmic surgical instruments are easier to use on avian patients than those manufactured for dogs and cats. A special avian microsurgical pack can be purchased through Sontec Instruments, Inc., Englewood, CO.

Specific avian equipment is useful and usually not a large investment. Incubators, digital gram scales (essential), acrylic perches for scales, examination boards, feeding needles, beak specula, and avian-specific Elizabethan collars are available through a number of companies that regularly exhibit at large veterinary conferences (Veterinary Specialty Products, Inc.,

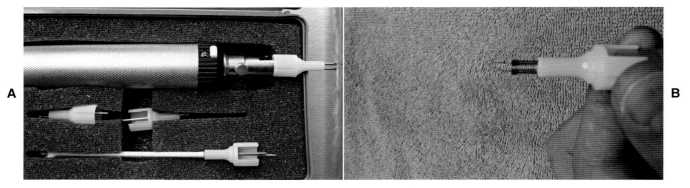

Figure 10-41 A and **B,** A battery-powered electrocautery unit is powerful and provides enough heat to aid in hemostasis of many vascular emergencies.

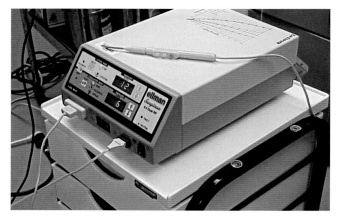

Figure 10-42 State-of-the-art radiosurgery is a must for any avian veterinary practice.

Mission, KS; Henry Schien, Inc., Port Washington, NY; and Lyon Electric Company, Inc., Chula Vista, CA).

Critical care feeding supplements made specifically for avian patients must be in stock when treating pet birds. Feeding supplements are manufactured for the debilitated patient as well as the newly hatched chick that needs a full-complement nutritional supplement. There are a number of commercially manufactured critical care feeding products available, but those manufactured by the Lafeber Company, Cornell, IL are excellent and highly recommended.

The initial phase of evaluating a patient's health is through a rapid external physical examination. If the patient appears to be severely debilitated or getting worse, the bird should be placed in a critical care unit. Any antibiotic, chelation agent, or fluid therapy should be initiated before the patient is placed into the incubator.

If it is determined the patient can withstand the stress of handling and treatment, then fluid therapy may be initiated. Normosol or lactated Ringer's solution can be administered SC, IV, IO, PO, or through the cloaca. Anatomic sites commonly used for IO catheter placement include the distal ulna (larger birds), proximal ulna, proximal tibiotarsal bone, and lateral femur (young and small birds). Placement of the IO catheter begins with proper site preparation. A 22-gauge, 1½-inch spinal needle is the catheter of choice in most psittacine

cases, although any size needle may be used, provided that a stylet is inserted into the needle before the IO catheter is placed into the medullary cavity of the bone.[24] When the IO catheter is placed in the distal ulna, the distal wing tip is flexed and the needle is inserted at a 45- to 60-angle; this angle is reduced once the catheter enters the cortex.[37] The needle should be advanced to the hub, stylet removed, and the catheter flushed with heparinized saline. The catheter should be capped with an injection port and managed as an IV catheter. An IO catheter requires more maintenance than an IV catheter and should be flushed 6 to 8 times a day to maintain patency. SC fluid therapy is not an effective method of rapid restoration of circulatory fluid volume. Adding hyaluronidase (Wydase, Wyeth-Ayerst Pharmaceuticals, Philadelphia, PA) to lactated Ringer's solution for SC fluid administration has been recommended as a method to increase the absorption rate of the fluid into the circulatory system.[38]

Environmental support has a significant impact on the success of many avian critical care cases.[24] Environmental support includes temperature and humidity control (in most cases, heat), oxygen supplementation and administration, and nebulization.[24] There are many avian intensive care units on the market, but the veterinarian should carefully examine the clinic's needs before purchasing this equipment.[24] When comparing avian intensive care units, cheaper is not always better. Important features that improve a unit's performance are digital temperature and humidity control, ease of cleaning and disinfecting, and durability.

An air sac breathing tube is sometimes needed to regain an appropriate air flow into the lower respiratory system if the mouth, glottis, or trachea is obstructed (Figure 10-43). An endotracheal tube (relative to the patient's size) is placed in the caudal thoracic air sac in the area of the last three or four ribs, just dorsal to the dorsal edge of the pectoral muscle.[24] The tube is placed through a stab incision that has been bluntly dissected through to the caudal thoracic air sac.[24] The tube is secured by inflating the cuff within the coelomic cavity (if the tube has a cuff) or suturing a tape butterfly, which has been applied to the tube, to the skin.[24] It has been my experience that to anesthetize or administer oxygen using an abdominal breathing tube requires a higher percentage of anesthetic agent plus an increased flow rate of oxygen.

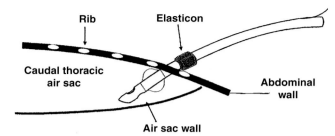

Figure 10-43 A properly placed air sac breathing tube will alleviate any respiratory compromise caused by partial tracheal obstruction.

Performing therapeutic techniques on avian species often means the difference between life and death. Knowing the proper techniques and formulas required for avian patients and using the proper equipment will result in treatment success.

THERAPEUTICS
Fluid Therapy

When determining the dehydration deficit of a psittacine patient, the veterinarian must estimate the percentage of deficit before calculating replacement fluid volumes.[24] Parameters applied to measure dehydration status in psittacine species include skinfold elasticity, corneal moisture, appearance of the globe, and packed cell volume.[24] Dehydrated psittacine chicks have wrinkled and reddened skin, with sunken faces and prominent eyes.[39] It is generally believed that in most cases of severe trauma or disease, a 5% to 10% dehydrated status should be estimated for the avian patient.[24] The estimated deficit should be replaced over a 48- to 72-hour period.[24] The recommended daily fluid maintenance formula for psittacine species is 100 ml/kg/day, and baby birds consume 2 to 3 times the maintenance fluid levels as adult patients.[24] Fluids should be warmed before administration and bolus fluids can be given with relative safety IO or IV over a 3- to 5-minute period.[24] Once the fluid deficit is replaced and the bird is eating and drinking normally for 2 or 3 days, the maintenance hydration therapy can be discontinued.[24]

Fluid therapy may be replaced through SC, IV, or IO administration. SC fluid replacement can be achieved using a 26- or 25-gauge needle attached to a syringe filled with a warmed crystalloid or colloidal agent. The sites usually preferred for SC administration are the featherless inguinal and/or axillary regions of most avian species. IV catheters are placed in the jugular vein of larger birds and median metatarsal of smaller birds. The distal ulna and proximal tibiotarsal bone are the recommended sites for IO catheter placement. Although IO catheter placement is easier in smaller birds, these catheters require more maintenance to prevent plugging. IO catheters have a delivery similar to the delivery of IV catheters and are much easier to place, especially in smaller species.

Nutritional Support

Species-specific and group-specific diets have been formulated for parrots, cockatiels, parakeets, canaries/finches, lories,

and mynahs/softbills. Feeding group- or species-specific diets to breeding birds may increase clutch size, increase fertility of breeding birds, increase the number of clutches per year, provide better hatchability, and yield healthier chicks that mature faster than birds that are fed lower quality diets. With the advent of powdered hand-feeding formulas, avian nutrition has arrived in the 21st century. Homemade batch formulas no longer need to be blended to adequately feed domestically raised companion bird species. Hand-feeding formulas are as easy as instant pancake mix: add warm water to the powder. With the instructions on the box, the amount needed can be reconstituted without waste or storage. All unused formula should be discarded to prevent bacterial contamination. Also, with warm water being used and the hand-feeding formula being "ready to eat," the need to microwave the formula is no longer necessary. By eliminating the microwave process, the likelihood of young birds sustaining thermal crop injuries is drastically reduced. There currently is debate on how often and when to feed young birds. No matter how advanced avian nutrition becomes, it still pales to properly fed parent-raised birds. In birds being fed by parents, the crops are always full. This is completely opposite of the hand-feeding techniques advocated by aviculturists and veterinarians over the past 25 years. It is recommended that birds should be fed approximately 10 ml/100 g body weight when their crop empties. Most hand-feeding owners will come very close to following the rule of feeding on an empty crop. Certain bird species, in particular macaws, often become stunted when hand-fed this way. There are specially formulated macaw formulas that should be used, but also macaws seem to thrive when their crop is maintained full and allowed to empty overnight. Hand-fed birds should be weighed daily, in the morning when the crop is empty before the first feeding. If the bird is not gaining weight, the formula may contain too much water or may be diluted with other ingredients, or the bird may not be fed often enough or may not be getting enough food at each feeding. Another problem with underdeveloped birds is that owners will "weaken" the formula to aid in digestion of a slow moving crop. Weakening the formula reduces the bird's nutritional intake, thereby compounding and disease problems a young bird may have. Diluting the formula may also have deleterious effects on the immune system.

As important as fluid replacement, nutritional supplementation must be considered for the debilitated avian patient.[24] To calculate the nutritional requirements for the avian patient, the following formula can be used with adjustment factors listed in Box 10-7:[24]

1. Calculate basal metabolic rate (BMR):
   BMR is K ($W^{0.75}$)
   Kcal = kilocalories (a constant) for 24 hours
   Kcal = 78 for psittacines
   W = weight of the bird in kilograms
2. Calculate maintenance:
   1.5 × BMR
3. Adjust maintenance requirements for stress
4. Kcal required/day ÷ Kcal/ml formula = amount of formula in ml required per day

---

BOX 10-7   Adjustments to Nutritional Maintenance for Stress (as Multiples of Maintenance Energy Requirements)

Starvation	0.5-0.7
Elective surgery	1.0-1.2
Mild trauma	1.0-1.2
Severe trauma	1.1-2.0
Growth	1.5-3.0
Sepsis	1.2-7.5
Burns	1.2-2.0
Head injuries	1.0-2.0

From Tully TN: Psittacine therapeutics, *Vet Clin North Am Exot Anim Prac* 3:59-90, 2000.

BOX 10-8   Commonly Used Antibiotics in Avian Veterinary Practice

1. Bacteriocidal—extended-spectrum penicillins; amoxicillin, ampicillin, carbenicillin, ticarcillin, piperacillin
2. Bacteriocidal—ß-Lactamase inhibitors/clavulanic acid; amoxicillin-clavulanate, ticarcillin-clavulanate
3. Bacteriocidal—first-generation cephalosporins; cefadroxil, cefazolin, cephalexin, cephalothin, cephradine
4. Bacteriocidal—third-generation cephalosporins; cefotaxime, ceftazidime, ceftiofur
5. Bacteriocidal—aminoglycosides; amikacin
6. Bacteriocidal—trimethoprim-sulfa
7. Bacteriocidal—fluoroquinolones; ciprofloxacin, enrofloxacin
8. *Bacteriostatic*—macrolides; erythromycin, tylosin
9. *Bacteriostatic*—tetracyclines; chlortetracycline, doxycycline, oxytetracycline, tetracycline
10. Other (cidal against anaerobes)—nitroimidazole; metronidazole

From Carpenter JW: *Exotic Animal Formulary*, ed 3, St Louis, 2005, WB Saunders.

The new formulated diets generally do not recommend supplementation because of the tendency of many owners to oversupplement, increasing the possibility of nutritional toxicosis. There is one supplement that may be of benefit to birds and can be given to young and old birds alike. This supplementation is an avian-specific probiotic formula. One of the common bacteria included in these probiotic formulations is *Lactobacillus* spp. Theoretically and scientifically, probiotic supplementation is supposed to aid digestion by inoculating the birds with favorable bacterial florae and protecting the intestinal tract against the colonization of pathogenic bacteria. Recommended conditions for probiotic supplementation include hand-fed birds, birds in a known stressed condition, birds on antibiotic therapy, and birds diagnosed with an illness. Birds that are extremely ill may need enteral feeding support. Products available through the Lafeber Company, Ordell, IL, that provide this critical care nutritional requirement include Critical Care®, Nutri-Support®, and Carbo-Boost®.

Antimicrobial Therapy

Care must be taken in the use of antibiotics, as antibiotic resistance can result from the overuse and abuse of effective antibiotic agents. Factors that must be considered before using antibiotic agents in avian patients include effectiveness of the agent against the specific bacterial organism being treated, ease of administration, stress on the patient, ability of the agent to reach therapeutic levels at the intended treatment site, and cost and availability of the drug. The best avian veterinary practices consider all available options, including relying on compounding pharmacies to create drug formulations that are no longer mass manufactured and to compound agents into forms and tastes that are easier to administer to avian patients. In addition to compounding pharmacies, regular pharmacies may compound certain drugs they have in their inventory or provide a compounded drug in the manufactured form so that a veterinary hospital does not need to maintain inventory for a drug that is rarely used. It is important to remember that just because a drug is rarely used does not mean that it is not a treatment option. Veterinarians should not be afraid to interact with professional pharmacists; they can not only provide drugs but also give advice on effective alternatives, new drug therapies, side effects associated with administration, and dosages.

A recommended text is *Exotic Animal Formulary,* 3rd edition, edited by J. W. Carpenter and published by Saunders. This is a complete exotic formulary listing dosages and references. When selecting an antibiotic, the veterinarian should know if it is bacteriocidal or bacteriostatic, how it is administered, if PO administration is the route of choice, how well it is absorbed through the gastrointestinal tract and disseminated through the body, how the dose varies depending on the species being treated, and what the major side effects are. Box 10-8 and Table 10-3 list antibiotics that are commonly used in avian veterinary practice. Although these are not complete selections, they give an overview of the types of agents used to successfully treat microbial infections in avian patients.

Although just a fraction of the antibiotic agents available, those listed in Box 10-8 are the most common to be used in avian pet medicine. It is useful and often recommended to use bacteriocidal agents when possible, but certain diseases respond better to agents that may be bacteriostatic (e.g., for *Chlamydophila psittaci,* the drug of choice is doxycycline). Disease-specific antibiotics also highlight the need for a proper diagnostic workup to definitively diagnose the illness in order to prescribe the correct treatment. Again, avian patients respond well to the proper treatment but die quickly if the proper treatment is not administered.

There are certain antimicrobial agents that are more effective when used to treat infection in specific areas of the body. The use of certain antimicrobials and their effectiveness in treating infections is an important consideration but should not overshadow the importance of culture and sensitivity, especially when treating avian patients.

Antimicrobial agents commonly used to treat bacteremia/ septicemia include synergistic aminoglycoside and penicillin or

TABLE 10-3	Dosages of Commonly Used Antimicrobials in Avian Practice	
Drug	**Dosage**	**Comment**
1. Amikacin	10-15 mg/kg IM, IV q8-12h	Most species
2. Amoxicillin/Clavulanate Clavamox®	125 mg/kg PO q6h	Psittacine species
3. Cefotaxime	75-100 mg/kg IM, IV q4-8h	Most species
4. Ciprofloxacin	15-20 mg/kg PO, IM q12h	Most species
5. Clindamycin	25 mg/kg PO q8h	Most species
6. Doxycycline	25 mg/kg PO q12h	Psittacine species
	25-50 mg/kg IM q5-7d × 5-7 treatments	
7. Enrofloxacin	5-10 mg/kg PO q12h	Most species
8. Metronidazole	50 mg/kg PO q24h × 5-7 days	Most species
9. Piperacillin/Tazobactam sodium Zosyn®	100 mg/kg IM q8-12h	Psittacine species
10. Ticarcillin/Clavulanic acid Timintin®	100 mg/kg IM q12h	Most species
11. Trimethoprim/Sulfadiazine Tribrissen®	20 mg/kg SC, IM q12h	Psittacine species
12. Trimethoprim/Sulfamethoxazole Bactrim®	20 mg/kg PO q8-12h	Psittacine species
13. Fluconazole	5-15 mg/kg PO q12h × 14-60 days or longer	Most species
14. Itraconazole	10 mg/kg PO q24h × 14-90 days with food	Psittacine species
		African grey parrots may be sensitive to drug

BOX 10-9	Speer's Nasal Flush

Mix 3.5 mg neomycin, 124.5 mg trypsin, and 10 mg amphotericin B with a 30-ml volume of a water-soluble suspension
Add 0.1 to 0.4 ml of this base solution to 10 to 20 ml of saline for direct flushing through the nares q24h.

---

cephalosporin therapy, enrofloxacin with amoxicillin, penicillins, and, for anaerobic infections, chloramphenicol, clindamycin, and metronidazole.[13]

Penicillins, cephalosporins, doxycycline, trimethoprim-sulfa, and fluoroquinolones are often used to treat aerobic soft tissue infections, whereas clindamycin or metronidazole is used to treat anaerobic soft tissue infections.[13]

Respiratory tract infections are one of the most common disease presentations among avian species. The drugs of choice for respiratory infections are penicillins, cephalosporins, tetracyclines, trimethoprim-sulfa, chloramphenicol, fluoroquinolones, doxycycline, macrolides, and, for anaerobic infections, clindamycin or metronidazole.[1] Antibiotics can be administered through nebulization techniques and nasal flushes (Box 10-9).

Another common disease presentation is gastrointestinal disorders. Trimethoprim-sulfa, fluoroquinolones, cephalosporins, amoxicillin, tetracyclines, neomycin, and metronidazole are commonly used for conditions that affect the gastrointestinal tract.[13]

Dermatologic presentations are treated with similar antimicrobial agents that veterinarians would use for other small companion animals: amoxicillin-clavulanate, cephalosporins, erythromycin, enrofloxacin, trimethoprim-sulfa, and lincomycin.[13]

Bone and joint infections are difficult to treat. As with any microbial infection, a culture and sensitivity will greatly aid in selecting the right antibiotic agent to use. Choices of antimicrobial agents to use for bone and joint infections include cephalosporins, extended-spectrum penicillins, fluoroquinolones, aminoglycosides, lincosamides, and, for anaerobic infections, penicillins with clindamycin and third-generation cephalosporins with clindamycin.[13] In difficult-to-treat musculoskeletal infections, antibiotic-impregnated polymethyl methacrylate beads (PMMA) can be used (Box 10-10).

Penicillins, cephalosporins, trimethoprim-sulfa, sulfisoxazole, fluoroquinolones, and tetracycline are all recommended for urinary tract infections.[13]

For central nervous system infections, it is important to choose an agent that crosses the blood barrier. The drugs of choice are chloramphenicol and fluoroquinolones.

Reproductive tract disorders are best treated with chloramphenicol, trimethoprim-sulfa, enrofloxacin, amoxicillin-clavulanate, and clindamycin against anaerobes.[13]

■ BANDAGING TECHNIQUES

Upon presentation to veterinary clinics, pet birds almost uniformly respond to the unfamiliar surroundings and manipulation by exhibiting stressful defense reactions, including vocalization, biting, increased blood pressure, increased heart rate, and other shock conditions. It is recommended that birds be handled gently, and if there is any indication of a life-threatening condition, the bird must be set down. Experience helps tremendously when making the critical decision of whether to continue the examination or set the bird down.

Dermal injury treatment, fracture stabilization, stabilization of fracture sites after internal orthopedic repair, joint injury treatment, and trauma prevention are common reasons bandages are used on avian patients. Bandages function to apply pressure to reduce dead space, swelling, edema, and hemorrhage; protect the wound from pathologic microorganisms; immobilize the wound and underlying fractures; protect the wound from desiccation and additional trauma from abrasions or self-mutilation; absorb exudates and help debride the wound surface; and provide patient comfort.[41] Although bandages may be less stressful to apply than internal fixation of a fracture, it is imperative that the proper application technique be used to prevent increased trauma to the affected area. Bandages that are applied incorrectly may not help the condition of the patient; if applied too tight, the bandage will restrict blood flow to the distal extremity, and if immobilization of the joints above and below the fracture is not achieved, the possibility of a nonunion increases significantly. Although it appears to be a simple technique, bandaging requires skill, proper materials, patience, a properly restrained patient, and an understanding of the forces to be controlled by the bandage.

Bandage materials used on avian patients include Vet-Wrap (3M Animal Care Products, St. Paul, MN), adaptic (Johnson & Johnson, New Brunswick, NJ), 4 × 4 and 2 × 2 gauze sponges, white cloth tape, cast padding, Hexcelite (Hexcel Medical Co., Dublin, CA), syringe cases, aluminum rods, and roll gauze. One of the most important aspects of bandaging avian patients is that most of the bandage materials listed do not come in sizes applicable to patients that weigh less than 300 grams, especially passerines that weigh less than 30 grams;

however, modification and manipulation of the bandage material mentioned is generally sufficient for proper application on the small avian patients. Vendors do not manufacture and sell specific splints for the different avian species or for animals the size of most pet birds. Therefore, veterinarians are required to use their skills at manufacturing splints out of Hexcelite, syringe cases, aluminum rods, or some other rigid material. To fabricate a syringe case splint, a Dremel tool is required to cut and shape the splint to the size of the anatomic area that needs to be immobilized. Hexalite is a thermal sensitive material that becomes malleable when placed in hot water and then hardens at room temperature in the shape of the injured anatomic area. Ultraviolet (UV) dental acrylic can be used in a similar manner as Hexalite, but it cures hard when exposed to the UV light generated by a UV gun. Eye protection must be worn by veterinarians and hospital staff when they use a UV dental acrylic curing instrument.

The owner of the bandaged avian patient must understand the importance of monitoring the bandage and affected area and bringing the pet to the required follow-up visits for reevaluation. Veterinarians, veterinary technical staff, and owners should monitor the bandage site for slippage of the bandage or splint, swelling distal to the bandage, non-use of the limb or a regression of ability to use a limb, irritation or picking at the bandage site, and tissue abrasions at contact surface sites with the bandage. If any of these conditions occur, the bandage should be removed, the area below and around the bandage evaluated, and the bandage reapplied if necessary.

Figure-of-Eight Wing Bandage

One of the most commonly used external coaptation bandages and, in my experience, one of the most incorrectly applied bandages is the figure-of-eight bandage (Figure 10-44). The figure-of-eight bandage is applied to the wing and can be used to immobilize fractures distal to the elbow, maintain the wing in position when an IO catheter is in place within the distal ulna, or treating dermal lesions. The supporting bandage material is dependent on the condition of the underlying tissue and/or bones. If there is a closed fracture involving the ulna or radius, underlying cast padding may be used to support the outer layer of nonstick wrap (Vet-wrap). If there is an incision, open wound or abrasion, the area is cleaned and treated, and a nonstick gauze pad (Adaptic) is placed over the affected area and supported with 2 × 2 or 4 × 4 gauze sponges held in place with an elastic gauze wrap (Kling®, Johnson & Johnson, New Brunswick, NJ) and an outer layer of nonstick wrap. These bandages may be changed daily or weekly depending on the injury and patient condition.

The difficulty in placing this wrap on the wing is keeping the bandage in place and incorporating the humerus in the bandage. Placement of the wrap should start at the axillary area where the wing attaches to the body. The bandage material is then brought over the dorsal surface of the wing toward the flexed carpal area. The wrap is then maneuvered under and around the ventral surface of the flexed carpal area, ending on the top of the wing. As the bandage material is brought back, caudally over the dorsal surface of the wing, the top part of

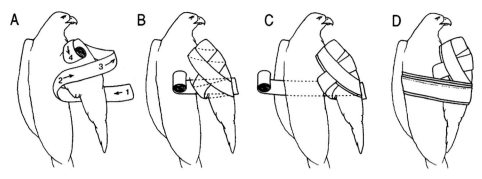

Figure 10-44 The figure-of-eight bandage is one of the most common and useful bandages placed on avian patients.

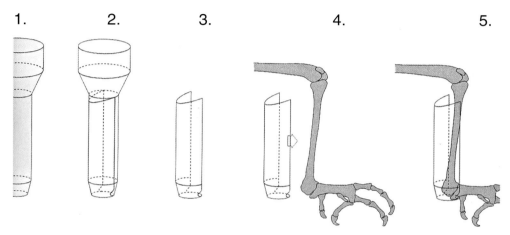

Figure 10-45 Easy application on lower leg fractures of small birds makes the syringe case splint a popular treatment choice.

the 8 is formed. Continue bringing the bandage material caudally and wrap under the primary feathers going back to the initiation point, completing the figure-of-eight. By wrapping the bandage in this manner, one can be assured of incorporating the humerus into this wrap. The figure-of-eight bandage is complete when the above instructions are repeated 3 or 4 times. If the humerus is to be stabilized, a body wrap can be incorporated into the bandage. Care must be taken, if a body wrap is used, not to make the bandage too tight, as it can hinder the patient's ability to breath. If the body wrap is placed too far caudal on the body, the patient's feet may have a tendency of getting caught in the bandage, or they may not be able to extend their legs. The nonstick bandage should be held in place with a small piece of adhesive tape.

Syringe Case Splint

The syringe case splint is an external coaptive device that is best used for birds that have been diagnosed with a tibiotarsal fracture or tarsometatarsal fracture (Figure 10-45). The syringe case and corresponding wrap help immobilize the joints and fracture site for healing to occur without surgical repair of the fracture. Surgical correction increases the possibility of collateral damage that may impair the function of the affected limb. A syringe case is selected based on the size of patient's leg that needs to be immobilized. Once selected, a Dremel tool with a

cutting bit is used to remove the flared top part of the syringe case and half of the barrel, leaving the flat base intact. If the splint is to be placed on a parrot that has been diagnosed with a tarsometatarsal fracture, notches can be etched on the side of the case where it comes into contact with the base, for rear toe placement. If the splint is to be placed on a passerine or raptor species that has been diagnosed with a tarsometatarsal fracture, then a hole can be made in the back of the syringe to accommodate the first digit. None of the modifications for toes have to be made for tibiotarsal fractures. For tibiotarsal fractures, the top of the back of the splint should be ground into a semicircular pattern to accommodate the flexor cruris medialis muscle. Cotton is glued on the base of the splint, and 4×4 gauze sponges are placed on the inside of the splint and over the back and held in place with nonstick bandage material (Vet-Wrap). This will soften the splint, thereby protecting the bird's skin from the sharp edges of the splint.

The feathers should be plucked where the splint will come into contact with the body part. Tape stirrups are placed on the lateral and medial aspects of the limb along the affected tibiotarsal or tarsometatarsal bone. Cast padding is then used to wrap the leg for increased immobilization. The splint is then applied over the cast padding and the tape stirrups taped to the side of the splint. Two pieces of adhesive tape are used to firmly attach the barrel of the splint to the leg. One of the most important points of properly applying this splint and assuring that it will remain in place is a cruciate tape pattern over the distal part of the limb as it rests in the base of the splint. This cruciate tape pattern goes over and around the splint before coming back over the top and back around on the opposite side. The limb should be securely in place and the fracture reduced as much as possible before applying the cruciate tape pattern. The splint and leg are then wrapped with a nonstick bandage material (Vet-Wrap), which is held in place with a piece of adhesive tape. The bandage should be reassessed regularly to check for swelling in the distal extremities and skin abrasions generated by the splint edges.

Tape Splint

The tape splint is a simple splint and is best used on birds that weigh less than 60 grams. Although some veterinarians use the splint in birds weighing up to 150 grams with supporting material placed under the tape, a simple tape splint works best on the lightest of avian patients.[42] The tape splint is recommended for the same type of fractures as those listed for syringe case splints. In lightweight birds, such as finches, canaries, and budgerigars, feathers do not have to be plucked over the tibiotarsal area to place the splint. An appropriate-sized piece of adhesive tape is placed under the leg, adhering the affected area to the tape with the joint above and below the fracture incorporated in the tape area. The tape is then folded over, allowing for extra tape to extend cranially and caudally from the leg. Hemostats are then used to press the tape together close to the leg, thereby immobilizing the fracture site.

Ball Bandage

A ball bandage is applied to the plantar surface of a bird foot. This bandage allows the bird to stand, with minimal or no pressure to the plantar surface of the foot. Applications for the ball bandage include infectious pododermatitis, lacerations, and protection of foot injuries/surgical sites during the healing process. An appropriate-sized piece of gauze or cast padding is placed on the plantar surface, allowing the toes to flex over the edges without touching the base. If there is a wound that needs to be treated, this step should take place before the gauze ball is put in place. While the toes are flexed over the "ball," a nonstick (Vet-Wrap) bandage material is used to wrap the foot, incorporating the ball.

Snowshoe Splint

This splint is also for foot injuries, in particular toe fractures and constricted toe syndrome cases. A tongue depressor is cut to the length of the foot including the claws. An electrocautery unit is used to create a hole in the tongue depressor where the (front and back) longest claws extend. The tips of the claws fit into the holes, helping to secure the foot onto the splint. Adhesive tape strips are then applied to the medial toes (front and back) and wrapped around the splint, securing the foot to the tongue depressor. The splint is completed with a nonstick (Vet-Wrap) bandage material being applied over the foot and splint. A small piece of adhesive tape holds the nonstick bandage material in place.

Duck Shoe Splint

Duck shoe splints are used with waterfowl that have foot injuries. Coat-hanger wire or small-gauge aluminum rod material is bent to the form of the waterfowl patient's foot, extending up the tarsometatarsal bone. The splint is padded with cast padding and wrapped in waterproof tape. The splint is applied to the extended foot, being held in place with adhesive tape. Two full width 1-inch adhesive tape strips are wrapped around the tarsometatarsal bone and the part of the splint that extends up the leg. The bandage is completed with nonstick tape applied over the foot, splint, and leg.

Wet-to-Dry Bandage

Wet-to-dry bandages are recommended for skin wounds that have to close by secondary intention, encouraging the natural healing mechanisms of epithelialization and contraction. These bandages are easy to apply, provide a means of debridement, allow the use of topical antimicrobial solutions, and provide a moist environment for eptithelialization.[43]

Although normal saline is the preferred wet solution, a weak solution of chlorhexidine diacetate (Nolvasan®, Fort Dodge, Labs Inc., Fort Dodge, IA) at approximately 0.1% in water for the primary layer of standard 4×4 gauze sponges may be used.[43] Chlorhexidine diacetate solutions of greater than 0.5% have been shown to retard granulation and inhibit epithelialization.[44] The secondary, absorptive, dry layer should consist of dry 4×4 gauze sponges. A nonstick (Vet-Wrap) bandage material is used for the tertiary layer to hold the first two layers in place. The bandage should be removed and reapplied daily until a healthy granulation bed forms. At that point the wetting agent can inhibit the progress of epithelialization and contraction.[43] To aid the healing process of the granulation bed, an occlusive, nonadherent bandage should be applied until epithelialization and contraction are complete.

■ SURGERY
Analgesia

Pain management has become an integral part of patient care within veterinary medicine. This also applies to avian patients and possibly has a significant impact of the successful conclusion to many surgical cases.

Radiosurgery

With the advent of new surgical technology in the form of laser (light amplification by stimulated emission radiation), there is a trend by veterinary practitioners and other health care professionals to disregard proven surgical equipment. The specific surgical equipment that does not have the glamour, or cost, associated with laser units is the dual-frequency Surgitron® (Ellman International, Inc., Hewlett, NY). The radiosurgery units have been part of medical operating rooms since the early 1960s, and with this history the radiosurgery units are more advanced and easier to use than in the past.

The most difficult concept regarding radiosurgery units for many veterinarians to overcome is the fact that radiosurgery is not electrocautery. As with any surgical instrument, improper usage of the radiosurgery unit or laser will result in tissue damage. In a comparison study of the use of a dual frequency Surgitron® to that of a CO_2 laser when used on human eyelid surgery, there was no apparent difference in the incision healing of the Surgitron-incised lid to that of the laser-incised lid.[45] This is not surprising given that the same basic cutting physiology is involved in either the Surgitron or laser equipment.

To fully understand the benefits of radiosurgery veterinarians must know the definition of some basic terms.[46]

1. *Electrocautery:* Radiosurgery is not electrocautery, and the two terms should not be interchanged. Electrocautery has been defined as a needle tip, wire tip, or scalpel heated to red-hot temperatures through the resistance of the device to the flow of low-voltage, high-amperage current.[46] No high-frequency radio waves are used with these instruments—only conductive heat.

2. *Radiosurgery:* This is the passage of fully filtered, high-frequency radio waves through tissue.[47] The radiosurgery unit is a radio-frequency generator that converts alternating current (AC) to direct current (DC) by a power supply with the electrosurgical unit that passes the DC current into a tuned coil capacitor that generates radio-frequency waves.[47] Radio waves are then passed through a high-frequency waveform adapter that alters the shape and magnitude of the wave to create different waveforms.[48] The waveforms are amplified and directed to the electrode; when this is applied to tissue, the electromagnetic field created heats up the intracellular fluid and volatilizes the cell.[47] When used correctly this cellular volatilization reduces trauma and will seal blood vessels up to 2 mm in diameter.[46]

3. *Laser surgery:* Photothermal interactions occur when laser light is absorbed by tissue and converted into heat, ultimately volatilizing the cell during incision. The CO_2 laser can coagulate blood vessels less than 0.6 mm in diameter.[49]

As with the radiosurgery surgery unit, it is easy to see the simplicity and benefits of using a technology that is time tested and improved. The many advantages of using the Surgitron® dual frequency unit include dual footswitch for cut and coagulation functions, three-button fingerswitch for waveform selection and activation, computerized "auto start-up test," a handpiece that allows for direct touch of the tissue with the electrode, different tips, and bipolar forceps for the different presentations seen in an avian practice.

The recommended frequency for incising epithelial, connective, and muscle tissue is 3.8 to 4.0 MHz.[50] The main modes on the Surgitron®, cut, cut/coagulation, and hemostasis are all 4.0 MHz. The cut setting has a waveform output of 90% cutting and 10 % coagulation, the cut/coagulation has s waveform output of 50% cutting and 50% coagulation, and the hemostasis has a waveform output of 10% cutting and 90% coagulation. The other commonly used setting, bipolar, is the same as the hemostasis waveform output, but the frequency is 1.7 MHz. With the new three-button fingerswitch, the surgeon can easily change settings.

To properly use the Surgitron®, the surgeon needs to follow a few specific recommendations from the company. These recommendations help protect the unit and allow for maximum effectiveness of radiosurgery by producing minimal tissue trauma. The finest wire electrode should be used when making incisions and the electrode maintained perpendicular to the tissue surface. A smooth incision stroke is recommended at a minimum rate of 7 mm/sec. To prevent lateral heat, the surgeon should wait 8 seconds between cutting strokes. The electrode tip should be clean and free of debris, and power to the electrode should not be applied until tissue contact is made. Power should be adjusted for each case and is set when no drag is noticed when the epithelial incision is being made. Nonflammable products should be used in preparation of a surgical site where radiosurgery will be used.

Radiosurgery has never been more state of the art than it is now. When used properly it has been shown in human procedures to be comparable to laser surgery. All avian veterinary practices should have one of these units as standard equipment.

■ZOONOSES

Despite the fact that zoonotic diseases are rare, bird owners should be informed and educated on the zoonotic illnesses associated with avian species. As with any disease, people in an immunocompromised state (e.g., organ transplant patients, AIDS patients, chemotherapy patients) should be especially careful and knowledgeable of the avian zoonotic diseases. A potential bird owner that is immune deficient is not only more susceptible to the diseases if exposed, but will often have a more severe infection. In some cases the diseases that are transferred from birds to humans can cause death. Bird owners seeking medical care should always mention to the physician that birds are in their household.

The most common zoonotic disease associated with pet birds is *Chlamydophila psittaci,* or psittacosis. This is an uncommon disease; fewer than 100 cases are reported in the United States each year.[21] *C. psittaci* can be found in birds that are not clinically ill. This subclinical condition will eventually lead to shedding and possible human exposure. Proper testing and treatment of birds that have been diagnosed with avian chlamydiosis is described earlier in the chapter. Humans that are diagnosed with psittacosis have periodic episodes of high fever and general flu-like symptoms. Tetracycline antibiotics are very effective in treating psittacosis.

Bird breeder's lung, or allergic alveolitis, is a condition of respiratory hypersensitivity to the feather dander and fomites produced by a single bird or many birds within an aviary. Bird owners with a history of lung disease or smoking are predisposed to the pulmonary inflammatory response associated with exposure to avian-derived fomites.

Other zoonotic diseases, rarely seen, include giardiasis, salmonellosis, and avian mycobacteriosis.[5] Knowledge of these diseases and risk of exposure to them will provide the bird owner a realistic perspective of the probability of infection. Other factors that will reduce the likelihood of human infection include proper veterinary care for the bird and normal immune status of the owner.

REFERENCES

1. King AS, McLelland J: *Birds: Their Structure and Function*, ed 3, London, 1984, Bailliere Tindall.
2. Lumeij JT: Gastroenterology. In Ritchie BW, Harrison GJ, Harrison LR, editors: *Avian Medicine: Principles and Application*, Lake Worth, Fla, 1994, Wingers.
3. Lumeij JT: Nephrology. In Ritchie BW, Harrison GJ, Harrison LR, editors: *Avian Medicine: Principles and Application*, Lake Worth, Fla, 1994, Wingers.
4. Clubb SL, Flammer K: The avian flock. In Ritchie BW, Harrison GJ, Harrison LR, editors: *Avian medicine: Principles and Application*, Lake Worth, Fla, 1994, Wingers.
5. Gallerstein GA: *The Complete Pet Bird Owner's Handbook*, Minneapolis, 2003, Avian.
6. Jones AK: Husbandry. In Harcourt-Brown N, Chitty J, editors: *BSAVA Manual of Psittacine Birds*, ed 2, Gloucester, UK, British Small Animal Veterinary Association.
7. Gerlach H: Bacteria. In Ritchie BW, Harrison GJ, Harrison LR, editors: *Avian Medicine: Principles and Application*, Lake Worth, Fla, 1994, Wingers.
8. Brooker BE: *Lactobacilli* which attach to the crop epithelium of the fowl, *Am J Clin Nutr* 27:1305-1312, 1974.
9. Gerlach H: Defense mechanisms of the avian host. In Ritchie BW, Harrison GJ, Harrison LR, editors: *Avian Medicine: Principles and Application*, Lake Worth, Fla, 1994, Wingers.
10. Joyner KL, Swanson JL: The use of a *Lactobacillus* product in a psittacine hand feeding diet: its effect on normal aerobic microflora, early weight gain and health, *Proc Annu Conf Assoc Avian Vet*, pp 127-137, 1988.
11. Coates ME: The influence of the gut microflora on digestion. In Boorman KN, Freeman BM, editors: *Digestion in the Fowl*, Edinburgh, 1976, British Poultry Science.
12. Eichinger E: *Lactobacillen* zur dekampfung von Enterobacteriacae in darmvon *Psittaciformes*, *DVG VII Tagung Volgelkrankheiten*, Munchen 231-234, 1990.
13. Carpenter JW: *Exotic Animal Formulary*, ed 3, St Louis, 2005, WB Saunders.
14. Abou-Madi N: Avian anesthesia, *Vet Clin North Am Exot Anim Pract* 4:147-168, 2001.
15. Paul-Murphy J, Ludders JW: Avian analgesia, *Vet Clin North Am Exot Anim Pract* 4:35-46, 2001.
16. Wyrick PB, Richmond SJ: Biology of *chlamydia*: reports from the symposium on avian chlamydiosis, *J Am Vet Med Assoc* 195:1507-1512, 1989.
17. Vanrompay D: Avian chlamydial diagnostics. In Fudge AM, editor: *Laboratory Medicine: Avian and Exotic Pets*, Philadelphia, 2000, WB Saunders.
18. Grimes JE: *Chlamydia psittaci* latex agglutination antigen and protocol improvement and psittacine bird antichlamydial immunoglobulin reactivity, *Avian Dis* 30:60-66, 1986.
19. Tully TN: Clinical aspects of companion bird chlamydial infections, *Semin Av Exot Pet Med*, 2:157-160, 1993.
20. Evans RT, Chalmers WSK, Woolcock PR et al: An enzyme-linked immunosorbent assay (ELISA) for the detection of chlamydial antibody in duck sera, *Avian Pathol* 12:117-124, 1983.
21. Compendium of measures to control *Chlamydophila psittaci* infection among humans (psittacosis) and pet birds (avian chlamydiosis), 2006, http://www.nasphv.org/Documents/Psittacosis.pdf, July 12, 2006.
22. Fudge AM: A review of methods to detect *Chlamydia psittaci* in avian patients, *J Avian Med Surg* 11:153-165, 1997.
23. Martin AA, Gubler PJ: West Nile encephalitis: an emerging disease in the United States, *Clin Infect Dis* 33:1713-1719, 2001.
24. Tully TN: *Psittacine* therapeutics, *Vet Clin North Am Exot Anim Prac* 3:59-90, 2000.
25. Clyde VL, Patton S: Diagnosis, treatment, and control of common parasites in companion and aviary birds, *Semin Av Exot Pet Med* 5:52-64, 1996.
26. Krautwald-Junghanns ME, Trinkhaus K: Imaging techniques. In Tully TN, Lawton MPC, Dorrestein GM, editors: *Avian Medicine*, Oxford, UK, 2000, Butterworth-Heinemann.
27. Ernst S, Goggin JM, Biller DS et al: Comparison of iohexol and barium sulfate as gastrointestinal contrast media in mid-sized psittacine birds, *J Avian Med Surg* 12:16-20, 1998.
28. Everett KDE, Bush RM, Anderson AA: Emended description of the order *Chlamydiales* proposal of *Parachlamydiaceae* fam nov and *Simkaniaceae* fam nov, each containing one monotypic genus, revised taxonomy of the family *Chlamydiaceae*, including new genus and five new species and standards for the identification of organisms, *Int J Syst Bacteriol* 49:415-440, 1999.
29. Scieux C, Grimont F, Regnault B et al: DNA fingerprinting of *Chlamydia trachomatis* by use of ribosomal RNA oligonicleotide and randomly cloned DNA probes, *Res Microbiol* 143:755-765, 1992.
29. Messmer T, Tully TN, Ritchie BW et al: A tale of discrimination: differentiation of *Chlamydiaceae* by polymerase chain reaction, *Semin Av Exot Pet Med* 9:36-42, 2000.
30. Lamberski N: A diagnostic approach to feather picking, *Semin Av Exot Pet Med* 4:161-168, 1995.
31. Lightfoot T: Feather plucking: causes and cures, *Proc Annu Mardi Gras Avicul Conf* 11:3-8, 2000.
32. Cooper JE, Harrison GJ: Behavior. In Ritchie BW, Harrison GJ, Harrison LR, editors: *Avian Medicine: Principles and Application*, Lake Worth, Fla, 1994, Wingers.
33. Romagnano A: Avian obstetrics, *Semin Av Exot Pet Med* 5:180-188, 1996.
34. Speer B: Clinical reproductive avian medicine, in foundations in avian medicine, *Proc Annu Conf Assoc Avian Vet*, pp 23-33, 1995.
35. Hudelson S, Hudelson P: Egg binding, hormonal control and therapeutic consideration, *Compend Cont Ed* 15:427-432, 1994.
36. Lamberski N, Daniel G: The efficacy of intraosseous catheters in birds, *Proc Annu Conf Assoc Avian Vet*, pp 17-19, 1991.
37. Griffin C, Snelling LR: Use of hyaluronidase in avian subcutaneous fluids, *Proc Annu Conf Assoc Avian Vet*, pp 239-240, 1998.
38. Clubb LS, Wolf S, Phillip A: Psittacine pediatric medicine. In Shubot RM, Clubb KJ, Clubb SL, editors: Psittacine aviculture perspectives techniques and research, Loxahatchee, Fla, 1992, Aviculture Breeding and Research Center.
39. Remple JD: A multifaceted approach to the treatment of bumblefoot in raptors, *J Exot Pet Med* 15:49-55, 2006.
40. Swaim SF, Wilhalf D: The physics, physiology and chemistry of bandaging open wounds, *Comp Cont Ed* 7:146-156, 1985.
41. Degernes LA: Trauma medicine. In Ritchie BW, Harrison GJ, Harrison LR, editors: *Avian Medicine: Principles and Application*, Lake Worth, Fla, 1994, Wingers.
42. King WW, Tully TN: Management of a large cutaneous defect in a moluccan cockatoo, *Proc Annu Conf Assoc Avian Vet*, pp 142-145, 1993.
43. Lee AH, Swaim SF, McGuire A, et al: Effects of chlorhexidine diacetate, povidone iodine and polyhydroxydine on wound healing in dogs, *J Am Anim Hosp Assoc* 24:77-84, 1988.
44. Niamtu J: Making waves, *Plastic Surg Prod* Oct:52-58, 2001.
45. Elkins AD: Optimizing the use of radiosurgery and all its varieties, *Vet Forum* April:50-56, 1998.
46. Altman RB: Radiosurgery (electrosurgery). In Altman RB, Clubb SL, Dorrestein GM, et al, editors: *Avian Medicine and Surgery*, Philadelphia, 1997, WB Saunders.
47. Sherman JA: *Oral Electrosurgery: An Illustrated Clinical Guide*, London, 1992, Martin Dunitz.
48. Bartels KE: Perspectives on the use of LASERS in veterinary medicine, *Laser Surgery Handbook*, 2000, AccuVet.
49. Maness WC, Roeber ES, Clark RE et al: Histological evaluation of electrosurgery with varying frequency and waveform, *J Prosthet Dent* 40:304-312, 1978.

Deborah Carboni
Thomas N. Tully, Jr.

CHAPTER 11

MARSUPIALS

■ INTRODUCTION

Marsupials are an interesting group of animals. These primitive mammals are being presented to veterinarians with increased frequency. This chapter will provide a review of common species found as both pets and in zoologic settings.

■ HUSBANDRY

Tammar Wallabies

Because tammar wallabies *(Macropus eugenii)* are small macropods, this species can be maintained within large groups in relatively small enclosures. As these animals browse heavily on grass, it is important that they have yards for periodic grazing. Tammar wallabies will eat bark they can access at the base of trees; therefore, tree guards made of wire are advisable. Pelleted food similar to what might be fed to domestic ruminants is often the primary diet component for these animals in captive settings. As stated, grass is advisable as a supplemental feed, but if grass is not available, alfalfa hay can be provided as an alternative.

The natural habitat of the tammar wallaby is low-growing and coastal scrub, eucalyptus species, woodland thickets, and sclerophyll forest. As such, it is important to provide shelter and places to hide, using branches and large, hollow concrete tubing in their yards.

The smaller size of the tammar wallaby makes it easier to catch than its larger counterparts. As with all exotic species, tammar wallaby captures should be conducted by experienced personnel and planned well in advance to minimize stress to the animal(s). An efficient capture will minimize the chance of injury that might otherwise occur from running into fences or other animals within the enclosure. A long-handled net can be used for the initial capture. Removal of the animal from the net is achieved by holding the base of the tail and holding the animal on its back. Animals can then be placed into a closed mesh bag. The bag should be as lightweight as possible to avoid any undue weight on the animal. Once restrained in the relative darkness of the bag, the animal will usually become calm, allowing for easier examination.

One of the most common reasons for examining these animals in captivity is to monitor breeding and pregnancy. Examination should be carried out while the animal is in a Hessian bag, again holding at the base of the tail and placing the animal on its back. The back legs should be free of the bag to prevent injury and allow better exposure of the pouch. The appearance of the pouch can be an indicator of the reproductive state of the animal. The pouch normally has a "dirty" appearance and is covered in a dark, tacky secretion. If the pouch appears moist and clean, then the female has likely been licking it in anticipation of an imminent birth. The presence of an elongated teat in an empty pouch indicates ongoing suckling of an "on foot" pouch young. Female tammars are capable of nursing two pouch young at the same time, one newborn and one on foot.

Fat-Tailed Dunnart

Fat-tailed dunnarts *(Sminthopsis crassicaudita)* can be maintained in windowless rooms with artificial light and at a constant temperature of 20° C to 24° C. Multiple rooms can be designated, each with a particular purpose. One room can have a reduced day length of 8 hours in preparation for stimulating males to breed. Other rooms to include are a nursery/maintain room and a breeding room—each with a 16-hour-day length.

299

Galvanized metal breeding cages (~50 × 35 × 20 cm) with hinged mesh tops, removable plate glass fronts, and metal base trays are advisable for this species. Nest boxes should be plastic (for ease of cleaning) and well ventilated, with shredded paper as a substrate. Animals that are able to eat on their own can be housed in standard laboratory rat cages. Plastic mouse wheels should be provided for breeding animals but not for nursing animals. It is essential to provide dry, clean autoclaved sand in cage trays for animals to groom themselves.

The natural diet of the fat-tailed dunnart is mainly comprised of invertebrate species (e.g., locusts, moths, cockroaches, centipedes, and scorpions) and vertebrates (e.g., small lizards and baby mice). In the laboratory setting, the dunnart can be fed canned pet food, dry cat food, and mealworms. Water and dry cat food should be fed ad libitum.

Restraint of the dunnart requires holding the tail and supporting the body. Brief restraint is accomplished by grasping the scruff of the neck. Pouch and health checks should not be conducted more than once a week to limit stress.

Brushtail Opossum

It is the habit of the brushtail opossum (*Trichosurus vulpecula*) to remain solitary, with the exceptions of the mating period and when nesting and feeding sites are limited. Cage styles include individual wire cages (1 m × 0.4 m × 0.4 m or 1 m × 0.4 m × 0.55 m) with mesh floors and a removable nest box (0.35 m × 0.2 m × 0.2 m), galvanized wire rabbit cages (0.5 m × 0.3 m × 0.55 m), and stainless steel wire cages (0.76 m × 0.6 m × 0.6 m). To ensure seclusion, solid sides can be provided with a drape over the cage front. Catch trays under cages should be cleaned and waste food removed once daily. Nest boxes should be cleaned at least once a week.

Group housing is possible for the brushtail opossum. Wire mesh pens with grass or concrete floors work well. Outdoor enclosures should be well built and impenetrable to birds or vermin. Enclosure sizes for breeding are approximately 11 m² for two animals, 16 m² for three to four animals, and 8 m² for up to seven animals. Identification of group-housed animals can be a challenge, and therefore individual animals should be identified by a small numbered metal ear tag or some other means of permanent identification. Opossums can maintain a body temperature of 36° C to 37° C in ambient temperatures from 10° C to 30° C. Yet, it is important that outdoor pens have shelters for the opossums to escape wind and rain. Nesting boxes or Hessian nesting sacks should be provided for each individual. Perches and branches will provide enrichment and reduce aggression. In particularly warm climates, ventilation and insulation may be required.

Opossums are hindgut fermenters, and as such, their digestive system is best equipped to handle a high-fiber diet. The cecum and proximal colon are well developed and serve as the primary sites of microbial fermentation. The brushtail opossum is predominantly an herbivore. In the wild, leaves, blossoms, and fruit from a wide range of tree species are consumed. Grass, clover, and broadleaf weeds also are part of their natural diet. They have been known to eat small birds, eggs, and

invertebrates as well. In the captive situation, a variety of fruits and vegetables, eucalyptus, and other leafy vegetation can be offered. Rabbit or stock feed pellets may be offered in a waterproof hopper, and water in a self-filling trough is appropriate for ad libitum administration in the outdoor environment. Opossums are susceptible to calcium toxicity and subsequent calcinosis; therefore, food with high calcium content should be avoided. Brushtails tend to be wasteful feeders, but on average, a 3.0 kg animal eats approximately 60 to 160 g of pellets daily. Adult live weights range between 1400 and 1600 g depending on diet, exercise, and genetic background.

Sugar Gliders

Sugar gliders (*Petaurus breviceps*) are best maintained in groups of two or more. Cage size should be appropriate to the number of animals being housed within the cage. For example, a 50 × 50 × 75-cm cage would accommodate two sugar gliders, and a 2 × 2 × 2-m aviary-type cage would hold up to six sugar gliders. Wire openings should be no greater than 2 × 2 cm. If no horizontal bars are present, vertical bars should be spaced no more than 6 mm apart. Galvanized wire should be avoided, as galvanization incorporates zinc and lead components, and therefore the potential for toxicity exists if these elements are consumed over time. Enrichment and use of cage space can be encouraged by providing tree branches and an exercise wheel 25 cm in diameter. It is important that the wheel is solid and not wire to avoid tail entrapment. In the wild, sugar gliders will hide in leafy nests found in the hollows of trees. This can be recreated in captivity by providing a hollow log or small wooden box. A 25 × 10 × 15-cm nest box with a 5-cm diameter entrance hole is appropriate for about six sugar gliders. The size of the nest box can be a determinant of group size in captivity. The nest box should be cleaned on a regular basis. A hinged top allows easy accessibility for capture and examination of the captive glider. It is important to note that sugar gliders will chew wooden structures, so nest boxes made of wood may need to be replaced.

A piece of cloth or sock placed in a nest box will provide comfort and security to a sugar glider. Owners may make the common error of using cedar or pine shavings. These wood products should be avoided because the aromatic oils in these products can prove to be toxic.

On average, owners will keep sugar gliders at temperatures between 64° F and 75° F (18° C to 24° C). However, this is the lower end of the normal ambient temperature for these animals; supplemental heat for these animals must be provided. Caution should be taken to prevent thermal burns that may occur with an additional heat source. Sugar gliders can withstand temperatures up to 88° F (31° C), but any warmer and hyperthermia is likely to result.

■ PERFORMING A PHYSICAL EXAMINATION

The diversity of marsupial species presented to the veterinary practitioner appears to be increasing. Before initiating a clinical

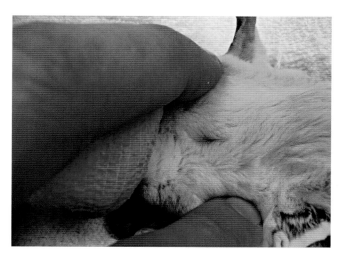

Figure 11-1 Male sugar glider, ventral chest gland.

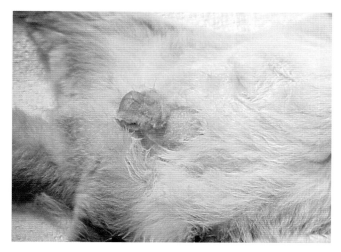

Figure 11-2 Pendulous scrotum of male sugar glider. The penis is actually located candal to the scrotum.

examination on any marsupial species, it is the responsibility of the practitioner to be familiar with the normal appearance and behavior of the species he or she is examining.

The sugar glider is gaining popularity as a companion animal and is one of the marsupials being presented more frequently to veterinary practice. In the wild, the sugar glider is known to inhabit the forests of Australia, New Guinea, and Tasmania. Its body averages 7 inches in length, with another 8 inches of tail.

The sugar glider has a thick, gray coat with a distinct black stripe running down its spine. Its ability to glide from tree to tree is assisted by a membrane of skin known as a *patagium,* which connects the lateral aspect of the forelimbs with the tarsi of the hindlimbs and forms a primitive wing. A bushy, squirrel-like tail acts as a rudder when the animal leaps through the air.

In the wild, sugar gliders are communal as a species. Each individual is marked with the scent of the dominant male in the group, and his scent is also used to mark territory (Figure 11-1). Sugar gliders will feed on sap, in particular, gum from the wattle tree, as well as fruit, nectar, and insects procured during flight. They can be aggressive animals and will attack small mammals if they perceive those mammals as a threat.

Sugar gliders breed readily in captivity, and as pets, sugar gliders can learn to recognize their owners. Young that are familiarized with their owners upon leaving the pouch should be encouraged to be "human oriented"; that is, the owners should have them riding in a small pocket, accepting hand-feeding, and accepting handling. Because these marsupials are inherently communal, singly housed sugar gliders may develop aberrant behavior patterns. To help reduce the development of aberrant behavior, a large cage should be used for housing to occupy the animal's time with climbing and gliding. An enclosed hiding area is also essential, to provide a sense of security.

Physical examination of the sugar glider can be a challenge to the veterinary practitioner, as they are usually intolerant of palpation and auscultation. Observation of the animal from a distance may offer the best opportunity for initial evaluation of respiration, musculoskeletal coordination, mental alertness, hair coat condition, sight and hearing acuity, and response to stimuli.

Owners should be briefed on the limitations of further examination without the benefit of inhalation anesthesia. If an owner should elect to forego general anesthesia, he or she should be informed, before the examination begins, of glider response under the duration and stress of restraint. The sugar glider is a nocturnal species and can be alarmed by sudden exposure to the bright lighting of an exam room. Although an owner may be familiar with the short chattering screams heard when a sugar glider is suddenly startled, they may be less accustomed to the more extensive vocalizations emitted upon restraint.

Though a sugar glider may be assessed to be physically healthy, it is essential to discuss nutrition, husbandry, and housing with the owner; an educated owner will contribute to the future health and well-being of the patient. If a sugar glider should arrive to the veterinary clinic in ill health, the owner must understand the necessity and benefit of a light plane of anesthesia to minimize added stress to the patient while the veterinarian is performing a thorough physical exam and diagnostic tests (e.g., radiographs, blood work). The full extent of medical problems that may be encountered with sugar gliders is still unknown to veterinary medicine. There are several common concerns of many new sugar glider owners.

Male sugar gliders have a scent gland on top of their heads; however, owners may report it as a bald spot and think it is the result of the animal's rubbing its head on the cage, nest box, or directly onto the female. These animals also have a scent gland on their chest (see Figure 11-1). Male sugar gliders, like other marsupials, have unique genitalia. The penis of these animals is bifurcated, and the scrotum is located cranial to the penis (Figure 11-2).

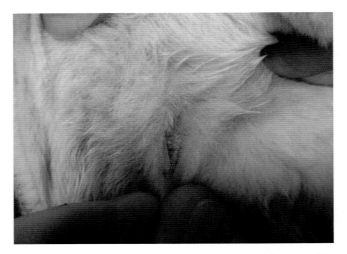

Figure 11-3 Marsupium of female sugar glider. (Courtesy Ms. Christina Legleu.)

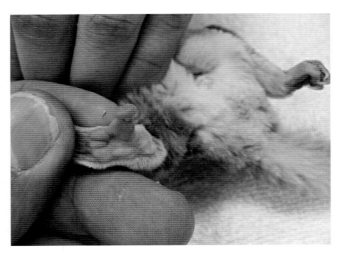

Figure 11-4 Rear foot of sugar glider. For complete examination, digits should be palpated for injury, infection, or the presence of foreign material.

Abdominal masses may indicate that a female glider is pregnant. The symmetry of these masses can reveal the number of young being carried by the female (Figure 11-3). Most pregnant sugar gliders give birth to one or two joeys. Gestation length is a mere 16 days, and once born, the joeys find their way to the pouch at the earliest stages of development. Joeys will remain in the pouch up to $2\frac{1}{2}$ months. Thereafter, the developing young will begin to venture from the pouch, returning primarily to nurse and for protection. The intermittent pouch life will last for a period of 1 to 2 months. The male glider is quite gentle and receptive to these newcomers of the nest box.

Reduced appetite or anorexia may be the result of any number of initiating factors. Stress is one of the more frequent causes of irregular eating patterns affecting sugar gliders. Sources of stress for a sugar glider can include environmental change; lack of a dark, secure hiding place; or absence of a companion. Illness or injury also may cause a decrease in appetite. Abnormal or damaged dentition should be a consideration of the practitioner presented with a glider having a depressed appetite. Cataracts or blindness cause obvious restrictions to eating as well. Dentition and ocular abnormalities have been known to occur in the offspring of obese parents. Blindness likely originates from the inadequate nutrition that was the predisposing factor for the obese condition of the parents rather than the actual obesity itself.

Rear leg paresis or paralysis has been noted within the species. The exact cause(s) remain undetermined, although reduced opportunity for exercise as a result of captivity may play a role. Nutritional deficiencies, such as inadequate protein intake, should be considered, and injections of vitamin B complex, vitamin C, vitamins A and D_3, vitamin E and selenium, and calcium may be administered to treat the condition.[1]

Sugar gliders appearing to miss landings, bounce off walls, or fall frequently may be suffering from one of several disease conditions. Rear limb ataxia, blindness, and obesity can all cause incoordination in gliders. Trauma resulting in long bone fractures, dislocations, or soft tissue trauma can have similar patient presentation.

Instability in, or absence of, normal stance should be investigated, commencing with a physical exam. General anesthesia of the patient should be used to ensure a thorough examination of the animal is obtained. Primary muscle bellies should be checked for asymmetry as a result of atrophy or swelling. Digits should be palpated for injury, infection, or foreign material (Figure 11-4). The appendages should be examined for joint symmetry and mobility, flexion and extension. The spinal cord should be palpated for deviation. Radiographs will serve to assist in determining soft tissue or skeletal injury. Appropriate nutrition and husbandry can often help to reduce the incidence of many of these locomotor abnormalities, and as such, client education is essential.

ANESTHESIA AND RESTRAINT
Manual Restraint of Macropods

The type of manual restraint selected for the macropod is dependent upon size. Animals up to 36 kg (80 lb) can be captured manually and then restrained by an experienced handler. The animal is initially caught by grasping the base of the tail with one or two hands. Once a handler gains control of the tail, the animal will tend to bounce upward, and this movement will provide an opportunity for the handler's arm to be placed around the animal's chest, just below the forelimbs. The animal can then be lifted up; however, hindlimb movement can injure veterinary personnel or the animal itself. The tail should be angled forward to prevent the ventral surface striking the handler or a hard surface. The goal of macropod restraint is to minimize any opportunity for the animal to gain leverage. The macropod then is tipped head first into a Hessian or denim bag for transport, weighing, examination, blood collection from the lateral tail vein, or the administration of chemical restraint.

Adult macropods of smaller size, 5 to 10 kg (11-22 lb), may be captured using a net on a long pole (1-2 m). The net should be composed of a fine mesh or solid cloth to prevent entanglement or leg injuries. Macropods sensing capture will often run along the fence line of an enclosure. A keeper can take advantage of this flight response by taking a position along the fence line. A space should be maintained between the fence line and the person that is poised to capture the animal. The capture pole with attached net is held parallel to the fence but behind the keeper. Other individuals then herd the selected animal along the fence line toward the net. As the animal passes between the keeper and the fence, the net is brought forward in front of the animal and the animal contained. Personnel involved with capture and restraint should be cautious not to overstress the animal, as stress may result in hyperthermia and subsequent exertional myopathy. If the macropod is not captured on the first attempt, consider postponement of the procedure or darting the animal. Once the animal is netted, basic clinical procedures can be performed. In animals that weigh 36 kg (80 lb) or greater, sedation by remote injection techniques is the safest approach for capture, reducing injury risk to both humans and animal.

Chemical Restraint of Macropods

Chemical restraint of macropods weighing less than 10 kg (22 lb), such as small wallabies, juvenile kangaroos, and wallaroos, may be accomplished with manual restraint and inhalation anesthesia. Anesthetic induction of smaller macropods is best accomplished using 5% isoflurane gas with a 1.5-L flow of oxygen delivered via a face mask. Larger animals require injectable anesthetic agents for chemical immobilization. A variety of these drugs have been used alone or in combination, including pentobarbital, thiopentone, phencyclidine-acepromazine, etorphine, etorphine-acepromazine, etorphine-methotrimeprazine, etorphine-ketamine, droperidol, droperidol-fentanyl, azaperone, alphaxalone-alphadolone, alphachloralose, diazepam, xylazine, ketamine, xylazine-ketamine, tiletamine-zolazepam, and medetomidine-ketamine.

Macropods are especially susceptible to trauma-related injuries and capture myopathy during restraint. The goal of chemical immobilization is a smooth and rapid induction and recovery, thereby reducing the incidence of trauma-related injuries.

Medetomidine-ketamine and tiletamine-zolazepam are two chemical immobilization combinations reported to be particularly effective. Both therapeutic combinations provide a rapid and smooth induction within 10 minutes. The advantage of medetomidine-ketamine over tiletamine-zolazepam is its reversibility with atipamezole. Dosages utilized for these combinations are species dependant. Doses of 40 μg/kg of medetomidine mixed with 4 mg/kg of ketamine administered intramuscularly (IM) have been found to be an effective combination when used on eastern gray kangaroos.[1] Ranges of 40 to 70 μg/kg of medetomidine with 4 to 7 mg/kg of ketamine have been found to be effective for red kangaroos, wallaroos,

Dorcopsis wallabies *(Dorcopsis macleayi)*, and Goodfellow's tree kangaroos *(Dendrolagus goodfellowi)*.[1] Atipamezole given at a dose 5 times the total mg of administered medetomidine has been found to be effective for reversal in the above-mentioned species.[1] A dose of 100 μg/kg of medetomidine and 5 mg/kg ketamine IM has been effective in immobilizing red necked wallabies.[1]

Tiletamine-zolazepam at a dose of 2 to 8 mg/kg is recommended for chemical immobilization of tree kangaroos.[1] In most macropods, however, the general dose range is 3 to 11 mg/kg IM.[1]

Other chemical combinations administered IM to immobilize macropods include xylazine and ketamine. If either medetomidine and ketamine or tiletamine and ketamine are selected as a combination, a supplemental injectable ketamine anesthetic may be administered as needed. Supplemental ketamine administration can be accomplished by placement of an intravenous (IV) catheter in the lateral tail or lateral saphenous veins.

Propofol offers the benefit of being an ultra–short-acting induction agent. An adverse side effect of propofol administration is an initial transient apnea. To reduce the risk associated with transient apnea, intubation is recommended when this agent is used. The standard mammalian dose of 6 to 8 mg/kg propofol is also the recommended dose for macropods and should be given slowly to effect. Alternatively, an animal can be premedicated with midazolam at 0.2 mg/kg, allowing a lower dose of 5 mg/kg of propofol to be given to effect.

If a surgical plane of anesthesia is desired, supplemental inhalation anesthetic (e.g., isoflurane), in addition to an injectable agent, may need to be supplied. Gas is delivered by a face mask and then followed by endotracheal intubation. The placement of an endotracheal tube is a challenge in macropods because of a narrow mouth opening. To aid in glottis positioning and endotracheal tube placement, the animal should be placed in dorsal recumbency with the head fully extended over the side of a table. By doing so, the glottis is aligned with the angle of the mouth, allowing easier passage of an endotracheal tube. Strips of gauze can be placed through and around the maxilla and mandible as an aid to open the mouth. A laryngoscope with a long blade (15 cm or 6 inches) is recommended to visualize the glottis as a straight, semirigid endotracheal tube is passed into the mouth. Visualization of the intubation procedure can be impeded by the tube and again is best performed utilizing the position described above. If intubation is unsuccessful, an alternative is to pass a smaller diameter tube first, such as a 6-Fr dog urinary polypropylene catheter. This smaller tube can be easily visualized as it is put into the trachea, thus confirming proper placement. The endotracheal tube is then passed over the catheter, which serves as a guide. The tube is secured by first tying a strip of gauze around the tube and then tying the remaining lengths of material behind the base of the skull. Both isoflurane and halothane inhalation anesthetics have been used successfully for macropod anesthetic induction and maintenance.

Manual Restraint of Sugar Gliders

The behavior of sugar gliders under manual restraint is often dependent on frequency of human handling. Sugar gliders that have been hand raised and/or frequently handled can be held in a small towel with cupped hands. Anyone holding one of these small marsupials should remain cautious because even a tame glider who is startled will attempt to escape. Many sugar gliders try to bite when being held. As such, restraint should include using the thumb and middle finger to hold the head and the index finger placed on top of it with the body being supported with the palm of the hand. Another method of restraint involves placement of a small, cloth bag over the handler's hand. It is important that the hand be on the inside of the bag or on the side with seams. The animal can then be cupped in the palm of the hand and the bag pulled off the hand and over the animal, thereby catching the animal in the bag. The seams of the bag will now be on the outside preventing any chance of the animal's entanglement in the frayed edge of a seam. The bag will provide a sense of security to the glider and help to keep it calm. It also provides a convenient way to weigh the animal as well as expose body parts for examination. The head alone can be exposed for masked anesthetic induction.

Sugar Glider Anesthesia

Anesthesia for sugar glider patients is best accomplished with inhalation agents (e.g., isoflurane). A medium- or large-sized mask can be used as an induction chamber, with isoflurane being delivered at a level of 5% and an oxygen flow rate of 1 L/min (Figure 11-5). Once induced, the animal can be transferred to a smaller face mask and maintained at 2% isoflurane (600-800 ml/L oxygen). Placement of an endotracheal tube (e.g., 14-16 gauge intravenous catheter) may be attempted, but it presents an obvious challenge in terms of the animal's size

and the possibility of tube blockage caused by the buildup of respiratory secretions.

Injectable anesthetics are rarely used to anesthetize sugar glider patients because inhalation agents have a much reduced risk and are easily provided. One study reported using tiletamine-zolazepam at doses ranging from 8.4 to 12.8 mg/kg IM with no adverse side effects.[1] However, tiletamine-zolazepam at 10 mg/kg has been associated with neurologic problems and death in squirrel gliders (*Petaurus norfolcensis*), so caution is advised with use of this drug.[1] Ketamine has also been used to induce anesthesia in gliders at a recommended dose of 20 mg/kg.[1] Acepromazine has been combined with butorphanol and given orally or with ketamine and given subcutaneously (SC) to maintain postoperative sedation and analgesia.

Manual Restraint of Opossums

The private practitioner or wildlife rehabilitator may be presented with a Virginia opossum (*Didelphus virginiana*) (Figure 11-6). Often, these animals have incurred vehicle or fight injuries, and as a result, attention and care must be taken in their restraint (Figure 11-7). Heavy gloves and towels should be used during the removal of the animal from its enclosure. These animals have particularly sharp teeth and, if not appropriately restrained, will turn quickly to bite. Similarly, opossums retain long claws and may scratch in a threatened situation. A firm grasp of the scruff of the neck and the base of the tail are essential in the movement of the animal. If assistance is available, these restraints can be divided between two individuals. However, if the handler is alone, the animal's head and neck should be held farthest from the handler and the base of the tail held as the primary means of support in the carriage of the animal. As in other species, the tip of the tail should never be held, as injury may result. Masked induction with 5% isoflurane and 1.5 L/min of oxygen followed by

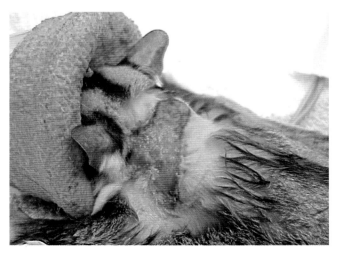

Figure 11-5 Anesthetized sugar glider: using face mask to examine degloving injury due to trauma associated with Elizabethan collar application.

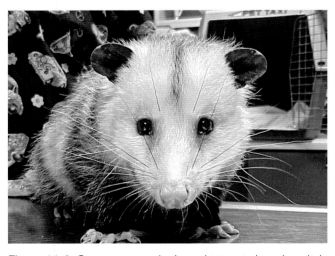

Figure 11-6 Opossums may be brought to veterinary hospitals as nonreleasable pets or injured wildlife.

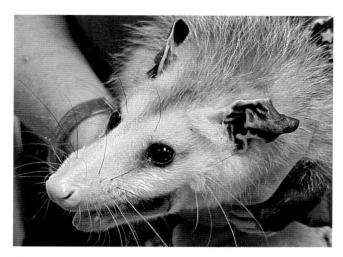

Figure 11-7 A firm grasp of the head is recommended for opossums that resist examination.

endotracheal intubation and a maintenance rate of 2% to 3% isoflurane and an oxygen flow rate of 1.5 L/min of oxygen is considered sufficient for basic examination, wound care, and diagnostics.

■ COMMON PRESENTATIONS BY SYSTEM

Respiratory System

Respiratory disease as a primary illness is rarely noted in marsupial species. Rather, respiratory conditions are more often associated with another disease process or as an opportunistic consequence. Similar to that of other companion animal species, diseases associated with the respiratory tract of marsupials may occur as a result of infectious disease (e.g., bacteria, viruses, parasites, fungi, yeast), neoplasia, and trauma. Diagnoses and treatments pursued for these disease processes should follow standard protocols.

TRAUMA

The marsupial with traumatic injury is one of the more frequent medical presentations encountered by the veterinary practitioner. Injuries sustained as a result of, for example, traumatic injury or vehicle impact, may directly result in impaired function to the head, neck, and thorax.

Traumatic injuries to the upper respiratory tract may involve fracture or laceration to the nares, turbinates, larynx, or trachea. Treatments for such injuries would not be unlike those pursued in companion animal medicine. If breathing itself is impaired, a tracheotomy can be performed and, if necessary, the tracheostomy tube left in place until healing occurs. Injuries involving the lower respiratory system, such as fractures to the ribs, may be accompanied by pneumothorax, diaphragmatic hernia, or collapsed lungs. Hemothorax is often associated with lacerated lungs or thoracic vessels. Treatment courses, again, follow those used in companion animals.

Trauma is often accompanied by shock. Pulmonary manifestations of shock include consolidation of tissue with increased risk of bacterial infection. Effects of shock on the lung are highly species specific. Some may experience acute respiratory distress syndrome or shock lung, which is characterized as pulmonary edema and decreased activity of alveolar macrophages.

FOREIGN BODIES

The foreign bodies most commonly found in the upper respiratory tract of marsupial species are the grass seed and grass awn. Over the course of eating, animals will accidentally inhale seeds, awns, or both. Grass seeds, in particular, will enter the nares of captive, grazing marsupial species, such as kangaroos, wallabies, and wombats. Wombats are susceptible to grass seed inhalation and present with unilateral purulent nasal discharge. Practitioners should be aware that marsupials that have contact with hay or straw, either as a bedding material or in an anesthetic recovery area, inadvertently inhale grass seeds.

Foreign bodies in the nares manifest in symptoms of unilateral purulent nasal discharge, sneezing, and persistent pawing at the nares. The offending foreign body must be visualized before removal. The animal first should be heavily sedated or placed under general anesthesia. An otoscope, rigid arthroscope, or endoscope can then be used to locate the foreign material. Removal is best achieved with alligator forceps. Antibiotics should be prescribed as a prophylaxis against bacterial infection. Clavulanic acid and amoxicillin (Clavamox) can be given to macropods and wombats at a dose of 12.5 mg/kg IM twice a day.[1] Alternatively, a Clavamox dose of 25 mg/kg can be given IM or SC once daily. The oral administration of Clavamox in macropods and wombats has been associated with yeast overgrowth in the gastrointestinal tract and subsequent diarrhea; therefore, if Clavamox is prescribed, treatment and patient response should be carefully monitored.

Diagnosis of foreign bodies within the lower respiratory tract of marsupials is infrequent when compared with the upper respiratory system. However, hand-raised marsupials are prone to aspiration of artificial milk formula and accompanying aspiration pneumonia. Aspiration of artificial milk is due most often to a juvenile marsupial receiving milk at too high a flow rate. The source of this high flow rate is usually an artificial teat with an opening that is too large. Squeezing a feed bottle or syringe feeding also can deliver milk in amounts the animal cannot accommodate. Attention to a patient's body temperature is essential, as hypothermia can predispose an orphaned marsupial to inhalation pneumonia as well. Animals with low body temperatures are sluggish and have a depressed swallow reflex, which can result in the inhalation of artificial milk formula.

VIRAL INFECTIONS

A poxvirus is associated with the development of papillomatous proliferations on the skin of macropods. The areas affected most often by these papillomatous proliferations are the head and extremities. The development of papillomas around the external nares and mouth may interfere with normal respiration. Marsupial species affected by this condition include tammar wallabies, Agile wallabies (*Macropus agilis*), swamp wallabies (*Wallabia bicolor*), eastern wallaroos (*Macropus robustus*), quokkas, red kangaroos (*Macropus rufus*), eastern gray kangaroos (*Macropus giganteus*), and western gray kangaroos (*Macropus fuliginosus*).[1] The disease itself is considered self-limiting, but if the growths impair an animal's ability to eat or breathe, surgical removal is an option.

An orbivirus was reported as causing death in Australian tammar wallabies during the summer months.[2] No premonitory signs were evident, and animals were usually found either comatose or dead. Diagnosis was based on history, serologic testing, and postmortem examination. Gross pathologic findings included marked pulmonary congestion and edema, hepatic congestion, and frequently, subcutaneous edema in the hindlimbs.[2] No effective treatment is currently available. Vaccine development for this orbivirus is currently in progress.

A herpesvirus has been established as the cause of death in a variety of marsupial species.[2] Clinical signs associated with this virus include respiratory rales, conjunctivitis, incoordination, and death.[2] Serologic testing is available, but a definitive diagnosis is often made when histopathologic examination of affected liver tissue reveals intranuclear inclusion bodies in hepatocytes. A viable treatment option has yet to be found.

BACTERIAL INFECTIONS

Although bacterial infection of the upper respiratory tract is uncommon in marsupial species, the koala appears to be most susceptible. Bacterial infections reported to cause rhinitis in the koala include *Bordetella bronchiseptica*, *Pseudomonas* spp., *Corynebacterium* spp., *Streptococcus* spp., *Escherichia coli*, *Micrococcus* spp., *Staphylococcus* spp., *Proteus* spp., *Pasteurella* spp., and *Enterobacter* spp.[1] In the koala, *Chlamydophila psittaci* has been implicated as a cause of nasal discharge.[1] Clinical signs of upper respiratory tract disease are not unlike those seen in mammalian species. Bilateral nasal discharge, sneezing, anorexia, and coughing are the more common signs encountered. Nasal discharge can be clear or mucopurulent in appearance. Pharyngitis and regional lymph node enlargement have been seen to occur. If *Chlamydophila psittaci* is suspected, specific guidelines should be followed for specimen collection, transport, and storage. The practitioner should be aware of the following:[1]

1. Wooden-shafted swabs are toxic to the *Chlamydophila psittaci* organism, so nontoxic aluminum-shafted plain cotton swabs should be selected.
2. The use of a *Chlamydophila psittaci*–specific transport medium is required.
3. Vigorous swabbing is required to obtain multiple host epithelial cells.
4. To ensure a maximal amount of organism is collected, two swabs should be taken of a suspect site and placed in the same vial of transport medium.

Swabs of the nasal mucosa can be analyzed with antigen enzyme-linked immunosorbent assay (ELISA) to assist in the diagnosis of chlamydiosis. Antigen ELISA kits are commercially available to practitioners. Antigen detection through direct immunofluorescence can also be performed with a commercial kit, but this technique appears less sensitive than the ELISA.[1]

Complement fixation tests can be used to detect antibody in serum but are less accurate than other tests available. Testing using polymerase chain reaction (PCR) technology is showing promise in the diagnosis of koala chlamydiosis.

The selection of an antibiotic in the treatment of rhinitis should be based on culture and sensitivity testing. The route of administration can be oral, parenteral, or through nebulization. Saline nebulization, in combination with systemic antibiotic therapy, appears particularly effective.

Effective treatments for chlamydiosis include doxycycline hydrochloride, 5 mg/kg every 7 days IM for 6 weeks; chloramphenicol, 30 mg/kg SC every 12 hours for 7 to 10 days; and oxytetracycline, 5 mg/kg SC every 7 days for a maximum of 4 injections.[1] Pseudoephedrine hydrochloride at a dosage of 1 mg/kg every 12 hours can be administered via nebulization or per os (PO) as a decongestant. The mucolytic, bromhexine hydrochloride given at a dosage of 2 mg/kg every 12 hours PO or through nebulization also can help to relieve clinical signs.[1] Supplemental feeding should be given to koalas when they are being treated with antibiotics, as antimicrobial effects of the therapeutic agents on the gastrointestinal flora have been associated with significant weight loss.

Bacterial pneumonias are commonly diagnosed in the koala. Organisms that have been identified as a causative agent of koala bacterial pneumonia include *Corynebacteria* spp., *Haemophilus* spp., *Bordetella bronchiseptica*, *Pseudomonas aeruginosa*, and *Streptobacillus moniliformis*. The animal may show signs of bilateral purulent nasal discharge, coughing, audible respiratory noises, and anorexia. Recommended diagnostic tests include culture and sensitivity and transtracheal wash. Thoracic radiography will often reveal advancement of disease and give indication to prognosis. Parenteral antibiotics are the treatment of choice and should be selected on the basis of culture and sensitivity results. Nebulization with an appropriate antibiotic can significantly contribute to patient recovery. Mucolytics can be used as a supportive measure and may be added to the nebulization cocktail. A vaccination for *Bordetella bronchiseptica* is available as a cell-free extract named Canvac-BB (CSL, Ltd., Parkville, Victoria, Australia). The vaccination protocol established for the koala is 2 doses SC 4 weeks apart and then annual boosters thereafter.

Necrobacillosis, commonly known as lumpy jaw, is a tooth root infection frequently encountered in captive macropods. Several factors are believed to foster the development of the disease, including overcrowding and poor husbandry—which lead to excessive fecal contamination, especially around feed stations—and a diet containing soft feed or awns. *Bacteroides (Dichelobacter) nodosus* and *Fusobacterium necrophorum*, usually acting synergistically, invade and cause infection. Other bacteria less commonly isolated from tooth root infections include *Actinomyces* spp. and *Corynebacterium* spp. Additional opportunistic bacteria will invade as an infection advances and may be the only organisms isolated when cultures are finally obtained. Primary clinical signs associated with necrobacillosis are swelling around the face and jaw, excessive salivation, loss of condition because of difficulty in eating, depression, and lethargy. Proptosis of the globe and squinting may be observed as a result of retrobulbar abscessation. A bacteremia may result, spreading organisms to other areas of the body, including the spleen, liver, stomach, bones, and lungs. Treatment of lumpy jaw is focused on removal of affected teeth and debridement of affected soft tissue. Clindamycin is the antibiotic of choice at a dose of 11 mg/kg PO (capsules or liquid) every 12 hours. Animals find the liquid formulation more palatable than capsules, and an injectable formulation exists but is expensive and restricted to IV use. Duration of treatment should be a minimum of 6 months because of the possibility of disease recurrence. Large doses of penicillin (150 mg/kg procaine penicillin and 112.5 mg/kg benzathine penicillin) every second day for approximately 2 weeks has also been recommended, but efficacy of this treatment course is unknown.[1]

Prevention of necrobacillosis focuses on providing appropriate diet and husbandry for captive animals. Overcrowding of macropod species should be avoided. Environments should be routinely cleaned to avoid the buildup of fecal material both on the ground and around food sources. A *Bacteroides nodosus* vaccine has been recommended at the following weights and doses: less than 5 kg, 0.2 ml SC; 5 to 10 kg, 0.25 ml SC; 10 to 20 kg, 0.5 ml SC; and more than 20 kg, 1 ml SC.[1] The skin over the ribs is the preferred site for recommended SC vaccine injection. Sterile abscesses have been reported at the vaccine injection sites. The vaccine schedule is 2 doses 4 weeks apart, then once a year.

Mycobacteriosis has been reported as a source of respiratory disease in marsupial species.[1] Tuberculosis caused by *Mycobacterium bovis* has had particular impact on the brushtail possum population in New Zealand. The disease is contracted from possums grazing in pastures frequented by infected animals (e.g., cattle, deer, or other possums). Discharge is emitted from the lymph nodes of these diseased animals and usually serves as the source of pasture contamination. Once a possum is exposed, the organism spreads throughout the body, targeting the lungs and other vital organs. Clinical signs associated with marsupial tuberculosis include dyspnea, depression, anorexia, and weight loss. Treatment of the wild brushtail possum is often not pursued because this animal is considered a pest species in New Zealand. The brushtail possum is viewed as perpetuating *Mycobacterium bovis* in cattle and deer herds in New Zealand, resulting in significant economic loss.

Mycobacteriosis has had a similar impact on captive tree kangaroos in the United States. It has been reported as a common cause of disease and mortality in three species of tree kangaroos in particular, including Matschie's (*Dendrolagus matschiei*), Goodfellow's (*Dendrolagus goodfellowi*), and Grizzled (*Dendrolagus inustus*).[1] *Mycobacterium avium* complex is the cause of more than 90% of infections diagnosed in captive tree kangaroos maintained in the United States. The apparent susceptibility of these animals is attributed to a cellular immune response comparatively lower than what is observed in eutherian mammals or other marsupial species. Clinical signs associated with mycobacteriosis in tree kangaroos include weight loss, dyspnea, lameness, abscesses, neurologic problems, and blindness. Definitive antemortem diagnosis is a challenge with the tree kangaroo, and signalment, history, clinical signs, radiology, and transtracheal washes are included as part of the recommended diagnostic regimen. The treatment protocol for infected tree kangaroos is amikacin, 3 mg/kg IM every 12 hours; rifabutin, 20 mg/kg PO every 24 hours; ethambutol, 20 mg/kg PO every 24 hours, and azithromycin, 20 mg/kg PO every 24 hours.[1] The duration of treatment can be quite long, with amikacin usually administered for 10 to 12 weeks and oral medications for 3 years or longer. Unfortunately, treatments have yielded poor results. The mycobacterial organism can often still be detected on cultures of transtracheal washes performed 3 or more years after treatment was initiated. Preventing animals from exposure to the organism is the best approach to controlling this organism. Captive tree kangaroos should not be housed near captive birds because of the risk of transmission posed by *Mycobacterium avium* complex.

FUNGAL INFECTIONS

One of the more common infections affecting the upper respiratory tract of marsupial species is cryptococcosis. Australian marsupials including brushtail possums, ringtail possums (*Pseudocheirus peregrinus*), striped possums (*Dactylopsila trivirgata*), Leadbeater's possums (*Gymnobelideus leadbeateri*), tammar wallabies, red-necked wallabies (*Macropus rufogriseus*), spectacled hare wallabies (*Largorchestes conspicillatus*), quokkas (*Setonix brachyurus*), and wombats and echidnas (*Tachyglossus aculeatus*) have been reported as having the disease.[1] The species that appears particularly susceptible, however, is the koala. The causative agent is the yeast-like fungi, *Cryptococcus neoformans var gattii*. The organism's close association with river red gums (*Eucalyptus camaldulensis*), mugga ironbarks (*Eucalyptyus sideroxylon*), and other red gum species results in extremely high koala exposure rates. Inhalation of the organism from a contaminated environment is believed to be the primary source of exposure. Clinical signs that have been observed in the koala include unilateral or bilateral nasal discharge, sneezing, and anorexia. The usual course of infection starts at the nares and progresses into the sinuses, with secondary lung involvement. Granulomatous formation may occur in the respiratory tract. Once the animal's respiratory system is infected and there is upper respiratory disease, the organism can infect the central nervous system (CNS) as well. With CNS infection, neurologic signs (e.g., seizures, blindness, behavior changes) may be observed. One of the primary diagnostic tests used to diagnose this disease is the microscopic examination of stained smears collected from the nasal cavity. Diff-Quik staining of the collected sample is easily performed and offers excellent visualization of the yeast-like organisms. India ink may be used as an alternative. Nasal discharge should be cultured, as the organism will grow on Saboraud's agar at 25° C and 37° C. A latex-cryptococcal antigen test (LCAT) is available to detect soluble cryptococcal capsular polysaccharide antigen in body fluid samples. The LCAT can be a particularly effective test when cryptococcosis is suspected, but the site(s) of infection is (are) unknown. Serial dilutions of serum are combined with a suspension of latex particles coated with hyperimmune rabbit serum, with titers of 1 : 2 or greater considered positive. The strength of a positive response can be an indicator of disease severity and, ultimately, prognosis for treatment response and recovery. The decline in LCAT titer is usually slower when compared with clinical improvement but can still be an effective tool in indicating treatment success and prognosis. Survey radiographs of the nasal cavities, sinuses, and lungs also will assist in localizing areas of infection, and survey computed tomography (CT) scans offer even more precision if available.

The recommended treatment protocol for cryptococcosis is fluconazole, 3 mg/kg PO every 24 hours for 30 to 60 days, with a loading dose of 6 mg/kg.[1] Amphotericin B is administered in approximately 50 to 60 ml of Hartmann's solution or 0.9% NaCl at a dose of 0.5 mg/kg SC every second day for 30 days because of the potential for renal toxicity that exists with amphotericin B.[1] Renal function should be checked every 2 weeks. If fluconazole is cost prohibitive, ketoconazole is an acceptable alternative. The dosage offered for ketoconazole is 10 mg/kg PO every 12 hours for 30 to 60 days.[1]

Aspergillus fumigatus has been implicated as a cause of mycotic pneumonia in the macropod. Itraconazole, fluconazole, and amphotericin B are considered to be effective drugs in the treatment regime. *Emmonsia*-like fungal spores have been detected in the lungs of common wombats (*Vombatus ursinus*) and southern hairy-nosed wombats (*Lasiorhinus latifrons*). As burrowing marsupials, they are suspected to inhale the soil-dwelling fungal spores, which then become lodged deep within the lungs, particularly in the alveolar lumen. Levels of infection were determined as being quite high, yet pulmonary responses were mild. Primary pathologic changes in the lungs were mild interstitial fibroplasias and collections of macrophages and leukocytes. The most severe lesions were assessed to be focal granulomas that contained the occasional giant cell. Overall, infection with *Emmonsia*-type fungal spores does not appear to produce any truly debilitating respiratory change.

NEOPLASIA

Primary neoplastic change occurs frequently in the koala and dasyurid species. Koalas, in particular, are susceptible to the development of craniofacial tumors. These tumors are limited to the upper respiratory tract, with subsequent distortion of the nasal cavity and paranasal sinuses that produce related clinical signs. Nasal discharge, facial distortion, and epistaxis are strongly indicative of the disease, but radiographs can significantly assist in determining a diagnosis. To distinguish a craniofacial tumor from a cryptococcal granuloma, a biopsy of the mass is recommended. Histologic examination reveals craniofacial tumors to be comprised of a mixture of cartilage and bone. Scattered areas or irregular compartments of hypertrophying chondrocytes are embedded in, or surrounded by, vascular and connective tissue. Different stages of calcification or ossification are also evident. Treatment of these tumors is at

best palliative, because recurrence is likely, even with complete surgical removal. Euthanasia should be considered in highly infiltrative or advanced cases.

Another common tumor occurring in the respiratory tract of the koala is mesothelioma. This neoplasm targets the serosal surfaces of body cavities, including the peritoneum and mediastinum. Labored breathing, anorexia, and abdominal distension are the predominant clinical signs associated with mesothelioma growth. Diagnosis is best achieved with thoracocentesis, abdominocentesis, or both, and cytologic testing of the collected sample and radiography. Nodules forming as a result of neoplastic change tend to be fibrous in content and have low cellularity. On histologic exam, mesothelial cells can be expected to predominate, with collagen fibers, ground substance, spindle cells, macrophages, lymphocytes, and neutrophils being present in smaller quantities.

PARASITES

The prevalence of toxoplasmosis is high. The causal agent is a protozoan parasite, *Toxoplasma gondii,* with the cat, serving as the definitive host. Oocysts are shed in the feces of cats and sporulate over a period of 3 to 4 days. Herbivorous marsupials become parasitized after ingesting hay or pasture contaminated with infective oocysts. *Toxoplasma* cysts embedded in animal tissues serve as the source of infection for carnivorous and omnivorous marsupials. The disease itself is multisystemic in effect, with interstitial pneumonia affecting the lungs of marsupial species.[1] Respiratory distress was observed in captive koalas during one reported outbreak.[1] Antemortem diagnosis of toxoplasmosis can be a challenge because of its acute onset and progression, but clinical signs and rising toxoplasma titers may be used to identify the disease. Because of the acute nature of the disease, IgM levels should be evaluated, as they represent an animal's primary immune response; IgG titers provide evidence of chronic or past exposure. The indirect fluorescent antibody method is used to detect both IgM and IgG immunoglobulins.

Treatment can be attempted using a potentiated sulfonamide, such as sulfadimethoxine, concomitantly with pyrimethamine. Clindamycin is another option at a dosage of 11 mg/kg twice daily PO or IM for at least 30 days.[1] Neither of these treatments has been shown to be very effective. Atovaquone (Wellvone) has been given at a dosage of 50 to 100 mg/kg PO every 24 hours for a minimum of 30 days, but response to this drug is also poor.[1]

Interstitial pneumonia in the koala has also been attributed to a parasitic infection (e.g., *Marsupiostrongylus* spp.). Histopathologic testing revealed nematodes both in the bronchioles and in distal airways. An infiltration of neutrophils, eosinophils, and mononuclear cells into alveolar walls was also observed. Giant cells around the distal airways and hyperplastic peribronchiolar lymphoid nodules were similarly noted. Parasites of this same genus have been reported to occur in wombats, eastern gray kangaroos, swamp wallabies, and brushtail possums.[3]

In the brushtail possums, *Marsupiostrongylus minesi* has been associated with severe bronchopneumonia.[3] Adult worms have been detected in the bronchioles of affected animals and larvae of the nematode also identified in lung tissue. Histopathologic examination is expected to reveal an inflammatory response, characterized by marked neutrophil infiltration, large numbers of macrophages, lymphoid foci, and extensive fibrinous debris.[3] The parasite and associated lesions are usually incidental findings on postmortem exam. As such, antemortem detection of the parasite is difficult.

Durikainema macropi is a small intravascular nematode found in marsupials. In addition to being identified in the lung, it has been identified in the liver, myocardium, and kidney of koalas. Prominent histologic changes include fibrin deposition and an intense inflammatory reaction characterized by eosinophils and lymphocytes. Ivermectin administered at a dose of 200 µg/kg PO, SC, or topically has been effective in treating marsupial species.[1] Toxicities in wallabies have been reported with the use of benzimidazole anthelmintics.[1]

Capillaria spp. have been recognized as a cause of enzootic bronchitis and bronchiolitis in captive rufous bettongs *(Aepyprymnus rufescens)* and long-nosed potoroos *(Potorous triadactylus)*. With infected animals, anorexia, weight loss, coughing, and dyspnea may be observed. Advanced clinical signs can assist in antemortem diagnosis of the disease, but definitive diagnosis is often made through postmortem examination. Bronchial washings of affected animals may contain trichenelloid eggs and a high number of neutrophils. Eggs may also be seen in fecal samples. Fenbendazole can be used as a treatment for *Capillaria* spp.–infected animals at a dose of 25 mg/kg PO every 24 hours for 5 days.[1] Treatment is generally effective in resolving clinical signs and eliminating eggs from the feces; however, mortalities can occur (likely from the bone marrow suppression associated with fenbendazole). Gross lesions at postmortem are generally confined to the lungs and consist of multiple yellow-gray, slightly raised granulomatous foci dispersed throughout the parenchyma. Squash preparations of these foci often reveal numerous eggs, larvae, and adult capillariid nematodes. Histopathologic samples of the lung frequently reveal congestion, alveolar edema, and emphysema.

Other parasitic infections that have been reported in marsupials include the lung mite in the cuscus and the filaroid nematode, *Breinlia mundayi,* in the swamp wallaby.[1] The latter causes fibrinous peritonitis, pleuritis, and pericarditis.

DIAGNOSTIC PROCEDURES
Radiology
Survey radiographs are an effective first step in evaluating the respiratory tract. Radiographic images can assist in the diagnosis of soft tissue and bone disease. Lung patterns may be helpful in the identification of respiratory disease (e.g., pneumonia). Cryptococcal granulomas in the anterior mediastinum will appear as a space-occupying lesion in the thorax. Fractured ribs and diaphragmatic hernias often are easily identified. If a diaphragmatic hernia is suspected, barium can be administered by nasogastric intubation to confirm diagnosis. Fluid in the thorax associated with mesothelioma in the koala is usually found through radiographic evaluation.

Endoscopy
Endoscopy allows direct visual inspection of the respiratory tract. Rigid endoscopes can be used to visualize and assist in the removal of foreign bodies from the interior nares of larger marsupials, such as wombats, kangaroos, and wallabies. Flexible endoscopes offer maneuverability, particularly in accommodating the limited mouth opening of larger macropods.

Computed tomography scans
Computed tomography (CT) is an effective diagnostic imaging tool that is becoming increasingly available to veterinary clinicians. CT scans are useful in locating soft tissue lesions, such as cryptococcal granulomas within the respiratory tract. Animals must remain motionless during scanning; therefore, a short-acting (10-15–minute) anesthetic given before the procedure is recommended for most marsupial patients.

Ultrasonography
Ultrasonography is not commonly utilized in respiratory medicine but can be helpful in evaluating pleural effusion or neoplastic processes.

Transtracheal aspiration
Transtracheal aspiration is performed in marsupials with a technique similar to that used for domestic animals. Sedation is recommended because restraint for the procedure can be challenging in marsupial species. A catheter is introduced between two tracheal rings, passed to the level of the tracheal bifurcation, and 2 to 3 ml of sterile saline is administered through the catheter into the trachea. The saline is then withdrawn and submitted for cytologic and bacteriologic examination. Alternatively, transoral aspiration may be attempted under sedation or inhalation anesthesia via an endotracheal tube.

Thoracocentesis
Thoracocentesis can be selected as a therapeutic or diagnostic measure. Sedation or inhalation anesthesia is required to perform this procedure in a safe and efficient manner. A standing position is not recommended. As in companion animals, the most productive collection site is the ventral third of the fourth to seventh intercostal space.

MICROBIOLOGY
Standard microbiologic techniques can be used to assist in the diagnosis of infectious disease. The species involved and clinical signs observed are important considerations when trying to identify the etiologic agent suspected to be a microorganism.

SEROLOGY
Latex cryptococcal antigen tests are available for the diagnosis of cryptococcosis in marsupials. A titer of greater than 1 : 2 is representative of active cryptococcal infection. Serologic tests for chlamydiosis, herpesvirus, toxoplasmosis, and orbivirus infections are available.

THERAPEUTICS

Antibiotics

Bacterial infections in the lungs of marsupials are usually attributed to Gram-negative bacteria. *E. coli, Klebsiella* spp., and *Pseudomonas* spp. are three bacteria commonly isolated from the respiratory tracts of marsupials. Initial antibiotic selection should be bacteriocidal with good coverage against Gram-negative bacteria. Antibiotics appropriate in the treatment of pneumonia include amikacin, 7.5 to 15.0 mg/kg IM every 12 hours; gentamicin, 2.5 to 3 mg/kg IM every 8 hours; and enrofloxacin 5 mg/kg PO, IM, or SC every 24 hours.[1]

Steroids

If aspiration pneumonia occurs in a marsupial species, corticosteroids should be administered as initial therapy. Dexamethasone or prednisolone at a dose of 1 mg/kg IV or IM reduces the amount of tissue reaction occurring in the lungs.[1] Antibiotic therapy should be initiated using any of the aforementioned antibiotic medications.

Prednisolone sodium succinate, a glucocorticosteroid dosed at 10 to 30 mg/kg IV, is considered the treatment of choice for the marsupial patient diagnosed with shock. Methylprednisolone sodium succinate (10-30 mg/kg IV) and dexamethasone sodium phosphate (5-10 mg/kg IV) also are effective glucocorticosteroid agents when treating the "shocky" marsupial patient.

Nonsteroidal antiinflammatory drugs

Nonsteroidal antiinflammatory drugs (NSAIDS) are a viable alternative to corticosteroids in the treatment of aspiration pneumonia. Flunixin meglumine given at a dose of 1.1 mg/kg IV or IM every 24 hours for 3 days has been very effective when used to treat the disease consequences of aspiration pneumonia in marsupials.[1]

Nebulization

Animals that are quiet and of a size as to be held in a small cage should be considered nebulization candidates. The antibiotics suggested for the treatment of pneumonia can be effectively administered into a nebulization chamber or by face mask.

Bronchodilators

Bronchodilators are often selected for marsupial patients showing signs of dyspnea. Two therapeutic agents frequently used are theophylline 10 mg/kg SC or IV every 12 hours or aminophylline 4 to 10 mg/kg SC or IV every 12 hours.[1]

Expectorants

Expectorants are rarely used as treatment for marsupial respiratory disease. If required, the combination of theophylline and glycerol guaiacolate, 1 ml/kg PO, can be administered every 8 hours.[1]

Antitussives

Antitussives are not often used, as treatment is typically aimed at the cause of a cough rather than the cough itself. One of the more common antitussives that is used is codeine, 1 to 2 mg/kg PO every 8 hours.[1]

Mucolytics

Mucolytics assist in the treatment of upper and lower respiratory tract disease. One of the more common mucolytics administered to marsupial patients is bromhexine hydrochloride. The average dose is 2 mg/kg PO or by nebulization every 12 hours for 5 days.[1]

Decongestants

Pseudoephedrine hydrochloride 1 mg/kg PO or by nebulization every 12 hours for 5 days is one of the decongestants most commonly chosen in the treatment of marsupial respiratory disease.[1]

Gastrointestinal System

There are numerous species of marsupials and a wide variation in dentition, including number of teeth, emergence and wear pattern, and potential for disease or disorder.

Rudimentary precursors of teeth have been determined to occur in some species of marsupials, for example, the short-tailed wallaby (*Setonyx biachyurus*) and the brushtail phalanger (*Trichosurus vulpecula*). However, in general, it is only permanent premolar 3 that is preceded by a deciduous tooth. In general then, the functional marsupial dentition can be thought of as a permanent one, with a basic dental formula of I 5/4, C 1/1, P 3/3, M 4/4 = 50.

In the superfamily *Didelphoidea,* the dental formula for the American opossum is I 5/4, C 0-1/1, P 3/3, M 4/4 = 48-50.[4] There are no diastemas along the upper and lower arcades, and adjacent teeth are in contact with one other. The buccal surfaces of the cheek teeth form a straight line. If there is crowding of teeth along the arcade, P3 will often be rotated mesially or lingually as a result. The lower incisors are all approximately the same size and not procumbent in position. The canines are comparably larger than the rest of the teeth, and each molar possesses three dental caniculi.

Possums, gliders, and phalangers comprise the diverse family *Phalangeridae.* The dental formula is equally varied: I 2-3/1-3, C 1/0-1, P 1-3 1-3/3, M 4/3-4 = 26-42. In the ringtailed possums *(Pseudocheirus),* the premolars of the upper arcade are different in size and of variable distance from each other. In the lower arcade, the first incisor is long and procumbent. Between the first incisor and premolar 3 of the mandibular arcade, there are numerous small teeth called "intermediate teeth." The total number of these intermediate teeth varies, and there remains the question as to whether any of them can be classed as canines.

In the oral cavity of the brushtail possum, the upper canines are naturally divided into a large mesial and small distal portion by grooves that separate the tips of the crown. A premolar, 1, and 3 are located on each maxilla. In *Trichosurus fuliginosis,* premolar 1 is comparable in size to the canine but may be absent as well. Premolar 1 is always present in the mountain possum *(Trichosurus caninus)*, but premolar 2 is frequently missing.

The length of the muzzle is seen to vary with the different species of the ring-tailed possum. In animals with longer muzzles, the upper incisors form a horseshoe-shaped arch, occluding at procumbent premolar 1. Following the mandibular arcade, a lengthy diastema is noted between procumbent incisor 1 and the cheek teeth. The canine and premolars 1 and 2 are absent; as such, there is no functional occlusion with the canine and premolar 1 of the upper arcades. In those with shorter muzzles, the spacing between the teeth is greatly reduced, and some teeth are in contact. There is no diastema along the mandible arcade, and the canine and premolar 1 are absent as well. Premolar 1 is likely absent as a result of minimized space. The first of the cheek teeth, therefore, is premolar 2, and it is usually in contact with recumbent incisor 1. Molars of all phalangerids are quadribucular, usually with rounded cusps.

The family Phasolarctidae has as its member the koala. An arboreal folivorous marsupial, it derives food, water, and shelter almost exclusively from selected eucalyptus trees. Over the course of evolution, the koala has developed specialized dentition and digestive processes to adapt to the toxic oils that are found in the leaves of the eucalyptus. The dental formula of the koala is I 3/1, C 1/0, P 1/1, M 4/4 = 30. Excessive tooth wear in older koalas can be the principal factor limiting the longevity of an otherwise healthy animal.

A higher incidence of opportunistic infections and neoplasia suggests the koala may be more immunodeficient compared with other eutherians. Primary or secondary oral infections (e.g., *Bordetella bronchiseptica, Pseudomonas aeruginosa,* and *Pseudomonas* spp.) with subsequent inflammation and lymph node involvement have been reported.[1] Culture and sensitivity testing is recommended before a definitive antibiotic treatment regime is selected. Mixed bacterial populations have been detected in oral ulcerations of the gingiva and tongue.

Oral thrush has been reported as being quite common in hand-raised young koalas. It may appear in the form of shallow erosions or as white curd-like accumulations. The causative agent, *Candida albicans,* is fungal in origin and Nystatin, given at a dose of 5000 IU/kg 3 times a day by mouth, is recommended as the treatment of choice.[1]

Wombats have developed their own unique adaption to an herbivorous diet. They maintain a single pair of upper and lower incisors that, like the remaining teeth in the mouth, are rootless.

PARASITES

Sarcocystis *spp.*

The determination of *Sarcocystis* spp. as a parasite of marsupials has early origins. Macroscopic cysts formed by protozoan parasites have been described in the gastrointestinal tracts of several macropodid marsupials. In the late 19th century, Raphael Blanchard performed a necropsy on a rock wallaby *(Macropus penicillatus),* and meronts/merozoites were detected within the connective tissue of the submucosa.[5] The organism was originally assigned the name *Balbiania mucosa.*[4,5] Labbé[6] and

Minchin[7] assigned it to the genus *Sarcocystis,* whereas Noller[8] placed it in the genus *Globidium.*[6-8] Mackerras went on to further designate it as *Globidium mucosae.*[9] Coutelen reexamined Blanchard's work and concluded the organism belonged to the genus *Sarcocystis.*[9,10]

Zwart and Strik located meront cysts in the upper small intestine of a Bennett's wallaby *(Macropus bennetti).*[11] They designated these meronts as *Globidium mucosum.* At the same time, several large coccidian oocytes were detected in the feces of this animal, and it was assumed they belonged to the same species as the meronts. *Globidium* then became synchronized with *Eimeria* when similar large oocysts were found in the gray kangaroo.[12]

However, as coccidia are host specific, the same species seldom are able to infect more than one host genus. The fact that Blanchard's meronts were in the large intestine and Zwart and Strik's in the small intestine would also indicate that they did not belong to the same species. Levine concluded that Blanchard's organism was a giant meront of *Eimeria* or similar coccidian, resembling *E. bovis* of the ox and *E. leuckarti* of the horse.[13]

Though the light microscopic examination for these organisms has been detailed, their taxonomy has remained uncertain.[14] O'Donoghue et al. reported detection of macroscopic protozoan cysts in the gastrointestinal walls of two unadorned rock wallabies and compared their ultrastructural characteristics with those of other cyst-forming protozoan parasites belonging to the phylum Apicomplexa.[14]

The cysts detected by O'Donoghue were predominantly in the forestomach, small intestine and colon, and occasionally in the cecum and esophagus.[14] The majority of the cysts were located within the muscularis externa, usually between the outer longitudinal and inner circular smooth muscle layers.[14] Several cysts were also located deep in the submucosa next to the muscularis externa in many of the organs examined.[14] Despite the differences in the locations of the cysts, all possessed similar morphologic features.[14] O'Donoghue et al. concluded that the macroscopic cysts recovered from the unadorned rock wallabies and the Bennett's wallabies belong to the genus *Sarcocystis* on the basis of ultrastructural characteristics, despite the apparently unusual location. Comparison of these findings with the earlier light microscopic descriptions of these organisms find them similar to those of the cysts originally detected in a brushtail rock wallaby by Blanchard[5] and Coutelen.[10] Therefore, it was recommended the species be classified as *S. mucosa.*[5,6]

The North American opossum is the definitive host for at least three pathogenic species of *Sarcocystis: S. neurona, S. falcatula,* and *S. speeri.*[15]

The apicomplexan, *Sarcocystis neurona,* is the primary cause of the neurologic disease in horses; it is known as equine protozoal myeloencephalitis. Horses are considered an aberrant host, as the meronts and merozoites are confined to the CNS, where the merozoites continually divide without encysting.[16]

The organism was first placed in the genus *Sarcocystis* because of ultrastructural and antigenic properties.[16,17] *Sarcocystis* spp. have an obligatory two-host life cycle, and the stage of the organism found in the CNS is likely not the stage in the horse that creates infection.[16]

In this heteroxenous life cycle, there is a sexual stage in the gastrointestinal tract of the definitive host (usually a predator or scavenger species) and a systemic asexual stage in the intermediate host (usually a prey species).[16] Sporocysts are passed in the feces of the definitive host and ingested by the intermediate host.[16] Sporozoites enter intestinal epithelial cells of the intermediate host and proceed through multiple stages of asexual reproduction.[16] This culminates in merozoites encysting in muscle cells to form sarcocysts—hence the genus name. Fenger et al. proceeded to use PCR screening of sporocysts from a variety of wildlife species in an effort to identify possible definitive host species.[16] The identity of the sporocysts was confirmed by sequencing the small subunit ribosomal RNA gene (SSURNA), as the gene contains regions that are species specific. Several opossum sporocyst samples were identified using the *S. neurona* SSURNA PCR assay, and these samples were further classified as *S. neurona* by the sequence of the complete SSURNA gene of the opossum sporocysts. Fenger's data were the first to establish the opossum as the definitive host of *S. neurona*.[16]

The means by which opossums become infected with *S. neurona* are unknown because neither the sarcocyst stage nor the intermediate host that harbors the sarcocyst stage is known.[18] Dubey et al. identified the sarcocyst stage of *S. neurona*, completing the life cycle, using domestic cats as experimental intermediate hosts.[18] Cats were fed *S. neurona* sporocysts from feces of a naturally infected opossum, and muscles from cats were fed to laboratory-raised opossums that later excreted *S. neurona* sporocysts.[18] Whether cats are a natural intermediate host remains to be determined.[18]

Sarcocystis flacatula is the second of the three known *Sarcocystis* spp. in the opossum in which that animal serves as the definitive host. It is unique in that it is currently the one species for which both the complete life cycle and natural intermediate host are known. *Sarcocystis falcatula* is thought to parasitize canaries (*Seinus* canaries), zebra finches (*Poephila gutta*), budgerigars (*Melopsittacus undulates*), grackles (*Quiscalus quiscula*), and sparrows (*Passer domesticus*). At the time of this writing, the most recently recognized *Sarcocystis* spp. in the opossum is *Sarcocystis speeri*; immunodeficient mice, have been identified as an experimentally intermediate host.[15]

In short, the complete life cycles of *S. neurona* and *S. speeri* are not known. For *S. neurona*, the true intermediate hosts and sarcocysts are unknown; the horse is considered an aberrant host, and only schizonts and merozoites have been detected in equine tissues.[17] For *S. speeri*, natural intermediate hosts are unknown.[15] Neither *S. neurona* nor *S. speeri* sporocysts have proven to be experimentally infective to budgerigars, relinquishing an association to *S. falculata*.[15,18]

Eimeria *spp.*

Eimeria-type species of coccidia are known to parasitize macropodid marsupials. Oocysts have been identified in the feces of Bennett's and red-necked wallabies, gray kangaroos, and red kangaroos. Barker et al. proceeded to classify coccidians occur-

ring in rock wallabies and from several species of potoroid marsupials. In further study of the coccidian fauna of the Macropodoidea, *Eimeria* spp. were identified as parasitic in wallabies and kangaroos of the genera *Setonix* (*S. brachyurus*), *Thylogale* (*T. billardierii,* the Tasmanian pademelon), *Wallabia* (*W. bicolor,* the swamp wallaby), *Lagorchestes* (*L. conspicillatus,* the spectacled hare-wallaby), and *Dendrolagus* (*D. lumholtzi,* Lumholtz's tree kangaroo).[19]

Besnoitia darlingi

In 1910, Darling presented a description of cysts in the tissue of an opossum, *Didelphis marsupialis,* captured in Panama. Darling classified these organisms as belonging to the genus *Sarcocystis* but noted several unique features. Schneider identified this same parasite from an opossum native to Panama. He reviewed the nomenclature associated with the organism and concurred the appropriate name for the organism was *B. darlingi,* as suggested previously by Minchow.[20]

Over the past 80 years, besnoitiosis has been recognized in opossums and certain American reptiles. It is a common parasite of the Virginia opossum in the United States. *B. darlingi* cysts have been reported in 1 opossum from Texas, 1 of 5 opossums from Lexington, Kentucky, 8 of 13 from Missouri and Illinois, 2 of 5 opossums from the Kansas City area, and 4 of 6 opossums from Indiana.[21]

Besnoita spp. are heteroxenous coccidian parasites of the family Sarcocystidae, which have a life cycle requiring intermediate and definitive hosts. The Virginia opossum has been determined as the intermediate host, whereas the domestic cat serves as the definitive host. Opossums may become infected with *B. darlingi* by ingesting food or water contaminated with oocysts excreted by cats, by ingesting infected tissues containing cysts through cannibalisms, or experimentally through intraperitoneal inoculation with tachyzoites.

Besnoitia cysts have been differentiated from other Sarcocystidae based on their characteristic thick wall that is composed of an outer fibrous component surrounding a thin rim of host cell cytoplasm.

Elsheika et al. examined Virginia opossums in Michigan during a 1-year period to document the presence of *B. darlingi* cysts.[22] Examination of cyst morphology, prevalence, seasonal variation, and tissue sites of isolation revealed the cysts were most prevalent in the summer, then the spring, and finally the fall. No cysts were noted in the winter months. Common locations of *B. darlingi* cysts in the body include ears, conjunctiva, tongue, abdominal muscles, diaphragm, stomach, heart, liver, kidney, lung, and spleen. Adult female opossums were particularly affected, but further studies of wildlife as definitive hosts are needed.

Stomach worms

Turgida turgida is a common stomach worm of the American opossum, reported in Florida, Louisiana, Texas, Georgia, Tennessee, North Carolina, Virginia, Illinois, Pennsylvania, New York, and Minnesota.[17]

In a survey of 96 opossums, larval *T. turgida* were most common in animals collected from May to August, perhaps because of the large number of insects available for consumption at that time of year and their role in transmission. Larvae of *T. turgida* were widely dispersed throughout the body, but adults tended to occur in one to three groups in the anterior near the fundus.

Small lesions observed in the stomach walls of all the opossums were considered the result of trauma associated with the attachment of worms. Eosinophilic material at the base and the sides of the lesions may have been a result of secretions from the parasites. *T. turgida* has been reported to perforate the stomach wall of opossums, suggesting that the size of the ulcer may be related to the number of adult worms present and the length of time the animals have been infected.

Physaloptera turgida is another noteworthy stomach worm known to occur in opossums. Worms, usually in immature stages, also pinpoint gastric ulcers.[23] Perforation of the stomach wall[24] and clinical signs such as profuse diarrhea, weight loss, partial gastric occlusion, and hemorrhagic enteritis have been associated with infection.[25]

Flagellates

Tetratrichomonas didelphis (family Trichomonadidae, subfamily Trichomonadinae) is a flagellate protozoan found in the intestine, cecum, and colon of the opossum, including *Didelphis marsupialis*,[26] *Lutreolina crassicaudatsa*,[27] and *D. albiventris*.[28] Its ability to survive and grow in the hostile, stressed environment of the gastrointestinal tract requires its ability to adapt to aerobic or anaerobic conditions and an abundance or absence of nutrients. The in vitro cultivation of *T. didelphis* is dependent on the resident microorganism, *E. coli*, as a growth-promoting partner. The phagocytosis of the bacteria by *T. didelphis* has been demonstrated on scanning electron microscopy by the presence of crater-like depressions on the surface of the protozoa, likely remnant endocytic channels following the ingestion and eventual intracellular degradation of bacteria.

Trichinella spiralis

Trichinellosis is a parasitic disease caused by the nematode, *Trichinella spiralis*. It is considered of public health importance as human infections are established by the consumption of insufficiently cooked meat, usually pork or bear.[29] Natural infection occurs most widely in *Carnivora*; however, *T. spiralis* has been reported in the orders Rodentia, Insectivora, Pinnipedia, Artiodactyla, Cetacea, Lagomorpha, Strigiformes, and Marsupialia.[30] The occurrence of *T. spiralis* in wildlife is important in respect to both agriculture and public health, because skinned carcasses of furbearers may be used to feed swine on smaller farms and because the meat of furbearers, for example, raccoons, muskrats, opossums and beaver, can provide food for some humans.[31] Additionally, it is important to note that pigs and rats maintained on swine farms have transmitted *T. spiralis* to the associated wild and feral animals.[32]

Other endoparasites

An array of helminth parasites, similar to those found in other mammals, have been found to infect the Virginia opossum.

Acanthocephala spp. possess an armed proboscis that usually becomes embedded in the mucosa and submucosa of the small intestine. Several ulcerations of the intestinal wall at the site of attachment will often result in perforation and subsequent peritonitis conceivable with extensive duration and severity.

The nematode, *Capillaria aerophilia*, is quite common in inducing parasitic change in the lungs of the opossums. Typically infecting the bronchioles and alveoli, the lesions can be recognized grossly as round, elevated yellow areas on the pleural surface. Dissection of the lesions reveals slender, coiled parasites or, on occasion, eggs.

Ectoparasites of opposums. Though extensive research has not been performed on ectoparasites that infest opossums, various arthropods have been documented. The fleas *Ctenocephalides felis* and *Polygenis gwyni*, the ticks *Dermacentor variabilis* and *Ioxdes scapularis*, and the macronyssid mite *Ornithonyssus wernecki* were determined to have the highest prevalence of occurrence in opossums surveyed in southeastern Georgia.[33] These parasites are of particular significance, as several are proven vectors of pathogens that cause zoonotic diseases. *C. felis* acts as a vector of *Rickettsia typhi*, the causative agent of murine (endemic) typhus.[34] *I. scapularis* is a vector of the Lyme disease spirochete.[35] *D. variabilis* can cause tick paralysis and is the principal vector in eastern North America of *Rickettsia rickettsii*, the causative agent of Rocky Mountain spotted fever.[33]

Anatrichosoma buccalis is a nematode known to affect the buccal mucosa of the Virginia opossum.[36] The female worms of *A. buccalis* deposit their eggs in tunnels created within the superficial layers of the buccal mucosa.[36] Eggs with well-developed larvae are released into the mouth as a result of sloughing of the surface epithelium and then leave the body by way of the digestive tract.[36] There is a rapid turnover in the mucosa, as individual lesions are seen to resolve in as little as 3 days.[36] A paucity in lesions may be attributed to a possible loss of infection, with subsequent reinfection or temporary cessation of egg laying by females.[36] Rarely have animals been found to be continuously negative for lesions, thereby indicating chronic infection.[36]

Cryptosporidium spp. causes enteric disease in animals and humans.[37] Cryptosporidiosis can be particularly severe in immunocompromised individuals,[37] resulting in a severe enterocolitis with no known effective treatment for infection.[37] Bilbies *(Macrotis lagotis)* are threatened Australian marsupials being bred in captivity as part of a recovery program to reintroduce the species to the southwestern region of Western Australia.[37] *Cryptosporidium muris* was detected in the feces of bilbies at one such captive-breeding colony.[37] The high density of bilbies at the facility may have predisposed the bilbies to stress and susceptibility to infection with *C. muris*.[37] *C. muris* is known to occur in mice, and it is suspected that the bilbies acquired infection from mice via fecal contamination of food and water.[37] Dimetridazole was used with questionable effectiveness, as the disease is self-limiting. *Cryptosporidium parvum* may also infect marsupials. Because this organism is zoonotic, strict hygiene should be practiced when managing infected animals.

Cardiovascular System

HEART

The study of the hearts of marsupial mammals offers useful information on cardiac structure and function in comparison with placental mammals. Marsupials have a heart that is ovoid and larger than most placentals, especially sedentary species. Marsupial hearts have large stroke volumes and beat considerably slower at rest, corroborating with a lower basal metabolic rate. However, at maximum performance, heart rates of marsupials are comparable to those of placental mammals. As a result, marsupials should be able to provide a supply of oxygen to the tissues at maximum performance at least as high as most athletic placental mammals. Indeed, maximal aerobic capacity of marsupials is considered to be equivalent to "athletic" placentals, with the red kangaroo reported as being among the most aerobic of all the mammals.[38]

CARDIOVASCULAR REFLEXES

A study of neural control of the cardiovascular system was compared in the newborn and adult opossum by measuring changes in blood pressure and heart rate following carotid arterial occlusion and vagal stimulation.[38] Results revealed that the newborn opossum baroreceptor mechanisms are as well developed as those in the adult.[38] The increase in blood pressure resulting from common carotid arterial occlusion was essentially the same in the newborn and adult opossum. However, the rise in blood pressure detected in the newborn was accompanied by a slight increase in heart rate, which would initially indicate that vagal control of the newborn heart is deficient to a degree. However, with vagal stimulation, both the newborn and adult demonstrated nearly identical vagal responses. Thus, vagal control in the newborn opossum appears to be almost as well developed as that of the adult. The results of this study would indicate that although the newborn opossum is incompletely developed for some time after birth, its neural development is adequate for control of their cardiovascular system.

COMMON DISEASE PRESENTATIONS
Bacteria

Leptospirosis. Leptospirosis is an infectious bacterial disease caused by pathogenic spirochetes belonging to the genus *Leptospira*. The zoonotic disease occurs worldwide, with human, domestic, and wild animal hosts affected. Leptospirae are divided into antigenically distinct serogroups and serovars.[39] The serogroup/type *L. interrogans* contains the five serovars most often identified in the United States, including *pomona, icterhemorrhagiae, canicola, hardjo,* and *grippotyphosa*. Small, mammalian wildlife are considered to be the most important reservoirs in nature, and each serovar has at least one primary maintenance/reservoir host. The serovar associated with a particular host can vary based upon geographic location.[39]

In maintenance hosts, infection with leptospira is endemic, and transmission between animals is through direct contact. Disease can be clinically recognizable in maintenance host, but most often these animals are subclinically infected. Following an initial, acute phase of infection, leptospires will localize and survive in the renal tubules of the kidney, being excreted in the urine of maintenance hosts for months to years.

Humans and domestic animals can be incidental or accidental hosts for leptospirosis, and though incidence is low, disease, when it does occur, can be severe. Leptospires are shed for a shorter duration in the urine of an incidental host and marked antibody titers may be detected in response to infection. In the incidental host, infections may be asymptomatic or evident as fever, jaundice, kidney and/or liver failure, and death. Diagnosis is most often made by dark field microscopy or special (silver) stains.

The transmission of leptospirosis from a maintenance host to an accidental host is through indirect contact. This involves the skin or mucous membranes of an accidental host being exposed to the tissues or urine of infected animals or to surface waters contaminated by their urine. The extent of transmission is dependent on several factors, including the degree of contact between host species, population density, and climate. Warm, wet weather enhances the survivability of leptospires in the environment. Regional and seasonal conditions characterized by high mean ambient temperature, increased rainfall, and alkaline soil pH appear to foster outbreaks of leptospirosis. The encroachment of human populations into wildlife habitats is resulting in the spread of infection from wildlife to humans and domestic animals.

Wildlife species are often reported to be potentially important reservoirs of *Leptospira* serovars, and certain marsupial species have been identified in this regard. Survey serologic testing was performed on opossums and other wildlife in southern Connecticut to determine the seroprevalence of five common *Leptospira* serogroups, represented by serovars *pomona, icterohemmorrhagiae, canicola, hardjo,* and *grippotyphosa*.[39] The opossums showed no reaction to any serovar in this five-antigen panel.[39] However, leptospirosis in Georgia opossums was associated most frequently with the serovar *ballum*.[39]

In New Zealand, the brushtail possum is considered to be the maintenance host for *Leptospira interrogans* serovar *balcanica*.[39] Disease is considered to be subclinical in these animals with no signs or biochemical changes suggestive of kidney damage evident and kidney lesions mild on examination. Lesions in the kidneys, if present, are usually mild. Infection is predominant in animals over 18 months of age, and prevalence of disease appears similar in both males and females.[39] Prevalence does vary, however, among habitats, with pastoral regions having a higher prevalence than forests.[39] Possum behaviors in pastoral habitats (e.g., larger home ranges, nest sharing, increased ground contact) are believed to have a higher occurrence of disease. Both social and environmental contact should be considered sources of transmission. The serovar *balcanica* has also been isolated from brushtail opossums in Australia.[39]

Bacterial endocarditis of the heart. Bacterial endocarditis has been identified in opossums in captivity. Valvular vegetative lesions generally seem to be the most striking gross lesions. Myocarditis generally appears as a focalized lesion, but in some cases lesions were seen to be diffuse. Bacterial cultures of vegetative lesions revealed a variety of bacteria, including *Proteus mirabilis, Salmonella bern,* alpha-hemolytic *Streptococcus,* and *E. coli*. The predominant bacteria were alpha- and beta-hemolytic *Streptococcus* spp., *Proteus* spp., and *Aerobacter* spp. Stress and/or diet may play contributing roles in the susceptibility of the captive opossum to bacterial infection. Diseases noted to occur concurrently with bacterial endocarditis are amyloidosis, pyelonephritis, and glomerulonephritis.[38] Amyloidosis may has been associated with captivity and associated diet and stress.[38] The association of amyloidosis to chronic infection and bacterial endocarditis has not been defined. Pyelonephritis potentially could serve as source bacteria for bacterial endocarditis. Glomerulonephritis has been associated with a hypersensitivity to bacteria in humans but has not been described in marsupial species.

Bacterial endocarditis has been experimentally induced in the opossum with injections of either *Streptococcus viridans* or *Staphylococcus aureus*.[38] Of animals injected with the former, approximately half developed bacterial endocarditis with the predominance of lesions of the left side of the heart.[38] All opossums injected with *Staphylococcus aureus* developed endocarditis. Lesions were smaller in size but were found in both left and right sides of the heart. The disease induced by *Streptococcus viridans* in captive opossums most closely resembles naturally occurring bacterial endocarditis in humans.[38]

Erysipelothrix rhusiopathiae. *Erysipelothrix rhusiopathiae* is a bacterial pathogen most commonly associated with swine, but it is known to occur in other animals and in humans. Lesions in swine include septicemia, arthritis, and endocarditis, but the most characteristic lesion is that of erysipelas or "diamond skin" disease, with its characteristic diamond pattern of skin necrosis. Similar lesions have been described in other animals. In humans, inflammatory lesions of the hands and fingers have been the most common findings; however, septicemia and endocarditis can also occur.

Erysipelothrix rhusiopathiae has been isolated in an opossum.[1] Signs and lesions were representative of a septicemia; no pathognomic lesions were identified.[40] Transmission of *E. rhusiopathiae* in the wild remains to be determined. However, the ready development of bacterial endocarditis in the captive opossum makes it a ready disease model for the study of *E. rhusiopathiae*–induced endocarditis.

Reproductive System

Marsupial reproduction is comparatively different to that of placental mammals. The bones and pouches (marsupium) distinguish marsupial mammals anatomically, yet it is important to recognize that not all marsupials have these distinctive structures. The sugar glider does not have marsupial bones but does have a pouch containing only two mammae.[41] The short-tailed opossum *(Mondelphis domestica)* has marsupial bones but no pouch.[41] The mammae vary in number and are arranged in a circle on the abdomen.[41] The Virginia opossum possesses marsupial bones, a pouch, and 13 mammae (Figures 11-8 and 11-9).[41] Wallabies, such as the tammar or Dama or Bennett's wallaby, have marsupial bones and pouches with two pairs of mammae near the base of the pouch.[41]

Wallabies can produce different types of milk in each mamma to accommodate joeys of different ages.[41] The milk in the teat of a newborn wallaby has a lower fat and protein

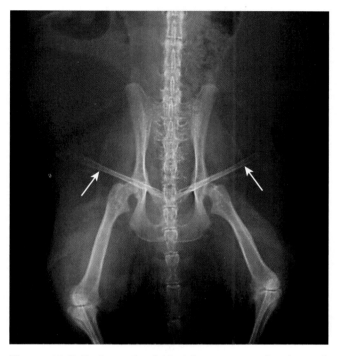

Figure 11-8 Radiograph of Virginia opossum showing epipubic (marsupial) bones *(arrows).*

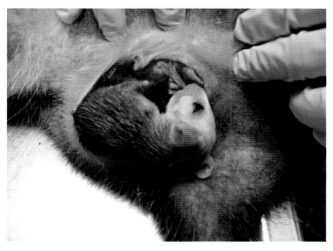

Figure 11-9 Young Virginia opossum in marsupium sucking on teat.

content that that of a teat used by the young who have already left the pouch and periodically return. While the newborn grows, the milk changes in content to suit the joey's needs.[41]

The development of passive and active immunity in marsupial young reveals general patterns as well. Study of normal pouch young of the quokka *(Setonix brachyurus)* reveals no prenatal transfer of antibody across the placenta. Maternal immunoglobulins are obtained from the gut of suckling pouch young until the end of pouch life. This significantly exceeds the 24- to 48-hour periods of intestinal absorption typically associated with placental species.[42] Further work in this regard has revealed that the passively acquired antibody has a short half-life of approximately 8 to 9 days and is almost entirely gone by 4 to 6 weeks. As a result, the quokka does not have the ability for active immunity and antibody production until at least 8 days after birth. The current presumption is that this active immunity response then proceeds to develop over the remaining duration of pouch life.[42] The active immune response of the Virginia opossum and passive immune responses of the tammar wallaby and brushtail opossum *(Trichosurus vulpeca)* have been found to be similar to those of the quokka. This would indicate that most marsupials follow a similar pattern. It is important, then, to be aware that an orphaned pouch-young will no longer be receiving passive maternal antibodies and that an underdeveloped active immune system will serve as its only protection.[42]

Dystocia is a rare event in marsupials, as the fetus is expelled early in gestation and then must proceed from the cloacal opening up to the pouch or abdominal area where it will firmly secure itself to a teat. The dam will lick a path from the cloaca to the entrance of the pouch or abdominal mammae. The skin lining the interior of the pouch is very soft and moist. At times when there are no young in the pouch, a brown, scaly secretion will be present. The dam will prepare the pouch for a fetus by thoroughly cleaning it a week before its birth.[41] When the fetus emerges from the urogenital opening into the cloaca, it is in an amniotic sac. The fetus must break free of this sac using its claws in an approximate time frame of 10 to 15 seconds. The fetus will appear with no visible eyes or ears, and it will be red in color. It then must climb unassisted through the mother's fur up to the pouch entrance or abdominal mammae. The entire journey of the joey to the pouch averages 5 minutes in the Macropodidae (kangaroos, wallabies).[43]

In addition to having claws, the fetus has an enlarged shoulder girdle to make the climb; both eventually regress, being replaced with skeletal structure typical for the species. This primitive shoulder girdle contains a continuous cartilaginous arc of primal elements known as the *metacoracoid*—a feature seen in reptiles and egg-laying mammals as well. Once the fetus attaches to the teat, the arc disperses and the shoulder girdle assumes its usual association with the sternum as seen in adult marsupials and placental mammals. The metacoracoid becomes the coracoid process of the scapula. The fetus is also seen to have a large tongue and prominent ridge on its upper palate, features which likely aid in suckling and remaining attached to the teat. The teat itself swells up inside the mouth of the fetus also ensuring a firm attachment. The fetus will remain

attached to the teat for approximately a third to half of its pouch life.[43]

Following parturition, the dam usually enters a postpartum estrus during which time breeding and fertilization occur. If the joey(s) which are presently in the pouch stay alive, there will be a pause in the development of the fertilized egg at the blastocyst stage when it will remain unimplanted until the pouch young have either died or finished suckling and departed the pouch. The blastocyst then proceeds in development and a new joey is born in a few weeks time. This hiatus in development is known as *fetal diapause*.

The anatomy of the reproductive tract of marsupials is quite different from that of placental mammals. The gastrointestinal tract, urinary ducts, and reproductive tract all share a common opening in the cloaca.[44] The female marsupial reproductive tract is comparatively smaller than that of a placental female. The proximal half of the tract consists of the ovaries, oviducts, and paired uterus bodies, while the distal portion is made up of two lateral, and a median or central, vaginal canals. With the exception of the potoroo, marsupials give birth through the median canal. The three vaginal canals join and create a urogenital sinus that contains the urethral opening before entrance into the cloaca.

At the time of parturition, the birth canal forms in the connective tissue between the median vaginal canal and the urogenital sinus. In most marsupials, this birth canal resolves and reforms with each birth. However, following the birth in kangaroos and wallabies, the birth canal becomes lined with epithelium and remains patent.

In sugar gliders, each ovary lies against the medioventral aspect of the uterus, near the junction of the uterus and oviduct. The oviduct itself begins as a large funnel and then continues as a convoluted tubule. Each uterus is fusiform in shape and elongates caudally into a narrow uterine neck. The necks of each uterus run parallel to each other for about 3 mm, ensheathed in a common tunic of connective tissue. Each neck then opens into a respective vaginal cul-de-sac at the os uteri, located ventrolaterally on the uterine papilla. A septum arises between each cul-de-sac at the uterine papillae. The median vaginal canal is short and the lateral canals quite long. By contrast, in opossums and marcopods, the median and lateral canals are almost equal in length. In the glider, the median vaginal canal and associated uterus merge with a lateral vaginal canal. Posterior to the bladder, the two merged lateral and median vaginal canals, as well as the urethra, unite to form the urogenital sinus.

The male reproductive system of possums and gliders is representative of other marsupial species. The penis of the male lies on the ventral aspect of the cloacal floor. It is bifid, or forked, and this is often mistaken as being abnormal by the uninformed owner (Figure 11-10). In Petaurids, each half has a ventral groove that extends from the base of the penis to a pointed tip. In marsupials, the scrotal pouch is external and located cranial to the cloacal opening. Within the scrotal pouch are paired testes and epididymides, which are connected by vas deferentia to the prostatic portion of the urethra. The prostate itself is large and disseminate, and one or more pairs of Cow-

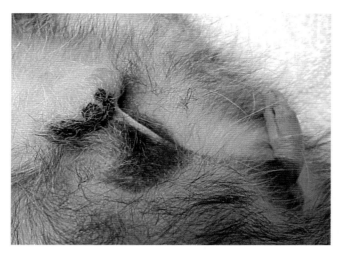

Figure 11-10 Scrotum and bifurcated penis of male opossum.

per's (bulbourethral) glands lie along the path of the urethra. In the sugar glider, there are two pairs of multilobed Cowper's glands that lie dorsal and lateral to the rectum. The duct of each Cowper's gland travels around the membranous urethra and enters its ventral surface near the crus of the penis. Male marsupials lack seminal vesicles and coagulating glands. Ampullae are usually absent as well. Male marsupials have been observed for the regulation of testicular temperature. Raising and lowering of the scrotal pouch and scrotal licking as a means of evaporative cooling have been observed as ways by which temperature is decreased.

Both male and female marsupials have cloacal glands. The white, oily secretion produced by these glands may be released in the urine or feces or at times when the animal is frightened. Male and female sugar gliders each possess three pairs of cloacal glands. One pair is anterior in location, with one gland on each side of the dorsal surface of the rectum near the cloaca. The ducts exiting each pair extend to the dorsal surface of the cloaca. A second pair takes a more posterior location, again with a single gland on each side of the dorsal surface of the cloaca. Short ducts empty the glands into the dorsal surface of the cloaca. Orientation of these ducts finds them near, but posterior to, the ducts of the anterior glands. The final pair of glands lies ventral to the posterior placed gland, with short duct drainage near the exterior opening of the cloaca. A glider will produce holocrine secretions from all three glands at times of fright, with the anterior paracloacal glands producing the largest amounts.

In mature males, the anterior glands are largest during breeding season. In captive animals, particularly females, the glands are quite small. In wild breeding and nonbreeding gliders, the ventral paracloacal glands are large in size. In wild females, they tend to be smaller in size, the largest being in lactating females. Captive females, by contrast, have larger glands than wild females.

The occurrence of spontaneous disease in the male and female reproductive systems is not a common one. Gross and histopathologic examination of the reproductive tracts of 150 male and female marsupials revealed a variety of lesions, though relatively few in number.[41] Metritis, uterine cysts, endometritis, uterine hemorrhage, and uterine metaplasia were found in six females. One mammary gland abscess, one ovarian cyst, and one mineralized ovary were also reported within the group. One female had edema while two others had adenitis of the urogenital sinus. Five males displayed testicular abnormalities: one testicular granuloma, one testicular cyst, one edematous testicle, one hydrocele, and one necrotic testicle were identified.[41] Adenitis, hypertrophy, and cysts were identified in three animals.[41]

Neoplasias affecting the genital tract have been diagnosed. Uterine leiomyoma, mammary gland papillary cystadenoma, and penile fibrosarcoma have been reported in marsupials.[41] Of particular note is the frequency with which pituitary adenomas with prolactinemia occur. These lesions are locally expansive rather than invasive, primarily affecting the adjacent neuroparenchyma. Often, within a tumor, are cyst-like spaces filled with hemorrhage, which stain strongly for prolactin. On clinical presentation, opossums diagnosed with pituitary adenomas exhibit a patchy endocrine alopecia.

Marsupials are susceptible to reproductive problems with one of the more common presentations being pouch eviction. This condition is often diagnosed in captive female marsupials. Possible etiologies of pouch eviction include overcleaning of the pouch, overcrowding of the fetus, an overexcited or panicking female, or the eviction of a yearling joey by a new joey. Accidental expulsion can occur in a stressed female if there is a loss of tone in the wall of the pouch.

In the absence of pouch infection, immediate remedies to pouch eviction should be considered. The joey can be replaced and a thin strip of surgical adhesive tape placed over the pouch entrance, closing the anterior and posterior lips of the entrance centrally. The dam should then be maintained in a relatively small, quiet, and dark area with minimal stimulation. Once the animal is calm, she can be transferred to her normal enclosure. Eventually, during the process of grooming, the tape can be removed. If the joey is again evicted, a potential alternative is to place two button sutures through the pouch, which would allow the dam accessibility to the joey and pouch interior without fully opening the pouch. With repeated evictions, consideration of fostering the joey becomes necessary. An evicted joey is susceptible to heat loss and dehydration, especially if it is still lacking fur. The joey should be transferred immediately to an incubator or heated environment with temperatures maintained between 88-90° F (32-33° C) for unfurred animals and 82-84° F (28-29° C) for furred joeys. Warmed gels or lotions can be used on the joey to maintain a moisture barrier and prevent dehydration in the unfurred orphan.

Infections of the pouch commonly occur in captive macropods. Macropods housed indoors with little exercise are especially susceptible to pouch infection. A variety of bacterial organisms have been cultured, with *Pseudomonas aeruginosa* being a frequent isolate. An odor from the pouch is often detected with these infections. On examination, the normal pink interior of the pouch will be brown in color and a thick

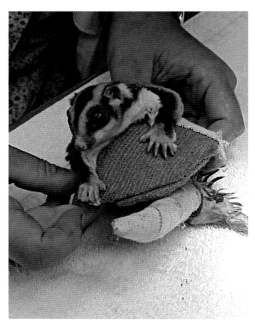

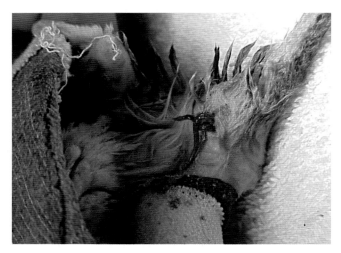

Figure 11-12 Mutilation and/or necrosis of the penis is frequently observed in the captive male sugar glider.

Figure 11-11 A body Elizabethan collar may be used to prevent sugar glider patients from traumatizing caudal abdominal injuries and surgical incision sites.

discharge present. The thick discharge should be removed and the pouch wall cultured. Dilute chlorhexidine should be used to gently cleanse the pouch. Once results of culture and sensitivity are received, appropriate topical and systemic antibiotics can be administered.

It is important for the practitioner to be cautious when selecting antibiotics to administer to herbivorous marsupials. Antibiotics with primarily a Gram-positive spectrum should be avoided. Antibiotics considered "unsafe" in herbivores include clindamycin, lincomycin, penicillin, ampicillin, amoxicillin/clavulanic acid, erythromycin, and first- and second-generation cephalosporins.[41] Any third-generation injectable cephalosporins should be used with caution.[41] Antibiotics classified as "safe" in herbivores are the fluoroquinolones, trimethoprim-sulfa combinations, sulfas, aminoglycosides, chloramphenicol, and metronidazole for anaerobes.[41]

Prostatitis has been described in the Virginia opossum exhibiting clinical signs of hematuria, localized pain, constipation, anorexia, and elevated rectal/cloacal temperature.[41] This condition has been similarly diagnosed in intact male sugar gliders, and a positive treatment response was achieved with broad-spectrum antibiotics, analgesics, antiinflammatories, and supportive care. Control of hormonal stimulation of the prostate can be attempted with the use of antihormonal medications, such as bicalutamide (Casodex; AstraZeneca, Wilmington, DE) (5 mg/kg PO q24h). In cases of severe prostatitis, castration should be considered to resolve the problem and reduce the likelihood of recurrence. An Elizabethan collar is recommended for sugar glider patients after the castration procedure to prevent trauma to the surgical site (Figure 11-11). Male gliders with signs of dysuria, stranguria, hematuria, and

congested/necrotic penis require examination for concurrent prostatitis and/or paracloacal gland involvement.

Mutilation or necrosis of the penis, or both, is observed frequently in the captive male sugar glider (Figure 11-12). An associated prostatitis, urinary tract infection, or both, may also be present. This disease condition of the penis has also been related to a self-mutilation syndrome seen in socially deprived or isolated captive males. An aggressive cagemate (male or female) may also be the initiating cause of the condition. On presentation, males will appear painful. Dehydration, distended bladders, or both, may be detected on physical exam along with swelling, hemorrhage, and variable necrosis of the penis. The condition can develop into a systemic infection; therefore, the treatment approach should consider this possibility. Broad-spectrum antibiotics, fluid therapy, a restraint device, and pain management are recommended. Cystocentesis, preferably under isoflurane anesthesia, is easily done on distended bladders. In some cases surgery may be required to remove the necrotic portion of the bifid penis and perform a urethrostomy. The limitations of anatomy and urethral swelling often require the use of microsurgery. A reduction in swelling and stabilization of the animal may be needed before surgery can be pursued. Unfortunately, despite the establishment of a patent urethra, these animals will often succumb to septicemia.

A Cushing-like syndrome has been reported to occur secondary to genital tract infections in female Virginia opossums.[41] Animals with this Cushing-like syndrome had a history of obesity, previous or current urinary tract infections, and periodic discharge from the genitourinary opening. These female opossums were also known to have had previous trauma resulting in abnormal urinary patterns: holding urine longer than normal or incomplete evacuation of the bladder. Though clinical signs were often similar to those reported in Cushing's disease of dogs, no primary lesions could be detected in the pituitary or adrenal glands. Fur became brown in color, and slight thinning to full alopecia was observed. All had some degree of depression, as well as variable anorexia and hindquarter weakness. Bloodwork changes included neutrophilia with a left shift and anemia, and urinalyses revealed high bacterial counts. Antibiotic therapy selection was based on culture and sensitivity results. Signs resolved with the initiation of therapy but returned once treatment was halted. It is theorized that urinary tract infections have the ability to spread to the genital system, particularly when the female is in delivery and the vaginal tract is patent. Once infection is established, metritis can, in turn, spread to the urinary tract. Ovariovaginal hysterectomy is the treatment of choice. Lateral canals must be removed to prevent those structures from serving as nidi for future infections.

SURGERY

Marsupial castration

In males, the scrotal stalk is located ventrally on the midabdomen and is narrow on appearance. An incision is made in the stalk skin close to the abdominal wall. The spermatic cord is bluntly dissected from the skin, clamped and ligated close to the body wall, and transected. A subcuticular pattern is used to close the incision. Postoperative analgesia is advised to reduce postoperative pain and the opportunity to cause damage to the surgical site.

Ovariohysterectomy and ovariovaginal hysterectomy

In females, the close involvement of the ureters with the genital tract can determine the spay approach selected. In obese females, it simply may not be possible to isolate the ureters. In this case, the ovaries and uterus can be removed, leaving the vaginal canals.

A standard midline entry incision is made through the inner wall of the pouch, avoiding the mammae. The ovaries should be isolated, the ovarian vessels ligated, and each ovary elevated. If the vaginal canals are to remain, the uterus can be clamped in preparation for pedicle ligation at the junction of the vaginal canals. Ligatures are then placed at the junction of the vaginal canals. If the vaginal canals are to be removed with the ovaries and uterus, then the vagina must be clamped just proximal to where the bladder empties into the urogenital sinus. As the canals are intimately related with the ureters, careful blunt dissection must be performed to separate the two. The vaginal canals may be removed best in sections, to avoid tearing or laceration of the ureters.

The abdominal incision can be closed in a similar manner as used in other mammals. If a pouch is involved, subcuticular sutures can be placed in the pouch wall. Sutures that are visible will likely be groomed out. Postoperative pain management is recommended.

Ophthalmology

KANGAROOS

Kangaroos have characteristic long upper eyelid lashes, and their iris is thick and brown throughout. The pupil is circular and can be dilated easily with tropicamide. Examination of the fundus will reveal a ventral and dorsal region, with the ventral fundus being heavily pigmented and usually dark brown in color. The practitioner may consider the ventral fundus equivalent to the nontapetal fundus in dogs. The dorsal fundus is typically lighter in color, and choroidal blood vessels may be visualized within the pigment. The dorsal fundus is equivalent to the tapetal fundus in dogs. The optic disc is located at the junction of the fundi. The disc is well vascularized, with a small vascular tuft often observed arising from the center. Myelination of the nerve fiber layer extends approximately two to three disc diameters from around the optic disc and is particularly prominent at the medial and lateral aspects of the disc.[1]

Conjunctivitis

Conjunctivitis frequently occurs in kangaroos, and foreign bodies are often the most common cause. Conjunctival blisters are indicative of a herpesvirus infection.

Corneal ulceration

Dehydration in young kangaroos increases their susceptibility to corneal ulceration. Dryness of the corneal surface as a result of dehydration is considered the most common initiating factor associated with corneal ulceration. Corneal ulcers may also occur from irritation caused by conjunctival foreign bodies or trauma from plant material. Healing of corneal ulcers in kangaroos is often characterized by a marked vascular response.

Kangaroo blindness syndrome

Kangaroo blindness syndrome (KBS) has been a persistent problem in the kangaroo populations of Australia over the past 20 years. Western gray kangaroos (*Macropus fulginosis*) are most often affected, but outbreaks have been reported in Eastern gray kangaroos and red kangaroos.[45,46] Male and female adult animals are most susceptible to KBS. Clinical signs of blindness are exhibited in kangaroos diagnosed with KBS; these signs typically include stumbling into objects (especially when startled) and demonstrating a high stepping gait. Examination of the eyes may reveal no or poor pupillary light reflexes and, in some cases, conjunctivitis.[45,46] If feed is readily available, animals should be able to maintain adequate body condition.

An arbovirus has been suspected as the cause of kangaroo blindness syndrome.[45,46] Kangaroos experimentally inoculated with strains of the virus develop initial ocular changes associated with the disease 5 weeks after exposure. Tropicamide may be used but does not completely dilate the pupils for ophthalmoscopic examination of KBS animals. Conjunctival hyperemia and aqueous flare may occur and are indicative of a mild uveitis. Blepharospasm may or may not be present.[45,46]

Examination of the fundus of one kangaroo revealed a pale area medial to the optic disc in the right eye and a linear pale area in the left eye.[45,46] These findings are characteristic of active retinal and/or choroidal inflammation. Four weeks after inoculation, lesions in the left eye became enlarged, and 10 weeks after inoculation, lesions in both eyes became pigmented and stabilized. One kangaroo receiving a second inoculation 4 weeks after initial inoculation developed distinct areas of pallor in the fundus, and the other developed a moderate anterior uveitis that obscured the fundus examination. On gross pathologic examination, retinas were pale and occasionally detached. Some retinas also showed small, white foci, 1 to 2 mm in diameter.[45,46]

The main histologic finding was a severe bilateral nonsuppurative panuveitis and retinitis with optic neuritis and secondary demyelination of the optic nerves. In approximately 45% of cases, a nonsuppurative meningoencephalitis was noted. The panuveitis was characterized by an infiltration of mononuclear cells, lymphocytes having the highest number. Inflammation in the choroid was particularly marked.[45] Severe degeneration and necrosis were evident in the retina, and in some cases, subretinal fluid accumulation resulted in retinal detachment. The optic nerves demonstrated perivascular lymphocytic cuffing and wallerian degeneration. Ellipsoids derived from the myelin sheaths of optic nerves were recognized, and some were observed to contain myelophages and axonal debris. The anterior and posterior segments of the eye often held inflammatory exudates comprised of protein-rich, edematous fluid, fibrin with many mononuclear cells, and occasional neutrophils.[45,46]

In almost half of the kangaroos examined, inflammation within the eyes was seen to extend to the brain as a nonsuppurative meningoencephalitis. Mononuclear cell infiltration of the meninges and Virchow-Robin spaces, focal gliosis, and patchy neuronal necrosis were found in animals that suffered from a nonsuppurative meningoencephalitis associated with KBS.[45,46] The optic tract itself contained axonal spheroids, vacuolation of the neuropil, and glial reaction. Pathologic examination of other tissues, including liver, lung, spleen, kidney, intestine, heart, and skeletal muscle, revealed no abnormal findings.

Vector-borne viruses have been implicated as the cause of the KBS epidemic because of the repeated isolation of Wallal and Warego serogroups of arbovirus from the eyes and brains of blind kangaroos.[45,46] Mosquitoes are proven vectors of Wallal virus and have been found where the disease is endemic. PCR testing found the DNA of both Wallal and Warego viruses in the mosquitoes *Culicoides austropalpalis, C. dycei,* and *C. marksi* during outbreaks. Blindness seems particularly prevalent in drought-affected areas.[45,46]

Cataracts

The development of cataracts has been associated with pouch-stage marsupials. Cataracts have been reported in some joeys fed cow's milk at an early age and those naturally raised. Cataracts progress quickly in joeys, maturing within a 1- to 2-week period. The difference between cow's milk and kangaroo milk is that the former contains lactose, whereas the latter is almost completely deficient of lactose.

Red and gray kangaroos have low levels of the liver enzymes normally responsible for the efficient metabolism of galactose in humans and other species. Specifically, many species of marsupials have been found to have low levels of activity of both erythrocytic galactokinase and galactose 1-phosphate uridyl transferase. It is suspected that depression of one or both of these enzymes is associated with the formation of cataracts in infant marsupials fed milk containing lactose. The galactose cataracts observed in kangaroos fed cow's milk is believed to be the result of both enzymes being depressed. This may allow accumulated galactose and galactose-1-phosphate to inhibit galactokinase activity in uridyl transferase deficiency. The stomach of immature marsupials has been identified as monogastric, which increases the absorption of galactose. This enhanced absorption, in combination with low levels of erythrocytic galactokinase and galactose-1-phosphate uridyl transferase activity, predisposes pouch marsupials to cataract formation. Older kangaroos, by contrast, possess a rumen-type stomach that can tolerate cow's milk, metabolizing galactose into volatile fatty acids using bacteria in the stomach.

Cataract surgery. Cataract surgery can be performed to remove galactose-induced cataracts in joeys fed cow's milk or spontaneous occurring cataracts seen in both joeys and older kangaroos. The eye can be accessed without the assistance of neuromuscular relaxants. The pupil is responsive to dilation with tropicamide 1%. The surgery itself is technically easy, and with soft lenses short phacoemulsification times can be achieved. In joeys with galactose cataracts, surgical removal of the lens will often reveal an opacification of the vitreous. A deep vitrectomy should be done to clear the inner eyeball of the vitreous body. Examination of the opacified vitreous reveals higher levels of galactose than seen in normal kangaroos.

In the first 1 to 2 weeks following surgery, there is minimal ocular inflammation. However, over the long term, many surgical patients develop glaucoma. A chronic uveitis may accompany the increased pressure within the globe. Intensive postoperative antiinflammatory therapy does not appear to preempt the occurrence of glaucoma. The postoperative increase in intraocular pressure that may occur following cataracts is difficult to control, and many kangaroos must then undergo globe evisceration or euthanasia. The potential for kangaroos to develop secondary glaucoma after cataract removal requires significant case review and owner consultation before a decision is made on whether to pursue cataract surgery.

Kangaroo age and total protein content

The ability to evaluate the age of kangaroos is essential in the management of wild populations. Body weight is one method used to evaluate age, but weight can vary based on environmental influences. Age can also be assessed based on limb, bone, and teeth measurements, but obviously these measurements are a challenge to obtain. Lens weight has been used to determine age in a kangaroo, but the total protein content of lenses provides an even more accurate estimation of age. The accumulation of protein within a lens is distinguished by two distinct linear growth phases: a rapid growth phase seen in pouch young and a slower growth phase associated with adults. The transition from one phase to another occurs at approximately 0.7 to 0.9 years, the usual time of weaning in the kangaroo.

Pox

A poxvirus is responsible for raised cutaneous lesions in kangaroos. The clinically evident wart-like lesions are usually located on the extremities of a kangaroo, particularly the feet, face, and tail. Lesions also affect the eyelids. The poxvirus is spread by biting insects, mosquitoes being the most common. Diagnosis is suggested by clinical appearance but can be confirmed by biopsy and histopathology. Kangaroo poxvirus is a self-limiting disease, but surgery can be performed to remove the lesions if they affect eyelid function.

Photosensitization

Photosensitization has been recognized in three red kangaroos after eating the toxic plant *Lantana camara*.[47] One kangaroo had scleral jaundice, whereas the other developed exudative dermatitis of the eyelids as well as opacity of the corneas 1 week following exposure.

Lumpy jaw

Lumpy jaw is common in kangaroo species and is typified by swelling around areas of the face and jaw (Figure 11-13). Multiple factors are believed to contribute to the development of lumpy jaw in kangaroos, including overcrowding and poor husbandry resulting in excessive fecal contamination, particularly around feed stations. An inappropriate diet of soft feeds and/or sharp plant awns may also be the primary cause of kangaroo lumpy jaw. *Bacteroides (Dichelobacter) nodosus* and *Fusobacterium necrophorum* serve as the main source of jaw infection, whereas *Actinomyces* spp. and *Corynebacterium* spp. are less commonly isolated bacterial pathogens. When culture samples are obtained for culture and sensitivity testing, other opportunistic organisms are likely to have invaded sites of infection, and as a result, it may be difficult to isolate the original organisms.

Ophthalmic signs may also be associated with cases of lumpy jaw. Proptosis of the globe from retrobulbar abscessation may be observed and is usually accompanied by blepharospasm. Complete or partial blepharospasm occurring unilaterally with a slight serous to purulent ocular discharge is another common ophthalmic presentation in kangaroo lumpy jaw. Animals that are diagnosed with blepharospasm will usually have infected teeth as well. Infection may be localized, involving only a few teeth, but no mobility in the teeth or gingival inflammation is usually observed. In more severe cases, loose teeth with purulent discharge, bone necrosis, and osteomyelitis are common findings. Ocular signs can be accompanied by mouthing with and without salivation, nasal discharge, and facial swelling.

Discomfort from ocular, facial, and oral involvement will contribute to a kangaroo with presenting signs of anorexia. The spread of bacterial organisms to the spleen, liver, stomach, and bones can result in abscessation and clinical signs associated with infection of these sites.

Surgery is recommended to drain retrobulbar infections, remove infected teeth, and debride other infected tissues.[48] Antibiotic therapy for a duration of 6 months or longer assists in the resolution of infection. Oral clindamycin syrup at a dosage of 11 mg/kg twice a day has been found to be effective in treating kangaroo lumpy jaw cases.[43] Clindamycin capsules are also available but have a bitter taste and are not palatable to most kangaroos. Lumpy jaw can recur following the conclusion of antibiotic therapy, so affected animals should be monitored on a regular basis. Some researchers support the use of a sheep footrot vaccination in kangaroos against *Bacteroides nodosus*.[43]

Prevention is key to the control of lumpy jaw in macropod populations. An appropriate diet and good husbandry are essential in reducing the incidence of this common kangaroo disease.

Tetanus

As with all animal species, tetanus in kangaroos is a fatal disease. The disease appears most often in kangaroos following a sudden rainfall. Macropods with tetanus may display prolapse of the third eyelid.

KOALAS
Chlamydial keratoconjunctivitis

Chlamydial infections have been widely implicated as the cause of clinical disease in urban, near-urban, and minimally disturbed koala populations.[49] *Chlamydia psittaci* strains 1 and 2 are the two types of this organism originally described as infecting koalas.[49] Since that time, *Chlamydia* has been renamed *Chlamydophila,* and the types 1 and 2 have been reassigned the names *Chlamydophila pecorum* and *Chlamydophila pneumoniae,* respectively.[49] The prevalence of chlamydial infections was examined in two free-range koala populations using genus-specific PCR technology and species-specific DNA probe hybridization.[50] One population had an infection rate of only 10%, whereas the other population had an 85% overall level of chlamydial infection.[50] Seven koalas were infected with *Chlamydophila pneumoniae,* but none in this group displayed clinical signs of illness.[50] By contrast, 5 of 24 koalas infected with *Chlamydophila pecorum* manifested ocular signs as a result of clinical infection.[50] These findings suggest that *Chlamydophila pecorum* may be more pathogenic in the koala than *Chlamydophila pneumoniae.*[50]

Topical oxytetracycline is the medical treatment of choice for chlamydial keratoconjunctivitis. In chronic stages of the disease, conjunctival hypertrophy develops and may advance to a point of obscuring the cornea. Surgical excision of the proliferating and granulating conjunctival tissue can serve to reduce the severity of the clinical condition. Conjunctival hypertrophy can also be minimized with subconjunctival injections of methylpredisone.

The use of systemic antibiotics in treating chlamydial keratoconjunctivitis has not been extensively reported. Antibiotics have been used for treatment of the urogenital form of the chlamydial infection. Oxytetracyline and erythromycin have been associated with wasting and death in koalas. At this time, doxycycline and azithromycin have not been documented as treatments for marsupial chlamydial infection. Systemic enrofloxacin has been administered as an oral paste at a dosage 5 mg/kg once daily for up to 60 days. Oral ciprofloxacin has

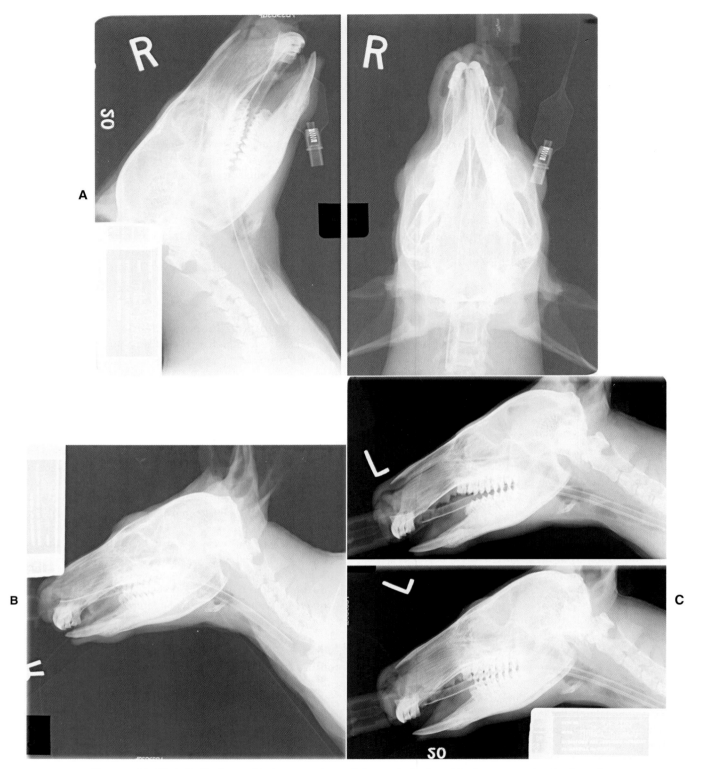

Figures 11-13 A-C: Radiographic images of a wallaby, typical of positioning to examine for fungal and bacterial infections involving the jaw and eye.

also been used in koalas at 10 mg/kg twice daily for 10 days. Many infections are accompanied by secondary *E. coli* infection, and as such, koalas should be treated with antibiotics that address both chlamydial and *E. coli* infections. The effectiveness of fluoroquinolones in the treatment of chlamydial keratoconjunctivitis of marsupials has not been determined. Malnutrition has been reported in koalas treated with systemic antibiotics; therefore, dietary protein supplementation is a recommended preventive measure. Vaccines have not been effective in producing immunity against marsupial chlamydial infection.

Keratitis

Marsupials may present with keratitis. Studies of free-range koalas found infections to be chronic and occur either in one or both eyes.[51] No specific cause could be determined and no clinical signs of *Chlamydophila* spp. infection were evident and serologic testing for koala chlamydiosis was negative.[51] Case work-up for marsupial keratitis should follow standard practice for domestic pets.

Cryptococcosis

Cryptococcus neoformans has been seen on occasion in the koala. The actual occurrence of *Cryptococcus* has been related to flowering of the eucalyptus tree, an inherent habitat and food source for the koala. Many animals affected by *Cryptococcus* spp. have dilated pupils as a result of optic neuritis. Blindness, a consequence of CNS infection, is another presentation for the disease. Treatment can be a challenge, as recurrence is common. Prognosis for affected animals is usually considered guarded.

Ocular lymphosarcoma

Lymphosarcoma is one of the neoplastic changes observed in koalas. Ocular involvement may be observed as masses in the eye, conjunctiva, or both. Retroviruses are believed to contribute to the development of lymphosarcoma although information remains nonspecific. Retroviruses are also suspected to have an immunosuppressive effect and may be precursors for other diseases such as chlamydial infections.

WALLABIES

The structure of the optic chiasm and retina has been compared in albino wallabies to those of normal pigmentation. The uncrossed pathway of albino wallabies was determined to be smaller than that of pigmented animals, and cell density in the retinal ganglion cell layer was reduced at the area centralis. Tammar wallabies have been determined to have dichromatic color vision and readily learn the relationship between presented colors as opposed to absolute hues. The tammar wallaby is also known to possess typical levels of mammalian rhodopsin, which allows animals the ability to see at night.

Conjunctivitis

Conjunctivitis has been observed in a captive gray dorcopsis (*Dorcopsis muelleri luctosa*) that had experienced a period of stress and then died.[52] On histopathologic examination, a diagnosis of herpesvirus was made.[52]

Toxoplasmosis

Toxoplasmosis in wallabies has been shown to produce a number of ocular lesions. Unilateral or bilateral cataract formation, as well as various degrees of keratitis, uveitis, chorioretinitis, and endophthalmitis, have been observed among affected animals. Wallabies with ocular toxoplasmosis often present with advanced cataracts and uveitis. Inflammatory reaction within affected eyes is considered to be mild and most evident in the anterior uvea. Less inflammation is observed in the inner retina and adjacent vitreous. No correlation has been established between the severity of chorioretinitis and cataract development or between the incidence of ocular lesions and serum antibody levels.

EASTERN BARRED BANDICOOTS

Ocular toxoplasmosis has been observed in Eastern barred bandicoots, with cataracts being a predominant clinical finding.[53] Fundic lesions included areas of chorioretinitis or loss of the small vascular tuft from the optic disc.[53] Statistical analysis showed bandicoots with toxoplasmosis titers greater than or equal to 1:64 were more likely to have ocular lesions.[53] Cataracts were more likely to occur in bandicoots with titers greater than or equal to 1:256 and greater than or equal to 1:152.[53]

BRUSHTAIL OPOSSUMS

Chronic meningoencephalitis and optic neuritis have been reported in brushtail opossums of Eastern and Southern Australia. The combination of these conditions result in a clinical syndrome commonly referred to as "wobbly opossums." Adult opossums are primarily affected, but cases are occasionally reported in both juvenile and pouch animals. Clinical signs are progressive, often spanning a period of weeks to months. Patients suffering with meningoencephalitis usually exhibit symptoms of depression, blindness, and ataxia. Opthalmologic findings include focal tapetal discoloration, a pale optic disc, or an optic disc that lacks the normal vascular tuft. Animals possessing these ocular changes are clinically blind and have dilated pupils. Wallerian degeneration and mild, nonsuppurative inflammation and retinal atrophy are often noted along the optic tracts of many opossums suffering from chronic meningoencephalitis. Chronic meningoencephalitis in brushtail opossums is considered to have a viral etiology.

Therapeutics

Blood-brain barrier. The choroid plexus marks the site of the blood-cerebrospinal fluid (CSF) barrier, part of the blood-CSF-brain barrier or blood-brain barrier, as it is commonly known.

The ability of a drug to permeate the blood-brain barrier can dictate its effectiveness and selection in both metherian and eutherian species. The blood-brain barrier is actually comprised of a series of permeability restriction mechanisms found at various interfaces between blood, CSF, and brain. It has been proposed that the exchange of molecules between blood, brain, and CSF decrease during development.

The opossum has been studied extensively in this regard, as it is born at a much earlier stage of brain development than are eutherian mammals, allowing changes in the barrier associated with development to be more thoroughly studied. Choroid plexuses of all four brain ventricles have been examined in the opossum. Epithelial changes occur throughout the course of the opossums' development with the choroidal epithelium changes from a pseudostratified to a cuboidal layer. Individual epithelial cells appear to undergo a similar maturation process though the timing of it varies between and within plexuses.

Microscopically, the number of mitochondria and microvilli increase, and structural changes are observed with the endoplasmic reticulum. By contrast, tight junctions between the choroidal epithelial cells show no detectable structural change with development. In general, cellular changes in the choroids plexus of the developing opossum resemble those observed in other species, validating the opossum as an excellent research model for mammalian choroid plexus development.[48]

REFERENCES

1. Johnson-Delaney CA: Marsupials. In *Supplement, the Exotic Companion Medicine Handbook for Veterinarians,* Lake Worth, Fla, 1997, ZEN.
2. Kirkland PD: Epidemic viral diseases of wildlife—sudden death in tammar wallabies, blind kangaroos, herpesviruses in pilchards—what next? *Microbiol Aust* 26(2):82-84, 2005.
3. Seebeck JH: Mammals of the western plains or; where have all the wombats gone? *J Aust Wildlife Research* 6:39-53, 1984.
4. Raillet A: *Éléments de Zoologie Médicale et Agricole,* Paris, Asselin et Houzeau, 1886.
5. Blanchard R: Note sur les sarcosporidies et sur un essai de classification de ces sporozoaires, *Bulletin de la Societe de Zoologie de France* 10:244-276, 1885.
6. Labbé A: Sporozoa. In Butschli O, editor: *Das Tierreich,* ed 5, Berlin, 1899, Friedlander.
7. Minchin EA: In Lankester ER, editor: *A Treatise on Zoology,* part 1, fasc 2, London, 1903.
8. Noller W: Klein Beobachtungen an parasitischen Protozoen. Zur Kenntrus der Darmprotozoen des Hamsters *(Eimeria falciformis var. cricetinov. Var.), Arch Protistenkd* 41:169-189, 1920.
9. Mackerras MJ: Catalogue of Australian mammals and their recorded internal parasites, *Proc Linnaean Soc New South Wales* 83:101-160, 1958.
10. Coutelen FR: *Annales de Parasitologie* 11:1-6, 1933.
11. Zwart P, Strik WJ: Globidiosis in a Bennett's wallaby, *Tijdschrift voor Diergeneeskunde* 89:138-143, 1964.
12. Reichenow E: *Doflein's Lehrbuch der Protozoenkunde,* ed 5, vol 6, Jena, 1953, G. Fischer Verlag.
13. Levine ND: What is "Sarcocysti" mucosa? *Ann Trop Med and Parasitol* 73:91-92, 1979.
14. O'Donoghue PJ, Obendorf DL, O'Callaghan MG et al: *Sarcocystis mucosa* (Blanchard 1885) Labbé 1889 in unadorned rock wallabies *(Petrogale assimilis)* and Bennett's wallabies *(Macropus rufugriseus), Parasit Research* 73(2):113-120, 1987.
15. Dubey JP, Lindsay DS: *Sarcocystis speeri* n sp (Protozoa: Sarcocystidae) from the opossum *(Didelphis virginiana)* 85:903-909, 1999.
16. Fenger CK, Granstrom DE, Langemeier JL et al: Identification of opossoms *(Didelphis virginiana)* as the putative definitive host of *Sarcocystis neurona, J Parasit* 81(6):916-919, 1995.
17. Dubey JP, Davis SW, Speer CA et al: *Sarcocystis neurona* n sp (Protozoa: Apicomlexa), the etiological agent of equine protozoal myeloencephalitis, *J Parasitol* 77:212-221, 1991.
18. Dubey JP, Saville WJA, Lindsay DS et al: Completion of the life cycle of *Sarcocystis neurona, J Parasitol* 86:1276-1280, 2000.
19. Barker IK, O'Callaghan MG, Beveridge I et al: Host parasite associations of *Eimeria* spp. (Apicomplexa: Eimeriidae) in rock wallabies, *Petrogale* spp. (Marsupialia: Macropodiadae), *Int J Parasitol* 18(3):353-363, 1988.
20. Schneider CR: Cross immunity evidence of the identity of *Besnoitia panamensis* from lizards and *B. darlingii* from opossums, *J Parasitol* 53(4):886, 1967.
21. Smith DD, Frenkel JK: *Besnoita darlingii* (Protozoa: Toxoplasmatinae): Cyclic transmission by cats, *J Parasitol* 63(6):1066-1071, 1977.
22. Elsheika HM, Mansfield LS, Fitzgerald SD et al: Prevalence and tissue distribution of *Besnoitia darlingii* cysts in the Virginia opossum *(Didelphis virginiana)* in Michigan, *Vet Parasitol* 115:321-327, 2003.
23. Nettles VF, Prestwood AK, Davidson WR: Severe parasitism in an opossum, *J Wildl Dis* 11:419-420, 1975.
24. Feldman DB, Moore JA, Harris MW et al: Characteristics of common helminthes of the Virginia opossum *(Didelphis virginiana)* from North Carolina, *Lab Anim Sci* 22:183-189, 1972.
25. Krupp JH: Treatment of opossums with *Physaloptera* infections, *JAVMA* 141:369-370, 1962.
26. Andersen FL, Reilly JR: The anatomy of *Tetratrichomonas didelphidis* (Hegner and Ratcliffe, 1927) comb nov from the opossum, *J Parasitol* 14:27-35, 1965.
27. Tasca T, De Carli GA, Glock L et al: Morphologic aspects of *Tetratrichomonas didelphis* isolated from opossum *Didelphis marsupialis* and *Lutreolina crassicaudata, Mem Inst Oswaldo Cruz* 96:265-271, 2001.
28. Tasca T, Indrusiak C, Glock L et al: Prevalence of *Tetratrichomonas didelphidis* from the opossum *Didelphis albientris* in the Botanical Garden, Porto Alegre, Rio Grande do Sul, Brazil, *Parasitol Dia* 25:132-134, 2001.
29. Stromberg BE: Trichenellosis. In Aiello SE, Mays A, editors: *Merck Veterinary Manual,* ed 8, New Jersey, 1998, Merck.
30. Zimmerman WJ, Hubbard ED: Trichiniasis in wildlife in Iowa, *Am J Epidemiol* 90:84-92, 1969.
31. Schad GA, Leiby DA, Murrell KD: Distribution, prevalence and intensity of *Trichinella spiralis* infection in furbearing mammals of Pennsylvania, *J Parasitol* 70:372-377, 1984.
32. Leiby DA, Gerhard AS, Duffy CH et al: *Trichinella spiralis* in an agricultural ecosystem, III. Epidemiological investigations of *Trichinella spiralis* in resident wild and feral animals, *J Wildl Dis* 24:606-609, 1988.
33. Pung OJ, Durden LA, Banks CW et al: Ectoparasites of opossums and raccoons in southeastern Georgia, *J Med Entomol* 31:915-919, 1994.
34. Azad AF: Epidemiology of murine typhus, *Annu Rev Entomol* 35:553-569, 1990.
35. Piesman J, Sinsky RJ: Ability of *Ixodes scapularis, Dermacentor variabilis,* and *Amblyomma americanum* (Acari: Ixodidae) to acquire, maintain, and transmit Lyme disease spirochetes, *J Med Entomol* 25:336-339, 1988.
36. Kinsella JM, Winegarner CE: A field study of *Anatrichosoma* infections in the opossum, *Didelphis virginiana, J Parasitol* 61(4):779-781, 1975.
37. Warren KS, Swan RA, Morgan-Ryan UM et al: *Cryptosporidium muris* infection in bilbies *(Macrotis lagotis), Aust Vet J* 81:739-741, 2003.
38. Dawson TJ, Webster KN, Mifsud B et al: Functional capacities of marsupial hearts: size and mitochondrial parameters indicate higher aerobic capabilities than generally seen in placental animals, *J Comp Physiol B* 173:583-590, 2003.
39. Johnson-Delaney CA: *Exotic Companion Medicine Handbook for Veterinarians,* Lake Worth, Fla, 1996, Wingers.
40. Lonigro JG, LaRegina MC: Characterization of *Erysipelothrix rhusiopathiae* isolated from an opossum *(Didelphis virginiana)* with septicemia, *J Wildlife Dis* 24(3):557-559, 1988.
41. Johnson-Delaney CA: Reproductive medicine of companion marsupials, *Vet Clin North Am Exot Anim Pract* 5:537-553, 2002.
42. McColl K, Wilks CR: Immune status of orphaned, pouch-young macropods. In Evans DD, editor: The Management of Australian Mammals in Captivity, *Proc Sci Meeting Australian Mammal Soc,* Healesville, Victoria, the Zoological Board of Victoria, Melbourne, pp 125-128, 1982.
43. Williams A, Williams R: *Caring for Kangaroos and Wallabies,* East Roseville, NSW, 1999, Kangaroo Press/Simon and Schuster, Australia.
44. Wallach JD, Boever WJ: *Diseases of Exotic Animals: Medical and Surgical Management,* Philadelphia, 1983, WB Saunders.
45. Hooper PT, Lunt RA, Gould AR et al: Epidemic of blindness in kangaroos—evidence of a viral aetiology, *Aust Vet J* 77(8):529-536, 1999.
46. Durham PJK, Finnie JW, Lawrence DA et al: Blindness in South Australian kangaroos, *Aust Vet J* 73:111-112, 1996.
47. Johnson JH, Jensen JM: Hepatotoxicity and secondary photosensitization in a red kangaroo *(Megaleia rufus)* due to ingestion of *Lantana camara, J Zoo Wildlife Med* 29(2):203-207, 1998.

48. McMenamin PG, Krause W: Development of the eye in North American opossum *(Didelphis virginiana)*, *J Anat* 183:343-358, 1993.

49. Girjes AA, Hugall AF, Timms P et al: Two distinct forms of *Chlamydia psittaci* associated with disease and infertility in *Phascolarctos cinereus* (koala), *Infect Immun* 56(8):1897-1900, 1988.

50. Jackson M, White N, Giffard P et al: Epizootiology of Chlamydia infections of two free range koala populations, *Vet Micro* 65:255-264, 1999.

51. Hirst LW, Brown AS, Kempster R et al: Keratitis in free-ranging koalas *(Phascolarctos cinereus)* on Magnetic Island, Townsville, *J Wildlife Dis* 28(3):424-427, 1992.

52. Callinan RB, Kefford B: Mortalities associated with herpes virus infection in captive macropods, *J Wildlife Dis* 17(2):311-317, 1981.

53. Beltiol SS, Jakes K, Le DD et al: First record of trypanosomes in Tasmanian bandicoots, *J Parasit* 84(3):538-541, 1998.

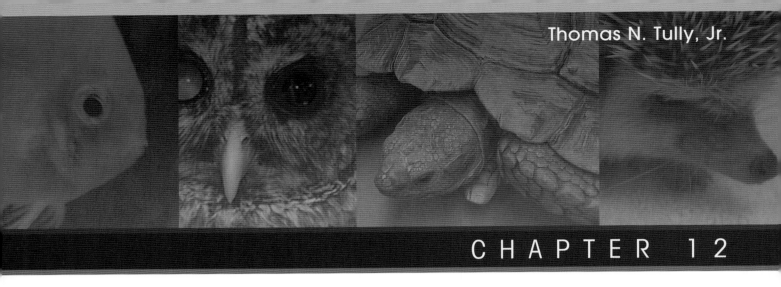

Thomas N. Tully, Jr.

CHAPTER 12

MICE AND RATS

This chapter, on mice and rats, contains information on the companion species that is useful for veterinarians treating the animals or providing information to the owners. Although similarities exist for mice and rats—in care, husbandry, diagnostic testing, and treatment—emphasis will be on the differences between the species.

MICE

Mice may be maintained as pets because of their size and playful nature. Although playful, mice can be aggressive to cagemates and owners. The aggressive nature often manifests as barbering and/or fighting with cagemates and biting their owners. Any potential owner should be educated on the aggressive nature of these small dynamos. Domestic mice *(Mus musculus)* and the African pygmy mouse (*Baiomys* spp.) are commonly sold for pets and are available in several varieties. The mice varieties sold in pet stores include white, black, or tan colored, satin hair coat (shiny), pied or spotted, and long-haired[1,2] (Figure 12-1). The size and ability of mice to escape quickly from the grasp of a human handler make these animals, as pets, better suited for older individuals. The timid nature of mice predispose these animals to biting if handled roughly, which commonly occurs with a young owner. Mice are nocturnal animals and may be a disturbance at night if maintained in a bedroom. Female mice produce less odor than males and therefore may be more desirable as pets. As mentioned earlier, male mice are territorial, and if placed with other male mice, may fight. Advantages of having mice as pets include their size, ability to be a good companion animal for the educated (regarding mouse behavior) owner, and adorable appearance.

Mice also rarely become infected with bacterial diseases, and their life span is approximately 2 years (Box 12-1).

■ BIOLOGY

The integument of mice is commonly associated with a number of disease presentations. A hair coat that has not been adequately maintained is often the first clinical sign associated with disease. Mice are fastidious with their grooming and, when healthy, maintain a very tidy hair coat. Common problems associated with a hair coat that is not maintained include general illness, parasitism (internal and external), aggression by cagemates as a result of psychological trauma, and infectious dermatitis.

Neoplasia is a disease condition that affects mice. There are some mouse strains in which mouse mammary tumor viruses have been identified that have a neoplasia incidence as high as 70%.[3] Tumor viruses, as well as a very short life span (up to 2 years), predispose these animals to cancer. Mammary adenocarcinomas and fibrosarcomas are the most common tumors that affect mouse mammary tissue.[4] Unfortunately, by the time many of these tumors are diagnosed, the malignant masses are large and ulcerated.[4] Fibrosarcomas may be hormonally induced, and the incidence of this disease process can be reduced through an ovariectomy at an early age. The small size of the female mouse often makes the ovariectomy surgery challenging for the veterinary surgeon.

Although relatively uncommon, urethral obstruction can occur in male mice as a result of preputial and/or bulbourethral gland infections.[4] Male mice suffering from an urethral obstruction may have a mutilated penis, a sign often associated with the disease process.

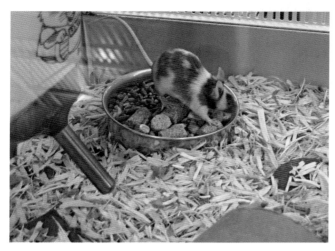

Figure 12-1 Mice are small companion animals that come in a variety of colors.

Mice are continuous, polyestrous rodents that should be bred in polygamous or monogamous setups because of the males' aggressive territoriality behavior.[2] When breeding mice that have been housed in a polygamous ratio, there may be one male with two to six females.[2] Females are removed from a polygamous cage before parturition, whereas the monogamous pair is maintained together with the young until weaning.[2]

■ HUSBANDRY

Environmental Considerations

Mice can chew out of enclosures; therefore, it is important that the housing be "mouse proof." If an animal escapes, the best way to capture the pet is to place food in the center of the room. Once it has been determined in which room the animal is staying, then it should be sealed and measures taken to look for the pet. Because mice are nocturnal animals, capture at night in a dark room with a flashlight may work best. This technique will work for capture of other small rodents and pocket pets too.

Mice are maintained in environments that are similar to other small rodents but require a thorough cleaning of their cage more often because of their malodorous urine. Ventilation is essential for small rodent housing to prevent irritation of the respiratory tract from ammonia vapors generated by urine. The recommended housing unit for mice is 12-15″ × 12-15″ × 6″ (length × width × height) for each adult mouse; females and young require 2 to 3 times the space listed.[2] The major considerations for selecting an enclosure for mice is that it be resistant to their escape and easy to clean. An open screen top of the enclosure is recommended for proper ventilation. Available rodent cages that fit this criterion are wire or metal mesh, plastic, and Plexiglas. If the plastic tube housing systems are used, there should be routine cleaning of the sections using hot water and a mild detergent. Owners should be informed of the small distance required for a mouse to escape and their ability to chew through plastic. An owner must always monitor the cage for possible escape avenues, especially if the animal has a predilection for modifying the cage opening through chewing. It is very important to provide cage toys and exercise opportunities for mice. The enclosure should be large enough to house not only food and water containers but also cage toys and an exercise wheel (Figure 12-2). Although not a cage toy, a hide box, in some form, should also be included for the psychological well-being of the animal. This hide box can be manufactured or a small cardboard container that has one end cut out. Mice like to hide and also sleep during the day. This piece of cage furniture will enable the mouse to sleep undisturbed during the daylight hours.

Mice, especially males, have odiferous urine. To prevent the buildup of urine and fecal material in the cage, commercially available paper rodent bedding or hardwood shavings should be used as a cage substrate. Although softwood (pine) and cedar shavings are available, the volatile oils that radiate from these substrates are irritating to small animals. These irritating

BOX 12-1 Basic Mice Information

Life Span	2 years
Body Weight	
Adult male	20-40 g
Adult female	25-40 g
Temperature, Pulse, and Respiration	
Rectal/body temperature	36.5°-38.0° C (98°-101° F)
Normal heart rate	325-780 beats/min
Normal respiratory rate	40-80 breaths/min
Amounts of Food and Water	
Daily food consumption	>15 g/100 g body weight/day
Daily water consumption	>15 ml/100 g body weight/day
Age at Onset of Puberty and Breeding Initiation	
Puberty females	28-40 days
Breeding initiation males	50 days
Breeding initiation females	50-60 days
Female Reproductive Cycle	
Estrous cycle	4-5 days
Gestation length	19-21 days
Litter size	10-12
Postpartum estrus	Fertile
Young production	8 months

Modified from Bihune C, Bauck L: Basic anatomy, physiology, husbandry, and clinical techniques. In Quesenberry KE, Carpenter JW, editors: *Ferrets, Rabbits and Rodents: Clinical Medicine and Surgery,* ed 2, St Louis, 2004, WB Saunders; Johnson-Delaney CA, Harrison LR: *Small Rodents: Exotic Companion Medicine Handbook for Veterinarians,* Lake Worth, Fla, 1996, Wingers.

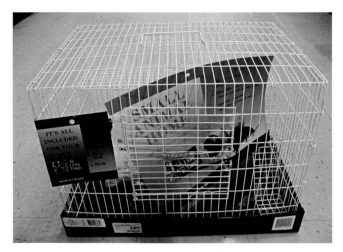

Figure 12-2 A typical mouse cage is made of wire and has room for a hide box and exercise wheel.

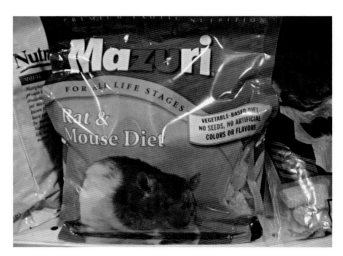

Figure 12-3 Commercial biscuit or pellet diets are nutritionally balanced and provide an excellent food source for pet mice.

compounds can cause dermal and respiratory inflammation, often leading to secondary bacterial infections.

Cardboard tissue tubes can be placed in a mouse enclosure; mice like to chew and run through these items. Because many fabrics have strong thread and elastic, it is not recommended to put clothes items in enclosures with animals that chew. Often mice will shred the clothing items, exposing thread and elastic that can become entangled around an extremity; this can lead to necrosis distal to the stricture. It is recommended to change the substrate within the enclosure at least twice a week—more often if there is a problem with odor or excessive excreta.

Temperature, humidity, and lighting within the enclosure should follow what is commonly maintained with the ambient conditions within the house. If the animals are housed outside or in an outbuilding, the temperature range should be 65° F to 85° F and humidity 30% to 70%, although the recommended humidity is on the higher end of the range provided.[2] Mice, especially males, are extremely territorial animals. If mice are housed alone, it is better to keep them separate, as introduction of new animals will often lead to aggression and fighting. To prevent aggression, fighting, and psychologically induced adverse behavior (e.g., barbering), a single mouse is recommended as a companion animal. For those who intend to breed the animals, enclosures with a single pair is necessary for reproductive success.

Nutrition

Because mice are commonly used as laboratory animals in investigations of human disease processes, much research literature is available on the recommended nutritional requirements of these animals. The benefit of these dietary studies is the availability of commercially produced diets that provide the recommended daily nutritional requirements of the mouse. The problem that most owners face is the multitude of dietary products available for mice and the lack of knowledge regarding which food to buy. Most new mouse owners think that

rodents eat seed-based diets. Although mice will happily eat seed, seed-based diets are lacking in a number of the nutritional requirements needed to maintain long-term health. Commercial rodent biscuits or pellets with more than 14% protein are the recommended diets for mice.[2] The commercial rodent biscuits or pellets are the only food mice need to obtain their required nutrients (Figure 12-3). Again, seed-based diets are not recommended, nor is a significant supplementation of fruits, nuts, vegetables, cheese, or other human foods (e.g., peanut butter). If a treat is to be given, yogurt or dried fruit treats manufactured specifically for rodents and/or mice should be provided 2 to 3 times a week. For younger mice, less than 3 weeks old, softer pellets are needed because babies start eating pellets and drinking water at 2 to 3 weeks of age.[2] A sipper bottle, placed on the outside of the cage, is easy to maintain and does not take any space within the enclosure. If the cage is plastic or Plexiglas, modifications will be needed to attach the sipper bottle on the outside of the cage. Most sipper bottles come with attachment hardware to attach to wire cages (Figure 12-4). Fresh bottled water is recommended for mice, although chlorinated tap water is acceptable. The water should be checked on a daily basis and clean water supplied at least every 2 days, if not every day.

■ PREVENTIVE MEDICINE
Quarantine

Quarantining an animal is important when a new animal is being introduced into a setting in which there is an established group. As with other animals, a 30-day quarantine period is recommended, along with a physical examination and fecal parasite check. Unfortunately, there is no time period that will screen 100% against potential infectious agents, and with mice, time is critical because their life span and reproductive time frame are so short. The animals should be quarantined in conditions similar to those in which they will be permanently maintained. Providing adequate food and water will

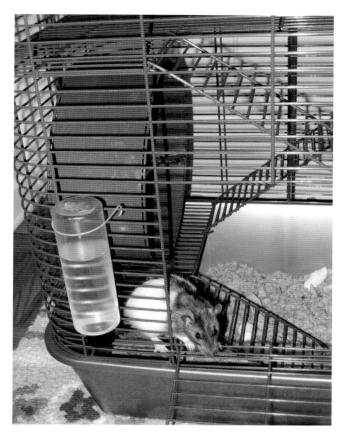

Figure 12-4 A sipper bottle attached to the outside of the cage is easy to fill and clean.

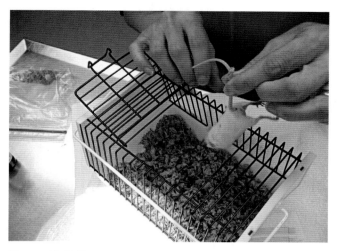

Figure 12-5 By grasping a mouse by the tail and slowly dragging over a cage, the mouse can be positioned for capture.

make for a smooth transition. It is imperative that the owner screen the new animal for diseases and watch for any signs of illness. The most common sign of clinical illness is a rough hair coat. The lack of grooming is most often related to the animal feeling depressed or sick, thereby not having the energy to perform routine behaviors. If a number of animals are being quarantined, sacrificing an apparently diseased animal is the most efficient way to determine a rapid definitive diagnosis. If it is a single or an expensive animal, routine diagnostic testing will be required.

To maintain oversight of breeding animals' health and reduce the exposure of young animals to infectious disease and parasites, routine screening of representative animals within the colony is recommended. In very large colonies, special caging (e.g., filter), food, and water may be necessary to prevent exposure to disease organisms.[2]

Routine Exams

Before a veterinarian examines a mouse, the examination table should be disinfected with either a dilute sodium hypochlorite or chlorhexidine solution. The examiner should always wash his or her hands and, if necessary, wear examination gloves to capture and restrain the patient. The difficulty with using latex gloves when examining a mouse is the small size of the patient

and its ability to twist and turn. The only way to restrain some mouse patients is without gloves. If gloves are not worn, the examiner's hands must be washed thoroughly after the examination is completed.

RESTRAINT

To catch a mouse, the tail should be grabbed with the thumb and forefinger, allowing the mouse to hold on to an object with their front feet (Figure 12-5). When the mouse securely attaches itself to an object, the opposite hand then grabs the dorsal skin in the cervical region while keeping the tail in a firm grasp.

If one is unable to adequately restrain a mouse while the animal is conscious, inhalant anesthesia may be used for sedation purposes. The animal should be placed in a small induction chamber and isoflurane gas permeated into the closed space. Once the animal has stopped moving, the enclosure top is removed and a nose cone placed on the anesthesia tube and placed on the patient's face. A syringe case can be modified as a nose cone for small rodents, including mice. Once the physical examination is complete, the nose cone is removed, allowing the patient to breath oxygen from the anesthesia unit.

HISTORY

Obtaining a detailed history of the mouse patient is very important, as it is with other animal patients that are brought to a veterinarian's office. It is important to get as much information from the owner as possible, even if it is a routine health examination.

Typical background information required includes how long the mouse been owned, where it was acquired, how often it is handled, and what the character of the feces and urine is. Husbandry questions should focus on the animal's housing and whether it is allowed to roam unobserved; cage location; type, size, and material of the cage; cage substrate, furniture, and toys; and the frequency with which the cage is cleaned and what disinfectant is used. When investigating the diet, the veterinarian should ask not only if pellets are fed and in what quantity, but also what the animal is eating and what the primary diet is. Supplemental offerings and frequency of feeding are important data for the case work-up. The veterinarian should find out about the water supply, how often the water is changed, and how much the animal drinks on a daily basis.

Because there are transmissible diseases among animals, the final questions should center on the other pets in the household, if new animals have been added to the family, and if the animals are housed together. A description of any previous problems and a complete chronological description of the presenting problem are needed to complete the history form.

PHYSICAL EXAMINATION

Before the animal is restrained, an observation should be made on the attitude, activity, and posture of the animal. The next step is to weigh the mouse in a basket on a digital gram scale. If possible, temperature, respiration, and pulse should be measured and any abnormalities in rate and/or character noted. The veterinarian should start the physical examination at the head, looking for any abnormalities. Eyes, ears, and nares are observed, looking for discharge or inflammation. The oral cavity is difficult to examine in mice because of the small opening and tendency for the buccal mucosa to encroach toward the middle of the mouth. A small speculum (e.g., modified paper clip) or an otoscope may be used to examine the oral cavity and cheek teeth. Mucous membranes help determine hydration status using capillary refill time and moisture. Body condition and abdominal palpation are important information that should be obtained. Lymph nodes and limbs are palpated before checking the nails and plantar surface of each foot. The patient should have a normal posture, be aware of its surroundings, and move properly. Any problems should be noted in the record. Finally, a dermatologic exam considers hair coat quality, alopecia, external parasites, and any skin abnormalities. All abnormal findings are written in the record for case review, differential diagnoses determination, diagnostic testing, and treatment considerations.

COMMON ABNORMALITIES FOUND ON PHYSICAL EXAMINATION

Most of the common problems noted during the physical examination of mice involve the skin and hair coat. As mentioned previously, an unkempt hair coat may point toward generalized illness or external parasitism. Abrasive lesions or pustules on the skin can be signs of external parasites or infectious dermatitis. If external parasites are a problem, the mouse may be uncontrollably scratching. Hair loss may be associated with barbering, either cagemate or self-induced, or with infection (e.g., ringworm). Although not common, *Trichophyton mentagrophytes* will cause hair loss in mice, from the face, head, and neck.[4]

Mice will commonly present with tumors and abscesses. The entire body of the mouse should be palpated for any evidence of masses. If a mass is identified, a fine needle aspirate is recommended for basic diagnostic evaluation. With most fine needle aspirate samples, the clinical pathology results are not very rewarding. If a diagnosis cannot be obtained through cytologic examination, a biopsy of the lesion is required, and if possible, an excisional biopsy is the procedure of choice.

As with many rodents, respiratory disease is commonly identified in mice. Mice may have presenting symptoms of dyspnea, sneezing, coughing, chattering, and sniffling if they have a respiratory infection. In cases where respiratory signs are observed, anesthetizing the animal to perform the physical examination is not recommended, and handling should be kept to a minimum. The two most common respiratory disease conditions in mice are Sendai virus and *Mycoplasma pulmonis*.[4] These two organisms are very difficult to identify through routine diagnostic measures, and obtaining samples significantly stresses the patient. If the animal is being examined for placement into a colony or breeding environment, sacrifice to identify the disease condition is recommended. If the animal is an individual companion animal, doxycycline treatment should be initiated. Although treatment with doxycycline will not clear the organism from the animal, it will reduce clinical disease and improve the quality of life. The treated animal should always be considered a carrier of these respiratory diseases if a definitive diagnosis cannot be obtained.

Male mice that are licking and/or mutilating their penis may be suffering from a urethral obstruction. Infection of accessory sex glands, young males with aggressive breeding activity, urolithiasis, and trauma may initiate this self-induced trauma to the penis.[4] *Pasteurella pneumotropica* is often isolated from accessory sex gland infections as well as subdermal abscesses.[4] Treatment for this organism may aid in the recovery of a mouse affected by urethral obstruction.

Diarrhea in mice is rare, but endoparasite examinations should be performed if the animal has diarrhea. Although pinworms are considered nonpathogenic in mice, *Syphacia obvelata* and *Aspiculuris tetraptera* may cause rectal prolapse due to straining in immunosuppressed individuals.[5] As with other animals, a tape test is the best way to identify these parasites. A tape test follows a procedure of pressing the sticky side of the tape against the rectum and perianal area and then examining the tape under a microscope for eggs and parasites.[5]

■ DIAGNOSTIC TESTING

Hematology

As with other pocket pets, blood collection from mice can be quite difficult. Approximately 0.5 to 0.7 ml/100 g body weight can be safely removed from a nonanemic healthy mouse.[2] The mouse patient should always be anesthetized for blood collection procedures. Usually inducing the animals in a closed chamber and maintaining the patients in a mask will allow the technician plenty of time to collect the blood sample. A small, 25-, 26-, or 30-gauge needle, usually placed on a 1-ml syringe, is recommended for collecting the blood. Recommended blood collection sites in a mouse are a warmed ventral tail vein

BOX 12-2	Retroorbital Blood Collection for Mice

1. Stabilize head at base of skull and point of jaw.
2. Occlusion of the jugular vein may distend the venous plexus.
3. Retract the dorsal lid of the eye with the index finger.
4. A microcapillary tube or small-bore Pasteur pipette is inserted at the medial canthus.
5. Once the tube is placed in the correct position, the tube can be gently rotated until the conjunctiva is punctured and the orbital venous plexus is penetrated.
6. The tube is filled by capillary action.
7. Slight pressure may be placed over the eye to aid in hemostasis after sample collection.
8. A volume of 0.2-0.3 ml may be collected from an adult mouse.

From Tully TN, Mitchell MA: *A Technician's Guide to Exotic Animal Care,* Lakewood, CO, 2001, American Animal Hospital Association Press.

or the tip of the tail.[2] Box 12-2 describes the technique used for retroorbital bleeding in mice. The retroorbital bleeding technique is commonly used in laboratory animal settings and is easily performed by an experienced veterinarian or veterinary technician.[5]

On smaller rodents, the saphenous vein or lateral vein of the tarsus may be used for multiple blood collections without the use of anesthesia. The patient must be properly immobilized in a restraint tube (35-ml syringe) with the leg extended and the skin held tight on the medial aspect of the thigh using the thumb and forefinger.[2] The taut skin on the lateral aspect of the thigh allows exposure of the saphenous vein. A 23-gauge needle is used to puncture the vein, and blood is collected in a microhematocrit tube as it flows from the vessel.[5]

Blood samples obtained from nail and ear clips are not considered appropriate diagnostic samples. Cardiac puncture is recommended only in terminal cases and when the animal is maintained under general anesthesia because of possible complications involving the lungs and heart vessels. Reference ranges for complete blood counts and serum biochemistry panels for mice are listed in Boxes 12-3 and 12-4.[1,2]

Bone Marrow Aspiration

Marrow samples may be obtained from the ilium, tibia, sternum, femur, or the bones of the proximal one third of the tail.[5] Preparation of the samples is consistent with that of other mammalian patients.

Urine Collection

Standard rodent cages can be used without substrate to collect urine and feces when the patient is hospitalized. After placing a rodent in a zip-lock bag, urination frequently occurs and the sample can be collected.[4] In a similar manner, urine can be collected over a disinfected stainless steel examination table.

BOX 12-3	Complete Blood Count Reference Ranges for Mice

Erythrocytes	$7\text{-}12.5 \times 10^6\ \mu L$
Hematocrit	36%-39%
Hemoglobin	10.2-18 mg/dl
Leukocytes	$6\text{-}15 \times 10^3\ \mu L$
Neutrophils	10%-40%
Lymphocytes	55%-95%
Monocytes	0.1%-3.5%
Eosinophils	0%-4%
Basophils	0%-0.3%
Platelets	$160\text{-}410 \times 10^6\ mm^3$
Serum protein	3.5-7.2 g/dl
Albumin	2.5-4.8 g/dl
Globulin	1.8-3 g/dl

BOX 12-4	Serum Biochemistry Reference Ranges for Mice

Serum glucose	62-175 mg/dl
Blood urea nitrogen	12-28 mg/dl
Creatinine	0.3-1.0 mg/dl
Total bilirubin	0.1-0.60 mg/dl
Cholesterol	26-82 mg/dl
Serum calcium	8.0-12.0 mg/dl
Serum phosphorus	3.0-6.0 mg/dl

BOX 12-5	Urinalysis Reference Values for Mice

Urine volume (ml/24 h)	0.5-2.5 ml
Specific gravity	1.034
Average pH	5.01
Protein	males proteinuric

From Bihune C, Bauck L: Basic anatomy, physiology, husbandry, and clinical techniques. In Quesenberry KE, Carpenter JW, editors: *Ferrets, Rabbits and Rodents: Clinical Medicine and Surgery*, ed 2, St Louis, 2004, WB Saunders.

The urine is voided while the animal is restrained and can be collected in a capillary tube for evaluation on urine reagent strips.[1] Urinalysis reference values for mice are listed in Box 12-5.

Diagnostic Imaging

Under most practice settings, the size of a mouse patient limits imaging capabilities to radiographs. Restraint is essential for quality diagnostic images and is even more important when patients weigh as little as 40 g. To obtain adequate restraint and prevent movement of the mouse patient during radiographic evaluation, sedation is required. As with all diagnostic procedures involving avian and exotic animals, an evaluation of the patient is required to determine its ability to withstand the stress associated with the assessment. If it is determined that the patient cannot withstand sedation, then it should be stabilized until it is deemed healthy enough for diagnostic imaging evaluation.

Sedating the mouse using an induction chamber and isoflurane anesthetic, as described for restraint, is necessary to obtain diagnostic films. High-speed, 300-mA machines with fine or detail-intensifying screens should be adequate for most small exotic mammal images. With mice, dental x-ray units that can focus at short distances may be advantageous for both isolation of focal anatomy and full body radiographs in extremely small patients. For extreme detail in small exotic mammal medicine, using a traditional radiography unit, the Min R mammography system (Eastman Kodak) with Min R single-intensifying screen cassettes, in conjunction with Min R single-emulsion film, has been recommended.[1] Digital radiography is bringing a new dimension to radiograph evaluations and detail. The secret to success in either traditional or digital radiographic imaging is to restrict patient movement during exposure. Two views, ventrodorsal and lateral, are recommend for mice patients. Again, because of a mouse patient's size, whole body radiographs are commonly obtained during the radiographic evaluation, even using dental radiographic equipment.

Microbiology

For the mouse patient in which microbiological testing is recommended, standard collection techniques used for other animals is appropriate. The difficulty when culturing mice is acquiring a representative sample of the suspect area that will provide diagnostic information. Sick mice often are extremely stressed when being examined or when diagnostic samples are being collected. It is also important to know what the common disease conditions are and the common etiologies associated with those clinical signs. With the most common respiratory conditions in mice, one is Sendai virus and the other a *Mycoplasma* sp. Both Sendai virus and *Mycoplasma* spp. will not be isolated using standard aerobic or anaerobic culture techniques. If in doubt on collecting, preserving, and/or shipping a microbiological sample, the diagnostic laboratory must be contacted for full instructions as they relate to mouse submissions.

Parasitology

Routine fecal parasite evaluations should be performed on small rodents when they are brought to the veterinary clinic for a health examination or an abnormal stool. Common protozoal organisms can be detected using a direct fecal examination, and mouse pinworms are commonly diagnosed using the sticky side of clear cellophane tape to make an impression of the perianal area. The anal tape test will aid in diagnosing *Syphacia* spp. The sticky surface will pick up any of the banana-shaped pinworm eggs that can be observed under a microscope.

Diagnosis of ectoparasites in small rodents is similar to that in other species listed in this text. The pelage tape test is performed by pressing clear cellophane tape against the pelt of a mouse, dorsally and ventrally, from the nose to the base of the tail. *Myobia* spp. and *Myocoptes* spp. can be diagnosed using the pelage tape test. A skin scraping of the affected area may also help in identifying ectoparasites. Diagnosis of intestinal parasites can be made by finding individual eggs during fecal examination or whole worms within the lumen of the small intestine during necropsy.[6]

Miscellaneous Diagnostics

Even though most of the diagnostic testing is performed through pathologic examination for mice, there are serologic tests available that can be run on a minimum of 50 µL of undiluted serum. Sound Diagnostics, Inc. (Woodinville, Washington) provides serologic testing on a number of common mouse diseases, including ectromelia virus, mouse hepatitis virus, mouse parvovirus, mouse minute virus, rotavirus, Theiler's murine encephalomyelitis virus, pneumonia virus of mice, reovirus 3, Sendai virus, *Mycoplasma pulmonis*, lymphocytic choriomeningitis virus, and mouse adenovirus. The serologic tests are done using enzyme-linked immunosorbent assay (ELISA) and, when indicated, are confirmed by indirect fluorescent antibody testing. Many of the diseases for which there are available serologic tests are beneficial in maintaining disease-free animals in laboratory settings or large breeding facilities. In cases of unknown disease conditions for the individual pet mouse, there are panels available that test for multiple diseases from a single serum sample. It is very important for the veterinary clinician to understand both the significance of any test that is being promoted for mice and how the results are interpreted.

■ COMMON DISEASE PRESENTATIONS

Infectious

Bacterial infections associated with dermatitis lesions and subcutaneous abscesses in mice are commonly caused by *Staphylococcus aureus*, *Pasteurella pneumotropica*, and *Streptococcus pyogenes*.[4] Acute and chronic respiratory infections may be caused by Sendai virus or *Mycoplasma pulmonis*.[4] Acute respiratory infections usually are associated with Sendai virus; adults live while neonates often die. Chronic respiratory infection, with clinical signs being pneumonia, suppurative rhinitis, and occasionally otitis media, may be the result of a *Mycoplasma pulmonis* infection.[4] Both infections should be treated using supportive care, whereas mycoplasmosis can be treated with enrofloxacin in combination with doxycycline hyclate for 7 days.[7]

P. pneumotropica has been associated with urethral obstruction caused by inflammation and swelling related to infection of accessory sex glands.[4] Although uncommon, *Trichophyton mentagrophytes* (ringworm) can cause alopecia of the face, head, and neck of mice.[4] In addition to the disease organisms mentioned in this chapter (which are the most common disease organisms identified in pet mice), there are other bacterial, fungal, and viral organisms that can cause disease in mice. Proper diagnostic protocol should always be followed to identify the causal agent. Once the cause is identified, the proper treatment can be initiated and control measures implemented to prevent other animals' exposure to the disease.

Parasites

ENDOPARASITES

Numerous parasites have been identified in mice. *Hymenolepis nana* (dwarf tapeworm) and *Cysticercus fasciolaris* (the larval stage of the cat tapeworm) can be isolated from these small rodents.[5] The dwarf tapeworm is often found in young mice that are dead or have severe gastroenteritis resulting in diarrhea. Diagnosis of the dwarf tapeworm can be made following either a fecal flotation exam or necropsy, when the adults may be found in the small intestine. Treatment for the dwarf tapeworm is with praziquantel.

The mouse pinworm *(Syphacia obvelata)* is a commensal oxyurid nematode that feeds on bacteria that inhabit the intestinal tract of mice.[6] Although these nematodes are nonpathogenic in most cases, an overwhelming number of them can cause severe irritation of the terminal gastrointestinal tract. These nematode parasites can be diagnosed using transparent tape and applying it to the rectal area. After removing the tape from the affected rectal area, it is placed on a slide and the ova may be viewed under a microscope. Ivermectin and fenbendazole have been used effectively in treating this parasite in mice.[6]

Giardia muris is a common protozoal parasite affecting mice.[5] This organism can be seen using a direct fecal examination of an affected patient's fecal material. Metronidazole is the treatment of choice for *Giardia* spp. infections in small rodents.

ECTOPARASITES

Myobia musculi, Myocoptes musculinis, Radfordia affinis, and *Psorergates simplex* are fur mites that can cause severe self-mutilation and hair loss in mice.[6] *Polyplax serrata* (house mouse louse) can cause anemia, pruritus, dermatitis, and death in severely infested mice.[6] Diagnosis of ectoparasites in mice is similar to that in other companion animal species (e.g., skin scraping, examining hair samples for nits). Treatment of ectoparasites can be accomplished with ivermectin and a topical miticide. As with other rodent species, there has been an increasing ectoparasite resistance to ivermectin treatment.

Nutritional Disease Problems

Because most rodent diets are manufactured in the form of pellets or small biscuits that provide all recommended nutrients, there are few nutritional disease problems diagnosed in pet mice. If mice are fed an all-seed diet, there could be nutritionally related consequences. A lack of vitamin A could result in roughened hair coat or skin lesions. A breakdown of the protective epithelial lining of the gastrointestinal and/or respiratory tract could predispose the mouse to secondary bacterial infections affecting those body systems. Nutritional deficiencies may also result in poor reproductive activity.

It is important to provide an adequate supply of fresh water and appropriate rodent food on a daily basis. Following these basic nutritional instructions should provide a nutritional basis for mice to live healthy lives.

Neoplasia

The average life span of a mouse is 2 years old. This short life span and aging process increase the prevalence of tumors in these small rodents. If an animal is over 18 months of age, neoplastic disease should be considered as a differential diagnosis, especially if an asymmetrical mass is present. The most common tumors diagnosed in mice are mammary adenocarcinomas and fibroadenomas.[4] Other tumor types are identified in mice, and if possible, the suspect tissue should be completely excised. Representative tissue sections should be submitted for histopathological evaluation. Although there are treatment options available for mice that have been diagnosed with neoplasia (e.g., radiation, chemotherapy), its small size does not allow it to withstand the stress and negative side effects of these healing modalities. In mice, the recommended treatment for neoplasia is removal of the affected tissue, if possible, to increase its quality of life.

Miscellaneous

The most common disease in mice colonies is barbering. Barbering is defined as the dominant mouse nibbling off the whiskers and hair around the face of the subservient cagemates.[5] The hair clipping is very close to the skin without causing skin lesions. This behavior is noted often among female mice, whereas male mice are more likely to fight.

Mice may injure themselves on cage furniture or poorly designed cages and sustain abrasions on the face or nose. Individual animals may show stereotypic behavior that results in abrasions and/or alopecia. Enrichment furniture and toys may help alleviate this initial cause of dermatologic abnormality.

■ THERAPEUTICS

The size of mice contributes to the difficulty in properly administering therapeutic medications. The scruff of the neck or caudal flank are the subcutaneous sites that may be utilized to administer medication, fluids, or both.[2] The semitendinosus, triceps, and epaxial muscles are commonly used for intramuscular injections, whereas intraperitoneal injections are used in extremely small animal species, including mice.[2] Intraosseous catheters are much easier to place in mice than are intravenous catheters. The tibial plateau and the greater trochanter are the sites of choice for intraosseous catheter placement in mice.[5]

Although there are many methods that may be used to administer medication in small mammals, oral treatment using a dropper or tuberculin syringe is the easiest to administer and the least stressful for the patient. Medication can be added to the food or water, but often the patient is anorexic or the medicated food or water is not palatable, in which case, the patient does not receive the treatment.

Although a relatively difficult procedure in mice, gastric gavage can be performed using a bulbed stainless steel feeding needle or flexible red rubber feeding tube. The length of the tube is premeasured, externally from the nares to the last rib, and marked. A water-based lubricant is applied to the feeding tube before it is inserted through the intradermal space toward the back of the oral cavity.[2] The tube should advance without difficulty until the premeasured mark is reached. Restraint of mice for this procedure is accomplished by pinching the dorsal neck skin fold and holding the body with the remaining free fingers. Both oral medication and nutritional supplementation can be administered through an oral gastric feeding tube.

Medication dosages for mice can be found in a number of formularies. Before administration of any therapeutic agent, the dosage should be checked twice and calculations thoroughly evaluated to make sure they are correct. Because mice are very small patients, any overdose of medication can have adverse consequences on the patient's recovery.

SURGICAL AND ANESTHETIC ASSISTANCE

Inducing and maintaining mouse patients under anesthesia can be very challenging. With the widespread use of isoflurane anesthesia in small animal practices, the previous problems associated with methoxyflurane and halothane anesthetic agents has been overcome. There are still concerns and differences in anesthetic protocol because of these animals' small size, but in general, isoflurane is a safe agent when used on a relatively healthy surgical candidate. Although there are doses of injectable agents for sedation, the small size of the mouse makes it difficult to respond to anesthetic crises that may appear during a diagnostic or surgical procedure. Therefore, inhalant anesthetic agents (e.g., isoflurane, sevoflurane) are recommended for anesthetizing mouse patients.

An induction chamber is used to induce the patients, and then they are maintained under gas anesthesia using a face mask. It may be possible to intubate a larger rodent, but it is very difficult in mice; under most conditions, a modified syringe case face mask is used.[5] To guard against aspiration of stomach contents in a patient that is not intubated, the veterinary surgeon should place the head and neck in a position slightly higher than the body.

Box 12-6 provides basic guidelines for proper techniques used in surgical preparation and surgical assistance in small mammals, including mice.[9]

Premedication and sedation doses for mice and rats are listed in Table 12-1. Although general anesthesia is not recommended under most circumstances, injectable doses are listed

---

BOX 12-6   Basic Guidelines for Mouse and Rat Surgery

1. Obtain an accurate body weight.
2. Know the appropriate preoperative fasting interval.
3. Properly dose and administer medication.
4. Minimize stress through premedication or minimal handling.
5. Prevent hypothermia by using external heat sources.
6. Administer oxygen when using injectable anesthetic agents.
7. Provide fluid therapy and maintain hemostasis during surgery.

From Tully TN, Mitchell MA: *A Technician's Guide to Exotic Animal Care,* Lakewood, CO, 2001, American Animal Hospital Association Press.

TABLE 12-1   Premedication and Sedation Drug Doses* for Mice and Rats

Drug	Mouse	Rat
Acepromazine	0.5-2.5	0.5-2.5
Diazepam	3.0-5.0	3.0-5.0
Midazolam	1.0-2.0	1.0-2.0
Xylazine	10-15	10-15
Atropine	0.05	0.05

From Tully TN, Mitchell MA: *A Technician's Guide to Exotic Animal Care,* Lakewood, CO, 2001, American Animal Hospital Association Press.
*All doses are mg/kg and should be given intramuscularly (IM) or subcutaneously (SC).

TABLE 12-2   Injectable Anesthetics* for Mice and Rats

Drug	Mouse	Rat
1. Acepromazine/ketamine	2.5-5/ 50-150	2.5-5/ 50-150
2. Xylazine/ketamine	5-10/50-200	5/90
3. Diazepam/ketamine	3-5/40-150	3-5/40-100
4. Tiletamine and zolazepam	50-80	50-80

From Tully TN, Mitchell MA: *A Technician's Guide to Exotic Animal Care,* Lakewood, CO, 2001, American Animal Hospital Association Press.
*All doses are mg/kg and should be given intramuscularly (IM).

---

in Table 12-2. Analgesia is important for patient recovery and should be administered before, during, and after surgery, depending on the patient's presenting symptoms and the procedure being performed. Table 12-3 lists analgesic drug dosages for mice and rats.

Surgical procedures that are performed on mouse patients require similar techniques to those used with larger animals. Veterinarians should follow the same protocol but remember that the surgical field is smaller and patient manipulation more delicate with patients that weigh less than 50 g.

TABLE 12-3	Analgesic Dosages* for Mice and Rats	
Drug	Mice	Rat
Butorphanol	1-5 q2-4h	2 q2-4h
Buprenorphine	0.05-0.1 q8-12h	0.05-0.1 q8-12h
Meloxicam	1-2 q 24h	1-2 q 24h

From Tully TN, Mitchell MA: *A Technician's Guide to Exotic Animal Care,* Lakewood, CO, 2001, American Animal Hospital Association Press.
*All dosages are mg/kg and should be given intramuscularly (IM) or subcutaneously (SC). Meloxicam can be administered orally.

ZOONOSES

Zoonotic diseases associated with mice maintained as pets are rare. Possibly the most commonly reported zoonotic condition associated with mice is an allergic reaction to their dander and urine. As with all animals, it is important that a handler wash his or her hands after interacting with a mouse. *Salmonella* spp. may colonize the intestinal tract of small mammals, including mice.[7] Contact with the feces or anus of a mouse may expose the handler to this enteric pathogen. Washing hands after handling a mouse will help prevent exposure to possible pathogenic organisms a mouse may carry. One can monitor the individual mouse and mice colonies for subclinical carriers of zoonotic organisms by culturing the terminal intestinal tract.

Mice are carriers of two potentially deadly viruses: the Hantaan disease virus and an arenavirus that causes lymphocytic choriomeningitis (LCM) in humans.[7] Mice that are propagated for sale in the pet trade are rarely if ever exposed to the Hantaan disease virus.[7] Lymphocytic choriomeningitis–infected mice generally show no clinical signs, although weight loss, photophobia, tremors, and convulsions may occur.[7] Humans are exposed to LCM through contaminated feces, urine, or a bite wound. Disease signs in humans infected with LCM are flu-like (e.g., malaise, headaches, fever, myalgia, arthritis).[7] Fatal aseptic meningitis or meningoencephalitis in humans infected with LCM is rare.

Hymenolepis spp. are cestodes found in mice that can infect humans if contaminated feces are ingested.[7] Rarely identified in pet mice, *Giardia* spp. are protozoan parasites that can cause severe gastroenteritis in humans. Because feces have to be ingested for someone to be exposed, it is more common for children to become infected with zoonotic intestinal parasites than for adults. Using proper sanitary practices after handling mice helps reduce exposure to zoonotic intestinal parasites and other potentially transmissible diseases. Although there are diseases listed in this zoonotic section that can be transmitted from mice to humans, the occurrence of this happening is extremely rare when commercially bred mice are purchased at reputable pet stores.

RATS

Rats, like mice, are common laboratory animals and are propagated for commercial sale in the pet trade and for use as reptile

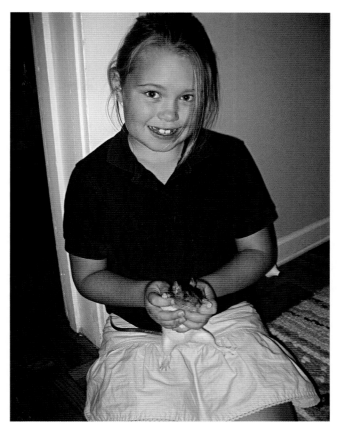

Figure 12-6 Rats make excellent companion animals, as they have a very interactive and curious personality.

food. The life expectancy of a rat is 2 to 3 years. Unlike mice, rats have excellent pet characteristics that include a charming personable disposition and extreme intelligence (Figure 12-6). The common rat species maintained as a companion animal is *Rattus norvegicus,* with the white rat and hooded rat being the most common variations. Although rats have an excellent temperament for companionship, they can inflict a serious bite if provoked. Also, as with other animal species, humans can be allergic to their hair, skin dander, and urine and salivary proteins.[2] Rats are not as territorial as other rodent species and are very social.

BIOLOGY

The integument of rats is commonly associated with a number of presenting symptoms of disease. As with mice, a rat's hair coat that has not been adequately maintained is often the first clinical sign associated with disease. Rats are fastidious with their grooming and, when healthy, maintain a very tidy hair coat. Common problems associated with a hair coat that is not maintained include general illness, parasitism (internal and external), aggression by cagemates as a result of psychological trauma, and infectious dermatitis.

Staphylococcus aureus infections initiated by self-trauma due to a fur mite infestation will manifest as ulcerative dermatitis.[4] The most common tumor in rats is a mammary-associated fibroadenoma.[4] Fibroadenomas rarely metastasize but are locally invasive and can grow to a large size.

A coronavirus is the etiologic agent behind sialodacryoadenitis which results in inflammation and swelling of the cervical salivary glands.[4] The most common disease presentations in rats involve the respiratory system. The three major pathogens that infect rat respiratory systems are *Mycoplasma pulmonis*, *Streptococcus pneumoniae*, and *Corynebacterium kutcheri*.[5] Respiratory disease in rats often produces "red tears" and a red nasal discharge. This red staining around the eyes and nose is not blood but porphyrins produced by an irritated harderian gland located behind each eye. The red staining at the nasal opening is due to the drainage of the porphyrins via the nasolacrimal duct.

Renal disease may present in older males in the form of chronic progressive nephrosis.[4] On necropsy, kidneys in affected animals are enlarged, appear pale, and have a pitted mottled surface.[4]

Rats are continuous, polyestrous rodents that should be bred in polygamous or monogamous systems.[2] When breeding rats that are housed in a polygamous ratio, it is recommended to have one male with two to six females.[2] Females are removed from a polygamous cage on day 16 of gestation, whereas the monogamous pair is maintained together with the young until weaning.[2]

Baseline rat physical information is listed in Box 12-7.

BOX 12-7 Basic Rat Information

Life Span	2-3 years
Body Weight	
Adult male	450-520 g
Adult female	250-320 g
Birth weight	5-6 g
Temperature, Pulse, and Respiration	
Rectal body temperature	99°-101° F
Normal heart rate	250-450 beats/min
Normal respiratory rate	70-115 breaths/min
Amounts of Food and Water	
Daily food consumption	10 g/100 g body weight
Daily water consumption	10-12 ml/100 g body weight
Age at Onset of Puberty and Breeding Life	
Sexual maturity, males	65-110 days
Sexual maturity, females	65-110 days
Female Reproductive Cycle	
Estrous cycle	4-5 days
Gestation length	21-23 days
Litter size	6-12

Modified from Bihune C, Bauck L: Basic anatomy, physiology, husbandry, and clinical techniques. In Quesenberry KE, Carpenter JW, editors: *Ferrets, Rabbits and Rodents: Clinical Medicine and Surgery,* ed 2, St Louis, 2004, WB Saunders; Johnson-Delaney CA, Harrison LR: *Small Rodents: Exotic Companion Medicine Handbook for Veterinarians,* Lake Worth, Fla, 1996, Wingers.

■ HUSBANDRY
Environmental Considerations

Rats, like mice, can chew out of enclosures; therefore, it is important that the housing be "rat proof" regarding the animal's ability to chew through the substance and escape into the house.

Rats are maintained in environments that are similar to those of other small rodents, but rats do not produce the quantities of odiferous urine associated with other rodents. For rats, large wire cages with easy-to-remove plastic bottoms are the optimal enclosure (Figure 12-7). The recommended housing unit size for rats is 15-20″ × 15-20″ × 7-10″ (length × width × height) for each adult rat, with females and young requiring 2 to 3 times the space listed.[2] Rats like to climb ramps and rope for exercise, so a cage that is taller than the listed requirements would be better suited for most singly housed animals. The major considerations for selecting an enclosure for rats, as with mice, are that it is resistant to their escape and easy to clean. An open screen top on the enclosure is recommended for proper ventilation. Available rodent cages that fit this criterion are wire or metal mesh, plastic, and Plexiglas. If the plastic tube housing systems are used, there should be routine cleaning of the sections using hot water and a mild detergent. An owner must always monitor the cage for possible escape avenues, especially if the animal

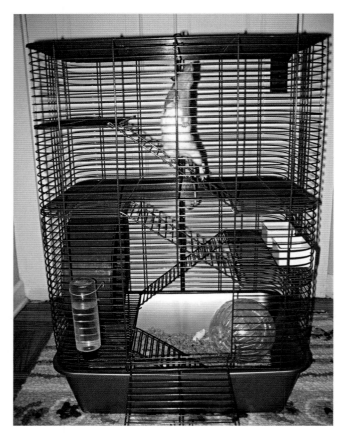

Figure 12-7 A pet rat's cage should have plenty of room for climbing and exercise.

has a predilection for modifying the cage opening through chewing. It is very important to provide cage toys and exercise opportunities for rats; therefore, the enclosure should be large enough to house not only food and water containers but also cage toys and an exercise wheel. Although not a cage toy, a hide box, in some form, should also be included, for the psychological well-being of the animal. This hide box can be a manufactured one or a small cardboard container that has one end cut out. Rats like to hide and also sleep during the day. By providing this piece of cage furniture or deep enough substrate for the rat to burrow, it will be able to sleep undisturbed during the daylight hours.

To prevent the buildup of urine and fecal material in the cage, commercially available paper rodent bedding or hardwood shavings should be used as a cage substrate (Figure 12-8). Although softwood (pine) and cedar shavings are available, the volatile oils that radiate from these substrates are irritating to small animals, especially because they are in very close contact with the material. These irritating compounds can cause dermal and respiratory inflammation, often leading to secondary bacterial infections.

Cardboard tissue tubes can be placed in a rat enclosure for chewing and play. Clothes items are not recommended in cages with animals that chew. Rats will shred the clothing items, exposing thread and elastic material that can become entangled around a rat's extremity, leading to necrosis distal to the stricture. It is recommended to change the substrate within the enclosure at least twice a week and more often if there is a problem with odor or excessive excreta.

Temperature, humidity, and lighting within the enclosure should follow what is commonly maintained with the ambient conditions within the house. For animals housed outside or in an outbuilding, the temperature range should be 65° F to 85° F.[2] The preferred light cycle for rats is 12 hours of light alternating with 12 hours of darkness.[2]

Nutrition

There have been a number of studies investigating the recommended nutritional requirements of rats. These studies have taken place because of the fact that rats are one of the most commonly used laboratory animals when investigating human disease processes. The benefit of these dietary studies is the availability of commercially produced diets that provide the recommended daily nutritional requirements of the rat. The problem that most owners face is the multitude of dietary products available for rats, and owners often buy seed-based diets. Like mice, rats will happily eat seed although seed-based diets are lacking in a number of the nutritional requirements needed to maintain long-term health. Commercial rodent biscuits or pellets with 20% to 27% protein are the recommended diets for rats. The commercial rodent biscuits or pellets are the only food rats need to obtain their required nutrients. Again, seed-based diets are not recommended, nor is a significant supplementation of fruits, nuts, vegetables, cheese, or other human foods (e.g., peanut butter). If a treat is to be given, yogurt or dried fruit treats manufactured specifically for rodents and/or rats should be provided 2 to 3 times a week (Figure 12-9). For younger rats, less than 3 weeks old, softer pellets are needed because babies start eating pellets and drinking water at 2 to 3 weeks of age.[2] A sipper bottle, placed on the outside of the cage is easy to maintain and does not take up space within the enclosure. If the cage is plastic or Plexiglas, modifications will be needed to attach the sipper bottle on the outside of the cage. Most sipper bottles come with attachment hardware to attach to wire cages. Fresh bottled water is recommended for rats, although chlorinated tap water can also be used. The water should be checked on a daily basis and clean water supplied at least every 2 days, if not every day.

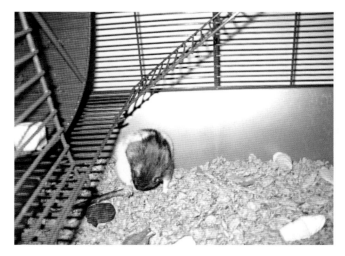

Figure 12-8 Paper substrate is nonirritating and makes an excellent environment base for a rat cage.

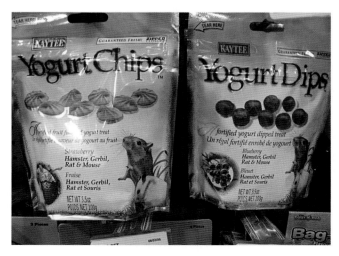

Figure 12-9 Specially produced treats are recommended for pet rats.

■ PREVENTIVE MEDICINE
Quarantine

Quarantining an animal is important for the pet owner who is introducing a new animal into a setting in which there is an established group. As with other animals a 30-day quarantine period is recommended, along with a physical examination and fecal parasite check. Unfortunately, there is no time period that will screen 100% against potential infectious agents, and with rats, time is critical because their life span and reproductive time frame is so short. Quarantining the introduced animals in conditions similar to those in which they will be maintained permanently, reduction of handling, and providing adequate food and water will make for a smooth transition. It is imperative that the owner screen the new animal for diseases and watch for any signs of illness. All rats that are captive, either as pets or in a breeding setup, should have no access to insects, wild rodents, or other animals. The most common sign of clinical illness is an unkempt hair coat. The lack of grooming is most often related to the animal feeling depressed or sick and thereby not having the energy to perform routine behaviors. If a number of animals are being quarantined, sacrificing an apparently diseased animal is the most efficient way to determine a rapid definitive diagnosis. If it is a single or an expensive animal, routine diagnostic testing will be required.

To maintain oversight of a breeding animal's health and reduce the exposure of young animals to infectious disease and parasites, routine screening of representative animals within the colony is recommended. In very large colonies, special caging (e.g., filter), food, and water may be necessary to maintain disease control.[1]

Routine Exams
DISINFECTION AND SANITATION

Before examining a rat, the examination table should be disinfected with either a dilute sodium hypochlorite or chlorhexidine solution. The examiner should always wash his or her hands and, if necessary, put on gloves before the capture and restraint of the patient. The difficulty with using latex gloves when examining a rat is the small size of the patient and its ability to twist and turn. Some rat patients can be restrained only if the examiner is not wearing gloves. If gloves are not worn, the examiner must thoroughly wash his or her hands, as with all cases, after the examination is completed.

To restrain a rat, the animal should be picked up with one hand being placed over the back and rib cage, restraining the head with the thumb and forefinger directly behind the jaws. The other hand is grasping the tail, stabilizing the animal (Figure 12-10). The skin on the dorsal cervical region may also be used, as with other rodents, to pick up the rat. A plastic sandwich bag can be modified as a restraint device for rats and small rodents. The rat's head is placed toward a bottom corner and the sides folded over the animal's back to limit movement.

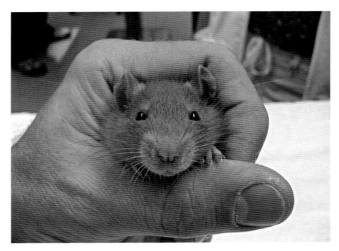

Figure 12-10 A rat should be restrained by supporting the body and grasping around the neck.

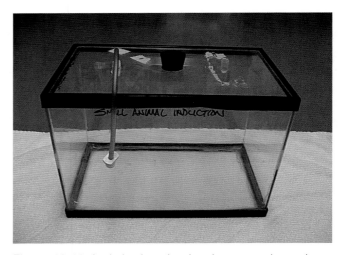

Figure 12-11 An induction chamber for companion rodents, most commonly used with isoflurane gas anesthesia.

If one is unable to adequately restrain a rat while the animal is conscious, an inhalant anesthetic may be used for sedation purposes. The animal should be placed in a small induction chamber and isoflurane gas permeated into the closed space (Figure 12-11). Once the animal has stopped moving, the enclosure top is removed and a nose cone placed on the anesthesia tube and placed on the patient's face. A syringe case can be modified as a nose cone for small rodents. After the physical examination is completed, the nose cone is removed and the patient is allowed to recover, breathing oxygen from the anesthesia unit.

Injectable agents are another form of sedation used with rats for examination and diagnostic sample collection purposes (see Table 12-2). A thorough assessment of the patient is necessary before using injectable drugs for sedation and anesthesia because of the inability of veterinarians or technicians to rapidly manipulate the effects of these treatments.

HISTORY

Obtaining a detailed history for the rat patient is very important. It is imperative to get as much information from the owner as possible as it relates to the patient's presenting problem, even if it is routine health examination.

Typical background information required for the rat patient includes how long the owner has had the animal, where it was acquired, how often it is handled, and the appearance of the feces and urine. Husbandry questions should focus on where the animal is housed, whether it is allowed to roam unobserved, where its cage is located; type, size, and material of the cage; cage substrate, furniture, and toys; how often the cage is cleaned and what disinfectant is used. When investigating the diet it is important to ask not only if pellets are fed and in what quantity, but also what the animal is eating and what its primary diet is. Supplemental offerings and frequency of feeding are very important data for the case work-up. The technician should find out about the water supply, how often the water is changed, and how much the animal drinks on a daily basis.

Because there are transmissible diseases among animals, the final questions should center on other pets in the household, if new animals have been added to the family, or if the animals are housed together. A description of any previous problems and a complete chronological description of the presenting problem are needed to complete the history form.

PHYSICAL EXAMINATION

Before restraining the animal, an observation should be made on its attitude, activity, and posture. The next step is to weigh the rat in a basket on a digital gram scale. If possible, temperature, respiration, and pulse should be measured and any abnormalities in rate and/or character noted. The physical examination starts at the head where the veterinarian should look for any abnormalities. Eyes, ears, and nares are observed for signs of discharge or inflammation. The oral cavity is difficult to examine in rats because of the small opening and tendency for the buccal mucosa to encroach toward the middle of the mouth. Rat incisors have a tendency to overgrow, so examination of the front teeth for normal occlusion and length is essential. A small speculum (e.g., modified paper clip) or an otoscope may be used to examine the oral cavity and cheek teeth. Mucous membranes help determine hydration status using capillary refill time and moisture. Body condition should be examined and abdominal palpation performed. Lymph nodes and limbs are palpated before checking the nails and plantar surface of each foot. The patient should have a normal posture, be aware of its surroundings, and move properly. Any problems should be noted in the record. Finally, a dermatologic exam considers hair coat quality, alopecia, external parasites, or any skin abnormalities. All abnormal findings are written in the record for case review, differential diagnoses determination, diagnostic testing, and treatment considerations.

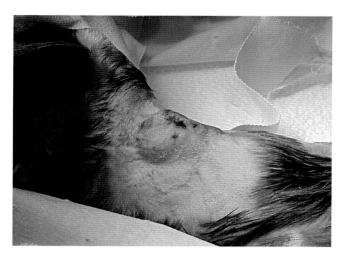

Figure 12-12 Fibroadenoma is the most common rat mammary tumor.

ABNORMALITIES COMMONLY FOUND ON PHYSICAL EXAMINATION

Respiratory disease is often the primary complaint offered by owners when presenting a sick rat to the veterinary hospital. Bacterial and viral pathogens can infect rats and are easily spread within breeding colonies because most of the organisms are transmitted by subclinical carriers. Ocular and nasal discharge is often observed in combination with dark red pigment. This pigment may be mistaken for blood by owners but actually is porphyrins produced by the harderian glands located behind the eyes. The irritation of the harderian glands causes the excessive production of porphyrins, which are secreted around the eye and down the nasolacrimal duct to the nose.

Rats have incisors that grow continuously. The continuous growth is not a problem for animals with normal occlusion. If the incisors do not line up, then there is a condition that leads to overgrowth of these teeth. The upper incisors will curve around, and if they are not cut, they will lodge in the dorsal aspect of the oral cavity. The ventral incisors will flare out from the oral cavity.

A common tumor found in older intact female rats is the mammary tumor. Mammary tumors can be large and extensive. Rat mammary tissue extends, on their ventrum, from the inguinal area to the thoracic inlet and up to their dorsal lateral body wall. The most common subcutaneous mammary tumor in the rat is a fibroadenoma (Figure 12-12).[4] Removing the ovaries at an early age reduces the incidence of the hormonally influenced tumor later in a female rat's life.

Swelling of the cervical salivary gland is caused by a virus. The etiologic agent of this condition is a coronavirus, sialodacryoadenitis virus, resulting in upper respiratory inflammation and the previously mentioned swelling of the cervical salivary and lacrimal gland.[4] There is no treatment for this highly contagious viral disease.

External and internal parasites may affect rats in the form of a rough hair coat or dermal lesions. Rats that are pruritic may cause abrasions or scratches that become infected with *Staphylococcus aureus* bacteria, leading to secondary ulcerative dermatitis.[4] Routine parasite examinations are necessary so that the veterinarian can identify parasitic infestations and administer treatment.

Rats can also present with neurologic, gastrointestinal, and urinary disease signs. A detailed history and examination will help direct the clinician toward a differential diagnosis list in which the appropriate diagnostic tests can be submitted to obtain a definitive diagnosis.

■ DIAGNOSTIC TESTING

Hematology

As with other pocket pets, blood collection from rats can be quite difficult. Approximately 0.5 to 0.7 ml/100 g body weight can be safely removed from a nonanemic healthy rat.[2] A rat patient should always be anesthetized for blood collection procedures, to reduce patient stress and movement. Usually inducing the animals in a closed chamber and maintaining the patients in a mask will allow the technician plenty of time to collect the blood sample.

Using a warmed ventral tail vein, 0.5 ml can be collected through a 23-gauge butterfly needle.[2] To collect from the tail vein, warm the distal two-thirds of the ventral aspect of the tail in a container of warm water for approximately 15 minutes.[2] The tail vein can be observed more clearly in the distal aspect of the tail. A 22- to 25-gauge butterfly needle is used, and free flowing blood can be collected directly into the microtainer tubes.[2] A tape bandage should be placed on the injection site to aid in hemostasis.

The easiest way to collect blood from many small mammals, including rats, is from the anterior vena cava. With the rat under general anesthesia, a 25-gauge, 1-inch needle attached to a 3-ml syringe is directed toward the umbilicus from the right side of the manubrium.[2]

Box 12-8 describes the technique used for retroorbital bleeding in rats and is not recommended for companion animals. The retroorbital bleeding technique is commonly used in laboratory animal settings and is easily performed by an experienced veterinarian or veterinary technician.

As with smaller rodents, the saphenous vein or lateral vein of the tarsus may be used for multiple blood collections without the use of an anesthetic. The patient must be properly immobilized in a restraint tube (35-ml syringe) with the leg extended and the skin on the medial aspect of the thigh held tightly between the handler's thumb and forefinger. The taut skin on the lateral aspect of the thigh allows exposure of the saphenous vein. A 23-gauge needle is used to puncture the vein, and blood is collected in a microhematocrit tube as it flows from the vessel.[2]

Blood samples obtained from nail and ear clips are not considered appropriate diagnostic samples. Cardiac puncture is recommended only in terminal cases and when the animal is maintained under general anesthesia because of possible complications involving the lungs and heart vessels.

BOX 12-8   **Retroorbital Blood Collection for Rats**

1. Stabilize head at base of skull and point of jaw.
2. Occlusion of the jugular vein may distend the venous plexus.
3. Retract the dorsal lid of the eye with the index finger.
4. With the middorsal approach, a microcapillary tube or small-bore Pasteur pipette is inserted midway along the superior border of the eye and advanced to the plexus located posterior to the globe.
5. Once the tube is placed in the correct position, the tube can be gently rotated until the conjunctiva is punctured and the orbital venous plexus is penetrated.
6. The tube is filled by capillary action.
7. Slight pressure may be placed over the eye to aid in hemostasis after the bleeding.
8. A volume of 0.5 ml may be collected from an adult rat.

From Tully TN, Mitchell MA: *A Technician's Guide to Exotic Animal Care*, Lakewood, CO, 2001, American Animal Hospital Association Press.

BOX 12-9   **Complete Blood Count Reference Ranges for Rats**

Erythrocytes	$5.4\text{-}8.5 \times 10^6 \ \mu L^3$
Hematocrit	37%-49%
Hemoglobin	11.5-16 mg/dl
Leukocytes	$6.6\text{-}12.6 \times 10^3 \ \mu L$
Neutrophils	$1.77\text{-}3.38 \times 10^3 \ \mu L$
Lymphocytes	$4.78\text{-}9.12 \times 10^3 \ \mu L$
Eosinophils	$0.03\text{-}0.08 \times 10^3 \ \mu L$
Monocytes	$0.01\text{-}0.04 \times 10^3 \ \mu L$
Basophils	$0.00\text{-}0.03 \times 10^3 \ \mu L$
Platelets	$150\text{-}460 \times 10^3 \ \mu L$
Serum protein	5.6-7.6 g/dl
Albumin	3.8-4.8 g/dl
Globulin	1.8-3.0 g/dl

From Bihune C, Bauck L: Basic anatomy, physiology, husbandry, and clinical techniques. In Quesenberry KE, Carpenter JW, editors: *Ferrets, Rabbits and Rodents: Clinical Medicine and Surgery*, ed 2, St Louis, 2004, WB Saunders; Johnson-Delaney CA, Harrison LR: *Small Rodents: Exotic Companion Medicine Handbook for Veterinarians*, Lake Worth, Fla, 1996, Wingers.

The collection of samples for diagnostic testing in rats is similar to that in other rodents. The reference ranges for complete blood counts and serum biochemistry panels are listed in Boxes 12-9 and 12-10.

Bone Marrow Aspiration

Marrow samples may be obtained from the ilium, tibia, sternum, femur, or the bones of the proximal one third of the tail.[5] Preparation of the samples is consistent with that of other mammalian patients.

BOX 12-10 | Serum Biochemistry Reference Ranges for Rats

Serum glucose	50-135 mg/dl
Blood urea nitrogen	15-21 mg/dl
Creatinine	0.2-0.8 mg/dl
Total bilirubin	0.20-0.55 mg/dl
Cholesterol	40-130 mg/dl
Serum calcium	7.2-13.9 mg/dl
Serum phosphorus	3.11-11.0 mg/dl
Alkaline phosphatase	56.8-128 IU/L
Alanine aminotransferase (ALT)	17.5-30.2 IU/L
Aspartate aminotransferase (AST)	45.7-80.8 IU/L

From Bihune C, Bauck L: Basic anatomy, physiology, husbandry, and clinical techniques. In Quesenberry KE, Carpenter JW, editors: *Ferrets, Rabbits and Rodents: Clinical Medicine and Surgery*, ed 2, St Louis, 2004, WB Saunders; Johnson-Delaney CA, Harrison LR: *Small Rodents: Exotic Companion Medicine Handbook for Veterinarians*, Lake Worth, Fla, 1996, Wingers.

BOX 12-11 | Urinalysis Reference Values for Rats

Urine volume (ml/24 h)	13-23 ml
Specific gravity	1.022-1.050
Average pH	5-7
Protein	<30 (mg/dl)

From Bihune C, Bauck L: Basic anatomy, physiology, husbandry, and clinical techniques. In Quesenberry KE, Carpenter JW, editors: *Ferrets, Rabbits and Rodents: Clinical Medicine and Surgery*, ed 2, St Louis, 2004, WB Saunders.

Urine Collection

Standard rodent cages can be used without substrate to collect urine and feces when the patient is hospitalized. By placing a rodent in a ziplock bag, urination frequently occurs and the sample can be collected. In a similar manner the urine in a rat can be collected over a disinfected stainless steel examination table.[1] The urine is voided while the animal is restrained and can be collected in a capillary tube for evaluation on urine reagent strips.[1] Urinalysis reference values for rats are listed in Box 12-11.

Diagnostic Imaging

Under most practice settings, the size of a rat patient limits imaging capabilities to radiographs. Restraint is essential for quality diagnostic images. To obtain adequate restraint and prevent movement of the patient during radiographic evaluation, sedation is required. As with all diagnostic procedures involving avian and exotic animals, an evaluation of the patient is required to determine its ability to withstand the stress associated with the assessment. If it is determined that the patient cannot withstand sedation, then it should be stabilized until it is deemed healthy enough for diagnostic imaging evaluation.

BOX 12-12 | Normal Radiographic Appearance of the Rat

1. Abdominal organs clearly identified
2. Food may be present in gastrointestinal tract
3. Gas may be present in gastrointestinal tract
4. Liver within rib area
5. Kidneys caudal to rib area
6. Heart and caudal lung lobes can be identified

From Johnson-Delaney CA, Harrison LR: *Small Rodents: Exotic Companion Medicine Handbook for Veterinarians*, Lake Worth, Fla, 1996, Wingers.

A rat can be sedated in an induction chamber following a technique similar to that described for mice. Because rats are larger than mice, they are easier to intubate. Using a special otoscope adapter, exposure is enhanced for endotracheal tube placement. High-speed, 300-mA machines with fine or detail-intensifying screens should be adequate for most small exotic mammal images. Dental x-ray units that can focus at short distances may be advantageous for both isolation of focal anatomy and full body radiographs in extremely small patients, including rats. For extreme detail in small exotic mammal medicine, using a traditional radiography unit, the Min R mammography system (Eastman Kodak) with Min R single-intensifying screen cassettes in conjunction with Min R single-emulsion film has been recommended.[1] Digital radiography is bringing a new dimension to radiograph evaluations and detail. The secret to success with either traditional or digital radiographic imaging is to restrict patient movement during exposure.[2] Two views, ventrodorsal and lateral, are recommend for rat patients. If there are rotational problems with the rat patient, a dorsoventral view may provide better imaging quality.[2] The patient should be taped to the cassette or positioning board with white cloth tape or masking tape. Taping the rat to the cassette or positioning board will aid in image consistency with that particular patient and among similar animals. In the lateral views, the dependent legs should be positioned cranial to the contralateral limbs.[1] Again, as with mice, whole body radiographs are commonly obtained for rat patients during the radiographic evaluation. Normal radiographic appearance of the rat patient is described in Box 12-12.

Microbiology

For the rat patient in which microbiological testing is recommended, standard collection techniques used for other animals are appropriate. With the most common respiratory conditions in rats being viral and bacterial organisms, it is important to try and aid the diagnostic laboratory in organism isolation through listing the potential pathogens. As always, if in doubt on collecting, preserving, and/or shipping a microbiological sample, the diagnostic laboratory should be contacted for full instructions regarding rat submissions.

Parasitology

Routine fecal parasite evaluations should be performed on small rodents when they are brought to the veterinary clinic for a health examination or an abnormal stool. Common protozoal organisms can be detected using a direct fecal examination. An anal tape test is useful for identifying *Syphacia* spp. in rats.

Diagnosis of ectoparasites in small rodents is similar to that in other species listed in this text. A skin scraping of the affected area or a pelage tape test (to identify *Radfordia* spp.) will usually yield the parasite. Diagnosis of intestinal parasites can be made by finding individual eggs in a fecal flotation of a macerated fecal pellet and in the lumen of the small intestine during necropsy.

Miscellaneous Diagnostics

There are serologic diagnostic tests available for rats through Sound Diagnostics, Inc. (Woodinville, Washington). Fifty μL of undiluted serum is needed to run one test or a rat infectious panel. Rat infectious diseases for which serologic tests are available include Kilham's rat virus, pneumonia virus of mice, rat parvovirus, rat coronavirus, *Mycoplasma pulmonis,* Toolan's H-1 virus, Sendai virus, Theiler's murine encephalomyelitis virus, cilia-associated respiratory bacillus, mouse adenovirus, and reovirus 3.

■ COMMON DISEASE PRESENTATIONS

Infectious

Staphylococcus aureus is the most common cause of ulcerative dermatitis in rats.[4] This organism is ubiquitous in most rat colonies and survives on the animals' skin. Unless there is a break in the skin, there is no infection or disease caused by the organism. In cases where there is a fur mite *(Radfordia ensifera)* infestation, rats become pruritic, developing lesions that seed the *S. aureus* organism.[4] The ulcerative dermatitis can be treated with an appropriate antibiotic through both systemic and topical application, cleaning the affected areas, and clipping the toe nails of the rear feet.

Mycoplasma pulmonis, Streptococcus pneumoniae, Corynebacterium kutscheri, Sendai virus, and cilia-associated respiratory bacillus have been isolated and identified as infectious agents causing rat respiratory disease.[4] With the respiratory pathogens, clinical signs can vary from mild dyspnea to severe pneumonia and death. Rats with mycoplasmosis are treated in much the same way as infected mice.

Sialodacryoadenitis virus is a highly contagious disease that causes rhinitis and inflammation of the cervical salivary and lacrimal glands.[4] There is no treatment for this viral disease, and supportive care is recommended for the affected patient.

There are other infectious diseases that can infect rats, as evidenced by the available serologic tests (e.g., Kilham's rat virus, pneumonia virus of mice, rat parvovirus, rat coronavirus,

Toolan's H-1 virus, Theiler's murine encephalomyelitis virus, mouse adenovirus, reovirus 3). These infectious diseases are diagnosed less commonly than those previously identified. Even so, veterinarians should be aware of the infectious disease organisms to which rat patients may be exposed and aware that tests are available for antemortem diagnosis.

Parasites
ENDOPARASITES

Specific intestinal parasites identified in rats include the dwarf tapeworm *(Hymenolepis nana),* pinworms *(Syphacia muris),* nematodes (specifically *Trichosomoides crassicauda),* and *Giardia muris.*[5] Diagnosis of intestinal parasites is important for the implementation of the appropriate treatment plan. Pinworms are diagnosed through the anal tape test, protozoan parasites (e.g., *Giardia muris*) through a direct fecal exam, and cestodes and nematodes from fecal flotation on macerated fecal pellets.[5] Once the parasite has been identified, proper treatment can be initiated and environmental recommendations applied to prevent exposure of other animals and reexposure of the patient being treated.

ECTOPARASITES

Rats do not appear as susceptible to ectoparasites as mice, but the following have been identified: *Ornithonyssus bacoti* (tropical rat mite), *Radfordia ensifera* (rat fur mite), *Demodex nanus* (demodex), *Polyplax spinulosa* (the spined rat louse), and fleas.[5] Diagnosis and treatments are similar to those recommended for mice although the dosages and duration differ.

Treatment of ectoparasites can be accomplished with ivermectin and a topical miticide. As with other rodent species, there has been an increasing ectoparasite resistance to ivermectin treatment.

Nutritional Disease Problems

Because most rodent diets are manufactured in the form of pellets or small biscuits that provide all recommended nutrients, there are few nutritional disease problems diagnosed in pet rats. It is also important to provide an adequate supply of fresh water and appropriate rodent food on a daily basis. If rats are fed an all-seed diet, there could be nutrition-related consequences. A lack of vitamin A could result in roughened hair coat or skin lesions. A breakdown of the protective epithelial lining of the gastrointestinal and/or respiratory tract could predispose the rat to secondary bacterial infections affecting those body systems.[2] Nutritional deficiencies may also result in poor reproductive activity. Vitamins B complex, C, and E plus selenium are recommended for treatment of female rats diagnosed with pregnancy toxemia.[2]

Rats, if fed a high quantity of human food, will develop dental plaque on the cheek teeth.[8] Proper diet, primarily rodent biscuits or pellets, will reduce the formation and buildup of dental plaque.[8] If left unattended, the excess plaque may lead to gum disease and dental caries. If caries develop within cheek teeth, the recommended treatment is removal of the affected teeth.[8]

Neoplasia

Rats are susceptible to tumors, most likely because of their short life span and physiologic predisposition. The most common subcutaneous tumor in rats is the fibroadenoma of the mammary tissue.[4] The mammary tumors can reach very large sizes and affect both males and females. To reduce the incidence of fibroadenomas, ovariohysterectomies are advocated at an early age in female animals. Whereas mammary tumors in mice are almost always malignant, rat mammary tumors are usually localized and respond to surgical resection.[4]

Miscellaneous

Rats have continuously growing incisors. Under normal anatomic conditions, the incisors maintain their length by grinding on their occlusive surface. If the position of the incisors is compromised, malocclusion will occur, causing overgrowth of their front teeth. The teeth, if left untrimmed, can cause trauma to the dorsal surface of the oral cavity (upper incisors) and the lower teeth extending outside of the mouth. In severe cases the teeth may adversely affect the animal's ability to eat. The teeth can be trimmed with a high-speed motor tool (e.g., Dremel®) with a cutting disk attachment.

A common disease in older male rats is chronic progressive nephrosis; the disease can also affect females.[4] The protein level in the urine commonly exceeds 10 mg/day and progressively increases as the animal ages.[4] The pathophysiology of chronic progressive nephrosis involves glomerulosclerosis with tubulointerstitial disease primarily affecting the convoluted proximal tubule.[4] The progression of the disease process may be slowed through a low-protein diet and anabolic steroid therapy.[4]

THERAPEUTICS

Fluid therapy can be given to rats through intramuscular, subcutaneous, intraperitoneal, and intravenous routes. Using a 25-gauge needle, a volume of up to 0.2 ml of fluid can be injected into the quadriceps muscle.[2] Up to 5 ml of fluid can be injected under the loose skin covering the neck or lateral body wall.[2] Intraperitoneal fluids should be administered while the rat is properly restrained to restrict movement. With one of the rat's hindlimbs extended, a 25-gauge needle is inserted into the center of the caudal quadrant of the abdomen, following the line of the extended leg.[2] Up to 5 ml of fluids can be given via the intraperitoneal route.[2] The most difficult method of providing fluids is intravenously to the lateral tail vein. To access the tail vein, warming the tail to dilate the vessel in warm water for approximately 15 minutes is required to aid in visualization.[2] The older the animal is, the more difficult it is to see the vessel through the tail skin.

Although there are many methods that may be used to administer medication in small mammals, oral treatment with

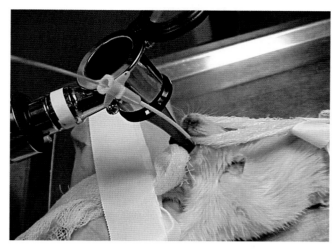

Figure 12-13 A modified otoscope head can aid in the intubation of rats.

a dropper or tuberculin syringe is the easiest for the veterinarian and least stressful to the patient. Medication can be added to the food or water, but often the patient is anorexic or the medicated food/water is not palatable, in which case, the patient does not receive treatment.

Both oral medication and nutritional supplementation can be administered through an oral gastric feeding tube to rat patients. The techniques described earlier for mice can also be applied to rats.

Medication dosages for rats can be found in a number of formularies. Before administration of any therapeutic agent, the dosage should be checked twice and calculations thoroughly evaluated to make sure they are correct.

SURGICAL AND ANESTHETIC ASSISTANCE

The same surgical and anesthetic techniques described for mice can be used for rats (see Box 12-6). Dosages for rat injectable anesthetic and sedative agents and analgesic treatment can be found in Tables 12-1 and 12-2.

Rats are larger than mice and can be intubated using a modified otoscope head (Figure 12-13). When using inhalant anesthesia, an intubated animal can be ventilated and there is less risk of aspiration from fluid that enters the oral cavity.

Surgical procedures that are performed on rat patients use similar techniques utilized on larger animals. Veterinary surgeons should follow the same protocols but remember that the surgical field is small and patient manipulation is delicate. The most common surgical procedures performed on rats are castration, ovariohysterectomy, and tumor (especially mammary tumor) removal.

ZOONOSES

Occurrences of humans becoming infected with zoonotic diseases associated with pet rats are uncommon. As with mice, an allergic reaction to rat dander and urine may be the most commonly reported zoonotic condition. As with all animals it is important that a handler always wash his or her hands after interacting with a rat. *Salmonella* spp. may colonize the intestinal tract of rats.[7]

There has been a human case of chorioamnionitis in which *Corynebacterium kutscheri* has been isolated.[7] This Gram-positive bacillus is routinely isolated from the nasopharynx of rats and therefore can be considered a zoonotic agent.

Streptobacillus moniliformis and *Spirillum minus* are organisms that initiate the disease called rat-bite fever.[7] A rat bite is required to seed the bacteria in a human, and after a 6- to 10-day incubation cycle, the human begins to show clinical signs associated with the disease (e.g., relapsing fever, chills, vomiting, myalgia, regional lymphadenopathy).[7]

Rats appear to be one of the primary rodent carriers of *Streptococcus pneumoniae*. The rodent develops respiratory disease through which the organism is shed and humans are exposed. Infected humans have respiratory and meningeal disease signs associated with *S. pneumoniae* illness.[7]

It should be mentioned that the rodent flea *(Xenopsylla cheopis)* transmits the plague organism *Yersinia pestis.*[7] It is wild rodents in which the plague organism is of most concern, but the disease is found worldwide, especially in the American Southwest. This is a very good reason why rats under the care of humans should have no access to wild animals.

Leptospira interrogans is transmitted from the infected urine of rats.[7] Again, restricting contact with wild rodents will reduce the risk of pet exposure. Humans infected with *L. interrogans* have chills and fever and often develop septicemic conditions that can lead to organ dysfunction.[7]

Hymenolepis sp. is a cestode found in rats, which can infect humans if contaminated feces are ingested.[7] *Giardia* sp. is a protozoan parasite, rarely identified in pet rats, that can cause severe gastroenteritis in humans.[7] Because feces have to be ingested for exposure, it is more common for children to become infected with zoonotic intestinal parasites than for adults. Proper sanitary practices after handling rats will help reduce humans' exposure to zoonotic intestinal parasites and other potentially transmissible diseases. All potential rat owners and current rat owners should know that the occurrence of zoonotic disease transmission is extremely rare when commercially bred rats are purchased from reputable pet stores.

REFERENCES

1. Bihune C, Bauck L: Basic anatomy, physiology, husbandry, and clinical techniques. In Quesenberry KE, Carpenter JW, editors: *Ferrets, Rabbits and Rodents: Clinical Medicine and Surgery,* ed 2, St Louis, 2004, WB Saunders.
2. Johnson-Delaney CA, Harrison LR: *Small Rodents: Exotic Companion Medicine Handbook for Veterinarians,* Lake Worth, Fla, 1996, Wingers.
3. Squartini F, Pingitore R: Tumours of the mammary gland. In Turusov US, Mohr U, editors: *Tumours of the Mouse,* ed 2, Lyon, 1994, International Agency for Research on Cancer.
4. Donnelly TM: Disease problems of small rodents. In Quesenberry KE, Carpenter JW, editors: *Ferrets, Rabbits and Rodents: Clinical Medicine and Surgery,* ed 2, St Louis, 2004, WB Saunders.
5. Tully TN, Mitchell MA: *A Technician's Guide to Exotic Animal Care,* Lakewood, Colo, 2001, American Animal Hospital Association Press.
6. Morrisey JK: Parasites of ferrets, rabbits, and rodents, *Semin Av Exot Pet Med* 5:106-114, 1996.
7. Mitchell MA, Tully TN: Zoonotic diseases. In Quesenberry KE, Carpenter JW, editors: *Ferrets, Rabbits and Rodents: Clinical Medicine and Surgery,* ed 2, St Louis, 2004, WB Saunders.
8. Crossley DA, Aiken S: Small mammal dentistry. In Quesenberry KE, Carpenter JW, editors: *Ferrets, Rabbits and Rodents: Clinical Medicine and Surgery,* ed 2, St Louis, 2004, WB Saunders.

Tiffany M. Wolf

CHAPTER 13

FERRETS

The ferret, *Mustela putorius furo,* has been domesticated for more than 2000 years. Its origin and early use are unclear, but historically it has been utilized for rabbit hunting and rodent control, particularly in the British Isles, Australia, and New Zealand. Ferrets have proven to be an important model in biomedical research, and much of what is known today about the ferret is based on this use. In recent years, its popularity as a household pet has risen dramatically because of its amicable nature, small size, and relative ease of housing and care. As the number of pet ferrets increase, so does the need for proper veterinary care. This chapter is written to familiarize the veterinarian with basic knowledge of ferret biology and care, medicine, and surgery.

■ BIOLOGY

The domestic ferret belongs to the order Carnivora and the family Mustelidae.[1] Other members of this family include the weasel, stoat, otter, mink, and skunk. The ferret is most closely related to, and may be a descendent of, the European polecat, *M. putorius,* or the Steppe polecat, *M. eversmanni.* It should not be confused with the North American black-footed ferret, *M. nigripes.* The name *Mustela putorius furo* was derived from the Latin words *putor* and *furonem,* meaning "stinky thief," and accurately describes its mischievous behavior and musky odor.

Ferrets have a long, slender body with short muscular legs, a long thin tail, small eyes, and short ears. The life span of the ferret is 5 to 8 years. They are very lively and active creatures, playing hard about 25% of the day and utilizing the remaining 75% for sleep. Ferrets are very curious and often investigate the smallest of spaces with ease, given their tubular-shaped,

flexible bodies. They may be vocal at times, eliciting a chirp with excitement during play, a hiss of warning when threatened, or a scream when a painful stimulus is experienced. Ferrets normally carry themselves as they walk with their torso elevated off of the ground in a slightly hunched posture. This posture is exaggerated during play, when they distinctly arch their backs, bringing their front and rear feet closer together, and move around with a characteristic bounce.

There are several color variations that can be found in the pet trade. The most common ferret color is the sable, characterized by dark guard hairs, mask, legs, and tail, and a cream-colored undercoat. Also quite common are the albino; the black-eyed white, with a white coat and dark irises; and the cinnamon, with beige guard hair, no mask, and a cream-colored undercoat. Silver ferrets, when young, have dark gray guard hairs, an indistinct mask, and some white present on the ventrum. As they age, the coat progressively turns to a black-eyed white variation. Varieties that have white paws are considered "mitts," and those with white heads and bibs are called "pandas." It has been reported that breeding silver mitts together or with black-eyed whites can produce offspring with congenital abnormalities.[1] A healthy ferret coat is shed twice a year, resulting in a long, thick winter coat and a shorter summer coat.

Ferrets measure 44 to 46 cm from nose to tail tip.[2] Males, also known as *hobs,* are larger than females, or *jills,* with the average male weight of 1 to 2 kg and the average female weight of 0.5 to 1 kg. The weight may be less in the neutered male or greater in the spayed female. There is a seasonal fluctuation in body weight of 40% loss in the summer and gain in the winter in intact animals.[3] Refer to Box 13-1 for additional physiologic data.

BOX 13-1	Normal Physiologic Values of the Ferret
Life span	5-8 yr[3]
Body temperature	100°-104° F[3]
Heart rate	180-250 beats/min[3]
Urine volume	26-28 ml/24hr[18]
Respiratory rate	33-36 /min[18]
Age of sexual maturity	6-12 months[18]
Gestation	42 ± 2 days[18]
Litter size	1-18 (average 8)[18]
Birth weight	6-12 g[18]
Eyes open	34 days[18]
Weaning	6-8 weeks[18]

Data collected from SA: Ferrets: Basic anatomy, physiology, and husbandry. In Hillyer EV, Quesenberry KE, editors: *Ferrets, Rabbits and Rodents: Clinical Medicine and Surgery,* Philadelphia, 1997, WB Saunders; and Fox JG: Normal clinical and biologic parameters. In Fox JG, editor: *Biology and Diseases of the Ferret,* ed 2, Philadelphia, 1998, Lippincott Williams and Wilkins.

BOX 13-2	Age of Tooth Eruption
Days	**Teeth**
20-28	Deciduous
50-74	Permanent
50	Upper and lower canines and 1st lower molars
53	1st upper molars
60	2nd, 3rd, 4th upper premolars and 2nd lower premolars
67	3rd lower premolars
74	4th lower premolar and 2nd lower molars

Data collected from Evans HE, An NQ: Anatomy of the ferret. In Fox JG, editor: *Biology and Diseases of the Ferret,* ed 2, Philadelphia, 1998, Lippincott Williams and Wilkins.

The musky odor of ferrets originates from the presence of a large number of sebaceous glands in the skin.[3,4] The number of these glands increases in the breeding season in the intact animal, resulting in a stronger body odor, yellow discoloration, and oiliness of the fur. The anal glands also produce a strong, pungent odor but are rarely expressed except when frightened or traumatized. The anal glands are usually removed at an early age in the United States at the breeding facility. Ferrets are unable to sweat because of a lack of sweat glands in the skin.[3,4] Overheated ferrets often flatten their bodies on a cool surface to dissipate body heat. Despite their musky odor, ferrets should be bathed no more than once or twice a month; otherwise, excessive drying of the skin and subsequent pruritus could result.

The head of the ferret is compressed dorsoventrally, elongated rostrocaudally, and lacks sutures in adults.[2] Like the dog, the zygomatic bones of the ocular orbits are open.[1,2] Ferrets have powerful jaws, large canines, and reduced molars. The mandibular teeth sit within the maxillary teeth when the jaws are closed, which allows for a shearing action when eating.[2] The dental formula of the ferret is: I-3/3, C-1/1, P-4/3, M-1/2. Box 13-2 gives the ages at which the permanent teeth erupt.

The spine of the ferret is long and flexible, with large vertebrae: numbers C7, T15, L5 (6 or7), S3, and Cd18.[2] There are 15 (sometimes 14) paired ribs, with 10 pairs attaching to the sternum and the last 5 pairs attaching to each other. The costochondral junction is usually swollen from rapid growth and can be palpated. The clavicle is reduced in the ferret. Each of the ferret's feet has five clawed digits. Unlike the cat, the claws are not retractable and require periodic clipping. In the hob, the glans of the penis contains a J-shaped os penis, which is attached at its base to the corpus cavernosum. The function of the corpus cavernosum is to stiffen the penis during intromission and possibly dilate the cervix.

The ferret heart is cone-shaped and lies between ribs 6 and 10. From a ventrodorsal view, the apex of the heart lies to the left of midline.[2] The ligament connecting the heart to the sternum is often heavily laden with fat, giving the heart a raised radiographic appearance from the lateral view. The ferret is also unique in having a single innominate or brachiocephalic artery arising from the arch of the aorta, rather than two carotid arteries.[5] Before the brachiocephalic artery's exit from the thoracic cavity, it branches into right and left carotid arteries that continue cranially along each side of the neck to supply the structures of the head. There are differing views as to whether or not this anatomic adaptation allows for continued blood flow to the head even when a ferret is turned 180 degrees.[3,5]

The respiratory tract of the ferret is also unique in several ways. The trachea, bifurcating at the fifth intercostal space, is quite long and large in diameter, characteristics that decrease the central airway and pulmonary resistance.[1] Ferrets also have a large total lung capacity and respiratory reserve compared with other animals of similar size. Even more interesting is that the airways grow in length and diameter with an increase in total body length.[1,2] This characteristic and the similarity of the tracheobronchial wall to that of humans makes it a good comparative model for respiratory research.[1,5]

The ferret's gastrointestinal tract differs from the dog and cat in the absence of a cecum, and that the jejunum, ileum, and ileocolic junction are not grossly identifiable.[2] The small intestine is approximately 182 to 198 cm in length, and the large intestine approximately 10 cm. The short length of the intestinal tract results in a gastrointestinal transit time of 3 to 4 hours. The liver is large relative to body weight, making up 4.3% of the body weight in the ferret, as compared with the dog liver, which makes up 3.4% of the dog's body weight.[2] The ferret liver is made up of six lobes: the right lateral, the right medial, the caudate, the quadrate, the left medial, and the left lateral. The pancreas is composed of two limbs: the right, extending along the descending aspect of the duodenum, and the left, situated between the stomach and the spleen. The spleen of the ferret varies greatly in size but normally measures 5.1 cm in length, 1.8 cm in width, and 0.8 cm in thickness.[2] It is readily palpable, and when enlarged, may extend from the left cranial abdomen across the midline and down along the right ventral abdomen caudally.

The kidneys of the ferret are bean-shaped, with the right kidney sitting more cranial than the left. The adrenal glands are closely associated with their respective kidneys, both of which are typically embedded in retroperitoneal fat. The left adrenal gland lies medial to the cranial pole of the left kidney, whereas the right adrenal gland may be found under the caudal border of the caudate lobe of the liver and is closely adhered to the caudal vena cava.[3] Accessory adrenal tissue has been found in some ferrets.[2] This characteristic and the anatomic location of the adrenal glands make complete adrenalectomy a difficult task.

The ferret prepuce is located on the ventral abdomen. The os penis can readily be palpated caudal to the prepucial opening. Hobs also possess a prostate that is situated around the urethra adjacent to the opening of the bladder.[2] This is important clinically, as enlargement of the prostate can restrict the flow of urine at this point. The vulva of female is located in the perineal region, ventral to the anus. In anestrus females, the vulva is only a slit-like opening, whereas hormonally active females have a swollen, fleshy vulva that may exhibit a thick, yellow vaginal discharge.

The ferret breeding season is from March to August, although artificial lighting may be used to induce year-round breeding.[3] Female ferrets are seasonally polyestrous, induced ovulators. They typically ovulate 30 to 40 hours after copulation. Gestation lasts 41 to 42 days; if fertilization does not occur, a pseudopregnancy may last 41 to 43 days. A physiologic consequence of prolonged estrus in unbred jills is bone marrow toxicity from the chronically elevated estrogen levels.

For further detail on the anatomy of the ferret, see Evans and An.[2]

■ HUSBANDRY
Housing

Ferrets may be housed singly or in groups, inside or outside of a house. When kept outdoors, however, they must be protected from extreme weather. Ferrets have difficulty tolerating temperatures above 90° F or below 20° F, and appropriate precautions must be taken to prevent their exposure to these extremes.[3] A multilevel wire cage with smooth or wire flooring is appropriate. Glass tanks are not recommended, as they do not provide adequate ventilation. A 24″ × 24″ × 18″ cage is a suitable sized enclosure for a ferret. A cage constructed out of a nonporous product is ideal for purposes of disinfection.

Because of their excretory habits, ferrets can be easily trained to use a litter box. This can be achieved in the cage and made readily available throughout the house when the ferret is allowed to roam free. Ferrets also enjoy a small, dark place to hide and sleep. Appropriate hide objects include a T-shirt, towel, hammock, or tent. Toys can offer great entertainment, but soft rubber or foam toys should be avoided as these objects are often the cause of foreign body obstruction. Polyvinyl chloride piping or cardboard tubes are great for play and exercise. Also, toys made of cloth, metal, hard plastic, or paper bags are safe for behavioral stimulation.

If ferrets are allowed to roam free in the house, the house should be ferret-proofed. This involves the obstruction of small places where they may escape, such as behind large appliances, inside of recliners, and within mattresses and furniture. These are often harmful places for ferrets where severe traumatic injuries may occur or soft foam might be ingested. Any other foam or rubber objects should be removed from the room as well. It is recommended that all free-roaming ferrets be supervised and suspect objects (e.g., recliners) inspected before use.

Nutrition

Ferrets are carnivorous and require a suitable diet. A diet that is high in good-quality animal protein and fat and low in complex carbohydrates and fiber is recommended. An adult, nonbreeding ferret has a dietary protein requirement of 30% to 40% and a fat requirement of 18% to 30%.[3] High-quality kitten or commercially prepared ferret food can be offered in a dry pelleted ration. Commercial dog and cat food should be avoided, as these do not have adequate protein levels and often contain plant-based proteins. The ingestion of a diet consisting of plant proteins can result in urinary calculi (see Nutritional Disease). There are several good-quality, commercially prepared ferret diets available, such as Marshall Farms Premium Ferret Diet (Marshall Pet Products, Wolcott, NY), Totally Ferret (Performance Foods, Inc., Broomfield, CO), Mazuri Ferret Diet (Purina Mills, Inc., Richmond, IN, and Zupreem Premium Ferret Diet (Premium Nutritional Products, Inc., Mission, KS). Fat may be supplemented through the use of Linatone (Lambert Kay, Cranbury, NJ), a commercially available fatty acid supplement. Treats may consist of pieces of meat or meat baby food. The sick ferret can be supplemented with Prescription Diet Canine/Feline a/d (Hill's Pet Products, Topeka, KS), Nutri-Cal (EVSCO Pharmaceuticals, Buena, NJ), or Glucerna (Abbott Laboratories, Columbus, OH), which are high-calorie, high-fat nutritional supplements. (See Therapeutics for further details on nutritional supplementation for the ill patient.) Ferrets that are prone to develop gastric hairballs can be given 1 to 2 ml of a cat laxatone 2 to 3 times a week as a prophylaxis. Water should always be made readily available. This can be accomplished via a heavy bowl or a sipper bottle. Fasting of ferrets for procedures requiring sedation or blood tests may be accomplished by withholding food for 4 to 6 hours. Extended fasts should be avoided, particularly in ferrets that have been diagnosed with insulinoma, to prevent severe hypoglycemia.

■ PREVENTIVE MEDICINE
Routine Exams

Owners should be educated early on about ferret preventative health care. It begins at an early age before the ferret even leaves the breeding farm with its initial vaccinations. It then becomes the owner's responsibility to complete the young ferret's early preventative health care, which consists of vaccination, heartworm prevention, and parasitic identification and treatment. These early visits to the veterinary clinic are great opportunities for veterinarians to educate owners about proper diet and husbandry. Owners should be encouraged to return annually for routine exams and subsequent vaccinations. The routine exam also creates opportunities for grooming (e.g., nail trimming) and identification and scheduling of necessary dental care. As the ferret ages, routine examination and even blood work, such as a complete blood count (CBC) and serum biochemistry panel, become important for the early detection of common, age-related diseases (e.g., insulinoma).

Vaccination

Ferrets are routinely immunized against canine distemper virus (CDV) and rabies virus. Ferrets are quite susceptible to CDV and there is a 100% mortality rate in unvaccinated ferrets infected with CDV.[6,7] There is little information available regarding natural rabies infection in the ferret; however, experimental studies have shown ferrets to be susceptible to infection with the virus.[8,9] Therefore, it is recommended to immunize them against rabies, particularly in rabies-endemic areas. As in dogs and cats, vaccination in ferrets is initiated in the presence of maternal antibodies and carried out to 14 to 16 weeks of age when maternal antibodies have waned and the ferrets' own immune system can be stimulated to develop protective antibodies. A recommended schedule for administration of the CDV vaccine is when the ferret is 6 to 8 weeks, 10 to 12 weeks, and 14 to 16 weeks of age; the rabies vaccine should be administered at the time of the last distemper vaccination. Thereafter, annual booster vaccines for CDV and rabies are recommended. The vaccines can be administered subcutaneously in the interscapular region of the body. Some municipalities have passed ordinances requiring intramuscular administration of the rabies vaccine.

A variety of CDV vaccines have been used in ferrets, including several types of modified-live virus vaccines and recombinant canary pox-vectored vaccines, but currently there are only two USDA-approved distemper vaccines for use in ferrets.[6-8,10] The first is a modified-live avian cell culture CDV vaccine, Fervac-D (United Vaccines, Inc., Madison, WI), and the other is a recombinant canary pox-vectored, subunit vaccine, Purevax (Merial, Duluth, GA). Canine combination vaccines or modified-live vaccines of ferret cell or low-passage canine cell origin should never be used in ferrets because of the occurrence of vaccine-induced distemper and death, particularly in sick or immunocompromised individuals.[6,8]

An inactivated rabies vaccine, Imrab (Rhone Merieux Inc., Athens, GA), is licensed for use in ferrets. There are differing regulations on rabies vaccination in ferrets within city, state, and local governments, and it is advisable for the veterinarian to contact these agencies for the current policies. At this time, the American Veterinary Medical Association policy (Model

Rabies Control Ordinance, http://www.avma.org/issues/policy/rabies_control.asp; March 17, 2006) for ferrets regarding vaccination, management of animals that have bitten humans, and exposure to rabid or suspect rabid animals is the same as that for dogs and cats.

Adverse reactions of the ferret to vaccination have been reported.[6,11,12] Anaphylactic reactions have been documented after ferrets received the Fervac-D vaccine and the Imrab vaccine, both in combination and alone.[6] Most of the ferrets experiencing an anaphylactic reaction did so after receiving the CDV vaccine, although there have been reports of reactions occurring in animals after administration of the rabies vaccine alone.[6,12] Currently there are no published reports of anaphylactic reaction with the use of the Pure-vax vaccine; however, there are anecdotal reports of similar anaphylactic reactions occurring. The specific component of these vaccines or which vaccine should be implicated as the cause of anaphylactic reactions in ferrets is still unknown.

Anaphylactic reactions to vaccination generally develop within 30 minutes of the injection. Clinical signs associated with a reaction include vomiting, diarrhea, hematochezia, generalized hyperemia (most evident on the nose, mucous membranes, and footpads), hypersalivation, and fever.[6,8,12] Less commonly, respiratory distress can develop. Treatment for a vaccine reaction should consist of dexamethasone (2 mg/kg SC), diphenhydramine (1 mg/kg SC or 0.5 mg/kg PO), and epinephrine (0.1 ml of a 1 : 1000 solution SC).[6] Supplemental oxygen should be administered as needed for dyspnea. Because anaphylactic reactions can persist for periods up to 24 to 48 hours, prolonged monitoring is recommended, with subsequent treatment with corticosteroids, antihistamines, or epinephrine as needed.[12] At the time of vaccination, owners should be advised to wait for 30 minutes after vaccination to monitor for the development of this type of reaction.

A recent report has suggested an association of the development of fibrosarcomas in ferrets with the vaccination site.[11] This is the first report of such an association in an animal other than the cat. Examination of fibrosarcomas that developed at the site of vaccination in ferrets revealed similar histologic, immunohistochemical, and ultrastructural characteristics to those reported in feline vaccine-associated sarcomas.

The projected benefits of vaccination must outweigh the adverse reactions in order for them to be considered a useful tool in preventative health care. As a whole, vaccination plays a vital role in reducing the level of infectious disease transmission in a population. However, due to the occurrence of adverse reactions, recommendations for vaccination must be made on an individual basis with the animal's age, immune status, and current health status in mind. Ferrets that have exhibited previous vaccine reactions should either receive no further CDV vaccine or receive a dose of diphenhydramine 15 minutes before vaccination, although there have been variable results with the latter option. An effective alternative CDV vaccine, which has not yet been found to elicit anaphylactic reactions, is Galaxy-D (Schering-Plough Animal Health Co., Omaha, NE), a modified-live primate cell culture CDV vaccine.[7] Duration of immunity induced by this vaccine in the ferret remains unknown, and use of Galaxy-D is extra-label in the ferret, requiring informed owner consent.

Quarantine

When a new ferret is brought into the household, a quarantine period is recommended before introducing it to other animals, particularly other ferrets. The purpose of the quarantine period is to identify and prevent transmission of infectious disease potentially carried by the new ferret. The duration of this period allows for the development of any clinical signs in a seemingly healthy ferret following entrance into the new household. Quarantine requires complete isolation of the ferret and its food, water, and cage supplies from other animals in the household for a period of at least 30 days. Proper hygiene such as hand washing, disinfection, and sanitation should be practiced during this period to avoid the transmission of any infectious organisms. The ferret also should receive physical and fecal examinations initially and vaccinations during quarantine. Should the new ferret exhibit any signs of sneezing, coughing, nasal or ocular discharge, fever, skin infection, diarrhea, or general unthriftiness, it should be brought to a veterinarian knowledgeable in ferret medicine immediately for a diagnostic work-up. In practice, these ferrets or any ferrets without a vaccination or medical history should be kept in strict isolation, as they can carry and transmit disease, such as canine distemper, to small animal patients. Precautions also should be made to prevent the transmission of any zoonotic disease from the ill ferret to the caretaker.

Disinfection

Routine disinfection in the veterinary clinic is important in preventing disease transmission and treating infection. Disinfection involves the killing of pathogenic microorganisms through physical or chemical means. Disinfectants are those chemical agents that are used on inanimate objects such as cages or feeding utensils, whereas antiseptics are those substances that may be used on living tissue for the treatment of open wounds or surgical scrub of the skin or mucous membranes. Sterilization is the complete removal of all living microorganisms from an object, an important application for instruments used for surgery or open wounds where there is a risk of infection. Techniques and agents should be chosen based on the nature and composition of the surface to be disinfected, the level of contamination and the degree of microbial killing desired, and the efficacy and safety of the disinfectant.[13] Sterilization should be performed on all surgical instruments through physical (moist or dry heat) or chemical (glutaraldehyde, ethylene oxide, 58% hydrogen peroxide) means. When using a disinfectant, veterinarians should always follow the manufacturer's recommendations on preparation and use to ensure efficacy and safety. Physical cleaning of any objects intended for disinfection improves the action of the disinfectant, as the killing power of disinfectants is significantly affected by the presence of organic matter. Antiseptics should be chosen based on their spectrum of action, residual effects, and tissue safety. Refer to Table 13-1 for information on commonly used antiseptics and disinfectants.

■ RESTRAINT

Physical Restraint

Healthy ferrets are lively and active creatures, and it is not in their nature to remain still for any prolonged period of time. Therefore, restraint of the ferret patient, either manual or chemical, is often necessary in the veterinary clinic. Restraint is also indicated for those ferrets with a tendency to bite or nip, such as young ferrets or those infrequently handled. For simple procedures, such as physical examination, grooming, and occasionally venipuncture, manual restraint is sufficient. For other procedures, such as venous catheterization or radiographs, chemical restraint is usually required.

Ferrets can be gently grasped under the thorax, allowing the caudal part of the body to rest in the opposite hand or hang freely. Fairly tractable animals can be restrained against the exam table with one hand over the neck and shoulders and the other hand over the hindquarters. With the animal in such a position, eyes, ears, nose, and skin can easily be examined, and vaccinations can be administered. More controlled restraint involves *scruffing,* or the grasping of the excess skin on the back of the neck, and allowing the caudal half of the body to hang freely. This technique of restraint is great for abdominal palpation. Scruffing often elicits a characteristic yawn from the ferret, aiding examination of the oral cavity or administration of oral medications. Another form of manual restraint involves supporting the length of the ferret's body along the handler's forearm while pressing its body snugly against the handler's body with the head of the ferret directed behind the handler's body.[4] This technique allows for easy administration of injections in the rear of the ferret's body. Alternatively, feeding the ferret a small amount of Nutri-Cal during a procedure can distract the ferret patient, aiding in restraint.

Chemical Restraint

When physical restraint is not sufficient to safely control the ferret for procedures, chemical immobilization can be a safe alternative. A variety of injectable drugs have been used alone or in combination for restraint or prolonged anesthesia, including ketamine, xylazine, acepromazine, medetomidine, diazepam, and Telazol (tiletamine and zolazepam; Fort Dodge Animal Health, Ft. Dodge, IA) (Table 13-2). Yohimbine and atipamizole are typically used for the reversal of sedation induced by xylazine and medetomidine, respectively. Chemical immobilization using any of these drugs should be restricted to healthy ferrets and avoided in sick and debilitated animals. Additionally, the use of any of these drugs alone is better suited for restraint to perform noninvasive procedures such as blood collection, whereas the ketamine combinations may be adequate for minor surgical procedures.

A ketamine/xylazine combination provides acceptable analgesia, muscle relaxation, duration, and a smooth recovery.[14]

TABLE 13-1	Disinfectants and Antiseptics Commonly Used to Treat Ferrets and their Environment		
Agent	**Use**	**Spectrum of action**	**Key characteristics**
Alcohols	Antiseptic/ disinfectant	Bactericidal	Safe; used alone or in combination; physical dirt inhibits action; cytotoxic
Aldehydes			
Formaldehyde	Disinfectant	Sporicidal	Poor penetration; noxious fumes
Glutaraldehyde	Disinfectant	Sporicidal	Organic matter slows action; good action against biofilms; used for sterilization of heat-labile instruments
Chlorhexidine	Antiseptic	Bactericidal/static, limited fungicidal and limited virucidal	Low toxicity; residual effects; unaffected by organic matter; used on skin wounds and mucous membranes; ototoxic to middle ear
Ethylene oxide	Disinfectant	Sporicidal	Gas sterilization of heat-labile equipment; toxic; mutagenic; carcinogenic; ocular and mucous membrane irritant
Halogens			
Chlorine	Disinfectant	Bactericidal, fungicidal, virucidal	Sodium hypochlorite used commonly; activity affected by organic matter, soap, or hard water; inexpensive
Iodine	Antiseptic/ disinfectant	Bactericidal, fungicidal, protozoacidal, somewhat virucidal and sporicidal	Activity affected by organic matter, soap or hard water; cytotoxic
Iodophors	Antiseptic	Bactericidal	Better penetration of organic matter; sustained release; used on skin wounds or mucous membranes; potential toxicity through use on large open wounds or in body cavities
Hydrogen peroxide			
3%	Antiseptic	Bacteriostatic	Wound irrigant; cytotoxic; poor antibacterial activity
58%	Disinfectant	Sporicidal	Plasma sterilization of heat-labile equipment; safe; expensive
Quaternary ammonia Compounds	Disinfectant	Bacteriostatic; particularly Gram-positive	Narrow margin of safety; high concentrations can cause skin irritation or burns; activity affected by organic matter
tris-EDTA	Antiseptic	Bactericidal; particularly Gram-negative (*Pseudomonas aeruginosa, Proteus vulgaris, Escherichia coli, Staphylococcus aureus*)	Potentiates effects of chlorhexidine in lavage solutions; inexpensive; decreases the minimum inhibitory concentration (MIC) for listed bacteria with select antibiotics in vitro

Data from Boothe HW: Antiseptics and disinfectants, *Vet Clin North Amer: Small Anim Pract* 28(2):233-248, 1998.

However, it is important to remember that this combination of drugs has been associated with cardiac arrhythmias and therefore should not be used in ferrets with cardiac disease. Use of the ketamine/xylazine combination also reduces certain hematologic parameters below baseline. The red blood cell count may be reduced by as much as 21%, hemoglobin concentration by 24%, hematocrit by 23%, and plasma protein by 15%. It has been suggested that these alterations may be due to sequestration of the blood in the spleen. Ketamine or Telazol may be used alone for restraint, but it is important to remember that these drugs may not lead to complete analgesia and muscle relaxation.[15] Both of these drugs also result in hypersalivation; therefore, the use of an anticholinergic such as atropine is beneficial, particularly when these drugs are used as preanesthetic agents. A medetomidine/ketamine/butorphanol combination provides prolonged anesthetic periods with acceptable analgesia and may be effectively reversed with atipamizole.[14]

The ideal choice for chemical immobilization in ferrets is gas inhalants. The benefit of using gas inhalants, such as isoflurane or sevoflurane, is that they are safe enough to use in healthy or sick ferrets, and the availability of these gas inhalants in most practices makes immobilization by gas anesthesia a convenient choice. Ferrets may be masked down or induced in a clear gas chamber. When utilizing either of these inhalants, the depth of anesthesia can be quickly adjusted by altering the concentration of the inspired gas. Sevoflurane has shown to provide better systolic arterial pressures and a lower heart rate than isoflurane.[14] Additionally, isoflurane can alter hematologic parameters by decreasing the hematocrit, hemoglobin concentration, and red blood cell count by 30% to 38%, and the plasma protein by 20% to 26%, likely by the same mechanism as the ketamine/xylazine combination. More detailed information on anesthesia of the ferret may be found in the Anesthesia section of the chapter.

TABLE 13-2 Dosages for Common Injectable Sedatives, Analgesics, Preanesthetics, Anesthetics, and Antagonists Used in Ferrets

Drug	Dosage	Use
Acepromazine	0.2-0.5 mg/kg SC, IM	sedative
	0.1-0.25 mg/kg SC, IM	preanesthetic
Atipamizole	0.4 mg/kg IM	alpha-2 antagonist
Buprenorphine	0.01 mg/kg SC, IM	analgesia
Butorphanol	0.05-0.1 mg/kg SC, IM	analgesia
Diazepam	1-2 mg/kg IM	sedative
Ketamine	10-20 mg/kg IM	sedative
	30-60 mg/kg IM	anesthetic
Ketamine/diazepam	25-35 mg/kg (K), 2-3 mg/kg (D) IM	anesthetic
Ketamine/medetomidine	5 mg/kg (K), 0.08 mg/kg (M) IM	anesthetic
Ketamine/medetomidine/butorphanol	5 mg/kg (K), 0.08 mg (M), 0.1 mg/kg (B) IM	anesthetic
Ketamine/xylazine	20-40 mg/kg (K), 1-4 mg/kg (X) IM	anesthetic
Medetomidine	0.08-0.1 mg/kg IM	sedative
Medetomidine/butorphanol	0.08 mg/kg (M), 0.1 mg/kg (B) IM	anesthetic
Naloxane	0.04-1.0 mg/kg IV, IM, SC	opioid antagonist
Telazol	12-22 mg/kg IM	anesthetic at higher dosage
Xylazine	1 mg/kg SC, IM	sedative
Yohimbine	0.5 mg/kg IM	alpha-2 antagonist

Dosages acquired from Marini RP, Fox JG: Anesthesia, surgery, and biomethodology. In Fox JG, editor: *Biology and Diseases of the Ferret*, ed 2, Philadelphia, 1998, Lippincott Williams and Wilkins.

PERFORMING A PHYSICAL EXAMINATION

The physical exam of the ferret should begin even before the animal is handled. Careful observation of the ferret's mentation, posture, and ambulation can be done while taking a history from the owner. Healthy ferrets often exhibit curiosity for the new environment, actively resisting restraint to explore the new surroundings. Ferrets with underlying disease may present with decreased activity, lethargy, or may even be recumbent. Assessment of body condition can be done at this time as well, taking note of any fluctuations in body weight with each visit. When this initial assessment is completed, the ferret can be minimally restrained for a basic exam. The body temperature should be taken before the start of the exam to prevent elevated recordings from increased body heat secondary to any struggle that may occur before obtaining the reading. Ferrets readily object to insertion of a rectal thermometer and restraint will be necessary. The normal body temperature range of a ferret is between 100° F and 104° F.[8]

The eyes, ears, nose, and oral cavity should be the initial anatomic features examined on the ferret. Symmetry of these areas should be noted. The eyes should be checked for pupil size, lens clarity, corneal abnormalities, and palpebral function. Cataracts causing distinct lens opacities can occur in both young and old ferrets, and retinal degeneration may be the cause of abnormal pupillary light response. Examination of the ears often reveals a dark brown, waxy build-up within the external ear canals. This can be normal for the ferret; however, should wax build-up be in excess or the ferret is reported to be scratching at the ears, microscopic exam of an ear swab should be performed to check for the ear mite, *Otodectes cynotis*. In the United States, the major breeding farm of ferrets tattoo the ferrets when they have been neutered and descented. This can be seen as two blue dots that are located on the ventral aspect of the right pinna. The nose should be examined for discharge, and the owner questioned about the ferret sneezing. Scruffing the ferret to elicit the characteristic yawn aids in oral examination. The mucous membranes should be pink and moist with a capillary refill time less than 2 seconds, indicating adequate hydration. It is important to examine the tongue and palate for evidence of ulcers or structural defects. Identification of the existence of any dental disease is important to the overall health of the ferret, with initiation of appropriate therapy and prophylaxis. Examination of the teeth may reveal broken canines. This is usually not a problem unless the broken teeth are dark in color or causing the ferret pain, as evidenced by anorexia or a diminished appetite. Tartar accumulation on the teeth is a common problem, particularly in ferrets that are fed a soft diet, and may be accompanied by gingivitis. Ferrets with moderate to severe tartar build-up should either have their teeth cleaned with a dental scraper or be scheduled for tartar removal with an ultrasonic scaler.

Following a thorough examination of the head, it is important to palpate all lymph nodes in the ferret. Lymphosarcoma, a common neoplasia of ferrets, can cause a (generalized) lymphadenopathy that can be readily detected upon palpation. A good lymph node evaluation should begin with palpation of the cranial most lymph nodes, the submandibular lymph nodes, and progress caudally, ending with the popliteal nodes. Ferrets accumulate fat in the subcutaneous areas of the neck, axillae, and inguinal region; therefore, it is important to differentiate between fat deposits and enlarged lymph nodes.

Palpation of the ferret abdomen can be done with relative ease and can yield important information about the patient's condition. The ferret should be held either with one hand under the thorax or by scruffing the neck while the other hand is used to palpate the abdomen. Palpation of the j-shaped stomach in the cranial abdomen should be performed carefully in ferrets presenting for anorexia or vomiting, as pain or further trauma may be elicited in animals presenting with foreign body obstruction. Sometimes the foreign body itself may be palpable as well. The spleen can be found in the left cranial abdomen. It is often enlarged, extending caudoventrally across the abdomen with the apex along the right side of the body. Enlargement of the spleen can occur in clinically healthy ferrets, but an irregular shape or masses on the spleen are considered abnormal and should be investigated further. The intestines are palpated for the presence of gas or thickened bowel loops. The mesenteric lymph nodes are also palpated for enlargement. An attempt should be made to palpate the adrenal glands lying medial to both kidneys, particularly in ferrets presenting with signs of adrenal gland disease. Normal adrenal glands typically cannot be palpated, and in obese ferrets it may be difficult to palpate enlarged glands because of the presence of retroperitoneal fat; however, significantly enlarged adrenal glands may be detected on palpation. The bladder can be palpated in the caudal abdomen and may be painful in ferrets that have urethral obstruction and/or bladder stones. Male ferrets presenting with a distended bladder due to urethral blockage will likely require drainage of the bladder before the prostate can be assessed. An enlarged prostate may be palpated caudal to the bladder in males with adrenal disease.

In male ferrets, the prepuce should be examined for erythema or swelling that may be associated with blockage of the distal urethra. The testicles of intact males should be examined and palpated, as testicular neoplasia can occur in the hob.[16] The vulva of jills should always be checked for swelling or discharge, a sign of estrus in intact ferrets and a sign of adrenal gland disease or remnant ovarian tissue in spayed females.

The skin and coat should also be examined for abnormalities. Dermal neoplasias, such as lymphosarcoma and mast cell tumors, may be identified as small, raised plaques or nodules, multiple or single in number. Examination for fleas or other external parasites should be performed at this time. Evidence of pruritus, such as erythema or minor excoriations in the interscapular region, may be secondary to external parasites or adrenal gland disease. Ferrets that are bathed frequently may also present with dry, pruritic skin.

Alopecia that is seasonally recurring or progressing from the caudal body cranially is the most common presenting problem associated with adrenal disease.

Auscultation of the heart and lungs should be done before completion of the physical exam. Labored breathing or increased respiration may be associated with primary lung disease or heart disease. The lungs should be assessed for abnormal sounds, such as harsh respiration, crackles, or wheezes, over all lung lobes. The heart can be auscultated at the level of the sixth and eighth intercostal spaces. In ferrets, the heart rate generally ranges between 180 and 250 beats per minute. The heart should be auscultated for arrhythmias, murmurs, or muffled heart sounds. Any of these can be indicative of primary heart disease, heartworm disease, or even the presence of pleural fluid. A respiratory sinus arrhythmia is common in the healthy ferret. Any ferrets with abnormal heart sounds or rhythms that are accompanied by clinical signs such as lethargy, anorexia, weight loss, or dyspnea should receive a complete cardiac work-up.

■ CLINICAL TECHNIQUES AND DIAGNOSTIC TESTING

Venipuncture and Hematologic Testing

Venipuncture is an important clinical technique that can be done with or without sedation. There are several sites for venipuncture that may be utilized depending on the volume of blood required for testing and the availability of assistants for restraint. Blood is assumed to be 5% to 7% of the ferret's body weight, and 10% of the ferret's blood volume may be safely withdrawn during a single collection.[17] Diagnostic laboratories performing hematologic tests on ferrets typically require only 0.5 to 2 ml of blood, whereas larger quantities are needed from ferrets serving as blood donors.

Blood may be collected from the cephalic or lateral saphenous vein using a 25- or 26-gauge needle and 1-ml syringe when quantities of less than 1 ml of blood are required. Restraint for venipuncture of the cephalic vein is similar to that of the cat or dog, with the head of the ferret securely restrained with one hand by an assistant to prevent biting during the procedure. A towel may be wrapped several times around the body to provide additional restraint. When utilizing the lateral saphenous vein for venipuncture, an easy technique involves the use of a 25- or 26-gauge needle without an attached syringe, collecting blood drop by drop directly from the hub of the needle into capillary tubes. This is a good site when serial glucose measurements are necessary. Topical Emla cream (AstraZeneca Pharmaceuticals, Westborough, MA) can be applied on the skin over the vein to provide local anesthesia during the collection process.

Larger quantities of blood should be withdrawn from the jugular vein or anterior vena cava. Again, the ferret may be restrained like a cat for jugular venipuncture, with the forelegs pulled forward from the body and the head extended, nose pointed upward. The jugular veins of the ferret lie more laterally than the cat. Overextension of the head should be avoided as this can reduce jugular vein distention. Another technique for jugular venipuncture involves positioning the towel-wrapped ferret into dorsal recumbency with its head extended.[14] While the ferret is distracted with Nutri-Cal, venipuncture can be performed using a 22- or 23-gauge needle bent at a 30-degree angle, attached to a 3-ml syringe. When collecting blood from the anterior vena cava, the veterinarian should consider sedating active ferrets with general anesthesia. This site should not be used in ferrets with bleedings disorders, because this vein is located within the thoracic cavity and does

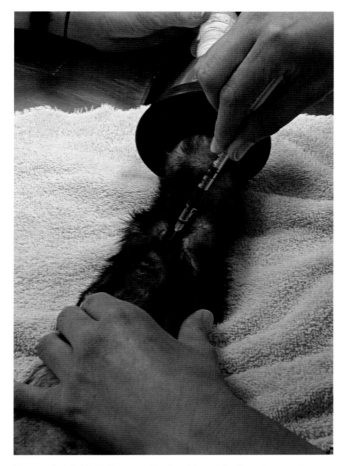

Figure 13-1 With the anesthetized ferret in dorsal recumbency, the anterior vena cava can safely be sampled.

BOX 13-3	Hematologic Values for the Ferret*	
Value	**Female**	**Male**
PCV (%)[18-20]	34.6-55	33.6-61
Hemoglobin (g/dl)[18-20]	11.9-17.4	12-18.5
Erythrocytes ($\times10^6$/mm^3)[18,19]	6.77-9.76	7.1-13.2
Reticulocytes (%)[18,19]	2-14	1-12
Platelets ($\times10^3$/mm^3)[18,19]	264-910	297-730
MCV (fl)[18]	44.4-53.7	42.6-52.5
MCH (pg)[18]	16.4-19.4	13-7.19-7
MCHC (g/dl)[18]	33.2-42.2	30.3-34.9
Leukocytes ($\times10^3$/mm^3)[18-20]	2.5-18.2	1.7-19.1
Neutrophils (%)[18-20]	12-84	11-82
Bands (%)[18,20]	0-4.2	0-2.2
Lymphocytes (%)[18-20]	12-95	12-73
Monocytes (%)[18-20]	1-8	0-9
Eosinophils (%)[18-20]	0-9	0-8.5
Basophils (%)[18-20]	0-2.9	0-2.7

*Combined values for adult female ferrets and for adult intact and castrated males from Fox JG: Normal clinical and biologic parameters. In Fox JG, editor: *Biology and Diseases of the Ferret*, ed 2, Philadelphia, 1998, Lippincott Williams and Wilkins; Thornton PC, Wright PA, Sacra PJ et al: The ferret, *Mustela putorius furo*, as a new species in toxicology, *Lab Anim* 13:119-124, 1979; and Lee EJ, Moore WE, Fryer HC et al: Hematological and serum chemistry profiles of ferrets (*Mustela putorius furo*), *Lab Anim* 16:133-136, 1982.

TABLE 13-3	Serum Biochemical Values for the Ferret*	
Value	**Female**	**Male**
Sodium (mmol/L)[18-20]	142-156	137-162
Potassium (mmol/L)[18-20]	4.2-7.7	4.1-7.3
Chloride (mmol/L)[18-20]	112-124	102-126
Calcium (mg/dL)[18-20]	8-10.2	8.3-11.8
Phosphorus (mg/dL)[18-20]	4.2-10.1	4-8.7
Glucose (mg/dL)[18-20]	85-207	62.5-198
Urea nitrogen (mg/dL)[18-20]	10-45	11-42
Creatinine (mg/dL)[18-20]	0-1	0.2-1.6
Protein (g/dL)[18-20]	5.1-7.2	5.3-7.4
Albumn (g/dL)[18-20]	2.6-4.1	2.8-4.2
Globulin (g/dL)[18]	2.2-3.2	2.0-4.0
A/G ratio (g/dL)[18]	1.0-1.6	0.8-2.1
Total bilirubin (mg/dL)[18,19]	0-1.0	0-0.1
Cholesterol (mg/dL)[18,19]	122-296	64-221
Alkaline phosphotase (U/L)[18-20]	3-62	11-120
Aspartate aminotransferase (U/L)[18,19]	40-120	28-248
Alanine aminotransferase (U/L)[18,20]	54-280	54-289
Carbon dioxide (mmol/L)[18,20]	16.5-27.8	12.2-28

*Combined values for female ferrets and intact and castrated male ferrets are from Fox JG: Normal clinical and biologic parameters. In Fox JG, editor: *Biology and Diseases of the Ferret*, ed 2, Philadelphia, 1998, Lippincott Williams and Wilkins; Thornton PC, Wright PA, Sacra PJ et al: The ferret, *Mustela putorius furo*, as a new species in toxicology, *Lab Anim* 13:119-124, 1979; and Lee EJ, Moore WE, Fryer HC et al: Hematological and serum chemistry profiles of ferrets (*Mustela putorius furo*), *Lab Anim* 16:133-136, 1982.

not allow for direct hemostasis by the clinician. With the ferret placed in dorsal recumbency, a 22- or 23-gauge needle, attached to a 1-to-6-ml syringe, is inserted at the junction of the first rib and the sternum (Figure 13-1). If you approach from the animal's left side, the needle should be directed toward the right elbow. If you approach from the animal's right side, the needle should be inserted parallel to the sternum. The anterior vena cava is superficial within the thoracic cavity and may often be located upon retraction of the needle. Always maintain a negative pressure draw, looking for a blood "flash" in the hub of the needle.

Diagnostic laboratories usually establish reference ranges for the tests offered for ferrets. Reference ranges for the ferret CBC and serum chemistry panel may be found in Box 13-3 and Table 13-3, respectively. Hematologic parameters for the ferret are very similar to those of the cat; however, the erythrocyte, hematocrit, and reticulocyte counts are generally higher in the ferret.[18] Ferrets also have a slower erythrocyte sedimentation rate; therefore, it is necessary to spin microhematocrit tubes for longer time periods than for dogs or cats. There is little information available on blood coagulation parameters in ferrets, although the prothrombin time has been reported to be 14.4 to 16.5 seconds.[18] As with other animals, there is an age-related decrease in the enzyme alkaline phosphatase due to a reduction in the bone isozyme when rapid growth has ceased.[18] Differential diagnoses for ferret patients that present with elevated liver enzymes include liver disease, exposure to ingested or environmental toxins, and Aleutian disease.[19] Creatinine is normally cleared from the blood much faster in ferrets than other mammalian species; thus, any elevation in creatinine is significant and should be pursued further.[20]

Urine Collection and Urinalysis

Urinalysis is useful for identifying urinary tract disease in the ferret. Urine can be collected from a voided sample, urethral catheter, or cystocentesis. When evaluating voided or catheterized samples, bacterial contamination is a possible complicating factor to consider. Although sometimes necessary in the blocked patient, catheterization, particularly in male ferrets, can be difficult. Samples acquired via cystocentesis are preferred, and in obstructed ferrets, where catheterization cannot be achieved, cystocentesis is necessary for immediate relief of a significantly distended bladder. With the ferret under anesthesia and positioned in lateral or dorsal recumbency, the bladder should be isolated between your index finger and thumb and the sample collected using a 22- to 25-gauge needle fastened to a 3- to 6-ml syringe; this is similar to the technique used for dogs and cats. Metabolism cages may also be used to collect 24-hour urine samples.

Catheterization of the ferret usually requires general anesthesia. Sterile technique is recommended to prevent the iatrogenic introduction of contaminants into the urinary tract. Again, male ferrets can be difficult to catheterize; this is because of the acute angle at which the urethra turns at the ischial arch. The presence of a urethral stone or prostatomegaly may make the procedure impossible without causing additional trauma. Care should be taken to prevent iatrogenic perforation of the urethra when passing the catheter through this turn at the ischial arch. With the ferret placed in dorsal recumbency, the penis is extracted from the prepuce, initiating the catheterization process. Magnification may be necessary to visualize the urethral opening on the ventral aspect of the penis. A needle with the bevel filed off can be inserted into the opening to flush and distend the urethra with saline to facilitate the introduction of the catheter into the urethra. A water-soluble lubricant also makes passage of the catheter easier. A 20- to 22-gauge, 8-inch jugular catheter, a 3.5-Fr red rubber tube, or a 3.0-Fr Slippery Sam Tomcat urethral catheter (Cook Veterinary Products, Eight Mile Plains, Queensland, Australia) may be used.[21] The latter option is preferred based on the size and rigidity of the catheter. An intravenous catheter stylet or sterile guitar string can be used to provide rigidity to the catheter; again, the veterinarian needs to be conscious not to traumatize the urethra during the passage of the catheter.[21]

Female catheterization is an easier technique. With the animal under general anesthesia, the female should be placed in ventral recumbency with the caudal body elevated. The urethral opening is located on the ventral floor of the vaginal vestibule, just cranial to the clitoral fossa. It may be visualized with an otoscope, endoscope, or a vaginal speculum. The catheter can be placed by sliding it along the ventral floor of the

TABLE 13-4	Normal Urinalysis Parameters for the Ferret	
Parameter	**Males**	**Females**
Volume (ml/24 hr)	8-48	8-140
pH	6.5-7.5	6.5-7.5
Protein (mg/dl)	7-33	0-32
Potassium (mmol/24 hr)	1.0-9.6	0.9-5.4
Sodium (mmol/24 hr)	0.4-6.7	0.2-5.6
Chloride (mmol/24 hr)	0.7-8.5	0.3-7.8

Data collected from Fox JG: Normal clinical and biologic parameters. In Fox JG, editor: *Biology and Diseases of the Ferret*, ed 2, Philadelphia, 1998, Lippincott Williams and Wilkins.

vagina, directed at an acute angle ventrally, until it enters the urethra.[21,22] Catheters that are placed for therapeutic purposes can be secured by suturing butterfly tape to the skin, and if necessary, catheters can be attached to a urine collection system. Ferrets should be closely monitored for entanglement of the tubing or disturbance of the catheter set.

Normal ferret urinalysis parameters can be found in Table 13-4. Protein is a common finding in ferrets, possibly due to high systolic pressure and thicker intrarenal arterial walls.[18] With this finding, however, the clinician should include genitourinary infection and Aleutian disease as differential diagnoses. Blood in the urine may be the result of iatrogenic trauma to the urethra during catheterization, cystitis, urethritis in males, or estrus in females. False positives for ketonuria in male ferrets have been reported with the use of urinalysis strips. The similarity in color of the dark urine produced by male ferrets and the reagent test strip is a possible explanation of the ketonuria false positive result.[17] Examination of urine sediment may reveal crystalluria in patients with blocked urethras or an accumulation of white blood cells in ferrets with urinary tract infection (Figure 13-2). An elevated urine pH has been associated with a diet high in plant proteins and is a good indication that diet correction may prevent crystalluria and subsequent urolithiasis.

Fecal Examination

Although intestinal parasitism is relatively uncommon in captive ferrets, the examination of feces as a diagnostic tool should not be overlooked considering the susceptibility of the ferret to a variety of gastrointestinal (GI) disorders. Due to the short GI transit times and the habit of ferrets to defecate in the same location within their cages, acquisition of a sample is not difficult. Often, restraint in the exam room is enough to stimulate defecation by the ferret patient. The color, quantity, and consistency of the fecal sample should be described in the record, as this may change according to the disease process present (e.g., green, mucoid diarrhea associated with green slime disease). Fecal exams for parasite identification may be performed at the time of the annual exam using a direct smear and a fecal flotation technique with sodium nitrate or a sugar solution. Further discussion of internal parasitism can be found in the section on infectious diseases. Ferrets that present with diarrhea should also have a fecal Gram stain done to evaluate

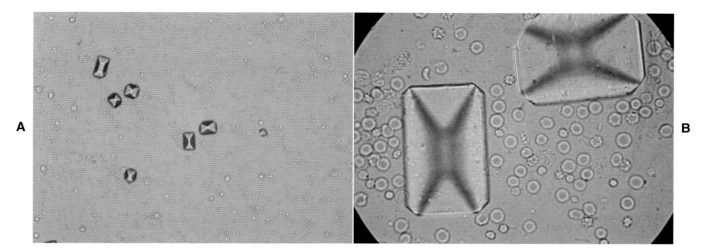

Figure 13-2 Struvite crystals are most commonly found in ferrets with crystalluria and can be identified easily with urine sedimentation. This finding is typically due to an improper diet containing high levels of plant-based proteins. **A,** Unstained (×100). **B,** Unstained (×400).

the sample for the presence of pathogenic microorganisms. If bacterial pathogens are suspected, a fecal culture should be pursued.

Diagnostic Imaging

Diagnostic imaging is very useful in the assessment of several disease processes in ferrets. Radiography is advantageous in the initial identification and assessment of common diseases, such as cardiac disease, splenomegaly, GI disease, urolithiasis, and prostatomegaly. Where questions may be left unanswered regarding GI disease through survey radiographs, the addition of contrast material becomes useful for the diagnosis of foreign body obstruction, bowel loop thickening, or even gastric ulceration. Ultrasonography has also proven useful in the further evaluation of certain disease processes such as cardiac disease, renal cysts, and adrenal gland disease.

Because radiographic techniques require an immobile patient, sedation is usually necessary. Ferrets' long cylindric bodies can make proper positioning for radiography challenging, but extension of the forelimbs cranially alongside the head and the rear legs caudally facilitate this endeavor. They can then be secured in place with medical tape for film exposure. The entire body of most ferret patients can fit on a large cassette film, reducing the number of radiographs required for many examinations. The radiographic settings preferred for all full body ferret radiographs are 50 kVp, 100 mAs, and 1/10 sec time. For contrast radiography, 4 to 6 ml of barium is the recommended oral contrast dosage. If gastric ulcers or a bowel perforation is suspected, an iodine-based contrast is recommended. Ferrets have a rapid GI transit time; therefore, films should be taken every half-hour to gain a complete assessment of the GI tract.

Ultrasonography in the ferret follows the same principles applied to the cat and dog. Although ultrasonography does not require sedation, a technique of distraction (e.g., Nutri-Cal treat) usually reduces any active resistance. A higher frequency transducer, such as a 10- or 11-MHz transducer, is recom-

mended to enhance the resolution of the image for the smaller ferret patient.[23]

Cytology and Microbiology

The use of cytology and microbiology as diagnostic tools can greatly improve the clinician's ability to identify and treat various ferret diseases. Impression smears or fine needle aspirates of masses or enlarged lymph nodes can aid in the identification of neoplastic disease, such as lymphosarcoma, before further work-up with biopsy and histopathology. Bone marrow aspiration and cytology are particularly useful in cases of anemia, thrombocytopenia, pancytopenia, and possible hematopoietic neoplasia (see Surgery). Obtaining culture and sensitivity results of any discharges, abscesses, or nonhealing lesions is very important for identifying a source of infection and the drugs that will provide the most effective treatment. Additionally, a Gram stain may be used to direct a clinician toward an appropriate antibiotic with which to initiate therapy until more definitive results are received.

Serology and Miscellaneous Tests

Serology can assist in the diagnosis of several important infectious disease processes in ferrets. The choice of serologic test is made based on a patient's possible exposure to infectious disease and the presence of associated clinical signs. Canine distemper virus can be tested by a fluorescent antibody test that is performed on conjunctival smears or scrapings, mucous membrane scrapings, or blood smears.[24] This test identifies CDV antigen within cells, but is only useful in the early stages of infection, and false negatives are possible. Influenza virus, another respiratory pathogen of ferrets, may be diagnosed serologically using an enzyme-linked immunosorbent assay (ELISA).[24] This test detects antibodies to the virus and may be an option for rapid diagnosis. Aleutian disease, a wasting disease of ferrets caused by a parvovirus, can be diagnosed by the demonstration of antibody titers to the disease as well as a hypergammaglobulinemia through serum protein electrophoresis.[25] There are two serologic tests used to diagnose Aleutian disease in ferrets: a counterimmunoelectrophoresis, with high specificity, and an immunofluorescent antibody test, having increased sensitivity.[25] Counterimmunoelectrophoresis, a screening test for the same disease in mink, also has the advantage of being rapid and inexpensive. Finally, ELISA tests used to detect the presence of heartworm antigen in dogs and cats can also be used to diagnose heartworm disease in ferrets (refer to Heartworm Disease for specific information).

COMMON DISEASE PRESENTATIONS

Ferrets are susceptible to many disease processes; some are diagnosed and treated similar to dogs or cats, whereas others are unique to the ferret. The preceding clinical techniques were provided as a guide to the practitioner in understanding and diagnosing these diseases. The following information will familiarize the clinician with specific ferret disease processes that are very common or limited to this species.

Infectious Disease

BACTERIAL DISEASE

Helicobacter *Gastritis*

There are several animal species that are affected by the gastric, spiral bacterium, *Helicobacter* spp., and ferrets are among those susceptible. Approximately 100% of ferrets in North America acquire *Helicobacter mustelae* at, or shortly after, weaning.[26] Ferrets have become important models for human infection of *Helicobacter pylori*. This bacterium colonizes the gastric mucosa and can cause gastritis and peptic ulcers. It has also been associated with gastric adenocarcinoma and mucosa-associated lymphoid tissue lymphoma.[26,27] Not all ferrets show clinical signs, despite the pathogenicity of this organism.

Ferrets younger than 2 years of age, or older ferrets that are stressed due to diet change or the presence of concurrent disease, are most likely to exhibit clinical signs of *Helicobacter* gastritis.[28,29] Clinical signs include bruxism, ptyalism, blood-tinged vomiting, diarrhea, melena, and chronic weight loss. Other common diseases that should be included as differential diagnoses for these clinical signs listed include foreign body obstruction, eosinophilic gastroenteritis, and proliferative bowel disease. A CBC may identify dehydration evidenced by an increased hematocrit or regenerative anemia from blood loss due to gastric ulcers. The identification of blood in the stool through a fecal occult blood test can also support a diagnosis of gastric ulceration. A positive diagnosis of this disease requires special media and culture techniques. Endoscopic biopsy may be utilized to acquire the necessary tissue sample to allow for the histologic demonstration of *H. mustelae* with the Warthin-Starry stain.[26]

Several therapeutic regimens exist for the treatment of *Helicobacter* spp. gastritis that use combinations of antibiotics, mucosal protectants, proton pump inhibitors, and H_2 receptor

TABLE 13-5	Treatment Combinations for *Helicobacter* Gastritis	
Drug	**Dosage**	**Route**
Combination 1[30]		
clarithromycin	25 mg/kg, BID	PO
omeprazole	0.7 mg/kg, SID	PO
metronidazole[a]	75 mg/kg, SID	PO
Combination 2[26]		
amoxicillin	30 mg/kg, BID	PO
metronidazole	20 mg/kg, BID	PO
bismuth subsalicylate	17.5 mg/kg, TID	PO
cimetidine[a]	10 mg/kg, TID	PO
Combination 3[26]		
enrofloxacin	8.5 mg/kg/day, divided twice	PO
colloidal bismuth subcitrate	12 mg/kg/day, divided twice	PO

[a]These drugs may be added preferentially by the practitioner.

antagonists (Table 13-5). Some of the therapeutic agents may be compounded to formulate a suspension that is not only easier to administer but more palatable through the addition of artificial flavorings. Metronidazole is best compounded to a 50-mg/ml meat-flavored suspension because of the drug's naturally bitter taste. During the initial stages of treatment, supportive care should not be overlooked. Fluids for the dehydrated patient and a highly palatable, easily digested diet such as Hill's Prescription Diet Canine/Feline a/d or Glucerna should be administered until the ferret regains its appetite. All of the listed regimens require long-term treatment of 3 to 4 weeks for complete recovery. Unfortunately, prior infection does not induce protection, and patients may become reinfected.[26]

Proliferative Bowel Disease

Proliferative bowel disease (PBD) is a GI disease that affects young ferrets, typically less than a year of age. *Desulfovibrio* sp., an intracellular *Campylobacter*-like organism, is the causative agent of ferret PBD and infects the ileum, the colon, or both.[28-32] *Desulfovibrio* sp. is closely related to, or is the same organism as, *Lawsonia intracellularis,* the etiologic agent of swine proliferative enteropathy.[32] Acute signs of this disease include colitis, diarrhea with flecks of blood, anorexia, and weight loss. Chronically affected ferrets may exhibit chronic diarrhea, tenesmus, and rectal prolapse. Neurologic signs, such as head tilt, ataxia, or tremors, may even be present in some cases.[31,33] On examination of a ferret with PBD, palpation of the abdomen may reveal a segmentally thickened colon and enlarged mesenteric lymph nodes. Other causes of GI disease should be ruled out; however, a presumptive diagnosis may be made based on history, clinical signs, and physical exam. PBD can be confirmed by histopathologic tests of tissue biopsies obtained from intestines or colon. The organism is identified using the Warthin-Starry stain and appears as comma-shaped organisms located in the apical regions of intestinal epithelial cells.[28] The preferred treatment is chloramphenicol, orally, subcutaneously, or intramuscularly at 50 mg/kg every 12 hours for 2 to 3 weeks.[29,31,33] If present, a rectal prolapse typically resolves with the antibiotic treatment, rarely requiring the application of a purse-string suture. When treated early in the disease process, most ferrets respond well; however, there are ferrets that do not survive despite implementation of the recommended treatment and supportive care.

Bacterial Pneumonia

Bacterial pneumonia is a common sequela to megaesophagus or to a primary viral disease (e.g., influenza). Primary bacterial pathogens include *Streptococcus zooepidemicus, Staphylococcus pneumoniae,* and groups C and D *Streptococcus.*[24] Other pulmonary bacterial pathogens found in ferrets include *Bordetella bronchiseptica, Listeria monocytogenes, E. coli, Pseudomonas aeruginosa,* and *Klebsiella pneumoniae.*[24] Overt clinical signs include labored breathing, cyanotic mucous membranes, nasal discharge, and fever. Harsh lung sounds, wheezes, or crackles may be heard on auscultation. A CBC often reveals a leukocytosis characterized by a neutrophilia with a left shift. An interstitial or alveolar pattern may be evident on radiographs. When aspiration pneumonia is present, the dependent lung lobes show evidence of change on radiographs, whereas primary airway disease produces a bronchial pattern. The most helpful diagnostic approach is a cytologic examination and culture of material obtained through a tracheal or lung wash. Cytologic examination typically reveals a septic inflammatory process characterized by degenerative neutrophils. The culture and sensitivity are important to ensure appropriate antibiotic selection. Until the clinician receives these results, initiation of a broad-spectrum antibiotic treatment regimen is warranted. Supportive care, including fluid therapy and nutritional support, is important in promoting the recovery of ferrets diagnosed with bacterial pneumonia.

Miscellaneous Bacterial Infections

Additional bacterial diseases of ferrets include abscesses, pyoderma, or urinary tract infections. For any disease presentation with a suspected bacterial etiology, a culture and sensitivity of the infection site are always recommended. If the bacterial infection is secondary to other disease processes, the primary disease should be identified and treated to prevent recurrence of the concurrent bacterial infection.

VIRAL DISEASE
Canine Distemper

Canine distemper is a highly fatal disease in ferrets, with a mortality rate of almost 100%. Fortunately, due to vaccination, preventative health, and client education, the disease is relatively uncommon.[7,10,34] Canine distemper is caused by a large, single-stranded RNA virus of the genus *Morbillivirus* and the family Paramyxoviridae. It is transmitted by aerosol exposure of infected body fluids and by direct contact with infected animals and contaminated fomites.[7,23,34] Canine distemper virus (CDV) is shed in conjunctival, nasal, and oral exudates, urine, feces, and skin dander. Transplacental transmission does not occur in the ferret.[34] Unvaccinated dogs and wildlife species (raccoons, mink, coyotes) are considered reservoirs of the virus.

Viremia may be detected 2 days postinfection and persists until neutralized by antibodies or death of the ferret.[7,34] The primary site of viral replication is within the respiratory epithelium and lymphoid tissue.[34] Replication may occur in the liver, kidney, gastrointestinal tract, bladder, and brain, following dissemination through peripheral blood leukocytes.

CDV is characterized by two classic phases of the disease.[34] The first and most common is the catarrhal phase, which occurs 7 to 10 days postinfection. This phase of the disease is characterized by anorexia, pyrexia, photosensitivity, and a serous nasal discharge. A fever will spike 3 to 5 days postinfection and last for several days. Also characteristic is an orange-tinged rash of the chin and inguinal areas.[24,34] As the disease progresses, the nasoocular exudate becomes mucopurulent, and a brown, crusted material accumulates around the eyes, lips, and nose. With the accumulation of this encrusted material and dehydration of the patient, the eyelids may become adhered. Hyperkeratosis of the footpads is an inconsistent clinical sign and may be difficult to appreciate, due to the small size of the ferret footpad.[34] Untreated cases may also develop a secondary bacterial pneumonia or other secondary disease processes. Melena may be observed early on, secondary to the stress of the disease process. Before death, the ferret's body temperature drops to a subnormal temperature. If the patient survives the catarrhal phase of CDV, a neurotropic phase will develop.[34] This phase of the disease is characterized by hyperexcitability, excess salivation, muscle tremors, convulsions, and coma.

A presumptive diagnosis may be made on the basis of a questionable vaccination history, clinical signs, and exposure to a potential source of CDV. Early in the course of the , with the presence of respiratory signs, influenza should be included as a differential diagnosis, whereas in the neurotropic phase of the disease, rabies must be a disease consideration for the patient. Diagnostic tests only lend support to a presumptive diagnosis of CDV infection, revealing a leukopenia on CBC and lung consolidation or congestion on radiographs.[24] The diagnostic test of choice to confirm the antemortem diagnosis is the fluorescent antibody test on a peripheral blood smear, buffy coat, or conjunctival scraping.[34] Unfortunately, the fluorescent antibody test is most useful in the first few days of infection and becomes less sensitive as the disease progresses.[24] Gross pathology is usually limited to nasoocular exudate, dermatitis, hyperkeratosis, and occasionally splenomegaly, pulmonic congestion, and consolidation.[34] Histologically, intracytoplasmic and possibly intranuclear inclusion bodies are present in the respiratory epithelial cells and bladder transitional epithelium. Fluorescent antibody staining of tissues can be used to confirm the diagnosis.

Ferrets with CDV infection have a grave prognosis. These patients should be isolated from other ferrets, monitored closely, and provided aggressive supportive care consisting of antibiotics, fluids, and force-feeding. There is no specific treatment for CDV. Prevention of infection or significant disease is accomplished through annual vaccination. Transmission and exposure can also be reduced through proper disinfection and quarantine. CDV is relatively labile and can be cleared from the environment using heat, drying, detergents, and common disinfectants.[24,34]

Influenza

Human influenza virus types A and B of the class Orthomyxoviridae infect ferrets, causing a respiratory disease similar to that of humans.[34] Ferrets are commonly used as animal models for flu research in humans because of this similar biologic response. In nature there are a number of influenza strains, exhibiting variable virulence.[24] The disease is generally mild in adults, characterized by upper respiratory signs, but is potentially fatal to very young kits.[24,34] Transmission of the virus occurs from human to ferret and ferret to human through aerosolization. Ferrets can transmit the virus at the height of the febrile state for 3 to 4 days.[24] The disease is commonly diagnosed in ferrets after the owner experiences a similar illness.

Influenza virus localizes in the nasal epithelium but may descend to cause pneumonia, which is a common problem in kits.[24,34] Clinical signs appear 48 hours after infection and include anorexia, malaise, pyrexia, sneezing, and a serous nasal discharge. Experimental infection has produced a biphasic febrile response and an increase in hemagglutination inhibiting (HI) antibodies.[34] The virus and antibodies can be found in the nasal secretions of the infected animal.

Diagnosis is based on history, clinical signs, and recovery in 4 to 5 days.[34] Rarely is viral isolation or HI antibody titer necessary to obtain a diagnosis. There is an ELISA diagnostic test available for rapid diagnosis of influenza A infection in ferrets.[24] Once a diagnosis of influenza is made, supportive therapy in the form of fluids and antibiotics should be implemented to treat the dehydrated patient and prevent secondary bacterial pneumonia. If needed, a pediatric cough suppressant (without alcohol) can be given at the pediatric dose on a per weight basis. Experimentally, the antiviral drug amantadine, at 6 mg/kg as an aerosol every 12 hours, has shown good results for treatment of the viral infection.[24] Drugs utilized to reduce pyrexia have shown variable results, as lowering the fever has been associated with higher viral shedding and a slower decrease in virus levels of the infected patient.[24] There is no vaccination; however, natural infection induces protective immunity that can last for at least 5 weeks postinfection.[34]

Epizootic Catarrhal Enteritis

Epizootic catarrhal enteritis is caused by a coronavirus and is characterized by an intestinal disease that is seen in resident ferrets 2 to 3 days after exposure to an infected ferret.[28] Older ferrets are most susceptible, whereas younger ferrets may be asymptomatic or present with only mild disease.[28,31] Transmission most likely occurs via direct contact or fecal/oral exposure. Infected ferrets exhibit a characteristic profuse, mucoid, green diarrhea from which this disease has obtained the nickname "green slime disease." Ferrets may also show signs of lethargy,

dehydration, and anorexia. A CBC is usually within normal limits, unless changes are present due to dehydration. Serum chemistry panel changes may include elevations in the liver enzymes, ALP and ALT, and elevations in BUN and glucose.[28,31] Morbidity may be high; however, with treatment, mortality may be kept to a minimum. Treatment is focused primarily on maintaining hydration while the immune system eliminates infection. Fluids can be administered via the subcutaneous, intravenous, or intraosseous route, depending on the severity of dehydration. Fluid volume should be calculated based on the fluid deficit and the daily fluid requirement of 75 to 100 ml/kg/day. Additional supportive therapy should consist of antibiotics to prevent secondary bacterial infection during the course of disease, as well as a critical care diet for nutritional supplementation. Ferrets with epizootic catarrhal enteritis should be kept in strict isolation from other ferrets, and proper disinfection of cages and cage items (food bowls, toys, litter pans) should be performed to prevent spread of the virus.

Aleutian Disease

The incidence of Aleutian disease has increased in recent years. It is a chronic progressive disease, caused by a parvovirus, first identified in mink with the autosomal recessive (aa) Aleutian (blue) coat color in 1940.[34] It was initially diagnosed in the ferret in the 1960s and called hypergammaglobulinemia, based on the major clinical feature associated with the disease. There are variable strains of the Aleutian disease virus (ADV) that display varying virulence and immunogenicity. Ferret strains are considered mutants of the mink ADV strains. Unlike mink, ferrets display a milder disease and may even be infected for years without exhibiting clinical signs.[34,35]

Transmission of ADV occurs ferret to ferret or mink to ferret through aerosolization of viral particles; direct contact with the urine, saliva, blood, or feces of infected animals; or via contaminated fomites.[34,35] Vertical transmission occurs in the mink but has not been positively identified in the ferret. All seropositive ferrets, regardless of clinical disease status, should be considered sources of infection.

Aleutian disease is an immune-mediated disease, characterized most commonly by the presence of a hypergammaglobulinemia. The severity of disease is dependent upon the origin of the ADV (ferret vs. mink). When mink are infected, ADV causes hypergammaglobulinemia, glomerulonephritis, arteritis, plasmacytosis, progressive wasting, and death within 5 months.[25] When ferrets are infected, the mink strain of ADV causes mild lesions and moderate increases in gammaglobulins, whereas the ferret strain of ADV causes a marked, persistent hypergammaglobulinemia and periportal lymphocytic infiltrates.[34] Glomerulonephritis and vasculitis are not as severe in the ferret as in mink, which may be due to lower levels of circulating viral antigen that results in a reduction in immune complex deposition.[34-36] Plasmocytic-lymphocytic infiltrates have been found in multiple organs, including the central nervous system.[34-36]

In some cases, death may occur without the development of clinical signs. ADV can cause chronic, progressive weight loss, cachexia, malaise, and melena.[25,34] Posterior paresis is the most consistent clinical sign.[34-38] Adults may clear the virus or become persistently infected without ever showing signs of disease.[25,34,35] Differentials for chronic weight loss should include neoplasia, cardiac disease, estrogen-induced anemia, and gastrointestinal disease (e.g., malabsorption, maldigestion, bacterial enteritis, eosinophilic gastroenteritis, proliferative bowel disease). The neurotropic form of CDV or rabies should also be considered in the presence of neurologic signs.

A presumptive diagnosis of ADV infection can be established based on a history of chronic weight loss and the presence of a hypergammaglobulinemia on serum protein electrophoresis, with gammaglobulins making up greater than 20% of the total protein.[34] Two tests are available to confirm a diagnosis of ADV: counterelectrophoresis and immunofluorescent antibody test.[25,34] Counterimmunoelectrophoresis is a popular screening test for the same disease in mink. It is a highly specific test, but unfortunately, it does not distinguish between strains of ADV and does not detect antibody to specific antigen of virus-infected cells.[35] Immunofluorescent antibody testing may be more sensitive.[25] PCR has also been utilized for the diagnosis of ADV.[34,36]

Because there is no treatment for ADV infection, prevention of the disease in ferret households is recommended. This can be accomplished through the testing of ferrets for the disease before introducing them into the household. Additionally, vaccination is contraindicated due to the immune-mediated effects of the disease and the inability of antibodies to neutralize the virus.[34] Ferrets that are identified as persistently infected should either be isolated or culled. Ferrets also should not be exposed to mink.

Rabies

Rabies is a disease of mammals caused by Rhabdovirus. There have been fewer than 20 cases of rabies reported in ferrets since 1954.[34] One of these cases occurred from the administration of a modified-live vaccine product that induced disease. There have been no reported cases of human rabies infection from exposure to an infected ferret. Additionally, there is a paucity of information of ferret vaccine history, clinical signs, or exposure to wildlife from the few reported cases of ferret rabies.

Experimental infection with rabies virus has induced ascending paralysis, ataxia, cachexia, fever, hyperactivity, bladder atony, tremors, and paresthesia.[9] Susceptibility to infection and development of clinical signs seems to be based on the inoculum dose. Although there was a lack of shedding of the virus in the saliva, isolation of the virus in the salivary glands was accomplished in a single ferret.[9,34]

Any unvaccinated ferret suspected of being infected with rabies virus should be euthanized and submitted to the state public health laboratory for confirmation. The diagnosis is based on direct immunofluorescent antibody testing of brain tissue. Vaccinated ferrets that inflict a bite to a human are required to undergo the same quarantine protocol as vaccinated dogs and cats. Because there is no treatment for this disease, prevention through vaccination is highly recommended. There are varying civic, county, and state laws regarding ferret ownership, and ferret owners should always inquire about the current ownership regulations, including vaccination requirements of their town, county, and state.

FUNGAL DISEASE

Fungal infection should be considered a top differential diagnosis for any persistent infections that are nonresponsive to antibiotics, particularly if other systemic signs, such as pyrexia, respiratory, or neurologic signs, are present. Histologic and cytologic examination and culture of discharge, tracheal washes, and cerebrospinal fluid samples can allow direct visualization and identification of the organism.

Pulmonary mycoses have been described in some ferrets exhibiting signs of coughing, wasting, lethargy, anorexia, lymph node enlargement, and oculonasal discharge. *Blastomycosis dermatitidis* infection has been diagnosed in ferrets in the southeastern United States, Mississippi River valley, and Ohio River valley.[24] In addition to pulmonary disease, *Blastomycosis* has also been involved in the development of multifocal granulomatous meningoencephalitis.[39] *Coccidioidomycosis immitis* has been diagnosed as an etiologic agent of pulmonary disease in the southwest United States.[24] Pulmonary signs tend to develop 1 to 3 weeks after infection with this organism.

Diagnosis of these fungal infections is based on clinical signs, radiographic changes, and identification of the organism. Radiographs may reveal multiple fungal granulomas throughout all lung lobes. A tracheal wash may be used to collect samples for cytologic examination. Culture of the wash may also be beneficial, particularly if the organism cannot be identified by microscopic examination of the wash. Although amphotericin B and ketoconazole have been used for the treatment of ferrets infected with these organisms, the prognosis is usually poor.[24]

The incidence of dermatophytosis seems to vary according to geographic location.[40] Both *Microsporum canis* and *Trichophyton mentagrophytes* have been diagnosed in ferrets. These organisms are transmitted by direct contact with infected animals or contaminated fomites, and infection has been associated with overcrowding. Dermatophytosis is much more common in young ferrets and is usually self-limiting. The skin and hair lesions are similar to those seen in other mammals, with small patches of alopecia and papules that spread peripherally, leading to crusting and erythematous pruritus. There may also be excoriations and secondary pyoderma due to associated pruritus.

Diagnosis is based on mycotic culture of a skin scrape or hair sample, or by biopsy of the lesion. Microscopic examination of the organisms grown in culture will reveal characteristic fungal arthrospores that allow for identification of the pathogen. *M. canis* will fluoresce under a Woods lamp in fewer than 50% of the cases.[40] Successful treatment of these cases requires clipping the hair surrounding the lesions and applying keratolytic shampoo, povidone-iodine, or chlorhexidine scrubs, and antifungal medications. Griseofulvin can be used at 25 mg/kg orally once a day for 21 to 30 days.[30,40] Adverse effects of griseofulvin treatment have not been reported in ferrets; however, it should not be used in breeding animals, and the CBC should be monitored every 2 weeks. As mentioned, this disease process is usually self-limiting and medical intervention is not always necessary. The environment will require disinfection to prevent reinfection of the organism.

Because dermatophytosis is a zoonotic disease, clients should be educated on the potential risk of infection.

Parasitic Disease
ECTOPARASITES

Ectoparasites can be common in pet ferrets, especially animals that are housed outdoors. Ferrets may become infested with *Ctenocephalides* spp. the same species of fleas that affects dogs and cats. Infestation may be acquired directly from another animal infested with fleas or exposure to an infested environment. Affected ferrets may experience mild to intense pruritus and develop erythremic papules or alopecia over the dorsal cervical and interscapular areas. Evidence of fleas may be noted as reddish-black "dirt" within the fur over the back, or fleas may be seen in the coat or around the face. Treatment involves eliminating the fleas on the ferret, in the environment, and on any other animals within the household. Compounds that are approved for use in cats may be used to treat flea-infested ferrets. Caution should be exercised when topical flea control is applied because toxic overdose to these small animals may occur. Organophosphates, dips, and Dichlorvos-impregnated collars should not be used because of the potential for toxicity. Frontline (Merial Limited, Duluth, GA) can be used topically as a flea preventative and treatment. To apply Frontline, a cloth should be sprayed and used to wipe down the ferret for treatment. Lufenuron (Program; Ciba Animal Health, Greensboro, NC), given at the cat dose, can also be used for treatment and is applied to the mid-dorsal region at the level of the shoulders.[40]

The ferret ear mite, *Otodectes cynotis,* is also commonly diagnosed in pet ferrets. This ear mite is directly transmitted between animals. Ferrets with ear mites may be subclinical, or they may shake their head or scratch at their ears. Although mite infestations are often associated with heavy brown, waxy otic exudate, this exudate is also found in mite-free ferrets. Microscopic examination of otic exudate can be used for diagnosis, allowing for direct visualization of the mites. When a diagnosis is made, all susceptible animals within the household should be treated. Ivermectin can be administered subcutaneously at 0.2 to 0.4 mg/kg every 14 days until resolution, or it can be used topically in each ear at a dosage of 0.5 mg/kg divided between the two ears.[40] To facilitate topical treatment, the ears should be cleaned before treatment. Tresaderm (Merck Agvet Division, Rahway, NJ)—a topical combination of thiabendazole, dexamethasone, and neomycin—can also be used, with a recommended treatment of 7 days application, 7 days off medication, and then 7 more days of treatment.[40,41]

Ferrets are also susceptible to *Sarcoptes scabiei,* acquiring the mite directly from infested animals or from a contaminated environment. There are two conditions described in ferrets, both of which are characterized by intense pruritus of the affected areas.[40,41] The first is a generalized form that consists of focal to generalized alopecia that may involve the face, the pinnae, and/or the ventrum. The second clinical presentation is localized, usually involving only the paws, which often appear inflamed, swollen, and crusted. Severe infestations can result in deformity of the nails or loss of the nails or toes. Diagnosis can be made by skin scrape, although false negatives are possible. Treatment should consist of ivermectin administered at a dosage of 0.2 to 0.4 mg/kg subcutaneously every 14 days until resolution.[40] Alternatively, weekly lime sulfur dips at a dilution of 1 : 40 may be used for up to 6 weeks.[40,41] Unfortunately, the use of lime sulfur dips will result in discoloration of the fur and a very strong odor. Prednisone and antibiotics can be added systemically or topically to alleviate pruritus and secondary dermal bacterial infections. All animals in the household should be treated and the environment should be decontaminated to ensure complete resolution.

Infestation with ticks and myiasis has been seen in ferrets housed outdoors. *Cuterebra* has been diagnosed in the subcutis of a ferret's neck.[40] It can be recognized by a swollen area containing an open pore. *Wohlfahrtia vigil,* the flesh fly, has been reported in commercially ranched mink and ferrets.[40,41] Mink kits of 4 to 5 weeks of age may be affected during the summer months. Eggs are laid on the face, neck, or flanks, where larvae bore into the subcutis and cause irritation. Infestation with *Hypodermis bovis* in the cervical area has also been documented in ferrets.[40,41] Myiasis treatment involves surgical removal of the larvae, debridement of the surrounding tissue, and topical application of antibiotics to the affected tissue.

ENDOPARASITES

Endoparasites are uncommon in pet ferrets; however, any ferret presenting with diarrhea should have a fecal exam performed. Juveniles are susceptible to coccidiosis or giardiasis infestation. *Isospora* and *Eimeria* species have been identified in ferrets.[41] Ferrets diagnosed with coccidiosis may be subclinical or present with diarrhea, lethargy, dehydration, or rectal prolapse. Coccidial infections are usually self-limiting, but ferrets may develop a chronic carrier state.[41] *Cryptosporidium* sp. has more recently been described in ferrets but is not associated with clinical disease.[41] It may cross species barriers, and ferrets acquire it by ingesting infective oocysts. It can be diagnosed by acid fast staining of the feces, with oocysts staining a bright pink, or by flotation in Sheather's sugar. Infection with the *Cryptosporidium* organism appears to be self-limiting and does not require treatment. Treatment of endoparasites involves the use of common anthelmintic drugs and should follow the published ferret dosages of these therapeutic agents.

HEARTWORM DISEASE

Ferrets are susceptible to natural infection by the filarial nematode *Dirofilaria immitis,* the etiologic agent of heartworm disease.[25] The parasitic larvae develop in, and are transmitted by, the mosquito, and infection is of particular concern for ferrets in endemic regions. Clinical signs of infection include dyspnea, cough, pale mucous membrane, lethargy, or anorexia. Muffled heart sounds or a grade II or III murmur may be heard on auscultation of heartworm-positive animals. Radiographs may reveal an enlarged heart, pulmonary congestion, pleural effusion, and possibly ascites. Echocardiography can be a definitive diagnostic test of heartworm disease, with the worms directly visualized as hyperechoic densities within the right atrium and ventricle.[42] Circulating microfilaria is uncommon in the ferret; however, a blood smear is necessary for diagnostic evaluation. Two ELISA diagnostic tests have been used successfully to identify circulating heartworm antigen in ferrets: the Snap Heartworm Antigen Test Kit (IDEXX Laboratories, Inc., Westbrook, ME) and Dirocheck Occult Heartworm kit (Symbiotics, San Diego, CA).[25,43] On necropsy, infected ferrets have been found to carry 1 to 10 worms, located in the right heart, the pulmonary artery, and the cranial and caudal venae cavae.

Treatment of ferrets with heartworm disease can be difficult because of the risk of fatal pulmonary thromboembolism. To reduce this risk, ferrets should be pretreated with heparin at a dosage of 100 U/lb of body weight once a day for 3 days before adulticide therapy and continued for an additional 2 to 3 weeks.[25,41] When heparin treatment is complete, aspirin should be initiated at 10 mg/lb once a day for 3 months. An alternative for heparin is prednisolone given at 2.2 mg/kg once a day for 3 months.[25] Adulticide therapy involves the administration of 0.22 ml/kg of thiacetarsemide (Capreolate) intravenously every 12 hours for 4 injections.[25,41] Heartworm prevention can be initiated 1 month after adulticide therapy is completed. A follow-up ELISA should be checked 3 months after treatment and at monthly intervals thereafter until negative results are achieved. During adulticide therapy, treatment for cardiac failure should also be considered depending on case presentation and patient response.

Ferrets living in heartworm endemic regions should be placed on yearly preventative medication. Oral ivermectin formulated for dogs (Heartguard-30; Merck Agvet Division, Rahway, NJ) can be administered once a month as a preventative.[25] One quarter of the smallest tablet should be given. The remainder of the pill should be discarded, as the drug deteriorates after the pill is broken. Alternatively, an oral suspension of ivermectin can be administered at the recommended dose of 6 μg/kg and up to 1 mg/kg orally once a month.[41] This can be accomplished by mixing 0.3 ml of 1% injectable ivermectin in 28 ml of propylene glycol, creating a concentration of 0.1 mg/ml.[25] A dosage of 0.2 ml/kg can be administered once a month, which will provide a prophylactic dosage of 0.02 mg/kg. The suspension should be protected from light and given a 2-year expiration date.

Nutritional Disease
UROLITHIASIS

The most common nutritional disease of ferrets is urolithiasis. This disease is often diagnosed in ferrets that are fed diets consisting of poor quality dog or cat food. These poor quality diets contain high levels of plant proteins that alkalinize the urine and predispose the animal to crystalluria and stone formation. The normal urine pH of ferrets ranges from 6.5 to 7.5, but ferrets that are fed high-quality, meat-based diets tend to have a pH around 6.0.[21,22] Magnesium ammonium phosphate (struvite) makes up the most commonly reported uroliths in ferrets (see Figure 13-2).[21,22] They can form anywhere in the urinary tract but are commonly found in the kidney,

bladder, and urethra. Nondietary causes of urolithiasis include urinary tract infection with urease-producing bacteria, also resulting in urinary alkalinization, or renal injury leading to increased mineral excretion.

Ferrets with urolithiasis exhibit signs consistent with urinary tract obstruction in other mammals. These signs may include stranguria, dribbling urine, frequent urination, hematuria, vocalization with urination, wet fur or skin irritation of the perineum or preputial areas, or frequent licking of the perineum or preputial areas. Some ferrets may show no initial signs of obstruction but show lethargy or inappetence. Palpation of the abdomen will reveal a distended bladder and may elicit vocalization from pain. Males present more commonly for urethral obstruction, as stones will often become lodged at the base of the os penis. Obstructed ferrets are at major risk for severe metabolic disturbances, bladder rupture, structural kidney damage, and even death. Steps should be taken immediately to alleviate the build-up of urine, in obstructed ferrets, through catheterization or cystocentesis.

Once the patient has been stabilized, a full diagnostic work-up can be done to identify the cause of urinary obstruction. Common differential diagnoses include urolithiasis, prostatomegaly, prostatic cysts, gross pyuria, and possibly neoplasia.[21] A CBC and serum chemistry panel should be performed to identify the presence of any infectious processes or metabolic abnormalities. Reliable urinalysis results are obtained from a sample acquired via cystocentesis and should include a gross exam for crystal identification and culture and sensitivity for bacterial identification. Radiographs are helpful in the diagnosis and location of uroliths and in ruling out other diseases, such as prostatomegaly. Ultrasonography can provide additional information when the patient presents with radiolucent stones, prostatomegaly, or prostatic cysts.

As mentioned previously, urinary obstructed patients should be immediately stabilized by urinary catheterization and correction of any metabolic disturbances. If catheterization cannot be accomplished, cystocentesis can be used for immediate reduction of the bladder. After the bladder has been reduced via cystocentesis, retrograde flushing of the urolith into the bladder can be attempted by placing a catheter partially into the urethra and pinching closed the prepuce while flushing the urethra with sterile saline. If catheterization is still not possible, a temporary tube cystotomy may be necessary.[21] Once the patient has been stabilized, a cystotomy can be performed for stone retrieval, either directly from the bladder or by anterograde flushing of the urethra to dislodge the calculi. Stones should then be submitted for analysis to determine the proper course of treatment and prevent further stone formation. Should removal of the stone be unsuccessful, a perineal urethrostomy is indicated.[21] This procedure should be performed caudal to the base of the os penis in males. A perineal urethrostomy is indicated only in the treatment of urethral obstruction caused by urolithiasis, as it will be unsuccessful in cases of prostatic disease. Renal uroliths may require unilateral nephrectomy.

Long-term treatment of urolithiasis requires the use of antimicrobial therapy for 10 to 14 days and a diet change to one that is higher in animal-based proteins. A commercially prepared ferret diet is specifically formulated to meet all of the dietary requirements of the species and is always recommended over any other diet option. High-quality cat or kitten diets also meet the need of high animal-based proteins and may be substituted. Urinary acidifiers are generally not necessary when a proper diet is initiated. Struvite-dissolving diets also do not work well for the medical treatment of urolithiasis, as it is unpalatable and does not contain sufficient protein for ferrets.[21]

Neoplasia

Ferrets were once thought to have a very low incidence of neoplasia. Although the true incidence is not known, the number of neoplastic cases has risen over the years.[16] This may be due, in part, to the recent increased popularity of the ferret as a pet and laboratory animal. Several etiologies have been proposed for the development of neoplastic diseases in the ferret, including genetic predisposition, early neutering at 5 to 6 weeks of age, the lack of a natural photoperiod, exposure to carcinogenic substances, as well as an infectious agent.[16,44-47] A variety of neoplastic diseases have been described in ferrets, but only a few are diagnosed with any regularity (e.g., adrenocortical cell tumors, insulinoma, lymphoma, cutaneous neoplasms).[44-48] Tumors have been found in most systems of the ferret body, including the gastrointestinal, reproductive, urinary, hematologic, lymphoid, endocrine, integumentary, nervous, and musculoskeletal systems.[16,47]

ADRENAL GLAND DISEASE

Adrenal gland disease is an endocrinopathic disease commonly found in ferrets in the United States, affecting middle-aged to older spayed or neutered ferrets. There is no sex predilection; males and females are equally affected. It is commonly diagnosed as adenoma, adrenocarcinoma, or adrenal hyperplasia.[33,49,50] Adrenal gland disease in ferrets differs from that of dogs in that the disease is characterized by the hypersecretion of sex steroids rather than cortisol. In ferrets, one or more sex steroids such as androstenedione, dehydroepiandrosterone sulfate (DHEA), estradiol, or 17-α-hydroxyprogesterone (17-OHP) will be elevated, whereas cortisol levels are usually within a normal range.[33,50,51] The early age at which ferrets are spayed and neutered in the United States has been associated with development of the disease later in life.[33,50-53] It has been proposed that at the early time of spaying and neutering, there are undifferentiated gonadal cells associated with the adrenal gland. The removal of the testicles or ovary and uterus allow for the chronic, unregulated stimulation of these remaining gonadal cells within the adrenal cortex by follicle-stimulating hormone (FSH) and luteinizing hormone (LH), resulting in ferret adrenal gland disease.

A common presentation for ferret adrenal gland disease is symmetric alopecia that begins with the caudal body and progresses cranially. Quite often in early stages, it may begin as a seasonal alopecia that eventually does not grow back after 2 to 3 seasonal cycles. Pruritis may be evidenced by the presence of erythema or papules in the dorsal neck or interscapular area. Muscle atrophy is another characteristic sign of this disease.

The elevated sex hormone levels also stimulate sexual behavior in males and produce a mild to significant vulvar enlargement in females, mimicking natural estrus. A mucopurulent discharge may be associated with the vulvar enlargement, and some female patients will develop a secondary vaginitis. Ferrets that are chronically affected can present with life-threatening, secondary disease, such as bone marrow toxicity in females (and males) (further described in Hyperestrogenism) and urinary obstruction in males due to prostatomegaly. The secondary prostatic disease may be cystic or hyperplastic, but it is hormone responsive and will typically resolve with treatment of the adrenal gland disease.[50,54] Palpation of enlarged adrenal glands is not always successful because of the abundance of fat that usually surrounds the glands in the retroperitoneal space. The left adrenal gland is palpated more often than the right and can be located craniomedial to the left kidney, whereas the right adrenal gland lies more on the midline and under the caudal extent of the liver.

The presumptive diagnosis of adrenal gland disease is based on the history and clinical signs and confirmed by demonstration of elevated sex hormones or ultrasound evaluation. Concurrent disease is often present, and a full work-up is indicated to determine the scope of illness. A CBC is usually normal in a ferret with adrenal disease unless bone marrow toxicity is present, in which case there will be evidence of anemia and pancytopenia. The serum biochemistry panel is somewhat more helpful in identifying the presence of concurrent disease, as an elevated alanine aminotransferase (ALT) may be the only change associated with adrenal gland disease. Radiographs are also indicated in ruling out additional disease, such as prostatomegaly or splenomegaly. Ultrasonography is useful for diagnostic support of adrenal gland disease, allowing the clinician to identify abnormalities in shape, size, or thickness of the adrenal glands.[55-57] It is important to note, however, that normal adrenal glands determined by ultrasound evaluation does not exclude disease.

The measurement of sex hormones may be used to confirm a diagnosis of adrenal gland disease. Plasma concentrations of 17-OHP, DHEA, and androstenedione are significantly higher in adrenal gland disease.[51] The Clinical Endocrinology Service of Comparative Medicine at the University of Tennessee College of Veterinary Medicine (Knoxville, TN) currently offers measurement of estradiol, androstenedione, and 17-OHP for the diagnosis of adrenal gland disease (Box 13-4). A volume of at least 0.5 ml of serum is required for testing and should be shipped frozen, overnight to the lab. Results are usually reported in about 1 week.

Options for the treatment of adrenal gland disease include medical or surgical therapy.[33,49,50,58] Surgical treatment also provides the opportunity to explore the abdomen and surgically correct any abnormalities noted. The left adrenal gland is more easily removed, as the right adrenal gland is located adjacent to the caudal vena cava. When a single gland is affected, unilateral adrenalectomy should be performed and the contralateral gland debulked if necessary. If disease is present in both adrenal glands, complete removal of adrenal tissue may be difficult. Because of the close proximity of the

Normal Reference Ranges for Sex Steroid Hormones Used to Evaluate Adrenal Gland Disease in the Neutered or Spayed Ferret*

Hormone	Range
Estradiol (pmol/L)	30-180
17-α-hydroxyprogesterone (nmol/L)	0-0.8
Androstenedione (nmol/L)	0-15

*Reference ranges are from the Clinical Endocrinology Service of the University of Tennessee College of Veterinary Medicine.

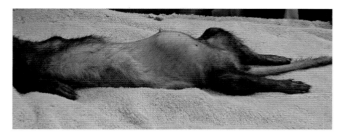

Figure 13-3 This 5-year-old male ferret with adrenal gland disease has a urethral obstruction secondary to prostatomegaly, resulting in a grossly distended bladder.

right adrenal gland to the caudal vena cava, a partial adrenalectomy of the right gland and a complete adrenalectomy of the left gland are recommended. This technique also reduces the need for postsurgical supplemental glucocorticoid therapy. The reported recurrence rate with development of disease of the contralateral gland following unilateral adrenalectomy is 17%, whereas recurrence following subtotal bilateral adrenalectomy is 15% 7 to 22 months after surgery.[49,58]

Alternatively, medical therapy is an option in the treatment of adrenal gland disease. Mitotane was previously recommended for this treatment; however, unlike canine Cushing's disease, ferret adrenal gland disease is nonresponsive. Leuprolide acetate, a long-acting gonadotropin-releasing hormone, is now recommended for the treatment of this disease in ferrets. It acts by suppressing the gonadotropins that are released by the pituitary gland, and it reduces elevated sex hormone levels and eliminates clinical signs.[53] A 3.75-mg, 30-day preparation of leuprolide acetate (Lupron Depot, TAP Pharmaceuticals, Inc., Deerfield, IL) can be administered at a dose of 100 μg intramuscularly every 30 days for ferrets weighing less than 1 kg, and 200 μg intramuscularly every 30 days for ferrets over 1 kg.[59] Injections must continue to be administered at regular intervals to prevent redevelopment of clinical signs. The use of this drug may be cost-prohibitive for some clients, and response to the drug has been variable. The differences in response may be a function of the type of disease process present, hyperplasia versus adenoma or adenocarcinoma, but this has not been evaluated. Additionally, the long-term safety and efficacy of Lupron administration has yet to be determined.

Males with adrenal gland disease that have partial or complete urinary obstruction from prostatomegaly require emergency intervention to empty the distended bladder (Figure 13-3). Manual expression, urethral catheterization, or cystocentesis should be cautiously attempted. As mentioned previously, prostatomegaly caused by adrenal gland disease is hormone responsive, and the prompt surgical removal of the affected gland will resolve urethral obstruction by the enlarged prostate in 24 to 48 hours. Leuprolide acetate has been successful in eliminating obstruction by reducing the sex hormone levels triggering enlargement of the prostate. Bicalutamide, an androgen blocker, has also been suggested at a dosage of 5 mg/kg orally once a day.[60]

The prognosis for ferrets with adrenal gland disease–associated alopecia is good, even without treatment. However, when adrenal gland disease leads to more severe complications, such as bone marrow toxicity, urethral obstruction, or metastasis, the prognosis becomes poor to grave if treatment is not initiated.

INSULINOMA

Insulinoma is a very common neoplastic disease of middle-aged to older ferrets, with males being slightly more susceptible than females.[50,61-64] It is a beta cell tumor of the pancreas that is characterized by hypersecretion of insulin, thus lowering blood glucose by driving glucose into the cells and decreasing hepatic gluconeogenesis and glycogenolysis. It causes an increase in the basal insulin level, and it is highly responsive to stimulation yet unresponsive to inhibitory mediators.[50]

Ferrets affected by insulinoma show signs of hypoglycemia, which may be variable depending on the degree of hypoglycemia and the rate of blood glucose decline. Early signs may be slow and insidious in their development and are not easily recognized by the owner. Such signs include a reduction in activity, weight loss, and difficult arousal from slumber. As the disease progresses and hypoglycemia worsens, more significant clinical signs develop, such as hypothermia, ptyalism, mental dullness, tremors, acute collapse, or a classic glassy-eyed appearance. Because ptyalism is associated with nausea, other diseases such as gastric ulcers or foreign body should be ruled out. Ferrets severely affected by low blood glucose may even have seizures or be comatose. Signs of acute collapse or unresponsiveness can be reversed temporarily with the application of a dextrose solution on the oral mucosa. Insulinoma may also be inadvertently identified in asymptomatic ferrets during the diagnostic work-up of disease processes.

A presumptive diagnosis of insulinoma is made based on the history, clinical signs, and the demonstration of hypoglycemia with a blood glucose test. Although insulinoma is much more common, other differentials for hypoglycemia should be considered, such as liver disease, sepsis, sample mishandling, or neoplasia.[62,63] The diagnosis of insulinoma is confirmed by biopsy and histopathology of affected pancreatic tissue.

The normal range for resting blood glucose in the ferret should be 94 to 207 mg/dl, while the fasting glucose should be 90 to 125 mg/dl.[50] Blood glucose measurements below

70 mg/dl are strongly suggestive of hypoglycemia. A 4- to 6-hour fast is helpful to determine a diagnosis; however, this is not recommended or necessary in animals showing clinical signs consistent with the disease. A human glucometer developed for diabetic patients facilitates measurement of blood glucose in practice, although these devices have not been validated for the ferret. Increased insulin levels and insulin : glucose ratio are also supportive of a diagnosis of insulinoma, but it is possible that ferrets with this disease may have normal insulin levels.[50,62,64] Additional parameters on a serum biochemical assay are typically within normal limits, with the exception of an elevated ALT. Radiography and ultrasonography are not helpful in the diagnosis of insulinoma in most cases, but they may assist in the identification of concurrent disease or metastasis.

Treatment of insulinoma may be accomplished medically or surgically. Medical treatment involves dietary management and the administration of prednisone, diazoxide, or octreotide, alone or in combination.[62] Prednisone acts by blocking peripheral uptake of glucose by cells and increasing hepatic gluconeogenesis. Initially it can be dosed at 0.25 mg/kg orally every 12 hours, but it can be increased up to 2 mg/kg every 12 hours as needed to control hypoglycemia. Prednisone has the unfortunate characteristic of a bitter taste, and ferrets tend to object to its administration. To improve palatability and acceptance, preparations containing alcohol should be avoided. Pediatric formulations of prednisone and prednisolone are available: the formulations Orapred (Lyne Laboratories, Inc., Brockton, MA) and Pediapred (Medeva Pharmaceuticals, Rochester, NY) work quite well. Smaller doses of prednisone can be used when diazoxide, a benzothiadiazine derivative, is added to the treatment plan. Diazoxide functions to antagonize the effects of insulin. It too has a broad dose range, which can be started at 10 mg/kg orally and divided twice a day, and increased to 60 mg/kg divided twice daily as needed.[30] Disadvantages associated with diazoxide include expense and gastrointestinal complications (e.g., vomiting and anorexia).[50] A 50-mg/ml suspension of diazoxide is available (Proglycem; Baker Norton Pharmaceuticals, Miami, FL), as well as 100-mg pills (Proglycem; Schering Canada, Inc., Pointe-Claire, Quebec, Canada), which can be compounded to a suspension at a lesser expense to the owner. The use of prednisone and diazoxide in combination should improve the blood glucose levels of the ferret in 24 to 48 hours. As neither drug slows or stops tumor growth, the dosages will need to be increased periodically as the disease progresses. Octreotide is a somatostatin analog that inhibits insulin secretion by the pancreatic tumor.[62] Because Octreotide requires subcutaneous injection every 12 hours; it is rarely used to treat ferrets diagnosed with insulinoma. Dietary management involves the feeding of meals high in protein and fat, 3 to 4 times a day. Simple sugars should not be offered. The blood glucose is measured daily until clinical signs are eliminated and weekly until the fasting blood glucose is within the normal range; drug dosages should be adjusted as needed. Thereafter, the affected ferret's blood glucose level should be rechecked every 3 months to ensure successful treatment.

Surgical treatment by nodulectomy or partial pancreatectomy is the preferred method of treatment. Unlike insulinoma in dogs, which is characterized by the presence of a single pancreatic mass, ferret insulinoma involves multiple nodules of the pancreas that may affect one or both lobes.[62,63] Because many of the nodules may be microscopic foci, nodulectomy combined with partial pancreatectomy can increase considerably the disease-free interval and survival times.[61] Metastasis is not uncommon in ferrets; local lymph nodes, liver, and spleen should be examined at the time of surgery for evidence of metastasis. Complications such as pancreatitis or iatrogenic diabetes are rare with surgical intervention.[61,62] It is important to note, that although the disease-free interval is increased with surgical therapy, recurrence is typically seen 7 to 10 months after surgery.[61-63] Medical therapy is usually chosen upon recurrence of the disease. The blood glucose should be measured immediately after surgery, at 1 month, and every 3 months thereafter to promptly initiate therapy with recurrence.

The average survival time with treatment following the diagnosis of insulinoma is 16 months.[61-63] Prognosis seems to be associated with the duration of clinical signs before diagnosis and initiation of treatment.[63] Ferrets with a longer duration of hypoglycemia tend to have a shorter disease-free interval and decreased survival times. Therefore, early recognition, diagnosis, and prompt treatment can make a difference in prognosis for ferrets with this disease.

LYMPHOMA

Lymphoma is the most common neoplastic disease affecting young ferrets. It is typically diagnosed in ferrets aged 6 months to 1 year and 3 to 5 years.[46] Numerous tissues are associated with this disease, including peripheral and visceral lymph nodes, spleen, liver, intestines, bone marrow, lung, and kidney.[47] In young ferrets, the disease has an acute onset and is characterized by a rapidly progressive, multicentric distribution of disease, commonly involving hematopoietic and lymphatic tissues, lung and kidney.[44,46] Adult lymphoma is more chronic and survival times tend to be greater. The cluster outbreaks that have occurred in juveniles have led to the suspicion that a viral agent, specifically a retrovirus, may play a role in the etiology of juvenile lymphoma, and is currently under investigation.[45] FeLV and ADV have been suggested as possible etiologic agents, but testing has not supported this theory.[45,46]

Nonspecific clinical signs are often associated with lymphoma in the ferret (e.g., anorexia, weight loss, lethargy).[44,47] Mediastinal lymphoma, a common finding in young ferrets, may result in dyspnea, coughing, or regurgitation (Figure 13-4). Adults may exhibit intermittent nonspecific signs that improve with corticosteroid use. Emesis, diarrhea, or tenesmus may be observed in ferrets with gastrointestinal or abdominal lymphoma, and the patient may have multiple palpable masses in the abdomen or peripheral lymphadenopathy. The peripheral lymph nodes are often surrounded by fat and should not be confused with enlarged lymph nodes that are a consequence of lymphosarcoma. Splenomegaly is a common finding and may be a result of neoplastic infiltrate or extramedullary hematopoiesis.

A CBC and serum biochemistry panel should be performed on any ferret suspected of having neoplastic disease. A CBC

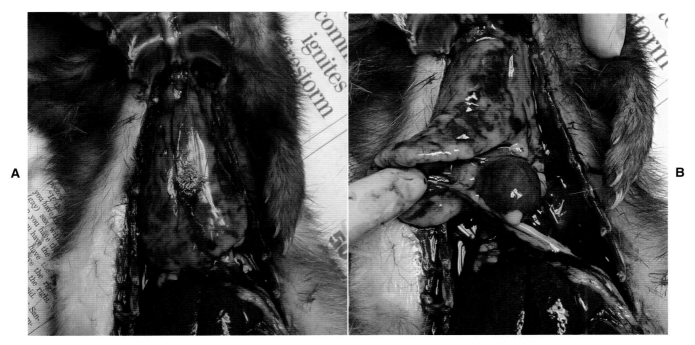

Figure 13-4 A, Approximately 80% of this ferret's thorax is occupied by mediastinal lymphoma. **B,** Note the significant reduction in lung space caused by the presence of the mass.

may reveal mild anemia and a normal or elevated white blood cell count. In young ferrets, a lymphocytosis is common, whereas in older ferrets, a lymphopenia is much more common.[44] The lymphocytosis generally exceeds 3500 cells/mm[3] or comprises greater than 60% of the total white blood cell count.[47] Less than 25% of lymphoma cases may be characterized as lymphoblastic leukemia.[46] Radiographs should be obtained from the dyspneic patient and are helpful in identifying the presence of a mediastinal mass, pleural effusion, or organomegaly (Figure 13-5). Fine needle aspiration and biopsy are quite useful for the definitive diagnosis of lymphoma. A fine needle aspirate should be performed on any masses or pleural effusion. The thoracic aspirate of pleural effusion allows for the differentiation between lymphoma, cardiac disease, pyothorax, or chylothorax. A bone marrow aspirate should be performed on any ferrets with evidence of leukemia, anemia, or atypical lymphocytes on the CBC. A peripheral lymph node biopsy or nodectomy with subsequent histopathologic evaluation of the tissue sample, particularly of the popliteal lymph node, is ideal for confirming a diagnosis of lymphoma in the ferret.[47] This can be beneficial in determining the diagnosis even if performed on a lymph node of normal size. Histopathologic examination of an enlarged peripheral lymph node may reveal lymphoid hyperplasia, which is often caused by viral infection or chronic antigenic stimulation. Histopathologic classification of ferret lymphoma cases are high grade, diffuse, small noncleaved, or immunoblastic in young.[44] Older ferret lymphoma cases have been classified as mixed cell immunoblastic (most commonly) or mature lymphocytic.

Once a definitive diagnosis of lymphoma has been made, a treatment protocol must be pursued. The ideal therapy is surgical removal of any solid masses combined with systemic che-

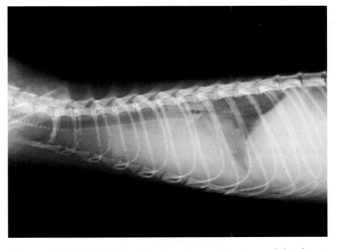

Figure 13-5 This is the lateral radiographic view of the ferret in Figure 13-4. The presenting clinical signs were lethargy and severe dyspnea.

motherapy. Young ferrets with multicentric distribution of disease typically respond poorly to chemotherapy and have short survival times.[44,46] Ferrets with concurrent disease have a greater risk of complications associated with chemotherapy. Additionally, those that have been previously treated with corticosteroids have a poor response to chemotherapy. The prognosis for ferrets with no overt clinical signs, but which were diagnosed based on chronic lymphocytosis and a positive lymph node biopsy, is variable.[47] Older ferrets probably respond better because the neoplasia has a slower growth rate.

Treatment should never be considered curative for a ferret patient diagnosed with lymphoma. Remission can be achieved with marked improvement or return to a clinically normal state.[47] Remission may be defined as resolution of organomegaly and a normal CBC. Biopsy, however, may show persistence of disease. Remission may last for 3 months to 5 years, during which time a patient's CBC should be monitored every 1 to 3 months.[47]

Protocols for chemotherapy for lymphoma are listed in Table 13-6. Before the initiation of chemotherapy a full patient evaluation should be made, consisting of a CBC, serum biochemistry panel, radiographs, and bone marrow aspirate. This allows for the complete assessment of the patient for risks associated with, and prognosis for, response to therapy. Patients with greater than 50% of the bone marrow composed of malignant cells are at a high risk for fatal complications from chemotherapy.[47] The client should be educated on the need for complete compliance, good nutritional support, and close monitoring of the patient. Side effects are dependent on the drugs that are used, but they are the same as those described in other species. Lethargy, posterior paresis, anorexia, vomiting, mild hair loss, dyspnea, and collapse are the most common side effects seen in ferrets. They may occur as soon as 1 to 2 days posttreatment or as late as 2 weeks posttreatment.[47] Veterinarians should always follow standard safety protocols when using antineoplastic drugs. Intravenous drug administration should be performed under anesthesia, using an indwelling catheter. To ensure patency, the catheter should always be flushed before drug administration, and extravasation should be managed according to procedures appropriate for the drug. With doxorubicin, the catheter should not be flushed with heparinized saline, as the heparin will cause the doxorubicin to precipitate out. The CBC should be evaluated no more than 24 hours before each treatment. Should the total white blood cell count drop below 1500/mm,[3] the PCV below 30%, or the patient become debilitated, treatment should be discontinued or postponed until the physiologic parameters return to normal.[47] The CBC should be rechecked 1 to 2 times a week until it has returned to normal limits. Additionally, nutritional support during chemotherapy is very important. The administration of Nutri-Cal, meat baby food, or Hill's Prescription Diet Canine/Feline a/d may be used as a nutritional supplement.

Patients that are poor candidates for antineoplastic therapy can be treated with glucocorticoids. This therapy would not be myelosuppressive and can potentially destroy sensitive tumor cells. Glucocorticoid medication can be given at a dosage of 0.5 mg/kg orally every 12 hours and increased as needed to control clinical disease signs.[47] Glucocorticoid therapy should not be used in asymptomatic ferrets, as there is the risk of resistance to treatment when signs develop and therapy is needed most. Herbal and homeopathic therapies have also been attempted with some success. A combination of vitamin C and Pau d'Arco has been used.[47] Vitamin C acts as an antioxidant and stimulates the immune system. The chelated, buffered, or ester form can be given at 50 to 100 mg/kg orally twice a day. Pau d'Arco also acts to support the

---

TABLE 13-6   **Chemotherapy Protocols for Lymphoma in Ferrets**

Protocol 1*[47]

Week	Day	Drug	Dosage
1	1	Prednisone	1 mg/kg PO q12h continued throughout treatment
	1	Vincristine	0.12 mg/kg IV
	3	Cyclophosphamide	10 mg/kg PO, SC
2	8	Vincristine	0.12 mg/kg IV
3	15	Vincristine	0.12 mg/kg IV
4	22	Vincristine	0.12 mg/kg IV
	24	Cyclophosphamide	10 mg/kg PO, SC
7	46	Cyclophosphamide	10 mg/kg PO,SC
9		Prednisone	Gradually decrease dose to 0 over 4 wk

From Brown SA: Ferrets: neoplasia. In Hillyer EV, Quesenberry KE, editors: *Ferrets, Rabbits and Rodents: Clinical Medicine and Surgery*, Philadelphia, 1997, WB Saunders.

Protocol 2**[33]

Week	Drug	Dosage
1	Vincristine	0.07 mg/kg IV
	Asparaginase	400 IU/kg IP
	Prednisone	1 mg/kg PO q24h, continued throughout therapy
2	Cyclophosphamide	10 mg/kg SC
3	Doxorubicin	1 mg/kg IV
4-6	Same as weeks 1-3, but discontinue asparginase	
8	Vincristine	0.07 mg/kg IV
10	Cyclophosphamide	10 mg/kg SC
12	Vincristine	0.07 mg/kg IV
14	Methotrexate	0.5 mg/kg IV

From Rosenthal KL: Ferrets, *Vet Clin North Am: Small Anim Pract* 24(1):1-23, 1994.

Protocol 3***[47]

Drug	Dosage
Doxorubicin	1 mg/kg IV q21 days for up to 5 treatments
Prednisone[#]	1 mg/kg PO q24h or divided q12h

From Brown SA: Ferrets: neoplasia. In Hillyer EV, Quesenberry KE, editors: *Ferrets, Rabbits and Rodents: Clinical Medicine and Surgery*, Philadelphia, 1997, WB Saunders.
*Check CBCs weekly during therapy, and every 3 months posttherapy with examination.
**Continue protocol in sequence biweekly after week 14.
***May be used for recurrence of disease following remission.
#Optional as concurrent therapy.

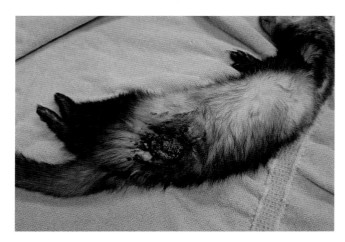

Figure 13-6 Histopathologic examination after complete surgical excision led to a diagnosis of this mass as a basal cell tumor. Metastasis and local regrowth of this type of tumor are rare in the ferret, and surgical excision yields a good prognosis.

immune system as a natural antibiotic. It can be administered at 3 to 5 drops orally every 12 hours.

CUTANEOUS NEOPLASMS

Cutaneous neoplasms are fairly common in ferrets, and a variety of tumor types have been described. Some of the more common cutaneous neoplasms include the basal cell tumor (Figure 13-6), mast cell tumor, fibrosarcoma and fibroma, sebaceous gland adenoma, hemangioma, and benign cystic adenoma.[47,48] These tumors are typically seen in middle-aged to older ferrets.[48] Areas where cutaneous neoplasms occur include the head, neck, shoulder, flank, legs, and feet. Biopsy and histopathology should be performed on all cutaneous masses to direct treatment and establish a prognosis. Some tumor types, such as basal cell and mast cell tumors, are benign and can be managed by complete surgical excision, with minimal risk of recurrence or metastasis. Others, such as adenocarcinoma, squamous cell carcinoma, or fibrosarcoma, have a greater tendency to metastasize and recur locally. Therefore, further evaluation, including CBC, serum biochemistry panel, and radiography, are warranted to fully assess the extent of disease.

Miscellaneous Tumors
CHORDOMAS

Chordomas are a common occurence in ferrets and originate from residual notochord tissue. They are typically round, smooth, firm masses that develop on the tail. This tumor type has also occurred at the atlantooccipital joint and C2-C3 vertebrae.[47] Chordomas are slow-growing tumors, but metastasis can occur. As with other neoplasms, a full evaluation should be performed to determine if metastasis has already occurred. The treatment of choice is surgical removal of the mass, which usually involves amputation of the tail cranial to the chordoma.

Miscellaneous Diseases
UROGENITAL DISORDERS
Hyperestrogenism

Jills are seasonally polyestrous, induced ovulators; thus, if they are not bred or artificially stimulated to ovulate, they will remain in estrus.[22] Ferrets are quite susceptible to the effects of estrogen, and those that remain in estrus for periods longer than a month are at great risk for developing estrogen-induced bone marrow hypoplasia.[21] Physical signs of hyperestrogenism are similar to those of adrenal gland disease and natural estrus, with ferrets exhibiting a fleshy, swollen vulva, with or without discharge, and bilateral symmetric alopecia. Ferrets with hyperestrogenism are typically much younger than those with adrenal gland disease, with the average age being 1 to 2 years. In the United States, where ferrets are generally spayed before leaving a breeding facility, hyperestrogenism is rare. It is possible that a spayed female with remnant ovarian tissue may present for hyperestrogenism.

When the bone marrow is affected in hyperestrogenism cases, ferrets will become lethargic, inappetent, and weak, and will show signs of pale mucous membranes and subcutaneous or mucosal hemorrhage (e.g., petechiation, ecchymosis). At the onset of estrus, the ferret's CBC will show a neutrophilia and thrombocytosis, but this will change to thrombocytopenia, leukopenia, and normocytic, normochromic, nonregenerative anemia when the bone marrow becomes affected.[21,22] Hyperestrogenism can be distinguished from adrenal gland disease based on age, history, clinical signs, and a response to the administration of hormones to stimulate ovulation.

Treatment of hyperestrogenism is ovariohysterectomy or surgery to search for and remove remnant ovarian tissue. Because of the significant anemia and thrombocytopenia associated with secondary bone marrow toxicity, surgery must be postponed in these ferrets until the ovaries have been stimulated to ovulate and the patient has been stabilized. A single injection of 100 IU human chorionic gonadotropin intramuscularly, repeated in 1 week if signs of estrus are still present after 3 to 4 days, will terminate estrus.[21,22,33] Alternatively, a single injection of gonadotropin-releasing hormone at 20 μg/kg intramuscularly or subcutaneously, also repeated in 1 to 2 weeks should signs of estrus persist, may be administered.[22] Treatment with antiestrogens such as tamoxifen citrate and clomiphene citrate should be avoided as they can have estrogenic effects in ferrets.[21,33] Treatment for bone marrow toxicity should include fluid therapy, iron and vitamin B supplementation, broad spectrum antibiotics, and enteral nutrition. Severely anemic and thrombocytopenic ferrets may require multiple whole blood transfusions. Once stabilized, the CBC should be rechecked with the patient in anestrus and again before surgery.

Ferrets not intended for breeding should be spayed to reduce or eliminate the risk of this disease. Prognosis for recovery of hyperestrogenism and bone marrow toxicity is dependent on the degree of anemia. If the PCV is greater than 20%, the patient has a good chance of recovery once the ovaries are stimulated to ovulate and surgery is performed. Ferrets with a

PCV below 15% have a grave prognosis, and aggressive medical intervention is required.

Prostatic Disease

Prostatic disease (e.g., prostatomegaly, prostatic cysts, and abscesses) is very common in male ferrets and is often secondary to adrenal disease.[21] Significant enlargement of the prostate can lead to urethral obstruction. Prostatic disease may go undetected until such signs of urinary obstruction or adrenal disease are noticed. In the normal ferret, the prostate is not palpable; however, when it is enlarged it can be palpated as a firm, soft tissue structure lying caudodorsally to the bladder. Treating the adrenal gland disease will often immediately correct the prostatic disease. Broad-spectrum antibiotics should be utilized in cases of prostatic abcessation. Grossly enlarged or infected prostates may require more aggressive intervention, such as surgical debulking or marsupialization for drainage of infected material.[21,22]

Renal Cysts

There is, in general, a low incidence of renal disease in the ferret; however, renal cysts are commonly diagnosed. Renal cysts may be one or more in number and affect one or both kidneys. Unlike polycystic disease in other animals and humans, the disease in ferrets has not been found to involve other organs.[21,22] Often cysts do not cause a problem for the ferret and will go undetected until found incidentally on palpation (one or more smooth masses on the kidneys) or ultrasound (one or more hypoechoic areas with smooth walls on the kidneys).[22] Renal cysts have also been identified during abdominal exploratory surgery or necropsy. Renal cysts may cause a problem when a significant amount of the normal renal architecture is disrupted by the size of the cyst. When polycystic disease is identified, a CBC, serum biochemistry panel, and urinalysis should be performed to determine the effects of the cysts. Just as in the dog and the cat, the urea nitrogen and creatinine are used to evaluate renal function. Creatinine, however, declines very quickly in the blood of ferrets; therefore, any elevation should be considered significant. Ultrasonography can be used to evaluate renal architecture, and intravenous pyelography can be used to evaluate renal function. There is no treatment available for bilateral renal cystic disease. If one kidney is compromised by the presence of renal cysts, a unilateral nephrectomy can be performed if the opposite kidney has adequate function. Those ferrets that show no ill effect from polycystic disease do not require medical or surgical intervention.

GASTROINTESTINAL DISORDERS
Foreign Body

Gastrointestinal foreign bodies are a common problem with ferrets, particularly in young animals that are allowed free roam of the household or have access to foam or soft rubber toys. Older ferrets present more commonly with obstructive trichobezoars.[28,31,33,65] Foreign body ingestion should always be a consideration in any ferret exhibiting signs of GI disease. Clinical signs may include diarrhea, anorexia, lethargy, and signs of nausea, such as pawing at the mouth or ptyalism. Vomiting is less common. Weight loss may occur if the obstruction is a chronic problem. On physical examination, the foreign object may be palpable, or the ferret may show signs of abdominal pain or discomfort with abdominal palpation. Radiographs may reveal evidence of gas or fluid in the stomach, a gas pattern in the intestines, or a radiopaque object present in the stomach or intestines. A barium series may provide additional support for a diagnosis.

The treatment of choice for foreign body removal is gastrotomy or enterotomy. A cat laxative can be attempted for the removal of trichobezoars, but surgical removal is preferred in these cases. Fluids and supportive therapy are necessary before surgery to stabilize the patient. The same principles for GI surgery and postoperative care in the dog and cat should be followed for the ferret. When a foreign body or trichobezoar is surgically removed, ferrets generally have no postoperative complications.

Eosinophilic Gastroenteritis

Eosinophilic gastroenteritis is a disease process of ferrets that is more commonly reported in young ferrets.[29] It is characterized by infiltration of the stomach wall, intestines, and mesenteric lymph nodes with eosinophils. As of yet, there is no confirmed etiology, but a food allergy has been proposed as a component of the disease process.[29,31,33] Chronic diarrhea that is nonresponsive to antibiotic therapy is a common clinical sign associated with eosinophilic gastroenteritis, as are weight loss and anorexia. On abdominal palpation, intestinal loops may feel thickened and mesenteric lymph nodes enlarged. A CBC will often reveal eosinophilia. Diagnosis is confirmed with gastric or intestinal biopsy and histopathologic examination. Other GI pathogens should be investigated, including internal parasites or *Helicobacter* spp., which may contribute to the development of the disease. Treatment in ferrets is similar to that used in dogs, cats, and humans with eosinophilic gastroenteritis and is focused on reducing the inflammatory process. Prednisone at 1.25 to 2.5 mg/kg orally once a day is the treatment of choice for ferrets diagnosed with eosinophilic gastroenteritis. After the first week, the frequency of administration can be reduced to every 48 hours until clinical signs have completely resolved.[29,31,33]

SPLENOMEGALY

Splenomegaly is a very common finding in ferrets. Often it is an incidental finding in a clinically normal ferret, and it can occur as a primary or secondary disease process. Primary diseases of the spleen that can result in enlargement include lymphoma, primary splenic neoplasia, and ADV. Splenomegaly can be an incidental finding with any disease process, including insulinoma, adrenal gland disease, cardiac disease, and dental disease. Therefore, a full diagnostic work-up should be done to rule out concurrent disease, particularly in middle-aged to older ferrets.

Clinical signs are often related to the primary disease. Occasionally, when a spleen is excessively large, signs of discomfort, such as inappetence or lethargy, may be present. The enlarged spleen can be easily palpated on physical exam, and any irregularities in shape should be noted. It is important to remember that the size of the spleen is not related to the severity of disease. A CBC and platelet count should provide a baseline of information and are important in ruling out lymphoma and hypersplenism. Hypersplenism is the excessive destruction of erythrocytes, leukocytes, and/or platelets and will be revealed as a cytopenia on the CBC.[25] For cases of suspected hypersplenism, a bone marrow aspirate is required, with results being normal or hypercellular. To adequately diagnose hypersplenism in the ferret, infection, neoplasia, and other causes of blood dyscrasias must be ruled out. Additional diagnostic tests to consider include radiographs, serum biochemistry panel (or at least a glucose level check), and urinalysis to rule out other disease processes, such as insulinoma or cardiac disease. A splenic biopsy can be helpful and should be obtained when surgery is required for a concurrent disease (e.g., insulinoma, adrenal gland disease). Histopathology often reveals extramedullary hematopoiesis and/or congestion in the absence of primary splenic disease.[25]

If no other abnormalities are identified and the ferret is determined to be clinically healthy, a record of the spleen size should be made, and subsequent evaluations should take place, at least on an annual basis. Splenectomy is not indicated in primary splenomegaly cases or cases of concurrently existing disease. When a concurrent disease process has been identified, treatment should be directed at the primary disease, not the organ response. A splenectomy is indicated for ferrets experiencing discomfort due to the enlarged spleen when no other disease process has been identified or there is risk of rupture. Splenectomy is also necessary for hypersplenism, splenitis, splenic neoplasia, torsion, rupture, or abcess.[25] Cases of hypersplenism may require whole blood transfusion before surgery to reduce intraoperative and postoperative hemorrhage. Supportive care such as B vitamins, antibiotics, and nutritional support should also be considered for the splenectomized ferret.

CARDIAC DISORDERS

Cardiac disease is common in middle-aged to older ferrets. Often ferrets may have a history of nonspecific signs, such as inappetence, weight loss, lethargy, or rear limb paresis. Some ferrets are subclinical, and cardiac disease is an incidental finding on annual exam. Physical exam findings of cyanosis, increased capillary refill time, jugular distension or pulses, abnormal femoral pulses, or hypothermia are dependent on the severity of disease.[25,66] Results of auscultation vary, depending on the type of disease process present, but can include tachycardia, muffled heart sounds, left-sided holosystolic murmur, right-sided murmur, gallop rhythm, or pulmonary crackles.[25,66] Animals in cardiac failure commonly have ascites, hepatomegaly, or splenomegaly.

A diagnosis of heart disease is made based upon history and clinical signs, physical exam findings, radiographic evidence, electrocardiography (ECG), and echocardiography. Radiographically a globoid heart is commonly present and may be accompanied by pleural effusion, pulmonary venous congestion, or a diffuse interstitial pattern. Additional findings may include hepatomegaly, splenomegaly and ascites. An ECG is helpful in the identification of arrhythmias and conduction disturbances. Ideally the ECG should be performed without the aid of anesthesia. The ECG can be accomplished more efficiently by removing the metal teeth of the clasps, to which ferrets actively object, and utilizing techniques of distraction such as a Nutri-Cal treat. Ferret ECGs on lead II have small P waves that are similar to cats and large R waves similar to dogs.[25] Additionally, the normal ferret ECG will contain short QT intervals and elevated ST segments. Abnormal findings may include, but are not limited to, sinus tachycardia, atrial or ventricular premature complexes, sinus bradycardia, tall and wide QRS complexes, and depression of the ST segment.[25,66] The presence of a second- or third-degree atrioventricular block is indicative of significant heart disease. Echocardiography, also best performed without sedation, is useful in the assessment of chamber size, shape, function, pleural and pericardial effusion, and cardiac or mediastinal masses. Color flow Doppler imaging allows for evaluation of valvular insufficiency by providing information on the direction of blood flow and the presence of turbulence.[25] Additional tests, such as a CBC and serum biochemistry panel, can provide information of concurrent disease. Microfilarial testing and heartworm antigen testing can be used to diagnose heartworm disease. Thoracocentesis not only has diagnostic value but may also offer temporary respiratory relief to ferrets with pleural effusion.

Dilated cardiomyopathy is the most commonly diagnosed cardiac disease in ferrets.[25] The cause of this disease is as yet unknown. Gross pathology reveals dilation of both atria and ventricles, and histopathology reveals multifocal myocardial degeneration, necrosis, and fibrosis. Treatment should be aimed at altering the heart rate, preload, afterload, and contractility. Hypertrophic cardiomyopathy is also diagnosed in ferrets. Ferrets with hypertrophic cardiomyopathy will have a thickened interventricular septum and a thickened left ventricular wall.[25] Histopathologically, these ferrets have fibrous connective tissue throughout the myocardium. The main objective of medical treatment is to improve diastolic function. The diagnosis of valvular disease in middle-aged ferrets is increasing.[25] In this disease process, valves become thickened and atria become dilated secondary to the developing valvular insufficiency. Myxomatous degeneration is a common histopathologic finding in valvular disease.[25] Another type of cardiac disease in ferrets is myocarditis, which is caused by toxoplasma-like organisms, ADV, sepsis, and heartworm disease.[25] There have been no reports of congenital cardiac disease or primary cardiac neoplasia in the ferret.

Treatment depends on the type of heart disease present and is based on treatment strategies in the dog and cat. Furosemide can be used safely in ferrets to alleviate fluid retention due to cardiac failure. The recommended dosage for furosemide is 2.5 to 4 mg/kg every 8 to 12 hours.[66] Digoxin, a positive inotrope, is integral to the treatment of dilated cardiomyopathy. The recommended initial dosage is 0.01 mg/kg orally every 24 hours and it should be increased to every 12 hours or decreased to once every other day, depending on the case. Just as in dogs and cats, serum digoxin levels should be checked 8 hours posttreatment to ensure that therapeutic levels are reached (0.8-2.0 ng/ml).[25] The dosage is based on an estimated 75% lean body weight.[30] Ferrets should be monitored for side effects that may be associated with digoxin therapy, such as cardiac arrhythmias, inappetence, vomiting, and diarrhea. Digoxin should not be used in ferrets that are azotemic or hypokalemic or have frequent ventricular arrhythmias. Nitroglycerin 2% ointment is also beneficial as a venodilator in the treatment of dilated cardiomyopathy. It can be applied to a shaved area of the skin on the inner thigh or pinna, 1/8 inch in size, every 12 to 24 hours.[25,30] ACE-inhibitors are used to reduce arteriolar and venous tone, to increase cardiac output, and decrease edema; however, ferrets are sensitive to their hypotensive effects and thus require close monitoring. After an initial low dose, the amount can be increased if there is no ill response (e.g., inappetence, lethargy). The recommended dosage for enalapril is 0.25 0.5 mg/kg orally every 24 to 48 hours.[30] Beta-adrenergic blockers and calcium channel blockers may be used for the treatment of hypertrophic cardiomyopathy. Their usage results in a decreased heart rate and increased diastolic filling. The recommended dose for atenolol is 6.25 mg orally every 24 hours, and propranolol is 0.2 to 1 mg/kg orally every 8 to 12 hours.[25,30] Diltiazem, a calcium channel blocker, is administered at a dose of 3.75 to 7.5 mg orally every 12 hours.[25] Side effects of diltiazem include arrhythmia, lethargy, and inappetence. Supportive care for the cardiac patient includes oxygen supplementation for dyspnea, restricted activity, and a low salt diet. The prognosis for ferrets with cardiac disease is guarded to poor, even with intensive medical treatment.

■ THERAPEUTICS

Fluid Therapy

The ill or debilitated ferret often requires fluid therapy as part of its supportive care. The accepted daily maintenance fluid requirement for the ferret is 75 to 100 ml/kg/day.[8,60] In addition to meeting the maintenance requirements, additional fluid doses should be calculated to replace ongoing losses and dehydration. Fluids can be easily administered subcutaneously in the ferret, with the fluid dose divided over 2 to 3 times a day. The loose skin over the neck, shoulder blades, and back are good places to administer subcutaneous fluids. Ferrets will often object to subcutaneous fluid administration, thus requiring adequate restraint. Severely debilitated animals may need intravenous or intraosseous fluid therapy administered continuously or 2 to 3 times a day. This can be accomplished with an infusion pump, a Buretrol device (Baxter Healthcare, Deerfield, IL), or a control flow regulator. The patient should be carefully monitored for fluid overload, which may result in

dyspnea, harsh lung sounds, or a heart murmur. Fluid overload is an important concern in cardiac patients that can quickly overhydrate.

Lactated Ringer's solution and Normosol are good options for fluid replacement in the ferret. Ferrets presenting for hypoglycemia may require the addition of 2.5% to 5% dextrose to the fluid therapy. Additional support can by provided to the debilitated patient through the addition of vitamin B or potassium to the fluids. The same protocols used in canine and feline medicine for the administration of these drugs should be applied to their use in the ferret.

Antimicrobials

Many of the same antimicrobial drugs of cats and dogs have been used safely in ferrets, and there are published drug dosages for ferrets. The same precautions and warnings for their use also apply to ferrets. An accurate body weight should be obtained from the ferret to properly dose the medications. The decision to use antimicrobials should always be based on diagnostic testing rather than empirical use. As with any animal, the results of culture and sensitivity diagnostic testing are ideal to identify the pathogenic organism and the appropriate antimicrobial drugs with which to treat the infection. When this is not available, the type of antimicrobial agent selected should be based on the spectrum of organism sensitivity, bioavailability, target tissue, and ease of administration.

Administration of the antimicrobial agents is sometimes a challenge. Injectable drugs are good for extremely ill patients. The quadriceps muscle is routinely used for intramuscular injections, but care should be taken to avoid the sciatic nerve. Intramuscular use should be limited because of the small muscle mass available for administration. Subcutaneous injections are another option available for administering treatment. Ferret skin can be quite tough, and scruffing is usually necessary for administration. Intravenous drugs are injected via the cephalic or saphenous veins with a 22- to 25-gauge butterfly catheter; however, anesthesia is almost always required if an indwelling catheter is not already in place.

When provided in a liquid form, oral medications are well suited for the ferret (Figure 13-7). Pills can be difficult to administer unless they are crushed and mixed with an oral supplement (e.g., Nutri-Cal) or treat. Liquid formulations that are bitter or unpalatable can also be a treatment challenge, as ferrets will readily object and excessively salivate. Pediatric formulations are much easier to give because their sweet taste increases palatability. The availability of compounding pharmacies and a variety of flavor additives offer additional options for liquid drug formulations that should be readily accepted by the ferret.

Emergency Drugs

The same drugs utilized for canine and feline emergencies may be used in the ferret when dosed by body weight. A complete physical assessment and history are necessary to determine an appropriate treatment plan. Initial diagnostic tests may also

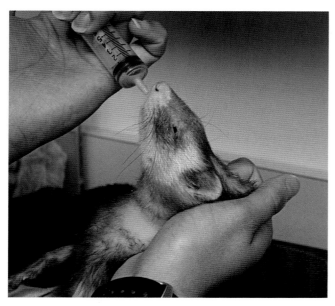

Figure 13-7 Scruffing the ferret with the nose directed upward facilitates the administration of oral medication.

facilitate the selection of a therapeutic option. When treating a ferret with life-threatening conditions, cardiopulmonary resuscitation may be necessary, and the same protocols used for cats should be followed. Cardiopulmonary stimulating drugs should be administered in conjunction with manual resuscitation. Epinephrine can be used to stimulate the heart beat at a dosage of 0.4 mg/kg diluted in saline and administered intratracheally or 0.2 mg/kg IV, IO, or intracardiac.[67] For the bradycardic patient, atropine is given at a dosage of 0.05 mg/kg IV or 0.10 mg/kg intratracheally.[67] Respiration can be stimulated using doxapram at 1 to 2 mg/kg IV.[30] Diazepam should be used to control seizures at an initial dose of 1 to 2 mg IV to effect.[30] Dexamethasone is appropriate for the treatment of shock, whereas nonsteroidal antiinflammatory drugs may be utilized for trauma.

Fluids are also very important when treating the emergency ferret case, particularly those suffering from shock or requiring CPR. An emergency fluid rate for the ferret is 70 ml/kg/hr.[67] Once the patient has been stabilized, the fluid rate can be reduced appropriately. Ferrets presenting in a hypoglycemic state characterized by collapse require immediate IV administration of dextrose. A slow bolus of 50% dextrose should be given until the ferret is responsive. The initial bolus dose should be followed up with the administration of fluid (e.g., LRS, Normosol) containing 5% dextrose and the initiation of prednisone to increase the blood glucose level. Blood glucose should be monitored regularly during treatment.

Close monitoring of the emergency patient for changes in its condition is required to determine treatment response. An external heat source is often needed to supplement and maintain a stable body temperature. Nutritional support should also be considered, as ill ferrets are often anorectic. Finally, analgesia should be provided, particularly with cases involving traumatic injuries, to reduce associated discomfort or pain.

Blood Transfusions

Ferrets lack detectable blood groups, an important consideration for patients (e.g., jills) with estrogen-induced bone marrow toxicity where multiple blood transfusions may be necessary. A study was conducted to test ferrets for naturally acquired or experimentally induced anti-erythrocyte antibodies, and no evidence could be found for the presence of anti-erythrocyte antibodies even after two blood transfusions from the same donors.[68] The results of the study showed that there was little risk associated with blood transfusion in the ferret for up to three transfusions from the same donor, even without cross-matching. It is unknown, however, whether antibodies are produced after multiple transfusions.

An anesthetized large male ferret with a known medical history is the best blood donor from which 6 to 12 ml of blood can be safely collected. An anticoagulant such as an acid-citrate-dextrose solution in a ratio of 1 ml anticoagulant to 6 ml of blood should be used.[8,68] A blood filter is not necessary, but a butterfly catheter introduced into the jugular vein facilitates blood collection from the donor and blood transfusion to the recipient. Infusion of the blood into the recipient should be done immediately under anesthesia by a slow bolus or infusion pump. A blood transfusion can also be administered via an intraosseous catheter.

Nutritional Support

Ill ferrets often are anorexic or have a reduced appetite and thus require nutritional support during hospitalization and treatment. The concern for the development of hepatic lipidosis or the exacerbation of hypoglycemia due to prolonged anorexia further emphasizes the need for nutritional supplementation. Enteral feeding is the preferred route of nutritional supplementation, and there are a variety of soft food preparations that can be administered via syringe. Hill's Prescription Diet Canine/Feline a/d is often used and is readily accepted by the ferret; this diet can be mixed with Glucerna, a human diabetic supplement, for additional calories. Nutri-Cal can also be used as a supplement but should be limited in ferrets with insulinoma because of its high sugar content and the risk of reflex hypoglycemia. Soft foods should be fed 3 to 4 times daily at a volume of 2 to 5 ml each feeding. Once the ferret is showing improvement in appetite, the critical care diet can be left in the cage for the ferret to eat ad lib. If the patient is to be fed this diet over a long period of time, a formulated ferret diet should be soaked until soft and mixed with the critical care diet to ensure that the ferret is receiving adequate nutrition.

Parenteral nutrition may be necessary for some ferrets that refuse syringe feeding or who suffer from GI disease characterized by maldigestion or malabsorption. A total nutrient admixture (TNA) of lipid, dextrose, amino acids, electrolytes, vitamins, and minerals can be compounded to provide parenteral nutrition.[67] Administration should be via infusion pump through a silicone elastomer or polyurethane jugular catheter (Cook Veterinary Products, Bloomington, IL).

SURGERY

Anesthesia

Producing anesthesia in the ferret is very much like that of the dog and cat. A preanesthetic work-up consisting of a physical exam, CBC, and serum biochemistry panel is recommended for all ferrets, to reduce or eliminate the risks associated with anesthesia when underlying disease is present. Like dogs and cats, ferrets should be fasted before an anesthetic procedure. Because of the rapid transit time of the ferret gastrointestinal tract, fasting should be no longer than 8 hours in the young ferret and 4 hours in the older ferret.[15] A shorter fasting time is of particular importance in middle-aged to geriatric ferrets because hypoglycemia secondary to insulinoma is a risk.

Either injectable drugs or gas inhalants may be used; however, gas anesthetic is preferred, particularly in the ill ferret. The ferret may be premedicated with a sedative or induced with a gas anesthetic via face mask or induction chamber. Induction via gas inhalant can be accomplished with flow rates of 5% isoflurane or 7% sevoflurane. Tracheal intubation is fairly easy in the ferret, and can be facilitated using a laryngoscope. Laryngospasm should not interfere with intubation; lidocaine can be used to minimize laryngospasms should they occur. A 2- to 3.5-mm endotracheal tube can be used and attached to a nonrebreathing system with a semi-open circuit. Most ferret patients are maintained on 3% isoflurane or 5% sevoflurane with an oxygen flow rate of 1 L/min.

An intravenous catheter should be placed in the ferret for any surgical procedure. The cephalic, lateral saphenous, or jugular veins may be accessed for intravenous catheterization. Ferrets have very tough skin, and a small stab incision adjacent to the vein may aid in placement of the catheter. Because of ferrets' small body size, fluid loss should be closely monitored and replaced as needed. Ferrets with insulinoma should receive fluids containing 2.5% to 5% dextrose to prevent hypoglycemia.

Because of their large surface area to volume ratio, ferrets can lose body heat very quickly under anesthesia and are subject to hypothermia. Close monitoring of the body temperature and maintenance of body heat throughout the anesthetic procedure is important to keep the patient stable and to decrease recovery time. Minimizing the duration of anesthesia will also minimize the loss of body heat. There are several different devices that may be used to maintain a ferret's body temperature during an anesthetic event, including a convective warm air blanket system, warm water circulating heating pad, heat lamp, or hot water bottle. Warm air will be trapped under the drapes and towels of a fully prepped surgical patient. Warm flush and intravenous fluids should also be used, when needed, to maintain body heat.

Close monitoring of the ferret during anesthesia can be accomplished in several ways. Depth of anesthesia may be assessed through the palpebral reflex or toe pinch. The cardiac rate and rhythm should always be monitored; monitoring is easily accomplished through the use of an ultrasonic Doppler, direct auscultation, or ECG. Pulse oximetry is also a good tool for monitoring the heart rate, as well as blood oxygen saturation.[14] This may be applied to the tail or any of the paws. It may be necessary, however, to shave the area of contact to ensure an accurate measurement.

Recovery from anesthesia is normally quite smooth. Again, even after anesthesia is discontinued, it is important to maintain body heat to reduce recovery time. Close monitoring and IV access should continue until the ferret completely recovers. Since analgesia provided by the anesthetic gas subsides once the vaporizer is turned off, supplemental pain management should be provided before recovery in the form of butorphanol or buprenorphine to provide postsurgical comfort for the patient. Flunixin meglumine can also be used pre- and postoperatively to reduce pain and inflammation associated with surgery.

Surgery

Surgery in the ferret follows the same guidelines and principles as that for the dog and cat. Many of the surgical procedures are carried out in the same manner, with slight alterations in technique to accommodate anatomic differences. In the United States, ferrets are typically descented and spayed or neutered at an early age at the facility where they are born; therefore, these procedures are not routinely performed in private practice. Intact ferrets should be spayed or neutered before 6 to 8 months of age if they are not intended for breeding. In female ferrets this practice reduces the risk of hyperestrogenemia, and in males it reduces aggression as well as the musky odor produced by the sebaceous glands. The technique for both of these procedures follows that for the cat.

Anal sacculectomy (descenting) can be done at the time of neutering. It is important to note that this procedure does not eliminate the musky odor produced by the sebaceous glands. The anal sacs are 10 to 20 mm in length and are located on either side of the anus at the 4 and 8 o'clock positions. The duct openings should be identified at the mucocutaneous junction, and a circumferential incision 2 to 3 mm from the opening should be made. The duct and sacs are removed utilizing sharp and blunt dissection, carefully avoiding rupture during the process. Should the sac rupture during the procedure, the site should be flushed with saline, and a close inspection for complete removal of any remaining material should be made. A draining tract can form at the site if the anal sac is not removed intact. The incisions can be left open or can be closed with a single 5-0 absorbable intradermal suture.

In middle-aged to older ferrets, surgery for the treatment of insulinoma or adrenal gland disease becomes much more common. Abdominal surgery in adult ferrets should include complete exploration of the abdominal organs for evidence of disease. Tissue biopsies should be collected from suspect organs. The pancreas should always be palpated, as nodules are often difficult to visually identify. If multiple small nodules are present on a lobe of the pancreas, a partial pancreatectomy is indicated. When larger, single nodules are identified, a nodectomy can be performed. Ferrets tolerate these procedures well and do not succumb to episodes of pancreatitis secondary to manipulation and trauma of pancreatic tissue.

The adrenal glands should always be palpated thoroughly at surgery. Both are located craniomedially to the kidneys; however, the right adrenal gland is also situated close to the caudal vena cava and below the caudal tip of the caudate lobe of the liver. Abnormal adrenal glands may be enlarged, irregular, firm, or discolored yellow or brown. The right gland is typically more difficult to remove due to its close proximity to the caudal vena cava. Removal of the adrenal glands can be done by bluntly dissecting the entire gland from the surrounding fat and ligating the adrenolumbar vessel, which is located on the ventral surface of the gland. Gel sponges can be placed to provide hemostasis for hemorrhage from the surrounding fat. When removing the right gland, care should be taken to avoid tearing the vena cava. Hemoclips can be applied to the longitudinal border of the vein as it borders the adrenal gland, allowing for safe trimming of the adrenal gland away from the vessel. Alternatively, the adrenal capsule can be incised and the gland removed from within.

Any tissues removed during abdominal surgery should be submitted for histopathologic examination. Again, complete examination of the entire abdomen for evidence of disease should be performed during any abdominal surgery. The abdomen can be closed using 4-0 absorbable suture for the linea and 5-0 absorbable suture for an intradermal layer. Skin sutures are not necessary. Ferrets usually do not chew at the incision, so further protection of the incision is not a concern. Follow-up evaluation of both the patient and the postoperative healing process should be scheduled 7 to 10 days following the procedure.

Bone marrow aspirates are indicated in ferrets with anemia, thrombocytopenia, or hematopoietic neoplasia. The procedure is similar to that used with cats. The iliac crest, proximal femur, and humerus are all bone marrow collection sites. After aseptic preparation of the proximal femur, a small stab incision can be made over the greater trochanter to facilitate placement of a 20-gauge, 1.5-inch spinal needle into the marrow cavity. While stabilizing the femur in one hand, the veterinary surgeon should direct the needle into the cavity just medial to the greater trochanter. Once the needle has been seated, a 6-ml syringe can be attached and used for aspiration. Negative pressure should be limited to prevent blood contamination of the sample.

■ ZOONOSES

There are certain diseases of ferrets that deserve recognition for their zoonotic potential. Some of these diseases were described previously in the chapter (e.g., influenza, rabies, *Sarcoptes scabei*, dermatophytosis, *Giardia*). Influenza is the only disease with documented ferret-to-human transmission.[69] However, influenza is more commonly transmitted from people to ferrets. There have been no documented cases of human-

acquired rabies from a ferret, but care must be taken when a suspect ferret rabies case is hospitalized. Client education of the zoonotic potential of infections such as scabies and ringworm is important, as these diseases are often treated at home. Handling should be restricted to those individuals providing treatment. Children and immunocompromised individuals should not handle the ferret during the course of treatment for scabies or ringworm. *Cryptosporidium parvum* is also a zoonotic concern, particularly for the immunocompromised pet owner, given its tendency to infect a variety of species. Ferrets are susceptible to several bacterial diseases (e.g., salmonellosis, listeriosis, tuberculosis, leptospirosis, campylobacteriosis), which may have zoonotic potential as well.[69] When treating an ill ferret, proper hygiene and disinfection should be a routine practice in the veterinary clinic so as to prevent disease transmission among animals and caretakers. Early recognition of disease and client communication are important steps in reducing the risk of transmission and ensuring prompt treatment to those already exposed.

REFERENCES

1. Fox JG: Taxonomy, history, and use. In Fox JG, editor: *Biology and Diseases of the Ferret,* ed 2, Philadelphia, 1998, Lippincott Williams and Wilkins.
2. Evans HE, An NQ: Anatomy of the ferret. In Fox JG, editor: *Biology and Diseases of the Ferret,* ed 2, Philadelphia, 1998, Lippincott Williams and Wilkins.
3. Brown SA: Ferrets: Basic anatomy, physiology, and husbandry. In Hillyer EV, Quesenberry KE, editors: *Ferrets, Rabbits and Rodents: Clinical Medicine and Surgery,* Philadelphia, 1997, WB Saunders.
4. Ball RS: Husbandry and management of the domestic ferret, *Lab Anim* 31(5):37-42, 2002.
5. Whary MT, Andrews PLR: Physiology of the ferret. In Fox JG, editor: *Biology and Diseases of the Ferret,* ed 2, Philadelphia, 1998, Lippincott Williams and Wilkins.
6. Greenacre CB: Incidence of adverse events in ferrets vaccinated with distemper or rabies vaccine:143 cases (1995-2001), *JAVMA* 223(5):663-665, 2003.
7. Wimsatt J, Jay MT, Innes KE et al: Serologic evaluation, efficacy, and safety of a commercial modified-live canine distemper vaccine in domestic ferrets, *Am J Vet Res* 62(5):736-740, 2001.
8. Quesenberry KE: Ferrets: Basic approach to veterinary care. In Hillyer EV, Quesenberry KE, editors: *Ferrets, Rabbits and Rodents: Clinical Medicine and Surgery,* Philadelphia, 1997, WB Saunders.
9. Niezgoda M, Briggs DJ, Shaddock J et al: Pathogenesis of experimentally induced rabies in domestic ferrets, *Am J Vet Res* 58(11):1327-1331, 1997.
10. Welter J, Taylor J, Tartaglia J et al: Vaccination against canine distemper virus infection in infant ferrets with and without maternal antibody protection, using recombinant attenuated poxvirus vaccines, *J Virol* 74(14):6358-6367, 2000.
11. Munday JS, Stedman NL, Richey LJ: Histology and immunohistochemistry of seven ferret vaccination-site fibrosarcomas, *Vet Pathol* 40:288-293, 2003.
12. Meyer EK: Vaccine-associated adverse events, *Vet Clin North Am: Small Anim Pract* 31(3):493-514, 2001.
13. Boothe HW: Antiseptics and disinfectants, *Vet Clin North Am: Small Anim Pract* 28(2):233-248, 1998.
14. Marini RP, Fox JG: Anesthesia, surgery, and biomethodology. In Fox JG, editor: *Biology and Diseases of the Ferret,* ed 2, Philadelphia, 1998, Lippincott Williams and Wilkins.
15. Mason DE: Anesthesia, analgesia, and sedation for small mammals. In Hillyer EV, Quesenberry KE, editors: *Ferrets, Rabbits and Rodents: Clinical Medicine and Surgery,* Philadelphia, 1997, WB Saunders.
16. Li X, Fox JG, Padrid PA: Neoplastic diseases in ferrets: 574 cases (1968-1997), *JAVMA* 212(9):1420-1406, 1998.

17. Moody KD, Bowman TA, Lang CM: Laboratory management of the ferret for biomedical research, *Lab Anim Sci* 35(3):272-279, 1985.

18. Fox JG: Normal clinical and biologic parameters. In Fox JG, editor: *Biology and Diseases of the Ferret,* ed 2, Philadelphia, 1998, Lippincott Williams and Wilkins.

19. Thornton PC, Wright PA, Sacra PJ et al: The ferret, *Mustela putorius furo,* as a new species in toxicology, *Lab Anim* 13:119-124, 1979.

20. Lee EJ, Moore WE, Fryer HC et al: Hematological and serum chemistry profiles of ferrets *(Mustela putorius furo), Lab Anim* 16:133-136, 1982.

21. Orcutt CJ: Ferret urogenital diseases, *Vet Clin North Am : Exot Anim Pract* 6(1):113-138, 2003.

22. Hillyer EV: Ferrets: urogenital diseases. In Hillyer EV, Quesenberry KE, editors: *Ferrets, Rabbits and Rodents: Clinical Medicine and Surgery,* Philadelphia, 1997, WB Saunders.

23. Williams J: Veterinary Clinical Sciences Department, Louisiana State University School of Veterinary Medicine, (personal communication), July 22, 2004.

24. Rosenthal KL: Respiratory diseases. In Hillyer EV, Quesenberry KE, editors: *Ferrets, Rabbits and Rodents: Clinical Medicine and Surgery,* Philadelphia, 1997, WB Saunders.

25. Stamoulis ME, Miller MS, Hillyer EV: Cardiovascular diseases. In Hillyer EV, Quesenberry KE, editors: *Ferrets, Rabbits and Rodents: Clinical Medicine and Surgery,* Philadelphia, 1997, WB Saunders.

26. Fox JG, Marini RP: *Helicobacter mustelae* infection in ferrets: pathogenesis, epizootiology, diagnosis, and treatment, *Semin Av Exot Pet Med* 10(1):36-44, 2001.

27. Johnson-Delaney CA: The ferret gastrointestinal tract and *Helicobacter mustelae* infection, *Vet Clin Exot Anim Pract* 8:197-212, 2005.

28. Paul-Murphy J: Ferret gastrointestinal disease overview, *Proc North Am Vet Conf* 15:895-896, 2001.

29. Bell JA: Ferrets: *Helicobacter mustelae* gastritis, proliferative bowel disease, and eosinophilic gastroenteritis. In Hillyer EV, Quesenberry KE, editors: *Ferrets, Rabbits and Rodents: Clinical Medicine and Surgery,* Philadelphia, 1997, WB Saunders.

30. Carpenter JW, Mashima TY, Rupiper DJ: *Exotic Animal Formulary,* ed 2, Philadelphia, 2001, WB Saunders.

31. Rosenthal KL: Management of ferret GIT disorders, *Proc North Am Vet Conf* 13:847-848, 1999.

32. Li X, Jingzhong P, Fox JG: Coinfection with intracellular *Desulfovibrio* species and coccidia in ferrets with proliferative bowel disease, *Lab Anim Sci* 46(5):569-571, 1996.

33. Rosenthal KL: Ferrets, *Vet Clin North Am: Small Anim Pract* 24(1):1-23, 1994.

34. Fox JG, Pearson RC, Gorham JR: Viral diseases. In Fox JG, editor: *Biology and Diseases of the Ferret,* ed 2, Philadelphia, 1998, Lippincott Williams and Wilkins.

35. Welchman D de B, Oxenham M, Done SH: Aleutian disease in domestic ferrets: diagnostic findings and survey results, *Vet Rec* 132:479-484, 1993.

36. Une Y, Wakimoto Y, Nakano Y et al: Spontaneous Aleutian disease in a ferret, *J Vet Med Sci* 62(5):553-555, 2000.

37. Wolfensohn SE, Lloyd MH: Aleutian disease in laboratory ferrets, *Vet Rec* 134(4):100, 1994.

38. Stewart JD, Rozengurt N: Aleutian disease in the ferret, *Vet Rec* 133(7):172, 1993.

39. Antinoff N: Ferrets: musculoskeletal and neurologic diseases. In Hillyer EV, Quesenberry KE, editors: *Ferrets, Rabbits and Rodents: Clinical Medicine and Surgery,* Philadelphia, 1997, WB Saunders.

40. Orcutt C: Ferrets: Dermatologic diseases. In Hillyer EV, Quesenberry KE, editors: *Ferrets, Rabbits and Rodents: Clinical Medicine and Surgery,* Philadelphia, 1997, WB Saunders.

41. Fox JG: Parasitic diseases. In Fox JG, editor: *Biology and Diseases of the Ferret,* ed 2, Philadelphia, 1998, Lippincott Williams and Wilkins.

42. Sasai H, Kato K, Sasaki T et al: Echocardiographic diagnosis of dirofilariasis in a ferret, *J Small Anim Pract* 41(4):172-174, 2000.

43. Smith P: Louisiana Veterinary Medical Diagnostic Laboratory, Louisiana State University School of Veterinary Medicine, (personal communication), Sept 8, 2004.

44. Erdman SE, Brown SA, Kawasaki TA et al: Clinical and pathologic findings in ferrets with lymphoma: 60 cases (1982-1994), *JAVMA* 208(8):1285-1289, 1996.

45. Batchelder MA, Erdman SE, Li X et al: A cluster of cases of juvenile mediastinal lymphoma in a ferret colony, *Lab Anim Sci* 46(3):271-274, 1996.

46. Erdman SE, Moore FM, Rose R et al: Malignant lymphoma in ferrets: clinical and pathologic findings in 19 cases, *J Comp Pathol* 106:37-47, 1992.

47. Brown SA: Ferrets: neoplasia. In Hillyer EV, Quesenberry KE, editors: *Ferrets, Rabbits and Rodents: Clinical Medicine and Surgery,* Philadelphia, 1997, WB Saunders.

48. Parker GA, Picut CA: Histopathologic features and post-surgical sequelae of 57 cutaneous neoplasms in ferrets *(Mustela putorius furo L), Vet Pathol* 30:499-503, 1993.

49. Weiss CA, Scott MV: Clinical aspects and surgical treatment of hyperadrenocorticism in the domestic ferret: 94 cases (1994-1996), *JAAHA* 33(6):487-493, 1997.

50. Rosenthal KL, Quesenberry KE: Ferrets: endocrine diseases. In Hillyer EV, Quesenberry KE, editors: *Ferrets, Rabbits and Rodents: Clinical Medicine and Surgery,* Philadelphia, 1997, WB Saunders.

51. Rosenthal KL, Peterson ME: Evaluation of plasma androgen and estrogen concentrations in ferrets with hyperadrenocorticism, *JAVMA* 209:1097-1106, 1996.

52. Shoemaker NJ, Schuurmans M, Moorman H et al: Correlation between age at neutering and age at onset of hyperadrenocorticism in ferrets, *JAVMA* 216(2):195-197, 2000.

53. Wagner RA, Bailey EM, Schneider JF et al: Leuprolide acetate treatment of adrenocortical disease in ferrets, *JAVMA* 218(8):1272-1274, 2001.

54. Coleman GD, Chavez MA, Williams BH: Cystic prostatic disease associated with adrenocortical lesions in the ferret *(Mustela putorius furo), Vet Pathol* 35(6):547-549, 1998.

55. Besso JG, Tidwell AS, Gliatto JM: Retrospective review of the ultrasonographic features of adrenal lesions in 21 ferrets, *Vet Radiol Ultrasound* 41(4):345-352, 2000.

56. Barthez PY, Nyland TG, Feldman EC: Ultrasonography of the adrenal glands in the dog, cat, and ferret, *Vet Clin North Am: Small Anim Pract* 28(4):869-885, 1998.

57. Neuwirth L, Collins B, Calderwood-Mays M et al: Adrenal ultrasonography correlated with histopathology in ferrets, *Vet Radiol Ultrasound* 38(1):69-74, 1997.

58. Weiss CA, Williams BH, Scott JB et al: Surgical treatment and long-term outcome of ferrets with bilateral adrenal tumors or adrenal hyperplasia: 56 cases (1994-1997), *JAVMA* 215(6):820-823, 1999.

59. Johnson-Delaney C: Ferret adrenal disease: alternatives to surgery, *ICE Proc* 1(pt 4):19-23, 1999.

60. William BH: Therapeutics in ferrets, *Vet Clin North Am Exot Anim Pract* 3(1):131-153, 2000.

61. Weiss CA, Williams BH, Scott MV: Insulinoma in the ferret: clinical findings and treatment comparison of 66 cases, *JAAHA* 34(6):471-475, 1998.

62. Caplan ER, Peterson ME, Mullen HS et al: Diagnosis and treatment of insulin-secreting pancreatic islet cell tumors in ferrets: 57 cases (1986-1994), *JAVMA* 209(10):1741-1745, 1996.

63. Ehrhart N, Withrow SJ, Ehrhart EJ et al: Pancreatic beta cell tumor in ferrets: 20 cases (1986-1994), *JAVMA* 209(10):1737-1740, 1996.

64. Hoefer HL: Ferret insulinoma, *Proc North Am Vet Conf* 14:1007-1008, 2000.

65. Hoefer HL: Gastrointestinal diseases. In Hillyer EV, Quesenberry KE, editors: *Ferrets, Rabbits and Rodents: Clinical Medicine and Surgery,* Philadelphia, 1997, WB Saunders.

66. Fox JG: Other systemic diseases. In Fox JG, editor: *Biology and Diseases of the Ferret,* ed 2, Philadelphia, 1998, Lippincott Williams and Wilkins.

67. Orcutt CJ: Emergency and critical care of ferrets, *Vet Clin North Am Exot Anim Pract* 1(1):99-125, 1998.

68. Manning DD, Bell JA: Lack of detectable blood groups in domestic ferrets: implications for transfusion, *JAVMA* 197(1):84-86, 1990.

69. Marini RP, Adkins JA, Fox JG: Proven or potential zoonotic diseases of ferrets, *JAVMA* 195(7):990-994, 1989.

Kristine M. Vennen
Mark A. Mitchell

CHAPTER 14

RABBITS

Domestic rabbits, *Oryctolagus cuniculus,* belong to the order Lagomorpha, and their ancestors are from Western Europe and northwestern Africa.[1,2] Unlike rodents, lagomorphs have a second set of maxillary incisors directly caudal to the first set. Pet rabbits have unique, lively, and affectionate personalities that make them ideal pets for mature children and adults. Handling pet rabbits when they are young will likely make them more comfortable with humans later in life. In contrast, wild rabbits, no matter their age, do not become comfortable with human interaction. Rabbit owners commonly seek medical attention for their rabbits and husbandry guidance from veterinarians.

■ COMMON BREEDS KEPT IN CAPTIVITY

There are as many as 50 different breeds of domestic rabbits.[3] However, many of the rabbits presented to private practice are mix breeds. Breed classification can be divided by size or fur type. The size classification is more helpful to the practicing veterinarian and can be divided into small breeds, less than 2 kg (e.g., Netherland dwarfs, lion head, mini-lop, and Dutch breeds); medium breeds, 2 to 5 kg (e.g., Rex, English, Angora, and Belgium hares), and large to giant breeds, more than 5 kg (e.g., New Zealand whites, English lops, British Giants, and Flemish Giants). The American Rabbit Breeders Association publishes information on the different breeds and various standards, and is an excellent resource for veterinarians (http://www.arba.net/).

Certain breeds are predisposed to health problems. For example, dwarf breeds, such as the Netherland rabbits, have short maxillae that make them more prone to nasolacrimal duct blockage and incisor malocclusion. In addition, dwarf breeds appear more susceptible to *Encephalocytozoon cuniculi* infections.[2] Dutch, Havana, tan, and French silver breeds are more likely to develop uterine neoplasia.[4] Because Rex rabbits have thin fur on the plantar surface of their feet, they are more susceptible to developing hock sores. Large and giant breeds are prone to developing arthritis and cardiomyopathies. British Giant and French lops are more likely to develop skin fold pyoderma under their dewlaps and in the perineum area, in addition to developing entropion.[2]

■ BIOLOGY AND PHYSIOLOGY

See Box 14-1.

Integumentary System

Rabbits have very thin and delicate skin that is covered with fine fur comprised of both a soft undercoat and stiff guard hairs. Care must be taken when clipping fur because the skin is prone to tearing. Unlike dogs and cats, rabbits lack footpads; instead, their feet are covered with thick coarse fur that protects the plantar and palmar surfaces of the feet. Because they lack footpads, rabbits should be provided soft padded areas within their enclosures. Rabbits have nonretractable claws, making declawing an inappropriate procedure. Certain breeds of female rabbits have a dewlap, which is analogous to a second chin. Female rabbits may pluck fur from the dewlap during the breeding season to build a nest. Male and female rabbits may have three types of scent glands, including a single chin gland, paired inguinal glands, and paired anal glands. The glands are used to mark the rabbit's territory.

BOX 14-1	Physiologic Parameters for Captive Rabbits

Life span	6-13 yr
Gestation	30-32 days
Ages of weaning	4-6 wk
Age of puberty	Small breeds 4-5 mo
	Large breeds 5-8 mo
Age of recommended neutering	Castration >3 mo, spay >5 mo
Temperature (rectal)	37.8°-39.4° F (100°-103° F)
Heart rate	130-325 beats/min
Respiratory rate	32-60

Sense Organs

Rabbits' ears represent a large amount of the animals' surface area. Because rabbits are low in the food web, these large ears serve an important function in assisting the animal with identifying potential predators. In addition, rabbits' ears are highly vascularized and serve an important role in thermoregulation via vasoconstriction and vasodilatation.[5] Rabbit ears are very sensitive and delicate and should never be used for restraint.

Rabbits have a wide field of vision, which is ideal for a prey species. With the lateral positioning of their eyes and their large corneas, rabbits have an overlapping field of vision of 190 degrees.[3] Although rabbits are visually acute within this region, they cannot visualize items below the horizon, including the area below their nose. Instead, rabbits use their highly sensitive vibrissae and lips as tactile structures to distinguish food items. Rabbits possess good night vision and some color vision. Rabbits have functional third eyelids that partially close with sleep or while under anesthesia.[5] A harderian gland is found at the base of the third eyelid. If this gland prolapses, then it may present as a mass under the third eyelid. Surgical intervention is recommended to replace the gland. Tear drainage from the eyes occurs via the nasolacrimal gland. There is a single lacrimal punctum located in the craniomedial aspect of the lower eyelid. The punctum empties into a cuniculus, leading to a lacrimal sac and continuing to the base of the maxillary incisor. At this point, the duct sharply changes direction, runs along the incisor root, and emerges in the nasal cavity in the ventromedial aspect of the alar fold.[2] Blockage of this duct is common in captive rabbits. Affected animals may have unilateral or bilateral epiphora. Rabbits have a large retrobulbar orbital venous plexus. When an enucleation is performed, this venous plexus must be ligated to minimize hemorrhage.

Musculoskeletal System

Rabbits have a light skeleton surrounded by a very well-developed muscular system, which makes the vertebrae and long bones susceptible to fractures. To minimize the likelihood of injury, the hindlegs should always be supported when transporting the rabbit. The number of vertebrae varies between breeds, from 12 to 13 thoracic and 6 to 7 lumbar vertebrae.[6] The epaxial and large muscles of the hindlimbs can be used for intramuscular injections.

Reproductive System

Female rabbits are classified as does, males as bucks, and neonates as kits. The onset of puberty occurs at approximately 4½ months of age; however, reproductive activity is generally dependent upon animal size, not age. In the dwarf breeds, sexual maturity occurs earlier than in larger breeds. The reproductive life of a rabbit is approximately 4 years.[1] Rabbits are induced ovulators. Their receptivity periods last approximately 14 to 16 days, followed by 1 to 2 days of nonreceptivity.[2] When females are ready to ovulate, they become restless, rub their chins, and assume a lordosis-like posture. Gestation lasts 31 to 32 days, and litters average 4 to 10 kits. As gestation or pseudopregnancy reaches the last 3 to 4 days, does initiate nesting behavior and line their nests with hair from the hip and dewlap.[3] During this period, does consume less food, which can cause an increased risk for pregnancy toxemia. Parturition usually occurs in the early morning and lasts less than 30 minutes. Kits generally only suckle 1 or 2 times a day and are not usually seen with the doe, especially in the wild. Weaning occurs at approximately 4-6 weeks of age.

Does have two separate uterine horns and two cervices. Rabbits do not have a uterine body. The cervices open into the vagina, along with the urethra, to form one common urogenital opening. Bucks have a hairless scrotum. The inguinal rings of the buck are open, which allows the testicles to ascend and descend into and out of the abdomen. Male rabbits do not have an os penis or nipples.

Urinary System

The kidneys of rabbits are located in the retroperitoneal cavity, and their position in the body cavity is similar to that in cats. The kidneys are generally covered in fat and can be palpated on the physical examination. The urinary bladder is located in the ventral body cavity, and it is ventral to the colon. Rabbits, like rodents, have a unique system for calcium metabolism. Serum calcium is reflective of dietary calcium, and the urinary system is the primary site of calcium and magnesium excretion. Rabbits that consume a high calcium diet will often have thick and creamy urine due to the formation of calcium carbonate precipitate. On average, rabbits produce 30 to 35 ml of urine daily. Rabbit urine may be straw-colored, yellow, or red. It is not uncommon for rabbit urine to have a turbid appearance. When a rabbit presents with "red" urine, it is important to differentiate whether the urine has blood or porphyrins. Porphyrins can be produced as a result of the ingestion of various vegetables, such as beet root, cabbage, broccoli, and dandelions, or as a result of stress.[2]

Gastrointestinal System

Rabbits have open-rooted teeth that grow continuously throughout their lives at a rate of approximately 10 to 12 cm a year.[1] The dental formula of the rabbit is $2 \times$ (2/1 I, 0/0 C, 3/2 P, 3/3 M). Directly caudal to the maxillary incisors is a second pair of small incisors called peg teeth, whose function is to protect the palate from injury against the sharp surfaces of the lower incisors. The buccal surface of the upper incisors' enamel is thicker and wears more slowly than the rest of the tooth, forming a chisel-like appearance. Caudal to the incisors is a space called the diasterna.[7] The cheek teeth are located caudal to the diasterna and are responsible for macerating and grinding food.

Rabbits have simple, glandular stomachs. Due to the positioning and well-developed nature of the cardiac sphincter, rabbits are unable to vomit.[8] Adult rabbits have a gastric pH of 1.5 to 2.2, whereas suckling rabbits have a higher pH of 5.0 to 6.5. The higher gastric pH in neonates is necessary for bacterial colonization of the intestinal tract. This elevated pH also makes suckling rabbits more susceptible to gastrointestinal disease. Dietary absences, especially during weaning, should be gradual, and foods high in sugars and starch should be avoided. Rabbits have a large cecum that acts as an anaerobic fermentation vat. The cecum has a complex and delicate population of microbes. The most common organisms found in the rabbit cecum are the Gram-positive *Bacillus* spp. In the cecum, fiber is broken down and separated. Rabbits are highly susceptible to antibiotic-induced enterotoxemia, especially when there is *Clostridium spiriforme* contamination in the environment. The rabbit's gastrointestinal tract is designed to eliminate fiber from the gut rapidly, in the form of hard feces, and digest the nonfiber portion of the diet, creating caecotrophs, which are reingested at a later time. Cecotrophs are covered with a thin mucus, which protects the volatile fatty acids, vitamins, and amino acids from the low pH of the stomach. Cecotrophs differ from feces in that they are soft, moist, usually stuck together, and are eaten directly from the anus.[8] The gastrointestinal transit time in rabbits is approximately 20 hours. Rabbits offered a diet deficient in fiber usually have increased gastrointestinal transit times.

The pancreas is found within the mesentery along the lesser curvature of the stomach and extends to the right side of the abdominal cavity to the level of the duodenum. The rabbit pancreas has both exocrine and endocrine functions.

The rabbit liver has a caudate lobe with a narrow stalk, which can displace on occasion. Rabbits have a gall bladder, and the primary function of this structure is to store bile. The rabbit liver performs many of the same functions that the liver plays in the dog and cat.

Respiratory System

Rabbits are obligate nasal breathers. A rabbit that presents for open-mouth breathing generally has a guarded prognosis. The respiratory rate of the rabbit is approximately 30 to 60 breaths per minute. In a healthy animal, the nose will move up and down approximately 20 to 120 times a minute. The thoracic cavity of the rabbit is small in comparison to that of nonlagomorph or rodent mammals. Rabbit lungs have four right and two left lung lobes.[3] Rabbits have an extremely narrow and long oral cavity. Because of these features, it can be difficult to visualize the glottis for intubation. Endoscopic examination provides the best visualization of the glottis for intubation. Inflammation of the upper respiratory tract increases the risk of anesthetic mortality in nonintubated animals.[4]

Cardiovascular System

Rabbits have a relatively small heart, and the average heart rate of the rabbit is 130 to 325 beats per minute.[9] Systolic blood pressure is approximately 90 to 120 mmHg. The right atrioventricular valve has only two cusps, and the aorta rhythmically contracts.[4] Rabbit veins are thin and susceptible to hematomas, so care must be taken with venipuncture.

■ HUSBANDRY
Environmental Considerations
ENCLOSURE SIZE

A rabbit enclosure should be large enough to provide a sleeping space, eating space, and latrine. Animals housed for long periods of time should also have ample room to exercise. The enclosure should be tall enough to allow the rabbit to sit up and not have its ears touch the top of the cage. In general, 3 square feet (sq ft) should be a minimum cage size for rabbits 2 to 4 kg, 4 sq ft for rabbits 4 to 4.5 kg, and larger rabbits require at least 5 sq ft.[5] Rabbits housed in hutches and cages should be allowed a minimum of 4 hours of exercise daily.[2] Indoor rabbits should be caged when they cannot be supervised, to decrease the likelihood of inappropriate chewing of carpet, electrical wire, or furniture. Cages should be cleaned daily to remove feces and urine. Gentle soap and hot water or a dilute bleach solution (1 : 32) should be used for cleaning. If bleach is used, then the cage should be cleaned in a well-ventilated area. Organic material should be removed before applying the bleach, to minimize the degradation of the bleach. The bleach or soap should have a minimum of 3 to 5 minutes of contact time on the cage to increase the killing potential of these products. It is important to clean, rinse, and dry off all detergents.

TEMPERATURE/HUMIDITY

Because rabbits are prone to heatstroke, they should be housed in temperatures ranging from 60° F to 75° F.[2] If rabbits are housed outdoors, they must have access to shade and clean water, and the shelter should protect them from the elements as well as from predators. Rabbits are prone to developing fur and skin problems when housed in environments with high humidity; therefore, these animals should be provided environments with low to moderate humidity (30%-60%).

LIGHTING

Rabbits show a diurnal rhythm for eating, activity, and even hematologic variation. Most feeding takes place from afternoon to evening. During foraging, rabbits commonly produce fecal pellets; in times of decreased intake, rabbits will actually ingest cecotrophs. In addition, hematologic parameters, such as the total white blood cell count, are lowest in the late afternoons and evenings. Although the eosinophils peak in early afternoon, the heterophils are highest in the late afternoon and early evening. Other changes can be seen with diurnal patterns, including changes in blood urea nitrogen, body temperature, and bile acid production.[2] Because much of the rabbits' behavior and physiology is regulated by diurnal patterns, it is important to provide a consistent light cycle. Although there are no specific lighting recommendations for rabbits, nonreproductive rabbits should be provided a 12-hour photoperiod, and breeding females should be provided 14 to 16 hours of light.[10]

SUBSTRATE

The ideal substrate for rabbits is grass hay; however, for indoor, caged rabbits, a foam rubber pad or a towel covered with newspaper and a thick layer of timothy hay can also be used.[2] Avoid wood shavings, which contain oils that can lead to hepatotoxicity.[2] Rabbits can easily be trained to use a litter box filled with straw, hay, or newspaper litter. It is important to keep any substrate clean and dry. If a rabbit is housed on a wire mesh floor, it is important that the mesh openings are no larger than 1×2.5 inches to prevent the feet from getting trapped and injured. In addition, it is also important to offer a solid, nonslip surface to provide rest off the mesh and prevent pododermatitis.[4]

ACCESSORIES

Most cat and bird toys can be used for rabbits. Because rabbits can chew these toys, it is important to be sure that they do not contain any toxins or small materials that can be ingested. Sticks or blocks of wood provide an excellent material for rabbits to file their teeth.

HOSPITALIZATION

In the veterinary hospital, rabbits should be housed in a cage with a nonslip surface on the bottom, such as a towel or thick bedding of fresh straw or hay. Rabbits should be hospitalized in a quiet, stress-free area within the practice, and protected from noises associated with dogs, cats, and ferrets. While in the hospital, rabbits should be offered fresh food and water, preferably what is being fed to them in their home environment. It is important to disinfect and dry the cage and accessories in contact with sick rabbits, using a dilute bleach, Roccal (Pfizer Animal Health, Kalamazoo, MI), or other hospital cleaner.

Nutrition

An average adult house rabbit should be offered ad lib grass hay, such as timothy, prairie, or oat brome; approximately 1 cup of leafy green vegetables; and, at most, $\frac{1}{4}$ cup of high-fiber (18%-22% to prevent obesity), low-protein (<18%) pellets per 2.2 kg (5 lbs) of body weight daily.[4,8] Examples of dark leafy greens include romaine lettuce, dandelion greens, Swiss chard, parsley, endive, kale, mustard greens, and carrot, beet, and turnip tops. Diets low in fiber, such as commercial, pelleted rations, may be associated with hypomotility, changes in the

gastrointestinal pH and microflora, wool block from increased hair consumption, and cheek tooth overgrowth.[7] Alfalfa hay should be avoided in adult animals, because of its high protein and calcium content, and instead, reserved for animals less than 6 months of age and for pregnant and lactating does with increased nutritional demands. When offering alfalfa hay to lactating does, slowly increase the amount over the first 5 days, as this will reduce the likelihood of milk overproduction and decrease the chance for the development of mastitis.[4] Any diet change should be gradual.

Rabbits ingest cecotrophs formed from fermentation of nonfiber ingesta; these cecotrophs contain volatile fatty acids, vitamins, amino acids, and microorganisms. Cecotrophs are ingested straight from the anus; consuming them allows for absorption of these nutrients that would be lost otherwise. They are covered with a mucus that protects them from breakdown from stomach acids.

Chlorinated water should always be in fresh and ample supply. Rabbits are very sensitive to water deprivation and therefore should experience no restriction. Rabbits generally drink 50 to 100 ml/kg/day.[2] Water should be offered in a nonleaking sipper bottle or in a heavy crock that cannot be tipped over. Rabbits that drink from crocks may develop "blue fur," which is a moist dermatitis of the dewlap that is associated with *Pseudomonas* infections.

■ PREVENTIVE MEDICINE

There are no U.S.-approved vaccines for domestic rabbits. It is recommended that all house rabbits receive an annual physical examination, and as they become geriatric (>4 years), a biannual examination is recommended. In addition to the annual examination, a serum chemistry panel, complete blood counts (CBCs), and fecal exams for parasites are also recommended annually. Ovariohysterectomy or orchiectomy should also be recommended for all nonbreeding rabbits to decrease aggression, decrease the incidence of scent marking with urine and feces, and avoid unwanted pregnancy, pseudopregnancy, and neoplasia.

When adding new rabbits into an existing population, it is always recommended to quarantine the new additions for a minimum of 90 days. Separating new arrivals can decrease the likelihood of introducing infectious diseases and parasites to a standing population of rabbits. Before the rabbits are released from quarantine, they should have a CBC and chemistry profile done, and have 3 to 5 negative (2 weeks apart) fecal examinations consecutively. The client should be made aware that even a 90-day quarantine may be insufficient to detect some infectious diseases.

Rabbits' enclosures should be cleaned on a daily basis. Organic material should be removed before disinfectant is applied. Fresh substrate should be offered either daily or as it is soiled. The cage may be disinfected with mild soap and water or a dilute bleach solution (1 : 32). The disinfectant should have a minimum of 3 to 5 minutes of contact time to increase the effectiveness of the compound. The solutions should be thoroughly rinsed away, and the surface of the cage dried

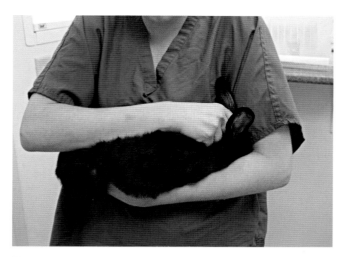

Figure 14-1 Proper restraint while transporting a rabbit. Notice the head is tucked in the crook of the elbow and the dorsum and feet are supported.

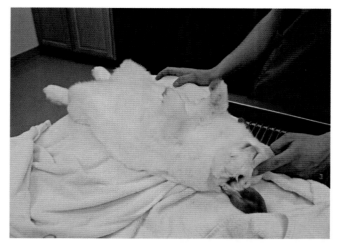

Figure 14-2 Rabbits placed in dorsal recumbency will enter a trance-like state that may facilitate simple procedures, such as taking radiographs.

completely. Roccal D or chlorhexidine (Fort Dodge Inc., Fort Dodge, IA) can also be used to disinfect rabbit enclosures.

RESTRAINT
Manual Restraint

Rabbit physical restraint needs to be carefully performed to avoid injury to the animal. Because rabbits have a well-developed muscular system and thin cortical bone, they are subject to vertebral and long bone fractures if restrained incorrectly. Because most skeletal injuries associated with incorrect restraint occur in the lumbar vertebrae, it is important to firmly restrain the hindlegs. Rabbits should be handled in a manner similar to cats; place one hand on under the forelimbs, and use the other hand to hold the rear legs against the body. Always place the rabbit onto a nonslip surface to ensure that it has good footing. To restrain the animal, lightly scruff the animal and support its dorsum with the same arm. The opposite arm is used to support the body and rear legs (Figure 14-1). It can be helpful to tuck the head of the rabbit into the crook of one's elbow to decrease the rabbit's vision, which can decrease the stress on the animal. Placing a rabbit in dorsal recumbency evokes an immobility response, which can be helpful during simple procedures. However, this response is performed by prey species under stressful or threatening conditions and may not be welcomed by all rabbits (Figure 14-2). The immobility response is characterized by a lack of spontaneous movement and a failure to respond to external stimuli. This restraint technique should only be used in those cases where chemical sedation is not desired.[2] A towel or blanket is usually necessary during the physical examination to cover the stainless steel exam table and to minimize slipping or kicking, which can lead to injury. In addition, a towel may be used to wrap the rabbit into a "bunny burrito" (Figure 14-3). The bunny burrito can be used to hold a rabbit for transport or to facilitate the examination of the head. Cat bags can also be

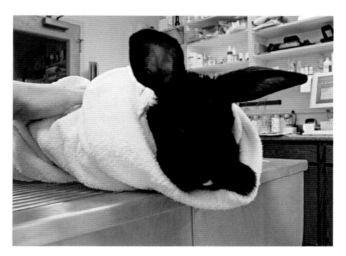

Figure 14-3 Rabbits can be wrapped firmly in a towel making a "bunny burrito." This technique can be used to facilitate an examination, nail trim, or other noninvasive procedure.

used to restrain rabbits. In addition to using these techniques for examination, they can also be used to administer medication, collect blood samples, or perform nail trims.

Chemical Restraint

Chemical restraint in rabbits should be used to decrease anxiety, and to provide sedation or immobilization for surgery. (The most common drugs used for premedication, sedation, and anesthesia are described later, in Anesthesia.) Isoflurane (Abbott Laboratories, Chicago, IL) or sevoflurane (Abbott Laboratories, Chicago, IL) can be used to anesthetize rabbits; however, in high stress animals, a premedication is usually recommended.

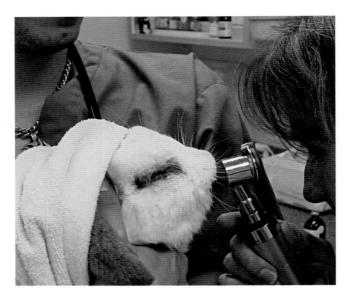

Figure 14-4 An oral examination can be performed using an otoscope.

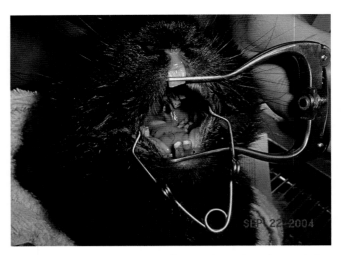

Figure 14-5 An oral examination performed under sedation enables the veterinarian to perform a more thorough exam.

PERFORMING A PHYSICAL EXAMINATION

Before beginning the "hands-on" examination, observe the rabbit at rest, paying close attention to the animal's mentation, how the rabbit is holding its body, if it has signs of respiratory distress, its nose movements, its gait, and fecal and urine output. Very relaxed and very ill rabbits' noses will be still. Note body condition for obesity, as well as signs of weight loss. When placing a rabbit on an exam table, be sure to offer it a nonslip surface such as a rubber mat or a towel. Routine physical exams should follow a thorough and consistent pattern, examining by system or from the head to the toes, being sure to examine everything in a similar manner to avoid overlooking a potential problem.

A thorough oral examination is an important component to any rabbit examination. Rabbits commonly present to the veterinarian with malocclusions of both incisors and cheek teeth. To examine the incisors, gently lift the lips for inspection. Be sure buccal surfaces are smooth (no horizontal ridges are present) and proper occlusion is met with mandibular incisors slightly caudal to the maxillary ones. A common noninvasive technique for examining the cheek teeth, which can be performed during every examination, is inserting an otoscope or vaginal speculum gently into the diasterna. Position the instrument caudally to visualize molars and premolars from both buccal and lingual surfaces (Figure 14-4). This technique does not provide the most thorough examination; however, it is relatively stress-free to the rabbit. If the rabbit is too stressed or uncooperative or a more thorough examination is necessary, lightly sedate the animal with an injectable sedative, or use isoflurane to get a better view. Once sedated, use a mouth speculum, mouth gag, or an endoscope to examine the molars (Figure 14-5). The most common locations for molar lesions are on the lingual surface of the mandibular cheek teeth and the buccal aspect of the maxillary teeth. The gingiva surrounding the molars should be at the level of the crowns except for the first mandibular cheek teeth in which the cranial aspect of the crowns will be more exposed. In addition to examining the teeth for overgrowth and malocclusion, it is important to inspect the oral mucosa and tongue for ulcerations and lacerations that may occur as a result of sharp points on teeth. The cheeks and jaws should be palpated for any swellings (e.g., abscesses) and the chin and dewlap examined for signs of drooling or slobbering. Abnormalities may be indicative of dental disease.

Rabbits should be given a thorough ophthalmic examination. Eyes should be closely examined for evidence of discharge, as ocular discharge is one of the most common ocular problems seen in veterinary practice. Purulent epiphora can be due to a variety of problems, including bacterial infection, corneal ulceration, a blocked nasolacrimal duct, or dental disease. The corneas should be clear and free from ulceration. A fluorescein stain should be done if ulceration is suspected. The anterior chamber should be examined closely. Hypopyon is a common finding in bacterial septicemia. The lens should be examined for clarity. Cataracts can occur as a result of congenital or traumatic causes. A fundic examination should be done to rule out retinal defects. *Encephalitozoon cuniculi* can cause retinal disease.

In addition to ocular discharge, it is important to evaluate the rabbit patient for nasal discharge. Rabbits are meticulous groomers and routinely use their front legs to clean their faces. Animals with nasal discharge routinely have secretions on their forelimbs. In rabbits, nasal discharge has been associated with upper respiratory infections, hypersensitivity (e.g., allergies), foreign bodies, and neoplasia.

An otoscope should be used to examine the ears on both sides of the tragus. Closely inspect the ears for evidence of pus, ceruminous discharge, and mites. With manipulation of the pinna and otoscope, it is possible to visualize deeper in the canal; however, it can still be difficult to visualize the tympanic membrane.

The legs should be palpated from a proximal to distal position. Limb fractures are common sequelae to inappropriate handling. Rabbits do not have footpads. Closely examine the plantar surface of feet for pododermatitis. Pododermatitis is a common problem in rabbits housed in metal-grate caging.

A rectal temperature should be taken during the examination. The body temperature of rabbits is generally between 100° F and 103° F (37.8° C to 39.4° C). To minimize the likelihood of measuring a falsely elevated temperature associated with stress, the body temperature should be collected early in the examination.

The integument should be thoroughly evaluated. Closely inspect the rabbit for alopecia or dandruff, especially near the shoulder blades. Palpate the mammary glands for abnormal masses. Mammary adenocarcinoma and mastitis are common findings in intact female rabbits. Evaluate the perianal area for urine scalding or fecal staining. This is very common in obese rabbits with redundant perianal tissue.

During the abdominal palpation, pay particular attention to the cranial left quadrant (e.g., stomach) and caudal lower quadrant (e.g., uterus, urinary bladder). A firm mass in the cranial abdomen may indicate a trichobezoar or delayed gastric emptying. A swelling or enlargement in the caudal quadrant of an intact doe may suggest pregnancy, pseudopregnancy, pyometra, or uterine adenocarcinoma. Cystic calculi can also occur and be palpated in the caudal abdominal quadrants.

Rabbits are obligate closed-mouth breathers. Open-mouth breathing in rabbits indicates an emergency situation. The heart and lungs should be ausculted. It is normal to hear the rapid movement of the air during inhalation and exhalation. These are usually referred to as sounds from the upper respiratory tract. An absence of these sounds can be associated with consolidation of the lungs. The respiratory rates of rabbits are generally more than 40 breaths per minute. The heart rate should be more than 180 beats per minute. To auscult the heart, place the stethoscope on the chest wall at the point of the elbow.

■ DIAGNOSTIC TESTING

Rabbits are prey species and have evolved to mask their illnesses. It is imperative that veterinarians working with these animals develop a thorough diagnostic plan to ensure success with diagnosing and treating a case. The following is a review of common diagnostic tests performed on rabbits.

Clinical Pathology

Venipuncture should be done with care, as rabbit vessels are delicate and prone to hematoma formation. The maximum volume of blood that should be collected at one time is 1 ml/100 g body weight.[9] Common sites for venipuncture include the jugular, lateral saphenous, cephalic and marginal ear veins. The jugular vein is the preferred site when a large sample is needed. To collect a jugular sample, the animal needs to be properly restrained. For restraint, a rabbit can be placed into a towel or a cat bag, and the neck gently extended

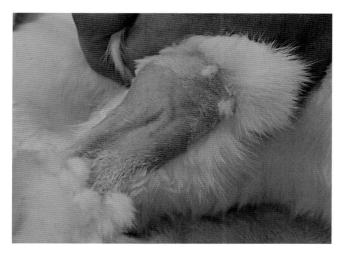

Figure 14-6 Shaving the lateral hindlimb will facilitate visualization of, and access to, the lateral saphenous vein.

in a manner similar to a cat; however, care should be taken not to extend the head too far. In some female rabbits, a large dewlap can reduce access to the jugular vein. Marginal ear veins can be used to collect blood samples with a 25- or 26-gauge needle. Generally, this site can only be used to collect small blood samples. This vein can also be used to place a catheter; however, catheterization can lead to vascular necrosis, thrombosis, and sloughing of the ear and should be avoided in breeds with small ears (e.g., dwarf breeds). The lateral saphenous vein is suitable for small- to moderate-sized blood samples (Figure 14-6). Placing alcohol over the venipuncture site or clipping the fur in that area can facilitate visualization of the vein. The cephalic vein can also be used to collect samples; however, this site is often reserved for intravenous catheter placement.

Hematology/Chemistry Panels

CBCs and serum chemistry panels should be performed in rabbits presenting for any disease process and as part of an annual exam. Rabbits have some unique hematologic differences in their CBC compared to other mammals. Healthy rabbits are primarily lymphocytic. Both small and large lymphocytes can be found in circulation. Rabbit lymphocytes are similar in appearance to this cell type in other vertebrates and are characterized by a deep blue cytoplasm, acentric nucleus, and high nuclear-to-cytoplasmic ratio. The acute inflammatory cell in rabbits is the heterophil. Although the function is similar to the neutrophil of other mammals, the staining characteristic of this cell type is different. Monocytes are the largest circulating white blood cell in rabbits and are characterized by diffuse nuclear chromatin, blue cytoplasm, and large, dark red granules in cytoplasm.[9,11] Eosinophils have large granules and a bilobed or horseshoe-shaped nucleus. Low-grade eosinophilia can be seen with chronic parasitism. Basophils are relatively common in rabbits and can represent up to 30% of the differential in healthy animals. Infections rarely cause elevated white blood cell counts (>15,000 cells/ml) in rabbits; however, several changes may be associated with an acute infection, including a low total number of white blood cells (<5000 cells/ml) with a normal differential or normal cell counts with a shift to heterophilia, thrombocytopenia, and nucleated red blood cells. Other reasons nucleated red blood cells may be found are endothelial changes and regenerative responses.

Rabbits, like rodents, have control over calcium excretion at the level of the kidney. Elevations in serum calcium can be attributed to an increase in dietary intake of the mineral or to renal disease; a reduction in serum calcium may be indicative of hypoalbuminemia, diarrhea, chronic renal failure, or hyperparathyroidism. Phosphorous can also increase with renal disease, but reduced levels can be seen with calcium excretion in the urine.

As with other mammals, creatinine levels can become elevated when reduced blood flow to the kidney occurs accompanied by a 50% to 70% loss of renal function. Blood urea nitrogen may also rise due to renal disease when 50% to 70% of kidney function is lost. There are a number of potential causes of renal failure in rabbits, including neoplasia, glomerular nephritis, and pyelonephritis. Elevations in blood urea nitrogen and creatinine can also occur with postrenal diseases (e.g., urethral calculi) and prerenal diseases (e.g., dehydration).

There are no liver-specific enzymes in rabbits. In many mammals, alanine aminotransferase is liver specific; however, in rabbits, this enzyme is found in both the liver and cardiac muscles. Aspartate aminotransferase is found in a number of tissues, including muscle (cardiac, skeletal, smooth), liver, kidneys, and pancreas. Elevations of both enzymes, however, should be considered suspicious and other testing done to rule out liver disease (e.g., liver biopsy). (See Table 14-1 for rabbit hematologic and serum chemistry reference ranges.)

The electrolytes reference ranges for rabbits are similar to those described for other mammalian vertebrates (see Table 14-1). Elevations in sodium and chloride can occur with dehydration or excess salts in the diet, whereas losses are generally associated with diarrhea or low dietary salt. Potassium levels may be low in animals with diets low in potassium or in animals that are starved. Total protein levels in rabbits can be higher compared to those levels found in other vertebrates.

Urinalysis

A urinalysis can provide a significant amount of information regarding a rabbit's health. Either a free-catch or cystocentesis urine sample can be used, but the cystocentesis sample is preferred. To perform a cystocentesis in a rabbit, a 22- to 25-gauge needle fastened to a 6-ml syringe is needed. The rabbit should be placed in dorsal recumbency. The bladder can be difficult to palpate; however, with care, it can be found cranial to the pelvis. The cystocentesis site should be disinfected with 70% isopropyl alcohol. The rabbit bladder should be stabilized between the index finger and the thumb, and the needle inserted along the ventral midline into the bladder. The consistency of the urine should be noted.

Urinary catheterization can be performed with a well-lubricated 9-French catheter inserted into the urethra.[11] Rabbit urine is generally straw-colored and clear to cloudy. If the urine

TABLE 14-1	Reference Hematologic and Serum Chemistry Values for Rabbits	
Parameter	**Range**	**Comments**
Erythrocytes ($\times 10^6/\mu l$)	4.9-7.8	Anisocytosis, polychromasia, low numbers of NRBCs, and Howell-Jolly bodies can be normal on rabbit blood smears for pet rabbits.
Hematocrit (%)	31-50	
Hemoglobin (g/dl)	10-17.4	
MCV (fl)	57.5-75	
MCH (pg)	17.1-23.9	
MCHC (%)	28.2-37	
Platelets ($\times 10^3/\mu l$)	250-650	
Leukocytes ($\times 10^3/\mu l$)	5.2-12.5	
Heterophils (%)	20-75	In healthy rabbits, heterophil-to-lymphocyte ratio is usually 1:1 or slightly lymphocytic.
Lymphocytes (%)	30-85	
Monocytes (%)	2-10	
Eosinophils (%)	0-5	
Basophils (%)	0-8	
ALP (U/L)	4-16	
ALT (U/L)	14-80	
AST (U/L)	14-113	
Bicarbonate (mEq/L)	16.2-38	
Bilirubin, total (mg/dl)	0-0.75	
BUN (mg/dl)	13-30	
Calcium (mg/dl)	5.6-14	
Chloride (mEq/L)	92-112	
Cholesterol (mg/dl)	10-80	
Creatinine (mg/dl)	0.5-2.5	
Glucose (g/dl)	75-155+	
LDH (U/L)	43-129	
Lipids, total (mg/dl)	243-390	
Phosphorous (mg/dl)	2.3-6.9	
Potassium (mEq/L)	3.6-6.9	
Protein, total (g/dl)	5.4-8.3	
Albumin (g/dl)	2.4-4.6	
Globulin (g/dl)	1.5-2.8	
Sodium (mEq/L)	131-155	
Triglycerides (mg/dl)	124-156	

Combined data from Carpenter JW, Mashima TY, Gentz EJ et al: Caring for rabbits: an overview and formulary, *Vet Med Rabbit Symposium: Rabbits Are Not Small Cats*, pp 348-380, April 1995; Harcourt-Brown F: *Textbook of Rabbit Medicine*, London, 2002, Elsevier; Mader DR: Basic approach to veterinary care. In Queensberry KE, Carpenter JW, editors: *Ferrets, Rabbits and Rodents: Clinical Medicine and Surgery*, St Louis, 2004, WB Saunders; Fudge AM: *Laboratory Medicine: Avian and Exotic Pets*, Philadelphia, 2000, WB Saunders.
ALP, alkaline phosphatase; *ALT*, alanine aminotransferase; *AST*, aspartate aminotransferase; *BUN*, blood urea nitrogen; *LDH*, lactate dehydrogenase; *MCH*, mean corpuscular hemoglobin; *MCHC*, mean corpuscular hemoglobin concentration; *MCV*, mean corpuscular volume; *NRBCs*, nucleated red blood cells.

BOX 14-2   **Reference Ranges for a Rabbit Urinalysis**

Specific gravity	1.003-1.036
pH	8.2
Crystals	Calcium carbonate monohydrate, anhydrous calcium carbonate, ammonium magnesium phosphate
Casts, cells, bacteria	None
WBC	Occasional
RBC	Occasional
Albumin	In young occasionally
Average urine production	130 ml/kg/day

From Mader DR: Basic approach to veterinary care. In Queensberry KE, Carpenter JW, editors: *Ferrets, Rabbits and Rodents: Clinical Medicine and Surgery,* St Louis, 2004, WB Saunders.

has a red appearance, then it is important to rule out blood in the urine from porphyrins. To differentiate hematuria from porphyrin pigmentation, use a urine dipstick or a woods lamp, as porphyrins will fluoresce. If a urinary tract infection is suspected, obtain a cystocentesis and submit a culture and sensitivity in addition to performing a complete urinalysis. Cloudy urine in rabbits is usually due to calcium excretion and the presence of crystals. The presence of crystals in the urine can make it difficult to identify bacteria on a cytologic test, and a culture should be performed if a bacterial cystitis is suspected. (See Box 14-2 for normal urinalysis values.)

Fine needle aspirates can be done to ascertain the histologic response of a mass. Although abscesses are a common finding in dermal and subcutaneous masses, neoplasia, granulomas (e.g., fungal), and hematomas can also occur. Rabbit abscesses are generally inspissated, so it is difficult to obtain much of a sample from a fine needle aspirate. The procedure for fine needle aspiration in a rabbit is similar to the technique described for domestic mammals. Using a local anesthetic can minimize the pain associated with the procedure. Applying topical EMLA cream (AstraZeneca LP, Wilmington, DE) over the fine needle aspirate site 20 to 30 minutes before performing the procedure can minimize the discomfort associated with the procedure.

Bone marrow aspirates should be performed when blood cell production problems are suspected. The proximal femur is the preferred site for sample collection. This procedure should be done with general anesthesia. A standard sterile preparation should be done to minimize the likelihood of introducing opportunistic skin pathogens. A spinal needle with a stylet should be used to perform the procedure. The needle should be inserted in the trochanteric ridge.

Diagnostic Imaging

Radiography is a useful diagnostic test in rabbit medicine. It is important to always take at least two radiographs (e.g., lateral and dorsoventral/ventrodorsal). Many times radiographs of the

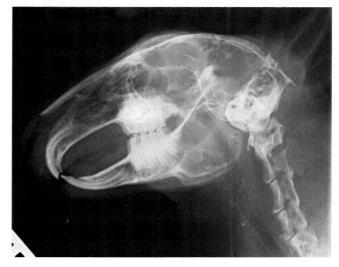

Figure 14-7 Normal lateral skull radiograph of a domestic rabbit.

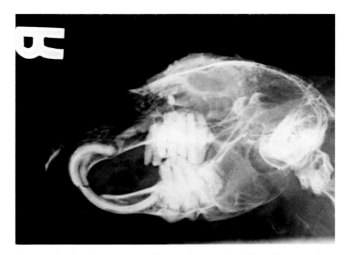

Figure 14-8 Contrast media can be instilled into the nasolacrimal duct to determine if the incisors are impinging on the duct.

abdomen or thorax can be taken with little or no sedation if the handlers are patient and careful. If more restraint is necessary, isoflurane or midazolam can be used to sedate or immobilize the patient. Skull radiographs are required to evaluate the roots of molars and incisors and should be taken in cases of suspected or known malocclusions. The most useful radiographic views for examining the teeth are rostrocaudal, dorsoventral, and lateral (Figure 14-7). In cases of ocular discharge, contrast media can be injected into the lacrimal duct to determine if any of the molar roots are impinging on the duct (Figure 14-8). Chronic cases of otitis or neurologic disease warrant evaluation of the tympanic bullae for radiographic changes. In cases of facial abscess, radiology can be used as a prognostic indicator; periosteal bone reaction decreases the prognosis for full recovery.

Abdominal radiographs can be used to assess the gastrointestinal, reproductive, and excretory systems. Survey radio-

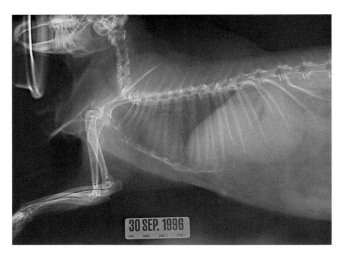

Figure 14-9 Normal thoracic radiograph. Note the small size of the thorax.

graphs can be useful for diagnosing ileus or gastric foreign bodies. Rabbits with severe generalized ileus carry a grave prognosis. Rabbits with trichobezoars are frequently anorectic. Therefore, the presence of a soft tissue mass in the stomach of an anorectic rabbit is highly suggestive of the presence of a gastric foreign body (e.g., trichobezoar). In cases where a gastrointestinal foreign body is suspected but not conclusive from survey radiographs, the veterinarian should consider doing a contrast study. Uterine adenocarcinoma should be considered in a differential list for any intact doe with a suspicious soft tissue mass in the caudoventral abdomen. Renal, urethral, and cystic calculi can generally be diagnosed from survey radiographs, although contrast studies are also needed in some cases.

Thoracic radiography is an important diagnostic test for ruling out respiratory and cardiac disease. The thoracic field of a rabbit is small in comparison with that of other mammalian vertebrates (Figure 14-9). However, radiograph interpretation is similar. Pneumonia, metastatic neoplasia, and trauma are common disease problems that can be diagnosed radiographically.

In addition to radiography, the other commonly used diagnostic imaging techniques can also be useful for assessing the rabbit patient. Ultrasound can provide excellent images of the abdomen and thorax and has been used to diagnose abdominal pathology, uterine disease, foreign bodies, excretory calculi, and cardiac disease. Success with ultrasound is based on the sonographer having a good knowledge of anatomy, so that he or she can interpret an image based on the position of the probe. A 7.5- to 10-mHz transducer is recommended for rabbit ultrasonography. Clipping the fur of the rabbit in the area of interest can also help improve the image by providing the contact between the skin and the probe; however, caution must be used when clipping the fur, as the skin tears easily. Echocardiography is an appropriate diagnostic aid in cases of suspected heart disease or in patients with audible murmurs. Echocardiographs should be conducted using a high-frequency

transducer (7.5-12 MHz) and high frame rate ultrasound machine.[4] Magnetic resonance imaging and computed tomography (CT) can prove invaluable in diagnosing certain conditions, including diseases associated with the sinuses, inner ear, cranium, and teeth. Although these tests are becoming more available, they still remain cost prohibitive for some clients.

Microbiology

Bacterial and fungal cultures are routinely collected to assist in the diagnosis of specific pathogens. Interpretation of the results, however, can sometimes require more art than science. It is important for veterinarians to recognize that the results they receive from their laboratories are based on what happens at the level of the culture plate. For example, although *Pasteurella multocida* is often considered a primary differential in many cases based on the animal's presentation, the culture results may suggest otherwise. *P. multocida* is a fastidious organism and may be outcompeted on a plate by other organisms (e.g., *Staphylococcus* spp.). Therefore, the interpretation of the results should be reviewed cautiously.

Rabbits can become bacteremic and develop an infection in practically any tissue. The most common sites of infection, however, are the urinary bladder, respiratory system, and integument. Urine cultures obtained from cystocentesis are preferred to those collected via free-catch. Rabbit urine should have a basic pH. If the urine pH becomes acidic, it will promote the growth of potential opportunistic pathogens. Most pathogens of the urinary tract are Gram-negative bacteria. Female rabbits are more susceptible because of their stouter urethras. In addition to urine cultures, deep nasal cultures for chronic respiratory disease and cultures of abscesses are considered routine. Deep nasal cultures usually require sedation, as the microculturette is advanced into the nasal passage up to the level of the medial canthus of the eye. When culturing an abscess, the best results are often obtained from sampling the abscess wall.[11] Samples collected from the nasal sinuses and abscesses often have a significant number of inflammatory cells associated with them. These cells can affect the results of a culture by reducing the number of organisms to the point where analytical sensitivity of culture cannot detect the bacteria. In some cases, serial samples may be needed to determine if an organism is a trace pathogen. Culturing microorganisms from rabbits is otherwise routine. If anaerobes are suspected, then the veterinarian should contact the laboratory to obtain the appropriate media for collection and transport.

Parasitology

Although rabbits are captive bred, and the expectation is that parasites would be absent or low in these animals, parasites remain a problem because few preventive health programs are instituted at the breeding population level. Endoparasites can be diagnosed using routine direct saline smears or fecal flotations. Direct saline smears are preferred for identifying protozoa, whereas a fecal flotation is preferred for finding nematodes, trematodes, and cestodes. Annual parasitological examinations include both techniques. Because parasites can be shed transiently, serial samples should be performed. Pooling fecal samples produced over the course of a week may reduce the likelihood of misclassifying a rabbit's parasitic status. For systemic parasitologic disease, serologic testing or histopathology is required. *E. cuniculi,* a microsporidian, is generally diagnosed antemortem via serology or postmortem via histopathology. *E. cuniculi* is shed in the urine and may also be diagnosed from direct visualization in a urine sample, but this is not analytically sensitive. *Eimeria steidae,* a hepatic coccidian, can be diagnosed antemortem via a fecal direct smear or postmortem via histopathology.

Ectoparasites are also common in captive rabbits. If ectoparasites are suspected, a routine dermatologic examination should be performed, including a skin scrape and mineral oil preparation of the fur. Microscopic examination of these samples can provide confirmation of the presence of these parasites. Multiple samples should be collected to prevent misclassification as negative, and samples should be collected along the edge of the lesion. A flea comb can be used to confirm the presence of adult fleas or flea dirt.

Miscellaneous Diagnostics
SEROLOGY

Serologic testing in rabbits is limited. The two most common serologic tests being used today are for *E. cuniculi* and *P. multocida.* As with any test, it is important to know the sensitivity and specificity of the assay to be able to be able to determine the value of the result. The interpretation of a single titer should be done cautiously. If a rabbit has a single positive titer, it suggests that the animal has been exposed to the infectious disease. To confirm that the animal has a current infection, a paired sample would need to be collected 2 to 3 weeks later. A two- to fourfold rise in the titer should be observed before concluding an animal is actively infected. However, in cases where the animal's first titer was already significantly elevated, a similarly high second titer may be used to confirm infection. If the titer is negative, then the animal may not have been exposed to the disease, or the result may have been a false negative. False negative results can occur during a peracute disease when a titer has not developed or when the immunoglobulin being measured (e.g., IgM or IgG) either has not been developed or has already passed. Serologic results should always be interpreted in combination with the animal's physical examination findings.

POLYMERASE CHAIN REACTION

Polymerase chain reaction (PCR) assays have improved veterinarians' ability to diagnose diseases. The PCR test provides a more sensitive method of characterizing the presence of an organism than culture. One shortcoming of PCR is that a specific assay needs to be developed for each disease in a species. If there generally is not a high demand for a test, it will not be developed. PCR tests are available for *E. cuniculi* and *P. multocida.*

■ COMMON DISEASE PRESENTATIONS
Infectious Disease
BACTERIAL DISEASE
Pasteurella multocida

Snuffles is a generic term used to describe upper respiratory tract infection in rabbits. Although a variety of opportunistic pathogens can cause this "disease," it is generally associated with *P. multocida.* This is unfortunate because it often leads to misdiagnosis. Snuffles is characterized by purulent nasal discharge, sneezing, and coughing or "snuffling." Affected animals may be weak, lethargic, and anorectic. Ideally, a deep nasal culture should be performed to determine which species of bacteria is responsible for the infection. Primary dental disease must be ruled out as a differential for purulent nasal discharge.

P. multocida is a Gram-negative organism. This bacterium is relatively fastidious and can be difficult to culture. *P. multocida* has been associated with multiple clinical diseases, including pneumonia, upper respiratory tract disease, abscesses, pleuritis, pericarditis, pyometra, orchitis, otitis media, neurologic disease, and ocular disease.

Both acute and chronic disease states can occur. In cases of acute pneumonia, animals can succumb within hours, whereas in chronic disease states, there may be limited or no overt clinical signs. Transmission of *P. multocida* can occur through direct contact with acutely infected animals, fomites, and via airborne bacteria. The pathogen generally is thought to enter the rabbit through the respiratory tract. *P. multocida* can be isolated from a healthy rabbit's respiratory tract; however, when epithelium and local defenses are disrupted, bacterial numbers can increase to levels at which an infection can occur. Conditions that predispose a patient to *P. multocida* infections include temperature change, presence of carrier rabbits, poor sanitation (causing increased ammonia fumes), reproduction status, and age.[13]

A thorough diagnostic work-up should be done because rabbits with other bacteria can exhibit the same clinical signs. Preferably, a diagnosis is made using PCR and paired serology; however, a single serologic sample and positive deep nasal culture may suffice.

A CBC may show an inflammatory leukogram, characterized by heterophils/neutrophils and monocytes, or may be within reference levels. Plasma biochemistry panels are generally within acceptable reference limits; however, if the animal is dehydrated, the panels may show electrolyte and protein disturbances. Radiographs often reveal soft tissue changes in the sinuses and lungs. Ideally, treatment should be based upon culture and antibiotic sensitivity results. Most cases of respiratory *P. multocida* infections can be treated with enrofloxacin (5 mg/kg PO BID × 14 days), ciprofloxacin (20 mg/kg PO SID × 10 days), injectable penicillin (24,000 U/kg SC/IM), or chloramphenicol (50 mg/kg PO BID).[4] For chronically infected animals, these treatments need to be extended until the clinical signs are no longer present and the serologic titers decrease. Reproductive disease can be managed by performing an orchiectomy or ovariohysterectomy and providing appropriate antibiotics. *P. multocida* abscesses can occur anywhere on the body and can be difficult to treat. An extensive review of abscess treatment can be found later in this chapter (see Abscesses).

Bacterial Dysbiosis

The microflora of rabbits is comprised of a variety of aerobic and anaerobic bacteria. This dynamic flora is what enables the rabbit to thrive on an herbivorous diet. Unfortunately, this microflora is extremely sensitive to several groups of orally administered antibiotics, including clindamycin, lincomycin, ampicillin, amoxicillin, amoxicillin-clavulanic acid, cephalosporin, penicillin, and erythromycin.[2] These antibiotics can lead to alterations in the microflora, resulting in fluctuations in the intestinal pH, an increase in volatile fatty acids, and proliferation of *Clostridium spiriforme*. The endotoxemia produced by this organism is responsible for the peracute death of rabbits. If there is no environmental exposure to endotoxin-forming bacteria, this condition will not occur. In general, oral antibiotics are also more likely to cause diarrhea than are parenterally administered antibiotics. Trimethoprim sulfa and enrofloxacin are considered two of the safest oral antibiotics and can be administered orally over extended periods of time. In comparison with oral penicillin, injectable penicillin can be used to treat disease with minimal risk of dysbiosis. Many veterinarians prescribe probiotics to minimize the risk for dysbiosis. Probiotics are comprised of bacteria considered to represent indigenous microflora. These anaerobic microbes are thought to compete for colonization sites within the intestines with pathogens, alter the microflora environment (e.g., pH fluctuations), and produce their own natural "antibiotics" to kill pathogenic bacteria. The true value of these products remains controversial; however, they do not appear to cause disease. Treatment for antibiotic dysbiosis is primarily focused on the provision of supportive care. Fluids should be given to correct losses associated with diarrhea. Calories should be provided to ensure gut motility. Offending antibiotics must be discontinued. Additional safe antibiotics (e.g., enrofloxacin) may be considered to minimize the likelihood of other opportunistic pathogens infecting the compromised epithelium.

Clostridium spp.

Clostridium piliforme, the causative agent of Tyzzer's disease, is a motile, Gram-positive, obligate intracellular bacterium. Infections caused by *C. piliforme* are commonly reported in compromised rabbits. Overcrowding, unsanitary conditions, inappropriate breeding conditions, and high ambient temperatures have all been associated with *C. piliforme* outbreaks. Transmission is via the ingestion of spores. Clinical signs shown by rabbits with acute disease can include watery diarrhea, depression, and sudden death. Weanlings (6-12 weeks) are most severely affected; however, this pathogen can cause disease in rabbits of any age. Adult rabbits usually develop a chronic disease course, which can lead to intestinal fibrosis, liver necrosis and stenosis, and myocardial disease.[2] Tissue

culture and serologic testing are available for diagnosis. Treatment is usually not successful but consists of providing supportive care.

Endotoxemia can be caused by *C. spiriforme*, *C. difficile*, and *C. perfringes*. These organisms can cause significant enteric pathology, and are often associated with a high number of mortalities. Weanling rabbits are most likely to be affected and may be more predisposed to disease development. Adults can develop clostridial enterotoxemia from inappropriate antibiotic administration, which was described previously.[2]

Escherichia coli

In neonatal rabbits, colibacillosis is associated with high morbidity and mortality. *E. coli* is a Gram-negative bacterium from the family Enterobacteriaceae. Members of this family are frequently associated with disease in vertebrates. The most severe disease occurs in rabbits that are 1 to 14 days of age. Affected animals show signs of profuse, watery diarrhea and staining of the abdominal and perineal areas. Dehydration is a common sequela. Intestinal coccidiosis may enhance *E. coli* proliferation by increasing the severity of the clinical signs.[2] A diagnosis can be made from a fecal culture of a pure isolate. A CBC and biochemistry panel should be done, and generally support a diagnosis of an inflammatory disease with dehydration. Treatment should be based on an antibiotic sensitivity profile from the culture. Supportive care, including fluids and calories, is required because of the poor reserves of neonatal rabbits. Generally, the goal of therapy is to quell the spread of disease and prevent additional losses, as clinically affected animals often succumb to the disease.

Miscellaneous Bacterial Diseases

Lawsonia intracellularis, *Salmonella* spp., and *Pseudomonas* spp. are also common pathogens in rabbits. *Lawsonia intracellularis* is a Gram-negative, spiral-shaped, intracellular bacterium that commonly infects weanling rabbits between 2 and 4 months of age. Affected animals present with profuse, watery diarrhea (e.g., wet tail). *Salmonella* spp. and *Pseudomonas* spp. can also cause enteritis in rabbits and are usually disseminated through contaminated food or water sources. Affected animals may present with diarrhea, pyrexia, dehydration, and weight loss. Some animals can become asymptomatic reservoirs. With virulent organisms, peracute death is common. Diagnosis is via culture and antibiotic sensitivity profile. A CBC can provide information regarding the animal's response to the infection, and a radiograph can provide information regarding intestinal motility. Ileus is a common sequela. Treatment should include supportive care and antibiotics.

Treponematosis (*Treponema cuniculi*), otherwise known as rabbit syphilis, is a sexually transmitted disease that is spread during birth from a doe to a kit. Affected animals often present with crusts on the mucocutaneous junction of the nose, lips, eyelids, and/or external genitalia. Does may abort kits, retain placentas, or develop metritis.[14] A diagnosis can be made from a scraping or biopsy. Serologic tests are also available to assist with diagnosis. Silver stain or dark field microscopy is necessary to identify the organisms. Injectable penicillin (40,000

U/kg IM SID × 3-5 days;[14] 40,000 U/kg IM q7days × 3 treatments)[15] is the treatment of choice.

Staphylococcus aureus is considered a component of the indigenous microflora of the nasal cavity, conjunctiva, and skin of rabbits; however, when the epithelial barrier of these structures is compromised, the pathogen can invade. Mammary glands, respiratory and ocular tissues, and the integument are common sites for *S. aureus* infections. *S. aureus* infections can lead to fatal septicemia. Diagnosis is based on culture and cytologic and histopathologic testing. Treatment should be based on the antibiotic sensitivity profile. Enrofloxacin (5 mg/kg BID) or trimethoprim sulfa (15 mg/kg BID) are both broad-spectrum antibiotics that can be used to manage the case while the sensitivity profile is pending.

Bordetella bronchiseptica is a Gram-negative bacterium that generally infects the upper respiratory tract of rodents and lagomorphs. Infection caused by *B. bronchiseptica* strikes primarily older animals. Clinical signs include sneezing and nasal discharge; rabbits can also serve as asymptomatic carriers. Culture is used to confirm diagnosis. Antibiotics should be given based on antibiotic sensitivity profile, and, again, enrofloxacin can be used for initially treating the animal.

VIRAL DISEASE

Rotavirus is a disease of neonatal rabbits. Affected animals are generally 4 to 6 weeks of age. In populations where this virus is endemic, there is generally a low morbidity in weanlings; however, if naive animals are exposed to the virus, then the disease course can be severe.[16] Rotavirus can cause severe changes to the intestinal villi, including blunting and fusing. Severe damage to the villi can result in inability to absorb nutrients and in loss of fluids.[17,18] There is no effective treatment. Affected animals should be given supportive care and broad-spectrum antibiotics. Quarantine is recommended to prevent introduction of the virus.

Enteric coronavirus causes disease in 3- to 10-week-old rabbits; it is characterized by the loss of the brush border of the enterocytes. Clinical signs in affected rabbits include lethargy, watery diarrhea, and abdominal swelling. Morbidity can reach between 40% and 60%. Death usually occurs within 24 hours of the onset of signs. Corona or corona-like virus can lead to pleural effusion disease or infectious cardiomyopathy. Infected rabbits may present for anorexia, weight loss, tachypnea, or sudden death. Mortality can exceed 75% of affected animals. Virus isolation from the feces and histopathology consistent with the disease are the two common methods of diagnosis. Affected animals should be provided supportive care and broad-spectrum antibiotics to combat opportunistic bacterial infections. This virus can be isolated from healthy adult rabbits. Because of this, quarantine and prescreening animals are recommended to prevent introduction of the virus into rabbitry.

Myxoma virus is a member of the poxvirus family. The virus group has two distinct geographic origins: South America and California. Myxoma virus is associated with a benign cutaneous fibroma in its natural hosts: *Sylvilagus bachmani* (wild brush rabbits in the western United States—the Califor-

nian type), and *S. brasiliensis* (the South American type). Both of the myxoma strains can cause lethal disease in the European rabbit.[3,16] Although rare, this virus has been found to cause high mortality in domestic rabbits from Oregon and California.[19] This virus is transmitted via mosquitoes and fleas. The clinical signs associated with myxomatosis in natural hosts include swelling of the eyelids, face, head and testes/scrotum, the production of a milky ocular discharge, 1-cm mucoid cutaneous nodules, pyrexia, lethargy, depression, and anorexia. Infected domestic rabbits may become lethargic, pyrexic, anorectic, and develop skin hemorrhages and seizures.[4] Death usually occurs within 14 days of clinical onset. Although the exact mechanism leading to the animal's demise is not well understood, it has been suggested that it is due to the proliferation of Gram-negative bacteria secondary to the immunosuppression caused by the virus. No effective therapy is known, and euthanasia is recommended.[15] Cross-immunity can be achieved using a live, attenuated, Shope fibroma virus vaccine. However, the vaccine does not provide full coverage and is safe only in healthy nonpregnant animals. Boosters should be administered at 6- to 12-month intervals in susceptible animals.[15]

Shope fibroma virus is a Leporipoxvirus and is related to the myxoma virus. Cross-immunity can be inferred between the viruses. Shope fibroma virus can cause localized, benign fibromas and generalized disease in newborn, wild rabbits. Outbreaks have been reported in rabbitries. Clinical signs include subcutaneous, nonattached, wart-like fibromas on the legs or feet and around the muzzle and eyes. In young rabbits, this virus has been associated with lethargy, reduced body condition, skin lesions, and edema.[20] Diagnosis is made from histologic samples. No treatment is available.

Shope papillomavirus is the causative agent in papillomatosis. This disease is generally found in wild cottontails from the midwestern United States. Domestic rabbits are susceptible to the disease, and outbreaks have been reported in rabbitries. Horny warts are the most common clinical finding, and they are generally found on the shoulders, abdomen, and neck. Oral papillomavirus can also lead to the development of papillomas on the ventral surface of the tongue; however, cross-immunity develops when the virus causes dermal lesions. Diagnosis is made based on histopathologic findings and viral isolation. There is no treatment for this virus. The virus can induce malignant neoplasia that is similar to squamous cell carcinoma.

Rabbit pox is a rare but highly contagious disease. Clinical signs include lymphadenopathy, fever, and dermatologic changes (e.g., crusts, nodules, papules). Death can occur in severe cases. Edematous changes may also be seen on the face, oral cavity, scrotum, and vulva. Diagnosis is via viral isolation and histopathology.[4] There is no treatment for this virus.

Rabbit calicivirus, formerly known as rabbit viral hemorrhagic disease, is a viral-induced hemorrhagic disease. This virus is primarily found in the eastern hemisphere. An outbreak in Mexico occurred in 1988; however, the virus has since been eradicated from that country. A single outbreak has been reported in the United States; the event occurred in Iowa.

Morbidity from this disease can be as high as is 70% to 80%, and mortality can approach 100%. The virus is spread directly from infected to noninfected rabbits. Infected rabbits may present for frank hemorrhage around the face and muzzle, tachypnea, cyanosis, abdominal distension, constipation, or diarrhea.[20]

FUNGAL DISEASE

The most common fungal infections of rabbits are associated with *Trichophyton mentagrophytes* and *Microsporum canis*. Clinical signs in infected rabbits are similar to those reported in infected domestic pets and include crusty erythematous alopecia that may or may not be pruritic. Lesions can occur anywhere on the body but are often found on the head, shoulders, and legs. Ringworm is most often diagnosed in young animals that have received inappropriate husbandry. A diagnosis can be made with a KOH preparation from a skin scrape or fungal culture.[21] Infected rabbits can be treated with weekly lime-sulfur dips, a topical povidone-iodine cleansing agent, and, in severe cases, griseofulvin (25 mg/kg PO BID × 30 days).[21] Because this disease is potentially zoonotic, clients should be advised to minimize handling during treatment. Rabbits can acquire ringworm from humans too, so clients should be advised to consult their clinician if they are the source of infection.

Parasitic Disease

ENDOPARASITES

Coccidial infections are common when rabbits are held at high densities under inappropriate husbandry conditions. Infections are more problematic in weanling rabbits. *Eimeria* spp. can infect both the intestinal tract and the liver *(E. steidae)*. The transmission of these protozoal parasites is via the fecal-oral route. Sporulated oocysts represent the infectious stage. Clinical signs associated with intestinal coccidiosis include inappetence, weight loss, dehydration, diarrhea (± hemorrhagic), and, in chronic cases, intussusception. Hepatic coccidiosis is considered a more serious disease. Rabbits infected with hepatic coccidiosis may have limited growth, diarrhea, weight loss, dehydration, ascites, hepatomegaly, icterus, and hepatic encephalopathy. Severe cases can result in death. A fecal flotation and direct smear or histopathology can be useful to confirm a diagnosis. Treatment may be accomplished using trimethoprim sulfadiazine (30 mg/kg PS or SC BID × 7-10 days), sulfadimethoxine (50 mg/kg PO once, then 25 mg/kg SID × 21 days), or sulfaquinoxaline (0.025% in feed or pellets).[14] Extended treatments may be required for some populations. If routine treatment is practiced, then the anticoccidial drugs should be rotated to minimize the likelihood of inducing resistance.

E. cuniculi is an obligate, intracellular, microsporidian protozoan.[22] The parasite is disseminated via contaminated urine. *E. cuniculi* is shed transiently and can live for 4 weeks at room temperature. Clinical signs can vary depending upon the organ or system affected and the severity and duration of the disease. This protozoan affects primarily the kidneys, eyes, and neuro-

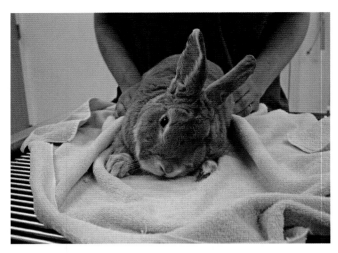

Figure 14-10 Head tilt in rabbit caused by *E. cuniculi*.

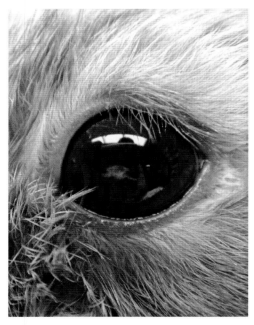

Figure 14-11 Lenticular changes associated with an *E. cuniculi* infection. (Courtesy Dr. David Guzman.)

logic system. Most infected rabbits present for vestibular disease. Clinical signs may include head tilt, hemiparesis, an inability to right itself, tumbling/rolling, seizures, ataxia, and paralysis (Figure 14-10). When *E. cuniculi* affects the neurologic system, the prognosis for recovery is grave. In some cases, rabbits show a reduction in vestibular signs but require life-long treatment. Without treatment, the quality of life is usually poor, and euthanasia is recommended. When the kidneys are affected, clinical signs may be absent because renal function is not usually altered. Cataracts and uveitis are common sequelae to ocular infections (Figure 14-11). Phacoemulsification is the treatment of choice for *E. cuniculi*–induced cataracts. Without treatment, the lens can rupture and induce a phacoelastic uveitis. Diagnosing *E. cuniculi* antemortem is usually done from the physical examination, hematology, and serology. Serology is generally only used to rule out *E. cuniculi* infection; however, a positive titer does not conclusively rule in disease. Albendazole, fenbendazole, or oxibendazole is generally used to minimize the inflammatory response associated with the infection.[4] Antibiotics that penetrate the blood-brain barrier (e.g., chloramphenicol) can be used to combat opportunistic infections. Diazepam can be used to control seizures. Although some corticosteroids have been used for treating *E. cuniculi,* they can cause immunosuppression and should be used with caution. The steroid's primary benefit is to increase the uptake of the respective antiparasitics. Life-long treatment is required to minimize the clinical signs associated with the disease.[23]

Baylisascaris procyonis, the raccoon roundworm, has been documented in rabbits and can be associated with fatal neurologic disease. Affected animals may present for torticollis, ataxia, and tremors.[24] Rabbits become infected from eating food or drinking water contaminated with raccoon feces. A diagnosis can be made from a serologic titer (exposure) or postmortem. Albendazole can be used to minimize the clinical disease associated with the parasites.

ECTOPARASITES

Cuterebra larvae, or bot flies, are common finding in rabbits housed outdoors. The larvae can be diagnosed easily by the presence of a small breathing hole. Infected rabbits generally have 1 to 5 bot larvae. The animal's fur may be matted around the breathing hole as a result of the rabbit licking in reaction to the pain associated with the larvae. Treatment requires surgical removal of the larvae. An incision should be made through the air hole, and the larvae extracted. The larval cyst should be removed to prevent secondary opportunistic infection. Care should be taken not to crush the larvae during extraction, as this can lead to anaphylaxis. Rabbits housed outdoors should be protected against flies by means of appropriate fly traps and cage screening.

Fly strike, or myiasis, is a common presentation for rabbits housed outdoors during the summer. Obesity, underlying dermatitis, and unsanitary conditions can predispose a rabbit to this condition. Aggressive wound debridement and maggot removal are required to treat affected rabbits. Ivermectin (0.2 mg/kg SC once) can be used to kill the maggots. Antibiotics may be used if the wound is large or there is a concern for systemic disease. Analgesics should be used during wound treatment to control pain. The dog flea *(Ctenocephalides canis)* and cat flea *(C. felis)* are the most common fleas found on rabbits. The fleas are found primarily along the dorsum between the shoulders and pelvis. Flea powder that is safe for kittens can be used for rabbits. Although not labeled for use in rabbits, lufenuron (Program, Novartis Animal Health Canada, Mississauga, Ontario) and Advantage (Bayer Animal Health, Agriculture Division, Shawnee Mission, KS) for cats have been used safely for rabbits. For rabbits that are 10 weeks of age and less than 4 kg, 0.4 ml of topical solution can be applied to the skin at the base of neck, as recommended for dogs and cats. Rabbits that are ≥4 kg can be treated with

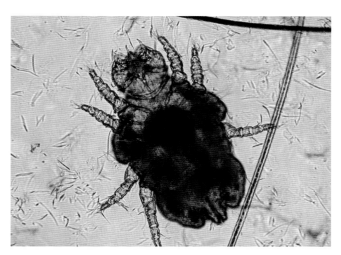

Figure 14-12 *Cheyletiella parasitovorax* is often described as "walking dandruff."

0.8 ml.[4] When treating the animal's environment, it is important to remove the rabbit and only return it once the chemicals are dry. Frontline (Merial Limited, Duluth, GA) should not be used on rabbits, as it can cause liver impairment.

Cheyletiella parasitovorax, an obligate, nonburrowing mite, is commonly referred to as "walking dandruff" (Figure 14-12). Clinical signs associated with an infection include mild pruritus, large flakes of white scales on limbs and neck, alopecia, and oily dermatitis. Infestations occur more commonly in young, obese, or otherwise immunosuppressed animals. A diagnosis can be confirmed from the microscopic examination of a skin scrape or scotch tape prep. Ivermectin (0.2-0.4 mg/kg SC × 3 treatments) is the treatment of choice.[4] Lime-sulfur dips and flea powder can also be used to treat affected rabbits. Cleaning the environment and treating other affected animals are also required to eliminate this parasite. This parasite can be zoonotic, so it is important to advise clients to take precautions when handling/treating affected animals.

Psoroptes cuniculi is the common rabbit ear mite. Affected animals can develop severe otitis externa. The external canal and pinnae can also have significant quantities of crusty exudates. The crusty exudate is the result of a hypersensitivity reaction to the mite and can cause a significant discharge and pruritus. One or both ears can be infested. Ear mites are transmitted by direct contact or contact with fomites. Mites can survive off the host for 21 days. *Psoroptes'* life cycle is 21 days. Ivermectin (0.4 mg/kg SC, ½ done in each ear) or selamectin (Revolution; Pfizer Animal Health, New York, NY) (6 or 18 mg/kg topically 1-2 times) can be used to eliminate mites.[25] Do not remove the crusts or clean the ears, as the skin under the crusts is ulcerated and painful. Prednisone (0.5 mg/kg PO BID × 5 days) or meloxicam (0.2 mg/kg PO BID × 5 days) may be used to reduce the otitis and provide pain relief.

Sarcoptes scabiei, the causative agent of scabies, can induce a crusty, pruritic dermatitis of the face, nose, lips, and external genitalia.[2] Diagnosis is via a deep skin scrape of the lesion. Ivermectin (0.4 mg/kg SC q14days × 3 treatments) or weekly lime-sulfur dips (1 : 40) and environmental clean-up can be

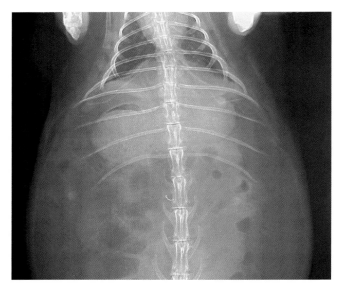

Figure 14-13 A history of anorexia and a radiograph showing soft tissue density in the stomach suggest the presence of trichobezoars in rabbits.

used to eliminate the mites. The mite is zoonotic, so clients should be instructed to wear gloves when handling/treating an infected animal.

Passalurus ambiguous, a pinworm, is considered by some to be commensal. This nematode is thought to play a role in the digestion of plant material. Clinical disease has been attributed to heavy burdens. Affected animals may be anorectic, lose weight, develop impaction, and be in poor condition. A diagnosis can be made from a fecal flotation. Fenbendazole (20 mg/kg PO SID × 5 days), thiabendazole (50 mg/kg PO q2wk-q3wk), or Piperazine (200-500 mg/kg/day PO × 2 days) can be used to treat affected animals.[3,5,15]

Haemodipsus ventricosus, the sucking rabbit louse, is rare in pet rabbits. Most cases occur in rabbits from poorly managed rabbitries. Affected animals can develop intense pruritus and anemia. Ivermectin (0.4 mg/kg SC q14days × 3 treatments) is the treatment of choice.[4]

Nutritional Disease

Hairballs, or trichobezoars, are most common in rabbits fed diets with inadequate fiber. Stress, barbering, and nest building have also been associated with the formation of trichobezoars. Anorexia, lethargy, diarrhea, small dry feces or an absence of feces, hair loss, and a palpable firm mass in the cranial abdomen are common findings in affected rabbits. A thorough history, physical examination, and survey radiographs (± contrast) are generally required to make a diagnosis. Endoscopy can be used to confirm a diagnosis. A history of anorexia in combination with a soft tissue density in the stomach is highly suggestive of gastric trichobezoars (Figure 14-13). Positive or negative contrast radiography can be used to help outline a trichobezoar. In most cases, medically managing a trichobezoar yields a higher treatment success than does surgery. However, there

are cases where surgical intervention is the only method that can be used to treat a trichobezoar. Treatment should focus on rehydrating the gastric contents through fluid administration and providing motility stimulants, analgesics, antibiotics, and nutritional support. Fresh greens and hay should be offered to animals that are still eating. Rabbits that are anorectic should be force-fed a critical care diet (Oxbow Pet Products, Murdock, NE) to prevent hepatic lipidosis. Fresh pineapple juice contains the enzyme bromelain, and this enzyme is thought to have ceratolytic properties (5-10 ml BID).[7] Papaya and prozyme may also be used to assist in the digestion of the trichobezoar. Metoclopramide or cisapride can be used to stimulate gastric motility; however, this should not be used if impaction is suspected. A broad-spectrum antibiotic, such as enrofloxacin or trimethoprim sulfa, is generally used to limit the overgrowth of bacterial pathogens. Analgesics, such as buprenorphine, flunixin meglumine, metacam, or carprofen, can be used to minimize the pain associated with the alterations in gastrointestinal motility. Without treatment, trichobezoars can lead to malnutrition and death or gastric rupture causing fatal peritonitis.[26] If the ingested material is synthetic (e.g., carpeting), surgery is usually required. The prognosis for cases going to surgery is generally considered guarded to grave; however, if the animal is stabilized before the procedure, then the likelihood for success is higher.

Obesity is a common problem in house rabbits and has been associated with high protein/fat pellets, free choice pellets, and restricted exercise. Obesity can increase the incidence of skin fold pyoderma, fecal staining of the perineum due to grooming difficulty, sore hocks, and an inability to acquire night feces. To prevent obesity, a rabbit should be provided a diet that is less than 18% protein, less than 10% fat, and more than 18% fiber. It is also important for clients to ensure their rabbits are given daily exercise.

Hepatic lipidosis in rabbits follows the same pathophysiologic response seen in other species. Obese or overweight animals are at higher risk of developing hepatic lipidosis than are those in good physical condition. If a rabbit becomes anorectic for any reason, such as dental disease, stress, illness, pregnancy, or postoperative complications, it can develop hepatic lipidosis. To minimize the likelihood of hepatic lipidosis from occurring in an anorectic rabbit, the veterinarian should provide a high-quality critical care diet (Oxbow). The underlying cause of hepatic lipidosis needs to be determined to break the cycle of anorexia and pathology.

Abnormal tooth wear can lead to laceration and ulceration of the tongue and buccal surfaces, which can lead to discomfort and difficulty chewing (Figure 14-14). There are a number of suspected etiologies attributed to the development of abnormal tooth wear, including genetics, anatomy, and nutrition. Feeding rabbits a pelleted diet can actually alter the natural movements associated with mastication by reducing the lateral, and increasing the vertical, jaw action.[7] The most common sites to find dental pathology (e.g., sharp points) are the lingual side of the mandibular teeth and the buccal surface of the maxillary teeth. Correcting these abnormalities is generally sufficient to get the rabbit eating again. With sedation, these

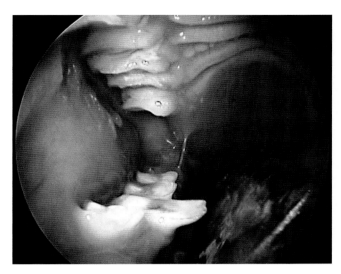

Figure 14-14 Lacerations on the tongue are a common sequela to cheek tooth malocclusion. (Courtesy of Dr. David Guzman.)

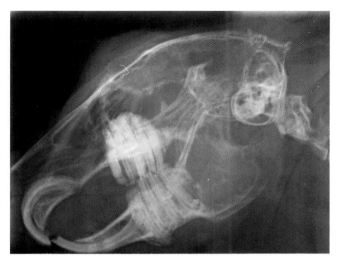

Figure 14-16 Dental disease as seen on radiographs. Note the cheek teeth elongation and the root pathology.

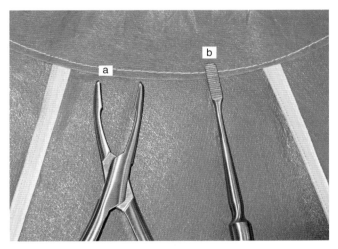

Figure 14-15 Rabbit dental instruments can be used to trim (a) and float (b) rabbit cheek teeth; however, care should be taken to limit secondary complications (e.g., tooth fracture, gingival hemorrhage).

sharp points can be floated or drilled down to appropriate length and angle to allow for a more natural bite (Figure 14-15). When evaluating the teeth of a rabbit, it is important to take radiographs to evaluate the tooth roots for any pathology (e.g., abscesses) (Figure 14-16). For chronic incisor overgrowth, removal is recommended. For cheek teeth abnormalities, removal of nondiseased teeth that oppose missing teeth or normal teeth left behind after the conspecific tooth is removed is not recommended unless essential, because they can be difficult to remove and possibly result in the fracture of an attached bone.

Neoplasia

Uterine adenocarcinoma is the most common neoplasia reported in female rabbits over 4 years of age. There is an increased incidence of this neoplasia (50%-80%) in Dutch, Havana, tan, French, and silver breeds.[27] Uterine adenocarcinoma is a slow-developing neoplasia; it can take 10 to 12 months for those tumors to metastasize from the uterine wall to surrounding peritoneal structures or lungs. The most common sites for metastasis include the liver, lungs, mammary glands, brain, and bones. Rabbits with uterine adenocarcinoma can present with a range of clinical signs, including hematuria, vaginal discharge, decreased fertility, increased kit mortality, depression, anorexia, dyspnea, and cystic mammary glands. A diagnosis can be made from a thorough history (e.g., age, intact), physical examination, CBC, chemistry panel, whole body radiographs, and ultrasound. It is often possible to palpate an enlarged uterus in rabbits with uterine adenocarcinoma. The neoplastic organ will palpate as a tubular structure in the caudoventral abdomen. An increased soft tissue density in the same area may be seen radiographically. Thoracic radiographs should be taken to assess the patient for metastasis. If metastasis to the lungs has occurred, then the prognosis is grave. If metastasis has not occurred, then an ovariohysterectomy is recommended. During the surgical procedure, the abdomen should be inspected for localized metastasis. Any suspect tissues should be biopsied.[4]

Mammary adenocarcinoma is another common neoplasia of adult (>3-4 years of age) rabbits.[4] These cases should be managed using the diagnostic plan described for uterine adenocarcinomas. Removing the affected mammary gland (local or radical) and the reproductive tract provides the best prognosis. Metastasis can be found in regional lymph nodes, lungs, or other organs. The incidence of mammary adenocarcinoma can be reduced significantly by performing ovariohysterectomies in rabbits before they are sexually mature. Some clinicians use different chemotherapeutics as adjunctive therapy to surgical treatment. Tamoxifen is a nonsteroidal, antiestrogen drug with antitumor effects that works by binding estrogen receptors.[28] The overall value of this drug in rabbits is unknown for spayed animals. However, clinicians using the protocol believe, subjectively, that survival is extended. If tamoxifen is used, the patient should be routinely monitored for changes in behavior, tumor size, and liver or CBC changes.

Although adenocarcinoma is the most common reported reproductive neoplastic condition in captive rabbits, uterine leiomyoma and leiomyosarcoma, vaginal squamous cell carcinoma, ovarian hemangioma, testicular seminoma, interstitial cell carcinoma, testicular adenocarcinoma, and teratoma have also been reported.

Lymphosarcoma, as in other mammalian species, is a commonly diagnosed neoplasia in rabbits. Urinary neoplasia rarely occurs; however, nephroma, lymphosarcoma, renal carcinoma, and urinary bladder leiomyoma have been reported. Primary neoplasia of the lungs is very rare. Carcinomas have been found to be associated with the nasal turbinates, causing an unresponsive nasal discharge. Thymomas have been reported in both juvenile and adult rabbits. Affected animals often present with tachypnea, dyspnea, and, occasionally, bilateral exophthalmos resulting from the interference of the blood flow to the heart. A thymomectomy can be performed via a median sternotomy.[4] Metastasis to the lungs is a common sequela for many different malignant neoplasias. Both teratoma and neurinoma affect the central nervous system of rabbits. Neoplastic conditions found to affect the digestive tract include adenocarcinoma, leiomyosarcoma, papilloma, and metastatic uterine adenocarcinoma. Surgical resection is the treatment of choice for those conditions. Bile duct carcinoma has been reported in rabbits; however, in these cases, surgery is not an option and metastatic disease carries a grave prognosis. Cutaneous neoplasias that have been reported in rabbits include the following: cutaneous lymphosarcoma, nonviral papilloma, basal cell carcinoma, squamous cell carcinoma, and sebaceous gland carcinoma. Malignant melanoma has been associated with ocular, abdominal, thoracic, and vertebral disease.[31]

Miscellaneous Diseases
DERMATOLOGY

Many different diseases or conditions, such as obesity, sore hocks, arthritis, poor diet, dental disease, urinary disease, and neurologic disease, can lead to secondary dermatitis. Moist dermatitis around the oral cavity is a common sequela to dental disease. Discomfort caused by tooth malocclusion can lead to drooling, and the chronic wetness associated with the drooling predisposes the animal to bacterial dermatitis. Skin fold pyoderma is a common problem in obese animals; the sites most commonly affected are the dewlap, perianal, and genital areas. Treatment for those conditions requires aggressive wound debridement. Fur from the affected area should be clipped to provide adequate exposure. The wound should be cleaned with a topical disinfectant (e.g., Betadine or chlorhexidine). To control bacterial infections, we recommend using a hyperosmotic solution (e.g., 50% dextrose). The wound should be liberally irrigated with the 50% dextrose solution. After 1 to 2 minutes, the wound should be irrigated with isotonic saline

to remove the dextrose. Extended contact with the dextrose can dry out the healing tissue. The procedure should be repeated at least three times, twice daily. In addition to this topical treatment, obese animals should be placed on a calorie-restrictive diet. This is best achieved by reducing the amount of pellets and providing (ad libitum) grass hay (e.g., timothy hay). Surgery may be required to remove excess skin folds. In cases of tooth malocclusion, the primary problem should be identified and corrected.

Dermal abscesses are a common presentation in rabbits and can occur anywhere on the body. Abscesses in rabbits are generally more caseous in nature than in other mammals. The thick, caseous nature of rabbit abscesses limits their drainage, and the use of standard Penrose drains is usually futile. Treating abscesses with (only) systemic antibiotics is ineffective, as the nucleus of the abscess in unaffected by the treatment. To effectively treat rabbit abscesses, the entire abscess (including the capsule) must be removed. In cases where the abscess and capsule are removed, the prognosis is good; however, in most cases the capsule is inherently attached to vital organs or bone and is difficult to remove. When it is impossible to extract the entire capsule, as much of the capsule should be removed as possible to avoid contact between caseous material and unaffected tissue. Culture and antibiotic sensitivity testing of the purulent material or capsule is recommended. Abscesses that cannot be completely removed should be left open for daily cleansing and debridement. When choosing a topical antibiotic therapy, be sure to select antibiotics that will not induce bacterial dysbiosis when the rabbit grooms itself. Penicillin (80,000 IU/kg) or ampicillin (20 mg/kg), although not to be given orally because of the potential for dysbiosis, can be used parenterally to treat local skin abscesses. In our experience, the application of honey to the abscess as a hyperosmotic has produced moderate success. The honey, in addition to acting as an antimicrobial, encourages a rabbit to groom or lick at the area and promotes drainage.[2] The honey also acidifies the area and promotes healing. Systemic oral antimicrobials and analgesics should also be considered when treating rabbit abscesses.[29] Antibiotic-impregnated polymethylmethacrylate (PMMA) beads can also be used to manage rabbit abscesses. Heat-stable antibiotics must be used to make PMMA beads. Amikacin 1.25 g/20 g methylmethacrylate, cefazolin 2 g/20 g methylmethacrylate, cephalothin 2 g/20 g methylmethacrylate, gentamicin 1 g/20 g methylmethacrylate, or tobramycin 1 g/20 g methylmethacrylate are all appropriate for PMMA beads.[30] Treating abscesses in rabbits can be frustrating and may require multiple procedures. In some cases, treatment is not successful, and amputation may be the only option. Owners should always be made aware of their pet's prognosis before treatment is initiated. Systemic antibiotics are appropriate for generalized abscesses. Antimicrobial treatment is ideally based on culture and antibiotic sensitivity testing. While testing is pending, abscesses can be treated with benzathine/penicillin G procaine (40,000 IU/kg SC SID × 14 days, then q48h × 2 weeks); enrofloxacin (5 mg/kg PO BID); or metronidazole (30 mg/kg PO BID).[30,35] The use of trimethoprim sulfa-dimethoxine should be avoided when there is caseous material present because the antibiotic is inactivated by pus.

"Sore hocks," or ulcerative pododermatitis, is caused by an avascular necrosis of the plantar surface of the rear feet. This is a painful, progressive disease that can be difficult to treat. Predisposing factors for this disease include breed (e.g., Rex), housing (e.g., metal grate flooring, concrete, carpet), lack of exercise, and obesity. Rabbits housed on an inappropriate flooring surface alter their weight distribution and bear the brunt of their weight on their metatarsus and hock instead of on the claws and plantar surface of the feet.[2] This shift in weight leads to the medical displacement of the superficial flexor tendon, which can exacerbate the condition.[2] Treatment is aimed at relieving the pressure on the affected area. A non-abrasive, dry surface should be provided. Providing an affected animal time during the day on a grass lawn or deep bed of hay is helpful. A thick foam rubber pad, towels, or newspaper substrate can also be used to minimize the likelihood of exacerbating this disease. Skin wounds can be managed using the technique described previously. Surgical skin glue can be used to protect the wounds. A padded splint can be used to alleviate any pressure on the lesions. Opportunistic infection should be managed with appropriate antibiotics. Analgesics (e.g., nonsteroidal antiinflammatories, opioids) should be used to alleviate discomfort. Underlying problems, such as obesity and inappropriate substrate, should be corrected. Surgery is usually not performed because there is no skin for closure.

Hypersensitivity reactions can occur immediately or days after an injection is given. Affected animals present with erythema and swelling around the face and extremities. Most animals heal without complication or with a need for topical therapy. Giving injections subcutaneously may reduce the occurrence of these reactions.[2] In severe cases, such as may occur with intramuscular injections, self-mutilation may occur.[21] Severe reactions can be managed with steroidal (prednisone, 0.5-1.0 mg/kg) or nonsteroidal (meloxicam, 0.3 mg/kg) antiinflammatories.

Alopecia is a common problem in captive rabbits and may result from self-mutilation, barbering, parasites, endocrine disease, or infectious causes. Self-mutilation is most common in rabbits after a traumatic experience or surgery. Barbering is the result of aggression between cagemates. If barbering is suspected, animals should be separated. Diagnosis of parasitic, infectious, or endocrine disease requires a complete diagnostic work-up. Treatment is dependent on the specific diagnosis.

Rectal papillomas can present as cauliflower-like masses extending from the rectum. Most of these masses do not cause a problem; however, occasionally these masses can cause frank hemorrhage or mild diarrhea. Surgical resection of the mass is required for treatment.

Rare dermatologic disorders of rabbits include sebaceous adenitis, nonpruritic scaling and alopecia, Ehlers-Danlos syndrome, and neoplasia (see Neoplasia). Infectious and parasitic diseases are frequently associated with dermatologic disease in rabbits (see Infectious Disease; Parasitic Disease).

DISEASES OF THE SENSE ORGANS

Ears represent a significant proportion of the surface area of a rabbit. Otitis externa is a common problem, and it is most often associated with a parasitic or bacterial predisposition. Parasitic infections were described previously (see Parasitic Disease).[32] Lop breeds are predisposed to developing bacterial otitis because of the flexion of the cartilage at the base of their ears. Rabbits with otitis externa may present for shaking, pruritus, erythematous pinna, malodor, and possible auricular discharge. Because otitis externa can be painful, care should be taken when manipulating the ears; we prefer to treat affected rabbits with systemic antibiotics and antiinflammatories rather than treating the ears topically. Bacterial cultures should be collected before treatment. Otitis externa can advance to otitis media or otitis interna. Otitis interna should be ruled out in rabbits with a head tilt. Radiographs and/or CT scans can be used to assess the tympanic bullae. In severe otitis cases, a permanent osteotomy may be required.[32] The most common causes of conjunctivitis in rabbits are bacterial infections (e.g., *Pasteurella*), trauma, and entropion. When evaluating rabbit eyes, the approach to the examination should be similar to that for other mammals. Unless trauma has been acknowledged in the history, a thorough work-up should be pursued, including a cytologic scraping and bacterial culture. For confirmed bacterial infections, topical antibiotics can be used. Treatment regimens may require three to four doses daily. Application of topical antibiotics three to four times a day in addition to removing the initial cause of conjunctivitis is recommended. Entropion is a common presentation in large breed and obese rabbits, and surgical resection is necessary for resolution.[21]

Epiphora can be associated with early signs of dental disease, causing the blockage of the nasolacrimal ducts, or it can occur secondarily to conjunctivitis or rhinitis. Any rabbit presenting with dacryocystitis, conjunctivitis, or epiphora should receive a thorough ophthalmic examination, in addition to skull radiographs, to evaluate the roots of the teeth. Because many cases of epiphora are the direct result of blocked or inflamed lacrimal ducts, the lacrimal punctum should be flushed with sterile saline to facilitate the removal of debris (Figure 14-17). The ducts can be flushed with antibiotics too if a bacterial infection is suspected.

Anterior uveitis can occur as a result of trauma, bacterial disease, or *E. cuniculi*–induced lens disease. Corneal ulcers are also somewhat common in rabbits housed with other animals. A fluorescein stain should be used to confirm the presence of an ulcer. Retrobulbar abscesses can be problematic; diagnosis and treatment should be based on culture and antibiotic sensitivity testing and aggressive antibiotic therapy instituted. In many cases, enucleation is required. Because of the large retro-orbital venous sinus, enucleation can be difficult.

NEUROLOGIC DISEASES

Vertebral luxation or fracture is a common finding in rabbits with a history of hind end paresis or paralysis. Rabbits have a highly developed muscular system and a relatively delicate vertebral column, making them more prone to fractures. The most common cause of these injuries is associated with inappropriate restraint (Figure 14-18). A diagnosis can be confirmed from a history, physical examination, and vertebral radiographs. The prognosis for these cases depends upon the extent of the lesions. With vertebral luxation, medical management may be attempted; however, it is usually not successful. Prednisolone sodium succinate (0.5 mg/kg IV) can be used to control edema in the spinal canal. In addition to the steroid treatment, cage rest and the manual expression of the bladder can be done.[21] Surgery can be attempted, but only by experienced surgeons.

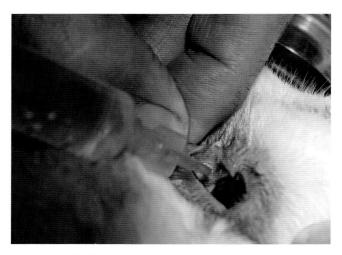

Figure 14-17 Flushing the nasolacrimal duct.

Rabbits with torticollis, difficulty righting, or abnormal locomotion (e.g., flipping over) generally have a central nervous system disorder. The three most common causes of head tilt in rabbits are *E. cuniculi* infection, trauma, and *P. multocida* infection. Although less common, listeriosis and aberrant larval migrans can also cause torticollis. Diagnosis is generally based on a thorough history, physical examination, radiographs, CBC, serology, and CT scans. Treatment can be difficult and prolonged. Enrofloxacin can be used to manage *P. multocida* and fenbendazole/albendazole to manage *E. cuniculi* infections.[21]

DISEASES OF THE MUSCULOSKELETAL SYSTEM

Splay leg or hip dysplasia is an apparent congenital condition seen in young rabbits. Affected rabbits present with an inability to abduct their legs, which prevents ambulation. Amputation is recommended if only one leg is affected.[14] Although this condition is thought to be genetic, environmental factors may also have some effect. In a recent study, rabbits housed on slippery surfaces had an increased incidence of splay leg compared with those housed with appropriate traction.[33] In severe cases, humane euthanasia is warranted.

DISEASES OF THE REPRODUCTIVE SYSTEM

Pyometra occasionally occurs in rabbits and is usually reported shortly after parturition. Affected rabbits may be asymptomatic or may show signs of anorexia, weight loss, vaginal discharge, hematuria, or infertility. Diagnosis is made based on history, physical exam, CBC, radiology, and ultrasound. Inflammatory leukograms are common. Survey radiographs

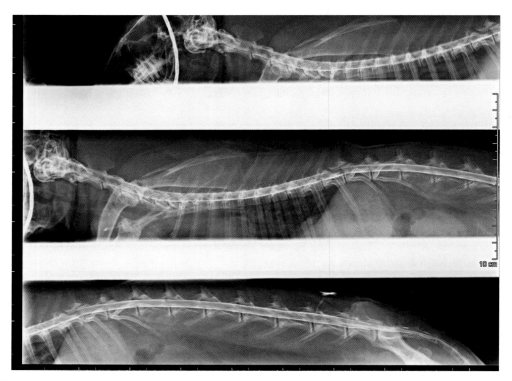

Figure 14-18 Vertebral injuries are common in rabbits that are not restrained properly. (Courtesy Dr. David Guzman.)

and ultrasound often reveal a fluid-filled soft tissue structure in the caudoventral abdomen. Affected animals should be provided supportive care (e.g., fluids, calories) to correct any deficiencies. Systemic antibiotics are warranted. Ovariohysterectomy is the treatment of choice.

Orchitis is relatively uncommon in captive rabbits because many animals are neutered at a young age. The disease is spread venereally, and can be caused by a bacterial infection. Clinical signs generally include enlarged testicles or epididymis and discomfort. Orchiectomy can be done in pet animals. Antibiotics may be used to treat breeding rabbits. The animal should be reevaluated before it is placed back into the breeding rotation.

Pregnancy toxemia is a problem that occurs in does at the end of gestation during nesting; these animals, especially obese Dutch, Polish, and English breeds, fast or have reduced caloric intake.[14] Clinical signs include weakness, depression, incoordination, coma, convulsions, or death. Fasting leads to ketoacidosis and shock. Treatment should be aimed at reversing ketoacidosis and providing both shock therapy and supportive care. Supportive care may include the provision of calcium gluconate, fluids, and nutritional support. Treatment is usually unsuccessful, so prevention is the key. Clients should attempt to reduce obesity in breeding does and monitor their caloric intake carefully during pregnancy.

Cystic uterine hyperplasia is a problem in aged, intact does. Clinical signs include hematuria, anemia, reduced activity, a firm irregular uterus, cystic mammary glands, and cystic ovaries. Diagnosis is via clinical signs, radiology, and ultrasound. Ovariohysterectomy should be recommended to treat this condition.[4]

Pseudopregnancy can occur in does and lasts, on average, 16 to 18 days. Toward the end of the pseudopregnancy, does will go through normal nesting behavior (e.g., pulling out hair to line nests) and will have mammary development. Pseudopregnancy can resolve spontaneously or lead to pyometra or hydrometra.[4] Ovariohysterectomy is the treatment of choice.

Dystocia and retained fetuses occur commonly in obese does, in cases where the fetus is too large for the doe's pelvic canal, or in does with uterine inertia. Clinical signs include nonproductive contractions and bloody to greenish-brown vaginal discharge. In nonobstructive dystocia, calcium gluconate and oxytocin may aid in the delivery of fetuses. In obstructive dystocia, a cesarean section is required. For prolonged dystocia events, the prognosis is guarded for both the doe and fetus.

Lactating or pseudopregnant does are prone to developing mastitis. Clinical signs in affected animals are similar to those observed in other animals and include pyrexia, swelling, blue coloration of teats, inappetence, and depression. Bacteria, such as *Staphylococcus* spp. and *Streptococcus* spp., are usually the causative agent. Without treatment, mastitis can progress to septicemia and death. Treatment includes surgical drainage or mastectomy, warm compresses, and appropriate antibiotics. Penicillin (40,000 U/kg IM BID × 5 days) has been used with success.[14]

Other reproductive problems that occur in rabbits are abortion-reabsorption, decreased fertility, prolapsed vagina, endometrial venous aneurysm, hydrometra, uterine torsion, cryptorchidism, testicular neoplasia, venereal spirochetosis, and cystic mastitis.

DISEASES OF THE EXCRETORY SYSTEM

The exact cause of urolithiasis in rabbits is unknown; however, diet, vitamin and mineral oversupplementation, and infections can be predisposing factors. Clinical signs are often nonspecific and include lethargy, inappetence, abdominal distension, urine scalding, perineal debris, and hematuria. A thickened bladder can sometimes be palpated on physical examination. A diagnosis can be made from radiographs and a urinalysis (e.g., crystals). A cystotomy is generally needed to treat urolithiasis. Reducing calcium in the diet may help decrease the likelihood of urolithiasis formation.

Cystitis is a common problem in does. Diagnosis is generally made from a cytologic examination (e.g., inflammatory cells and bacteria) and bacterial culture and sensitivity. Opportunistic Gram-negative bacteria are the most common isolates. Treatment is ideally based on culture and antibiotic sensitivity results.

Renal failure can occur in rabbits as a result of hypercalciuria (e.g., mineralization) or infectious agents (e.g., *E. cuniculi*). Clinical signs include polyuria and polydypsia, weight loss, inappetence, anemia, and lethargy. Diagnosis can be made based on radiology, chemistry panel, CBC, and urinalysis. An inverse calcium-to-phosphorus (Ca : P) ratio is generally indicative of renal failure. Survey radiographs may reveal mineral densities in the kidneys. Isosthenuria, in the face of an inverse Ca : P ratio, on a urinalysis can be used to confirm a diagnosis. Confirmation can be made via renal biopsy. Treatment should focus on monitoring fluid levels.

Renal cysts, or renal polycystic kidney syndrome, have been reported in New Zealand white rabbits. Most affected rabbits have nonspecific clinical signs. Animals with clinical disease generally are lethargic and anorectic. Polycystic disease can be associated with hypercalcemia, hypercreatinemia, and arterial mineralization.[34]

E. cuniculi can cause renal disease in rabbits. Early in the disease course, the parasite causes segmental, granulomatous, interstitial nephritis, which can be seen as irregular depressions on the surface of the kidneys. However, interstitial fibrosis can occur late in the disease. Many times these changes do not cause a reduction in kidney function. (For more information about *E. cuniculi,* see Parasitic Disease.)

"Red urine" is a common problem in rabbits. In these cases, veterinarians must determine whether a sample is red because of the presence of blood or porphyrin pigment. Blood indicates a breakdown in the epithelial barrier and is common with cystitis, uroliths, and neoplasia. The presence of porphyrin pigment is associated most with stress, dietary changes, or both. A thorough history will often provide insight into whether a recent stress event or dietary change occurred. A urinalysis should be done to determine if a color change in the urine is based on blood or pigment. The presence of red blood cells is diagnostic. Disease rule-outs for animals with blood in their urine include neoplasia (e.g., adenocarcinoma), endometrial aneurysms, urinary or reproductive tract polyps, cystitis, pyelonephritis, urolithiasis, disseminated intravascular coagulopathy, and lead toxicosis.

DISEASES OF THE GASTROINTESTINAL SYSTEM

Dental disease, as previously mentioned, is common in pet rabbits. Clinical signs can vary, but generally include difficulty with prehension of food, anorexia, cachexia, dacryocystitis, abnormal facial swelling, and excessive salivation. Incisor malocclusion has been attributed to congenital factors, such as mandibular prognathism, and is seen at an increased rate in rabbits less than 1.5 kg or certain breeds (e.g., Netherland dwarf rabbits).[2] Animals that suffer traumatic injuries to the jaws are also more susceptible to developing tooth malocclusion. Abnormal incisor growth can lead to the blockage of the nasolacrimal duct, resulting in epiphora. Incisor malocclusion can also lead to molar malocclusion, causing further dental complications. Trimming incisors is the primary method for correcting malocclusion, and this can be done using a high-speed Dremel tool (Dremel, Racine, WI) or dental drill (Figure 14-19). Incisors grow at a rate of 3 mm per week when the opposing incisor is present and 1 mm per day when there is no tooth opposition. Therefore, trimming should be done at approximately 3-week intervals when there is a malocclusion or no opposing incisor. Toenail clippers have been recommended for trimming incisors; we do not recommend this, as toenail clippers have been associated with tooth fracture. Where there is severe malocclusion, complete incisor extraction is recommended. This is a relatively easy procedure; however, it does require patience. Aggressive, rough manipulation of the teeth can lead to tooth fracture and, again, pain and discomfort. (This procedure is discussed in detail in Surgery.) If the entire root and germinal tissue are not removed, the teeth can regenerate, requiring additional surgery.

Cheek teeth or molar malocclusion is characterized by crown elongation and the development of hooks and points. Coronal overgrowth (due to incisor overgrowth or poor occlu-

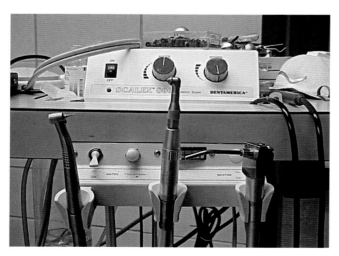

Figure 14-19 High-speed dental tools are recommended for trimming rabbit teeth.

sion) requires not only that the spikes be removed but also that the crowns be reduced and the angulation be corrected for ideal occlusion. Maxillary cheek teeth and all but the first mandibular cheek teeth can be reduced to the level of the gingiva; however, this is not always necessary. In some cases, removing the points is sufficient. The gingiva naturally exposes the cranial aspect of the first mandibular cheek tooth. Ideally, when trimming or floating the cheek teeth, the procedure should be done with power equipment (e.g., flat fissure bur) to ensure rapid tooth removal without damaging the surrounding tissue. The use of rasps or clippers can create friction and rock the teeth, causing periapical and periodontal damage. For this reason, these tools are not recommended or should be used with extreme caution. Extraction of the cheek teeth is much more complicated than removal of the incisor and more traumatic to the rabbit. (Crossley DA, personal communication) When several extractions are required, it is best to perform multiple procedures to minimize the pain and discomfort to the animal. For example, extracting the teeth on one side of the jaw will allow the animal to still use the opposite side to process its food. (Cheek tooth extraction is discussed in detail in Surgery.)

Incisor and cheek tooth root elongation can result in an overall deterioration of the tooth quality. Affected animals often present with epiphora, mandibular swelling, or nasal discharge. If left undiagnosed and untreated, root elongation can lead to abscess formation and osteomyelitis. Dental or skull radiographs can be used to evaluate the roots of the teeth, and if any are diseased, extraction should be considered.

Mucoid enteropathy is a poorly understood condition that causes both constipation and diarrhea, especially in young rabbits. The etiology of this disease is unknown, but it may be associated with a reduction in cecal pH. Feeding rabbits a diet that is high in fiber appears to control cecal pH and reduce the likelihood of this disease. Because the etiology of this disease is unknown, treatment is based on providing supportive care, antibiotics against opportunistic bacteria, and probiotics.

Rabbits are susceptible to a number of different infectious and parasitic diseases, many of which affect the gastrointestinal system. (A review of those diseases can be found in Infectious Disease.)

DISEASES OF THE RESPIRATORY SYSTEM

Upper respiratory tract disease (URTD) is a common presentation in rabbits. Affected rabbits often present with rhinitis and sinusitis. There are numerous potential causes of URTD in rabbits, including bacterial infections (e.g., *P. multocida*, *B. bronchiseptica*, and *Staphylococcus* spp.), foreign bodies, dental abscesses, and myxomatosis. Rabbits with URTD are often anorectic, as they cannot smell or locate their food. Serous to purulent nasal discharge is common. Epiphora is also a common finding. Many rabbits with clinical disease have *snuffles*. This is a generic term used to describe clinical signs, but it is attributed primarily to pasteurellosis. It is important to recognize that snuffles is nonspecific and may be associated with any of the previously mentioned causes. Rabbits with URTD often have "wet" forelegs as a result of the chronic nasal discharge. In severe cases of URTD, when a rabbit cannot move air through its nasal passages, it becomes dyspneic and breathes with an open mouth. Hematologic testing (e.g., CBC), culture and antibiotic sensitivity testing, radiographs, and endoscopy may be required to diagnose a specific cause of URTD. Treatment should be based on a specific diagnosis. Animals that are dehydrated and anorectic should be provided fluids and caloric support.

In rabbits, lower respiratory tract disease is primarily associated with bacterial disease. Gram-negative bacteria (e.g., *P. multocida, B. bronchiseptica, Klebsiella* spp.) are the most common cause of pneumonia in rabbits. Although not as common, Gram-positive bacteria *(Staphylococcus aureus)* have also been associated with pneumonia. Viral diseases are not well-studied but likely play a limited role. Primary lung neoplasia can occur, but it is not common. Rabbits are more likely to develop secondary metastasis. Rabbits with pneumonia may present in either an acute or chronic disease state. Rabbits with acute pneumonia are often acutely depressed, lethargic, and anorectic. The rabbits may or may not have audible respiratory sounds (e.g., wheezing, crackling). On physical examination, the rabbit may be febrile, have nasal discharge, and have auscultable respiratory wheezing or crackling. With chronic pneumonic presentations, the rabbit may appear clinically normal (e.g., walking pneumonia) but may have abnormal lung sounds. Beyond the physical examination, a CBC, survey radiographs, tracheal wash with cytologic examination and culture and antibiotic sensitivity profile, and endoscopic examination can be used to diagnose the pneumonic condition and establish a prognosis. Pneumonia in rabbits generally carries a poor to grave prognosis. Treatment should be based on the diagnostic results. Fluoroquinolones and potentiated sulfonamides are excellent first-choice antibiotics, as they have excellent distribution to the lungs.

CARDIAC DISEASE

Cardiac disease is a problem being encountered with increased frequency in captive rabbits. The primary reason for this is improved husbandry and the resultant increased longevity. Rabbits with cardiac disease may be dyspneic, tachypneic, exercise intolerant, lethargic, and depressed and have edematous extremities. A complete diagnostic work-up is required to characterize the status of the patient and provide the client a prognosis. Beyond a physical examination and careful cardiac auscultation, suspect cardiac cases should have an electrocardiogram done to determine if there are any abnormal arrhythmias, survey radiographs to evaluate heart and great vessel size, and an echocardiogram to assess the valves, muscle thickness, and cardiac function. A CT scan or MRI can also be done to evaluate the heart in more detail.

Cardiomyopathy can occur in all breeds, but it occurs at a higher incidence in giant breeds.[2] Affected animals often develop myocardial fibrosis. A number of different causal factors have been associated with cardiomyopathy in rabbits, including bacterial and corona-virus infections and vitamin E deficiency. Arteriosclerosis is also a common finding in rabbits fed a vitamin D and calcium-rich diet. Although a diagnosis

of arteriosclerosis is most often made at necropsy, in some cases, a diagnosis can be made from survey radiographs. An increased mineralized density in the aorta is the most common radiographic finding.

Congestive heart failure is common in middle-aged to geriatric rabbits. Rabbits with congestive heart failure should be stabilized and the excess burden on the heart controlled. Furosemide (1-4 mg/kg IV or IM) and 2% nitroglycerine ointment ($\frac{1}{8}$ strip on the ear) can be used to eliminate excess fluid and improve contractility.[4] In cases of pleural effusion, a thoracocentesis may be performed. After the animal's immediate condition is stabilized, further work should focus on diagnosing the cause of the congestive heart failure. Because rabbit cardiac drug doses are empirical and frequently inaccessible, doses for cats or ferrets can be used.[4] It is important to monitor rabbits for adverse effects to cardiac drugs, as would be done in domestic pets.

HEAT STROKE

Rabbits are extremely sensitive to elevated environmental temperature, especially when combined with high humidity. Because rabbits are unable to sweat, and panting is inefficient for them, they rely on the large surface area of the ears to serve as the site of evaporative cooling. Rabbits with heat stroke may present for lethargy, lateral recumbency, dyspnea, cyanosis, diarrhea, hyperthermia (>104° F), and seizures. Heat stroke carries a grave prognosis. Cooling a hyperthermic rabbit too quickly can lead to iatrogenic hypothermia, which can exacerbate the physiologic shock the animal experiences. In addition to cool water baths, 70% isopropyl alcohol can be applied to the ears and extremities to facilitate body cooling. An intravenous catheter should be placed, and fluids should be provided to maintain the intracellular and extracellular fluid balance. Antiinflammatories (e.g., meloxicam and carprofen) should be administered to minimize the catastrophic effects of the inflammatory response. Parenteral antibiotics are warranted to minimize the impact of opportunistic infections. Because some of the deleterious effects associated with heat stroke are not immediately apparent (e.g., cell death resulting from fluid shift), veterinarians should monitor animals closely for 7 to 14 days after the presentation.

■ THERAPEUTICS

Many of the therapeutics used to treat dogs and cats can also be used to manage rabbit patients, which reduces the burden of maintaining an appropriate rabbit pharmacy for the veterinarian. However, in some cases, it may be necessary for the veterinarian to obtain rabbit-specific formulations, that are flavored (e.g., fruity) or more specific to the needs of the rabbit. Fortunately, there are a number of compounding pharmacies that can assist with designing specific formulations for these animals. The following section is an introduction to the therapeutics commonly used to treat rabbits in captivity. (For a more extensive list, see Carpenter, JW: *Exotic Animal Formulary,* St. Louis, 2005, WB Saunders.)

Fluid Therapy

Rabbits that are dehydrated require immediate attention. The redistribution of fluids that results from dehydration can lead to a number of internal changes. One of these changes, occurring when fluid is resorbed from the intestinal tract, can lead to reduced intestinal motility and catastrophic changes to the microflora.

The maintenance fluid rate for rabbits is 80 to 100 ml/kg/day. For rehydration the rate can be increased to 10 to 20 ml/kg/hr over the first few hours.[9] In addition to providing the maintenance fluids for an anorectic rabbit, the veterinarian should also estimate and correct the animal's fluid deficit. Skin elasticity, mucous membrane moisture, capillary refill time, femoral pulse, positioning of the globe, and packed cell volume and total solids concentration are useful indicators for assessing dehydration. Slowed skin elasticity and tacky mucous membranes generally suggest an animal is 3% to 5% dehydrated. Those findings, in combination with a decreased capillary refill time, increased packed cell volume and total solids, and increased "thready" pulse, suggest 5% to 8% dehydration. All of these findings, in combination with the presence of sunken eyes, suggest an animal is more than 8% dehydrated. It is essential that the fluid deficit be replaced promptly (e.g., over 24 hours) to reestablish the fluid balance between the extra- and intracellular spaces.

When selecting fluids for replacement, it is important to consider the rabbit's physiologic status. Animals with elevated osmolalities should be provided hypotonic fluids to prevent worsening the fluid dynamics. Normasol (293 mOsm/L), lactated Ringer's (273 mOsm/L), and 0.9% saline (308 mOsm/L) represent isotonic crystalloids that can be used for fluid replacement. Dextrose (253 mOsm/L) can also be used, especially if the animal is hypoglycemic or if there is a need to rapidly replace the intracellular space. Animals that are hypoproteinemic may require colloid fluid replacement. Colloids can be used to offset the loss of oncotic pressure that can occur with hypoalbuminemia. Rabbits that are anemic may also require a blood transfusion or oxyglobin, a synthetic hemoglobin replacement. All rabbit patients should be monitored closely during fluid replacement so that neither fluid overload nor insufficient fluid replacement occurs. Pulmonary edema, ascites, and/or anasarca may occur in animals provided excess fluids. Animals provided insufficient fluids will remain clinically dehydrated. In these cases, the fluid deficit should be reevaluated and the appropriate fluid volume provided.

Fluids can be delivered per os (PO), subcutaneously (SC), intravenously (IV), intraosseously (IO), or intraperitoneally (IP). The route of administration should be based on the needs of the rabbit. If the animals is mildly dehydrated and has a functional gastrointestinal tract (e.g., no diarrhea), then fluids should be provided PO. This represents the natural route of fluid administration. For mildly dehydrated animals that will not tolerate PO fluids or have diarrhea, SC fluids are recommended. SC fluids can be administered on the dorsum between the scapulae or over the lateral body wall. Animals that are moderately to severely dehydrated should be given fluids IV

or IO. The primary IV sites we use are the cephalic, lateral saphenous, or auricular veins. The site for catheter placement should be sterilely prepared before catheter placement. The largest bore catheter that can be fitted comfortably into the vein should be used. For most large breeds, a 20- or 22-gauge catheter can be used, whereas a 24-gauge or 26-gauge catheter may be required for smaller breeds. A smaller bore catheter should be used for the auricular vein. The peripheral site for IO catheter placement is the femur. A surgical preparation using a disinfectant (e.g., Betadine or chlorhexidine) should be done to minimize contamination at the catheter site. A local anesthetic should be used to minimize the discomfort associated with the procedure. The trochanteric fossa is the landmark for catheter insertion. A spinal needle should be used for the procedure, as it has a stylet and will prevent the needle from being clogged with a bone core. The IO route is preferred in cases where the animal is severely dehydrated and the veins are collapsed. IP fluids are generally reserved for moderately dehydrated rabbits when IO or IV catheters are not available or for juvenile rabbits. To administer these fluids, place the rabbit in dorsal recumbency and insert the needle in the caudal abdomen. The needle should be inserted at a 20- to 30-degree angle to the body. Aspirating before delivering the fluids should ensure that the needle is not in the viscera.

Antimicrobial Therapy
ANTIBACTERIAL AND ANTIFUNGAL AGENTS

Antimicrobial therapy is ideally based on culture and antibiotic sensitivity testing. When selecting an antimicrobial for a rabbit, it is important to avoid those compounds that may predispose the rabbit to dysbiosis, such as lincomycin, ampicillin, amoxicillin, amoxicillin-clavulanic acid, cephalosporins, clindamycin, penicillins, and erythromycin. Because most infections in rabbits are associated with opportunistic Gram-negative bacteria, initial antibiotic selection should be based on broad coverage against these bacteria. Enrofloxacin and trimethoprim-sulfadiazine are two excellent first-choice antibiotics. For a complete list of antibiotic compounds, see Box 14-3. A list of common antifungal compounds can be found in Box 14-4.

Antiparasitic Therapy

Rabbits are susceptible to a number of endo- and ectoparasites. The most common endoparasites are coccidia and nematodes. The drugs and doses commonly used to treat these parasites are found in Box 14-5. Ectoparasites, including mites and lice, are also common.

Nonsteroidal Antiinflammatories

Nonsteroidal antiinflammatories (NSAIDs) are routinely used to manage inflammation and pain in rabbits. Some of their most common uses include treating musculoskeletal pain associated with trauma, arthritis, soft tissue pain from dental disease, and gastric stasis. Historically, flunixin meglumine was

BOX 14-3 **Antibiotic Agents Commonly Used to Treat Bacterial Infections in Rabbits**

Chloramphenicol	30 mg/kg PO BID
Ciprofloxacin	10-20 mg/kg PO BID
	Ophthalmic 0.3%: 1 drop BID-TID
Enrofloxacin	5 mg/kg PO, SC, IM, IV BID[35]
Metronidazole	20 mg/kg PO BID
	40 mg/kg PO SID × 3 days
Penicillin	40,000-60,000 IU/kg SC, IM SID × 5-7 days
Penicillin G, benzathine	42,000-60,000 IU/kg SC, IM q48h
Penicillin G procaine	42,000-84,000 IU/kg SC, IM SID
Rifampin/clarithromycin	R-40 mg/kg; C-80 mg/kg PO BID
Silver sulfadiazine	Topical SID; safe if ingested
Sulfadimethoxine	10-15 mg/kg PO BID
Trimethoprim sulfadimethoxine	30 mg/kg PO BID

From Carpenter JW, Mashima TY, Rupiper DJ: *Exotic Animal Formulary*, ed 2, Philadelphia, 2001, WB Saunders.
BID, twice a day; *IM*, intramuscular; *IU*, international unit; *IV*, intravenous; *PO*, per os; *SC*, subcutaneous; *SID*, once a day; *TID*, three times a day.

BOX 14-4 **Antifungal Drugs Commonly Used to Treat Rabbits**

Clotrimazole	Topical
Fluconazole	25-43 mg/kg IV slowly BID
Ketoconazole	10-40 mg/kg PO SID × 14 days
Lime-sulfur dip (2%-3%)	Topical q 5-7 days × 4 wk
Miconazole	Topical SID × 2-4 wk

BID, twice a day; *PO*, per os; *SC*, subcutaneous; *SID*, once a day.

BOX 14-5 **Antiparasitic Drugs Commonly Used to Eliminate Parasites in Rabbits**

Drug	Dosage	Parasite
Albendazole	7.5-20 mg/kg PO SID	Nematodes; E. cuniculi
Ivermectin	0.4 mg/kg SC q7days × 2-3 wk	Nematodes, ectoparasites
Fenbendazole	20 mg/kg SID	E. cuniculi
	10 mg/kg PO, repeat in 14 days	Nematodes
Lime-sulfur dip (2%-3%)	Topically q7days × 4 wk	Ectoparasites
Sulfadimethoxine	10-15 mg/kg PO BID	Coccidia

BID, twice a day; *PO*, per os; *SC*, subcutaneous; *SID*, once a day.

BOX 14-6 **Nonsteroidal Antiinflammatory Drugs Commonly Used to Manage Inflammation and Pain in Rabbits**

Meloxicam	0.3 mg/kg PO SID
	0.2 mg/kg IM or SC SID
Flunixin meglumine	1-2 mg/kg IM or SC BID; limit to 3 days to minimize gastric ulcer formation
Carprofen	2-4 mg/kg SC SID
	1.5 mg/kg PO BID
Ketoprofen	3 mg/kg IM or SC BID

BID, twice a day; *IM*, intramuscular; *PO*, per os; *SC*, subcutaneous; *SID*, once a day.

the only compound available for rabbits. This drug serves an important purpose in managing pain, but it has to be used judiciously because of the potential for gastric ulcer formation. The newer generation NSAIDs (e.g., carprofen and meloxicam) are more selective and less likely to cause complications. A list of commonly used NSAIDs and their doses can be found in Box 14-6.

Steroids

The use of steroidal compounds is controversial in rabbits. In the past, steroids have been recommended for managing inflammation associated with neurologic disease (e.g., trauma or *E. cuniculi* infection) or shock. However, hydrocortisone has been found to cause significant immunosuppression in rabbits.[36] Because of the high likelihood for immunosuppres-

sion, steroids should be used judiciously. We generally reserve their use for the treatment of spinal disease (prednisone sodium succinate, 1 mg/kg IV) and dermatologic conditions (e.g., flea bite allergy or extreme hypersensitivity) (prednisone, 0.5-1 mg/kg SID to BID, taper dose).

Cardiac Drugs

Long-term therapy for heart disease may require treatment with diuretics (furosemide, 1-4 mg/kg IM) and other compounds required for a particular cardiac disease presentation. The use of cat and ferret dosages for cardiac drugs is advocated. Monitoring for drug side effects should be done as in feline medicine.

Emergency Drugs

Rabbits that develop respiratory or cardiac arrest should be treated immediately with the appropriate emergency drugs. Dopram may be used for respiratory arrest, whereas epineph-

BOX 14-7 **Emergency Drugs Commonly Used to Treat Rabbits**

Epinephrine	0.2 mg/kg IV or IT
Furosemide	1-4 mg/kg IM
Hetastarch	20 ml/kg IV
Lactated Ringer's solution	10-20 ml/kg/hr
Lidocaine	1-2 mg/kg IV

IM, intramuscular; *IT*, intratracheal; *IV*, intravenous.

rine should be administered during cardiac arrest. A list of commonly used emergency drugs and their doses is listed in Box 14-7. Rabbits have atropinases, so the use of atropine is not commonly recommended. Glycopyrrolate can be used to help manage bradycardia; however, it is important to consider that this compound can increase the viscosity of tracheal secretions and impede the airflow to the lungs. Intubating and ventilating animals can minimize this risk.

Transfusions

In cases of severe anemia (PCV < 10%) or acute blood loss (20%-25%), a blood transfusion is recommended. The blood volume of a rabbit is estimated to be between 55 and 65 ml/kg.[37] Cross-matching for transfusion in rabbits is not necessary for a first-time recipient.[37] The donor must be healthy and must not have a history of infectious disease or neoplasia. A healthy blood donor can have up to 10 ml/kg of blood collected. The jugular vein is the recommended site for blood collection from the donor rabbit. The blood should be collected with a citrate anticoagulant that is mixed with blood at a rate of 1 : 3.5 (citrate : donor blood). The blood transfusion should be done within 4 to 6 hours of collection at a rate of 6 to 12 ml/kg/hr.

Nutritional Support

Anorexia in rabbits should be treated as an emergency. When rabbits stop eating, physiologic changes can occur in the gastrointestinal tract (e.g., mucosal atrophy) that alter the gastrointestinal permeability. From this, a cascade of events can occur (e.g., reduced motility, decreased water absorption, pH alterations, microbial flora changes) that lead the animal into a life-threatening situation. The first step in managing these cases should be to restimulate the gastrointestinal tract, and the second step is to diagnose the cause of the anorexia. Providing nutritional support is the best method for restimulating the gastrointestinal tract. Motility modifiers can also be used, but these should be given only when there is no concern for a gastric or small intestine foreign body (e.g., trichobezoar).

The preferred method for administering nutritional support to mild or moderately ill animals is syringe feeding. In more severe cases, an orogastric tube or nasogastric tube should be

placed. A 3.5- to 5.0-French pediatric feeding tube can be used as a nasogastric tube. Before placing the tube, it should be marked to estimate the distance between the nare and the stomach. Placement can be achieved by inserting the tube through the ventral medial nasal meatus and advancing it ventromedially. The rabbit's head should be maintained in a natural position during the procedure to facilitate passage of the tube. Placement of the tube should be evaluated using survey radiographs. Once placed, the tube can be secured to the skin covering the nasal bones using suture. A pharyngostomy or gastrotomy tube can also be placed to facilitate feeding.

Enteral diets used for dogs or cats are not appropriate for use in rabbits. The domestic pet enterals are based on the nutritional needs of omnivores (dogs) and carnivores (cats) and will not meet the needs of an herbivore (rabbit). Oxbow critical care for herbivores (Oxbow Pet Products, Murdock, NE) is our preferred enteral. High-fiber Ensure or Ensure plus (Ross Laboratories, Columbus, OH) can also be used, but, again, these are not considered ideal. Although less complete, a variety of other pelleted rations, leafy greens, and vegetable baby foods can also be used as enterals.[9] Label directions should be followed closely to ensure that the rabbit receives the appropriate quantity of calories. In cases where homemade diets are used, calorie content of the enteral constituents should be estimated or determined using available resources in the literature or on the Internet. The provision of nutritional support should continue until the rabbit is free-feeding on its own.

■ SURGERY

Preoperative and Postoperative Considerations

Although fasting is not necessary in rabbits because they cannot vomit, eliminating access to food 1 to 2 hours before inducing anesthesia minimizes the amount of food in the oral cavity and improves the direct visualization of the larynx for intubation. We recommend performing presurgical blood work to determine the physiologic status of the rabbit patient. This information can be used to provide the client with a prognosis related to the anesthetic procedure. Any rabbit with preexisting respiratory disease should be thoroughly evaluated before it undergoes a procedure. Rabbits have a small lung capacity, and any pulmonary disease can have a negative impact on the anesthesia event.

Postoperative considerations for rabbits include minimizing the likelihood for anorexia, providing analgesia and antibiotics (when necessary), and monitoring fluid therapy. Thermal support should be provided until the rabbit has recovered and can maintain a normal body temperature. Rabbits should be recovered in a quiet area. Excessive noise or commotion can lead to increased stress (e.g., increased cortisol), immunosuppression, and decreased healing. Animals should be offered their normal food for a prolonged stay and a comfortable substrate in their cages.

Anesthesia

Anesthetic selection should be based on the procedure being performed. For example, in a case where a localized abscess needs to be lanced, a local anesthetic (e.g., lidocaine, prilocaine) and an opioid can be used to perform the procedure. Many veterinarians anesthetize rabbits using only inhalant anesthesia. Rabbits can be induced using a face mask or induction chamber. We prefer to induce rabbits with additional compounds before we provide inhalants, because it more effectively relaxes the animal for intubation. A benzodiazepam (e.g., diazepam, midazolam) and opioid are routinely used to provide relaxation and analgesia before inducing the animal. Other commonly used veterinary anesthetics (e.g., ketamine HCl, medetomidine, acepromazine) and analgesics can also be used for induction or as maintenance anesthetics. Doses for these compounds can be found in Tables 14-2, 14-3, and 14-4. One compound that should be avoided is Telazol (Fort Dodge Animal Health, Fort Dodge, IA), as it has been shown to cause severe renal tubular necrosis in rabbits.[38]

We recommend intubating rabbits for any procedure that requires general anesthesia. When an animal is intubated, it gives the anesthetist more control over the patient. Rabbits that are not intubated and experience respiratory arrest are rarely recovered. Intubating rabbits can be difficult. These animals have long, narrow oral cavities, which restrict direct visualization of the larynx. Several techniques have been described for intubating rabbits. Blind intubation using a 2.0

TABLE 14-2 Induction and General Anesthetics for Rabbits

Agent	Dose (mg/kg)	Route	Sedation	Analgesia
Acepromazine	1 mg/kg	IM	++	*
Diazepam/midazolam	0.5-2 mg/kg	IV, IM	+ to ++	*
Fentanyl (can cause respiratory depression; can be partially reversed with buprenorphine)	0.2-0.5 mg/kg	IM	+ to +++	+ to +++
Glycopyrrolate	0.01 mg/kg	IV		
	0.1 mg/kg	SC, IM		
Ketamine	10-50 mg/kg	IM	++ to +++	+
Medetomidine (reversible with atipamizole)	0.1-0.5 mg/kg	IM	+ to +++	+
Xylazine (reversible with atipamizole 1 mg/kg or yohimbine 0.2 mg/kg IV)	2-5 mg/kg	IM	+ to ++	+
Propofol (light anesthesia; can cause apnea, use with caution in un-intubated patients)	3-6 mg/kg	IV		

From Harcourt-Brown F: *Textbook of Rabbit Medicine*, London, 2002, Elsevier; Flecknell P: *Laboratory Animal Anaesthesia*, ed 2, San Diego, 1996, Academic Press.
IM, intramuscular; *IV*, intravenous; *SC*, subcutaneous.
*, none; +, minimal; ++, moderate; +++, heavy.

TABLE 14-3 Analgesics Commonly Used for Captive Rabbits

Agents	Dose (mg/kg)	Route	Comments
Buprenorphine	0.01-0.05	IV, SC	Analgesia for 6-12 h; for acute soft tissue, GI, and urogenital pain
Oxymorphone	0.05-0.2	IM, SC	q8-12h
Butorphanol	0.1-0.5	IM, SC, IV	Analgesia lasts 2-4 h; can be used with acepromazine to deliver sedation
Fentanyl	0.2-0.3	IM	
Carprofen	2-4	SC	q24h
	1.5	PO	q12h
Meloxicam	0.2	IM, SC	q12h
	0.3	PO	
Flunixin meglumine	1-2	IM, SC	q12h
Ketoprofen	3	IM, SC	q12h

From Harcourt-Brown F: *Textbook of Rabbit Medicine*, London, 2002, Elsevier; Heard DJ: Anesthesia, analgesia, and sedation of small mammals. In Queensberry KE, Carpenter JW, editors: *Ferrets, Rabbits and Rodents: Clinical Medicine and Surgery*, St Louis, 2004, WB Saunders; Paul-Murphy J, Ramer JC: Urgent care of the pet rabbit, *Vet Clin North Am Exot Anim Pract* 1(1):125-152, 1998.
IM, intramuscular; *IV*, intravenous; *PO*, per os; *SC*, subcutaneous.

TABLE 14-4	Common Anesthetic Combinations Used to Anesthetize Rabbits		
Agents	Dose (mg/kg)	Route	Duration/anesthesia
Medetomidine Ketamine Butorphanol	0.2 mg/kg 10 mg/kg 0.05 mg/kg	SC, IM	Anesthesia 30-40 min; recovery 1-4 h
Fentanyl Midazolam	0.3 ml/kg 0.5-2 mg/kg	IM IV	Anesthesia 20-40 min with good muscle relaxation; recovery 1-2 h
Ketamine Xylazine	20-35 mg/kg 3-5 mg/kg	IM/IV	Anesthesia 25-35 min; recovery 1-2 h
Ketamine Diazepam	20-35 mg/kg 1-5 mg/kg	IM/IV	Anesthesia 20-30 min; recovery 1½ h

From Harcourt-Brown F: *Textbook of Rabbit Medicine*, London, 2002, Elsevier; Flecknell P: *Laboratory Animal Anesthesia*, ed 2, San Diego, 1996, Academic Press.
IM, intramuscular; *IV*, intravenous; *PO*, per os; *SC*, subcutaneous.

to 2.5 outside diameter (OD) endotracheal tube can be done, but it can be associated with laryngeal trauma.[9] To perform the procedure, the head should be elevated and neck stretched. The endotracheal tube should be gently lowered into the trachea. This technique requires patience and skill. Practicing this technique on recently expired rabbits is one way of obtaining experience with this procedure. Our preferred method for intubating rabbits is via an endoscope.[39] A 2.7-mm rigid endoscope can be used to directly visualize the larynx and ensure passage of the tube into the trachea. In those cases where laryngospasms limit access to the trachea, lidocaine can be applied topically.

Rabbits should be monitored closely during a surgical procedure. An ultrasonic Doppler, ECG, and/or pulse oximeter can be used to monitor the heart rate and rhythm during the procedure. A respiratory monitor can be used to monitor respirations. We prefer to use a ventilator during rabbit procedures to ensure that the rabbit is receiving an appropriate dose of anesthesia and oxygen. The ventilator also ensures that the animal is respiring. A capnograph can be added in line to measure carbon dioxide levels and determine the rabbit's respiratory efficiency. In addition to the capnograph, the pulse oximeter can provide additional blood gas information by providing an estimate of oxygen saturation levels. Rabbits should be provided thermal support during a procedure, and its body temperature should be measured throughout the procedure. Routine anesthetic monitoring during a procedure is essential to a veterinarian's success and will limit the occurrence of anesthetic deaths.

Surgical Procedures

The majority of the surgical procedures performed on rabbits are associated with the reproductive tract, gastrointestinal tract, and integument. Of course, a rabbit can develop a need for surgical procedures on other systems as well, but, in our experience, they are less common. When faced with the need to perform a surgery on a rabbit, the veterinarian must identify the specific anatomic features that will be affected by the procedures and familiarize himself or herself with any specific

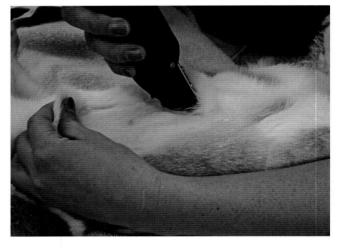

Figure 14-20 When shaving rabbit fur for a surgical procedure, be careful to avoid tearing the delicate skin.

indications on tissue handling methods. In cases where there are no specific descriptions for a surgical procedure in rabbits, veterinarians may rely on those surgical descriptions reported in canine and feline surgery.

When preparing a rabbit for surgery, it is important to adhere to strict aseptic techniques. Because rabbit skin is thin and tears easily, care should be taken when clipping the fur. We generally clip the fur with a small, battery-powered clipper or shave the fur with a razor. Holding the skin tight during fur removal can help reduce the likelihood of tearing the skin (Figure 14-20). There are a variety of methods that can be used to aseptically prepare a surgical site. Chlorhexidine and Betadine are excellent disinfectants. We generally use physiologic saline instead of alcohol during the preparation because it does not act as a heat sink, lowering the rabbit's body temperature.

The surgical instruments used for domestic pet surgery can also be used for rabbit surgery. Because of the small size of some dwarf rabbit breeds, ophthalmic instruments can also be beneficial. Microscopic loupes are helpful when manipulating fine tissues. Radiosurgery can be used to provide hemostasis during a procedure and minimize tissue trauma.

REPRODUCTIVE SURGERY

Orchiectomy or ovariohysterectomy should be recommended for rabbits when the pet owner has no interest in reproducing the animal. This prevents unwanted pregnancies in mixed gender populations, reduces the risk for certain neoplastic conditions, and can reduce the likelihood for certain behaviors (e.g., aggression in males). It is generally recommended that males be castrated after 3 months of age and females be spayed after 5 months. The procedure can be performed at an earlier age if deemed appropriate, such as may be the case in large, mixed colonies, but this may affect the growth of the animal (e.g., smaller size).

Orchiectomy

The inguinal canals of a rabbit are open throughout the animal's life. Therefore, a male rabbit can actively move its testicles between the scrotum and body cavity. Because the inguinal canals remain open, it is important to either perform a closed orchiectomy, or to close the inguinal canal after performing an open orchiectomy. If the inguinal canals are left open, it is possible for the animal to herniate omentum or bowel into the scrotal area.

There are two approaches that can be taken when making an initial incision. Either a prescrotal incision can be made, similar to that made for the dog, or scrotal incisions can be made, similar to those recommended for the cat. When performing the scrotal approach, each testicle is removed through a separate incision. If the tunic is not incised, a closed procedure can be done. At least two sutures should be placed on the cord in case a suture fails. Once ligated, the cords can be replaced into the scrotum, and the scrotum closed with an absorbable suture using a subcuticular pattern. Tissue glue can also be used to complete the skin closure. For the prescrotal incision, each testicle must be retrograded out of the incision. The same technique described earlier can be used for the orchiectomy, or a suture can be placed around the tunic at the cranial aspect of the incision, an open castration done, the remnant cord directed cranially past the suture placement, and the suture ligature tied down to close the canal. Again, a subcuticular closure or tissue glue can be used to close the skin incision. The animal should be monitored postoperatively for any swelling or discharge in the area of the incision or scrotum.

Ovariohysterectomy

An ovariohysterectomy should be recommended for any female rabbit not intended for breeding. It is recommended that the procedure be done when the animal is young (<5 months of age) because the amount of intraabdominal fat can increase dramatically with age and will reduce the surgeon's visibility. The incision for a rabbit ovariohysterectomy should be made from cranial to the pelvis to the umbilicus. The incision may need to be extended in some cases. Care should be taken when entering the peritoneal cavity, as the urinary bladder and/or

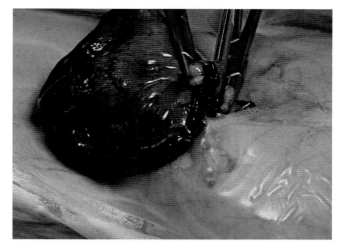

Figure 14-21 A rabbit reproductive tract. Note the two cervices.

cecum may be directly under the body wall. The ovaries are located in the same location as would be expected for a cat or dog. The ovaries can generally be grasped by hand, but a spay hook may be needed for some large breeds. Once the ovary is in hand, the ovarian pedicle should be identified. Circumferential sutures (at least two) should be placed around the pedicle, and the pedicle incised. The ovary and uterine horns should be gently grasped and elevated from the body cavity. Rabbits have two separate uterine horns, each with its own cervix (Figure 14-21). Each uterine horn should be ligated just cranial to its cervix. A circumferential and transfixation suture can be used to ligate the uterine horn. The large uterine vessels running parallel to the uterine horns should also be ligated at this time. Closure for an ovariohysterectomy is routine. The body wall, subcutaneous space, and subcuticular space can be closed with absorbable suture in a continuous pattern.

TEETH EXTRACTIONS

Incisor removal in rabbits should be done under general anesthesia. The gingival surfaces surrounding the base of the incisors should be thoroughly cleaned and disinfected. The peg teeth (second upper incisors) should be removed first. A dental elevator can be inserted in a 360-degree manner around the base of the tooth to separate the periodontal ligament. The tooth, when loose, can be gently extracted. For the large primary incisors, the elevator or incisor luxator blade can be used to perform the same procedure (Figure 14-22). Care should be taken when manipulating the tooth to prevent fracture. Once the tooth is loosened, gently rock it and pull it in the direction of the natural curvature. If the pulp tissue is not removed with the tooth, curette the socket with a sterile probe to destroy any remaining germinal tissue. If there is evidence of infection, treatment should include flushing with a disinfectant and the provision of systemic antibiotics.

Cheek teeth extractions can be done in a similar manner to incisor extractions. Anesthetize the patient, clean and disinfect

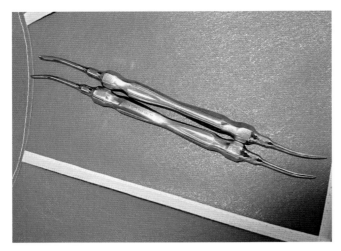

Figure 14-22 Incisor tooth elevators can be used to facilitate extraction.

the teeth and gingiva, and use a molar luxator to break down the periodontal fibers that secure the tooth to the bone. Molar forceps can be used to extract the cheek teeth. Mandibular cheek teeth extraction can also be performed via surgical access from the ventrolateral border of the mandible. In this case, the teeth are elevated from the apical end.

GASTROINTESTINAL SURGERY

In cases where gastric foreign bodies (e.g., carpet or hair) cannot be successfully treated medically, surgery should be attempted. However, it is important that owners be informed that the prognosis for gastrotomies in rabbits is poor. The prognosis can be improved if the surgical procedure is performed before the animal's condition worsens (e.g., hepatic lipidosis, bowel rupture). Before the surgical procedure is attempted, it is important to correct any fluid deficits or nutritional anomalies (e.g., hepatic lipidosis).

The approach to a gastrotomy in rabbits is similar to that described for domestic animals. An incision should be made that extends from the umbilicus to just caudal to the xiphoid process. The entire abdominal cavity should be explored, and any abnormalities noted. Biopsies of the liver may be collected to assess the status of the organ. The stomach should be isolated and surrounded with moist lap pads. Two stay sutures should be placed in the greater curvature of the stomach and an incision made in the avascular region between the greater and lesser curvature. The gastric contents should be removed using a sterile spoon. Once emptied, the stomach should be lavaged. The pylorus should be palpated to confirm its patency. The stomach should be closed using a two-layer inverting pattern with absorbable monofilament suture (3-0 or 4-0). The abdomen should be lavaged with warm saline before being closed. Closure of the body wall, subcutaneous space, and subcuticular space are routine. Intestinal resection and anastomosis and enterotomies are similar to other small animals.

INTEGUMENTARY SURGERY
Lateral Ear Canal Resection

Otitis can be a chronic, frustrating disease in rabbits. Pet owners often become disillusioned with the constant medical treatments required to care for their pets. In cases where medical management is not successful, surgery should be considered. Lateral ear resection has been found to provide relief to both the rabbit patient and the pet owner. The approach to the lateral ear resection is similar to that described for dogs. For the procedure, the rabbit should be placed in lateral recumbency. Two parallel incisions should be made at the base of the ear that follow into the line of the pinna. The skin and subcutaneous tissue should be dissected free and reflected rostrally to reveal the vertical canal. An additional two parallel incisions are made into the lateral wall of the vertical canal. The cartilage should be carefully dissected to avoid the auricular veins. The dissection should continue to the level of the horizontal ear canal. Once exposed, the flap of cartilage is removed and the cartilage of the horizontal and vertical canals is sutured to the surrounding subcutaneous and skin tissues using absorbable suture. Rabbits should be maintained in the hospital for a minimum of 5 to 7 days to ensure that the surgical site is disinfected daily and does not dehisce.[32]

In severe, chronic cases of otitis interna, when rabbits have nystagmus, head tilt, and radiographic abnormalities in the bulla(e), a total ear canal ablation and tympanic bulla(e) osteoectomy can be performed. For the procedure, the rabbit should be placed in lateral recumbency and the area around the base of the ear clipped and prepped. The skin at the base of the ear should be incised, and the lateral wall of the ear canal dissected away from the subcutaneous tissue without entering the canal. During the dissection process, it is important to remain close to the auricular cartilage to avoid damaging the rostral and caudal auricular veins. Next, the horizontal tract of the ear canal should be dissected down to the junction of the tympanic bulla. At that point, the canal should be transected. The opening of the tympanic bulla should be widened (using needle drivers), debrided, and flushed. The subcutaneous tissue surrounding the ablated vertical canal should be closed with 3-0 absorbable suture. After closing the subcutaneous sites, the surgeon should close the tissue surrounding the bulla by marsupializing the opening to the bulla. This will allow for postoperative flushing.[32]

■ZOONOSES

Zoonotic diseases are not commonly associated with rabbits. Although not generally considered an important disease of domestic or wild rabbits, rabies has been diagnosed in several pet rabbits. The clinical course of rabies in rabbits is nonspecific, but affected animals are generally depressed and weak and exhibit paralytic signs. In areas where rabies is endemic and prevalent, rabbits housed outdoors need to be protected from exposure to mesopredators (e.g., raccoons, foxes, coyotes) that may serve as rabies vectors.[40] Additionally, *E. cuniculi, Cheyletiella,* ringworm, *Pasteurella* sp., *Salmonella* sp., tularemia, and *Mycobacterium* spp. have zoonotic potential to humans, especially in immunocompromised individuals.

REFERENCES

1. Carpenter JW, Mashima TY, Gentz EJ et al: Caring for rabbits: an overview and formulary, *Vet Med Rabbit Symposium: Rabbits Are Not Small Cats,* pp 348-380, April 1995.
2. Harcourt-Brown F: *Textbook of Rabbit Medicine,* London, 2002, Elsevier.
3. Hillyer EV: Pet rabbits, *Vet Clin North Am Small Anim Pract* 24(1):25-64, 1994.
4. Paré JA, Paul-Murphy J: Disorders of the reproductive and urinary systems. In Queensberry KE, Carpenter JW, editors: *Ferrets, Rabbits and Rodents: Clinical Medicine and Surgery,* St Louis, 2004, WB Saunders.
5. Harkness JE: Rabbit husbandry and medicine, *Vet Clin North Am Small Anim Pract* 17(5):1019-1044, 1987.
6. Greenway JG, Partlow GD, Gonsholt NL et al: Anatomy of the lumbosacral spinal cord in rabbits, *JAAHA* 37:27-34, 2001.
7. Crossley DA: Oral biology and disorders of lagomorphs, *Vet Clin North Am Exot Anim Pract* 6:629-659, 2003.
8. Jenkins JR: Feeding recommendations for the house rabbit, *Vet Clin North Am Exot Anim Pract* 2(1):143-151, 1999.
9. Paul-Murphy J, Ramer JC: Urgent care of the pet rabbit, *Vet Clin North Am Exot Anim Pract* 1(1):125-152, 1998.
10. Suckow MA, Brammer DW, Rush HG et al: Biology and diseases of rabbits. In Fox JG, Anderson LC, Loew FM, Chrisp CE, editors: *Laboratory Animal Medicine,* ed 2, San Diego, 2002, Academic Press.
11. Benson KG, Paul-Murphy J: Clinical pathology of the domestic rabbit, *Vet Clin North Am Exot Anim Pract* 2(3):539-551, 1999.
12. Fudge AM: *Laboratory Medicine: Avian and Exotic Pets,* Philadelphia, 2000, WB Saunders.
13. Johnson JH, Wolf AM: Ovarian abscesses and pyometra in a domestic rabbit, *JAVMA* 203(5):667-669, 1993.
14. Gentz EJ, Harrenstien LA, Carpenter JW: Dealing with gastrointestinal genitourinary and musculoskeletal problems in rabbits, *Vet Med* April 1995:365-372, 1995.
15. Meredith A: Skin diseases of rabbits, *Irish Vet J* 56(1):52-56, 2003.
16. Thouless ME, DiGiacomo RF, Deeb BJ et al: Pathogenicity of rotavirus in rabbits, *J Clin Microbiol* May 1988:943-947, 1988.
17. Schoeb TR, Casebolt DB, Walker VE et al: Rotavirus-associated diarrhea in a commercial rabbitry, *Lab Anim Sci* 36(2):149-152, 1986.
18. Harris IE: Rabbits: medicine and other veterinary aspects, *Aust Vet Prac* 18(1):6-10, 1988.
19. Kerr PJ, Best SM: Myxoma virus in rabbits, *Rev Sci Tech* 17(1):256-268, 1998.
20. DiGiacomo RF, Mare CF: Viral diseases. In Manning PJ, Ringler DH, Newcomer CE, editors: *The Biology of the Laboratory Rabbit,* ed 2, San Diego, 1994, Academic Press.
21. Harrenstien L, Gentz EJ, Carpenter JW: How to handle respiratory ophthalmic, neurologic and dermatologic problems in rabbits, *Vet Med* April 1995:373-380, 1995.
22. Harcourt-Brown FM, Holloway HKR: *Encephalocytozoon cuniculi* in pet rabbits, *Vet Rec* 152:427-431, 2003.
23. Pilny AA: *Encephalitozoon cuniculi*-associated phacoclastic uveitis in a dwarf rabbit, *Exot Health* 3:2, 2004.
24. Kazacos KR, Reed WM, Kazacos EA et al: Fatal cerebrospinal disease caused by *Baylisascaris procyonis* in domestic rabbits, *JAVMA* 183(9):967-971, 1983.
25. McTier TL, Hair JA: Efficacy and safety of topical administration of selamectin for treatment of ear mite infestation in rabbits, *JAVMA* 223(2):322-332, 2003.
26. Lee KJ, Johnson WD, Lang CM: Acute peritonitis in the rabbit *(Oryctolagus cuniculus)* resulting from a gastric trichobezoar, *Lab Anim Sci* 28(2):202-204, 1978.
27. Queensberry K: Nutritional and gastrointestinal diseases of rabbits, *Intern Med: Small Companion Anim Proc* 306:61, 1998.
28. *Physicians' Desk Reference,* ed 58, Montvale, NJ, 2004.
29. Taylor M: A wound packing technique for rabbit dental abscesses, *Exot DVM* 5(pt 3):28, 2003.
30. Carpenter JW, Mashima TY, Rupiper DJ: *Exotic Animal Formulary,* ed 2, Philadelphia, 2001, WB Saunders.
31. Weisbroth SH: Neoplastic disease. In Weisbroth SH, Flatt RE, Kraus AL editors: *The Biology of the Laboratory Rabbit,* New York, 1974, Academic Press.
32. Capello E: Surgical treatment of otitis external and media in pet rabbits, *Exot DVM* 6(pt 3):15, 2004.
33. Owiny JR, Vandewoude S, Painter JT et al: Hip dysplasia in rabbits, *Comp Med* 51(1):85-88, 2001.
34. Maurer KJ, Marini RP, Fox JG et al: Polycystic kidney syndrome in New Zealand White rabbits resembling human polycystic kidney disease, *Kidney Int* 65:482-489, 2004.
35. Broome RL, Brooks DL, Babish JG et al: Pharmacokinetic properties of enrofloxacin in rabbits, *Am J Vet Res* 52(11):1835-1841, 1991.
36. Nagornev VA, Zubzhiskii IuN, Pigarevskii PV et al: [Effect of hydrocortisone on the development of experimental atherosclerosis in rabbits] [Article in Russian], *Biull Eksp Biol Med* 90(10):407-409, 1980.
37. Flecknell P: *Laboratory Animal Anaesthesia,* ed 2, San Diego, 1996, Academic Press.
38. Doerning BJ, Brammer DW, Chrisp CE et al: Nephrotoxicity of Tiletamine in New Zealand White rabbits, *Lab Anim Sci* 42(3):267-269, 1992.
39. Worthley SG, Roque M, Helft G et al: Rapid oral endotracheal intubation with a fibre-optic scope in rabbits: a simple and reliable technique, *Lab Anim* 34:199-201, 2000.
40. Karp BE, Ball NE, Scott CR et al: Rabies in two privately owned domestic rabbits, *JAVMA* 215(12):1824-1827, 1999.

J. Jill Heatley
M. Camille Harris

CHAPTER 15

HAMSTERS AND GERBILS

■ COMMON SPECIES KEPT IN CAPTIVITY

Hamsters and gerbils are members of Rodentia, the largest order of mammals. Their name is derived from the Latin term *rodere,* meaning "to gnaw."

Hamsters

In addition to the golden or Syrian hamster *(Mesocricetus auratus),* which is the most common hamster used in research and maintained as a pet, there are several other species that the clinician may encounter. These include the Siberian or Djungarian hamster *(Phodopus sungorus),* the Chinese or striped hamster *(Cricetulus griseus),* the common black-bellied or European hamster *(C. cricetus),* and the gray Armenian hamster *(C. migratorius).* Hamsters are members of the family Muridae, subfamily Cricetinae, and comprise five genera dispersed across Europe and Asia.[1] In total there are 24 species of hamster in five genera found across Europe and Asia. Of these species in the wild, the golden hamster *(M. auratus),* of northwestern Syria, and *Calomyscus hotsoni* are endangered, and *M. newtoni* is considered vulnerable.[1]

The golden hamster is the largest of the common pet species, with an average body weight of 120 g. The golden hamster was originally described from a single specimen collected in 1839. In 1930, a female and her young were found in Syria, taken to Israel, and then bred and distributed to England and the United States.[1] All golden hamsters in captivity today descended from these original 13 hamsters captured in Syria. The golden hamster is nocturnal, solitary, and known for its pugnacious tendencies. Today, captive golden hamsters are primarily found in the wild-type or reddish-golden brown

hair coat with gray-white ventrum. Other coat color variations are the result of genetic mutation and include cinnamon, very dark brown, cream, white, piebald, albino, and long-haired "teddy bear" hair coats.[2]

Other hamster species commonly found in the pet trade are the Chinese hamster and the Siberian or dwarf hamster. Chinese hamsters were brought to the United States in 1948 and domesticated and reproduced in captivity beginning in 1949-1952.[3] Chinese hamsters, also known as striped back hamsters, are dark brown and smaller than Syrian hamsters. These hamsters are aggressive, solitary, and nocturnal with a body weight of 30 to 35 g; males are larger than females. Chinese hamsters have the lowest number of chromosomes (11; 2N = 22) of any lab animal but are difficult to breed in captivity.[3] Chinese hamsters are used as lab animal models for cytogenetics, diabetes mellitus, and toxicology research investigations.

Siberian hamsters are dwarf hamsters with an average body weight of 40 g. These hamsters have a gray pelage dorsally with a dorsal midline black stripe and a white ventrum. Also known as the Dzungarian hamster, this species is relatively tame and nonaggresive compared with other hamsters. Unlike Syrian hamsters, this species is colonial and can be housed in family groups.[4] Male hamsters will attend to the young. Dzungarian hamsters are used for research of photoperiod, the pineal gland, and thermoregulation.

Gerbils

The Mongolian gerbil *(Meriones unguiculatus),* more correctly called the Mongolian jird, is also known as the clawed jird, the sand rat, or the desert rat.[5,6] This gerbil is one of 95 species and 14 genera in the order Rodentia, family Muridae, subfamily Gerbillinae, which are all correctly called gerbils.[6] Gerbils are the world's largest group of rodents adapted to arid environments, which range from Africa though the Middle East to Asia.[6] Of the 95 extant species of gerbils, 18 are endangered and 4 species are vulnerable to extinction.

M. unguiculatus, the common captive species of gerbil, is a burrowing diurnal rodent with crepuscular tendencies (Figure 15-1). This is a hot-desert-dwelling, social species native to Mongolia and northeast China. Agouti is the "wild type" and most common pelage color, but gerbil pelage color may also be black, gray, piebald, blue, Burmese, Himalayan, silver, or white.[4] Agouti animals have darkly pigmented skin with a light

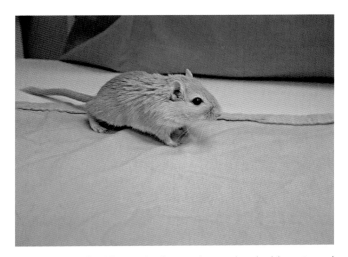

Figure 15-1 Gerbils can be interesting and amicable pets and come in a wide range of coat colors.

buff to white ventrum and mixed white, yellow, and black hairs dorsally, giving the animal a mixed brown appearance.[5] Adult *M. unguiculatus* weigh 70 to 150 g, and males are 5% to 10% heavier than females.[4,5] The Libyan gerbil, *M. libycus,* is also maintained as a pet and has similar attributes. Most gerbils live about 2 to 3 years, but a 5-year life span may occur; females tend to live longer than males.[5,7]

■ BIOLOGY
Unique Anatomy and Physiology

Hamsters and gerbils are rodents and have common dentition: I 1/1, C 0/0, PM 0/0, M 3/3.[8] The crown-to-length ratio of upper to lower incisors is 1 : 3.[8] The lack of canines and premolars creates a gap between the molars and incisors called the *diastema.* The incisors are open rooted and grow continuously, whereas the molars are not open rooted. Rodents cannot sweat or pant; they dissipate excess heat primarily through their tail and ears.[8] Thus, they are susceptible to heat stress and require controlled environmental temperatures. Both hamsters and gerbils are polyestrous. Gender determination is based on an increased anogenital distance in the male (Figure 15-2). The penis of rodents, including the hamster and gerbil, has a baculum (os penis). In general, the anatomic and physiologic parameters of gerbils and the golden hamster are similar (Table 15-1).

Hamsters

Multiple texts, including an anatomic atlas, are available for detailed study of the anatomy of the hamster.[9] The following

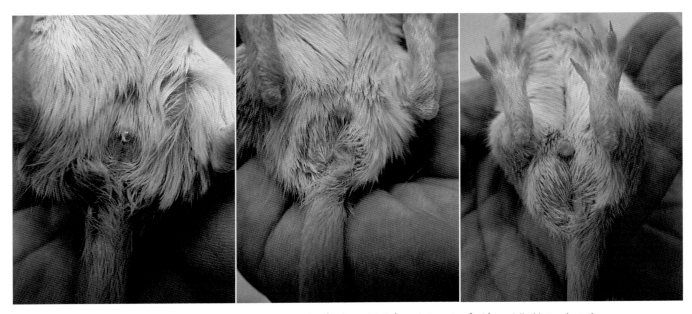

Figure 15-2 External genitalia of the male *(right, middle)* and female *(left)* gerbil. Note that the anogenital distance of the female is shorter than that of the male. The adult male can also be determined by the presence of testicles in the scrotum *(right),* but the frightened gerbil may retract the testicles from the scrotum *(middle).*

TABLE 15-1	Biodata of Hamsters and Gerbils		
Parameter		Hamster	Gerbil
Body temperature (° C)		37-38	38-39
Respiratory rate (breaths/min)		38-110	85-160
Blood volume (ml/100 g body weight)		6.5-8.0	7.7
Heart rate (beats/min)		310-471	260-600
Adult body weight (g)			
Male		87-130	46-131
Female		95-130	50-55
Life span (mo)			
Average		18-24	24-39
Maximum		36	60
Food consumption/100 g body weight/day (g)		8-12	
Water consumption/100 g body weight/day (ml)		8-10	
Preferred environmental temperature range (° C)		21-24	18-22
Preferred environmental relative humidity (%)		40-60	45-55

Data from Battles A: The biology, care and diseases of the Syrian hamster, *Vet Compend Cont Ed* 7(10):815-825, 1985; Harkness J, Wagner J: *The Biology and Medicine of Rabbits and Rodents,* ed 4, Baltimore, 1995, Lippincott Williams and Wilkins; Bihun C, Bauck L: Basic anatomy, physiology, husbandry and clinical techniques. In Quesenberry KE, Carpenter JW, editors: *Ferrets, Rabbits and Rodents: Clinical Medicine and Surgery,* ed 2, St Louis, 2003, WB Saunders.

TABLE 15-2	Reproductive Data for the Hamster and Gerbil		
Parameter		Hamster	Gerbil
Breeding onset			
Male		70-98 days	70-85 days
Female		42-70 days	65-85 days
Cycle length		4 days	4-6 days
Gestation		15-16 days	24-46 days
			Lactating 27-48 days
Postpartum estrus		No	Yes
Litter size		5-9	3-7
Birth weight		2 g	2-3 g
Weaning age		20-25 days	20-26 days
Breeding duration		10-12 mo	12-17 mo

Data from Battles A: The biology, care and diseases of the Syrian hamster, *Vet Compend Cont Ed* 7(10):815-825, 1985; Harkness J, Wagner J: *The Biology and Medicine of Rabbits and Rodents,* ed 4, Baltimore, 1995, Lippincott Williams and Wilkins; Motzel S, Wagner J: Mongolian gerbils: care, diseases and use in research. In Dahm L, J MB, editors: *Laboratory Animal Medicine and Science, Series II,* Seattle, 2001, University of Washington; Bihun C, Bauck L: Basic anatomy, physiology, husbandry and clinical techniques. In Quesenberry KE, Carpenter JW, editors: *Ferrets, Rabbits and Rodents: Clinical Medicine and Surgery,* ed 2, St. Louis, 2003, WB Saunders.

anatomic description should be considered only a summary of clinical anatomy of the Syrian hamster. The body of the Syrian hamster is short and stocky, about 15 to 20 cm long.[2] Adult weights range from 110 to 140 g, with females being larger, on average, than males.[2] Hamsters have short legs, thick fur, large ears, prominent dark eyes, long whiskers, and sharp claws. The paws of the front limbs of hamsters are modified hands with five digits. This adaptation affords dexterity for food and bedding manipulation.[1] The rear foot has three toes.[3]

Hamsters have sebaceous "hip" glands on either flank which are used to mark territory and stimulate mating behaviors.[4] These dark brown patches are covered by the fur and are larger in males than in females.[4] In the sexually aroused male, these glands become readily visible as secretions cause the overlying fur to become matted.[3]

Hamsters have a movable mandibular symphysis which may not close during the hamster's life span.[4] The molars may retain food particles and are prone to dental caries.[4] Newborn hamsters have fully erupted incisors for use in nursing.[4] Cheek or buccal pouches of the hamster are used for storage and transport of food and bedding. These pouches evaginate from the lateral cheek at the diastema and extend alongside the head and neck to the scapulae.[1,4] These thin walled, highly distensible, muscular sacs measure 35 to 40 mm × 4 to 8 mm × 20 mm and are lined with stratified squamous epithelium and are well vascularized.[4] To empty these pouches, hamsters squeeze the cheek pouch contents forward with the paws.[1] Regurgitation or vomition is unlikely in these species because of a limiting ridge at the junction of the esophagus and stomach. The hamster stomach has squamous and glandular portions and some fermentation occurs in the squamous forestomach.[4]

Gender determination, as in other rodents, is based on an increased anogenital distance in the male. In addition, the adult female has a more blunt posterior and 6 pairs of nipples, whereas the male has a more pronounced posterior bulge because of the testes in the scrotum.[1,2] Reproductive characteristics of the hamster are summarized in Table 15-2.

The brain has a smooth cerebrum with generalized areas of function and large olfactory bulbs. Hamsters have acute hearing and olfaction, thus communication is achieved through sounds audible to the human ear, through ultrasound, and through scent.[1] Hamsters recognize other like individuals through scent and receptive mates by odor. Figures 15-3 and 15-4 overview the important anatomic features of the hamster.

Gerbils

Gerbils are characterized by their long fully furred tail, strong claws for burrowing, and elongate muscular hindlimbs for leaping and standing upright.[4,5] The body and tail each range from about 11 to 15 cm in length, with the body being a bit longer than the tail.[5] Gerbils have multiple anatomic adaptations to help them avoid predation. The large middle ear enables them to hear low-frequency sounds, such as the owl wing beat.[6] Gerbils have a wide field of vision because of the dorsal placement of their large eyes.[6] The tail tip has a contrasting color of fur, which may distract predators; furthermore, the tail may be detached from the animal or degloved by the predator while allowing the gerbil to escape. This characteristic tail slip is of particular importance to the veterinarian; avoid holding gerbils by the distal tail to avoid tail degloving or amputation in the exam room.

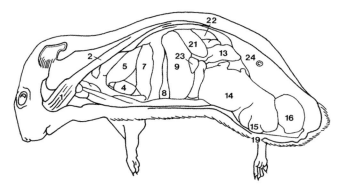

Figure 15-3 Lateral anatomic diagram of the internal anatomy of the adult male Chinese hamster *(Cricetus griseus).* (Reprinted with permission from Gabrisch K, Grimm F, Isenbugel E et al, editors: *Diagnostic Radiology of Exotic Pets,* Philadelphia, 1991, WB Saunders.)

1. Retractor bursae buccalis muscle	13. Fat pad and head of epididymis
2. Fat pad	14. Testes
3. Heart	15. Tail of epididymis
4. Left lung	16. Bladder
5. Right lung	17. Penis
6. Diaphragm	18. Preputial orifice
7. Liver	19. Anus
8. Proventriculus	20. Spleen
9. Glandular stomach	21. Kidneys
10. Jejunum	22. Pancreas
11. Cecum	23. Acetabulum
12. Vesicular gland	24. Scrotum

The gerbil does not sweat and produces extremely concentrated urine as an adaptation for living in arid environments.[6] The relatively large adrenal glands may also be adaptive for arid environments.[4] All gerbils have a tan hairless elliptical area in the midventral abdomen that is a scent marking gland. This prominent abdominal pad is composed of large sebaceous glands that are responsive to testosterone and are therefore larger in the male.[4] The female gerbil has two pairs of thoracic teats and two pairs of inguinal teats. Gerbils have a thoracic thymus, which persists into adulthood.[4] The internal anatomy of the gerbil is detailed in Figures 15-5 and 15-6.

Like other rodents, the gender is determined in gerbils by anogenital distance, which is greater in the male. The increased prominence of the scent marking gland and the darkly pigmented scrotum is also helpful in sexing adult males.[5] The neonatal gerbil may be gender determined based on the increased anogenital distance and the more prominent genital papilla of the male.[5] Gerbils have 7 cervical, 13 thoracic, 6 lumbar, 4 sacral, and 7 or more coccygeal vertebrae (C7, T13, L6, S4, Cy7+). The gerbil has a nonglandular forestomach, lined with keratinized squamous epithelium, and a glandular stomach.

Gerbils form lifelong monogamous pair bonds. Male gerbils need not be removed from the enclosure when the litter is born, as aggression may ensue upon his reintroduction. Gerbils are polyestrous spontaneous ovulators with an estrous cycle of 4 to 6 days. Gestation in the gerbil can be prolonged by delayed implantation of postpartum estrus.[5] For a summary of reproductive characteristics of the gerbil, refer to Table 15-2.

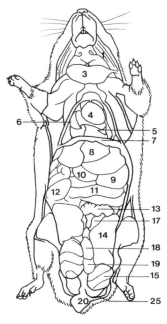

Figure 15-4 Ventral anatomic diagram of internal anatomy of the adult male Chinese hamster *(Cricetus griseus).* (Reprinted with permission from Gabrisch K, Grimm F, Isenbugel E et al, editors: *Diagnostic Radiology of Exotic Pets,* Philadelphia, 1991, WB Saunders.)

1. Retractor bursae buccalis muscle	13. Fat pad and head of epididymis
2. Fat pad	14. Testes
3. Heart	15. Tail of epididymis
4. Left lung	16. Bladder
5. Right lung	17. Penis
6. Diaphragm	18. Preputial orifice
7. Liver	19. Anus
8. Proventriculus	20. Spleen
9. Glandular stomach	21. Kidneys
10. Jejunum	22. Pancreas
11. Cecum	23. Acetabulum
12. Vesicular gland	24. Scrotum

Wild gerbil reproductive behavior differs from that of other rodents. These animals live in large social groups of up to three adult males, up to seven adult females, and numerous subadults and juveniles in a single burrow system. Territories are strictly maintained, food is communally foraged and stored, and strange gerbils are chased away. However, the stable territorial group of gerbils that breed only among themselves would be subject to a variety of genetic problems associated with inbreeding. To avoid this issue, the female gerbil in estrus leaves her territory and mates with a male from another gerbil community.[6] The female then returns to her own burrow where she raises her offspring along with her relatives.

■ HUSBANDRY

Enclosures for hamsters and gerbils should be easy to clean, be lightweight, and have a plastic bottom and sides deep enough to contain bedding. Additionally, these enclosures should be well ventilated. A large door or doors should be provided for

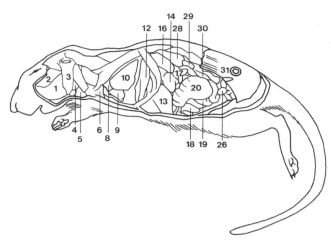

Figure 15-5 Lateral diagram of internal anatomy of the female gerbil *(Meriones unguiculatus).* (Reprinted with permission from Gabrisch K, Grimm F, Isenbugel E et al, editors: *Diagnostic Radiology of Exotic Pets,* Philadelphia, 1991, WB Saunders.)

1. Masseter muscle
2. Facial nerve
3. Parotid gland
4. Mandibular lymph nodes
5. Mandibular salivary glands
6. Thymus
7. Clavicle
8. Left atrium/auricle
9. Left ventricle
10. Left lung
11. Right lung
12. Diaphragm
13. Liver
14. Stomach
15. Greater omentum
16. Spleen
17. Pancreas
18. Jejunum
19. Ileum
20. Cecum
21. Testes
22. Fat pad and head of epididymis
23. Tail of epididymis
24. Penis
25. Vesicular gland
26. Bladder
27. Anus
28. Left kidney
29. Ovary
30. Uterus
31. Acetabulum

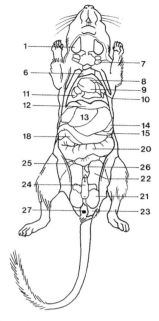

Figure 15-6 Ventral diagram of the anatomy of the male Mongolian gerbil *(Meriones unguiculatus).* (Reprinted with permission from Gabrisch K, Grimm F, Isenbugel E et al, editors: *Diagnostic Radiology of Exotic Pets,* Philadelphia, 1991, WB Saunders.)

1. Masseter muscle
2. Facial nerve
3. Parotid gland
4. Mandibular lymph nodes
5. Mandibular salivary glands
6. Thymus
7. Clavicle
8. Left atrium/auricle
9. Left ventricle
10. Left lung
11. Right lung
12. Diaphragm
13. Liver
14. Stomach
15. Greater omentum
16. Spleen
17. Pancreas
18. Jejunum
19. Ileum
20. Cecum
21. Testes
22. Fat pad and head of epididymis
23. Tail of epididymis
24. Penis
25. Vesicular gland
26. Bladder
27. Anus
28. Left kidney
29. Ovary
30. Uterus
31. Acetabulum

removal of the animal from the cage. Small plastic heavy dishes are recommended for food and sipper bottles for water. Water deprivation is a common problem in pet rodents and should be avoided by inspection of sipper bottles or water containers daily for function, water level, and cleanliness. Although sipper water bottles are preferred, they can leak and become blocked with air bubbles, food material, or bedding material.

Exercise wheels and spherical exercise balls can be provided for exercise. Hamsters are well known for using exercise wheels, with female hamsters running up to 10 km/night.[8] Long-haired hamsters should have their hair trimmed to avoid entanglement in their exercise wheels. Spherical exercise balls are also favored by the hamster, but owners should protect the hamster from stairs, direct sunshine, small children, and other pets.

Materials such as recycled paper products, compressed wheat straw, citrus litter, aspen, oak, and corncob by-products can be used as bedding. Pine shavings are the most popular bedding material. Corncob by-products are excellent for gerbils and dwarf hamsters. Cedar shavings can cause increased liver enzymes in rats and mice, facial dermatitis in gerbils, and hair loss and respiratory disease in some rodents. Some of these adverse clinical signs and diseases are associated with the aromatic oils and terpenes of cedar shavings.

Hamsters

Hamsters are relatively asocial and are best maintained as a solitary animal. Thus, housing groups of hamsters or introducing a new hamster into another hamster's cage is not recommended, as cagemate trauma will likely result. Hamsters are escape artists and can chew through wood, soft metal, and plastic. The enclosure therefore must be well constructed, have rounded corners and be securely fastened. A dark place to hide (e.g., a can) is recommended.[3] Adequate space for an adult hamster's enclosure is 20″ × 20″ × 6-10″ in height.[3] A 12-hour light cycle is preferred, and a light cycle of 14 hours light and 10 hours dark is optimal for reproduction.[2] The hamster should have an environmental temperature of 65° to 70° F (18.3° to 21.1° C) or 71° to 75° F (21.6° to 23.8° C) for young.[3]

Gerbils

Gerbils are social animals and prefer to be maintained in family groups. However, care should be taken not to introduce a single gerbil into an established group, or aggression will likely ensue. Gerbils like to burrow in bedding and will use toys and wheels. Glass tanks make excellent enclosures, but gerbils are strong jumpers, so a secure lid should be provided. Gerbils often return to the enclosure if they escape. Gerbils may be fed from the floor of the enclosure and sipper bottles should be placed low enough to be accessed. Gerbils should be provided a sand bath or sand substrate to avoid oily fur and an environment of less than 50% humidity.

■ NUTRITION

In the wild, hamsters as a group are mainly herbivorous but may also eat insects, lizards, frogs, mice, young birds, and snakes. The wild diet is comprised mainly of seeds, shoots, root vegetables, and leaves and flowers of items such as wheat, barley, millet, soybeans, peas, potatoes, carrots, and beets.[1] Hamsters like to store food and bedding: A single hamster was found to have stored 90 kg of plant material.[1] Smaller materials are carried in the cheek pouches, but large materials are carried with the incisors for storage in the burrow.

Wild gerbils are opportunistic vegetarians and eat primarily seeds, fruits, leaves, stems, and roots. However, they may also eat insects, snails, reptiles, and even other small rodents. Most gerbils take their food back to their burrow for storage before consuming it. One Mongolian jird was documented to have 20 kg of seeds stored in its burrow.[6]

Hamsters and gerbils have similar dietary requirements in captivity and should be given a diet with a minimum of 16% protein and 4% to 5% fat. However, gerbils may require dietary protein of 20% or more. Formulated diets in pellet and block form are recommended for both hamsters and gerbils. Occasional treats should be limited to those high in protein and low in fat. Seed-based diets should not be fed exclusively to hamsters, as they are prone to osteoporosis.[8]

Hamsters eat about 12 g of feed and 10 ml water for every 100 g of body weight daily and are coprophagic.[3] Newborn hamsters begin eating on their own at 7 to 20 days of age. Hamsters should be fed from the floor rather from a hopper to avoid both lesions around the nares and neglect of pups. Gerbils eat about 8 g of feed per day. Young gerbils begin eating solid food at about 14 days of age. Because gerbils are physiologically adapted to arid regions, they only consume about 4 ml of water per day and produce very little urine.

■ PREVENTIVE MEDICINE
Quarantine

Annual or semiannual examination and fecal flotation are the minimum health maintenance recommendations for hamsters and gerbils. No vaccines are currently labeled for use in hamsters and gerbils.

Hamsters, by nature, are solitary animals and should be maintained in this manner for optimum health and reduced likelihood of injuries. Thus, a strict quarantine period, except for handling the new hamster last, is generally not necessary. In the case of the gerbil, new animals should be maintained separately and cared for last, after handling other animals, during a 30-day quarantine period. Animals should be observed for food and water intake before being introduced into the group.

Further, a physical examination and the results of serial fecal assays (e.g., flotation and direct smear) should be free of signs of infectious disease before a new animal enters the group. New entries should be monitored carefully for barbering and appropriate food intake as they acclimatize to the new environment.

DISINFECTION AND SANITATION

Hamsters and gerbils should be kept in a clean environment to avoid disease problems. Food and water containers should be cleaned with dilute soap weekly and washed free of debris on a daily basis. Enclosures should be thoroughly cleaned on a weekly basis, by removing all bedding and cleaning the enclosure with soap and hot water. Solid plastic cages should be cleaned more regularly as they have less ventilation. Inspection and removal of solid and liquid wastes should occur on a daily basis. As a general rule, if one can smell the enclosure, it must be cleaned. Many rodents suffer mortality and morbidity from ammonia build-up and improperly cleaned or maintained enclosures.

■ RESTRAINT

The goal of manual restraint is to avoid harming or stressing the rodent while minimizing the risk to the handler. Handling should be firm, yet calm and decisive.

Manual Restraint of Hamsters

Hamsters are agonistic in nature and may bite if roughly handled, startled, awakened, or injured.[4] Do not surprise or startle the hamster before handling.[2] Wake the hamster gently if it is sleeping, as they are deep sleepers.[4] One effective method for restraint is to place the hamster on a flat surface and cover it with the palm of your hand, with your thumb near the hamster's head.[2] The loose skin over the back should be firmly grasped with all the fingers, lifting the hamster. If the skin is taut over the abdomen and chest, the hamster will be securely held, although the eyes may bulge with this over-the-back grip. Hamsters may also be picked up by the scruff over the dorsal

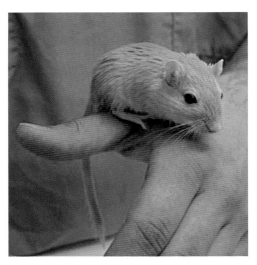

Figure 15-7 Most gerbils are relatively docile and easily handled for physical examination.

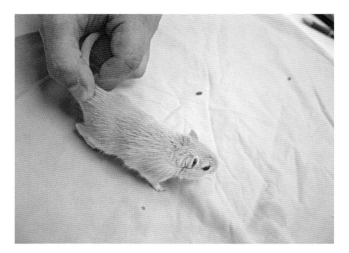

Figure 15-8 Initial gerbil restraint is facilitated by catching the gerbil by the base or proximal-most aspect of the tail.

cervical area and shoulders.[4] When scruffing the hamster, beware of the extensive cheek pouches and excessive loose skin of this animal, which facilitate the hamster's ability to turn and bite the handler.

Manual Restraint of Gerbils

Gerbils are generally docile animals, require minimal restraint, and can be picked up and loosely cupped in one hand (Figure 15-7).[8] However, the excited, threatened gerbil will rhythmically thump its rear foot and may bite. Gerbils can be restrained similarly to the hamster, with back or scruff techniques. The initial capture of a gerbil may be facilitated by grasping the base of the tail (Figure 15-8). Tail degloving or detachment can occur as an antipredator mechanism and is more likely to occur when the tail is grabbed distally or the animal is young. Grasp the base of the tail with one hand and then use the forefinger and thumb to gently pin down the head.

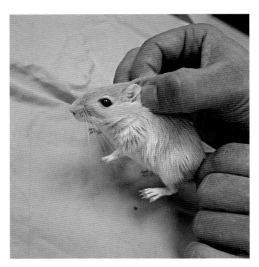

Figure 15-9 The gerbil is then scruffed over the neck and shoulders after the head is pressed gently against the surface to facilitate this grip.

With the remaining fingers, grasp the loose skin along the neck and back and use the little finger to hold the tail (Figure 15-9). Alternately, the docile gerbil may be scooped up in the palm.

Chemical restraint of hamsters and gerbils is discussed in detail in Anesthesia. However, for short procedures such as venipuncture, other sample collection and radiography, I prefer isoflurane anesthesia administered via face mask.

■ PERFORMING A PHYSICAL EXAMINATION

Much of the examination process should occur before restraining the hamster or gerbil. While the animal is in the enclosure, evaluate the quantity and consistency of the feces and urine. Examine the animal for any outward signs of parasitism (e.g., hair loss, unthrifty, greasy fur). Observe the water and food containers for appropriate diet type and cleanliness. Evaluate the bedding in the enclosure and check for any inappropriate sharp edges in the enclosure. For physical examination, place the animal on a padded surface in a room free from extraneous noise and other animals. Then, observe the behavior and respiratory rate. The pugnacious nature of the hamster makes adequate restraint necessary for a full physical examination. As gerbils are prone to seizures, the physical examination should be done quickly to avoid stress.

Obtain an accurate weight of the animal with a gram scale accurate to 1 gram. The rectal temperature of a gerbil or hamster is not readily obtained because of the large size of most commercial thermometers. However, should one choose to attempt this procedure, a flexible plastic thermometer should be used. The hamster or gerbil should then be examined in a systematic manner, from head to tail. The normal anatomy of the species being examined should be noted. Auscultation of both the thorax and abdomen is best evaluated when the animal is less stressed. A small pediatric or neonatal stethoscope will facilitate this assessment. Listening without a stethoscope to the respirations of the animal may also be of benefit.

Any lesions of the skin and pelage should be noted and the lymph nodes and mammary glands palpated. Abdominal palpation may reveal masses, and fecal or urine staining may represent gastrointestinal disease, urinary tract infection, or reproductive tract disease. The plantar surface of each foot should be examined for pododermatitis and trauma.

Full oral or ophthalmic examination is challenging and may require anesthesia. Generally the areas of the mouth in rodents are very sensitive, to aid in food discrimination. Because many rodents are resistant to mouth or lip manipulations, the oral examination is performed last. In the docile rodent, the incisors may be directly visualized. Viewing the molars with an otoscopic cone may be attempted in the awake animal, but generally only flashes of white and pink are visualized. Anesthesia is highly recommended for a full oral evaluation, which may include rigid endoscopy.

Common abnormalities found on the physical examination include diseases affecting the eyes, and the integumentary, respiratory, and gastrointestinal systems.[10] Common disease presentations that affect small pet rodents include trauma, coma, respiratory disease, skin scald, malocclusion, and diarrhea or other gastrointestinal disturbances.[7]

Diseases of the integument of hamsters and gerbils include ectoparasitism, endocrine disease, trauma, sore nose, neoplasias, and abscesses. Demodectic mange and other mites and lice cause hair loss in hamsters and gerbils. Symmetric hair loss of the flanks, hyperkeratosis, and hyperpigmentation of the skin are associated with adrenal disease in the hamster.[10] Trauma from cagemates occurs both to hamsters and gerbils and involves the fur and skin, especially of the urogenital region in males.[10] Gerbils can also develop "sore nose," a facial dermatitis of unknown etiology. Neoplasias and abscesses affecting the skin may also be diagnosed.

Ophthalmologic diseases are common in hamsters and gerbils. Transient cataracts may develop secondary to anesthesia; ocular lubrication and closure of the eyelids during anesthetic episodes may limit this occurrence and prevent iatrogenic corneal injuries.[10] Exophthalmos occurs in hamsters and is due to trauma, infection, and inappropriate restraint. Correction of the initiating cause and the proptosis in a timely manner is required for a good prognosis with these cases.[10]

Respiratory disease is probably underreported in the hamster and gerbil because of the lack of overt clinical signs. Radiographic examination is indicated if respiratory disease is suspected, because it is a more sensitive indicator of lung and cardiovascular disease than is auscultation in these diminutive patients. It is emphasized that radiographs and the anesthesia necessary for appropriate positioning should be attempted only in the stabilized patient.

Gastrointestinal disease, especially diarrhea, is a common clinical symptom in small rodents, and the prognosis for these cases is guarded. Differentials for diarrhea in hamsters and gerbils include Tyzzer's disease, dysbiosis, salmonellosis, colibacillosis, proliferative ileitis, listeriosis, coccidiosis, and cryptosporidiosis. Dependent upon the organism of infection, diagnosis may be challenging and treatment may be unrewarding. (For more information regarding treatment, see Bacterial Diseases Found in Hamsters and Gerbils.) For the anorectic gerbil

or hamster, incisor malocclusion and dental caries in the hamster should be considered as differential diagnoses. Tooth root abscesses may also occur, resulting in facial or jaw deformity.

Other miscellaneous diseases less commonly affect the hamster. Renal amyloidosis is common in geriatric hamsters, in which the patient presents with polyuria and weight loss. Smothering of the young occurs when a female hamster perceives a threat and uses the cheek pouches to protect the young. Hamsters may develop clinical signs compatible with hyperadrenocorticism (e.g., weight loss, polydipsia, polyuria, polyphagia, alopecia, hyperpigmentation). Gerbils have epileptiform seizures triggered by novel stimuli. This inherited trait first manifests in the weanling gerbil but may be outgrown. Head tilt is often caused by otitis media or interna, with the common cause being bacterial infection in both hamsters and gerbils. Heat stroke may occur in both hamsters and gerbils, especially when these animals are placed in an inappropriate environment, enclosure, or both.

■ DIAGNOSTIC TESTING

Clinical Pathology

Excellent, detailed reviews of the hematology of the gerbil and hamster exist and should be consulted when more than a brief clinical summary, as provided here, is necessary for patient diagnosis (Tables 15-3 and 15-4).[11-13]

Hamster

Erythrocytes of the normal adult hamster may show polychromasia or be nucleated about 2% of the time. Castration may decrease circulating erythrocytes in the hamster by 25% to 30% because of the resultant testosterone decrease. This condition has been alleviated with testosterone administration, but the clinician should be aware of this cause of a decrease in packed cell volume to differentiate it from continuing blood loss due ligature failure of castration.

Hamsters are a lymphocytic species with small and large lymphocytes comprising 60% to 80% of the circulating white blood cells. Hamster neutrophils may also be referred to as heterophils. Although the morphology of the neutrophil and lymphocyte varies slightly from other rodents, the form of the eosinophil, basophil, and monocyte of the hamster are similar to those of other rodents. Bone marrow constituents and coagulation values for hamsters have been established and published.[11]

Hibernation of the hamster causes a variety of hematologic changes, including an increased erythrocyte life span and resultant increased erythrocyte count and hemoglobin concentration, along with a decrease in platelets. The total white blood cell count decreases to 2500 cell/µl in the Syrian hamster and 100 cells/µl in the European hamster. The neutrophil-to-lymphocyte ratio also changes to 1 : 1. After hibernation, a neutrophilic leukocytosis normally occurs, with 70% to 90% neutrophils and a total white blood cell count of 10,000 to 20,000 cell/µl.

TABLE 15-3	Ranges of Hematologic Values for the Gerbil and Hamster			
Parameter (unit)	Gerbil	Syrian hamster	European hamster	Djungarian hamster
RBC ($\times 10^6$/µl)	7-9	3.96-10.3	6.04-9.10	4.4-9.1
PCV (%)	35-52	32.9-59	44-49	36.5-47.7
Hb (g/dl)	10-17.9	10-19.2	12.4-15.9	10.7-14.1
MCH (pg)	16.1-19.4	20.2-25.8	18.6-22.5	15.5-19.1
MCV (fL)	46.6-60	64.0-77.6	58.7-71.4	53.6-65.2
MCHC (%)	30.6-33.3	27.5-37.4	26.4-32.5	27-32
Platelets ($\times 10^3$/mm^3)	432-830	200-590	–	–
WBC ($\times 10^3$/mm^3)	4.3-21.6	3.0-15	3.4-7.6	2.7-9.6
Neutrophils (%)	2-41	17-35.2	3.5-41.6	14.8-23.6
Lymphocytes (%)	32-97	50-96	50-95	68.1-84.8
Eosinophils (%)	0-4	0-5	0-2.1	0.3-3.1
Basophils (%)	0-2	0-5	0-0.2	0-0.5
Monocytes (%)	0-9	0-5	0-1	0-2.4

Data from Harkness J, Wagner J: *The Biology and Medicine of Rabbits and Rodents,* ed 4, Baltimore, 1995, Lippincott Williams and Wilkins; Moore D: Hematology of the Syrian (Golden) hamster *(Mesocricetus auratus).* In Feldman BF, Zinkl JG, Jain NC, editors: *Schalm's Veterinary Hematology,* ed 5, Philadelphia, 2000, Lippincott Williams and Wilkins; Moore D: Hematology of the Mongolian gerbil *(Meriones unguiculatus).* In Feldman BF, Zinkl JG, Jain NC, editors: *Schalm's Veterinary Hematology,* ed 5, Philadelphia, 2000, Lippincott Williams and Wilkins; Ness RD: Rodents. In Carpenter JW, editor: *Exotic Animal Formulary,* ed 3, St Louis, 2005, WB Saunders. *Hb,* hemoglobin; *MCH,* mean corpuscular hemoglobin; *MCHC,* mean corpuscular hemoglobin concentration; *PCV,* packed cell volume; *RBC,* red blood cell count; *WBC,* white blood cell count.

TABLE 15-4	Serum Biochemical Values of the Hamster and Gerbil	
Analyte (unit)	Gerbil	Syrian hamster
ALT (IU/L)	–	22-128
AP (IU/L)	–	99-186
AST (IU/L)	–	28-122
Bilirubin, total (mg/dl)	0.2-0.6	0.1-0.9
Glucose (mg/dl)	50-135	37-198
Calcium (mg/dl)	3.7-6.2	5.3-12
Phosphorous (mg/dl)	3.7-7	3.0-9.9
Creatinine (mg/dl)	0.6-1.4	0.4-1
Urea nitrogen (mg/dl)	17-27	12-26
Protein, total (g/dl)	4.3-12.5	5.2-7.0
Albumin (g/dl)	1.8-5.5	3.5-4.9
Globulin (g/dl)	1.2-6.0	2.7-4.2
Triglycerides	–	72-227
Cholesterol (mg/dl)	90-150	55-181
Sodium (mEq/L)	141-172	128-144
Potassium (mEq/L)	3.3-6.3	3.9-5.5

Data from Harkness J, Wagner J: *The Biology and Medicine of Rabbits and Rodents,* ed 4, Baltimore, 1995, Lippincott Williams and Wilkins; Ness RD: Rodents. In Carpenter JW, editor: *Exotic Animal Formulary,* ed 3, St Louis, 2005, WB Saunders.

Gerbil Hematology

Lipemic serum is common in gerbils older than 13 months, independent of gender. Although unconfirmed, the addition of sunflower seeds to the diet may predispose gerbils to lipemia. Circulating reticulocytes, stippled erythrocytes, and polychromasia are common in adult and juvenile gerbils; these conditions may be due to the relatively short life span of their erythrocytes, 9 to 10 days.

Gender and age significantly affect gerbil hematology. Neonatal gerbils have a variety of hematologic anomalies that are considered normal and that spontaneously resolve at about 8 weeks of age: erythrocyte macrocytosis, panleukocytosis, and a red blood cell count that is half of the adult value. Male gerbils tend to have a higher mean corpuscular volume (MCV), hemoglobin, hematocrit (HCT), and mean corpuscular hemoglobin concentration (MCHC). Male gerbils also have a higher total white blood cell count based on a higher absolute number of lymphocytes, resulting in a 6 : 1 lymphocyte-to-heterophil ratio in the male, compared with a 3 : 1 ratio in the female gerbil.

Diagnostic Sample Collection

In the pet rodent, clinical sampling usually requires anesthesia. Options for venipuncture in the hamster and gerbil include the retroorbital venous plexus, cardiac puncture, and toe nail clip. These methods are generally avoided except in the research setting, based on pain and the risk of morbidity or mortality of the animal as well as sample artifacts associated with the collection method. More appropriate options for use in the clinical setting include jugular, cranial vena cava, saphenous, cephalic, or tail vein venipuncture. The cephalic, saphenous, and tail veins may be collected after sterile lancet puncture and open collection or via small-gauge preheparinized needle placement with open collection from the hub. Small microtainer tubes with a variety of anticoagulant additives are available for this purpose (Figure 15-10). Volume of blood collected for diagnostic tests should not exceed 10% of the blood volume, or approximately 8.0 ml/kg of body weight.

Urinalysis

Hamster urine has a normal pH range of 5.1 to 8.4 and is milky and turbid due to the normal crystal concentration of

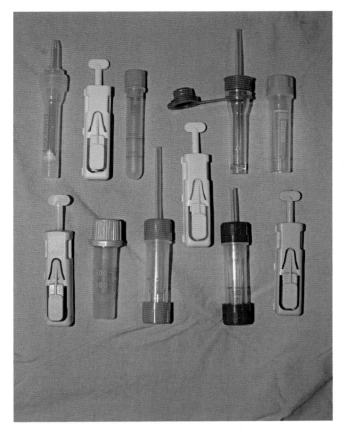

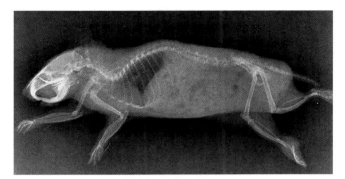

Figure 15-11 Lateral radiographic whole body view of an adult female golden hamster *(Mesocricetus auratus).* (Reprinted with permission from Gabrisch K, Grimm F, Isenbugel E et al, editors: *Diagnostic Radiology of Exotic Pets,* Philadelphia, 1991, WB Saunders.)

Figure 15-10 Microtainers with a variety of anticoagulant additives and lancets in a variety of styles are available for blood sampling of hamsters and gerbils.

the urine.[4] Hamsters produce up to 7 ml of urine per day, and urinary protein levels are normally high.[4]

Diagnostic Imaging

Radiographic imaging is facilitated by anesthesia for appropriate positioning and relaxation of muscle tone in these species. Small tape strips modified to stirrups around the limbs facilitates extension of the limbs for appropriate positioning. The radiographic technique for use in the hamster may be modified slightly for the gerbil. A tabletop technique with a focal film distance of 40 in (102 cm) for extremities and 38 in (97 cm) for whole body views is recommended.[14] With these settings, an mAs of 6.4 and a kVp of 54 are recommended for imaging the skull and an mAs of 7.5 and a kVp of 52 for imaging elsewhere.[14] Fine or mammography cassettes and film or dental film and cassettes are recommended to obtain maximum detail in these diminutive patient's radiographic images.[15]

An atlas of normal Syrian hamster radiographic anatomy with and without contrast has been published.[14] Individual organs may be poorly defined in the radiographic images (Figure 15-11). In the normal Syrian hamster, the apex of the heart points caudoventrally and to the left (Figure 15-12).[16] In the golden hamster, the abdomen is large in comparison with the thorax and filled with the voluminous gastrointestinal tract. In those cases in which there is significant gas in the

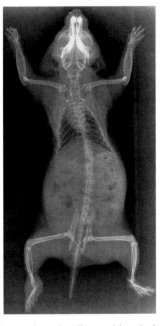

Figure 15-12 Ventrodorsal radiographic whole body view of a normal adult female golden hamster *(Mesocricetus auratus).* The heart's apex points caudolaterally to the left within the thorax. (Reprinted with permission from Gabrisch K, Grimm F, Isenbugel E et al, editors: *Diagnostic Radiology of Exotic Pets,* Philadelphia, 1991, WB Saunders.)

intestines, radiographic contrast is poor. The kidneys are situated dorsally, near the first lumbar vertebral body, and may be faintly visible on survey radiographs.

Clinical presentations of the Syrian hamster suited to diagnostic radiographic imaging include impaction of the cheek pouches, bloat, and abdominal masses.[16] Extreme dilation of the cheek pouches, gaseous distension of intestinal loops and abdominal distension, and displacement of the gastrointestinal tract or other organs by a peritoneal mass (mass effect) may be observed radiographically in these cases.[16]

Survey radiographs can also be useful in evaluating gerbils with similar clinical presentations. Both lateral and

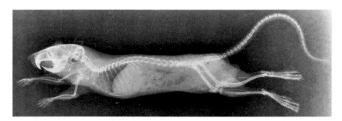

Figure 15-13 Lateral radiographic whole body view of a normal adult male Mongolian gerbil *(Meriones unguiculatus)*. (Reprinted with permission from Gabrisch K, Grimm F, Isenbugel E et al, editors: *Diagnostic Radiology of Exotic Pets,* Philadelphia, 1991, WB Saunders.)

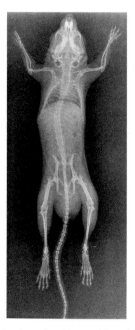

Figure 15-14 Ventrodorsal radiographic whole body view of a normal adult male Mongolian gerbil *(Meriones unguiculatus)*. (Reprinted with permission from Gabrisch K, Grimm F, Isenbugel E et al, editors: *Diagnostic Radiology of Exotic Pets,* Philadelphia, 1991, WB Saunders.)

ventrodorsal/dorsoventral images should be taken (Figure 15-13 and 15-14). In gerbils, the thorax is large, compared with that of other rodents.[16] The liver and gastrointestinal tract are located relatively cranially in the abdomen because of the abdominal fat pads, which extend from the os penis to the umbilical region.[16] The liver and gastrointestinal tract of the male gerbil are located cranially in the abdomen because of the scrotal fat pads, which extend from the os penis to the umbilical area.

Ultrasound using a small pencil type probe is clinically useful in these animals, as are computed tomography (CT) and magnetic resonance imaging (MRI). However, economic concerns and the lack of normal imaging studies currently limit the demand for these procedures for rodent patients in the clinical setting.

Parasitology

Diagnostic tests used to evaluate hamsters and gerbils for parasites are similar to those for small companion animals. Gastrointestinal parasites are uncommon in hamsters and gerbils. However, a fecal flotation and direct smear are recommended for the annual/semiannual physical examination. A perianal tape preparation is also recommended to check for pinworms.

Miscellaneous Diagnostic Tests

Diagnostic tests using blood serum and polymerase chain reaction (PCR) technology are available for a variety of viruses to which the hamster is susceptible, including lymphocytic choriomeningitis virus, Sendai virus, mouse pneumonia virus, hamster polyomavirus, and hamster parvovirus.

■ COMMON DISEASE PRESENTATIONS

Infectious Diseases

BACTERIAL DISEASES

Tyzzer's Disease

Tyzzer's disease, caused by infection of the gastrointestinal tract with *Clostridium piliforme,* has been described in gerbils and hamsters.[8] Compared with mice and rats, gerbils and hamsters suffer increased mortality when infected with Tyzzer's disease. Gerbils are particularly susceptible; hence, this is a common disease in gerbils. This disease is not observed in immunocompetent hamsters. Clinical signs in hamsters are nonspecific and are often associated with the generally ill rodent; these signs include death, without premonitory signs; or an unkempt, scruffy pelage; depression; dehydration; and diarrhea. In the gerbil, the most common clinical signs are death with or without diarrhea, general signs of illness as described for the hamster, or death after a short illness. Gross necropsy generally reveals multiple necrotic hepatic foci and, if present, intestinal lesions. Gerbils may contract this disease from contaminated bedding. This disease may be precipitated by environmental factors, such as overcrowding, high environmental temperature, heavy parasite load, and poor diet. Treatment may be unrewarding but is based on supportive care and appropriate antimicrobials (see Table 15-8).

Proliferative Ileitis

Proliferative ileitis or "wet tail" is a diarrheic disease of hamsters that may occur at any age. The etiologic agent is the intracellular bacterium *Lawsonia intracellularis,* which causes a similar disease in pigs and ferrets.[8] Treatment of diarrheic disease of the hamster should include correction of fluid deficits and electrolyte imbalances, antibiotic administration, and nutritional support. Antibiotic treatment options include tetracycline, enrofloxacin, and trimethoprim sulfa. Symptomatic treatment for diarrhea with bismuth subsalicylate may also be indicated for protracted clinical signs. Owners should be advised of serious sequelae that may accompany this disease (e.g., obstruction, intussusception, and rectal prolapse).

Miscellaneous Bacterial Infections

Dysbiosis is associated with overgrowth of *Clostridium difficile* in hamsters. (For details of causes and treatment of dysbiosis in hamsters, see Table 15-8.)

A variety of pathogenic bacteria have been isolated from the diseased respiratory tract of hamsters. Cilia-associated respiratory bacillus infection causes mild disease in Syrian hamsters but produces clinical disease in the South African hamster *(Myostromys albicaudatus)*.[17] *Streptococcus pneumoniae* is commonly associated with respiratory disease in hamsters. Hamsters can harbor *Corynebacterium kutscheri* and *Pasteurella pneumotropica* without apparent clinical disease.[4] All of these bacteria may subclinically affect the respiratory systems of hamsters and other rodents and can progress to pneumonia. Hamsters are resistant to *Bordetella bronchiseptica* infection.

Clinical signs of bacterial pneumonia in hamsters include a purulent rhinitis and blepharitis, with a poor prognosis.[8] Streptococcal and other bacterial pneumonias may be transmitted from children to hamsters. The clinical diagnosis can be supported by the finding of Gram-positive diplococci in nasal or ocular discharge.

Pyometra has been described in pet hamsters, with ovariohysterectomy being the treatment of choice. Hamsters are prone to dental caries of the molars, especially if *Streptococcus mutans* is present.[4]

Hamsters often present with bacterial pyoderma and cutaneous abscesses, which manifest clinically as moist dermatitis or skin ulceration, most often of the head. Mite infestation, trauma, bite wounds, rough cage surfaces, and soiled or abrasive bedding may all contribute to the development of this disease.[18] These bacterial infections involve *Staphylococcus aureus* most commonly, but also *Streptococcus* spp., *Actinomyces* spp., *P. pneumotropica,* and *Mycobacterium* spp.[18] Treatment should include correction of the cause of bacterial infection, surgical removal of abscesses, and appropriate antibiotic treatment based on culture and sensitivity results.

The large ventral abdominal marking gland of the aged gerbil may become inflamed and infected. Infection must be differentiated from a neoplastic process that also commonly affects the gland. Treatment of the infected gland includes local debridement and topical antibiotic application.

Facial Eczema (Sore Nose)

Facial eczema, sore nose, and nasal dermatitis are synonyms for the syndrome of facial lesions in gerbils.[8] This clinical syndrome is caused by an increase in harderian gland secretions, which are irritating to the skin. Erythematous lesions begin adjacent to the nares and progress to alopecia and then to moist dermatitis of the region. The lesions may be secondarily infected by *Staph. aureus* or *Staph. xylosis.* Facial eczema can be prevented by providing appropriate (low) humidity, access to a sand bath, and not using wood shavings with volatile oils (e.g., pine, cedar). Treatment should include cleansing of the face. For severely affected patients, topical or systemic application of antibiotics is warranted.

VIRAL DISEASES

Viral diseases of clinical significance in the hamster are rare, and no viral diseases have been reported to occur in the gerbil.

Lymphocytic Choriomeningitis virus

Lymphocytic choriomeningitis virus (LCMV) is a disease that is uncommon in young hamsters and is caused by an RNA arena virus.[19] However, pet and laboratory hamsters can transmit this virus to humans.[16] Hamsters can persistently shed large amounts of the virus in the urine. In experimentally infected hamsters, variations in clinical disease are based on viral strain, animal strain, and age at time of infection. Hamsters infected in utero or perinatally and those hamsters born to viruric dams become persistently but subclinically infected or may develop a chronic wasting disease and multiorgan inflammation. About half of these hamsters clear the infection. Hamsters infected as young adults have no clinical signs, but viremia and viruria can persist up to 6 months postinfection. Diagnosis is made based on PCR, finding LCMV serum antibodies, or evidence of the virus in tissues. Because LCMV is a zoonotic agent, infected or exposed hamsters should be euthanized and submitted for necropsy, and enclosures and cage furniture should be disinfected or discarded. Owners must be informed about the zoonotic risk of this disease and advised to consult their physician if their pet has been diagnosed with this disease.

Polyoma Virus

Hamster polyoma virus is a DNA oncogenic virus that causes neoplasms in young and adult hamsters.[19] Young hamsters develop multicentric lymphoma involving the mesenteric lymph nodes and abdominal viscera, whereas adult hamsters develop trichoepithelioma. Gross, cytologic or histologic findings consistent with lymphoma or epithelioma are consistent with viral infection. However, confirmation requires histologic verification and PCR diagnostic testing of infected tissues.

Parvovirus

Hamster parvovirus can cause decreased litter size in reproductively active hamsters and clinical signs in 2- to 4-week-old offspring. Young hamsters have dome-shaped crania, a potbelly, testicular atrophy, and their incisors become discolored and malformed and fall out. Experimentally, some hamsters also developed multisystemic hemorrhagic disease. Confirmation of the clinical diagnosis requires PCR of the affected tissues.

Miscellaneous Viral Infections

Diagnostic and histologic evidence of many other viruses has been reported in hamsters without apparent clinical signs.[19] Seropositive results for Sendai virus and pneumonia virus of mice, both RNA viruses of the Paramyxoviridae family, are common in hamsters. Although no clinical signs or lesions have been described in seropositive animals when naturally infected, experimental infection results in the development of clinical signs including rhinitis, bronchitis, and neonatal death. Seroconversion to other viral diseases of rodents, such as reovirus 3 and simian virus 5, also occurs in hamsters without apparent clinical signs. Inclusions of adenovirus and cytomegalovirus have been reported in hamsters without documented clinical disease. The clinical implications of these findings are unknown at this time.

FUNGAL DISEASE

Fungal disease in the hamster and gerbil is rare. Dermatophytosis (ringworm) can be caused by a variety of fungi (*Microsporum* spp. or *Trichophyton* spp.) but rarely infects the Syrian hamster or the Djungarian hamster and has not been reported in the Mongolian gerbil.[20] Although this fact is not clinically relevant, hamsters are experimentally susceptible to *Sporothrix schenckii*.[20] Appropriate antifungal treatment and counseling of the owner about the zoonotic potential of dermatophytes should be instituted when a confirmed diagnosis is made.

Parasites
ENDOPARASITES

Hamsters can be infected by the pinworm of mice *(Syphacia obvelata),* the pinworm of rats *(S. muris),* and the pinworm of hamsters *(S. mesocriceti).* As commensals of the rodent cecum, these oxyurid nematodes feed on bacteria. *Syphacia* spp. have a direct life cycle and a prepatent period of 8 to 15 days. Transmission may occur by the fecal-oral route, by retrograde infection via deposition of embryonated ova on perineal skin, or via aerosolization. Oxyuriasis is diagnosed by identification of parasite ova in fecal flotation or in perineal tape impressions. High parasite loads can cause decreased activity, weight loss, rectal prolapse, rectal irritation with self-mutilation, impaction, and intussusception. Pinworm infestations are more common in the young, immunocompromised, or male hamsters.[4] For treatment of oxyurids in hamsters, see Table 15-5. Environmental cleaning for removal of pinworms is a necessary part of the treatment plan to prevent reinfestation.

The most significant endoparasite affecting hamsters is *Hymenolepis nana,* the dwarf tapeworm. Usually found in the small intestine, *H. nana* segments can be identified in the feces. This cestode can infect rodents, such as mice, rats, and hamsters, as well as nonhuman primates and humans. Infections are usually benign in hamsters, but large parasitic loads may be associated with intestinal obstruction and death.[3] *H. nana* can have a direct or indirect life cycle and is capable of autoinfection, especially in humans. The indirect life cycle is of variable length, with the intermediate hosts identified as fleas or flour beetles. The direct cycle is about 15 days. Treatment must be accompanied by frequent bedding changes and cage cleanings to prevent reinfestation. Owners should be educated about the risks of being infected with this zoonotic tapeworm.

Hamsters may also be infected with *H. diminuta.* It affects the upper small intestine, whereas *H. nana* affects the lower small intestine. Morphologically, this tapeworm is relatively large when compared to *H. nana,* but the zoonotic risk of this cestode is low.[21] Liver cysts of *Cysticercus fasciolaris,* the intermediate stage of *Taenia taeniaeformis,* have been found in hamsters. Hamster exposure to *T. taeniaeformis* occurs when

the feces of dogs or cats, the definitive hosts, contaminate hamster food.[21]

PROTOZOANS IN HAMSTERS

Few enteric protozoans of hamsters have pathogenic significance, but in aged hamsters with concurrent systemic disease (e.g., amyloidosis), chronic giardiasis *(Giardia muris)* can adversely affect the animals' health. In affected hamsters, chronic diarrhea and emaciation are noted, along with classic pathologic lesions of giardiasis, such as enterotyphlocolitis, plasma cell and lymphocyte infiltration of the intestinal lamina propria, and thickening of the small intestine and cecal walls.[21] Diagnosis of giardiasis is made by identification of cysts on fecal flotation or direct smear using warmed saline or Lugol's iodine. Whereas *G. mesocricetus* and *G. muris* have had no documented transmission to humans, *Giardia* spp. lack host specificity and have a direct life cycle.[22] Therefore, owners, especially immunocompromised individuals, should be educated about the zoonotic risk of giardiasis.

Although *Cryptosporidium* spp. were found in a Syrian hamster that died from proliferative ileitis, this disease was likely opportunistic based on histopathologic findings.[23] Cryptosporidiosis is unlikely to occur in hamsters but upon diagnosis, owners of an affected hamster should be educated about the potential zoonotic risk associated with this organism.[22]

PROTOZOANS IN GERBILS

Several pinworms *(Syphacia obvelata, S. muris, Dentostomella translucida)* infect gerbils, but none has been associated with clinical disease.[21] Experimentally induced infection of *Giardia lamblia* in gerbils has been reported. The helminth *Hymenolepis nana* has been associated with dehydration, mucoid diarrhea, and debilitation in gerbils. Diagnosis and treatment of these parasites in gerbils are similar to diagnosis and treatment of the affected hamster. Both *G. lamblia* and *H. nana* have zoonotic potential; therefore, owners of affected gerbils should be informed of this potential risk.

ECTOPARASITES IN HAMSTERS

Although present in clinically normal hamsters, large numbers of demodectic mites found on a skin scraping, accompanied by clinical signs, provides a presumptive diagnosis of demodectic mange. As in dogs and cats, primary disease considerations should be investigated when demodectic mange has been diagnosed. Acariasis is often seen in older hamsters affected with hyperadrenocorticism. Clinically, demodectic mange causes a nonpruritic alopecia with scales and crusts along the back, neck, and rump.[21] The two species of demodectic mites of hamsters are *Demodex aurati,* which is elongate and lives in hair follicles and sebaceous gland canals, and *D. criceti,* which is short and stubby and is found in epidermal pits.[24] If several hamsters are affected, it is best to sample the males because they usually have a larger parasitic burden.[21] The sarcoptic mange mites, *Notoedres notoedres* and *N. cati,* can cause intense pruritus in hamsters. These mites burrow in the stratum corneum and cause scabby lesions on the ears, muzzle, limbs, and perineal and genital areas.[21] Clinical signs and the

TABLE 15-5 **Antiparasitic Agents for Use in Hamsters and Gerbils**

Drug	Dose*	Route	Regimen	Indications
Amitraz	1.4 ml/L	Topical dip	q14 days ×3-6	Demodex spp. Not recommended in young animals
Fenbendazole	20	PO	q24h × 5 days	G, H
	50	PO	q24h × 5 days	G, H: Giardia spp.
Ivermectin	0.2-0.5	SC, PO	q14 days × 3	H
	0.3-0.5	SC	q7 days until clinical signs resolve	H: demodectic, notoedric mange
	0.2-0.4	SC	q10 days × 3 or until clinical signs resolve	G: demodectic mange
Lime-sulfur dip	Dilute 1 : 40	Topical Dip	q7 days × 6	G, H: dermatophytosis, adjunct for acariasis
Malathion	3%-5% powder	Dust	3/wk × 3 wk	G, H
Permethrin	5% solution or 0.25% dust	Cotton ball in cage	4-5 wk	G, H
Piperazine citrate	2-5 mg/ml	Drinking water	On 7 days, off 7 days, on 7 days	G, H: pinworms, tapeworms
Praziquantel	6-10	PO		G, H: tapeworms
Pyrantel pamoate	50	PO	q24h × 5 days	G, H: nematodiasis
Pyrethrin powder	0.5%	Topical Dust	3×/wk × 3 wk	Ectoparasites
Pyrethrin shampoo	0.5%	Shampoo	1/wk × 4 wk	G, H
Quinacrine HCL	75		q8h	G, H: giardiasis
Sulfadimethoxine	50, 25	PO	50 once, then 25 q24h × 10-20 days	G, H: coccidiostat
	75	PO	7-14 days	G, H: coccidiostat
Sulfamerazine	1-5 mg/ml	Drinking water	q24h for several weeks	G, H: coccidiostat
Sulfaquinoxaline	0.1%	Drinking water	q24h for several weeks	G, H: coccidiostat
Thiabendazole	100	PO	q24h × 5 days	G, H

Data from Adamcak A, Otten B: Rodent therapeutics, *Vet Clin North Am Exot Anim Pract* 3(1):221-237, 2000.
G, gerbil; *H*, hamster; *IM*, intramuscular; *IP*, intraperitoneal; *IV*, intravenous; *PO*, per os; *prn*, as needed; *SC*, subcutaneous.
*mg/kg, unless otherwise stated.

presence of mites on microscopic examination of a skin scraping are diagnostic.[18] Ivermectin, frequent bedding changes, and environmental disinfection are the treatments of choice for these mites (Table 15-5). Both of these mites may require more than 2 or 3 treatments, and response and continued treatment should be based on continued skin scrape evaluations. Environmental sanitation should be emphasized to prevent reinfestation. Lime-sulfur dips may also be of use in clinical cases refractory to ivermectin treatment.

The hamster can have a transient infestation of the tropical rat mite, *Ornithonyssus bacoti*, or the northern fowl mite, *O. sylvarium*.[21] Clinical signs associated with these two parasites are limited to pruritus and bites. The transient nature of a northern fowl mite infestation allows only frequent bedding and cage changes as necessary for treatment.[18] However, owners should be informed that the bite of the northern fowl mite can cause pain, pruritus, and erythematous papular skin lesions in humans.[25]

ECTOPARASITES IN GERBILS

A gerbil infested with the demodectic mite (*Demodex meroni*) will present with clinical signs of alopecia, hyperemia, ulceration, scaly skin, and secondary bacterial pyoderma.[26] Predisposing factors, such as age and systemic disease, should be investigated after a definitive diagnosis is made by microscopic examination of a skin scraping.[18] Several other mite species have been observed on gerbils without apparent clinical signs. Because some of these mites can cause disease in humans, they are included here, and owners should be warned of the mild risk of zoonotic disease. *Tyrophagus castellani*, the copra itch mite, has been an incidental finding on gerbils.[21] *T. castellani* is a stored-products mite that feeds on fungi living on stored dried coconut kernels used for the production of coconut oil. This mite has been associated with cutaneous and respiratory allergies in workers from Italy.[25] *Liponyssoides sanguineus*, the house mouse mite, has been seen on gerbils and in their cage bedding.[27] The house mite spends most of its time in the bedding, only crawling onto the gerbil to blood feed. The house mite can bite humans, resulting in reddened papules and pruritus. Further, this mite can transmit *Rickettsia akari*, the causative agent of rickettsial pox, a zoonotic disease.[25] If these mites are identified in gerbils, frequent bedding changes and cage cleanings are warranted.

Nutritional Disease

Gerbils fed a rat or mouse diet rather than a gerbil diet can develop periodontal disease, obesity, and diabetes.[8] Hamsters are likely to develop nutritional secondary hyperparathyroidism if fed a predominantly seed or unbalanced diet.

Clinical signs of cystic calculi or cystic bladder stones in the hamster include hematuria, stranguria, dysuria, incontinence, anorexia, and pain. If urolithiasis is diagnosed, owners need to be warned about the common recurrence of cystic calculi. A dietary history should be obtained because calculi are often diet related and may respond to dietary management.

Neoplastic Disease in Hamsters

The incidence of neoplastic disease in the Syrian hamster is only 4%.[4] However, for hamsters over 2 years old, the incidence of neoplasia may approach 50%, although most tumors are benign.[4] Hamsters have a variety of tumors reported (Table 15-6); the system most commonly affected by tumors is the endocrine system, followed by lymphoreticular, dermatologic, and gastrointestinal systems.[4]

The most common tumors of the hamster are carcinomas or adenomas of the adrenal cortex. Clinical signs of adrenal tumors in the hamster are alopecia, behavior change, and skin hyperpigmentation.[29] The incidence of adrenal tumors is 14.5% overall, with 1.7% in hamsters less than 1 year old, 35.5% in hamsters in their second year, and 40% in hamsters older than 2 years.[29] Treatment of adrenal tumors in three related teddy bear or long-haired hamsters with metapyrone and op-DDD resulted in clinical improvement for only one of the hamsters.[29] Benign follicular thyroid tumors have occurred in hamsters with known iodine deficiency.[4]

Three clinical variants of lymphoma—multicentric, cutaneous, and epizootic—exist in hamsters.[8] The multicentric form occurs in adult hamsters and affects the thymus; thoracic, mesenteric, and superficial lymph nodes; spleen; and liver. The cutaneous form resembles mycosis fungoides and causes lethargy, anorexia, weight loss, patchy alopecia, and exfoliative erythroderma in adult hamsters. The epizootic form occurs in young hamsters and is caused by hamster polyoma virus. These animals develop skin tumors, appear thin, and develop palpable abdominal masses or enlargements of the mesenteric, axillary, or cervical lymph nodes. Treatment of lymphoma in hamsters remains anecdotal and is based on companion mammal regimens, with medication administered subcutaneously, orally, or intraperitoneally.

Reproductive tumors of the golden hamster are uncommon but include tumors of the ovaries and uterus. Ovarian tumors are usually benign in hamsters and gerbils while uterine tumors are often malignant.[30] Thecoma, granulosa cell tumors, leiomyomas, and endometrial polyps have been reported.[29] Uterine adenocarcinoma is common in Chinese or striped hamsters older than 100 weeks of age. Clinical signs of vaginal hemorrhage and a radiographically enlarged uterus may be observed in cases of hamster uterine adenocarcinoma.[29]

Hamsters rarely present with skin tumors, but the most common skin tumor of the hamster is melanoma. This tumor is seen in males, likely because of the enlarged hip glands in the male hamster.[29] Cutaneous mastocytoma of the head and neck occurs with about a 10% incidence in Russian or Djungarian hamsters, and basal cell tumors have also been reported in this species. Djungarian hamsters have a midventral sebaceous gland that should not be considered abnormal anatomy.[29] Male reproductive tumors, tumors of the urinary system, and tumors of the central nervous system are rare but have been identified.[4]

Neoplastic Disease in Gerbils

The neoplastic incidence in gerbils over 2 years of age is high (8.4%-26.5%).[4,29] This incidence includes wild-caught animals as well as the first generations bred in the laboratory.[29] Tumors of the female reproductive system, especially ovarian tumors, are most common, followed by those of the skin and subcutis.[4,29] Although not a neoplastic disease, cystic ovaries are also common in the female gerbil. Tumors of the ventral, abdominal scent gland account for a large percentage of the tumors of the skin reported in this species. The neoplastic scent gland of the gerbil may appear grossly inflamed or ulcerated, predisposing the affected tissue to secondary bacterial infections. Benign adenomas also occur; therefore, it is important to differentiate normal ventral abdominal gland from ulcerated tumors.[29] Melanomas of the ear, foot, and base of the tail have also been reported in the gerbil. Tumors that have been identified in the gerbil are listed in Table 15-6.

Endocrine Disease

Whereas adrenocortical neoplasia in the hamster is common, clinical signs resulting from Cushing's disease in the hamster are rarely noted. Diagnosis of adrenocortical disease in the hamster relies on observance of the clinical signs as seen in the dog: polydipsia, polyuria, polyphagia, alopecia, hyperpigmentation, and increased serum concentration of cortisol and alkaline phosphatase. Although hamsters can respond to exogenous adrenocorticotropic hormone administration, they secrete both cortisol and corticosterone. Reference ranges of serum cortisol are 0.5 to 1.0 mg/dl in the adult healthy male and female hamster.[31] Thus, appropriate diagnosis is somewhat empirical. Treatment with op-DDD and metapyrone have been attempted with equivocal results.[31]

Miscellaneous Disease in Hamsters

Amyloidosis of the liver and kidneys is associated with weight loss in the aged hamster and is the leading cause of death in laboratory hamsters.[31] Factors that contribute to the development of amyloidosis in hamsters include crowding and gender. Compared with male hamsters, female hamsters have a higher incidence, increased severity, and earlier age of onset of amyloidosis. Although no reports of this disease exist in pet hamsters, expected clinical signs include edema and ascites due to

TABLE 15-6 **Tumors of the Gerbil and Hamster**

System	Tumor	Mongolian jird (gerbil)	Hamster
Endocrine	Adrenal cortical adenoma	X	X
	Adenocarcinoma	X	X
	Follicular thyroid	X	X
	Pancreatic islet cell carcinomas	X	X
	Thymoma		X
	Pituitary chromophobe adenoma		
	Parathyroid		
Lymphoreticular/hemopoietic/ splenic	Lymphoma/lymphosarcoma	X	X
	Splenic hemangioma	X	X
	Splenic histiocytic sarcoma	X	
Skin	Cutaneous lymphosarcoma	X	X
	Cutaneous hemangiosarcoma	X	X
	Basal cell carcinoma	X	
	Melanoma	X	
	Sebaceous adenoma	X	
	Fibrosarcoma	X	
	Squamous cell carcinoma	X	
	Aural cholesteatoma (keratoma)		
Gastrointestinal/hepatic	Adenoma		X
	Cheek pouch fibroma		X
	Papilloma	X	X
	Adenocarcinoma	X	X
	Cholangioma		X
	Hepatic lymphangioma		X
	Hepatocellular carcinoma		
	Histiocytic sarcoma of the liver		
Reproductive	Cervical carcinoma		X
	Vaginal squamous cell carcinoma	X	X
	Thecoma	X	X
	Granulosa cell	X	X
	Dysgerminoma	X	X
	Teratoma	X	X
	Lutein cell tumor	X	X
	Leiomyomas	X	X
	Endometrial polyp		X
	Adenocarcinoma		X
	Seminoma		
	Teratoma		
	Prostatic adenomas		
Urinary	Urinary hemangioma	X	
	Renal hemangiosarcoma	X	
Musculoskeletal	Osteosarcoma	X	
Nervous	Astrocytoma (glioma)	X	

From Battles A: The biology, care and diseases of the Syrian hamster, *Vet Compend Cont Ed* 7(10):815-825, 1985; Harkness J, Wagner J: *The Biology and Medicine of Rabbits and Rodents,* ed 4, Baltimore, 1995, Lippincott Williams and Wilkins; Greenacre C: Spontaneous tumors of small mammals, *Vet Clin North Am Exot Anim Pract* 7:627-651, 2004.

hypoproteinemia resulting from hepatic and renal insufficiency. The prognosis in these cases would be guarded and treatment is supportive.

Cardiomyopathy occurs in the aged hamster, older than $1\frac{1}{2}$ years.[31] Clinical signs include tachypnea, lethargy, anorexia, and hypothermic extremities. Treatment is based on that for dogs and cats and may include digoxin, diuretics, angiotensin enzyme inhibitors, calcium channel blockers, and prophylactic anticoagulants (see Table 15-10 later in this chapter). There is little information available to determine the short- or long-term effectiveness of cardiac therapy in hamsters.

Miscellaneous Disease in Gerbils

From 20% to 40% of captive gerbils develop spontaneous, "reflex, stereotypic epileptiform (tonic-clonic)" seizures.[31] Seizure activity may be initiated by sudden stress, handling, or introduction to a new environment. This is an inherited trait caused by a deficiency in cerebral glutamine synthetase. Seizure-prone and seizure-resistant strains have been bred for laboratory use. Onset of seizure activity usually occurs at about 2 months of age and lasts until the animal reaches 6 months of age. The seizure response to handling can be substantially mitigated by frequent handling in the first 3 weeks of life. Seizures can vary in severity from a cessation of activity and pinnae and vibrissae twitching to myoclonic convulsions followed by tonic extensor rigidity. A refractory period of up to 5 days can follow severe seizures. Treatment is not recommended; fatality due to seizure is rare and most gerbils suffer no permanent damage. Treatment with diphenylhydantoin is not recommended, as deaths associated with its administration have occurred in gerbils.[31]

■ THERAPEUTICS

All drugs administered to rodents are used in an extralabel manner, as no drugs are currently approved for use in rodent species. Few drugs have pharmacokinetic studies performed in rodents to guide dosage regimes; therefore, all doses must be considered anecdotal. Dosages can be based on allometric scaling; however, this is no substitute for pharmacokinetic data, which accounts for the animal's size and metabolic rate as well as many other complex physiologic processes, such as hepatic metabolism, renal filtration, and excretion rates. Clients should be advised of the extralabel manner in which these animals are routinely treated.

Medication Administration Considerations in Hamsters and Gerbils

Route of administration for rodents are guided by temperament, size, and restraint methods. Parenteral administration of drugs is generally limited to subcutaneous, intramuscular, intraperitoneal, or intraosseous routes (Table 15-7).

For intraperitoneal access in the rodent, hold the rodent in dorsal recumbency with the head below the abdomen and the hindlimb in extension. Inject into the caudal abdomen on the side of the extended leg.[28] In the gerbil, intraperitoneal injection into the right side is preferred, to avoid iatrogenic injection or trauma to the cecum, liver, and spleen. The intramuscular route of administration is restricted in hamster and gerbil patients because of their small size and muscle mass. The muscles of the caudal thigh are avoided because of their proximity to the sciatic nerve. Inadvertent injection of irritating substances in this area may result in lameness or self-mutilation of the area.[8]

Intravenous administration in the hamster and gerbil is limited to a single injection into the tail vein, which is functionally absent in the short-tailed hamster and which is fully furred and subject to degloving in the gerbil. This procedure is therefore limited to the anesthetized gerbil. The cephalic, saphenous, or jugular vein can be catheterized with sedation or anesthesia for fluid and drug administration, but these methods are difficult to perform. Intraosseous fluid and drug administration is an alternative that provides vascular access and ease of maintenance. Generally, the intraosseous catheter is placed in the proximal aspect of the tibia or femur.[28]

Medication administration via food or water may be problematic in the hamster and gerbil. Most rodents are unlikely to ingest feed with an unfamiliar taste or smell. Thus, medication of food or water may result in nontherapeutic drug levels or, even worse, reduced intake of food or water in the ill rodent. In most cases oral medication via gastric lavage or oral syringe is preferred over food or water medication. Nebulization has not been extensively investigated in rodent species but has been beneficial to small rodents that present with respiratory disease treated by the authors.

Fluid Therapy

Hamsters and gerbils who go into cardiopulmonary arrest secondary to hypovolemic shock can be treated with shock fluid doses of 65 to 80 ml/kg for the hamster and 60 to 85 ml/kg for the gerbil.[32] If hypovolemic shock is not the cause of the cardiopulmonary arrest, a combination of crystalloids (10-15 ml/kg at rapid infusion) and colloids (5 ml/kg Hetastarch over 5-10 min) is recommended for fluid resuscitation.[33] Preoperative subcutaneous fluid administration of 4% dextrose at 10 ml/kg has been advocated for the small rodent.[34] Controlled infusion using a syringe driver or fluid pump (e.g.,

TABLE 15-7	Details Recommended Routes for Drug Administration in Gerbils and Hamsters				
Route	**Species**	**Site**	**Maximum volume**	**Needle gauge**
Intramuscular	Gerbil and hamster	Quadriceps, gluteals	0.1 ml/site	23-26
Intraperitoneal	Gerbil	Lower right quadrant of abdomen	2-3	22-26
	Hamster		3-4	
Intravenous	Gerbil	Lateral tail veins	0.2-0.3	25-26
Intragastric	Gerbil	Stomach	3-5 ml/100 g BW	18-22; 3-4 cm*
	Hamster	Stomach	3-5 ml/100 g BW	18; 4-4.5 cm*
Subcutaneous	Gerbil	Neck, back	2-3	21-26
	Hamster	Neck, back, abdomen	3-5	

*Bulbed feeding needle.
BW, body weight.

BOX 15-1 **Rehydration of Hamsters and Gerbils Based on Hypovolemic Presentations**

Blood Volume Lost	Fluid Recommendations
5%-10%	Balanced crystalloids at three times the estimated volume of blood loss
10%-20%	Colloids (e.g., hetastarch, plasma)
20%-30%	Whole blood transfusion

Medfusion 3 2010i, Medexing, Duluth, GA) is recommended because the volume of fluids to be administered is small. Maintenance fluid rates of 5 to 10 ml/kg/hr are appropriate for these small patients.[35] For the hemorrhaging patient, the packed cell volume and total solids determination do not immediately reflect severity of blood loss. Blood loss greater than 20% of blood volume (i.e., 1.2 ml for the gerbil, 1.4 ml for the hamster) may be dangerous.[36] Therefore, general guidelines for fluid selection have been developed (Box 15-1).[35]

Although technically challenging in small rodents, vascular access should be obtained prior to anesthetic induction for fluid resuscitation and emergency drug therapy. Intraosseous catheters, (e.g., spinal needles, small-gauge needles), can be placed in the proximal femur or tibia.[37] Potential vascular catheterization of the hamster is best accomplished with placement of a 27- to 30-gauge needle in the lateral tarsus, cephalic, lingual, or dorsal penile vein.[38] Using a 25-gauge needle, sites often used for vascular access in the gerbil include the lateral tail, saphenous, and metatarsal veins.

Antimicrobial Agents

Antibiotic-associated enteritis or antibiotic-associated clostridial enterotoxemia or dysbiosis commonly occurs in rodents, causing severe, even fatal, gastrointestinal tract disease. Hamsters are one of the most susceptible species to this syndrome, whereas gerbils are relatively more resistant.[13,28] The bacterial flora of most rodents is Gram positive, with the hamster's normal intestinal flora being predominantly *Lactobacillus* spp. and *Bacteroides* spp. The most common mechanism of antibiotic-associated enteritis is via disruption of normal enteric bacterial flora or dysbiosis; however, other mechanisms, such as disruption of gastrointestinal ion transport and disruption of muscular function, can also occur.[39] Dysbiosis occurs as normal bacteria are killed by antibiotics; this leads to overgrowth of abnormal flora, particularly *E. coli* and *Clostridium* spp. This bacterial growth lowers intestinal pH, creating a favorable environment for continued growth of these inappropriate bacteria. In the hamster, *C. difficile* overgrowth is more common, and treatment with cephalosporin or lincomycin can result in patient death.[39] Other drugs associated with dysbiosis in hamsters are the penicillins, including ampicillin and amoxicillin, clindamycin, erythromycin, vancomycin, bacitracin, oral gentamicin, and tylosin.[13]

Cases of dysbiosis warrant a guarded prognosis. Treatment consists of fluid therapy, supportive care, nutritional support, and some specific therapies. Administration of *Lactobacillus* spp. in a probiotic preparation (see Table 15-10 later in this chapter) and cholestyramine, a strongly basic anion exchange resin that binds the toxins of enterotoxemia, may alleviate clinical signs.[28] Transfaunation may also be considered to replace normal gastrointestinal flora. Balanced appropriate antibiotic therapy, metronidazole therapy, motility modifiers, and antiendotoxin therapy may also be indicated.

Administration of streptomycin, dihydrostreptomycin, and procaine in hamster and gerbils is contraindicated.[28] These drugs are toxic to these species and death ensues shortly after administration. Death is caused by the neuromuscular blocking action of these drugs (Table 15-8).[28]

Emergency Drugs

Emergency drug dosages should be calculated before any anesthetic event. Although no specific dosages have been calculated for hamsters and gerbils, recommendations can be made based on weight (Tables 15-9 and 15-10).[41]

Cardiopulmonary Resusitation CPR

The general resuscitation rules of **ABC**—establishing an **a**irway, **b**reathing for the patient, and **c**ardiac stimulation—apply in the gerbil or hamster in cardiopulmonary arrest. If intubation proves difficult, emergency airway access of these small rodents can be obtained by tracheostomy, wherein an over-the-needle catheter is inserted between the tracheal rings.[42] Positive-pressure ventilation with 100% oxygen is provided at 20 to 30 breaths/min.[41] External chest compressions or circumferential cardiac compressions at a rate of at least 100/min produce blood flow by the cardiac pump and increase cardiac output in small mammals. An intraosseous or intravenous catheter should be placed to provide vascular access. (Shock fluid dosages were listed earlier, in Fluid Therapy.) The amount of time before the onset of severe neurologic damage is shorter in small rodents because of their high metabolic rate.[41]

Small mammals go into decompensatory shock, manifested by normal or slow heart rate, severe hypothermia, weak pulse, and depression.[33] Because hypothermia plays a significant role in shock and extremely small animals are more predisposed to a drop in core body temperature, re-warming must be part of the resuscitation plan. During the critical recovery period, patients should be placed in a dark, warm environment for monitoring. Supportive care provided while the patient is anesthetized should be continued until the patient has fully recovered. Anesthetic agents, blood glucose levels, and thermoregulation should be considered when recovery is prolonged.

For humane euthanasia of hamsters and gerbils, cardiac injection of euthanasia solution is recommended.[42]

Nutritional Support and Hospital Diets

Nutritional support is needed not only in the anorectic gerbil or hamster but also in the gerbil or hamster that is eating but

TABLE 15-8	Antibiotics for Use in Hamsters and Gerbils		
Antibiotic	**Dose (mg/kg)**	**Regimen**	**Indication/species**
Amikacin	0.5-1.0 IM	q12h	G, H: renal toxicity can occur
	2-5 SC, IM	q8-12h	H, G
	10-20 SC, IM total daily dose divided	q8-24h	G
	10-15 SC, IM, IV total daily dose divided	q8-24h	G
Ampicillin	20-100 PO, SC total daily dose divided	q8h	PO may be associated with dysbiosis; G: *S. pneumoniae* pneumonia
Chloramphenicol palmitate	50 PO	q12h	G, H
	50-200 PO	q8h	G, H
Chloramphenicol succinate	20-50 SC	q6-12h	G, H
	50 SC	q12h	G, H: proliferative ileitis, dermatitis, skin abscesses
Chlortetracycline	20 IM, SC	q12h	H
Ciprofloxacin	7-20 PO	q12h	G, H
Doxycycline	2.5-5.0 PO	q12h	G, H Do not use in young or pregnant animals
Erythromycin	20 PO	q12h	H*: proliferative ileitis
	0.13 mg/1 ml drinking water	q24h	H*: proliferative ileitis May cause enterocolitis
Gentamicin	2-4 SC, IM	q8-24h	G, H
	5 SC, IM	q24h	G, H
Metronidazole	20-60 PO	q8-12h	G, H
	7.5 mg/70-90 g body weight PO	q8h	G, H Anaerobes, add sucrose to increase palatability
Neomycin	0.5 mg/1 ml drinking water	q24h	H
	100 PO	q24h	G, H: proliferative ileitis
Oxytetracycline	10 PO	q8h	G
	0.8 mg/1 ml drinking water	q24h	G
	16 SC	q24h	H
	0.25-1.0 mg/1 ml drinking water	q24h	H
Sulfadimethoxine	10-15 PO	q12h	G, H
Sulfamerazine	0.8 mg/1 ml drinking water	q24h	G
	1 mg/1 ml drinking water	q24h	H
Sulfamethazine	0.8 mg/1 ml drinking water	q24h	G
	1 mg/1 ml drinking water	q24h	H
Sulfaquinoxaline	1 mg/1 ml drinking water	q24h	G, H
Tetracycline	10-20 PO	q8-12h	G, H
	20 IM, PO	q24h	G
	20 IM, PO	q4h	G
	0.4 mg/1 ml drinking water	q24h × 10 days	H: proliferative ileitis
	30 mg PO	q6h	H: proliferative ileitis
	2-5 mg/1 ml drinking water	q24h	G: Tyzzer's disease, *Mycoplasma* spp. pneumonia
Trimethoprim sulfa	15-30 PO, SC, IM	q12h	H, G Tissue necrosis may occur when given SC
Tylosin	2-8 PO, SC, IM	q12h	H*
	10 PO, SC, IM	q24h	G, H: proliferative ileitis
	0.5 mg/1 ml in drinking water	q24h	G, H*
Vancomycin	20 mg/kg		H: *Clostridium difficile* enteritis, treatment for 3+ mo

Data from Johnson-Delaney C: Small rodents. In Harrison LR, editor: *Exotic Companion Medicine Handbook,* Lake Worth, Fla, 1998, Zoological Education Network; Ness RD: Rodents. In Carpenter JW, editor: *Exotic Animal Formulary,* ed 3, St Louis, 2005, WB Saunders; Adamcak A, Otten B: Rodent therapeutics, *Vet Clin North Am Exot Anim Pract* 3(1):221-237, 2000; Morrisey JK, Carpenter JW: Formulary. In Quesenberry KE, Carpenter JW, editors: *Ferrets, Rabbits and Rodents: Clinical Medicine and Surgery,* St Louis, 2004, WB Saunders.

G, gerbil; *H,* hamster; *IM,* intramuscular; *IP,* intraperitoneal; *IV,* intravenous; *PO,* per os; *prn,* as needed; *SC,* subcutaneous.

*Use with caution. Toxicity, enteritis, and other problems have been reported with use of this drug in this species. Discontinue drug use if enteritis, diarrhea, anorexia, or other gastrointestinal signs occur. Consider concomitant administration of probiotics when using this drug.

TABLE 15-9 Emergency Drugs for Use in the Hamster and Gerbil Based on Weight

Drug (conc.)	Dose (mg/kg)	25 g	50 g	100 g	200 g
Epinephrine					
Low (1:10,000) (0.1 mg/ml)	0.01	0.0025 ml	0.005 ml	0.01 ml	0.02 ml
High (1:1000) (1 mg/ml)	0.1	0.0025 ml	0.005 ml	0.01 ml	0.02 ml
Atropine (0.54 mg/ml)	0.05	0.0025 ml	0.005 ml	0.01 ml	0.02 ml
Lidocaine (20 mg/ml)	2	0.0025 ml	0.005 ml	0.01 ml	0.02 ml
Calcium (100 mg/ml)	30	0.0075 ml	0.015 ml	0.03 ml	0.06 ml
Vasopressin (20 units/ml)	0.8*	0.001 ml	0.002 ml	0.004 ml	0.008 ml
Naloxone (0.4 mg/ml)	0.05	0.003 ml	0.006 ml	0.012 ml	0.025 ml
Flumazenil (0.1 mg/ml)	0.02	0.005 ml	0.01 ml	0.02 ml	0.04 ml
Yohimbine (2 mg/ml)	0.2	0.003 ml	0.005 ml	0.01 ml	0.02 ml

* units/kg

TABLE 15-10 Miscellaneous Drugs for Use in the Hamster and Gerbil

Drug	Dose (mg/kg)	Route, regimen	Indication	Species
Atropine	10	SC q20 min	Organophosphate overdose	G, H
Cimetidine	5-10	PO, SC, IM q6-12h		G, H
Cisapride	0.1-0.5	PO q12h	Motility enhancer	G, H
Dexamethasone	0.1-0.6	IM	Antiinflammatory	G, H
Doxapram	5-10	IV	Respiratory stimulant	
Digoxin	0.05-0.1	PO q12h	Dilated cardiomyopathy	H
Furosemide	5-10	IV, SC q12h		G, H
LRS	50-100 ml/kg	q24h IV, SC, IP	Maintenance fluid supplementation	G, H
	10-25 ml/kg	IV bolus over 5-10 min	Critical hypovolemic shock	
Lactobacilli		PO, 2h pre- or 2h postantibiotic administration. Give during and 5-7 days after antibiotic administration	Normal flora maintenance; prevention of dysbiosis	G, H
Loperamide HCL	0.1	PO q8hr. Give in 1 ml water	Antidiarrheal	G, H
Metoclopramide	0.2-1.0	PO, SC, IM q12h	Motility modifier	G, H
Naloxone	0.01-0.1	IP, IV	Respiratory stimulant	G, H
Oxytocin	0.2-3.0 IU/kg	IV, IM, SC	Milk let down, parturition induction, uterine involution	G, H
Prednisone	0.5-2.2	IM, SC		G, H
Vitamin A	2 mg/1 g feed	In food daily		H
Vitamin B	0.002-.02 ml/100 g	IM, SC	Hamster cage paralysis	G, H
Vitamin B complex	0.02-0.2 ml/kg	IM, SC		G, H
Vitamin E/selenium	0.1 ml/100-250 g body weight	SC	Hamster cage paralysis	G, H
Vitamin K₁	1-10	PO prn	Coumarin rodenticide toxicity	G, H
Xenodyne		Swab affected area prn		

Data from Johnson-Delaney C: Small rodents. In Harrison LR, editor: *Exotic Companion Medicine Handbook,* Lake Worth, Fla, 1998, Zoological Education Network.
G, gerbil; *H,* hamster; *IM,* intramuscular; *IP,* intraperitoneal; *IV,* intravenous; *PO,* per os; *prn,* as needed; *SC,* subcutaneous.

continuing to lose weight and body condition. Nutritional support diets appropriate for herbivores are commercially available (Critical care for herbivores, Oxbow Pet Products, Murdoch, NE). However, pureed baby food (e.g., spinach, apples, carrots) mixed with a slurry of moistened rabbit or rodent pellets and yogurt containing active cultures may also be used. Adding honey to the slurry may increase palatability.

Analgesia in Hamsters and Gerbils

The use of preemptive analgesics, such as opioids and nonsteroidal antiinflammatory drugs (NSAIDs), reduces the amount of anesthetic required to maintain a surgical plane, decreases peripheral inflammation, and inhibits noxious stimuli from reaching the central nervous system (Table 15-11).[43] However, because injectable anesthetics cannot be dosed to effect,

TABLE 15-11	Analgesics, Anesthetics, and Premedicants for Use in the Hamster and Gerbil			
Drug	**Dose***	**Route**	**Regimen**	**Comments**
Acepromazine	0.5-1.0	IM	Once	H only
Acetaminophen	1-2 mg/ml	Drinking water	Mix fresh daily	G, H: Analgesia
Atropine	0.05	SC, IM	Once	Premed G, H
Aspirin	100-150	PO	q4h	G, H
Buprenorphine	0.05-0.1	SC, IV	q6-8h	Analgesia G, H
Butorphanol	1-5	SC	q4h	Analgesia G, H
Carprofen	5	SC	q12h	G, H
Diazepam	1-5	IM, IP, IO, IV	Once	G, H: Premed, seizures
Flunixin meglumine	2.5 mg/kg	SC	q12h	G, H: Analgesia
Glycopyrrolate	0.01-0.02	SC, IM	Once, prn	G, H: Premed
Ketamine/ diazepam	40/1-2	IM	Once	G, H: Restraint/light sedation
Ketamine/medetomidine	100/250 µg/kg	IP	Once	Surgical anesthesia
Ketamine/xylazine	50/2	IP	Once	G
	50-100/5-10	IP	Once	H
				Muscle necrosis if given IM
Meloxicam	1-2	IM, SC, PO	q24h	G, H: Analgesia
Midazolam	3-5	IM, SC	Once	G, H: Premed
	1-2	IM		G, H: Short-acting sedative
Naloxone	0.01-0.1	SC, IP	Once or prn	G, H: Narcotic reversal
Oxymorphone	0.2-0.5	SC, IM	q6-12h	G, H: Analgesia
Tiletamine/zolazepam (Telazol)	50-80	IP	Once	G, H: Anesthetic induction and maintenance; immobilization
				G: Prolonged recovery
Telazol/xylazine	30/10	IP	Once	H: 30 min of surgical time
				Causes muscle necrosis if given IM
Xylazine	5-10	IM, SC, IP	Once	G, H: Premed
				Causes muscle necrosis if given IM

Data from Harkness J, Wagner J: *The Biology and Medicine of Rabbits and Rodents,* ed 4, Baltimore, 1995, Lippincott Williams and Wilkins: Adamcak A, Otten B: Rodent therapeutics, *Vet Clin North Am Exot Anim Pract* 3(1):221-237, 2000; Heard DJ: Anesthesia, analgesia, and sedation of small mammals. In Quesenberry KE, Carpenter JW, editors: *Ferrets, Rabbits and Rodents: Clinical Medicine and Surgery,* St Louis, 2003, WB Saunders; Cantwell S: Ferret, rabbit, and rodent anesthesia, *Vet Clin North Am Exot Anim Pract* 4(1):169-191, 2001; Morrisey JK, Carpenter JW: Formulary. In Quesenberry KE, Carpenter JW, editors: *Ferrets, Rabbits and Rodents: Clinical Medicine and Surgery,* St Louis, 2004, WB Saunders; Flecknell P: Analgesia of small mammals, *Semin Av Exot Pet Med* 7(1):41-47, 2001; Hrapkeiwicz K, Stein S, Smiler K: A new anesthetic agent for use in the gerbil, *Lam Anim Sci* 39(4):338-341, 1989; Curl J: Ketamine-xylazine anaesthesia in the Djungarian hamster *(Phodopus sungorus), Lab Anim* 22:309-312, 1988.

G, gerbil; *H,* hamster; *IM,* intramuscular; *IP,* intraperitoneal; *IV,* intravenous; *PO,* per os; *prn,* as needed; *SC,* subcutaneous.
*mg/kg, unless otherwise stated.

preemptive analgesia may be inappropriate for use in these anesthetic protocols. Postoperative analgesia should be provided, however. Multimodal analgesia is still preferred, whether an inhalant or an injectable anesthetic protocol is used. Combinations of analgesics from different classes increase the effectiveness of the analgesia and, in general, decrease the required dosages for the administered agents. Concurrent administration of short-term rapid-acting analgesics (e.g., buprenorphine) and long-term slow-acting drugs (e.g., NSAIDs) has been recommended.[43]

■ANESTHESIA

Patient Monitoring and Supportive Care

The large surface area to body mass ratio of these patients makes them highly susceptible to hypothermia, so thermoregulatory support is essential.[46] Hypothermia can be prevented by increasing ambient temperature, decreasing surgical and anesthesia time, warming parenteral fluids and flush, wrapping the body in insulating materials (e.g., plastic bubble wrap), and using circulating warmwater pads.[38] Convective heaters (e.g., Bair® Hugger Warming Unit, Augustine Medical, Eden Prairie, MN) are effective in maintaining core body temperature, but temperature monitoring is essential to avoid overheating the patient.[47]

Ophthalmic ointment and eyelid closure should be attended to before surgery is performed. Xylazine, used both in combination and alone (see Table 15-11), has been identified as a causative agent of acute reversible cataracts in rodents; however, prevention can easily be achieved with eyelid closure during anesthesia.[48] Because dissociative anesthetics decrease tearing and the palpebrae remain open, ophthalmic ointment should be applied to protect the eyes.

Response to painful stimuli, such as a pinch of the toe, tail, or ear, should be absent in small animals in a surgical plane of anesthesia. Whereas the respiratory rate will decrease at a surgi-

From Bailey J, Pablo L: Anesthetic monitoring and monitoring equipment: application in small exotic pet practice, *Semin Av Exot Pet Med* 7(1):53-60, 1998.

BOX 15-2	Allometric Equations for Hamsters and Gerbils
Heart rate (beats/min)	$241 \times BW(kg)^{-0.25}$
Respiratory rate (breaths/min)	$53.5 \times BW(kg)^{-0.26}$
Tidal volume (ml)	$7.69 \times BW(kg)^{1.04}$

cal plane of anesthesia, the depth of respiration should be similar to that of the awake patient. Palpebral reflex and some jaw tone will remain. Loss of corneal reflex suggests the patient is hazardously deep, and appropriate measures are required to improve the animal's condition.[46]

Allometric equations can approximate resting values to use when monitoring vital signs in anesthetized small rodents (Box 15-2).

Cardiovascular monitoring during surgery is best achieved through the use of a Doppler ultrasonic flow probe. Contact sites for small mammals include the ventral aspect of the tail base, carotid, femoral and auricular arteries, and directly over the heart. Unfortunately, the small size of hamsters and gerbils precludes an accurate measurement of indirect blood pressure.[46] Pulse oximetry is accurate in small mammals for hemoglobin saturation levels greater than 85%.[35] The transmission probe may be placed on the foot pad, ear, tongue, or proximal tail. Thermoregulatory monitoring and support is essential in these small patients, with established rectal temperatures for hamsters being 98.6° to 100.4° F and gerbils being 98.6° to 102.2° F.[32]

Anesthetic Premedication

General anesthesia and recovery time can be reduced by preanesthetic administration of tranquilizers and sedatives. Consider parasympatholytics to prevent bradycardia if the rodent is to be anesthetized with a ketamine/α_2-adrenergic agonist combination. Parasympatholytics also decrease secretions and prevent vagally mediated bradyarrhythmias. Atropine is rapidly eliminated from the rodent body based on its metabolism; therefore, glycopyrrolate is considered a more effective anticholinergic agent for use in these species.[49]

Sedatives indicated for use in the hamster and gerbil include acepromazine, diazepam, midazolam, and xylazine. These drugs also provide increased depth of anesthesia, decreased muscular tone, and provide some pain control. While acepromazine may be used for tranquilizing the healthy hamster, it is contraindicated for use in the epileptic gerbil.[38] Benzodiazepines such diazepam and midazolam provide a mild tranquilizing effect with minimal cardiopulmonary effects; thus they are viable tranquilizer selections for the debilitated patient and can also increase muscle relaxation and anesthetic duration. α_2-adrenergic agonists such as xylazine medetomidine have the added benefit of being reversible. Tolazoline may be the most effective reversal agent for α_2 agonists in hamsters and gerbils, as it is in rats.[50]

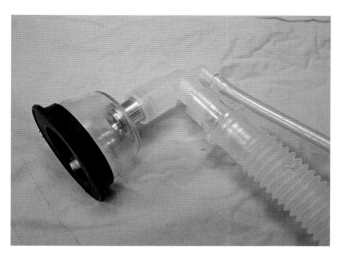

Figure 15-15 Small anesthetic mask with a fresh gas inlet *(right, smaller tube)* and gas scavenging hose *(left, larger hose)*. This system can be used in anesthesia of gerbils and hamsters without intubation.

Parenteral Anesthesia
DRUG ADMINISTRATION

Routes of administration in small rodents include intraosseous (IO), intraperitoneal (IP), subcutaneous (SC), intravenous (IV), and intramuscular (IM). Intraperitoneal injections should be given in the lower left abdominal quadrant after aspirating the syringe to ensure that the injection does not infiltrate a blood vessel or organ.[4] Avoid the intramuscular administration of anesthetic agents, as significant muscle necrosis has been reported with their administration.[4]

Injectable anesthetic regimens for hamsters and gerbils are covered in Table 15-11. Injectable anesthetic regimens in gerbils are generally avoided because of fatality and prolonged recoveries.[35,43,44] Ketamine combinations may not provide a surgical plane of anesthesia and can cause fatality in gerbils. Therefore, inhalant anesthesia is preferred in this species. A variety of injectable anesthetic regimens have been used in the hamster, but isoflurane anesthesia is still the preferred agent.

Inhalation Anesthesia
ANESTHETIC EQUIPMENT

Nonrebreathing systems, such as the Bain coaxial or a modified T-piece, are indicated for anesthetizing small rodents.[51] The minimum fresh gas flow rate is about 100 to 200 ml/kg/min in the gerbil and hamster. Small balloons used as rebreathing bags allow for visualization of respiration.[35] A face mask is often used to maintain inhalant anesthesia in these patients because intubation is challenging and stressful. If intubation is not elected, the mask should have a fresh gas line inlet and a waste gas line outlet (Figure 15-15).[35]

While intubation provides for assisted ventilation, administration of inhalants reduces the incidence of upper airway obstruction; small endotracheal tubes are easily occluded, and the opacity of catheters prevents visualization of obstruction by fluid condensation, mucus, or blood. Intubation can be challenging in these diminutive patients. For hamsters, a 16-gauge over-the-needle catheter or a tomcat urinary catheter can serve as an endotracheal tube.[35] A similar or smaller sized tube may be appropriate for gerbils.

INHALANT ANESTHETICS

Isoflurane and sevoflurane are the most common inhalants used in small mammals. Sevoflurane provides a more rapid induction and recovery but is more expensive.[35] The average minimum anesthetic concentration (MAC) for small mammals is 1.5% for isoflurane and 2.8% sevoflurane.[46] Maintenance settings for surgical anesthesia are approximately 25% above MAC. Thus, for surgical maintenance, the expected vaporizer setting would be 1.8% for isoflurane and 3.5% for sevoflurane, although premedication and hypothermia will decrease MAC and, consequently, vaporizer flow rates.

■ SURGERY
Preoperative and Postoperative Considerations

Because of small rodents' propensity toward respiratory and renal disease, a thorough physical examination, complete blood count, plasma biochemical analysis, urinalysis, and whole-body radiographs are recommended before surgery is perfomed.[30] The exam findings and diagnostic results can then be used to classify the patient's physical status as defined by the American Society of Anesthesiology.[38] The patient should be physiologically stable, so any abnormalities (e.g., dehydration, anemia, hypoglycemia) should be corrected prior to induction.[35]

The rodent's inability to vomit, due to a ridge at the gastroesophageal junction, and limited glycogen stores contraindicate preoperative fasting of these species. Blood glucose values should be monitored pre- and postoperatively. If the length of anesthesia exceeds 30 minutes, consider adding 5% dextrose to the maintenance crystalloid solution to prevent hypoglycemia.[38]

INSTRUMENTATION

Microsurgical instruments are recommended for small rodent surgery based on their standard length of 5 to 7 in, rounded handles, and appropriate counterbalance. Ophthalmic instruments are not recommended because they are shorter, making body cavity manipulations difficult.[52] Minimally a rodent surgical pack should include a microsurgical needle holder, scissors, thumb forceps, No. 15 and No. 11 scalpel blades, small gauze pads (2 × 2 in), sterile cotton-tipped applicators, suture scissors, hemostats, and other instruments of a standard pack. The bulb syringe of an ophthalmic pack, for lavage, as well as small hemostatic clips and the applicator are also recommended. Magnification provided by binocular magnification loupes or an operating microscope will improve visualization and should be considered a necessity for small rodent surgery.[52] The use of clear adhesive plastic drapes are recommended because they decrease heat loss, decrease weight on the patient's respiratory system, and improve respiratory monitoring.[30]

Common Surgical Procedures
ORCHIECTOMY

Orchiectomy is indicated for prevention of breeding, retained testicle(s), severe testicular trauma, nonresponsive orchitis or epididymitis, behavioral modification, and abscessation or neoplasia involving the testicle or epididymis.[34] Castration before puberty may prevent aggression and decrease urine marking behaviors.[30] Reproductive anatomy of hamsters and gerbils is similar to that of cats and dogs, except for their large open inguinal canals.[53] Thus, a closed castration technique or an abdominal approach to castration is recommended.[4]

The closed castration technique is similar to that described for the cat. Anesthetize and restrain the patient in dorsal recumbency, clip the fur, and perform a standard sterile preparation of the area without alcohol. A small incision (1-1.5 cm) is made through the skin and vaginal tunic on both sides of the scrotum. A standard open castration technique is used. The pedicles may be tied in an overhand knot or, preferably, ligated with an absorbable suture material. The testis, gubernaculum, epididymis, and fat are removed. The tunic and skin may be closed with simple interrupted 4-0 or smaller synthetic absorbable suture. Suturing is necessary because the inguinal canals are larger than the testes of hamsters and gerbils. Complications of orchiectomy in the rodent include hematoma formation, self-trauma, and infection, which may result from excess activity or sexual activity. Although sexual activity will cease 2 weeks postoperatively, sexual behavior may persist for several weeks.[30]

OVARIOHYSTERECTOMY

An ovariohysterectomy is indicated for decreasing the risk of mammary neoplasia, prevention of reproduction, pseudopregnancy, ovarian or uterine neoplasia, cystic ovaries, pyometra, dystocia, uterine aneurysm, and, possibly, behavioral modification.[30] Pyometra in the hamster must be differentiated from the normal mucoid, odorous discharge of estrus. Cystic ovaries of the hamster or gerbil may cause compression of abdominal organs, decreased nutrient intake, and respiratory compromise. These cysts should be drained before they are surgically removed.[30]

The ovariohysterectomy surgical technique for hamsters and gerbils is routine because reproductive tract anatomy of these species is similar to that of dogs and cats, with two uterine horns and one cervix. The ovaries lie within a large fat pad at the caudal pole of the kidneys. The ovaries are easily exteriorized because of long suspensory ligament attachments. The oviduct encircles the ovaries cranially, and the ovarian vessels run medial to the ovaries and uterine horns.[36]

Anesthetize and restrain the patient in dorsal recumbency. Clip and prepare the patient with a standard surgical scrub without alcohol. A 1- to 2-cm ventral midline incision is then made between the umbilicus and pubis. This long incision eases visualization of ovarian vessels.[53] If the ventral abdominal sebaceous gland interferes with the incision, make the incision lateral to this gland and use blunt dissection to expose the linea alba. Exteriorize one of the uterine horns, which are found dorsal to the bladder. Identify the vessels within the mesovarium and make an opening through the avascular mesovarium. The surgeon should then ligate the uterine horn and vessels with a synthetic 4-0 or 5-0 absorbable suture or hemostatic clips. It is important to identify and ligate vessels that may be hidden in the abundant fat of the mesometrium. Distal to the ligature, transect the mesovarium, suspensory ligament, and vessels. This procedure is repeated for the other uterine horn. Bluntly dissect the broad ligament on each side to the level of the uterine body. Double ligate the uterus cranial to the cervix with transfixing sutures or hemostatic clips. Transect the uterus and check ovarian and cervical stumps for hemorrhage. Avoid major manipulation of the gastrointestinal tract during surgery because rodents, especially hamsters, are prone to adhesion development.[34] Routine closure of the abdominal body wall and subcutaneous layers is performed. Subcuticular sutures and/or tissue adhesive may be used for skin closure.

CESAREAN SECTION

Cesarean section is indicated for dystocia or uterine inertia. The patient should be stabilized preoperatively, and medical therapy of calcium and oxytocin should be considered if an obstruction is not present. Position the patient in dorsal recumbency with the body tilted so that the viscera fall away from the thoracic cavity. The midline abdominal incision should avoid vascular mammary and uterine tissues. Remove the fetus close to the cervix and attempt to remove the placenta with it. Clamp and transect the umbilicus, clear the neonate's airways, and stimulate breathing of the neonate by administering doxapram if necessary. Close the uterus with a double-layer inverting suture pattern. If uterine contractions are not observed before closure, administer oxytocin (1-2 IU/kg IM or IV) to assist with uterine involution. Lavage the abdomen with warm isotonic saline and use a routine closure for the abdomen and skin.[34]

CYSTOTOMY

The surgical procedure of cystotomy is indicated for urolithiasis, urine scald, and neoplasia. Preoperatively, the urinary system should be assessed by the standard diagnostics of urinalysis, urine culture, and radiographs. The cystotomy procedure is routine in hamsters except that the suture is smaller and gentle tissue handling is essential. A ventral midline incision is made through the linea alba from the umbilicus to the pubis. The bladder is located and, if necessary, emptied by cystocentesis. The exposed abdominal viscera should be packed with moist gauze sponges. If necessary, stay sutures may be placed in the bladder cranial and caudal to the incision site. An incision is made in the bladder, and it is explored while avoiding the trigone area. Uroliths are removed and samples obtained for culture and histopathologic testing, if needed. Flush the bladder with warm isotonic saline and catheterize the urethra to ensure patency. The thin bladder wall is closed with single inverting pattern with 6-0 or smaller synthetic, monofilament absorbable suture. Following irrigation of the abdominal cavity, closure of the abdomen is routine. Postoperatively, ensure the patient is urinating properly. If not, the urethra should be catheterized for up to 72 hours.

MAMMARY GLAND NEOPLASIA EXCISION

Mammary neoplasia has been identified in the Syrian hamster, Russian hamster, and the gerbil.[29] Such tumors are usually benign in the hamster and malignant in the gerbil. In both the hamster and gerbil, unlike in the rat, the mammary tissue is confined to the ventrum. Treatment includes tumor excision and removal of associated mammary tissue.[30,34] The subcutaneous tissue associated with the tumor is often highly vascularized. Vessels should be ligated with sutures or hemostatic clips to avoid hemorrhage. Radiosurgery or the use of a laser may be useful when removing these tumors. Use of a local block for analgesia will help prevent postoperative self-trauma. Closure of the subcutaneous and subcuticular layers is routine.

ABSCESSES

Abscesses result from trauma, bite wounds, and hematogenous infection. The aggressive hamster is more likely to develop abscesses than is the nonaggressive hamster. Diagnosis is based on fine needle aspirate and cytology of the abscess, revealing neutrophilic inflammation. Facial or limb abscesses indicate radiographic evaluation for osteomyelitis. The rodent abscess is usually thick-walled and filled with caseous, purulent material. The treatment of choice is complete excision of the abscess and its capsule. Culture and sensitivity testing should be submitted and broad-spectrum antibiotics administered, pending results. Antibiotic-impregnated polymethylmethacrylate beads may be inserted to fill in the defect. Care must be taken not to use more than a single appropriate dose; otherwise, the animal is at risk for toxicity. Closure of the subcutis and skin is then routine.

DENTAL DISEASE

Hamsters commonly develop periodontal disease and dental caries. Clipping the teeth may result in abscessation secondary to iatrogenic longitudinal fractures.[34] Facial abscesses near the eyes may be caused by a tooth root abscess. Recommended treatment is irrigation, drainage, debridement, and curettage of the abscess, along with extraction of the affected tooth. Radiographs should be taken before surgery to assess the patient, as osteomyelitis warrants a guarded prognosis. Extraction may be less challenging than expected, because decay loosens the tooth root. The socket should be flushed thoroughly with isotonic saline and packed with doxycycline gel to provide an antibiotic depot. Postoperatively, appropriate systemic antibiotics should be administered and abscess samples submitted for culture and sensitivity. Regular recheck examinations postoperatively are necessary to assess possible complications such as tooth regrowth, tipping of adjacent teeth into extraction site, and fistula formation.[30,34,54]

EVERTED CHEEK POUCH IN HAMSTERS

The cheek pouches of hamsters may spontaneously evert and should not be mistaken for tumors. There is a high likelihood of eversion recurrence if tack sutures are not placed. Under general anesthesia, the pouch is inverted using a cotton-tipped applicator. A monofilament, nonabsorbable 4-0 or smaller suture is placed full thickness, percutaneously, and snug but not tight against the skin. Food need not be withheld. Remove the suture in 2 weeks. This treatment is definitive; recurrence has not been reported.[30,52]

TAIL TRAUMA IN GERBILS

The long tail of gerbils is loosely covered with thin skin and prone to degloving injury. Degloving of the tail can occur when the gerbil is inappropriately picked up or restrained, or when the gerbil's tail is wedged in the cage or mutilated by a cagemate. Although the tail will slough off on its own, surgery is warranted because of the associated pain and risk of denervation causing additional self-mutilation.

Under general anesthesia, amputation is performed with the patient in ventral recumbency as the tail is suspended away from the body with tape. A local analgesic block is administered using 0.01 ml bupivacaine or lidocaine via injection at the base of the tail. Following surgical preparation, an incision is made in healthy skin proximal to the degloved section. The skin edges are trimmed to healthy normal tissue, and the tail is disarticulated between the two most cranial coccygeal vertebrae visible. Bleeding from coccygeal vessels can be controlled with cautery or ligatures, although cautery should be minimal to prevent self-trauma postoperatively. Closure is in two layers, with absorbable 5-0 or 6-0 suture used to close the subcutis and suture or tissue adhesive applied for skin closure.[30,34,52,54]

EXCISION OF ABDOMINAL MASSES

The reproductive tract, liver, and kidneys of hamsters are commonly affected by cystic masses. The presence of any abdominal mass should be an indication for abdominal exploratory surgery. Successful resection of the mass will improve the patient's quality of life and should be discussed with the owner.[30,52]

PROLAPSED BOWEL IN HAMSTERS

Prolapsed bowel is a common sequela to proliferative ileitis but may also occur due to parasitism or other cause of diarrhea. Surgery is imperative if the necrotic bowel or small intestine is prolapsed. A prolapse is rectal if a small probe such as a lubricated cotton-tipped applicator cannot be passed on either side of the prolapsed tissue. If the probe can be passed, the bowel is prolapsed. Vital rectal tissue can be reduced with a small cotton-tipped applicator. The tissue is maintained in place with a 5-0 nonabsorbable purse-string suture in the anal ring. The suture is maintained while the underlying condition is treated medically, and the patient is stabilized for 3 to 5 days. Resection and anastomosis is indicated when necrotic rectal tissue is prolapsed. Prolapsed bowel is often associated with an intussusception, so abdominal exploratory and resection and end-to-end anastomosis is indicated. The critical condition of these patients relegates the prognosis for survival to poor.[30,52]

ENUCLEATION

Enucleation is indicated for intraocular or retrobulbar neoplasia, abscess, corneal perforation, nonresponsive hypopyon,

glaucoma, uveitis, or keratitis. Proptosis is common in rodents, which lack a third eyelid. Unless treatment is initiated within a few hours of the injury, the eye may be unsalvageable. Buphthalmos in rodents has been associated with an intrathoracic mass, so thoracic radiographs are indicated preoperatively. Rodents have a large venous orbital sinus surrounding the eye muscles, which may cause significant intraoperative hemorrhage, and a harderian gland caudal to the globe. The transconjunctival approach to rodent enucleation is recommended unless the tissue is infected; if the tissue is infected, a transpalpebral approach is used. With transconjunctival approach, tissues are dissected close to the globe, and tissue is left within the orbit to prevent a postoperative sunken appearance. In the transpalpebral approach, no tissue is left in the orbit because tissues are dissected close to the orbit. To control infection and prevent the sunken appearance postoperatively, an antibiotic-impregnated polymethylmethacrylate bead can be placed in the vacated orbit.[30,34]

■ZOONOSES

The overall zoonotic risk to pet owners of captive-bred hamsters and gerbils is low. However, a number of zoonotic pathogens can occur in these species, and the clinician should be familiar with the etiologic agents, clinical signs, appropriate diagnostics, and treatment and prevention recommendations for these diseases. The potential for rodents to carry zoonotic disease is minimized by eliminating exposure to wild rodents, eliminating parasitic infestation, and screening for viral agents. Important zoonotic diseases are generally limited to salmonellosis and hymenolepiasis in the gerbil and these two diseases as well as *Acinetobacter* spp., dermatophytosis, and lymphocytic choriomeningitis virus in the hamster.[13] Additional zoonoses of historical and other importance will also be reviewed.

Bacterial Zoonoses

Rickettsial pox is a mite-borne disease of humans first recognized in New York City in 1946. Even though fewer than 1000 cases are reported in the United States annually, the clinician should be aware of this risk to gerbil owners.[55] The house mouse mite that carries the causative agent of rickettsial pox is not pathogenic to gerbils, but it is to humans. *Rickettsia akari* is a spotted fever group rickettsia that is similar to *R. rickettsii*, the causative agent of Rocky Mountain spotted fever. In humans, rickettsial pox is a mild, nonfatal disease. Within 48 hours of being bitten by *L. sanguineus*, a nonpruritic erythematous papule develops at the bite site and progresses to a vesicle and then to an eschar. Lesions primarily occur on the face, trunk, and extremities. Eschar formation is usually concomitant with systemic disease and clinical signs of fever, headache, muscle aches, malaise, sweats, and chills. Most cases resolve within 10 days, but headaches may persist for another 2 weeks. Physicians may prescribe antibiotics to alleviate clinical signs.[25]

Salmonellosis is a bacterial disease caused by a variety of *Salmonella* spp., which are Gram-negative aerobes. Although rare in gerbils and hamsters, *Salmonella* Enteritidis and *S.* Typhimurium are the most common serotypes recovered from rodents. Clinical signs in the rodent can vary from subclinical signs to anorexia, weight loss, enteritis, lymphadenopathy, and septicemia. Clinical signs in humans are similar and include headaches, nausea, vomiting, abdominal pain, enteritis, and septicemia. Salmonellosis can be acquired from direct or indirect contact, and incubation in humans varies from about 6 to 48 hours. Strict hygiene as well as hand washing after handling of hamsters and gerbils should prevent transmission of this disease.

Viral zoonotic disease in rodents is rare. Important viral zoonotic diseases that may affect the hamster and gerbil are limited to lymphocytic choriomeningitis virus, Hantaan disease, rabies virus, and more recently, monkey poxvirus. Because all rodents are considered susceptible to Hantavirus, domestic rodent colonies are screened for this disease. In humans, Hantavirus pulmonary syndrome, first recognized in 1993, can cause mortality and is transmitted by inhalation of infected rodent urine, droppings, or saliva. Rabies virus antibodies have been found in various rodent species.[56] Rabies viral vaccination is not recommended for rodents. Domestic rodents should not be maintained outside or allowed contact with wild rodents that may be carrying these rare diseases. The susceptibility of hamsters and gerbils to monkey poxvirus remains unknown, but common sense dictates that these species be considered susceptible to the disease. Humans may become infected with monkeypox through contact with tissue or fluid of infected animals. A monkeypox vaccine is available for use in people.[56] To prevent exposure to monkeypox virus, hamsters and gerbils should not be mixed with other species of rodents.

The hamster can serve as a reservoir for the RNA arenavirus, lymphocytic choriomeningitis virus. This rare disease may be transmitted in rodents horizontally and vertically and to humans through exposure to contaminated feces, urine, or rodent bite.[56] Rodents may be asymptomatic or develop clinical signs of weight loss, tremors, convulsions, or photophobia. Humans may suffer flu-like symptoms including malaise, headache, fever, myalgia, arthritis, and very rarely, fatal aseptic meningitis or meningoencephalitis.[56] Captive hamsters are screened for this disease, but humans with high risk, such as those in lab animal colonies, should wear gloves for protection. Upon definitive diagnosis of this disease, affected and exposed hamsters should be euthanized, and cages, cage furniture, and bedding should be discarded.

Parasitic Zoonoses

Parasitic zoonoses of the hamster and gerbil are rare. Cryptosporidiosis is rare in hamsters and gerbils. The pathogen *Cryptosporidium parvum* is nonhost specific and poses a disease risk to the immunocompromised human. *Giardia lamblia, G. mesocricetus,* and *G. muris* may affect gerbils and hamsters. In humans clinical disease affects primarily the gastrointestinal

tract (diarrhea), but joint synovitis and allergic reactions may also occur. Transmission is via the direct fecal-oral route, and diagnosis is achieved by direct fecal examination. Appropriate hygiene and sanitation measures will prevent exposure to the parasite. Treatment will alleviate signs and control disease in humans and animals.

Hymenolepiasis is caused by the cestodes *Hymenolepis nana* or (rarely) *H. diminuta,* which have worldwide distribution. Hymenolepiasis is common in children because of the fecal-oral route of transmission, but fecal contamination of food by rodents may also provide exposure to the disease. Most human infections come from other humans, and the role of rodents in the epidemiology of hymenolepiasis is not well known but probably limited. Risk factors for children are human fecal contamination of the environment, poor hygiene, lack of drinking water, and presence of another infected person in the home. Symptoms in children are nonspecific and include decreased appetite, abdominal pain, irritability, weight loss, and flatulence. A positive fecal examination provides the diagnosis. In humans, a single dose of praziquantel is effective for 80% of infections but should be accompanied by an improvement in environmental hygiene.

Other Zoonoses

Fungal disease of the hamster and gerbil is rare. However, *Trichophyton* spp. (especially *T. mentagrophytes*) and *Microsporum* spp. may affect both rodents and humans.[56] Affected animals may be asymptomatic or suffer pruritus and excoriation, alopecia, and circular areas of crusting and scale. Humans with dermatophytosis may have lesions similar to those of rodents. Clients should be instructed to consult their physician for treatment, which is curative, and be advised of appropriate treatment for their rodent.

Allergic reactions to rabbits and rodents in humans have up to a 15% occurrence.[56] Human clinical signs include respiratory, dermatologic, and ophthalmic manifestations of anaphylaxis. Hamsters and gerbils are among the least irritant of small animal antigens to humans. Antihistamine therapy and other treatment of people with recognized allergies is indicated, along with avoidance of the offending antigen.

REFERENCES

1. Feaver J, Zhibin Z: Hamsters. In MacDonald D, editor: *The Encyclopedia of Mammals,* New York, 2001, *Facts on File.*
2. Gibson SV, Brady AG: Hamsters: use in research. In *Laboratory Animal Medicine and Science, Series II,* Seattle, 2000, University of Washington.
3. Battles A: The biology, care and diseases of the Syrian hamster, *Vet Compend Cont Ed* 7(10):815-825, 1985.
4. Harkness J, Wagner J: *The Biology and Medicine of Rabbits and Rodents,* ed 4, Baltimore, 1995, Lippincott Williams and Wilkins.
5. Motzel S, Wagner J: Mongolian gerbils: care, diseases and use in research. In Dahm L, J MB, editors: *Laboratory Animal Medicine and Science, Series II,* Seattle, 2001, University of Washington.
6. Schlitter DA, Agren G: Gerbils. In MacDonald D, editor: *The Encyclopedia of Mammals,* New York, 2001, *Facts on File.*
7. Johnson-Delaney C: Small rodents. In Harrison LR, editor: *Exotic Companion Medicine Handbook,* Lake Worth, Fla, 1998, Zoological Education Network.

8. Bihun C, Bauck L: Basic anatomy, physiology, husbandry and clinical techniques. In Quesenberry KE, Carpenter JW, editors: *Ferrets, Rabbits and Rodents: Clinical Medicine and Surgery,* ed 2, St Louis, 2003, WB Saunders.

9. Popesko P, Rajtova V, Horak J: *A Colour Atlas of Anatomy of Small Laboratory Animals,* St Louis, 2002, WB Saunders.

10. Daviau J: Clinical evaluation of rodents, *Vet Clin North Am Exot Anim Pract* 2(2):429-445, 1999.

11. Moore D: Hematology of the Syrian (Golden) hamster *(Mesocricetus auratus).* In Feldman BF, Zinkl JG, Jain NC, editors: *Schalm's Veterinary Hematology,* ed 5, Philadelphia, 2000, Lippincott Williams and Wilkins.

12. Moore D: Hematology of the Mongolian gerbil *(Meriones unguiculatus).* In Feldman BF, Zinkl JG, Jain NC, editors: *Schalm's Veterinary Hematology,* Philadelphia, 2000, Lippincott Williams and Wilkins.

13. Ness RD: Rodents. In Carpenter JW, editor: *Exotic Animal Formulary,* ed 3, St Louis, 2005, WB Saunders.

14. Silverman S, Tell L: *Radiology of Rodents, Rabbits and Ferrets,* St Louis, 2005, WB Saunders.

15. Stefanacci JD, Hoefer HL: Radiology and ultrasound. In Quesenberry KE, Carpenter JW, editors: *Ferrets, Rabbits and Rodents: Clinical Medicine and Surgery,* ed 2, St Louis, 2004, WB Saunders.

16. Gabrisch K, Grimm F, Isenbugel E et al: *Diagnostic Radiology of Exotic Pets,* Philadelphia, 1991, WB Saunders.

17. Schoeb T: Respiratory diseases of rodents, *Vet Clin North Am Exot Anim Pract* 3(2):481-496, 2000.

18. Ellis C, Mori M: Skin diseases of rodents and small exotic mammals, *Vet Clin North Am Exot Anim Pract* 4(2):493-542, 2001.

19. Kasuba C, Hsu C, Krogstad A et al: Small mammal virology, *Vet Clin North Am Exot Anim Pract* 8(1):107-122, 2005.

20. Pollock C: Fungal diseases of laboratory rodents, *Vet Clin North Am Exot Anim Pract* 6:401-413, 2003.

21. Percy D, Barthold S: *Pathology of Laboratory Rodents and Rabbits,* ed 2, Ames, 2001, Iowa State Press.

22. Fox J, Newcomer C, Rozmiarek H: Selected zoonoses. In Fox J, Anderson LC, Loew FM, Quimby FW, editors: Laboratory Animal Medicine, San Diego, 2002, Academic Press.

23. Davis A, Jenkins S: Cryptosporidiosis and proliferative ileitis in a hamster, *Vet Pathol* 23:632-633, 1986.

24. Timm K: Pruritus in rabbits, rodents, and ferrets, *Vet Clin North Am Small Anim Pract* 18(5):1077-1091, 1988.

25. Mullen G, O'Connor B: Mites *(Acari).* In Mullen G, Durdin L, editors: *Medical and Veterinary Entomology,* San Diego, 2002, Academic Press.

26. Schwartzbrott S: Demodicosis in the Mongolian gerbil *(Meriones unguiculatus), Lab Anim Sci* 24:666-668, 1974.

27. Levine J, Lage A: House mites infesting laboratory rodents, *Lab Anim Sci* 34:393-394, 1984.

28. Adamcak A, Otten B: Rodent therapeutics, *Vet Clin North Am Exot Anim Pract* 3(1):221-237, 2000.

29. Greenacre C: Spontaneous tumors of small mammals, *Vet Clin North Am Exot Anim Pract* 7:627-651, 2004.

30. Bennett RA, Mullen HS: Soft tissue surgery. In Quesenberry, KE, Carpenter JW, editors: *Ferrets, Rabbits and Rodents: Clinical Medicine and Surgery,* St Louis, 2003, WB Saunders.

31. Donnelly TM: Disease problems of small rodents. In Quesenberry KE, Carpenter JW, editors: *Ferrets, Rabbits and Rodents: Clinical Medicine and Surgery,* St Louis, 2004, WB Saunders.

32. Antinoff N: Small mammal critical care, *Vet Clin North Am Small Anim Pract* 1(1):153-175, 1998.

33. Lichtenberger M: Principles of shock and fluid therapy in special species, *Semin Av Exot Pet Med* 13(3):142-153, 2004.

34. Redrobe S: Soft tissue surgery of rabbits and rodents, *Semin Av Ex Pet Med* 11(4):231-245, 2002.

35. Heard DJ: Anesthesia, analgesia, and sedation of small mammals. In Quesenberry KE, Carpenter JW, editors: *Ferrets, Rabbits and Rodents: Clinical Medicine and Surgery,* St Louis, 2003, WB Saunders.

36. Harkness J: *Essentials of Pet Rodents: A Guide for Practitioners,* Lakewood, Colo, 1997, American Animal Hospital Press.

37. Anderson N: Intraosseous fluid therapy in small exotic animals, *Kirk's Current Veterinary Therapy XII,* 1995.

38. Cantwell S: Ferret, rabbit, and rodent anesthesia, *Vet Clin North Am Exot Anim Pract* 4(1):169-191, 2001.

39. Rosenthal KL: Therapeutic contraindications in exotic pets, *Semin Av Exot Pet Med* 13(1):44-48, 2004.

40. Morrisey JK, Carpenter JW: Formulary. In Quesenberry KE, Carpenter JW, editors: *Ferrets, Rabbits and Rodents: Clinical Medicine and Surgery,* St Louis, 2004, WB Saunders.

41. Costello M: Principles of cardiopulmonary cerebral resuscitation in special species, *Semin Av Exot Pet Med* 13(3):132-141, 2004.

42. Briscoe J, Syring R: Techniques for emergency airway and vascular access in special species, *Semin Av Exot Pet Med* 13(3):118-131, 2004.

43. Flecknell P: Analgesia of small mammals, *Semin Av Exot Pet Med* 7(1):41-47, 2001.

44. Hrapkeiwicz K, Stein S, Smiler K: A new anesthetic agent for use in the gerbil, *Lab Anim Sci* 39(4):338-341, 1989.

45. Curl J: Ketamine-xylazine anaesthesia in the Djungarian hamster *(Phodopus sungorus), Lab Anim* 22:309-312, 1988.

46. Bailey J, Pablo L: Anesthetic monitoring and monitoring equipment: application in small exotic pet practice, *Semin Av Exot Pet Med* 7(1):53-60, 1998.

47. Orcutt C: Use of convective heaters with exotic patients, *Exot DVM* 2(pt 3):47-48, 2000.

48. Calderone L, Grimes P, Shaley M: Acute reversible cataract induced by xylazine and by ketamine-xylazine anesthesia in rats and mice, *Exp Eye Res* 42:331-337, 1986.

49. Olson M, Vizzutti D, Morck D et al: The parasympatholytic effects of atropine sulfate and glycopyrrolate in rats and rabbits, *Can J Vet Res* 57:254-258, 1993.

50. Komulainen A, Olsen M: Antagonism of ketamine-xylazine anesthesia in rats by administration of yohimbine, tolazoline, or 4-aminopyridine, *Am J Vet Res* 52:585-588, 1991.

51. Lerche P, Muir W, Bednarski R: Nonrebreathing anesthetic systems in small animal practice, *JAVMA* 217:493-497, 2000.

52. Bennett R: Preparation and equipment useful for surgery in small exotic pets, *Vet Clin North Am Exot Anim Pract* 3(3):563-585, 2000.

53. Jenkins J: Surgical sterilization in small mammals: spay and castration, *Vet Clin North Am Exot Anim Pract* 3(3):617-627, 2000.

54. Crossley DA: Small mammal dentistry: dental anatomy and dental disease. In Quesenberry KE, Carpenter JW, editors: *Ferrets, Rabbits and Rodents: Clinical Medicine and Surgery,* St Louis, 2003, WB Saunders.

55. Krussel A, Comer JA, Sexton DJ: Rickettsial pox in North Carolina: a case report, *Emerg Infect Dis 2002* (Available from http://www.cdc.gov/ncidod/EID/vol8no7/01-0501.htm.).

56. Mitchell MA, Tully TN: Zoonotic diseases. In Quesenberry KE, Carpenter JW, editors: *Ferrets, Rabbits and Rodents: Clinical Medicine and Surgery,* St Louis, 2004, WB Saunders.

J. Jill Heatley

CHAPTER 16

HEDGEHOGS

■ COMMON SPECIES KEPT IN CAPTIVITY

Hedgehogs are members of the order Erinaceomorpha, family Erinaceidae, subfamily Erinaceinae. The 12 species from 5 genera are widespread throughout the Old World (e.g., Africa, Europe, and Asia),[1] though they are not found in central Asia, including India, Nepal, Pakistan, Tibet, and western equatorial Africa. Hedgehogs are classified based on the shape and pattern of their spines, ear length, and skull morphology.[2] Commonly encountered species include *Atalerix albiventris,* also known as the white-bellied or four-toed African pygmy hedgehog from central Africa, and *Erinaceous europaeus,* the European hedgehog of western Europe. The *Atalerix* genus has other members, including Pruner's hedgehog *(A. pruneri),* the Algerian hedgehog *(A. algirus),* Sclater's hedgehog *(A. sclateri),* and the Cape hedgehog *(A. frontalis).*[3] Other hedgehog genera include the desert hedgehogs *(Paraechinus* spp.) from the Middle East and North Africa; the long-eared hedgehogs *(Hemiechinus* spp.) from Asia, India, and North Africa; and the Daurian hedgehogs *(Mesechinus* spp.) from China. Hedgehog classification, however, is somewhat confusing, as some consider the *Atalerix* genus part of the *Erinaceus* genus.[3,4] Of these hedgehog species, only the African pygmy hedgehog *(A. albiventris)* and the European hedgehog *(E. europaeus)* are considered acceptable—based on temperament—as pets.[5] There are currently no hedgehog species considered vulnerable to extinction; however, the Cape hedgehog listed in CITES appendix 2 is rare. Decline of this species may have been caused by loss of habitat, or its popularity as a local delicacy and pet.[2,3,6]

Reviews of disease and rehabilitation of the European hedgehog are readily available, as this is the most thoroughly studied of the hedgehog species.[7-11]

This chapter will focus on the African pygmy hedgehog, as it is the most common species encountered in the North American pet trade. Importation of the European hedgehog and other species of hedgehogs is strictly controlled. However, information known from hedgehog species in general will be included where the generality applies to this species. The importation of the African pygmy hedgehog to the United States has been prohibited since 1991 because of their potential to carry foot-and-mouth disease.[12] This species is native to central Africa, from Senegal to Sudan and Zambia, in an area stretching from the southern part of the Sahara to the Congo and into East Africa. The African pygmy hedgehog has even been found on Mount Kilimanjaro at elevations of 1800 m.[3] Color varieties found in the pet trade include the standard colored quill, "salt and pepper," and the all-white quilled "snowflake."

■ BIOLOGY AND BEHAVIOR

Antipredator defenses include not only the spiny pelage, but the ability to roll into a tight ball to protect the feet, face, and soft underbelly. Hedgehogs possess a protein, erinacin, which can be extracted from their muscles and inhibits the hemorrhagic and proteolytic activity of venom.[1,13] However, the *in vivo* protection this affords hedgehogs, although the stuff of folktales, remains unknown and may be incomplete and individually variable. Nonetheless, this attribute, along with their protective spines, likely gives hedgehogs the ability to attack and eat snakes.

Hedgehogs are predominantly solitary creatures. These animals have relatively small eyes; therefore, it is believed that they rely on olfactory and auditory cues for communication.[2] Thus, vocalizations of *A. albiventris* are multiple and varied (Box 16-1).[2,14-15] Hedgehogs have a well-developed sense of

433

BOX 16-1 African Pygmy Hedgehog (Atalerix albiventris) Vocalizations

Sound	Description
Snorting/huffing Hissing/grunting	Aggressive or warning sounds produced by sharp vibrating exhalations through the nostrils. Generally made when the animal is disturbed, when it encounters another animal, or when it is in the process of rolling up.
Screaming	A severe distress call given when the animal is in distress or pain.
Twittering/whistling	High-pitched sounds of neonates. Whistling stimulates contact by the dam.
Clucking	High-pitched contact call of the dam to neonates, also made by courting males.
Snuffling	Made as hedgehogs search for food.
Inaudible sounds	Hedgehogs can make and hear sounds in the 40- to 90-kHz range, above the range of human hearing.

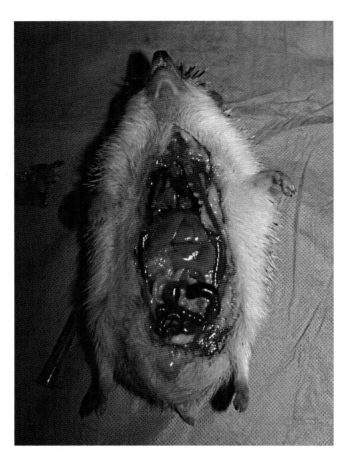

Figure 16-1 Internal anatomy of a diseased hedgehog *(Atalerix albiventris)*. Note the enlarged discolored liver, the dark bowel, and the enlarged spleen. This animal was diagnosed with myeloproliferative disease.

smell to find food and get information about others of their species.[2]

Anting, or anointing, is a feature of all hedgehog species. In this strange behavior, the hedgehog encounters a substance, may lick or chew the substance, and then begins to hypersalivate to produce copious foamy saliva which is then slathered onto the spines of the flank and back with the tongue. Food bits may be found on the quills from this behavior. Direct contact with a substance is not necessary to elicit this behavior, which is commonly caused by anesthetic gases as well as perfume. This behavior has also been induced by strong smelling substances such as cigarettes, glue, toad skin, leather, creosote, cat food, fish, wool, various plants and vegetables, foxes, and other hedgehogs.[2,13,16] The true purpose of anointing remains unknown, but theories explaining its purpose in the hedgehog include reduction of skin parasites, predator deterrence, mate attraction, and communication among conspecifics by imparting an odor to each animal in its home range.[2,16] This behavior can occur in the African pygmy hedgehog as early as 15 days of age.

The African pygmy hedgehog is nocturnal in captivity but will emerge from its nest during the day.[3] In the wild, these creatures will rest by day, curled underneath matted grass, leaf litter, or in a rock crevice or hole in the ground.[6] These resting places are changed daily unless the animal has a litter or is in hibernation or torpor. In nature, hedgehogs are active and gain weight in the rainy season and enter hibernation when the weather is cool and dry, from about June to September. During this period, animals may remain torpid for up to 6 weeks but emerge in periods of warm weather.[6] In captivity, hibernation is not considered physiologically necessary for African pygmy hedgehogs. African pygmy hedgehogs are an adaptable species and have been found in a wide variety of habitats, such as grassland, scrub, savannah, and even suburban gardens.[6] However, they are generally absent from areas of extreme heat or cold, such as deserts, marshes, and dense forest.

Hedgehogs tend to be solitary in the wild and will travel several miles per night to find food or mates. Males do not partake in parental care, and litters disperse soon after weaning. Although hedgehogs are not generally territorial, they avoid each other to prevent direct competition.

■ UNIQUE ANATOMY AND PHYSIOLOGY

The African pygmy hedgehog has a variety of unique anatomic features that make clinical examination and treatment challenging (Figure 16-1).

Integumentary System

The most characteristic feature of the hedgehog is the spiny pelage.[1] In common with all hedgehogs except the long-eared

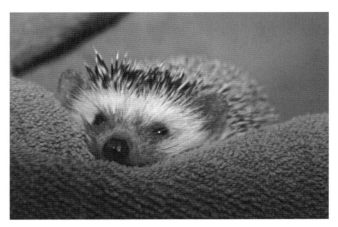

Figure 16-2 The normal variegated spines of the African hedgehog *(Atalerix albiventris).*

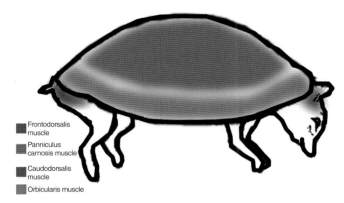

Frontodorsalis muscle
Panniculus carnosis muscle
Caudodorsalis muscle
Orbicularis muscle

Figure 16-3 The muscles used for curling the body and spine control in the hedgehog.

genera, the African pygmy hedgehog has a narrow spineless tract on the crown of the head, which runs rostrocaudally for about 2 cm and is about 0.5 cm wide.[15] Spines cover the dorsum of the body overlying a thin epidermis, a thick dermal fibrous layer, and a loose layer of fat and subcutaneous tissue that is poorly vascularized. Spines give way to true, white hair on the ventrum and legs, whereas the muzzle and feet are essentially hairless. Hair and sebaceous glands are absent in the spined region; however, sweat glands and sebaceous glands are present in the haired regions and on the soles of the feet.[16]

At birth, hedgehogs are equipped with white soft spines that harden within a few hours.[3] A second set of harder darker spines emerges 2 days after birth.[3] The spines of the adult wild type African pygmy hedgehog are white at the base and tip with a central dark black or brown band (Figure 16-2). This band coloration is darker or lighter depending on the animal's native geographic range.

The quills or spines are not detached easily, are firm, measure from 0.5 to 2 cm, are relatively uniform in length and diameter, and have needle-sharp unbarbed quill tips.[17] The average adult hedgehog carries about 5000 spines, which are predominantly in telogen.[13,17] Spines may last up to 18 months and are individually replaced.[16] These spines are modified hair, each filled with a spongy matrix inside the outer fibrous cortex.[17,18] At its insertion into the skin, the base of the spine tapers and then forms a cup-shaped bulb that is embedded in the skin.[17,18] This structure allows force applied to the spine by a blow or fall to be transferred into the spine, causing it to bend at the base rather than transferring force into the hedgehog.[19] These spines may be difficult to remove, as traction causes them to break midshaft.[17]

Musculoskeletal System

Whereas most hedgehogs have five toes on all feet, the African pygmy hedgehog only has four toes on the pes; the hallux is absent.[15] Hence, it is also known as the four-toed hedgehog.[2]

The toenails are highly curved caudally and are round in cross section.[16] Another anatomic trait of the hedgehog is a distally fused radius and ulna.[16] The normal stance is plantigrade, with the ventrum held slightly off the ground.[16] Hedgehogs can run at up to 2 m/sec, but they usually walk slowly with a toddling or waddling gate.[2]

The most interesting feature of the hedgehog musculoskeletal system is the complex of muscles that erect and position the spines and curl the hedgehog into a ball (Figure 16-3). This complex of muscles consists of the *frontodorsalis* and *caudodorsalis* muscles, which move the spines down over the rump and forehead; the *panniculus carnosus* muscle, which rolls up the hedgehog; and the *orbicularis* muscle, which pulls the mantle of spines together as a drawstring. In the fully curled position, only a 1-cm diameter ventral opening is left that is not covered by spines. In this completely balled up position, the head, ventrum, and feet are not visible. If only somewhat disturbed, the hedgehog will just use the frontodorsalis and caudodorsalis muscles to pull the spines forward and down on the forehead and down and back over the rump. The position affords protection to the face and rump and still allows the hedgehog to see and hear. The rump is an area where hedgehogs are likely to be bitten by other hedgehogs, and the position of the spines forward over the face allows the hedgehog to ram other hedgehogs or attackers with the forward-facing spines. When engaging all the muscles of rolling, the hedgehog curls into a spiny ball and generally vibrates and hisses. If necessary, the hedgehog can stay in the position of a spiny ball for hours.

Reproductive System

The sex of African hedgehogs can be determined by their external anatomy. Males have a prepuce located midway along the ventral abdomen. The penis is spineless and has lateral horns on either side of the meatus, making it resemble a snail's head.[20] The male hedgehog lacks a scrotum, but the testicles are palpable in the subcutaneous para-anal recesses.[20] The male hedgehog is generally accepted to have multilobed seminal vesicles, a bilobed prostate and paired Cowper's glands as accessory sex glands.[15] Hedgehog sperm normally have an offset or eccentrically positioned tail.[20]

The vulva of the female is located close to the anus, resulting in a decreased anogenital distance similar to rodent species. Female *A. albiventris* have three pairs of mammae. The urethra opens into the distal vagina several millimeters from the vulva.[16] The large, thin-walled vagina is always patent, located within the abdominal cavity, and is flanked on each side by large, fan-shaped glands homologous to the Cowper's gland of the male.[16] The female hedgehog has a bicornuate uterus and a single muscular cervix; there is no uterine body.[20] Short (7.5 mm) fallopian tubes emerge from each side of each uterine horn, and the mesosalpinx and ovarian bursa are relatively fat laden.[20] The ovaries are held within a tough peritoneal capsule. Reproductive and other biological characteristics of the African hedgehog are summarized in Box 16-2.

Alimentary Tract

The teeth and lips are a characteristic morphological feature of the hedgehog.[24] In all hedgehogs the first upper two molars are low and cusped, the labial styles are reduced to a cingulum, and the first two lower molars are subrectangular.[24] Hedgehogs are adapted for an omnivorous diet with stronger jaws and blunter teeth than most insectivores, along with brachydont or closed rooted teeth.[15] Short incisors, canines, and prominently cusped molars grip and penetrate food, whereas the flattened crowns and multiple cusps of the molars crush the food.[25] The upper incisors are separated by a wide gap into which the blunt, forward-projecting lower incisors fit (Figure 16-4). When a hedgehog bites down, the lower incisors scoop and lift the insect to the upper incisors, which impale the prey.[2] Hedgehogs can also inflict a similar bite on the handler. The dental formula of *A. albiventris* is I 3/2 C1/1 P3/2 M3/3 for a total of 36 teeth.

BOX 16-2 **Biological and Reproductive Characteristics of the African Pygmy Hedgehog (*Atalerix albiventris*)**

Parameter	*Atalerix albiventris*
Life expectancy	Wild 1-4 yr, captive 5-10 yr, average 3-8 yr
Male adult weight	500-600 g
Female adult weight	250-400 g
Rectal temperature	36.1°-37.2° C (97°-99° F)
Body length	17-25 cm (7-9 in)
Heart rate	180-280 beats/min
Respiratory rate	25-50 breaths/min
Preferred enclosure temperature	24°-27° C (75°-80° F)
Male sexual maturity	2-6 mo
Female sexual maturity	6-8 mo
Ovulation	Induced
Gestation period	32 days
Milk composition	Fat 25.5 g/100 g, protein 16 g/100 g, trace carbohydrates
Litter size	1-7 young (average 3)
Birth weight	8-13 g
Eyes open	13-16 days
Weaning age	4-6 wk, eating solid foods starting week 3
Tooth eruption	
Deciduous	Starts day 18, all erupted by 9 wk
Permanent	Begins at 7-9 wk

Data from Smith AJ: Husbandry and medicine of African hedgehogs, *J Small Exot Anim Med* 2(1):21-28, 1992; Smith AJ: Husbandry and nutrition of hedgehogs, *Vet Clin North Am Exot Anim Pract* 2(1):127-141, 1999; Bedford J, Mock O, Nagdas S et al: Reproductive characteristics of the African pygmy hedgehog *Atalerix albiventris, J Reprod Fertil* 120:143-150, 2000; Smith AJ: Neonatology of the hedgehog (*Atalerix albiventris*), *J Small Exot Anim Med* 3(1):15-18, 1995; Larson RS, Carpenter JW: Husbandry and medical management of African hedgehogs, *Vet Med* Oct: 877-890, 1999; Carpenter JW: Hedgehogs. In Carpenter JW, editor: *Exotic Animal Formulary*, ed 3, St Louis, 2005, WB Saunders.

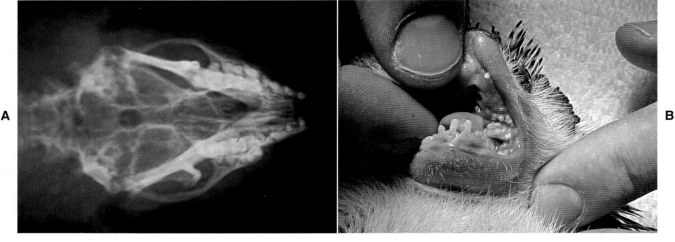

Figure 16-4 Radiographic view of an African hedgehog skull **(A)** and photographic view of the incisors of the African hedgehog *(Atalerix albiventris)* **(B)**. Note the normal gap between both the upper and lower incisors and the slight forward projection of the lower incisors.

The hedgehog gastrointestinal tract is relatively short and simple, as in other insectivores, with a 12- to 16-hour transit time.[15] The stomach is simple, but a vomit response is present.[16] The colon in noncomplex, and there is no cecum. Hedgehogs have anal glands, but they are not well developed.[2]

Neurology and Special Senses

The small cerebrum of the hedgehog suggests that the learning ability of this animal may be somewhat less than that of the rodent or carnivore. However, hedgehogs can recognize their owner and understand simple commands if trained.[16] Hedgehogs have relatively small eyes for their body size, and the retina contains only rod cells, thus allowing only for discrimination of some colors with bright lighting.[15] Hearing of the hedgehog is particularly sensitive to high-frequency sounds. These senses may be used for location and capture of prey but can also elicit a defensive posture in the hedgehog.[15] Olfaction is the best developed special sense in the hedgehog. The hedgehog olfactory lobes of the brain and the vomeronasal organ are well developed. Olfactory cues are used by hedgehogs in orientation, navigation, intraspecific communication, predator detection, prey and food detection, and as the signal for initiating the self-anointing behavior.[2,15]

■ HUSBANDRY

The enclosure for a hedgehog should be smooth walled and high enough to prevent escape of these agile climbers. Options include heavy plastic storage bins and 20-gallon or larger glass tanks. A minimum floor size of 2′ × 2′ per hedgehog is recommended, and the enclosure should be tall enough that the outstretched hedgehog cannot get its feet over the top. Avoid wire flooring, as small hedgehog feet may become caught in the wire and result in toe or foot trauma or fracture. Hedgehogs should be allowed out of their enclosure daily for exercise, but the area should be "hedgehog proof." Remove all loose fibrous materials that might wrap around hedgehog feet, cords that may be chewed, and small objects that may be ingested. Clear plastic exercise balls for the ferret or guinea pig allow exercise without free access. However, exercise balls should be cleaned after each use.

Appropriate substrate should be provided. A soft absorbent material, such as shredded newspaper, recycled newspaper product, pelleted cat or bird litter, or other materials, such as crushed corncobs or alfalfa pellets of about a 3″ depth, is recommended to provide an environment for the animal to dig and explore. Aromatic wood shavings, especially cedar, should be avoided because their volatile compounds can cause dermatitis of the ventrum and feet. For a natural display, wood chips, sphagnum moss, or soil may be used; however, these are generally avoided because they are difficult to clean. Potted plants may also provide hiding places and increase humidity, but a hedgehog enclosure is not particularly healthy for the potted plants. Avoid plants with toxic leaves, stems, flowers, berries, or roots. Avoid terry cloth towels or other fabrics, as the hedgehog may ingest these fibers or entangle its feet,

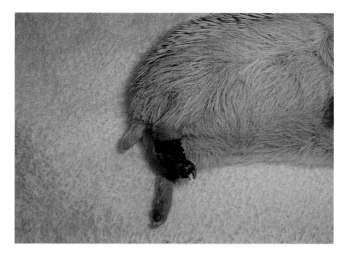

Figure 16-5 This hedgehog was presented for lameness of a few days duration. Carpet fibers caused annular constriction of the limb and necessitated amputation.

resulting in necrosis of the foot and necessitating amputation (Figure 16-5). Change the bedding frequently and spot-clean daily to avoid dermatitis and other problems of urine and fecal soiling of the cage. Hedgehogs can be taught to use a litter box, but one should avoid clumping or clay litter, which attaches to the perineal and preputial areas. Litter attached to these sensitive areas may cause urinary or fecal blockage.

A nest box or hide box that is only slightly larger than the animal is also necessary. The hide box should consist of a nontoxic large hollow object, not easily uprooted, that has smooth edges and is easily disinfected or replaceable. Options include modified cardboard boxes, flower pots, or large PVC pipe (4-6″ diameter) with one end cap. Other cage furniture can include a shallow pan of water for bathing and swimming and commercially available hedgehog exercise wheels. Large rocks may also serve as cage furniture for hedgehogs to wear down their nails. All cage furniture should be easily disinfected and cleaned on a regular basis.

Maintenance of hedgehogs on a reverse day-night light cycle allows owners to better observe and interact with their pets on a regular basis. This is not necessary, however, and potential owners should be aware that hedgehogs will generally be more active at dawn and dusk. Temperature should be maintained between 24° C and 27° C (75° F to 80° F). Below this temperature, hedgehogs' activity level will decrease and their immune system may be compromised, predisposing them to infection. Should the ambient temperature fall below 18° C (65° F), hedgehogs will go into torpor. African pygmy hedgehogs have no apparent need to hibernate in captivity. Heat can be provided with an under-tank heater or heating pad set on low and placed under $\frac{1}{2}$ to $\frac{1}{3}$ of the container or a heat lamp over part of the tank to provide a temperature gradient. A hygrometer/thermometer can best monitor enclosure conditions and is therefore recommended.

Housing Multiple Hedgehogs

Hedgehogs are solitary animals in the wild and are easily maintained as single pets in captivity. If multiple animals are housed together, each animal should have least one hide box. Animals that have been raised together may tolerate each other better as adults, but as a rule only a single male is kept per group. Housing multiple adult males together may result in fighting and a disproportionate food intake. Males can damage each other with their teeth and spines.[4] Hedgehogs often bite cagemates on the hind legs in the area without spines.[16] Groups of up to three females with a male, a harem, or without a male are best. However, fighting can arise between either sex, and any new addition to an established group should be closely monitored.[26] Zoonotic disease transmission has occurred more than once from herds of hedgehogs.[12] Housing a group of hedgehogs demands attention to appropriate sanitation.

Should one choose to own multiple hedgehogs, permanent identification is highly recommended, especially if they cohabitate or interact with each other. Identification of hedgehogs can be accomplished by a number of methods. Ear tags and tattoos have been used but are discouraged, as these markings are obscured when the hedgehog rolls up. Microchipping is the preferred method of identification. Microchips can be placed in the subcutaneous dorsal fat pad between the shoulders (between the spines) as for many small mammals. Anesthesia can facilitate appropriate placement. Animals may also be identified in a semipermanent fashion, by marking the spines with nontoxic permanent markers or nontoxic fabric paint.[4,16,22] Both spine markings and the transponder microchips have the advantage of accessibility when the animal is in its defensive posture.

Hospitalization

For hospitalization of the debilitated patient, a quiet, warm 27° C to 29° C (80° F to 84° F), humid environment should be provided, with low lighting and minimal noise. The enclosure should be smooth sided and allow for heat and humidity control and have bars closely spaced enough to prevent escape or limb trauma. A smooth-sided incubator works well to achieve and maintain hospitalization parameters while also keeping the patient secure. A hide box can consist simply of a cardboard box or an upside-down cat litter box with a suitable access hole. Supplemental oxygen may be provided to the moribund animal while in the incubator or via face mask.

■ NUTRITION

The exact dietary requirements for hedgehogs have not been determined. Few accounts exist for the diet of the wild African hedgehog (Box 16-3).[6,15] However, the African hedgehog has been maintained and bred successfully in captivity on a variety of diets (Box 16-4). As in other species, caloric and nutritional requirements probably vary based on age, reproductive status, gender, and activity level. Nutritional recom-

| BOX 16-3 | Dietary Items of the Wild African Hedgehog |

Invertebrates	Vertebrates	Plants
Ants	Frogs	Roots
Earthworms	Lizards	Fungi
Slugs	Snakes	Fruit
Beetles	Bird eggs	
Snails	Chicks	
	Small rodents	

mendations should be adjusted based on these factors. In all wild hedgehogs, insects constitute the bulk of the diet; however, plant material, vertebrates, eggs, mollusks, and carrion are also consumed.

In captivity, hedgehogs have a tendency to become obese. Further, a predominantly captive insect diet, high in fat and with an inappropriate calcium-to-phosphorous ratio, may also increase the likelihood of secondary nutritional hyperparathyroidism. A base diet of reduced calorie, small kibble cat or dog chow provides an appropriate calcium-phosphorous balance while limiting caloric intake. A commercially available hedgehog diet can also form the base of the diet but should not be used as the sole diet because it is unknown whether the total nutritional requirement of the hedgehog is met. Preliminary studies show that fiber improves fecal quality and that hedgehogs are able to break down fiber.[27] Thus, small amounts of mixed fruits and vegetables and occasional live insects, especially those with chitinous exoskeletons, should form a regular part of the hedgehog's diet. Intake of dry kibble and insects with chitinous exoskeletons may also improve dental and gingival health. Hedgehogs develop food preferences; therefore, it is recommended that one offer a variety of foods early in life (Box 16-4). Avoid giving nuts or grains, which may become lodged in the gingival tissue and/or oral cavity, and milk, which may cause diarrhea.[28]

Hedgehogs can learn to drink water from a sipper bottle but should be offered water in an open dish until consumption from the sipper bottle is confirmed. Bowls for food and water should be shallow and heavy or attached to the enclosure because hedgehogs often overturn them in their natural rooting behavior. Food and water containers should be cleaned and refilled daily.

The amount of food required to feed an animal will change based on their physiologic need. Generally, a 500-g adult male hedgehog will eat about 2 to 3 tsp of the base diet, 1 tsp of the fruit and vegetable mix, and 1 tsp of invertebrate offerings or other protein source. Adult females require less protein than adult males, whereas young may eat an adult portion and lactating or pregnant females may need more than these portions. The hedgehog should be weighed on a regular basis to avoid overfeeding and obesity. Feed only what the hedgehog will eat overnight. (Appropriate diets for orphan hedgehogs are discussed in Reproduction System.)

BOX 16-4   **Components of the Captive Hedgehog Diet**

Base	Invertebrate	Vegetable	Fruit	Other
Dry kitten food	Earthworm	Spinach	Apple	Cooked egg
Dry low-calorie cat food	Mealworm	Kale	Banana	Wheat germ
Dry low-calorie dog food	Waxworm	Leaf lettuce	Grape	Evaporated milk
Ferret chow	Crickets	Carrot	Raisin	Cottage cheese
Hedgehog chow	Grasshoppers	Tomato	Papaya	Pinky mice
Bird of prey diet		Yam	Orange	Meat baby food
Insectivore diet			Melon	
Feline diet			Blueberries	

Hospital Diets

Hospitalized hedgehogs should be offered a high-quality diet, as described in the previous section, and weighed daily. The patient should be fed its normal diet. In the case of the anorectic hedgehog, or the hedgehog that is losing weight, additional measures may be necessary to assure adequate nutritional intake. Syringe feeding of a high-caloric, wet, cat or dog food, powdered, high-energy, carnivore diet or human enteral diets with sweet flavoring added can be tried. Placement and maintenance of nasogastric or esophagostomy tubes is problematic because of the small size and defensive nature of this species. However, pharyngostomy tubes have been placed with success in this species, using methods applied to the feline patient.[28]

■ PREVENTIVE MEDICINE

Quarantine

When introducing a new animal into a group of hedgehogs, it is advisable to keep the introduced hedgehog in a separate enclosure for at least 30 days. This "new" animal should be cleaned, fed, and handled last each day. During the quarantine period, observe the animal daily for signs of illness and monitor the animal's weight, fecal consistency, and activity. Before introducing the hedgehog to the herd, a physical examination must be performed, and results of a complete blood count, fecal flotation, smear, and culture should show no abnormalities. Monitor the new animal's weight and ability to interact within the group. Supervised play, where the new hedgehog is gradually introduced behind a screen or while closely observed, may facilitate the acclimation process.

Health Maintenance

The short life span, propensity for this species to hide illness, and common incidence of neoplasia and other degenerative diseases necessitate a semiannual physical examination (see Performing a Physical Examination) in this species, including examination with isoflurane anesthesia. Owners should be instructed to transport the hedgehog in a small, sturdy, top-opening carrier and to bring food container labels, food samples, substrate samples, and fresh fecal samples. Routine examination should include a full physical examination. A review of the hedgehog's husbandry and diet, as well as the potential for zoonoses, should be included in the initial consultation with the owner. A fecal flotation and smear are also recommended in the young healthy hedgehog. The hedgehog should be accurately weighed to the gram and the owner advised about the tendency of this species to become obese. If the hedgehog is owned by a family with young children, elderly adults, or immunocompromised individuals, fecal culture for *Salmonella* spp. and dermal fungal culture are also recommended. In the geriatric hedgehog, a complete blood count, chemistry panel, and ECG are recommended.

Currently, there are no vaccines labeled for use in hedgehogs. However, the wild African hedgehog has been found to be serologically positive for exposure to *Leptospira* spp.[29] Rabies and Morbillivirus infection closely related to distemper have been diagnosed in the closely related European hedgehog.[12,29] Because hedgehogs are generally not housed in mixed gender groups, castration or ovariohysterectomy is not generally requested or recommended. Nevertheless, castration and ovariohysterectomy can be performed without incident.[30,31] Although the incidence of uterine tumors and mammary tumors is a concern, the effect of early age ovariohysterectomy on tumor reduction is unknown (see Surgery). Fleas and ticks are not generally a problem in captive African pygmy hedgehogs, but mite infestations can be severe. Several monthly antiparasitic products have been used in hedgehogs without apparent ill effects (see Ectoparasites and Table 16-3) and therefore may be used in the multiple hedgehog household.

Nails quickly become overgrown or ingrown, making examination and trimming necessary on a regular basis. This will likely require anesthesia, but owners and veterinarians can also try placing the hedgehog on a small screen. Most hedgehogs will uncurl to climb the screen and the nails can then be trimmed through the screen.[28]

Dental disease is also a common problem and may be controlled though the choice of diet (hard crunchy foods rather than soft canned foods). The addition of an abrasive substance to the diet, such as charcoal or insects with a chitinous exoskeleton, may also help promote periodontal health.[15,32] Enzy-

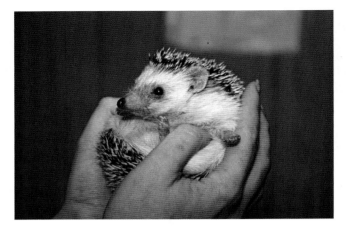

Figure 16-6 Only the tamest of hedgehogs can be handled in this manner without some discomfort to the handler.

matic pet dentifrice applied to a treat (e.g., malt, chicken, or fish flavors) or tartar control treats for companion mammals have also been recommended to maintain hedgehog dental health.[16]

RESTRAINT

Although a tame, even-tempered hedgehog can be handled without protection (Figure 16-6), the spines can cause discomfort at best and pain, disease, or an allergic reaction at worst. Hedgehog quills can spread a variety of fungi and cause hives in humans. Generally, double gloving with latex examination gloves for examination of hedgehogs is sufficient protection, but light leather or cloth gloves also work well for minor exams. A heavy terry cloth towel also works well for a short examination or for restraint for subcutaneous injections.

Manual Restraint

Many methods of manual restraint are described for the hedgehog patient, which alludes to the fact that none of these methods works particularly well. Even the most even-tempered of hedgehogs will roll or become difficult to handle after only minor manipulation. Chemical restraint is almost always necessary to perform a complete physical examination, including cardiac auscultation, oral examination, and abdominal palpation. However, for completeness, methods for handling and restraining the hedgehog and coaxing the hedgehog out of its ball without the help of chemicals are detailed below.[15,16]

- Scruff the hedgehog before it rolls into a ball.
- Place the hedgehog in a shallow pan of warm water (less than 2 cm deep), keeping the mouth and nose well above water.
- Leave the hedgehog undisturbed on a flat surface for a few minutes.
- Support the hedgehog in a normal standing position, and gently rock up and down in a see-saw fashion.
- Stroke the spines of the rump backward, against the grain or direction of the spines.
- Hold the hedgehog's head down over a surface to tempt the hedgehog to unroll and extend toward the surface.

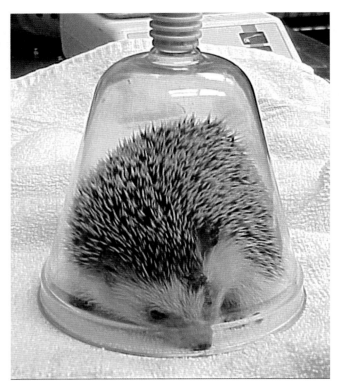

Figure 16-7 Anesthetic induction of the African pygmy hedgehog *(Atalerix albiventris)* is readily accomplished with a standard dog face mask.

- Bounce the animal gently in your hands.
- Blow on the animal with a hair dryer on the cool setting.
- Wearing light leather gloves, unroll the hedgehog by grasping on the back and gathering the skin folds and spines into the hand. Gently but firmly roll the muscular mantle outward. Upon visualizing the head, place the finger under the chin to prevent the animal from rerolling. Continue unrolling the hedgehog by gathering the skin and spines over the back into the hand until the animal is fully unrolled.
- Place digital pressure on the back of the neck when the snout is visualized to prevent the head from tucking back in.

ANESTHESIA

Isoflurane anesthesia administered via small induction chamber (Figure 16-7) and then via face mask or endotracheal tube is an effective and safe restraint protocol in the African hedgehog *(A. albiventris)*. Hedgehogs should be fasted for 4 to 6 hours before any anesthetic procedure of a duration greater than 20 minutes to reduce gastric volume.[33] A cuffed or uncuffed endotracheal tube with an internal diameter of 2 mm or less, a 14- to 16-gauge over the needle catheter with the needle stylet removed, or a small feeding tube can be used for the small glottis.[16,34] Intubation may be accomplished via direct visualization or with the aid of a rigid endoscope. Atropine may be administered as a preanesthetic agent to avoid hypersalivation

TABLE 16-1 Pain Control, Antiinflammatory, Preanesthetic, Anesthetic, and Chemical Restraint Agents for Administration in African Hedgehogs (*Atalerix albiventris*)

Drug	Dose (mg/kg)	Route	Comments/Indications
Acepromazine	0.1-1.0	SC, IM, PO	Sedative, combine with ketamine; hypotension may occur if used alone; atropine pretreatment may alleviate this effect
Atipamezole	0.3-1.0	IM	Reversal of medetomidine
Atropine	0.01-0.05	IM, SC	Preanesthetic to avert hypersalivation
Buprenorphine	0.01-0.5 q6-12h prn	IM, SC	Analgesia
Butorphanol	0.05-0.4 q6-12h prn	SC, IM, PO	Analgesia
Carprofen	1.0 q12-24h	PO, SC	Antiinflammatory, analgesia
Diazepam	0.5	1.0 IM, IV, PO	Mild sedative; may combine with ketamine for anesthetic induction; seizure control; above 2 mg/kg is PO dose
Dexamethasone	0.1-1.5	SC, IM, IV	Antiinflammatory
Depo-Medrol	1.0-5.0	SC, IM	Antiinflammatory
Enflurane	To effect	Inhalation	Induction and maintenance of anesthesia
Fentanyl	0.1	SC	Combine with medetomidine and ketamine for reversible anesthesia; reverse with naloxone
Flunixin meglumine	0.03-1.0 q8-24h	IM, SC, PO	Nonsteroidal antiinflammatory; arthritis, chronic inflammation; nephrotoxic in other hedgehog species
Isoflurane	3%-5%, to effect 0.25%-3%, to effect	Inhalation	Induction of anesthesia Maintenance of anesthesia
Ketamine	5.0-25.0	IM	Combine with xylazine or medetomidine for anesthesia
Medetomidine	0.05-0.2	IM, SC	Combine with ketamine and or fentanyl; can provide light to heavy sedation when used alone or anesthesia when paired with ketamine and/or fentanyl
Meloxicam	0.2 q24h	PO, SC	Nonsteroidal antiinflammatory, analgesic
Methylprednisolone	1.0-2.0	SC	Antiinflammatory
Naloxone	0.16	IM	For reversal of fentanyl
Prednisolone	2.5 q12h prn 1.0 q12h prn	PO, SC, IM	Allergies Antiinflammatory
Prednisone	2.5 q12h	PO, SC, IM	Antiinflammatory
Sevoflurane	To effect	Inhalation	Anesthesia induction and maintenance
Tiletamine/zolazepam	1.0-5.0	IM	Sedation, anesthesia; prolonged or difficult recovery; margin of safety questionable
Triamcinolone	0.2	SC, IM	Antiinflammatory
Xylazine	0.05-1.0	IM	Combine with ketamine
Yohimbine	0.5-1.0	IM	Reversal for xylazine

Data from Larson RS, Carpenter JW: Husbandry and medical management of African hedgehogs, *Vet Med* Oct: 877-890, 1999; Carpenter JW: Hedgehogs. In Carpenter JW, editor: *Exotic Animal Formulary*, ed 3, St Louis, 2005, WB Saunders; Lightfoot TL: Therapeutics of African pygmy hedgehogs and prairie dogs, *Vet Clin North Am Exot Anim Pract* 3(1):155-172, 2000; Morrisey JK, Carpenter JW: Formulary. In Quesenberry KE, Carpenter JW, editors: *Ferrets, Rabbits and Rodents: Clinical Medicine and Surgery*, St Louis, 2004, WB Saunders; Pye G: Marsupial, insectivore and chiropteran anesthesia, *Vet Clin North Am Exot Anim Pract* 4(1):211-238, 2001; Association of Exotic Mammal Veterinarians: Guide to small mammal analgesics, *Exot Mamm Med Surg* 2(2):10-11, 2004.
IM, intramuscular; *IV*, intravenous; *PO*, per os; *prn*, as needed; *SC*, subcutaneous.

during induction.[35] A variety of injectable anesthetic protocols have been used and recommended in the African pygmy hedgehog and other hedgehog species (Table 16-1). No controlled study of hedgehog anesthesia has yet been performed, so all anesthetic regimens must be regarded as anecdotal and guided by clinician preference and drug availability.

PERFORMING A PHYSICAL EXAMINATION

Subdued light and avoidance of high-pitched sounds may facilitate the examination process by relaxing the hedgehog.[15,16] Provide a padded high-traction surface, such as a cloth towel, for the animal to stand or ambulate on during the examination. A clear acrylic ferret tunnel or small anesthetic induction chamber can be used for an initial "hands-off" examination. Adequate time should be allowed for the observational exam, which should take place in a quiet room to allow the hedgehog to interact, undisturbed, with the environment. A brief physical examination can be done with manual restraint. The normal unrolled hedgehog's posture will include a ventrum that is completely raised from the ventral surface. Crouching or otherwise allowing the ventrum to touch the examination surface can be a sign of weakness or wariness. Generally a good examination of the quilled skin can be done with minimal restraint. The normal hedgehog's skin is somewhat dry and flaky, but excessive skin debris, quill loss, or erythema and crusting require a dermatologic diagnostic work-up (Figure 16-8). Diagnostic tests regarding quill loss (e.g., quill pluck, skin scrape, tape preparation) may be pursued with only minimal

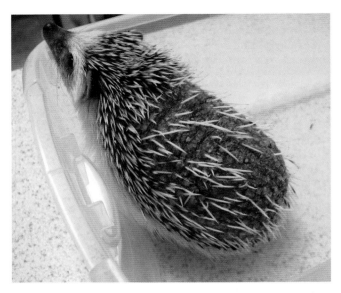

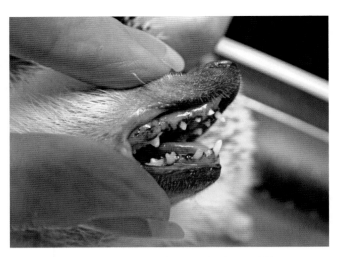

Figure 16-9 Petechiation of the gingiva in an African pygmy hedgehog *(Atalerix albiventris)*.

Figure 16-8 African pygmy hedgehog with severe quill loss due to mite infestation. (Courtesy Dr. Chris Griffin.)

restraint, as the hedgehog becomes fairly immobile when assuming its defensive posture. However, a complete physical examination will often require anesthesia.

During the physical examination, proceed as one would for a companion animal, but pay attention to the following areas as these are likely to have problems in the hedgehog. Auscult carefully, retracting the spine-covered skin dorsally as necessary, and consider performing an ECG while the animal is anesthetized.[35] Pneumonia and cardiomyopathy are common problems associated with this species. The heart should beat regularly without murmur, and the femoral pulse should be palpable. Examine the eyes closely, as trauma to the eyes, proptosis, and neoplasia commonly affect this area. The nose should be moist.[16] The ears are normally crust free and have smooth edges. Examine the oral cavity completely, as hedgehogs are prone to oral neoplasias (e.g., squamous cell carcinoma) and periodontal disease. The teeth should be white, the incisors gapped, and the gingiva similar to other companion mammals in texture, appearance, and color (Figure 16-9).

Examine the ventrum and palpate beneath the quilled skin for any lumps or bumps. Normal lymph nodes are difficult to palpate. The abdominal contour is normally flat when the unconscious hedgehog is in ventral recumbency.[16] Icterus may be most easily visualized in the axillary areas as a yellow color of the skin.[16] Neoplasias affecting the dermis are common in the hedgehog, as are external parasites. Closely examine the feet, as annular fiber constriction and ingrown toenails are often diagnosed etiologies of lameness. Examine the prepuce, anus, vulva, perineum, and testicles, located subcutaneously in para-anal recesses, for swelling, asymmetry, discharge, or foreign material that may lead to blockage and neoplasia. Lastly, perform a thorough abdominal palpation for the presence of masses, fluid, or organomegaly. Multiple types of neoplasia, along with hepatic lipidosis and kidney disease, are common in the African pygmy hedgehog. Consider perform-

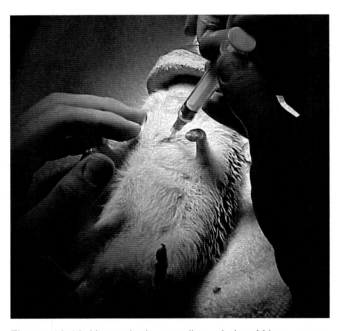

Figure 16-10 Hematologic sampling of the African pygmy hedgehog *(Atalerix albiventris)* can be accomplished via the cranial vena cava while the hedgehog is anesthetized with isoflurane.

ing any initial diagnostic tests while the animal is still anesthetized.

■ DIAGNOSTIC TESTING
Clinical Pathology
HEMATOLOGY

Blood sample collection from the hedgehog can be challenging and generally requires sedation or anesthesia. I prefer the vena cava for blood sampling, which is performed similarly to the technique used in the ferret (Figure 16-10). However, caution is advised in that the hedgehog heart is located more cranially in the thorax than is the ferret heart. The jugular vein may be difficult to visualize, especially in the obese hedgehog, but it is located in the same thoracic inlet region as in other companion mammals. Small blood samples of 1 ml or less may be obtained from the femoral, lateral saphenous, and cephalic veins, which are located in a position similar to that in other mammals. Caution is advised when accessing the femoral vein, as laceration of the femoral artery can result in morbidity and mortality in the debilitated hedgehog. The diminutive size of the cephalic and saphenous veins commonly limits the volume and quality of the sample that can be collected from these sites because of venous collapse and clotting of the sample in the syringe. These problems can be combated via an open collection of blood into the hub of a 25-gauge needle, which in turn is collected into a heparinized hematocrit tube (a method described for ferrets), or use of preheparinized tuberculin syringe fitted with a 25- or 26-gauge needle. To preheparinize the syringe, draw a small amount of heparin into the needle and syringe and then forcefully expulse it from the syringe and needle prior to venipuncture. These methods do not guarantee a sample from any site mentioned, but they give the clinician options. Blood samples can be placed into the appropriate Microtainer tube (Microtainer, Becton Dickinson and Company, Franklin Lakes, NJ) based on the test desired. Hematologic methodology is then performed as for other small mammals. While toenail clips and retroorbital blood collection methods have been described in the hedgehog, these collection techniques are debatably inhumane and therefore are not recommended for use in the pet except in terminal situations.

Urine may be collected for urinalysis by placing the hedgehog in a clean plastic or stainless steel container (the hedgehog modification of free catch) or by cystocentesis via ventral percutaneous approach or by catheterization while the hedgehog is anesthetized. An African pygmy hedgehog reference range for this diagnostic remains unknown; however, these animals would be expected to have acidic urine with a lack of white blood cells, neoplastic cells, red blood cells, or crystals.[22]

The respiratory tract may be sampled for cytologic or microbiologic analysis via percutaneous insertion of a needle or sterile catheter into the trachea for a transtracheal wash.[4] A transtracheal wash will generally require heavy sedation or anesthesia.

A true reference range for African hedgehogs for any clinicopathologic data, consisting of a data set for clinically healthy animals, has not been constructed. Values encountered in both ill and clinically normal hedgehogs have been used to construct the average and standard deviation values for the values given in Table 16-2. No range is given, as this is not clinically useful information. Further, whether data from these values are normally distributed is not known. Obviously all actions by the clinician must be guided by the picture of the entire patient and clinician experience with this species rather than relying solely on diagnostic test data.

Diagnostic Imaging
RADIOGRAPHY

Radiographic positioning in all but the moribund hedgehog patient requires anesthesia. Radiography may be accomplished

with extremity film and standard tabletop methods. Mammography plates and dental film may increase detail, especially for oral or foot lesions. The spines of the dorsum may hinder radiographic detail, especially in the ventrodorsal view. On the lateral view, the spines and associated dorsal elastic skin may be retracted dorsally and held in place with a large plastic spring clip manufactured for resealing chip bags.[16] This method can facilitate lateral positioning and increase radiographic internal detail on the lateral radiographic view. Positioning can be further facilitated by small tape stirrups placed on the feet and taped to the film cassette after extension of the legs.

Ultrasound examination is best accomplished with the patient anesthetized or sedated and can be used to evaluate abdominal or subcutaneous masses and cardiac function and to obtain fine-needle aspiration samples of suspect masses.[40] Heavy sedation or anesthesia may be required to perform a thorough ultrasound examination. Normal size for hedgehog organs has not been determined, but the contralateral organ can be used for comparison. Clinical cases and baseline information have not been published regarding the use of bone scans, computed tomography (CT), and magnetic resonance imaging (MRI) in the African pygmy hedgehog. Cost currently limits the clinical application of these diagnostic modalities in the hedgehog for most clinical cases.

Microbiology

Normal or expected microbiologic flora of the African hedgehog skin, alimentary tract, and reproductive tract has not been determined in the African pygmy hedgehog. Clinical judgment must be used when interpreting cultures of these areas and should be correlated with clinical signs associated with disease.

Parasitology

The African pygmy hedgehog is susceptible to both endoparasitism and ectoparasitism. Speciation of parasites of the African hedgehog is in its infancy. Mites are a common external parasite infestation, but fleas, myiasis, and ticks may also occur. Internal parasites, although relatively rare in the captive African hedgehog, include cestodes, nematodes (including those of the lung and gastrointestinal tract), trematodes, and protozoans. External parasitism can be diagnosed based on clinical signs, physical examination, and skin scrape or tape preparation. Internal parasitism diagnosis is based on finding parasitic ova or protozoa in the fecal flotation or in a direct smear of feces. The owner should be asked to bring a fresh fecal sample to the office for parasite screening when examination visits are scheduled.

▬ MISCELLANEOUS DIAGNOSTICS

No other diagnostic tests are routinely used in the African pygmy hedgehog. However, the clinician is urged to pursue appropriate diagnostic tests as for other companion mammals when needed and available. The African pygmy hedgehog is a mammal, and diagnostic tests used for companion mammals should be applicable, with the caveat that appropriate interpretation of the results is necessary and the norms for this species generally remain unknown. Thus, supplemental diag-

TABLE 16-2 Clinicopathologic Data for the African Hedgehog

Measurement	Unit	Average value	Standard deviation
Hematocrit	%	36	7
Red blood cell count	$\times 10^6\,\mu l$	6	2
Hemoglobin	g/dl	12.0	2.8
Mean corpuscular volume	fl	67	9
Mean corpuscular hemoglobin	pg	22	4
Mean corpuscular hemoglobin concentration	g/dl	34	5
Platelets	$\times 10^3\,\mu l$	226	108
White blood cell count	$\times 10^3\,\mu l$	11	6
Neutrophils	$\times 10^3\,\mu l$	5.1	5.2
Lymphocytes	$\times 10^3\,\mu l$	4.0	2.2
Monocytes	$\times 10^3\,\mu l$	0.3	0.3
Eosinophils	$\times 10^3\,\mu l$	1.2	0.9
Basophils	$\times 10^3\,\mu l$	0.4	0.3
Alkaline phosphatase	IU/L	51	21
Alanine aminotransferase	IU/L	53	24
Amylase	IU/L	510	170
Aspartate aminotransferase	IU/L	34	22
Bilirubin, total	mg/dl	0.3	0.3
Blood urea nitrogen	mg/dl	27	9
Calcium	mg/dl	8.8	1.4
Chloride	mEq/L	109	10
Cholesterol	mg/dl	131	25
Creatine kinase	IU/L	863	413
Creatinine	mg/dl	0.4	0.2
Gamma glutamyl transferase	IU/L	4	1
Glucose	mg/dl	89	30
Lactate dehydrogenase	IU/L	441	258
Phosphorous	mg/dl	5.3	1.9
Potassium	mEq/L	4.9	1.0
Protein, total	g/dl	5.8	.7
Albumin	g/dl	2.9	.4
Globulin	g/dl	2.7	.5
Sodium	mEq/L	141	9
Triglycerides	mg/dl	38	22

From Ivey E, Carpenter JW: African hedgehogs. In Quesenberry KE, Carpenter JW, editors: *Ferrets, Rabbits and Rodents: Clinical Medicine and Surgery,* St Louis, 2004.

nostics, while advised, should not be the sole basis for diagnosis or rule-out of disease in this species but may support a clinical diagnosis.

COMMON DISEASE PRESENTATIONS

Relatively few reports of disease in the African hedgehog exist. However, the clinician is urged to perform the appropriate diagnostic tests, based on the clinical signs, in order to arrive at a diagnosis.

Infectious

BACTERIAL

Respiratory infections in the hedgehog have been attributed to *Pasteurella* spp., *Bordetella bronchiseptica,* and *Corynebacterium*

spp.[4,41] Clinical manifestations of respiratory infection include rhinitis, laryngitis, tracheitis, pneumonia, and mortality. Clinical signs of respiratory disease are similar to those in other species (e.g., nasal discharge, increased respiratory noise, dyspnea) but also include lethargy, inappetence, and sudden death.

Periodontal disease, often associated with a bacterial component, is a clinical entity in both wild and captive hedgehog species.[32] As with other insectivores, the addition of abrasive items to the diet, such as charcoal or bone, and antibiotic treatment are recommended to prevent and treat periodontal disease, respectively.[32] As a prophylaxis for tartar accumulation, the use of a hard kibble rather than a moist food is recommended. Abscessed and fractured teeth can cause anorexia and weight loss.[4] Dental prophylaxis, periprocedural antibiotics, and tooth extraction may be necessary to treat more severe dental disease.

Salmonella Tilene has been reported to cause enteritis in the African pygmy hedgehog.[42,43] However, hedgehogs may also be subclinical carriers. European hedgehogs have also been reported to be infected with a variety of other *Salmonella* spp. (*S. Enteritidis, S. Typhimurium*); thus, the African pygmy hedgehog should be considered susceptible to these bacteria as well. Clinical signs of Salmonellosis in the hedgehog may include anorexia, mucoid diarrhea, dehydration, and weight loss. Should salmonellosis be suspected, the clinician is urged to obtain a culture and serotype because of the public health issues. Special enrichment media may be necessary for culture of *Salmonella* spp.; therefore, veterinarians should consult with the diagnostic laboratory before shipping the sample. Hedgehog owners must be advised of the zoonotic potential of this organism and take appropriate precautions when handling infected or suspected carrier animals. Treatment of the hedgehog with bacterial enteritis includes fluid and nutritional support as well as broad-spectrum parenteral antibiotic administration, pending culture and sensitivity results.

VIRAL

Few viruses have been reported in the African pygmy hedgehog. African pygmy hedgehogs are susceptible to foot-and-mouth disease (FMD), a reportable, foreign animal disease in the United States.[12] The ban on the importation of these animals decreases the probability of an FMD case in the United States. However, the practitioner should be aware that the hedgehog infected with FMD has the typical vesicular lesions of the tongue, snout, and feet associated with the disease in cattle. Fatal herpes simplex virus type 1 infection has been reported in an adult African pygmy hedgehog.[44] Initially, clinical signs were limited to posterior paresis, which was diagnosed as intervertebral disk disease. Treatment with an immunosuppressive dose of steroids resolved the paresis, but the animal then suffered from anorexia and died. The owners had oral sores consistent with herpes simplex virus type 1 infection and possible cross-contamination occurred between the owner and the hedgehog. Retroviral particles have been found in two cases of multicentric lymphoma in sibling hedgehogs.[45] However, the significance of this finding on the general hedgehog population is unknown. Papillomas found in African pygmy hedgehogs have been postulated to have a viral origin, but this has not been proven.[4] The African pygmy hedgehog is also susceptible to Crimean-Congo hemorrhagic fever, which is a zoonotic disease of the Middle East, Asia, and Eastern Europe.[12]

More viral diseases have been documented in the European hedgehog, and logic dictates that the African hedgehog be considered susceptible to these diseases. Viral diseases isolated from the European hedgehog include rabies from a neurologic hedgehog in Budapest; a paramyxovirus closely related to canine distemper and found in several apparently healthy hedgehogs; and tickborne encephalitis virus, Tahyna virus, and Bhanja virus.[12]

FUNGAL

Dermatophytosis is a common clinical disease in the African pygmy hedgehog. *Trichophyton mentagrophytes* var erinacei,

Arthroderma benhamiae var erinacei, and *Microsporum* spp. have all been isolated the African pygmy hedgehog. Most of these isolates have documented zoonotic potential with the possibility of causing serious human clinical signs.[46-48] Although hedgehogs may harbor fungi without significant clinical signs, clinical dermatophytosis of the hedgehog may present as crusting pruritic dermatitis of the face, pinnae, and body and quill loss.[16,36] Diagnosis may be made by fungal culture, skin scrape, or tape preparation, and microscopic examination of the resultant sample can be done with a lactophenol blue mount. Treatment should consist of topical and/or systemic antifungal therapy (see Table 16-5). Owners should be counseled regarding the zoonotic potential of these organisms and urged to seek medical care should lesions consistent with "ringworm" be reported.

Other reported fungal diseases of the hedgehog are limited to candidiasis. One case of intestinal infection and one case of footpad invasion have been reported in the African pygmy hedgehog.[49,50] Diagnosis of candidiasis can be made by cytologic or histopathologic examination of the lesion. Treatment includes both topical and systemic antifungal therapy.

Parasitic
ECTOPARASITES

Ectoparasitism is often diagnosed in African pygmy hedgehog patients. In the wild, tick, flea, and mite infestation are common in the various hedgehog species.[13] However, in captivity, maggot, flea, and tick infestation are rare. If ticks or fly larvae are found on the pet hedgehog, they can be manually removed. Fleas of the European hedgehog can infest the African hedgehog, but cat and dog fleas generally do not infest African pygmy hedgehogs. This species predilection likely occurs because of the hedgehog's low body temperature.[36] For treatment the practitioner can choose from a variety of topical or systemic flea control agents (Table 16-3). Topical shampoo and powder products for approved use in kittens appear safe for hedgehogs.[16]

Acariasis, or mite infestation, is a common problem of the African pygmy hedgehog. The identification of these mites is not complete, but they are generally accepted to be *Caparinia* spp., *Chorioptes* spp., or *Notoedres* spp. In one study of wild African hedgehogs, three mites were found with differing incidences and pathogenicities (Figure 16-11).[51] *Notoedres oudesmani,* a sarcoptic mite, was sporadically found, but it usually infected male hedgehogs and caused high mortality. *Caparinia erinacei,* a psoroptic mite, was identified on most animals but had low pathogenicity. *Rodentopus sciuri,* a hypodermid mite, was found on about half the animals studied, but clinical signs associated with its presence were minimal.

Clinical signs vary greatly as some animals may have subclinical infestation without evidence of pruritus, whereas others may scratch or rub themselves against stationary objects. Anorexia, lethargy, seborrhea, quill loss, overly flaky skin, and white or brown mite droppings at the base of the quills and on the face are commonly observed in affected animals. Diag-

TABLE 16-3	Antiparasitics for Use in African Pygmy Hedgehogs		
Drug	**Strength, Dosage**	**Route**	**Indication**
Amitraz	0.3%, q7-14days	Dip	Mite infestation
Fenbendazole	25 mg/kg	PO	Repeat treatment as necessary based on patient parasite status
Fipronil	1 pump/ hedgehog	Spray	Fleas, mites; safety unknown
Ivermectin	0.2-0.5 mg/kg once q7-14days × 3-5 treatments	PO, SC	Nematodes Mites
Imidacloprid	½ puppy/kitten dose every month	Topical quilled areas behind head	Fleas
Levamisole	10 mg/kg q48h; repeat prn up to 14 days	SC	Lung worms; therapeutic margin of safety may be small
Lime-sulfur dip	2.5%, q5-7days	Spray or dip	Mites, bacterial and fungal dermatopathies
Lufenuron	½ puppy kitten dose every month	PO	Fleas
Metronidazole	25 mg/kg q12h, 3-7 days	PO	Intestinal protozoans, flagellates
Permethrin	1%, once	Topical, apply fine mist	Mites
Praziquantel	7 mg/kg q14days	PO,SC	Cestodes (tapeworms), trematodes (flukes)
Selamectin	6 mg/kg	Topical	Fleas, mites
Sulfadimethoxine	2-20 mg/kg q24h for 2-5 days, off 5 days, repeat for 5-7 days	PO, SC, IM	Coccidia

Data from Carpenter JW: Hedgehogs. In Carpenter JW, editor: *Exotic Animal Formulary,* ed 3, St Louis, 2005, WB Saunders; Lightfoot TL: Therapeutics of African pygmy hedgehogs and prairie dogs, *Vet Clin North Am Exot Anim Pract* 3(1):155-172, 2000; Morrisey JK, Carpenter JW: Formulary. In Quesenberry KE, Carpenter JW, editors: *Ferrets, Rabbits and Rodents: Clinical Medicine and Surgery,* St Louis, 2004, WB Saunders.

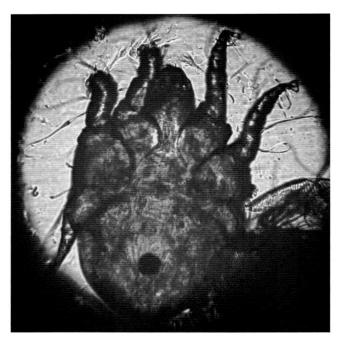

Figure 16-11 Chorioptes-like mite recovered from an African pygmy hedgehog with severe quill loss. (Courtesy Dr. Chris Griffin.)

nosis is confirmed by finding the mites and or their eggs (nits) microscopically from skin scrapings. Treatment for mite infestation, regardless of the species, is similar, and response to treatment, including environmental sanitation, guides therapy (see Table 16-3). Treatment with ivermectin, permethrin, or

amitraz has been successful in cases of mite infestation. Owners and practitioners should be vigilant about environmental sanitation, and all hedgehogs and their habitats should be treated simultaneously.

Ear mites *(Otodectes cynotis)* are occasionally diagnosed in the captive African pygmy hedgehog.[16] Affected animals may scratch at their ears. Diagnosis is made by finding the mites or their eggs microscopically from a swab of the brown waxy crust generally found in the external ear canal. Treatment is similar to that recommended for ear mite infestation in cats.

ENDOPARASITES

Numerous species of nematodes, cestodes, and protozoa have been identified in the wild African hedgehog. However, gastrointestinal parasitism in the captive African hedgehog is rare. Nonetheless, a fecal flotation and direct smear are recommended in any hedgehog exhibiting gastrointestinal clinical signs and for the semiannual physical examination. Treatment should be instituted in case these parasites are found (see Table 16-3).

Lungworm infestation can cause pneumonia in African pygmy hedgehogs but is rarely diagnosed in the domestically raised hedgehog.[16] Similarly, a fatal case of Chagas' disease, likely caused by insect ingestion by an outdoor hedgehog, and cryptosporidiosis, in a neonatal African pygmy hedgehog in a zoo, have been reported.[52,53] The diagnosis of cryptosporidiosis was made upon histopathologic examination and after the animal was found dead without apparent premonitory signs. Diagnosis of Chagas' disease was determined by finding

Trypanosoma spp. on the blood smear. Clinicopathologic abnormalities included a mature neutrophilia, monocytosis, elevated creatine phosphokinase (18,532 IU/L), hematuria, and proteinuria (500 mg/dl). No specific treatment was attempted, and this animal died 7 days after clinical signs developed. If specific treatment is attempted in these cases, it should be based on current recommendations described for companion mammals and humans. The zoonotic potential of cryptosporidiosis should be considered, and if a diagnosis has been confirmed, the owner should be informed about exposure.

Nutritional Disorders

Nutritional diseases of the hedgehog are generally limited to obesity and periodontal disease. In brief, the hedgehog's diet should be limited to what it can eat overnight, and the animal should be weighed weekly to avoid obesity. Further, the base diet of adult hedgehogs should consist of a low-calorie, dry kibble dog food to prevent weight gain and promote dental health.

Neoplasia

The African pygmy hedgehog appears particularly prone to neoplasia. A number of reviews are available detailing the specifics of the numerous reported cases.[40,54] About 30% of hedgehogs have neoplasia upon necropsy, and about 10% have multiple tumors that may be clinically undetected.[55,56] Except in cases of reproductive tumors, gender does not affect tumor incidence. As in other animals, geriatric hedgehogs are predisposed to neoplastic disease and the 2-year-old hedgehog should be considered geriatric. Yearly or semiannual examinations of the geriatric hedgehog should include the appropriate diagnostic work-up for neoplasia, and owners should be informed about this issue during their first visit. The systems most likely to be affected by tumors in descending order are the integumentary, hemolymphatic, gastrointestinal, and endocrine systems.[55] A viral component has been implicated in some tumors, but most appear spontaneous.[45] Table 16-4 details the organ system and tumors found, along with other pertinent details of the neoplasms documented in this species. Treatment of these tumors has not been clinically studied, but a few anecdotal reports exist of treatments that are generally extrapolated from mammalian protocols.[36]

Diseases of Noninfectious, Unknown, Degenerative, or Multiple Etiologies
CARDIOVASCULAR DISEASE

According to a published report, the incidence of cardiomyopathy in the captive African hedgehog is 38%.[57] Affected hedgehogs are more likely to be male and geriatric, but disease has been documented as early as 1 year of age. Death may occur without clinical signs, but overt disease is observed in the majority of cases. Clinical signs are referable to cardiac and lung dysfunction, as well as general illness (e.g., heart murmur, moist rales, dyspnea, dehydration, anorexia, weight loss, and lethargy). Cardiomegaly, hepatomegaly, pulmonary edema, and/or congestion, hydrothorax, ascites, and pulmonary or renal infarcts are common gross necropsy findings associated with hedgehog cardiovascular disease. Concurrent pathology often occurs with cardiovascular disease in the hedgehog, including renal tubular necrosis and vascular infarct. The cause of cardiomyopathy in hedgehogs remains unknown, although diet, toxins, stress, and genetics are possible contributing factors.

The type or types of cardiomyopathy in the captive African hedgehog have not yet been determined, and normal values for echocardiographic measurement remain unknown in this species. A fractional shortening of more than 25% and a cardiac wall thickness of 1.5 mm have been reported anecdotally for the normal hedgehog.[16] Radiographic evaluation may suggest cardiomegaly based on cardiac silhouette size and a dorsally displaced trachea when compared with a normal hedgehog. Pulmonary radiographic evidence of disease may include pleural edema, pleural effusion, or evidence of aerophagia.[16] A minimum database of a complete blood count, plasma chemistry panel, and urinalysis are indicated in cardiovascular cases to assess for the presence of renal disease or organ infarct, which may affect prognosis and treatment options.[57] Treatment with enalapril, furosemide, and/or digoxin should be considered in cases with heart disease, although the long-term prognosis is guarded.[16]

URINARY TRACT DISEASE

Based on a necropsy survey, hedgehogs have a 50% prevalence of renal disease.[56] Urolithiasis, cystitis, nephrosis, intrarenal calcinosis, renal calculi, nephritis, nephrocalcinosis, tubular necrosis, glomerulosclerosis, renal infarcts, and glomerulonephropathy have been diagnosed in hedgehogs.[16,58] The cause for this high prevalence of renal disease in unknown, but genetic or dietary factors may contribute. Diagnosis should be based on urinalysis and plasma chemistry panels. However, true normal values of the African hedgehog remain unknown, and clinical experience should dictate treatment and prognosis.

MUSCULOSKELETAL DISEASE

Bone cysts should be considered a differential diagnosis for masses of the mandible, along with neoplasia and trauma to the musculoskeletal system.[58] Prognosis is favorable after removal of the cysts. Fractures, especially of the long bones and feet, may occur when animals trap appendages in cage furniture or in inappropriate enclosure flooring. External coaptation and internal fixation are viable methods of repair, but the method must be able to withstand the normal defensive posture.[4] Palpation under sedation or anesthesia along with radiography should be performed to assess the type of fracture or other bone diseases and possible repair options. Pain control should be considered in all cases of bone involvement, and antibiotic therapy is indicated in open or contaminated fractures or lesions. Excisional biopsy with histopathologic exami-

TABLE 16-4   Neoplasms of the African Pygmy Hedgehog by Organ System

Organ System	Neoplasm	Organ affected	Metastases
Integument	Mast cell tumor	Skin	Rare, usually locally invasive
	Mammary tumors	Mammary gland	Y
	Squamous cell carcinoma	Junction of quilled and unquilled skin.	Rare, usually locally invasive
	Neurofibroma	Skin	Likely based on clinical signs
	Fibrous histiocytoma	Skin	N
Vascular/hemolymphatic	Lymphosarcoma	Multicentric or gastrointestinal	Y
	Myeloproliferative disease/ myelogenous leukemia	Lymphatic and hemopoietic organs	Y
	Hemangioma	Eye	N
		Ventricle wall	N
Neuroendocrine	C-cell carcinoma	Thyroid	N
	Follicular adenoma	Pituitary	N
	Adenocarcinoma	Parathyroid	N
	Adenoma	Pancreas	N
	Adenoma	Adrenal	N
	Islet cell tumor	Upper GI tract	Locally invasive
	Cortical carcinoma	Nerve sheath	Y
	Pheochromocytoma		N
	Neuroendocrine		Y
	Schwannoma		N
Musculoskeletal	Osteosarcoma	Multicentric	Y
		Bone	N
		Subcutaneous	N
Gastrointestinal	Squamous cell carcinoma	Oral	Rare, usually
	Fibrosarcoma plasmacytoma	Oral	Locally invasive
	Acinic cell carcinoma	Intestinal	Locally invasive
	Hepatocellular carcinoma	Eye, retrobulbar	Locally invasive
	Adenocarcinoma	Liver	Locally invasive
		Stomach	Y
		Colon	Y
Reproductive	Granulosa cell tumor	Uterus	N
	Adenoma/adenosarcoma	Uterus	Locally invasive
	Leiomyosarcoma	Uterus	N
	Adenocarcinoma	Uterus	N
	Adenoleiomyosarcoma	Uterus	N
	Spindle cell tumor	Vagina	N
	Neurofibrosarcoma	Testicular tunic	Unknown
Respiratory	Bronchoalveolar carcinoma	Lung	Y
	Squamous cell carcinoma	Lung	N

Data from Greenacre CB: Spontaneous tumors of small mammals, *Vet Clin North Am Exot Anim Pract* 7:627-651, 2004; Heatley J, Maulden G, Cho D: Neoplasia in the captive African hedgehog *(Atalerix albiventris), Semin Av Exot Pet Med* 14(3):182-192, 2005.

nation is warranted in cases of skeletal disease without a history of trauma to confirm a neoplastic or degenerative process. A packed cell volume and total solids determination are minimally recommended in these cases to assess a patient's fitness for anesthesia and surgery.

Osteoarthritis and myositis due to cellulitis also occur in the hedgehog. Other differentials to be considered in the lame hedgehog include annular fiber constriction of the limb or digit, ingrown toenails, pododermatitis, or neurologic disease.

GASTROINTESTINAL DISEASE

Pyloric and intestinal obstructions of the stomach and intestines occur in the hedgehog and may be caused by rubber, hair, or carpet fibers, among other things.[16] Clinical signs are similar to those in other small mammals and include acute anorexia (with or without vomiting), lethargy, and collapse. Intestinal mesenteric torsion resulting in fatality has also been reported.[16]

Diarrhea is a common presenting complaint of hedgehogs, and differentials include inappropriate dietary components (such as milk), recent dietary change or dietary indiscretion, malnutrition, toxicosis, liver disease, infectious or parasitic causes of diarrhea, or systemic disease. Hematochezia should be clearly defined from urinary or vaginal bloody discharge in these cases.

Hepatic lipidosis and obesity are common disease syndromes in the captive African hedgehog. Obesity is the most likely cause of hepatic lipidosis, but nutritional imbalance, starvation, toxicosis, pregnancy, and infectious and neoplastic diseases have also been noted as contributing factors.[16] Clinical signs stem from hepatic dysfunction and include lethargy, inappetence, icterus, diarrhea, or signs of hepatic encephalopathy. Diagnosis can be supported by hepatic enzymes, plasma bilirubin, and bile acids test results. Radiography may reveal an enlarged liver, and an ultrasound-guided aspirate can provide a noninvasive diagnosis. Caution should be exercised when obtaining diagnostic samples of the diseased liver, as a dysfunctional liver may result in prolonged clotting times. Treatment is supportive with fluids and a low-protein, low-fat, high-energy, easily digestible diet. Milk thistle or other nutraceuticals may be beneficial in cases of hepatic disease.

NEUROLOGIC DISEASE

Neurologic diseases of the hedgehog are rare but include trauma, torpor, parasitic migration, toxicosis, infarcts, malnutrition, postpartum eclampsia, neoplasia, otitis media, rabies, polioencephalomalacia, and wobbly hedgehog syndrome.[16,22,36] Wobbly hedgehog syndrome has been reported in African and European hedgehogs, primarily in animals 2 to 3 years of age. Clinically, wobbly hedgehog syndrome is characterized by muscle atrophy and hindlimb ataxia, which progresses to tetraparesis, although animals with only forelimb signs or generalized paresis have also been diagnosed with disease. Death occurs 18 to 25 months after onset of clinical signs.[16] Diagnosis is via histologic lesions of axonal swelling, degeneration of the ventral spinal cord tracts, and degeneration of axons and myelin in the white matter of the brain, in the spinal cord, and in the peripheral nerves. A definitive cause has not been found for this syndrome, but possible causes include viral agents, genetic factors, nutrition or autoimmune syndromes.

OPHTHALMIC DISEASE

Proptosis and orbital cellulitis has been reported in eight male and female African pygmy hedgehogs ranging in age from 2 to 24 months.[59] Concurrent neurologic disease was present in two hedgehogs with clinical signs of circling to one side, progressive weakness, reluctance to stand, and lateral recumbency on the ipsilateral side and proptosis on the contralateral side.[59] Degenerative neurologic disease was found in these two hedgehogs: One hedgehog had leukopolioencephalopathy, myelopathy, and Wallerian degeneration of spinal nerves, and the other hedgehog had vacuolar myeloencephalopathy. Incipient anterior subcapsular cataracts were also present in one hedgehog. Fat occupied about $\frac{2}{3}$ of the orbit in an obese hedgehog.[59] Orbital cellulitis, corneal perforation, and panophthalmitis were the predominant findings in the eyes of all reported cases. In most cases of eye disease in the hedgehog, the retina, lens,

uvea, and retina were extruded through the perforated cornea, and periorbital tissues were markedly inflamed. No definitive cause was found for these cases, but trauma seems a likely cause and the shallow orbit of hedgehogs may predispose them to orbital disease. Additionally, these cases occurred in Canada, where even indoor the temperature and humidity may be inappropriate for maintaining hedgehogs. All bacteria found were considered opportunistic invaders. Before proceeding with enucleation, lateral tarsorrhaphy may be a viable option for managing these cases, in order to maintain the globe. Surgical replacement of the globe with a prosthetic was not considered a viable option based on the shallow orbit. A complete ophthalmic examination via isoflurane anesthesia is recommended in all suspected cases of hedgehog ocular abnormalities. Culture and appropriate treatment should be initiated early and aggressively in cases of hedgehogs exhibiting these clinical signs.

OTIC DISEASE

Clinical signs of *otitis externa* in the hedgehog include sensitivity of the area and purulent discharge and malodor from the ear.[16] Tick and mite infestation may predispose hedgehogs to *otitis externa,* and bacterial and yeast infections should be included as possible causes. Diagnosis is based on cytology and/or culture of the exudate from the affected ear.

Crusty ear edges, or pinnal dermatitis, is a common finding in captive and wild African pygmy hedgehogs (Figure 16-12).[16,46] Skin secretions accumulate at the ear margins, resulting in a ragged crusted ear edge.[16] Multiple factors have been associated with this syndrome and include dermatophytosis, acariasis, nutritional deficiency, low-humidity conditions, and dry skin.[16,46]

◼ THERAPEUTICS

No efficacy, safety, or toxicity studies of any drug have been performed in the African pygmy hedgehog. All drug dosages listed in this chapter must be regarded as anecdotal.

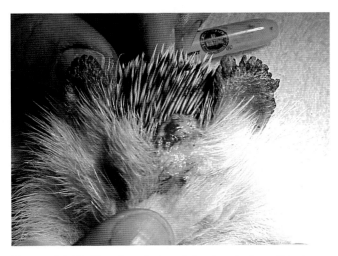

Figure 16-12 Pinnal and dorsal forehead dermatitis in an African pygmy hedgehog *(Atalerix albiventris).*

Approximately 50% of the hedgehog's body weight is composed of the poorly vascularized spines and the dorsal subcutaneous fat associated with the subdermal tissue.[4] Therefore, subcutaneous injection in the conscious hedgehog is generally deposited into adipose tissue, which may alter drug uptake or distribution. However, this method of administration is readily achieved, even when the hedgehog is in its defensive posture, and guarantees that the entire dose is administered although the drug distribution rate in unknown.[36] Clinically this site is considered a viable route of administration for fluids and drugs for subcutaneous use, and absorption may be improved with the administration of hyaluronidase (see Table 16-7).

The oral administration of medications is generally the preferred route of treating the stable hedgehog. Fruit-flavored medications may be readily accepted, especially in the affable hedgehog. The addition of sweetened grape juice to medication immediately before administration, to improve palatability, has been advocated.[36] Mealworms or waxworms injected with medications may also be readily accepted. With oral administration, choose medication flavorings carefully, as some tastes may be poorly accepted or cause hypersalivation. Upon hypersalivation, the anointing behavior will occur, resulting in the medication being slathered onto the spines. Similarly, things applied to the spines may be advertently lapped from them, causing unexpected oral ingestion by the hedgehog patient.

Hedgehogs are avid groomers, and Elizabethan collars are not an option in this species. Topical medications, especially those that are distasteful or noxious to the hedgehog may be rapidly removed and inadvertently ingested and lapped along the dorsal spines.[18] Only topical medications that are washed away after application or those suitable for oral ingestion are recommended for use. In general, light coatings of any topical medication are recommended, and topical treatment should be limited whenever possible. Active lavage with topical antimicrobial solution suffices for lathering and massaging medications into the skin and can effectively exfoliate and flush the skin.[36] Medications applied to the extremities can be covered with bandages.[16]

Vascular access can be challenging in the hedgehog because the vessels are relatively small and the legs are short and easily covered by the spiny muscular mantle, causing catheter displacement when the hedgehog exhibits its normal defensive posture. However, the cephalic vein can be accessed with an insulin syringe or 26-gauge needle for bolus fluid administration. Generally this route of fluid administration requires anesthesia. Intraosseous catheter placement is preferred for vascular access because of ease of placement and maintenance of vascular access. Intraosseous catheters can be placed in the proximal femur through the trochanteric fossa or into the proximal or distal tibia.[16,22] A 20- or 22-gauge hypodermic needle alone may be used; however, I prefer using a 1″ spinal needle, as the stylet prevents the catheter from plugging with bone or cartilage. This system may be used for fluid, colloid, or antibiotic administration via slow bolus or syringe pump infusion. Any drug that can be given intravenously in other species should

be considered for intraosseous administration in the critical hedgehog. However, basic or acidic drugs or those that are very concentrated should be diluted before being administered.

Fluid Therapy

Fluids may be given intravenously, subcutaneously, or intraperitoneally. Up to 100 ml/kg may given in the dorsum underneath the loose spines if divided in several sites. However, fluid absorption from this site may take several hours to complete. Appropriate choice of fluid type and fluid rate is based on extrapolations from companion mammals and clinician preference. Caution is advised in determining fluid rates, and animals should be monitored throughout fluid therapy for hydration status, urinary output, and other fluid loss, as cardiomyopathy and renal disease are prevalent in this species. Clinical use of colloids or blood transfusions in this species has not been reported and may be necessary in very critical cases.

Antimicrobials

Hedgehogs are insectivores with relatively short, uncomplicated gastrointestinal tracts. Therefore, antibiotic selection is not limited as in rabbits or rodents (Table 16-5). The omnivorous nature of the hedgehog and lack of hindgut fermentation allow the use of many drugs commonly used in dogs and cats.[36] No pharmacokinetic data are available for antibiotic use in hedgehogs, so all drugs listed here must be considered anecdotal.

Emergency Drugs

See Table 16-6.

Miscellaneous Drugs

See Table 16-7.

■ SURGERY
Preoperative Considerations

A full physical examination, including gender determination, facilitated by isoflurane anesthesia is recommended prior to performing any surgical procedure in the hedgehog.[33] This same anesthetic procedure can be used to facilitate sampling for a complete blood count and plasma chemistry panel, which are also recommended prior to any surgical procedure. Plans for fluid therapy, pain control, and thermal support should be established for the African pygmy hedgehog prior to any prolonged anesthetic event. Perioperative antibiotics should be considered when the procedure involves the mouth or other aspects of the alimentary tract. Emergency cardiopulmonary resuscitation drugs dosages can be extrapolated from other small mammals (see Table 16-6). Calculations should also be made on a per-patient basis, and drugs should be readily avail-

TABLE 16-5 **Antimicrobials and Antifungals for Administration in the African Hedgehog (*Atalerix albiventris*)**

Antibiotic	Dose/Frequency	Route	Indication
Amikacin	2.5-5.0 mg/kg q8-12h	IM	Gram-negative infection
Amoxicillin	15 mg/kg q12h	PO, SC, IM	Palatable to most hedgehogs
Amoxicillin/clavulanate	12.5 mg/kg q12h	PO	Palatable to most hedgehogs
Ampicillin	10 mg/kg q12h	PO, IM	Gram-positive infection
Ceftiofur	20 mg/kg q12-24h	SC	Gram-positive infection
Cephalexin	25 mg/kg q8h	PO	Palatable to most hedgehogs
Chlorhexidine			
Solution	0.1-0.05% dilution prn	Topical to affected area	Soak or lavage for wound treatment
Shampoo	2%-3% prn q2-7days	Topical to affected area	Bacterial, fungal dermatitis
Chloramphenicol	30-50 mg/kg q6-12h	PO, IM, IV, SC	Acute salmonellosis; palatable; human idiosyncratic reactions
Ciprofloxacin			Broad-spectrum antibiotic
Clindamycin	10-15 mg/kg q12h	PO	Anaerobic infection, dental disease; generally unpalatable, mix with favorite food
Enrofloxacin	2.5-10 mg/kg q12h	PO, SC, IM	Broad-spectrum antibacterial
Erythromycin	10 mg/kg q12h	PO, IM	Penicillin-resistant Gram-positive cocci; *Mycoplasma* spp., *Pasteurella* spp., and *Bordetella* spp. infections
Gentamicin			
Injectable	2 mg/kg q8h	SC, IM	Gram-negative infection; nephrotoxic, rarely indicated
Ophthalmic drops	1-2 drops q4-12h	To affected eye	Corneal ulcer, conjunctivitis
Griseofulvin	25-50 mg/kg q24h	PO	Dermatophytosis
Itraconazole	5-10 mg/kg q12-24h	PO	Fungal infections
Ketoconazole	10 mg/kg q12h	PO	Yeast/fungal infections
Metronidazole	20 mg/kg q12h	PO	Anaerobes
Mucopiricin (2%)	Light coating q12-24h prn	Topical to affected area	Bacterial dermatitis, skin wounds
Nystatin	30,000 IU/kg q8-24h	PO, topical to affected area	Superficial yeast infections
Oxytetracycline	25-50 mg/kg q24h 5-7 days	PO, in food	Bordetellosis
Panalog cream, nystatin, neomycin, thiostrepton, triamcinolone	Light coating q12-24h prn	Topical to affected area	Bacterial/mycotic dermatitis, allergic dermatopathy, antiinflammatory; long-term use of steroid may slow healing
Penicillin G	40,000 IU/kg q24h	IM	
Piperacillin	10 mg/kg q8-12h	SC	
Sulfadimethoxine	2-20 mg/kg q24h	IM, SC, PO	Gram-negative bacteria; nephrotoxic
Terramycin ophthalmic ointment	Match head or less q6h-q12h	Affected eye(s) or conjunctiva	Corneal ulcer, conjunctivitis
Tresaderm: thiabendazole, dexamethasone, neomycin	1-2 drops or enough drops to contact affected area q12h	Topical to affected area or ear canal	Bacterial or mycotic dermatitis, otitis externa, antiinflammatory; prolonged use may slow healing due to steroid
Trimethoprim sulfa	30 mg/kg combined q12h	PO, SC, IM	Respiratory infections; palatable to most hedgehogs
Triple antibiotic ophthalmic ointment; bacitracin, neomycin, polymyxin	Match head or less q6h-q12h	Affected eye(s) or conjunctiva	Corneal ulcer, conjunctivitis
Tylosin	10 mg/kg q12h	PO, SC	Mycoplasmosis, clostridiosis; IM administration causes muscle necrosis

Data from Carpenter JW: Hedgehogs. In Carpenter JW, editor: *Exotic Animal Formulary*, ed 3, St Louis, 2005, WB Saunders; Lightfoot TL: Clinical examination of chinchillas, hedgehogs, prairie dogs, and sugar gliders, *Vet Clin North Am Exot Anim Pract* 2(2):447-469, 1999; Morrisey JK, Carpenter JW: Formulary. In Quesenberry KE, Carpenter JW, editors: *Ferrets, Rabbits and Rodents: Clinical Medicine and Surgery*, St Louis, 2004, WB Saunders; Delaney CJ: Hedgehogs. In Delaney CJ, editor: *Exotic Companion Medicine Handbook*, Lake Worth, Fla, 1998, Zoological Education Network.
IM, intramuscular; *IV*, intravenous; *PO*, per os; *prn*, as needed; *SC*, subcutaneous.

TABLE 16-6	Shock and Emergency Drug Dosages for Use in the Hedgehog (*Atalerix albiventris*)			
Agents	**Dose**	**Route**	**Comments/Indications**	
Dexamethasone	1-4 mg/kg	IV, IM, SC	Shock, spinal trauma	
Prednisolone	10 mg/kg	IM, SC	Shock, spinal trauma	
Atropine	0.05-0.2 mg/kg	SC, IM	Bradycardia	
Epinephrine	0.003 mg/kg	IV	Cardiac arrest	
Doxapram	2-10 mg/kg	IV, IP	Respiratory stimulant	
Glycopyrrolate	0.01-0.02 mg/kg	SC	Bradycardia	

Data from Ness RD: Rodents. In Carpenter JW, editor: *Exotic Animal Formulary*, ed 3, St Louis, 2005, WB Saunders.
IM, intramuscular; *IP*, intraperitoneal; *IV*, intravenous; *SC*, subcutaneous.
These dosages are extrapolated from other small exotic mammal doses.

TABLE 16-7	Miscellaneous Drugs for Use in the African Pygmy Hedgehog (*Atalerix albiventris*)		
Drug	**Dosage Regime**	**Route**	**Comments**
Calcium glubionate	23 mg/kg q12-24h	PO	Palatable
Calcium gluconate	0.5-50 mg/kg	IM	Fracture repair, hypocalcemia
Cimetidine	10 mg/kg q8h	PO	Gastric ulcers
Enalapril	0.5 mg/kg q12h	PO	Cardiac insufficiency, vasodilator
Erythropoietin	100 U/kg q2-3days	SC	Chronic anemia, anemia of renal disease
Furosemide	1-5 mg/kg q8h	PO, SC, IM	Diuretic for edema
Hyaluronidase	100-150 U/L of fluid	Add to fluids	Facilitates absorption of subcutaneous fluids
Iron dextran	25 mg/kg	IM	Anemia
Lactobacilli	2.5 ml/kg q24h	PO	Restoration of gastrointestinal flora
Lactulose	0.3 ml/kg q8-12h	PO	Hepatic disease/encephalopathy
Metoclopramide	0.2-0.5 mg/kg prn	PO, SC	Vomiting, regurgitation
Sucralfate	10 mg/kg q8-12h	PO	Gastrointestinal ulcers
Theophylline	10 mg/kg q8-12h	PO, IM	Bronchodilator
Vitamin A	400 IU/kg q24h ×10 days	IM	Dermatopathy, excessive quill loss
Vitamin B complex (small animal formulation)	1 ml/kg once	SC, IM	CNS signs, paralysis of undetermined etiology, anorexia
Vitamin C	50-200 mg/kg	PO, SC	Vitamin C deficiency, infection, gingival disease
	1 g/L	Drinking water	Change daily

Data from Carpenter JW: Hedgehogs. In Carpenter JW, editor: *Exotic Animal Formulary*, ed 3, St Louis, 2005, WB Saunders; Lightfoot TL: Therapeutics of African pygmy hedgehogs and prairie dogs, *Vet Clin North Am Exot Anim Pract* 3(1):155-172, 2000; Morrisey JK, Carpenter JW: Formulary. In Quesenberry KE, Carpenter JW, editors: *Ferrets, Rabbits and Rodents: Clinical Medicine and Surgery*, St Louis, 2004, WB Saunders.
CNS, Central nervous system; *IM*, intramuscular; *IV*, intravenous; *PO*, per os; *SC*, subcutaneous.

able during the procedure and anesthetic event. Every effort should be made to maintain the hedgehog in an appropriate environment preoperatively to expedite the recovery process (see Hospitalization). Thermal support should be provided via a convective air blanket, a circulating water heating pad, and/or a heat lamp intraoperatively and an incubator postoperatively.

For preoperative, anesthetic, and pain management options, see Anesthesia under Restraint; see also Table 16-1. Common surgical procedures are limited to mass removal, dental prophylaxis, or tooth removal and exploratory laparotomy. Teeth

may be scaled, polished, and fluoridated, as one would in the companion mammal.[60]

For surgical preparation, saline is preferred to prepare the epithelial surface rather than alcohol to limit heat loss of the patient. Spines may be removed with steady traction at the base and will regrow postoperatively. Alternately, the dermal spine processes may be clipped. Adherent, Betadine-impregnated clear plastic drapes, such as those used for ophthalmic surgeries, facilitate patient visualization to monitor anesthetic depth, limit drape motion without the use of traumatic surgical clamps, and reduce the weight of the drape on the patient. Small ophthalmic instruments are ideal for use in these patients, but the skin can be relatively thick so a cutting needle may be necessary to close an incision. Absorbable suture (3-0 or 4-0) is preferred for vessel ligation and incision closure in this species. Subcuticular suture patterns and tissue glue facilitate skin closure while limiting patient access to the suture line.

Orchidectomy and ovariohysterectomy are not commonly requested but can be performed.[30,31,40] Indications for ovariohysterectomy in the hedgehog are prevention of offspring, prevention of disease of the reproductive tract, or removal of a diseased reproductive tract.[33] Ovariohysterectomy is performed as for the cat or dog. Indications for castration of the hedgehog include prevention of offspring, decrease of aggression, and removal of diseased testicles.[33] The male African pygmy hedgehog has no scrotum, likely because a pendulous scrotum is unnecessary based on the animal's low body temperature and low profile to the ground. The testicles can be easily palpated subcutaneously in the para-anal recess.[20] Orchidectomy is a simple matter of a skin incision and a closed castration with two ligatures. A preferred technique is placing one transfixation ligature and then placing one encircling ligature more distally on the vascular pedicle. Closed castration is necessary, as hedgehogs have an open inguinal ring.[33] However, should an open castration be inadvertently performed, the inguinal ring should be closed before the skin is closed to avoid herniation of abdominal contents.

Exploratory laparotomy and lumpectomies are performed based on standard small animal surgical technique. However, if the muscles of rolling are involved in the incisional closure, they should be closed in a separate layer with an appropriate suture pattern and orientation for muscle. Strong contractions of these muscles may make this area prone to dehiscence.[7] Muscle relaxants and sedatives could be considered as an adjunct to wound or incisional healing in this area.

Wound Care

Treatment of epidermal wounds in the hedgehog may be necessary due to male-male intraspecific interaction, interspecific altercations, constriction of limbs with encircling fibers, overgrown nails, abscesses, and neoplasia.[4,18] Although general wound care in hedgehogs is guided by principles used in companion mammals, hedgehog behavior mandates some modifications. Hedgehogs often resort to self-mutilation, and as Elizabethan collars are not an option in this species, timely wound closure should be the primary concern, with subcuticular sutures recommended.[18] Hedgehogs tolerate bandaging and splinting although anesthesia will likely be required to apply and change bandages.[4] Animals may also be dipped in topical disinfectants as an adjunct for wound care.[4]

■ ZOONOSES

A variety of zoonotic diseases have been reported in African hedgehogs (Table 16-8). Etiologic agents include bacteria, fungi, viruses, and allergens. Zoonotic diseases commonly reported in hedgehogs, transmission routes, clinical signs of the zoonotic pathogen in hedgehogs and in people, diagnostic recommendations, as well as recommendations for control and eradication of the etiologic agent, will be reviewed in this section. Treatments for hedgehogs with these diseases, where applicable, is discussed under Common Disease Presentations.

Salmonella spp. is the primary zoonotic disease of concern in African pygmy hedgehogs.[12] Affected hedgehogs can present with anorexia, diarrhea, and weight loss, or may be asymptomatic carriers of the pathogen. African hedgehogs can transmit *Salmonella* serotype Tilene, a serotype rarely encountered in humans. Direct contact with hedgehogs is not necessary to contract the organism. Most cases have been reported in children, and many cases have been associated with hedgehog breeding herds. Other bacteria, such as *S.* Typhimurium, *S.* Enteritidis, *Yersinia pseudotuberculosis, Y. pestis, Mycobacterium marinum,* and *M. avium intracellulare,* have also been reported in other hedgehog species.[12,48] Antibodies to *Coxiella burnetii* (Q-fever), *Chlamydophila* spp. (ornithosis), *Toxoplasma gondii* (toxoplasmosis), and *Leptospira* spp. (leptospirosis) have also been isolated in other hedgehog species.[12,29] Until proven otherwise, African hedgehogs should be considered susceptible to these diseases. In the case of bacterial agents, a client can reduce the risk of infection by avoiding direct contact with feces and by washing their hands after handling pets and before handling food. Similarly, hedgehogs should be kept in a clean, sanitary environment, and ill hedgehogs should be separated and receive veterinary attention in a timely manner.

African pygmy hedgehogs can be subclinical carriers of *Trichophyton mentagrophytes* var. *erinacei, Microsporum* spp., and *Arthroderma benhamiae*, and are therefore zoonotic transmitters of these fungi.[12,46] In the hedgehog, lesions are similar to that of other species. Dry, scaly skin with loss of hair and spines is common. Transmission can occur after only a few minutes of contact. In humans, inflammatory and pruritic eruptions can be severe and commonly occur on the wrist and hands as areas of contact with the hedgehog, although lesions of the legs and abdomen have also been reported. The lesions may resolve spontaneously 2 to 3 weeks after onset, but topical or systemic treatment of the affected human may be necessary.

Two case reports of candidal infection of the footpads and intestine, respectively, of the African Pygmy hedgehog have been reported.[49,50] No human cases of candidiasis associated with hedgehogs have been reported. Therefore, the zoonotic potential of transmission of this organism is unknown but should be considered possible.

The African pygmy hedgehog appears susceptible to Crimean-Congo hemorrhagic fever, a zoonotic and often fatal disease of the Middle East, Eastern Europe, and Asia. This disease is generally contracted though contact with blood or tissues of infected animals or people or by tick bite. Although the African Pygmy hedgehog is susceptible to Crimean-Congo hemorrhagic fever, their role as an amplifying host in unknown.

TABLE 16-8	Zoonotic and Potentially Zoonotic Agents of the African Pygmy Hedgehog (*Atalerix albiventris*)			
	Bacterial	**Viral**	**Fungal**	**Protozoal**
Zoonotic agents of *Atalerix albiventris**	*Salmonella* Tilene	Human herpesvirus 1	*Trichophyton mentagrophytes* var. *erinacei* *Microsporum* spp.	–
Potential zoonotic agents of *Atalerix albiventris*†	*Yersinia pseudotuberculosis* *Mycobacterium marinum* *Chlamydophila psittaci* *Coxiella burnetii* *Yersinia pestis*	Tickborne encephalitis Crimean-Congo hemorrhagic fever Tahyna virus Bhanja virus Paramyxovirus Rabies virus	*Candida albicans*	*Cryptosporidium* spp. *Toxoplasma gondii*

*Agents found in *Atalerix albiventris* and cause of disease in humans or other species.
†Agents found in other hedgehog species or agents with zoonotic potential.

The closely related South African hedgehog *(Atalerix frontalis)* does not serve as an amplifying host. However, hedgehogs can act as a host to immature stages of the tick species that harbor the virus. Many other types of viruses, including arboviral tick-borne encephalitides and paramyxoviruses of the Morbillivirus group, have been documented in other hedgehog species based on susceptibility, antibody titers, or viral isolation. Rabies has also been documented in a hedgehog in Budapest. Prudence dictates that the African pygmy hedgehog be considered susceptible and a possible carrier of these viruses.

Herpesvirus infection has been documented in the African pygmy hedgehog.[44] The affected animal developed acute posterior paresis; it improved with steroid administration but developed anorexia and died 2 weeks later.[44] Human herpes virus 1 was isolated from the animal's diseased liver. Although no definitive link was established, the hedgehog owner reported that several family members suffered periodically from "cold sores," and this was postulated to be the source of infection for the hedgehog. Whether the hedgehog should be considered a dead end host or a possible carrier of this virus remains unknown.

Although not a direct health threat to humans, both African and European hedgehog species are susceptible to foot-and-mouth disease virus.[12] Hedgehogs may play a role in local spread of this disease, as the full cycle may occur between hedgehog and infected cattle in both African and European species.[62,63] Affected hedgehogs develop typical vesicular lesions on the tongue, snout, and feet.[12]

Acute intestinal cryptosporidiosis of unknown species caused death in a juvenile African pygmy hedgehog (Table 16-8).[44] Large numbers of the organisms in various development stages were found in the lower jejunum. The affected hedgehog was a 1-month-old male that had shown no clinical signs before being found dead. As a waterborne organism, this organism is a health threat to immunocompromised individuals.

REFERENCES

1. Symonds MR: Phylogeny and life histories of the *"Insectivora"*: controversies and consequences, *Biol Rev* 80:93-128, 2005.
2. Wroot A: Hedgehogs. In Macdonald D, editor: *The Encyclopedia of Mammals,* New York, 1984, Facts on File.
3. Grzimek B: Hedgehogs (Family *Erinaceidae*), *Grzimek's Encyclopedia of Mammals,* New York, 1989, McGraw-Hill.
4. Smith AJ: Husbandry and medicine of African hedgehogs, *J Small Exot Anim Med* 2(1):21-28, 1992.
5. Mori M, O'Brien SE: Husbandry and medical management of African hedgehogs, *Iowa State Univ Vet* Spring:64-72, 1997.
6. Nowak R: African hedgehogs. In Nowak R, editor: *Walker's Mammals of the World,* ed 6, Baltimore, 1999, Johns Hopkins University Press.
7. Isenbugel E, Baumgartner R: Diseases of the hedgehog. In Fowler ME, editor: *Zoo and Wild Animal Medicine: Current Therapy,* ed 3, Denver, 1993, WB Saunders.
8. Barbiers R: *Insectivora* (hedgehogs, tenrecs, shrews, moles) and *Dermoptera* (flying lemurs). In Fowler ME, Miller RE, editors: *Zoo and Wild Animal Medicine,* St Louis, 2003, WB Saunders.
9. Lewis C, Cusdin P, Norcott M et al: Normal haematological values of European hedgehogs *(Erinaceus europaeus)* from an English rehabilitation centre, *Vet Rec* 151(19):567-569, 2002.
10. Stocker L: Hedgehogs. In Stocker L, editor: *Practical Wildlife Care,* Oxford, 2000, Blackwell Science.
11. Keymer I, Gibson E, Reynolds D: Zoonoses and other hedgehogs *(Erinaceus europaeus):* a survey of mortality and review of literature, *Vet Rec* 28:245-249, 1991.
12. Riley PY, Chomel BB: Hedgehog zoonoses, *Emerg Infect Dis* 11(1):1-5, 2005.
13. Rondinini C: Hedgehogs and moonrats. In MacDonald D, editor: *The Encyclopedia of Mammals,* New York, 2001, Facts on File.
14. Gregory M: Observations on vocalization in the central African hedgehog, *Erinaceous albiventris,* including a courtship call, *Mammalia* 39:1-7, 1975.
15. Smith AJ: Husbandry and nutrition of hedgehogs, *Vet Clin North Am Exot Anim Pract* 2(1):127-141, 1999.
16. Ivey E, Carpenter JW: African hedgehogs. In Quesenberry KE, Carpenter JW, editors: *Ferrets, Rabbits and Rodents: Clinical Medicine and Surgery,* St Louis, 2004.
17. Elliot MW, Dunstan RW, Slocombe RF: A comparative study of the morphologic features of the porcupine, hedgehog, and *echidna* quills and quill follicles, *Annual Members Meeting, AAVD and ACVD,* Las Vegas, Nev, 1996.
18. Hernandez-Divers SM: Principles of wound management of small mammals: hedgehogs, prairie dogs, and sugar gliders, *Vet Clin North Am* 7:1-18, 2004.

19. Wroot A: Hedgehogs and moonrats: spines and curling in hedgehogs. In MacDonald D, editor: *The Encyclopedia of Mammals,* New York, 2001, *Facts on File.*

20. Bedford J, Mock O, Nagdas S et al: Reproductive characteristics of the African pygmy hedgehog *Atalerix albiventris, J Reprod Fertil* 120:143-150, 2000.

21. Smith AJ: Neonatology of the hedgehog *(Atalerix albiventris), J Small Exot Anim Med* 3(1):15-18, 1995.

22. Larson RS, Carpenter JW: Husbandry and medical management of African hedgehogs, *Vet Med* Oct:877-890, 1999.

23. Carpenter JW: Hedgehogs. In Carpenter JW, editor: *Exotic Animal Formulary,* ed 3, St Louis, 2005, WB Saunders.

24. Corbett G: The family *Erinaceidae:* a synthesis of its taxonomy, phylogeny, ecology, and zoogeography, *Mamm Rev* 18:117-172, 1988.

25. Crossley DA: Small mammal dentistry, part I: dental anatomy and dental disease. In Quesenberry KE, Carpenter JW, editors: *Ferrets, Rabbits and Rodents: Clinical Medicine and Surgery,* ed 2, St Louis, 2004, WB Saunders.

26. Hoefer HL: Hedgehogs, *Vet Clin North Am Small Anim Pract* 24(1):103-111, 1994.

27. Graffam WS, Fitzpatrick MP, Dierenfeld ES: Fiber digestion in the African white-bellied hedgehog *(Atalerix albiventris):* a preliminary evaluation, *J Nutr,* 128(12 suppl):2671-2673, 1998.

28. Simone-Freilicher EA, Hoefer HL: Hedgehog care and husbandry, *Vet Clin North Am Exot Anim Pract* 7:257-267, 2004.

29. Sebek Z, Sixl W, Reinthaler F et al: Results of serological examination for leptospirosis of domestic and wild animals in the Upper Nile province (Sudan), *J Hyg Epidemiol Microbiol Immunol* 5:161-178, 1989.

30. Lightfoot TL: Clinical techniques of selected exotic species: chinchilla, prairie dog, hedgehog, and chelonians, *Semin Av Exot Pet Med* 6(2):96-105, 1997.

31. Mikaelian I, Reavill D: Spontaneous proliferative lesions and tumors of the uterus of captive African hedgehogs *(Atalerix albiventris), J Zoo Wildl Med* 35(2):216-220, 2004.

32. Clarke DE: Oral biology and disorders of chiroptera, insectivores, monotremes, and marsupials, *Vet Clin North Am* 6:523-564, 2003.

33. Lightfoot TL, Bartlett L: *Exotic Companion Animal Surgeries,* Lake Worth, Fla, 1999, Zoological Education Network.

34. Heard DJ: Anesthesia, analgesia and sedation of small mammals. In Quesenberry KE, Carpenter JW, editors: *Ferrets, Rabbits and Rodents: Clinical Medicine and Surgery,* ed 2, St Louis, 2004, WB Saunders.

35. Lightfoot TL: Clinical examination of chinchillas, hedgehogs, prairie dogs, and sugar gliders, *Vet Clin North Am Exot Anim Pract* 2(2):447-469, 1999.

36. Lightfoot TL: Therapeutics of African pygmy hedgehogs and prairie dogs, *Vet Clin North Am Exot Anim Pract* 3(1):155-172, 2000.

37. Morrisey JK, Carpenter JW: Formulary. In Quesenberry KE, Carpenter JW, editors: *Ferrets, Rabbits and Rodents: Clinical Medicine and Surgery,* St Louis, 2004, WB Saunders.

38. Pye G: Marsupial, insectivore and chiropteran anesthesia, *Vet Clin North Am Exot Anim Pract* 4(1):211-238, 2001.

39. Association of Exotic Mammal Veterinarians: Guide to small mammal analgesics, *Exot Mamm Med Surg* 2(2):10-11, 2004.

40. Greenacre CB: Spontaneous tumors of small mammals, *Vet Clin North Am Exot Anim Pract* 7:627-651, 2004.

41. Raymond J, Williams C, Wu C: Corynebacterial pneumonia in an African hedgehog, *J Wildl Dis* 34:397-399, 1998.

42. Seattle-King County Dept. of Public Health: African pygmy hedgehog-associated salmonellosis, *Morbid Mortal Wkly Rep* 44(24):462-463, 1994.

43. Craig C, Styliadis S, Woodward D: African pygmy hedgehog-associated *Salmonella tilene* in Canada, *Can Commun Dis Rep* 23(17):129-132, 1997.

44. Allison N, Chang T, Steele K et al: Fatal herpes simplex infection in a pygmy African hedgehog *(Atalerix albiventris), J Comp Pathol* 126:76-78, 2002.

45. Peauroi J, Lowenstein L, Munn R et al: Multicentric skeletal sarcomas associated with probable retrovirus particles in two African hedgehogs *(Atalerix albiventris), Vet Pathol* 31:481-484, 1994.

46. Gregory M, English M: *Arthroderma benhamiae* infection in the Central African hedgehog *Erinaceus albiventris, Mycopathologia* 55(3):143-147, 1975.

47. Takahashi Y, Haritani K, Takizawa K et al: An isolate of *Arthroderma benhamiae* with *Trichophyton mentagrophytes* var *erinacei* anamorph isolated from a four-toed hedgehog *(Atalerix albiventris)* in Japan, *Nippon Ishinkin Gakkai Zasshi* 43(4):249-255, 2002.

48. Rosen T: Hazardous hedgehogs, *South Med J* 93:936-938, 2000.

49. English M, Gregory M, Spence J: Invasion by *Candida albican* of the footpads of the Central African hedgehog *(Erinaceus albiventris), Mycopathologia* 55(3):139-141, 1975.

50. Campbell T: Intestinal candidasis in an African hedgehog, *Exot Pet Pract* 2(79):79, 1997.

51. Gregory M: Mites of the hedgehog *Erinaceus albiventris* Wagner in Kenya: observations on the prevalence and pathogenicity of *Notoedres oudesmansi* Fain, *Caparinia erinacei* Fain and *Rodentopus sciuri* Fain, *Parasitol* 82(1):149-157, 1981.

52. deMaar TW, Kassell NL, Blumer ES: Chagas' disease in an African hedgehog, *AAZV,* Proceedings of the American Association of Zoo Veterinarians and American Association of Reptilian and Amphibian Veterinarians, Pittsburgh, PA. 1994.

53. Graczyk TK, Cranfield MR, Dunning C et al: Fatal cryptosporidiosis in a juvenile captive African hedgehog *(Atelerix albiventris), J Parasitol* 84(1):178-180, 1998.

54. Heatley J, Maulden G, Cho D: Neoplasia in the captive African hedgehog *(Atalerix albiventris), Semin Av Exot Pet Med* 14(3):182-192, 2005.

55. Raymond JT, Garner MM: Spontaneous tumors in hedgehogs: a retrospective study of fifty cases, *Joint Conf AAZV, AAWV, ARAV,* and *NAZWV,* Orlando, Fla, Sept 18-23, 2001.

56. Done L, Dietze M, Cranfield M et al: Necropsy lesions by body systems in African hedgehogs *(Atalerix albiventris):* clues to clinical diagnosis, *Annu Meeting AAZV,* Oakland, Calif, 1992.

57. Raymond J, Garner M: Cardiomyopathy in captive African hedgehogs, *J Vet Diagn Invest* 12(5):468-472, 2000.

58. Buergelt CD: Histopathologic findings in pet hedgehogs with nonneoplastic conditions, *Vet Med* 97:660-665, 2002.

59. Wheler CL, Grahn BH, Pocknell AM: Unilateral proptosis and orbital cellulitis in eight African hedgehogs *(Atalerix albiventris), J Zoo Wildl Med* 23(2):236-241, 2001.

60. Delaney CJ: Hedgehogs. In Delaney CJ, editor: *Exotic Companion Medicine Handbook,* Lake Worth, Fla, 1998, Zoological Education Network.

61. Ness RD: Rodents. In Carpenter JW, editor: *Exotic Animal Formulary,* ed 3, St Louis, 2005, WB Saunders.

62. McLauchlan J, Henderson W: The occurrence of foot and mouth disease in the hedgehog under natural conditions, *J Hyg* (Cambridge) 45:474-479, 1947.

63. MacCaulay J: Foot-and-mouth disease in non-domestic animals, *Bull Epizoot Dis Afr* 1(2):143-146, 1963.

Shannon M. Riggs

CHAPTER 17

GUINEA PIGS

■ COMMON SPECIES KEPT IN CAPTIVITY

Guinea pigs, *Cavia porcellus,* are members of the Caviidae family of the order Rodentia. Guinea pigs are native to mountainous regions of South America where they were domesticated as long as 3000 years ago. Wild species of guinea pigs, or *cavies,* still inhabit Columbia, Peru, Venezuela, Argentina, Brazil, and Paraguay. Domesticated cavies in these countries are used for food. In the wild, guinea pigs live in small groups and, therefore, are often more comfortable in the presence of other guinea pigs when maintained as companion animals.

Extensive breeding has resulted in numerous varieties of coat color and characteristics. The most common breeds are the American (or English) which has a short, smooth coat and the multicolored Teddy (Figure 17-1); Abyssinian (Figure 17-2), which has a medium length coat in a whorled pattern; and the Peruvian, which has a very long, smooth coat.

■ BIOLOGY

Guinea pigs have wide bodies with short limbs. A distinctive anatomic characteristic of species in the family Caviidae is the number of digits on the front and rear feet (4 digits front feet and 3 digits rear). Tails are usually very short or absent. The guinea pig has a short, flat nose, laterally placed eyes, and hairless external pinnae. Adult guinea pigs usually weigh between 700 and 1200 g, with the males being slightly larger than females. The average life span of the companion guinea pig is approximately 5 to 7 years.

The dentition of the guinea pig is described as aradicular hypsodont (e.g., all teeth have a relatively long crown and are "open rooted").[1] The maxilla is slightly wider than the mandi-

ble, and the occlusal angle of the premolars and molars is marked compared to other rodent species. The dental formula of the guinea pig is 2(I 1/1, C 0/0, PM 1/1, M 3/3) = 20. The maxillary incisors are much shorter than those set in the mandible. The molars and premolars are not easily visualized without special instrumentation because of the small size of the oral cavity and tendency for the involution of the buccal surface.

Females are sexually mature at 6 weeks of age, whereas males on average reach puberty approximately 4 weeks later. Gestation is long, when compared to other rodents, at 68 days.[2] As a result of this long gestation period, young are precocial when born. Juvenile pigs usually eat solid foods by 4 or 5 days of age.[3] Litter sizes range from 1 to 6, with an average of 3 to 4 young.[2] A female guinea pig should deliver her first young before she is 6 months of age. If birth has not occurred before 6 months of age, the pubic symphysis becomes mineralized, with future pregnancies resulting in an inability of the sow to naturally deliver the babies. Female guinea pigs that become pregnant after 6 months of age invariably require cesarean section deliveries.

■ HUSBANDRY
Housing

Guinea pigs are best housed in well-ventilated, wire-sided cages with solid bottoms. Wire-bottom cages may also be used; however, care must be taken to ensure that the mesh is small enough that a limb cannot become entrapped. An area of solid flooring should be provided, as uninterrupted time on wire mesh may predispose the guinea pig to pododermatitis. Adequate space is needed in the enclosure for the guinea pig to

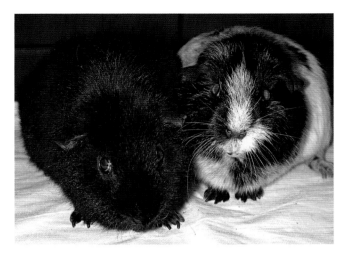

Figure 17-1 Two common guinea pig breeds: Teddy *(left)* and American *(right).*

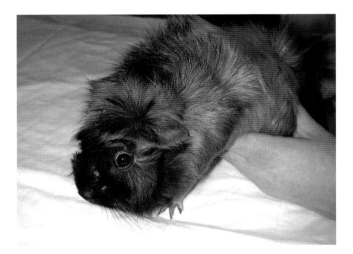

Figure 17-2 Abyssinian guinea pig.

move about unencumbered with enough space for a hide box. Hide boxes or a secluded space is required for prey species (e.g., rodents) to reduce stress that may lead to disease problems. Substrate products that contain aromatic oils (e.g., cedar and pine shavings) should not be used, as they can act as contact and respiratory irritants. Appropriate bedding materials include recycled newspaper products, shredded paper, and aspen shavings. The enclosure should be cleaned thoroughly on a regular basis (e.g., 2 times per week) because unsanitary conditions predispose the guinea pig to pododermatitis, respiratory, and other health problems. If housed indoors, guinea pig enclosures do not require a cover, as these animals do not typically jump or climb. However, the sides of the enclosure should be high enough to prevent escape (approximately 25 cm).[2] Heavy food containers are recommended to make dumping of the receptacle more difficult. All food containers should be easy to

disinfect and cleaned regularly, as guinea pigs have a habit of soiling their food bowls. Most guinea pigs readily accept drinking water from a sipper bottle, which will decrease spillage and will keep feces, urine, and bedding from contaminating the water.

These animals, native to the Andes Mountains, are very susceptible to hyperthermia and should never be housed in temperatures greater than 80° F. High humidity can also exacerbate a guinea pig's sensitivity to elevated temperatures by increasing the heat index. All animals are very sensitive to environmental and/or nutritional changes. Therefore, if changes have to be made, gradual exposure of the animal to the changes is recommended.

Diet

An appropriate guinea pig diet includes a formulated, pelleted diet for that species, high-quality hay (e.g., timothy, orchard grass, oat) ad libitum, and ample fresh vegetables. As the animal's food intake is more dependent on volume consumed rather than calories consumed, a pet fed a predominantly pelleted diet (higher nutritional concentration) has a tendency to become obese. Fruits and grains, if they are offered at all, should comprise a very small portion (<10%) of the total diet and offered only as treats.

Because guinea pigs lack the enzyme L-gulonolactone oxidase, they are unable to synthesize ascorbic acid from glucose. Therefore, guinea pigs require supplemental vitamin C in their diets. Although commercial guinea pig pellets are manufactured with vitamin C, the supplement often degrades rapidly, especially if the pellets are subjected to high heat and humidity. Vitamin C placed in drinking water also degrades rapidly and should be changed daily. To ensure that a guinea pig is receiving a proper amount of vitamin C, it is necessary to supplement a diet of pellets and hay with plenty of fresh foods or often a specifically manufactured vitamin C supplement tablet (Oxbow, Inc., Murdock, NE). Many green, leafy vegetables, such as kale, mustard greens, dandelion greens, parsley, and many others, are excellent sources of ascorbic acid (Box 17-1). The vitamin C requirement of an adult, nonbreeding guinea pig is 10 mg/kg/day.[2,3]

■ PREVENTIVE MEDICINE

In the United States, guinea pigs are not routinely vaccinated for infectious diseases. However, owners should be encouraged to have annual examinations that include an oral examination and a complete blood count. Being prey species in the wild, guinea pigs are adept at hiding illness, and routine evaluations by a qualified veterinarian may help in detecting abnormalities early.

Many health problems of guinea pigs are related to improper husbandry. During a routine veterinary visit, the owners should be asked to provide a detailed description of the animal's housing environment, including substrate, frequency of cleaning, ambient temperature, and exercise time. The diet history is also important. Owners should be asked not only

BOX 17-1	Vitamin C Content of Selected Fruits and Vegetables

Vegetables	mg vitamin C/100 g
Red bell pepper	190
Parsley	133
Kale	120
Broccoli	93.2
Brussels sprouts	85
Mustard greens	70
Turnip greens	60
Cauliflower	46.4
Dandelion greens	35
Cilantro	27
Romaine lettuce	24
Sweet potato	22.7
Carrot	9.3
Fruits	**mg vitamin C/100 g**
Kiwi	98
Strawberry	56.7
Orange	53.2
Cantaloupe	42.2
Apple	5.7

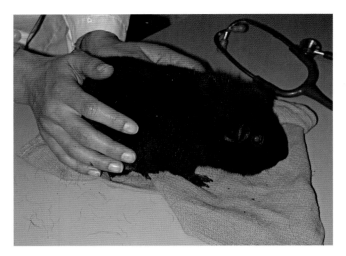

Figure 17-3 Restraint of a guinea pig patient for examination.

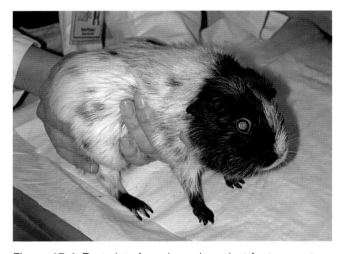

Figure 17-4 Restraint of a guinea pig patient for transport.

what the guinea pig is offered, but also in what proportions and of what foods the animal actually eats.

RESTRAINT

Most guinea pigs are quite docile and do not require aggressive restraint. Often a hand on the animal's dorsum is adequate to restrain a guinea pig patient on the examination table (Figure 17-3). When transporting a guinea pig, support the body with one hand under the thorax and abdomen while placing the other hand on the back to prevent the patient from falling or jumping (Figure 17-4).

If chemical restraint is required, gas anesthesia with isoflurane or sevoflurane is generally well tolerated. Anesthetic gases can be delivered via mask or induction chamber. Mild sedation can be achieved with an intramuscular injection of a combination of midazolam (0.2-0.5 mg/kg) and butorphanol (0.2-0.5 mg/kg) intramuscularly.

PERFORMING A PHYSICAL EXAMINATION

Guinea pigs often do not exhibit clinical signs early in a disease process. Therefore, a thorough physical examination can be extremely useful in determining the overall health status of the animal. Before beginning a physical examination, it is important to observe the animal before it has been stressed by restraint. A healthy guinea pig should be alert and aware of its

surroundings. As guinea pigs are often shy animals, they may attempt to hide or escape. The examiner should use a thorough, systematic approach to focus on the respiratory character and rate, posture, and attitude of the animal. It is also important to have any instruments (e.g., transilluminator, stethoscope, thermometer, blood-collecting supplies) that may be necessary to decrease the amount of handling time for the patient.

Obtaining an accurate body temperature, heart rate, and respiratory rate is best accomplished at the beginning of the examination, as these parameters will invariably change with handling. An accurate weight should be obtained using an electronic gram scale. A "hands-on" physical examination should begin with the head; the veterinarian should assess the eyes for symmetry or discharge and check that the external pinnae of the guinea pig are hairless, as normal. The external ear canals often contain a small to moderate amount of dark,

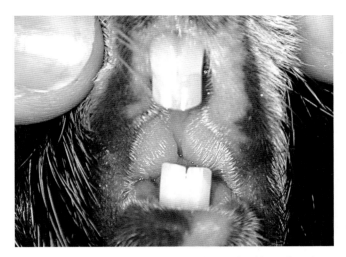

Figure 17-5 The oral cavity of a guinea pig. Note the abundance of soft tissue that obscures visualization of the molars and premolars.

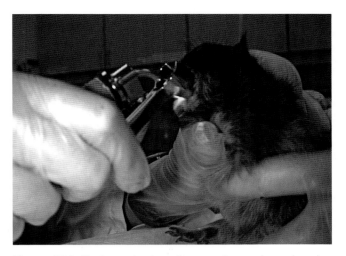

Figure 17-6 Oral examination of a conscious guinea pig using a human nasal speculum on a transilluminator base.

ceruminous debris. The nasal planum should be dry and flat, whereas palpation of the ventral mandible may reveal deformities secondary to overgrowth of molar and premolar apices.

The guinea pig coat varies somewhat with breed but, in general, should be smooth and shiny. Guinea pigs often have a mild to moderate amount of dark sebaceous debris on the skin of the dorsum. Older male guinea pigs may develop a focal accumulation of this debris at the base of the vertebral column, which may be referred to as the "grease gland."[4]

Thoracic auscultation and abdominal palpation can be performed as in other patients. Heart and respiratory rates will vary depending on the degree of stress a patient experiences. As pulse and respiratory rates can be very rapid, careful auscultation is necessary to detect subtle abnormalities (e.g., murmurs, crackles, wheezes). Auscultation of gut sounds is also an important part of the guinea pig physical exam. A healthy guinea pig should have 1 to 2 borborygmi per minute. The practitioner should keep in mind that stress will decrease gastrointestinal (GI) motility; therefore, a stressed animal will often have a decrease in borborygmi. Structures normally found on abdominal palpation include kidneys, urinary bladder, cecum, and intestines. Fecal pellets are often palpable in the colon. Careful examination may reveal the presence of abnormalities such as GI distention, masses, or, in females, ovarian cysts. Limbs and joints should be carefully evaluated because thickened or painful joints may be indicative of a vitamin C deficiency.

A complete oral examination is an important part of the guinea pig exam. Because of the potential stress associated with the oral exam, this evaluation should be reserved for the end. The oral cavity of the guinea pig is very narrow with a small opening, making visualization difficult (Figure 17-5). Instruments such as an otoscope with cone or a human nasal speculum will increase visualization of the caudal oral cavity (Figure 17-6). However, many dental lesions may be overlooked using these methods, and anesthesia is often required to adequately determine oral health.

DIAGNOSTIC TESTING

Venipuncture

Obtaining blood samples from guinea pigs for routine diagnostics is a challenging procedure. Peripheral venipuncture sites available for most mammals (e.g., lateral saphenous vein and cephalic vein) are difficult to visualize in guinea pigs and only allow for the collection of small sample volumes. The jugular vein may be used; however, the short neck of the guinea pig and poor tolerance of the aggressive restraint by the patient restrict the availability of this site for blood collection. Often to obtain an adequate blood sample, it is necessary to anesthetize the patient. Once anesthetized, the large central vessels may be accessed with less stress on the patient and phlebotomist. Acceptable venipuncture sites while the patient is anesthetized include the cranial vena cava (Figure 17-7), femoral vein (Figure 17-8), and jugular vein.

Hematology

Baseline blood work is an important tool in the routine monitoring of health as well as in the diagnosis of disease. A complete blood count is essential for assessing red blood cell and white blood cell parameters (Box 17-2).

Guinea pigs have heterophils rather than neutrophils as the predominant circulating granulocyte. Heterophils lack myeloperoxidase, the enzyme that causes purulent, liquid exudates. Therefore, the debris contained in guinea pig abscesses is often found to be very thick and caseous, a fact that must be understood when treating these conditions. A normal guinea pig white blood cell differential will consist of primarily heterophils and lymphocytes, usually with a greater proportion of lymphocytes. The remaining leukocyte types (e.g., monocytes, eosinophils, basophils) are normally present in very low numbers. Early stages of a guinea pig's inflammatory response are often characterized by a shift in the differential white cell ratio (e.g., increased heterophils, decreased lymphocytes) rather

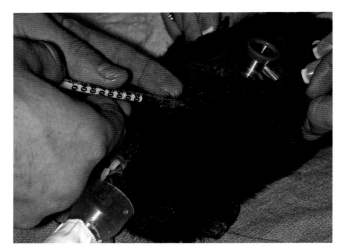

Figure 17-7 Blood collection via the cranial vena cava in an anesthetized guinea pig.

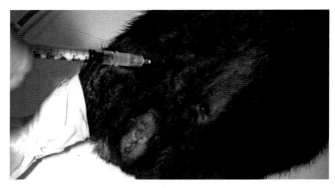

Figure 17-8 Blood collection via the femoral vein in an anesthetized guinea pig.

than an increase in total leukocyte count. This ratio shift makes evaluating the entire leukogram essential for health evaluation (Box 17-3). The platelet count is also an important marker of inflammation in guinea pigs and other small mammal species. Large increases in the platelet count (>1,000,000/μl) can be seen without an increase in the total white blood cell count.

A cell type that is unique to guinea pigs is the Kurloff cell. These large lymphocytes contain a cytoplasmic inclusion (e.g., a Kurloff body). Kurloff cells are noted most often in the peripheral blood of reproductive age females, although they are also identified in male guinea pigs. The number of circulating Kurloff cells will increase in response to exogenous estradiol and testosterone administration, although the effects were more dramatic with estradiol administration.[7,8] Other studies have shown the disappearance of Kurloff cells in spayed female and castrated male guinea pigs.[8] The function of the Kurloff cell is not completely understood, and these cells appear to lack lysosomes. At this time, there is no evidence that the Kurloff cell has phagocytic activity.[8] The activity of Kurloff cells appears to most closely correlate with that of natural killer cells found in other species.[7]

BOX 17-2 **Hematologic Parameters for Guinea Pigs**

Hematologic Parameter	Reference Interval
PCV (%)	30-50
RBC ($\times 10^6$ cells/μl)	4-11
Hb (g/dl)	11-17
MCV (fl)	70-95
MCHC (%)	25-40
MCH (pg)	23-27
WBC ($\times 10^3$ cells/μl)	6-17
Heterophils (%)	20-60
Lymphocytes (%)	30-80
Monocytes (%)	1-10
Eosinophils (%)	0-7
Basophils (%)	0-3
Platelets ($\times 10^3$ cells/μl)	300-600

Data from Quesenberry KE, Donnelly TM, Hillyer EV: Biology, husbandry, and clinical techniques. In Quesenberry KE, Carpenter JW, editors: *Ferrets, Rabbits, and Rodents: Clinical Medicine and Surgery*, ed 2, St Louis, 2003, WB Saunders; Carpenter JW: Hematologic and serum biochemical values of rodents. In Carpenter JW, editor: *Exotic Animal Formulary*, ed 3, St Louis, 2005, WB Saunders; Campbell TW: Mammalian hematology: laboratory animals and miscellaneous species. In Thrall MA, editor: *Veterinary Hematology and Clinical Chemistry*, Baltimore, 2004, Lippincott Williams and Wilkins.
Hb, hemoglobin; MCH, mean corpuscular hemoglobin; MCHV, mean corpuscular hemoglobin concentration; MCV, mean corpuscular volume; PCV, packed cell volume; RBC, red blood cell count; WBC, white blood cell count.

BOX 17-3 **Example of an Inflammatory Leukogram in a Guinea Pig**

Hematologic Parameter	Value
HCT (%)	43
WBC ($\times 10^3$ cells/μl)	13.1
Heterophils ($\times 10^3$ cells/μl/%)	7.8/59.3
Lymphocytes ($\times 10^3$ cells/μl/%)	3.4/25.9
Monocytes ($\times 10^3$ cells/μl/%)	1.2/8.8
Eosinophils ($\times 10^3$ cells/μl/%)	0.7/5.4
Basophils ($\times 10^3$ cells/μl/%)	0.09/0.7
Platelets ($\times 10^3$ cells/μl)	694

Clinical Chemistries

Plasma biochemical analysis is necessary for evaluation of organ function as well as plasma glucose and proteins. It is important to interpret the results of a chemistry panel in conjunction with history, physical exam findings, and the results of other diagnostic tests. Reference intervals for biochemical parameters are shown in Box 17-4.

Urinalysis

Urinalysis is a useful diagnostic test in guinea pigs with signs of upper or lower urinary tract disease. Urine samples may be

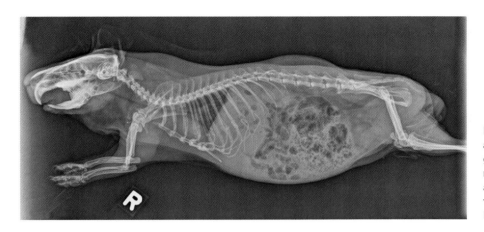

Figure 17-9 Right lateral radiograph of a guinea pig. Note the moderate overgrowth of the apices of the mandibular molars and premolars, remodeling of ribs, and large amount of ingesta within the GI tract. (Courtesy University of California–Davis.)

BOX 17-4	**Plasma Biochemical Parameters for Guinea Pigs**

Biochemical Parameter	Reference Interval
Sodium (mEq/L)	120-150
Potassium (mEq/L)	4-8
Chloride (mEq/L)	90-115
Glucose (mg/dl)	60-125
Blood urea nitrogen (mg/dl)	9-32
Creatinine (mg/dl)	0.6-2.2
Calcium (mg/dl)	8-12
Phosphorous (mg/dl)	3-8
Total protein (g/dl)	4-7
Albumin (g/dl)	2-5
Globulin (g/dl)	2-4
Creatine kinase (IU/L)	0-300
Aspartate transferase (IU/L)	30-70
Alkaline phosphatase (IU/L)	60-110
Bilirubin (mg/dl)	0-1
Cholesterol (mg/dl)	20-50

Data from Quesenberry KE, Donnelly TM, Hillyer EV: Biology, husbandry, and clinical techniques. In Quesenberry KE, Carpenter JW, editors: *Ferrets, Rabbits, and Rodents: Clinical Medicine and Surgery,* ed 2, St Louis, 2003, WB Saunders; Carpenter JW: Hematologic and serum biochemical values of rodents. In Carpenter JW, editor: *Exotic Animal Formulary,* ed 3, St Louis, 2005, WB Saunders; Campbell TW: Mammalian hematology: laboratory animals and miscellaneous species. In Thrall MA, editor: *Veterinary Hematology and Clinical Chemistry,* Baltimore, 2004, Lippincott Williams and Wilkins.

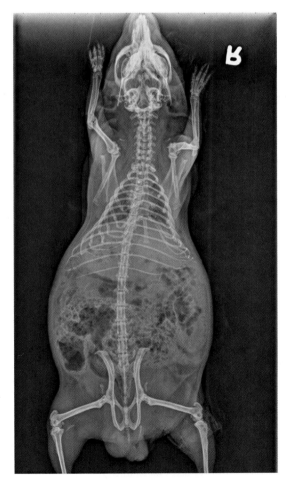

Figure 17-10 Ventrodorsal radiograph of the same guinea pig pictured in Figure 17-9. (Courtesy University of California–Davis.)

obtained by free catch, floor catch, or cystocentesis. If urine is to be cultured, it is ideal to use the cystocentesis method of collection. Ultrasound guidance and/or mild sedation of the patient will aid the veterinarian and/or veterinary technician in obtaining the urine sample.

The urine of guinea pigs is typically yellow to amber in color, but it may be darker and more orange depending on the patient's diet. Pigments in the urine can sometimes be mistaken for hematuria, so differentiation is important. Because guinea pigs are herbivores, the pH of guinea pig urine is alkaline, usually 8.0 to 9.0. Crystalluria may be seen but is not a normal finding. If crystals are found in a urine sample, the guinea pig patient should be examined for urinary calculi.

Imaging

Whole body radiographs may provide a large amount of information for the veterinarian treating an ill patient. Both lateral and ventrodorsal (or dorsoventral) views should be obtained (Figures 17-9 and 17-10). To minimize rotation, care should

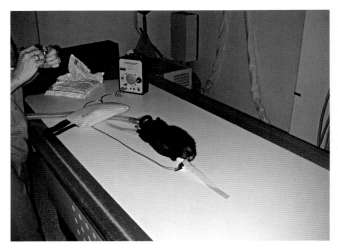

Figure 17-11 Positioning of an anesthetized guinea pig patient for a right lateral radiograph.

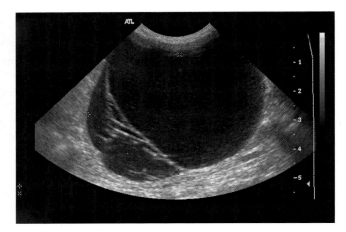

Figure 17-12 Ultrasound image of a large ovarian cyst in a mature female guinea pig. (Courtesy University of California–Davis.)

TABLE 17-1	Guidelines for Radiographic Techniques for Selected Radiographic Studies in Guinea Pigs	
Anatomic location	mA	kVp
Whole body	5.0	44
Extremities	7.5	54
Skull	6.0	48-53

From Silverman S, Tell LA: Radiology equipment and positioning techniques. In Silverman S, Tell LA, editors: *Radiology of Rodents, Rabbits, and Ferrets: An Atlas of Normal Anatomy and Positioning*, St Louis, 2006, WB Saunders. *kVp*, kilovolt peak; *mA*, milliampere.

be taken to extend the limbs symmetrically when positioning the patient. Because guinea pigs have stocky builds with short limbs, and because they resent aggressive restraint, sedation or anesthesia is helpful in obtaining diagnostic radiographs as well as in reducing the patient's stress (Figure 17-11). Table 17-1 is a guideline for radiographic techniques used in common small mammal radiographic studies.

Dental malocclusion is a common disease problem in guinea pigs. Radiographs of the skull are helpful in assessing the degree of malocclusion as well as potential bone involvement. In addition to lateral and dorsoventral views of the skull, right and lateral oblique views can help to localize lesions. Magnified views of the skull can be obtained by placing the patient on an elevated platform under the x-ray beam without changing the distance between the x-ray cassette and beam.

Ultrasound is another imaging modality that is very useful in the diagnosis of common guinea pig disease processes, such as ovarian cysts (Figure 17-12) and urinary tract calculi. As with radiographs, sedation or anesthesia can assist in reducing patient stress and improve the quality of images. Guinea pigs

often have a large amount of gas accumulation in the GI tract, which obscures the ultrasound image, sometimes making this imaging technique of limited value.

Advanced imaging techniques, such as computed tomography (CT) and magnetic resonance imaging (MRI), are useful tools in the diagnosis of disease in guinea pig patients. Limitations of these modalities include limited availability, expense, and decreased image quality compared with that of larger patients. MRI has the added limitation of requiring a significant amount of time (often >45 min) under anesthesia with limited monitoring ability.

Regardless of the present limitations, veterinarians should be aware that these techniques are available and that reference material exists that depicts normal anatomy.[9] As guinea pig owners continue to demand high-quality care for their pets, these imaging techniques will likely become more commonplace in small mammal practice for these patients.

Microbiology

Microbiologic samples can be obtained for diagnosis of various guinea pig infections. Exudates from nasal or ocular secretions can be examined for abnormal flora. Some bacterial organisms (e.g., *Bordetella bronchiseptica*) are difficult to culture. Laboratories need to be advised as to the organisms in question so they can perform more specific diagnostic tests to obtain organism identification.

Abscesses are another disease condition that may require culture for proper treatment. Because guinea pigs form caseous abscesses, the purulent debris itself is typically not useful for bacterial isolation. For the best chance of identifying organisms within an abscess, a portion of the abscess capsule should be submitted to the laboratory. Both aerobic and anaerobic bacterial cultures should be requested, especially if it is suspected that the abscess may have originated from a dental problem.

Parasitology

Roundworms and coccidia are seen in guinea pigs and can be identified by fecal flotation or fecal direct smear, as in other species. Cryptosporidiosis has also been reported.[10] Identification of *Cryptosporidium* organisms usually requires acid-fast staining or immunofluorescent antibody testing in addition to fecal flotation.

Ectoparasites (e.g., mites, lice, fleas) commonly infest guinea pigs. Visualization of the parasites and/or their waste, as well as skin scrapings, microscopic examination of hair follicles, and tape preparations can be useful in the identification of these parasites.

■ COMMON DISEASE PRESENTATIONS

Gastrointestinal

ENTEROTOXEMIA

The term *enterotoxemia* refers to the overgrowth of toxin-producing bacteria in the GI tract, particularly *Clostridium difficile*. This can occur with stress, an abrupt change in diet, GI stasis, or inappropriate antibiotic administration. The GI flora of guinea pigs is predominantly Gram positive, and administration of antibiotics with a primarily Gram-positive spectrum (e.g., beta-lactam antibiotics, macrolides, lincosamides) can lead to the depletion of normal gut flora, allowing colonization by opportunistic bacteria (e.g., Gram-negative organisms, *Clostridium* spp.).

DENTAL DISEASE

The dentition of the guinea pig is described as *aradicular hypsodont,* meaning all teeth grow throughout the animal's life and are open-rooted.[1] The dental formula of the guinea pig is I 1/1, C 0/0, P 1/1, M 3/3. The mandible of these animals is wider than the maxilla. The occlusal angle of the molars and premolars in the guinea pig is quite severe when compared with that of rabbits and other rodents (Figure 17-13). Guinea pigs lack the layer of yellow enamel present on the rostral surface of the incisors in most other rodents.

Dental malocclusion is a common disease process in guinea pigs. The development of malocclusion can be the result of multiple etiologies or a combination of factors (e.g., improper diet, genetics, trauma). Incisor malocclusion alone is rare in guinea pigs, so a thorough oral examination is necessary to determine the presence of cheek teeth malocclusion. When the molars and premolars do not occlude properly, overgrowth of the crowns and reserve crowns takes place. With improper wear, sharp points can form on the buccal aspects of the maxillary cheek teeth and the lingual aspects of the mandibular cheek teeth. The mandibular cheek teeth can overgrow to such an extent that they entrap the tongue, making eating and drinking difficult (Figure 17-14).

Clinical signs can include inappetence or dysphagia, decreased fecal output, ptyalism, poor coat quality, and leth-

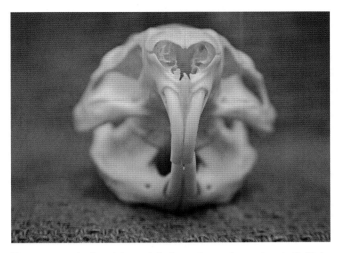

Figure 17-13 Cranial-caudal view of a guinea pig skull. Note the lack of yellow enamel on the cranial surface of the incisors and the severe occlusal angle of the premolars and molars.

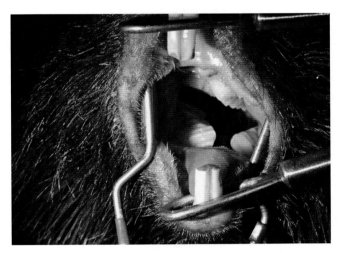

Figure 17-14 Guinea pig with malocclusion. Note the severe overgrowth of the mandibular premolars and molars, causing entrapment of the tongue. (Courtesy Michelle G. Hawkins, VMD, DABVP [Avian].)

argy. Abscesses commonly occur at the apical aspects of overgrown molars and premolars. Because the premolars and molars are elodont (open-rooted), it is possible that these teeth can overgrow and impinge on the nasolacrimal duct, causing ocular and nasal discharge. The reserve crowns can also overgrow into the nasal cavity, where oral bacteria may be seeded, causing rhinitis and sinusitis.

Diagnosis of dental disease is based on physical and oral examination findings. Careful palpation of the ventral mandible and maxilla may reveal bony protuberances corresponding to overgrowth of the apical surfaces of the cheek teeth. Proper instrumentation is very important for adequate visualization of the oral cavity. Dental speculums and pouch dilators are invaluable aids in obtaining a good view of the molars and premolars (Figure 17-15). However, many abnormalities can

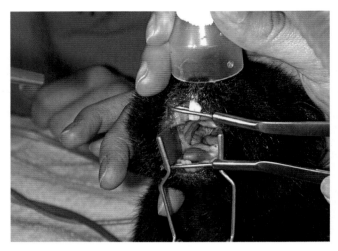

Figure 17-15 Oral examination of an anesthetized guinea pig aided by the use of incisor dilators and pouch dilators.

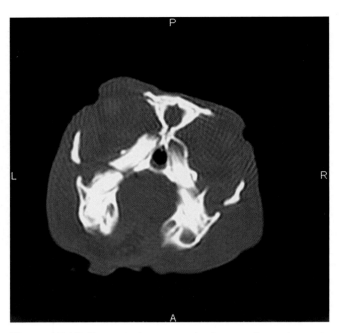

Figure 17-17 Computed tomography image of a guinea pig with mild to moderate malocclusion of the premolars and molars. (Courtesy University of California–Davis.)

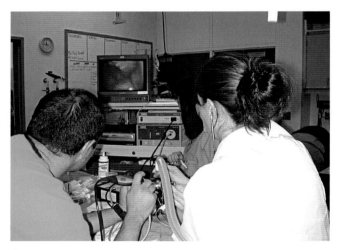

Figure 17-16 Examination of the oral cavity of an anesthetized guinea pig using a rigid endoscope.

be overlooked in a conscious animal, so anesthesia is often required to obtain a thorough oral examination. Visualization of the oral cavity and occlusal surfaces can be facilitated by the use of an endoscope (Figure 17-16). Most endoscopes available in veterinary practice have a degree of angulation of the field of view, allowing greater focal area. Abnormal oral examination findings may include an uneven occlusal surface or angle of the cheek teeth, formation of sharp points with or without associated ulceration of the oral mucosa, food impaction, and abnormal spaces (diastema) between teeth. Imaging, including routine radiographs, magnified skull radiographs, and computed tomography can be incorporated to better evaluate the extent and seriousness of the process (Figure 17-17). Radiographic studies should include dorsoventral, lateral, and right and left oblique views.

Treatment is centered on restoring a normal occlusal plane to the teeth, a procedure that should be performed while the

animal is under general anesthesia. Unstable animals should be provided with supportive care before the anesthetic event. A high-speed surgical dental handpiece can be used to restore a normal occlusal plane and to reduce any sharp points. Handheld trimmers are not acceptable, as they tend to crush teeth and can cause fractures and pulp exposure.[1] Dremel tools are also not considered acceptable because the small size of the guinea pig oral cavity will not allow for appropriate trimming. With any dental instruments, care should be observed to minimize oral soft tissue trauma.

When a guinea pig is diagnosed with dental malocclusion, it is important to convey to the owners that this will be a lifelong problem for their pets. With many cases, routine occlusal adjustments will be necessary for the remainder of the animal's life.

TYZZER'S DISEASE (C. PILIFORME)

Tyzzer's disease is the common term for bacterial enteritis caused by *Clostridium piliforme*. Infection with this organism is more commonly described in small rodents such as mice and hamsters, although it has also been described in guinea pigs as well as other mammalian groups.[11] Tyzzer's disease often presents acutely, with signs such as diarrhea, depression, and poor coat quality, often progressing rapidly to death. Transmission is via the fecal-oral route. Guinea pigs can be infected with *C. piliforme* without showing clinical signs. Animals that are carrying the organism but showing no signs of illness have still been found to shed organisms.[12] Animals that carry the organism and then become immunocompromised (e.g., stress, immunosuppressive drug therapy) often develop clinical disease.

Clostridium piliforme is an intracellular bacterium that will not grow on routine culture media, so antemortem diagnosis is difficult. Tyzzer's disease begins as an intestinal infection, but later spreads to the liver hematogenously, causing areas of necrosis.[11,13] Positive identification of the organism on necropsy requires examination of hematoxylin and eosin or silver staining of affected tissues.

Treatment should consist of fluid and nutritional support as well as appropriate antibiotic therapy. Unfortunately, the progression of the disease is rapid, making treatment unrewarding. Prevention is key, focusing on owners' reducing housing stress, providing a proper diet, and maintaining a clean environment.

CRYPTOSPORIDIOSIS

Cryptosporidiosis has been described as causing disease in guinea pigs in a laboratory setting.[10] Diagnosis was made histologically from affected animals that lost weight, had diarrhea, and suffered an acute death. *Cryptosporidium* organisms were found in the brush border of the intestinal tract from the duodenum to cecum, with associated inflammation.[10]

CORONAVIRUS

Suspected coronavirus infection has been described in young guinea pigs.[14] Clinical signs in affected animals included anorexia, weight loss, and diarrhea.[14] Approximately half of the affected animals in the reported outbreak recovered.[14] Necropsies performed on animals that died or were euthanized showed lesions consistent with coronavirus infection resulting from an acute to subacute necrotizing enteritis involving primarily the distal ileum.[14] Coronavirus-like virions were identified on transmission electron microscopy of feces collected from the lower GI tract at necropsy.[14]

SALMONELLOSIS

Outbreaks of salmonellosis have occurred in guinea pig colonies. Some of the organisms that have been isolated include *S. enteritidis*, *S. dublin*, *S. florida*, *S. poona*, and *S. bredeney*.[15,16] Salmonellosis has been described to affect guinea pigs in acute and chronic disease processes. With acute salmonellosis, guinea pigs often die after a brief illness characterized by nonspecific signs of illness and diarrhea.[15] Usually only a few pathogenic abnormalities are found at necropsy, and confirmation of a diagnosis is dependent on culture of affected tissues.

Chronic salmonellosis is a wasting disease, lasting several weeks. Splenomegaly, hepatomegaly, and mesenteric lymphadenopathy are common postmortem findings in affected animals.[15] Guinea pigs that recover can remain chronic, intermittent shedders of *Salmonella* organisms.

YERSINIA PSEUDOTUBERCULOSIS

Yersinia pseudotuberculosis causes several disease syndromes in guinea pigs.[15,17] The most common presentation affects the mesenteric and colonic lymph nodes, infiltrating these lymph nodes with caseous nodules. Clinically, affected guinea pigs will lose weight, have diarrhea, and develop a generalized lymphadenopathy. Transmission of the disease can be either vertical or horizontal.

Musculoskeletal
HYPOVITAMINOSIS C

As stated previously, guinea pigs require dietary supplementation of ascorbic acid because they lack the enzyme L-gulonolactone oxidase necessary for synthesis of this compound. Although diets formulated for guinea pigs are supplemented with ascorbic acid, it is important to remember that it breaks down very rapidly, usually within the first 90 days after production. If a guinea pig is not receiving vitamin C supplementation in its diet, the veterinarian can assume that the diet is deficient in this important nutrient.

Ascorbic acid is a necessary component of collagen, and deficiencies are often noted as manifestations of abnormal collagen synthesis.[13] Clinical signs of hypovitaminosis C can include lameness, hemorrhage, lethargy, anorexia, poor coat quality, and bruxism.

Diagnosis of hypovitaminosis C is based largely on clinical signs and history. Radiographs will reveal changes to the costochondral junctions and widening of the epiphyses of long bones. Recommended treatment includes fluids and nutritional support, pain control, and parenteral vitamin C supplementation. Attention should also be paid to improvement of the guinea pig's diet at home.

In addition to causing skeletal and cartilage abnormalities, vitamin C deficiency has been known to reduce immune function. In vitro, vitamin C deficiency was demonstrated to cause a reduction in migration of macrophages in guinea pigs.[18]

Urogenital
DYSTOCIA

Dystocia most frequently occurs in primiparous sows that are bred after approximately 6 months of age. At this time, the symphysis between the pubic bones becomes fused and will not expand to allow the passage of fetuses. Cesarean section must be performed in these cases to save the sow and the young. Factors other than age that can predispose a sow to dystocia include large fetuses in relation to sow size, uterine inertia, and obesity.[13]

URINARY CALCULI

Urolithiasis occurs commonly in pet guinea pigs, and the common clinical signs associated with the disease include stranguria and pollakiuria, vocalizing when urinating, and hematuria. The underlying cause(s) of this condition is not completely understood but is likely associated with a genetic predisposition and/or the presence of a high-calcium diet. Other less common underlying etiologies associated with urinary calculi formation include ureteral neoplasms (e.g., papilloma).[19] Calculi are primarily composed of calcium carbonate, although magnesium ammonium phosphate hexahydrate and calcium phosphate calculi will also occur.[20] Radiographic or ultrasonic imaging can be used to confirm the location of the urinary calculi, which may be present in the renal pelvis, ureters, urinary bladder, or urethra (Figure 17-18). Urinary tract calculi often require surgical removal. Ideally, once

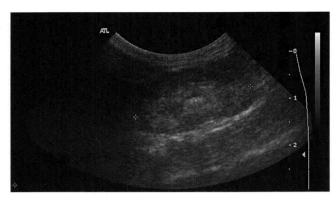

Figure 17-18 Ultrasound image of a calculus in the right renal pelvis of a guinea pig. (Courtesy University of California–Davis.)

removed, the calculus and/or a portion of the bladder wall should be cultured. It may also be helpful to analyze the composition of the stone to help determine ways of preventing recurrence.

OVARIAN CYSTS

Ovarian cysts are a common finding in middle-aged to older female guinea pigs. This disorder has a reported prevalence of 76% in female guinea pigs aged 1.5 to 5 years.[13,21] Multiple cysts can be present on one or both ovaries. Clinical signs related to cystic ovaries can include abdominal distention, lethargy, and anorexia related to the space-occupying nature of the cysts. Ovarian cysts that are actively producing hormones can produce bilaterally symmetrical alopecia of the flanks.

Ovarian cysts can be quite large (up to several centimeters) and can often be identified on physical examination. Abdominal ultrasound is the most useful diagnostic tool for a definitive diagnosis. The most definitive treatment for cystic ovaries is ovariectomy or ovariohysterectomy, curing the current problem and preventing recurrence. In animals where surgery is not a viable option, ultrasound-guided percutaneous aspiration of ovarian cysts can be performed as a palliative treatment. However, without removal of the ovaries, the cysts will recur, requiring repeated procedures.

PREGNANCY TOXEMIA

Pregnancy toxemia typically occurs in pregnant sows during the last 2 weeks of gestation. As with other species, pregnancy toxemia is the result of a negative energy balance and the metabolism of fat. Sows that experience pregnancy toxemia are typically overweight and become anorexic. Clinical signs include lethargy, dyspnea, and anorexia, usually progressing to death within a few days.[13] Therapy of affected sows should center on providing nutritional support, correcting electrolyte imbalances, and preventing opportunistic infections. Prognosis is generally considered poor, as many sows fail to respond to treatment.

REPRODUCTIVE NEOPLASMS

Neoplasia of the reproductive tract is not commonly reported in guinea pigs, but several tumor types have been described. Of the described reproductive neoplasms, the vast majority occur in female guinea pigs. Uterine leiomyoma (often associated with ovarian cysts)[22] and leiomyosarcoma, ovarian teratoma, and granulosa cell tumor are reported neoplasms of the reproductive tract.[21] Diagnosis, as in any other patient, should be based on the results of cytologic or histopathologic sampling. Benign neoplasms may be resolved with ovariohysterectomy, but further diagnostics to determine the extent of local invasion should be performed before surgery takes place. A thorough diagnostic work-up, including imaging techniques (e.g., abdominal ultrasound, thoracic radiographs), should be performed to look for metastases of malignant tumor types.

MYCOPLASMA CAVIAE

Mycoplasma caviae has been isolated from the reproductive tracts of guinea pigs.[15] These guinea pigs are often unaffected by the organism, but metritis has been suspected to be associated with infection. As with other species, *Mycoplasma* spp. is suspected to cause reproductive problems (e.g., abortion and decreased fertility).

Respiratory
PNEUMONIA

Respiratory disease is a common presenting complaint in guinea pig patients. Clinical signs can vary from sneezing and upper respiratory signs to severe dyspnea and death.

Bordetella bronchiseptica is one of the most common respiratory bacterial agents associated with pneumonia in guinea pigs.[15] Many guinea pigs are carriers of the organism, which will cause clinical disease if the animal is stressed. A thorough history, obtained from the patient's owner, often reveals interactions with other species that are also subclinical carriers of *B. bronchiseptica* (e.g., rabbits, dogs).[13] Clinical signs noted in guinea pigs infected by the *Bordetella* organism include nasal discharge, dehydration, tachypnea, and lethargy.[23] Diagnosis should be based on clinical and radiographic signs and history. Confirmation of the diagnosis can be determined with enzyme-linked immunosorbent assay (ELISA) and indirect immunofluorescence diagnostic tests, or culture of exudates.[24] Treatment/preventive options for *B. bronchiseptica* infections in guinea pigs include an autogenous bacterin vaccine as well as three commercially available vaccines for *Bordetella* spp. (porcine *B. bronchiseptica* and human *B. pertussis*), which were found to offer some protection against the development of bronchopneumonia in experimentally infected guinea pigs.[25]

STREPTOCOCCUS PNEUMONIAE

Streptococcus pneumoniae can cause pleuropneumonia, pleuritis, and peritonitis in guinea pigs.[26] Serologic detection of *S. pneumoniae* antibodies using ELISA have been described in previously published papers.[26] On postmortem examination, lesions found to be associated with *S. pneumoniae* infection included pleuritis, pleural effusion, lung abscessation, otitis media, pericarditis, and others.[20]

Streptococcus pneumoniae was also identified from septic arthritis lesions in a group of guinea pigs.[26] Five guinea pigs in a laboratory colony demonstrated multiple enlarged joints from which pure cultures of *S. pneumoniae* were isolated. Several other individuals in this colony had previously died with typical *S. pneumoniae* lesions (e.g., pleuritis, pericarditis) and lesions consistent with hypovitaminosis C. The group with septic arthritis also had scorbutic changes on necropsy.[26]

STREPTOBACILLUS MONILIFORMIS

Streptobacillus moniliformis, the causative agent of rat-bite fever in humans, was isolated from a laboratory guinea pig with pneumonia. This organism is of particular importance because of its zoonotic potential.[27]

ADENOVIRUS

Adenovirus has been shown to cause necrotizing bronchopneumonia in guinea pig populations, although it can also produce a transient, subclinical infection.[28,29] Clinical signs include depression and dyspnea, but guinea pigs often die acutely without clinical signs.[30] Identification of adenovirus DNA from diseased lung tissue was achieved using a polymerase chain reaction technique in one study.[28] Development of this PCR assay for identification of the virus has determined that the guinea pig adenovirus is distinct.[28] Histopathologic examination of affected tissues of animals infected with adenovirus will reveal the presence of characteristic intranuclear inclusion bodies.[29]

BRONCHOGENIC PAPILLARY ADENOMA

The most commonly reported neoplasm of the respiratory tract in guinea pigs is bronchogenic papillary adenoma. The prevalence of the tumor is as high as 30% in guinea pigs over the age of 3 years.[13] Given the relatively more common occurrence of pneumonia in guinea pigs, bronchogenic papillary adenoma can often be misdiagnosed. For this reason, thoracic radiographs of guinea pigs with respiratory disease are highly recommended.

YERSINIA PSEUDOTUBERCULOSIS

Yersinia pseudotuberculosis can cause septicemic pneumonia in guinea pigs.[15] Death usually occurs rapidly, after the development of coughing and dyspnea. At necropsy, severe congestion of the lungs is found grossly and through histologic evaluation of the tissues.

Integument
ECTOPARASITES

Trixacarus caviae are sarcoptoid mites that commonly affect guinea pigs (Figure 17-19). Affected guinea pigs are intensely

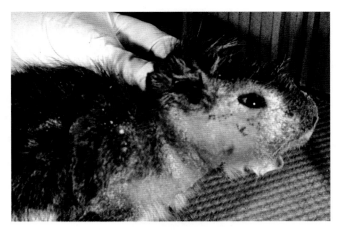

Figure 17-19 A guinea pig patient with severe *Trixacarus caviae* infestation. (Courtesy Stephen D. White, DVM, DACVD.)

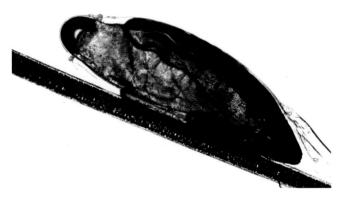

Figure 17-20 Microscopic view of an egg of the louse *Gliricola porcelli* adhered to a shaft of hair. (Courtesy Stephen D. White, DVM, DACVD.)

pruritic, sometimes to the extent of seizure development. As with other mite infestations, diagnosis is based on the identification of the parasites on skin scrapings. Once definitive diagnosis has been made, treatment with ivermectin and selamectin (6 mg/kg q2-4wk) is usually effective. *Chirodiscoides caviae* are fur mites diagnosed in guinea pigs. Because it rarely causes clinical disease, treatment is usually unnecessary.[20,31]

Gyropus ovalis and *Gliricola porcelli* are species of lice that are commonly identified in guinea pigs (Figure 17-20). Infested guinea pigs may be pruritic, but are usually unaffected.[20] Guinea pigs severely infested with these mites may demonstrate poor coat quality and alopecia.

DERMATOPHYTES

Patchy hair loss without associated pruritus may be attributed to dermatophytosis, most commonly *Trichophyton mentagrophytes*[2] (Figure 17-21). Lesions are circular and scaled and usually occur on the face and head.[20] The diagnosis of dermatophytosis is made by a positive fungal culture. Because of the zoonotic potential of these fungal organisms, care should be

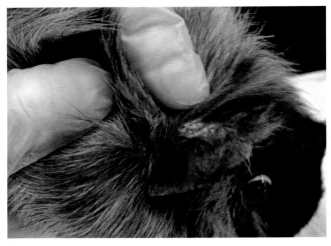

Figure 17-21 A guinea pig with a crusted area on the dorsal pinna consistent with dermatophytosis. A *Trichophyton* organism was cultured from the site.

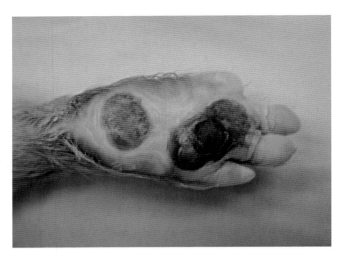

Figure 17-22 Severe, ulcerative pododermatitis in a guinea pig. (Courtesy Michelle G. Hawkins, VMD, DABVP [Avian].)

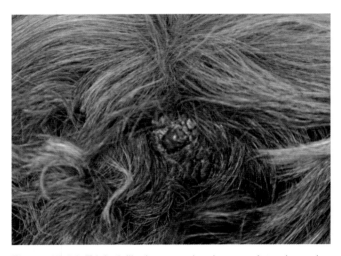

Figure 17-23 Trichofolliculoma on the dorsum of a guinea pig.

taken when handling guinea pig patients suspected of having dermatophytosis.

CERVICAL LYMPHADENITIS

Streptococcus zooepidemicus Lancefield's group C is the causative agent of cervical lymphadenitis. This disease will cause severe swellings of the lymph nodes in the cervical region in guinea pigs. Affected guinea pigs will frequently exhibit no other clinical signs but may become septicemic, with lesions affecting the heart, lungs, kidney, and skin.[20] The most effective treatment for cervical lymphadenitis is complete surgical excision of the affected lymph nodes, followed by appropriate antibiotic therapy based on culture and sensitivity testing. Lancing and draining the abscesses is often not curative, as the abscesses form thick capsules that harbor organisms, leading to recurrence.

Yersinia pseudotuberculosis has also been shown to cause cervical lymphadenitis in guinea pigs.[17] Although the affected guinea pigs are usually not ill, the concern is that rupture of the abscesses will release large amounts of this potentially zoonotic organism into the environment. Another potential causal agent of cervical lymphadenitis is *Streptobacillus moniliformis.*[32]

One report exists of a cervical mass, initially believed to be cervical lymphadenitis, which was histologically determined to be a thyroid papillary adenoma.[33] The mass was apparently nonfunctional and the guinea pig appeared otherwise healthy, but surgical resection was curative.

PODODERMATITIS

Guinea pigs housed in cages with wire flooring are predisposed to developing ulcerated lesions on the plantar surfaces of their feet. Mild lesions may appear as hyperemic, swollen areas of the weight-bearing surfaces. These lesions can progress to ulcerations with secondary infections (Figure 17-22). Vitamin C deficiency has also been considered a predisposing factor for

the development of pododermatitis, as affected animals may be in pain and reluctant to move, resulting in the development of pressure sores.[20] Ulcerated, infected lesions should be managed with appropriate antibiotics and antiinflammatory drugs, but the focus of treatment should be improving husbandry (e.g., providing appropriate flooring/bedding, vitamin C supplementation).

TRICHOFOLLICULOMA

Trichofolliculomas are the most common cutaneous tumor seen in guinea pigs.[20] These benign tumors often occur on the dorsum and are typically round and hairless (Figure 17-23).

CUTANEOUS VASCULAR MALFORMATION

Another cutaneous abnormality that has been described in guinea pigs is cutaneous vascular malformation.[34] The lesion described was a raised, ulcerated plaque on the animal's flank, which bled intermittently. Ultimately, the cutaneous vascular malformation resulted in fatal hemorrhage. Histologically, the lesion was described as an expansile mass extending into the skeletal muscle and consisting of multiple vascular spaces of varying sizes. These vascular spaces were lined with endothelial cells.

Neoplasia

Compared to the incidence of neoplasia in other mammalian species, the incidence of neoplasia in guinea pigs appears low or is underreported. However, there have been several reported cases of neoplasia in guinea pigs. As more guinea pig owners seek quality veterinary care for their pets, reports of neoplasia will increase.

LYMPHOMA

Lymphoma is the most commonly reported neoplasia in guinea pigs.[20] Clinical signs associated with guinea pig neoplasia include lymphadenopathy, splenomegaly, and hepatomegaly. Leukemic and aleukemic forms of guinea pig lymphoma have been identified.

THYROID CARCINOMA

Thyroid carcinoma has been reported in an adult guinea pig that demonstrated multiple masses in the ventral cervical region.[35] As there was no evidence of neoplastic disease elsewhere on postmortem examination, this was considered a primary tumor.

MESOTHELIOMA

Mesothelioma has been reported in the abdomen of an adult guinea pig.[36] The guinea pig had died of complications associated with pneumonia, and the mesothelioma was diagnosed through a necropsy examination. The mass consisted of diffuse nodules on the serosal surfaces of numerous organs in the abdominal cavity.

Miscellaneous
HEAT STROKE

Guinea pigs are native to cooler regions of South America and are therefore relatively intolerant of temperatures above 80° F, lower if the environment is also humid. Guinea pigs should be housed in well-ventilated enclosures at temperatures between 65° and 75° F to prevent heat stress.

Clinical signs of heat stress include rapid, shallow respirations, lethargy, poor peripheral perfusion, and ptyalism.[13] Treatment includes reducing the animal's core body temperature with cool water baths or applying alcohol to the feet and ears; in addition, fluid therapy (either intravenous or subcutaneous) is recommended to improve perfusion. The prognosis for this condition is guarded.

INCLUSION-BODY CONJUNCTIVITIS

Chlamydophila psittaci has been identified as a disease-causing agent in guinea pigs; it usually causes a mild, self-limiting conjunctivitis. This intracellular bacterial disease usually occurs in young guinea pigs 4 to 8 weeks of age but has been reported in adults as well.[37] In one outbreak, the typical conjunctival abnormalities were present with other, more significant, clinical signs, such as rhinitis, abortion, and pneumonia.[38] A definitive diagnosis can be achieved through Giemsa staining, immunofluorescent antibody testing of conjunctival scrapings, and serologic testing.[37]

PROLIFERATIVE UROCYSTICA AND ADENOMA

Guinea pigs have been reported to develop pathologic changes related to ingestion of Forssk fern.[39,40] In these studies, guinea pigs fed fresh fern developed hematuria and hemorrhage of the bladder wall.[40] One guinea pig fed dried fern developed proliferative urocystica and adenoma of the bladder, a finding sometimes considered precancerous in human patients. This guinea pig did not show clinical signs associated with the bladder abnormalities.[39]

RABIES

Rabies virus infection is uncommon in rodent species, but it has been described and should be considered a differential diagnosis for an ill guinea pig with suspect contact to wildlife, especially raccoons. A recent report of a rabies in a privately owned guinea pig described abnormal behavior (biting the owner) 26 days after the guinea pig had possible interactions with a raccoon.[41] In this guinea pig, rabies virus antigen was detected by immunofluorescent antibody testing in the sublingual salivary gland, tongue, and buccal tissues, implying that the guinea pig could have transmitted the virus via a bite wound.

■ THERAPEUTICS
Fluids

Sick guinea pigs are often anorexic and therefore dehydrated. Restoration of normal hydration status is crucial for the successful treatment of many disease processes. Replacement of fluid deficit and maintenance of normal hydration can be achieved by administering crystalloids substances through subcutaneous, intraperitoneal, intravenous, or intraosseous routes. Because of the difficulty in placing and maintaining catheters in peripheral veins and bones, the most common route for fluid administration is subcutaneous.

Subcutaneous fluid administration is generally well tolerated. Fluids are administered under the skin of the cranial, dorsal thorax (Figure 17-24). Butterfly catheter needles are useful because they allow the patient to move around without pulling out the injection needle. Maintenance fluid rates for guinea pigs are 80-100 mL/kg/day.

Feeding

Another important aspect of management for the sick guinea pig is nutritional support. Anorexic guinea pigs can experience a change in their normal GI flora in as little as 8 to 12 hours. This change of GI flora can lead to ileus, colic, overgrowth of

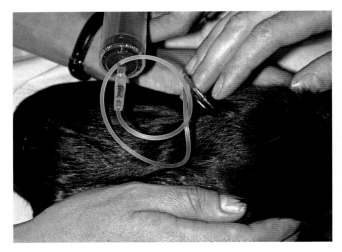

Figure 17-24 Subcutaneous fluid administration to a guinea pig using a butterfly catheter.

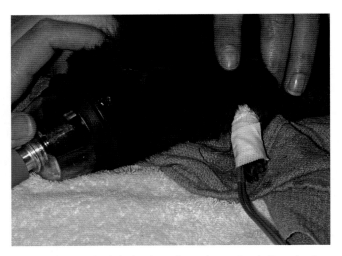

Figure 17-25 Mask induction of a guinea pig. A Doppler has been placed on the right forelimb to monitor heart rate.

pathogenic bacteria, and enterotoxemia. Commercial products are available that are palatable and high in fiber. These products help to maintain gut motility (Oxbow Critical Care for Herbivores, Oxbow Hay Company, Murdock, NE).

Patients will often eat directly from a dish or 60-ml catheter tip syringe. For patients that are more resistant to eating, a technique that is useful, in my experience, is to remove the plungers from 1-ml or 3-ml syringes and fill them individually using a catheter tip syringe. Although this method may seem tedious, it allows the delivery of small boluses of food to be incrementally dispensed.

Antibiotics

The GI tract of guinea pigs can be very sensitive to the effects of certain classes of antibiotics. The GI flora of guinea pigs is primarily Gram positive, and administration of antibiotics with a primarily Gram-positive spectrum can result in overgrowth of Gram-negative and anaerobic organisms. Enteral administration of penicillins (e.g., amoxicillin, ampicillin), macrolides (e.g., erythromycin, lincomycin), and first-generation cephalosporins can result in overgrowth of opportunistic pathogens.[20] Ampicillin administered subcutaneously at doses of 8 and 10mg/kg three times a day resulted in mortality rates of 20% and 30%, respectively, in a group of guinea pigs. At necropsy, *Clostridium difficile* was cultured from the ceca of all fatalities.[42] Twenty-five percent of guinea pigs administered 100 mg/kg of cefazolin, a first-generation cephalosporin, intramuscularly died of enterocolitis after several injections.[43] All antibiotics should be used with caution in guinea pigs because of the possibility of disruption of the GI flora (Table 17-2).

■SURGERY
Anesthesia

Guinea pigs can be induced using isoflurane or sevoflurane administered by mask or induction chamber (Figure 17-25).

For lengthy or potentially painful procedures, preanesthetic medications may be used before induction of the inhalant anesthetic agent. As a preanesthetic, an injectable combination, midazolam (0.2-0.5 mg/kg) and butorphanol (0.2-0.5 mg/kg), has been used with success. The administration of premedications will also decrease the stress of induction. Isoflurane and sevoflurane are both acceptable inhalant anesthetics for guinea pigs. The advantage of sevoflurane is that it does not appear to have as noxious a scent as isoflurane, thereby reducing breath holding during induction and producing a smoother anesthetic episode. After induction, the inhalant anesthetic may be switched to isoflurane if cost is an issue. Guinea pigs should not be fasted more than 2 to 3 hours before anesthesia. Because these animals are hindgut fermenters, withholding food for longer periods of time may disrupt GI flora.

Careful monitoring during anesthesia is essential. The number of respirations must be visually monitored for depth and character. Heart rate and rhythm should also be monitored continuously using a pediatric stethoscope or Doppler unit, which can be placed on a peripheral artery. Changes in heart rate or respiratory rate can occur rapidly, so it is advantageous to have precalculated doses of emergency drugs (e.g., glycopyrrolate, epinephrine, atropine, dopram) drawn and available for use before anesthetic induction.

Intubation

Intubation of guinea pigs is generally considered to be very difficult. The long, narrow oral cavity makes visualization of the glottis difficult. The soft tissues of the tongue and soft palate are continuous in the caudal oropharynx, leaving only a small aperture, the *palatal ostium*. Intubation must be performed through this opening in the mucosal tissues. Several techniques have been described for visualizing the glottis to assist with intubation. These usually involve alterations of laryngoscope blades so that they may be introduced into

TABLE 17-2 Selected Drug Dosages, Dosing Frequencies, and Routes of Administration

Drug	Route(s) of administration	Dose(s)[44-46]	Dose frequency
Analgesic/anesthetic agents			
Atropine	IM	0.1-1.0 mg/kg	–
Buprenorphine	SC, IV	0.05 mg/kg	q8-12h
Butorphanol	SC, IM	0.4-2.0 mg/kg	q4-12h
Carprofen	PO, SC	1-4 mg/kg	q12-24h
Diazepam	IM	0.5-3.0 mg/kg	–
Glycopyrrolate	SC, IM	0.01-0.02 mg/kg	–
Ketamine	IM	10-44 mg/kg	–
Ketamine/diazepam	IM	20-30 mg/kg(K)/1-2 mg/kg(D)	–
Ketamine/midazolam	IM	5-10 mg/kg(K)/0.5-1.0 mg/kg(M)	–
Ketoprofen	SC, IM	1 mg/kg	q12-24h
Midazolam	IM	1-2 mg/kg	–
Nalbuphine	IM	1-2 mg/kg	q3h
Antibiotic agents			
Chloramphenicol	PO, SC, IM, IV	20-50 mg/kg	q6-12h
Ciprofloxacin	PO	5-20 mg/kg	q12h
Enrofloxacin	PO, SC, IM	5-15 mg/kg	q12h
Metronidazole	PO	25 mg/kg	q12h
Trimethoprim-sulfa	PO, SC, IM	15-30 mg/kg	q12h
Antifungal agents			
Griseofulvin	PO	5-25 mg/kg	q24h
Itraconazole	PO	5 mg/kg	q24h
Ketoconazole	PO	10-40 mg/kg	q24h
Antiparasitic agents			
Fenbendazole	PO	20 mg/kg	q24h
Ivermectin	SC	0.2-0.4 mg/kg	q7-14days
Lime sulfur dip	Topical	–	q7days
Metronidazole	PO	25 mg/kg	q12h
Praziquantel	PO, SC, IM	5-10 mg/kg	q10-14days
Selamectin	Topical	6 mg/kg	q28days
Sulfadimethoxine	PO	25-50 mg/kg	q24h
Miscellaneous agents			
Cimetidine	PO, SC, IM, IV	5-10 mg/kg	q6-12h
Cisapride	PO	0.1-0.5 mg/kg	q8-12h
Diphenhydramine	PO, SC	5-7.5 mg/kg	–
Epinephrine	IV	0.003 mg/kg	–
Furosemide	PO, SC	2-10 mg/kg	q12h
Lactated Ringer's	SC, IV	50-100 ml/kg	q24h
Metoclopramide	PO, SC, IM	0.2-1.0 mg/kg	q12h
Sucralfate	PO	25-100 mg/kg	q8-12h
Vitamin C	PO, SC, IM	10-100 mg/kg	q24h

IM, intramuscular; *IV,* intravenous; *PO,* per os; *SC,* subcutaneous.

the oral cavity without traumatizing the delicate buccal mucosa.[47,48]

Another possible intubation technique utilizes a stethoscope altered so that an appropriately sized endotracheal tube can be affixed to the end. The endotracheal tube is then inserted into the caudal oropharynx. The anesthetist will then listen through the ear pieces of the stethoscope for expiration.

The tube is then gently introduced into the trachea. This technique requires practice to perfect but, once the procedure has been performed several times, is a reliable way to intubate guinea pigs. Application of a small amount of lidocaine to the *rima glottis* can ease intubation. Rigid endoscopes and otoscopes, when available, are also very helpful in visualizing the glottis for intubation.

Ovariohysterectomy

Indications for an ovariohysterectomy procedure in guinea pigs include routine sterilization, dystocia, and reproductive tract disease (e.g., neoplasia, muco/hydro/pyometra, ovarian cysts). In general, the surgical approach and technique are similar to those used with domestic species. The patient is placed in dorsal recumbency, and a ventral midline incision is made through the *linea alba*. Care must be taken upon entering the abdomen to avoid incising the large cecum, which is often situated along the ventral body wall. The body of the uterus can be located dorsal to the bladder. The ovaries lie caudally and laterally to the kidneys and are 6 to 8 mm in length.[49] The abdomen of the guinea pig is deep, and the ovaries can be difficult to exteriorize. Care must be taken to avoid tearing the short ovarian vessels. Once the ovaries are removed, the uterus is ligated and transected in a manner similar to that used with other mammals.

Ovariectomy

Another method of sterilization that is reported in guinea pigs is ovariectomy. The incidence of uterine disease compared with ovarian disease in guinea pigs is quite low. The approach for removal of the ovaries is through small incisions of the dorsal-lateral body wall caudal to the last rib. The advantage of this approach is that the sensitive GI tract is not manipulated to reach the structures to be excised.

Orchiectomy

Orchiectomy is typically performed to prevent reproduction, to decrease undesirable sexual behavior, and to treat reproductive tract disease. The orchiectomy procedure in guinea pigs is performed by making an incision through the scrotum over each testicle. A closed technique or open technique, whereby the vaginal tunic is incised, may be performed. Although herniation of abdominal contents through the inguinal canal does not commonly occur with open castration, it is still advisable to close the inguinal ring if this technique is used. The incisions may be closed with either an intradermal suture pattern or with tissue glue.

Suture Reaction

Reactions to suture material are relatively common in guinea pigs after surgical procedures. These reactions can vary in severity from mild local irritation to abscessation. Suture materials that cause a large amount of inflammation, such as chromic gut, should never be used in guinea pigs. In general, monofilament suture materials that are degraded by hydrolysis are preferred.

REFERENCES

1. Verstraete FJM: Advances in diagnosis and treatment of small exotic mammal dental disease, *Semin Av Exot Pet Med* 12(1):37-48, 2003.

2. Flecknell PA: Guinea pigs. In Beynon PH, Cooper JE, editors: *Manual of Exotic Pets,* Cheltenham, Gloucestershire, 1991, British Small Animal Veterinary Association.

3. Harkness JE: Biology and husbandry: guinea pigs. In Harkness JE, editor: *A Practitioner's Guide to Domestic Rodents,* Lakewood, Colo, 1993, American Animal Hospital Association.

4. Quesenberry KE, Donnelly TM, Hillyer EV: Biology, husbandry, and clinical techniques. In Quesenberry KE, Carpenter JW, editors: *Ferrets, Rabbits, and Rodents: Clinical Medicine and Surgery,* ed 2, St Louis, 2003, WB Saunders.

5. Carpenter JW: Hematologic and serum biochemical values of rodents. In Carpenter JW, editor: *Exotic Animal Formulary,* ed 3, St Louis, 2005, WB Saunders.

6. Campbell TW: Mammalian hematology: laboratory animals and miscellaneous species. In Thrall MA, editor: *Veterinary Hematology and Clinical Chemistry,* Baltimore, 2004, Lippincott Williams and Wilkins.

7. Eremin O, Coombs RRA, Ashby J et al: Natural cytotoxicity in the guinea-pig: the natural killer (NK) cell activity of the Kurloff cell, *Immunol* 41:367-378, 1980.

8. Revell PA: The Kurloff cell, *Int Rev Cytol* 51:275-314, 1977.

9. Silverman S, Tell LA: Radiology equipment and positioning techniques. In Silverman S, Tell LA, editors: *Radiology of Rodents, Rabbits, and Ferrets: An Atlas of Normal Anatomy and Positioning,* St Louis, 2006, WB Saunders.

10. Gibson SV, Wagner JE: Cryptosporidiosis in guinea pigs: a retrospective study. *JAVMA* 189(9):1033-1034, 1986.

11. Wobeser G: Tyzzer's disease. In Williams ES, Barker IK, editors: *Infectious Diseases of Wild Mammals,* ed 3, Ames, Iowa, 2001, Blackwell.

12. Motzel SL, Riley LK: Subclinical infection and transmission of Tyzzer's disease in rats, *Lab Anim Sci* 42:439-443, 1992.

13. O'Rourke DP: Disease problems of guinea pigs. In Quesenberry KE, Carpenter JW, editors: *Ferrets, Rabbits, and Rodents: Clinical Medicine and Surgery,* ed 2, St Louis, 2003, WB Saunders.

14. Jaax GP, Jaax NK, Petrali JP et al: Coronavirus-like virions associated with a wasting syndrome in guinea pigs, *Lab Anim Sci* 40(4):375-378, 1990.

15. Rigby C: Natural infections of guinea pigs, *Lab Anim* 10:119-142, 1976.

16. Haberman RT, Williams FP: Salmonellosis in laboratory animals, *J Natl Cancer Inst* 20: 933-947, 1958.

17. Paterson JS: The guinea pig or cavy, *The UFAW Handbook on the Care and Management of Laboratory Animals,* ed 4, Edinburgh and London, 1972, Churchill Livingstone.

18. Ganguly R, Durieux MF, Waldman RH: Macrophage function in vitamin c-deficient guinea pigs, *Am J Clin Nutr* 29:762-765, 1976.

19. Steiger SM, Wenker C, Zeigler-Gohm D et al: Ureterolithiasis and papilloma formation in the ureter of a guinea pig, *Vet Radiol Ultrasound* 44(3):326-329, 2003.

20. Quesenberry KE: Guinea pigs, *Vet Clin North Am Small Anim Pract* 24(1):67-86, 1994.

21. Bishop CR: Reproductive medicine of rabbits and rodents. In Speer BL, editor: *The Veterinary Clinics of North America, Exotic Animal Practice: Reproductive Medicine* 5:3, Philadelphia, 2002, WB Saunders.

22. Greenacre CB: Spontaneous tumors of small mammals. In Graham JE, editor: *The Veterinary Clinics of North America, Exotic Animal Practice: Oncology* 7:3, Philadelphia, 2004, WB Saunders.

23. Trahan CJ, Stephenson EH, Ezzell JW et al: Airborne-induced experimental *Bordetella bronchiseptica* pneumonia in strain 13 guinea pigs, *Lab Anim* 21:226-232, 1987.

24. Wullenweber M, Boot R: Interlaboratory comparison of enzyme-linked immunosorbent assay (ELISA) and indirect immunofluorescence (IIF) for detection of *Bordetella bronchoseptica* antibodies in guinea pigs, *Lab Anim Sci* 28:335-339, 1994.

25. Matherne CM, Steffen EK, Wagner JE: Efficacy of commercial vaccines for protecting guinea pigs against *Bordetella bronchiseptica* pneumonia, *Lab Anim Sci* 37(2):191-194, 1987.

26. Matsubara J, Kamiyama T, Miyoshi H et al: Serodiagnosis of *Streptococcus pneumoniae* infection in guinea pigs by an enzyme-linked immunosorbent assay, *Lab Anim* 22:304-308, 1988.

27. Kirchner BK, Lake SG, Wightman SR: Isolation of *Streptobacillus moniliformis* from a guinea pig with granulomatous pneumonia, *Lab Anim Sci* 42(5):519-521, 1992.

28. Pring-Åkerblom P, Blažek K, Schramlová J et al: Polymerase chain reaction for detection of guinea pig adenovirus, *J Vet Diagn Invest* 9:232-236, 1997.

29. Butz N, Ossent P, Homberger FR: Pathogenesis of guinea pig adenovirus infection: *Lab Anim Sci* 49(6):600-604, 1999.
30. Harris IE, Portas BH: Adenoviral bronchopneumonia of guinea pigs, *Aust Vet J* 62(9):317, 1985.
31. Lumeij JT, Cremers HJWM: Anorexia and *Chirodiscoides caviae* infection in a guinea pig *(Cavia porcellus), Vet Rec* 119:432, 1986.
32. ILAR: A guide to infectious diseases in guinea pigs, gerbils, hamsters, and rabbits, part II, diseases outlines, *Inst Lab Anim Res News* 17:ID7-ID15, 1974.
33. LaRegina MC, Wightman SR: Thyroid papillary adenoma in a guinea pig with signs of cervical lymphadenitis, *JAVMA* 175(9):969-971, 1979.
34. Osofsky A, De Cock HEV, Tell LA et al: Cutaneous vascular malformation in a guinea pig *(Cavia porcellus), Vet Dermatol* 15:47-52, 2004.
35. Zarrin K: Thyroid carcinoma of a guinea pig: a case report, *Lab Anim* 8:145-148, 1974.
36. Wilson TM, Brigman G: Abdominal mesothelioma in an aged guinea pig, *Lab Anim Sci* 32(2):175-176, 1982.
37. Deeb BJ, DiGiacomo RF, Wang SP: Guinea pig inclusion conjunctivitis (GPIC) in a commercial colony, *Lab Anim* 23:103-106, 1989.
38. Schmeer VN, Weiss R, Reinacher M et al: Verlauf einer *Chlamydien-bedingten* "Meerschweinchen-Einschluß Körperchen-Könjunktivitis" in einer Versuchstierhaltung, *Zeitschrift für Versuchsteirkunde* 27:233-240, 1985.
39. Somvanshi R, Sharma VK: Proliferative urocystica and adenoma in a guinea pig, *J Comp Pathol* 133:277-280, 2005.
40. Somvanshi R, Sharma VK: Preliminary studies on *Christella dentate* (Forssk) fern toxicity in guinea pigs, *J Lab Med* 5:6-15, 2004.
41. Eidson M, Matthews SD, Willsey AL et al: Rabies virus infection in a pet guinea pig and seven pet rabbits, *JAVMA* 227(6):932-935, 2005.
42. Young JD, Hurst WJ, White WJ et al: An evaluation of ampicillin pharmacokinetics and toxicity in guinea pigs, *Lab Anim Sci* 37(5):652-656, 1987.
43. Fritz PE, Hurst WJ, White WJ et al: Pharmacokinetics of cefazolin in guinea pigs, *Lab Anim Sci* 37(5):646-651, 1987.
44. Ness RD: Rodents. In Carpenter JW, editor: *Exotic Animal Formulary,* ed 3, Philadelphia, 2005, WB Saunders.
45. Morrisey JK, Carpenter JW: Formulary. In Quesenberry KE, Carpenter JW, editors: *Ferrets, Rabbits, and Rodents: Clinical Medicine and Surgery,* ed 2, St Louis, 2003, WB Saunders.
46. Plumb DC: *Veterinary Drug Handbook,* ed 4, Ames, Iowa, 2002, Iowa State Press.
47. Blouin A, Cormier Y: Endotracheal intubation in guinea pigs by direct laryngoscopy, *Lab Anim Sci* 37(2):244-245, 1987.
48. Turner MA, Thomas P, Sheridan DJ: An improved method for direct laryngeal intubation in the guinea pig, *Lab Anim* 26:25-28, 1992.
49. Breazile JE, Brown EM: Anatomy. In Wagner JE, Manning PJ, editors: *Biology of the Guinea Pig,* New York, 1976, Academic Press.

Shannon M. Riggs
Mark A. Mitchell

CHAPTER 18

CHINCHILLAS

COMMON SPECIES KEPT IN CAPTIVITY

There are two species of chinchilla that are kept in captivity: *Chinchilla laniger* (or *lanigera*) and *C. brevicaudata*.[1,2] *C. laniger* is the species commonly kept in captivity in the United States. Originally imported into the United States to provide a commercial fur, these long-lived rodents make excellent pets.

BIOLOGY
Unique Anatomy and Physiology

Chinchillas are native to the semiarid mountainous areas of South America, particularly the countries of Peru, Argentina, Bolivia, and Chile.[1,2] Most of the chinchillas kept in the United States are descendants of a small group of animals imported into California in the 1920s.[1] Because of overhunting for its beautiful coat, the chinchilla is believed to be nearly extinct in the wild. Wild-type chinchillas have a silver-gray coat with black ticking. Today, there are a number of different coat color variations that have been developed as a result of the fur, show, and pet chinchilla trades. Because the captive chinchillas found in the United States originated from a very small number of animals, a genetic component is suspected in many of the commonly seen disease processes.

Adult chinchillas usually weigh between 400 and 800 g, females being slightly larger than males. Relative to other rodent species, the life span of the chinchilla is long, sometimes nearing 20 years of age.[1] Chinchillas are naturally nocturnal, but they can adapt to a more diurnal lifestyle.

Chinchillas are unique-looking animals with a short body, large head, delicate limbs, large hairless ears, and a bushy tail.

Chinchillas have the longest gestation period of any commonly kept rodent species (110 days). Young, of which there are one to six (average two), are precocial. Chinchillas become sexually mature at 7 to 9 months of age.

HUSBANDRY
Creating an Appropriate Habitat
ENCLOSURE SIZE

Chinchillas are active animals, requiring a relatively large enclosure. The enclosure should be large enough to provide an area for eating, sleeping, exercising, and eliminating wastes (a latrine). Cages with multiple levels are preferred, as they provide additional room for the animals to exercise. Chinchilla cages are generally constructed of wire. Any other materials being considered for a cage should be "chew proof." When considering a wire cage, it is important to select a structure that will not entrap limbs. The floor of the cage should be solid. If the bottom of the cage is also wire, a section of solid flooring should be provided to prevent pododermatitis. Chinchillas tend to be somewhat timid, so it is essential to provide ample space for hiding. Hide boxes should be constructed of materials that can be cleaned easily (e.g., polyvinyl chloride pipes) or can be disposed of (e.g., cardboard boxes). Wooden hide boxes are not recommended, as they are difficult to disinfect and are commonly chewed on by chinchillas.

TEMPERATURE/HUMIDITY

Because of their dense hair coat, chinchillas are not tolerant of temperatures greater than 80° F (26.7° C). That said, chinchillas should be housed indoors throughout the summer. In hot weather, owners should be encouraged to operate the home's air conditioner to maintain an appropriate temperature for their chinchilla. If this is not possible, alternatives might include using electric fans or placing plastic bottles filled with ice in the chinchilla's enclosure.

LIGHTING

Chinchillas are naturally a nocturnal animal, although they easily adapt to a diurnal lifestyle. These animals should be provided a 12-hour photoperiod (12 hours light, 12 hours darkness). Although there is no published evidence for this, these animals likely benefit from natural unfiltered sunlight. If they are housed indoors, full-spectrum lighting may be beneficial.

SUBSTRATE

A layer of soft bedding should be provided on the floor of the cage to absorb waste and decrease pressure on the plantar surfaces of the feet. Recycled paper products, shredded newspaper, and aspen shavings are the substrates of choice. Cedar and pine shavings should be avoided, as the aromatic oils in these substrates can act as contact and respiratory irritants. The enclosure should be cleaned thoroughly on a regular basis, at least 2 times per week. Unsanitary conditions can predispose the chinchilla to pododermatitis, respiratory problems, and other health problems.

ACCESSORIES

Shelter Box

Chinchillas should be provided shelter areas within their enclosure. Non-treated wooden boxes may be used, but may eventually need to be replaced if the animal chews on the box.

Dust Baths

To maintain proper coat health, chinchillas must be provided with a dust bath 2 to 3 times per week for 10 to 20 minutes (Figure 18-1). The dust used for these animals is a volcanic ash, and commercial brands are readily available. It is important to remove the dust bath from the chinchilla's enclosure after the bathing period. If the dust bath is not removed, chinchillas tend to bathe excessively, and the prolonged exposure to dust can cause ocular and respiratory irritation.

■ NUTRITION

Diet

Chinchillas are native to an area of the world that contains sparse vegetation, primarily consisting of grasses. The recommended nutritional composition of a chinchilla diet is 16% to 20% protein, 2% to 5% fat, and 15% to 35% bulk fiber.[3] An appropriate chinchilla diet should be comprised of a high-quality hay (e.g., timothy, oat, or orchard grass), chinchilla pellets, and an assortment of dark leafy vegetables (e.g., romaine lettuce, mustard greens, collard greens). Some veterinarians recommend rabbit or guinea pig pellets for chinchillas; however, these pellets are shorter in length than those recommended for chinchillas and are more difficult for these animals to hold. Fruits, grains, and raisins may also be provided as

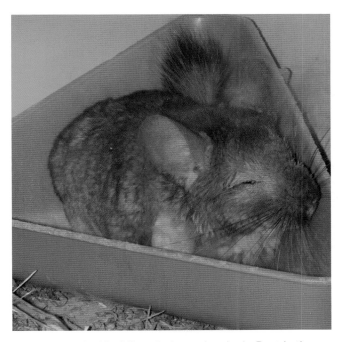

Figure 18-1 A chinchilla enjoying a dust bath. Dust baths are essential for chinchillas' skin maintenance and coat health. (Courtesy Michelle G. Hawkins, VMD, DABVP [Avian].)

treats on an occasional basis, but they should comprise less than 5% of the animal's diet. Chinchillas should be provided ad lib access to water in a hanging water bottle.

■ PREVENTIVE MEDICINE

Quarantine

Newly acquired animals should be quarantined from established animals for a minimum of 30 days. This recommendation should be considered a minimal quarantine period, as certain diseases could remain latent for more than 30 days. All quarantined animals should be thoroughly examined and screened using baseline diagnostics (e.g., complete blood count, plasma biochemistries, and a fecal exam). During the quarantine period, the animal's appetite, demeanor, and fecal output should be monitored closely.

Routine Exams

Chinchillas are not routinely vaccinated for infectious diseases in the United States. However, owners should be encouraged to have an annual examination performed on their pets, including a thorough oral examination and blood work. Being a prey species, chinchillas are adept at hiding illness, and a routine evaluation by a qualified veterinarian may help in detecting abnormalities early.

Many health problems of chinchillas are directly related to improper husbandry. During a routine veterinary visit for chinchilla patients, owners should be asked to provide a detailed description of the animal's environment, including cage size and type, substrate, frequency of cleaning, ambient temperature, and exercise time. Information pertaining to the animal's diet, feeding frequency, and bowel movements is also important to obtain.

Disinfection and Sanitation

Chinchilla enclosures, food bowls, water bottles, and cage accessories should be sanitized using a standard disinfection protocol. Sodium hypochlorite is the preferred disinfectant (dilute 5.25% solution 1 : 32). It is important to thoroughly rinse the enclosure and accessories before replacing them in the cage. The cage should be allowed to dry in a well-ventilated area.

◼ RESTRAINT
Manual Restraint

Chinchillas are relatively docile and usually do not require aggressive restraint; however, they are capable of quick bursts of activity. A chinchilla that is dropped may injure itself, so appropriate restraint is necessary when examining or transporting these animals. In general, the more a chinchilla is restrained, the more it tends to struggle, so a "less is more" approach should be used. A chinchilla should be restrained by supporting the weight of the body with one hand under the thorax and grasping the base of the tail with the other hand (Figure 18-2). Chinchillas should never be scruffed or handled roughly. Rough handling can result in "fur slip" or the loss of a patch of fur at the site where the animal was grasped. This lost fur can take several months to grow back (see Dermatologic Conditions).

Chemical Restraint

Chinchillas that are fractious or must be anesthetized can be given either parenteral or inhalant anesthetics. We prefer inhal-

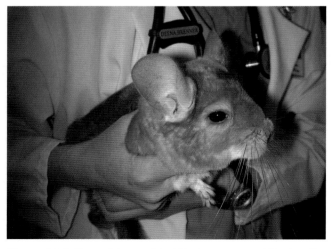

Figure 18-2 Restraining a chinchilla for transport. The handler has control of both the pelvic and thoracic limbs to prevent the patient from jumping and injuring itself.

ants for these animals, although the parenterals can be used as preanesthetics to limit the concentration of inhalant required for a procedure. Chinchillas can be induced via a face mask with isoflurane or sevoflurane (Abbott Laboratories, North Chicago, IL). In general, an induction rate of 3% to 5% isoflurane (per 1 L oxygen) or 5% to 7% sevoflurane (per 1 L oxygen) is required. Chinchillas, like other rodents, are difficult to intubate because of their long, narrow oral cavity. We prefer to intubate these animals using an endoscope. A rigid 2.7-mm endoscope can be used to visualize the airway and direct the endotracheal tube into place. The endotracheal tube size required for a chinchilla can vary, although 2.0 to 4.0 outside diameter tubes are generally acceptable. Once the chinchilla is intubated, the endotracheal tube should be secured and the animal maintained on the inhalant. In general, chinchillas can be maintained at 1.5% to 3.0% isoflurane (per 0.5-1 L oxygen) or 3.0% to 5.0% sevoflurane (per 1 L oxygen). Many of the parenteral anesthetics used for domestic pets can also be used for chinchillas. (For a complete list of parenteral agents please refer to Anesthesia; see also Table 18-6).

◼ PERFORMING A PHYSICAL EXAMINATION

A physical examination should include both a hands-off and a hands-on review of the animal. For the hands-off exam, particular attention should be paid to the respiratory rate and character, attitude, and posture. Animals with respiratory compromise or neurologic disease should be handled carefully during the hands-on examination. It is important to always measure the animal's body temperature before performing the complete physical exam. A chinchilla's body temperature is generally lower (96° to 99° F [35.5° to 37.2° C]) than that found in other domestic mammals. Because chinchillas have such a dense hair coat, their body temperature can increase dramatically over the course of a physical examination, and this should be taken into consideration. Otherwise, the physical exam should be approached in a thorough, systematic manner, as in any mammalian patient. Thoracic auscultation and abdominal palpation can be performed as in other patients. Auscultation of gut sounds is also an important part of the chinchilla physical exam. A healthy chinchilla should have 1 to 2 borborygmi per minute.

A complete oral examination is another important facet of the chinchilla physical exam. This should be reserved for the end of the examination, as it can be rather stressful for the patient. As is the case for most rodent species, the cranial surface of the incisors is covered with a layer of yellow to orange enamel (Figure 18-3). The oral cavity of the chinchilla has a small opening and is very narrow and long. In most cases, an otoscope with cone or a human nasal speculum is required to fully examine the molars and caudal aspect of the oral cavity. In most cases, the oral exam can be performed on an alert animal; however, anesthesia may be required when the animal is difficult to restrain, appears to be experiencing pain, or requires a more detailed oral exam.

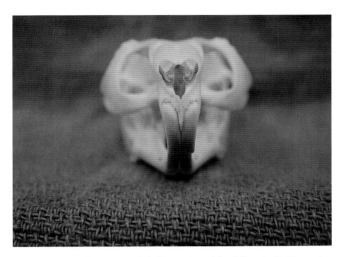

Figure 18-3 Rostrocaudal view of a chinchilla skull. Note the normal orange coloration of the enamel on the rostral surface of the incisors.

BOX 18-1 Hematologic Parameters for Chinchillas

Hematologic Parameter	Reference Interval
PCV (%)	30-55
RBC ($\times 10^6$ cells/µl)	5-10
Hemoglobin (g/dl)	9-15
WBC ($\times 10^3$ cells/µl)	6-16
Heterophils (%)	25-50
Lymphocytes (%)	10-70
Monocytes (%)	0-5
Eosinophils (%)	0-5
Basophils (%)	0-2
Platelets ($\times 10^3$ cells/µl)	300-600

Data from Quesenberry KE, Donnelly TM, Hillyer EV: Biology, husbandry, and clinical techniques of guinea pigs and chinchillas. In Quesenberry KE, Carpenter JW, editors: *Ferrets, Rabbits, and Rodents: Clinical Medicine and Surgery*, ed 2, St Louis, 2003, WB Saunders; de Oliveria Silva T, Kruetz LC, Barcellos LJG et al: Reference values for chinchilla *(Chinchilla laniger)* blood cells and serum biochemical parameters, *Ciência Rural*, 35(3):602-606, 2005.
PCV, packed cell volume; *RBC*, red blood cell count; *WBC*, white blood cell count.

Common Abnormalities Found on the Physical Examination

As with any species, it is important to always perform a thorough physical examination to minimize the likelihood of misclassifying the disease state of a patient. Therefore, veterinarians working with an animal should avoid the trap of only examining the system(s) that a client mentions during the history and instead examine the entire animal. There are a number of potential abnormalities that may arise during a physical examination. In many cases, an animal may present with multiple, unrelated problems. The primary problems found on a chinchilla examination include teeth malocclusion, otitis externa, heat stroke, upper and lower respiratory disease (e.g., pneumonia), penile fur ring, pododermatitis, and fur slip.

◼ DIAGNOSTIC TESTING

Hematology

Venipuncture in chinchillas can be difficult for the veterinarian and stressful for the patient. Many of the peripheral vessels that are accessible in dogs and cats are very small in chinchillas and do not allow for the collection of adequate volumes of blood for routine testing. Access to larger vessels, such as the jugular vein, requires somewhat aggressive restraint, which may not be appropriate in a sick or stressed animal. It is often preferable to perform venipuncture under sedation or anesthesia in these patients; however, veterinarians must carefully consider the benefits of obtaining diagnostic samples against the risk of anesthesia for each individual patient.

When a large blood sample is required (e.g., for complete blood count and plasma biochemistry panel), the jugular, cranial vena cava, or femoral vein can be used. These sites are best accessed under anesthesia, as restraint is stressful and excessive struggling by the patient may cause laceration of these large vessels. A 25-gauge needle fastened to a 1-ml or 3-ml syringe can be used to collect the sample. If small quantities of blood are required (e.g., blood glucose or PCV/TS [packed cell volume and total solids determination]), blood can be collected from the cephalic or lateral saphenous veins. When sampling these smaller veins, a 25- or 27-gauge needle fastened to a 1-ml syringe can be used. Insulin syringes may also be used. Using a smaller syringe will help minimize the likelihood of collapsing the blood vessel. When placing the sample into a blood storage tube, it is important to remove the needle before discharging the sample to prevent hemolysis.

Hematologic testing is an important diagnostic tool in chinchilla medicine. Because these prey species can mask their illness, veterinarians must rely on hematologic and other diagnostic tests to fully assess their patients. Box 18-1 presents reference intervals for chinchillas.

The most common leukocyte in the chinchilla is the lymphocyte. The second most common circulating granulocyte is the heterophil. Heterophils lack myeloperoxidase, the enzyme responsible for liquefying purulent material. Therefore, chinchilla abscesses tend to be very thick and caseous. The remaining leukocyte types—monocytes, eosinophils, and basophils—are normally present in very low numbers. During an inflammatory response in a chinchilla, the early stages are often characterized by a shift in the differential (e.g., increased heterophils, decreased lymphocytes) rather than an increase in absolute leukocyte count, so evaluation of the entire leukogram is essential. The platelet count can also serve as an important marker of inflammation in chinchillas. Large increases in the platelet count (>1,000,000/µl) may be seen without an increase in the total white blood cell count, indicating an inflammatory process.

Plasma biochemistries can provide important information regarding the physiologic status of a chinchilla. As with any patient, it is important to interpret the results of a chemistry

Plasma Biochemical Parameters for Chinchillas

Biochemical Parameter	Reference Interval
Sodium (mEq/L)	130-170
Potassium (mEq/L)	3-7
Chloride (mEq/L)	110-130
Glucose (mg/dl)	80-125
Blood urea nitrogen (mg/dl)	10-40
Creatinine (mg/dl)	0.8-2.3
Calcium (mg/dl)	8-15
Phosphorous (mg/dl)	4-8
Total protein (g/dl)	5-8
Albumin (g/dl)	2.5-4.0
Globulin (g/dl)	3.5-4.2
Creatine kinase (IU/L)	0-300
Aspartate transferase (IU/L)	15-100
Alkaline phosphatase (IU/L)	10-70
Bilirubin (mg/dl)	0.6-1.3
Cholesterol (mg/dl)	40-300

Data from Quesenberry KE, Donnelly TM, Hillyer EV: Biology, husbandry, and clinical techniques of guinea pigs and chinchillas. In Quesenberry KE, Carpenter JW, editors: *Ferrets, Rabbits, and Rodents: Clinical Medicine and Surgery,* ed 2, St Louis, 2003, WB Saunders; de Oliveria Silva T, Kruetz LC, Barcellos LJG et al: Reference values for chinchilla *(Chinchilla laniger)* blood cells and serum biochemical parameters, *Ciência Rural,* 35(3):602-606, 2005.

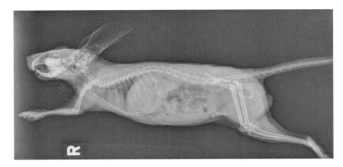

Figure 18-4 A right lateral radiograph of a chinchilla. Note the small size of the thorax and the large size of the abdominal cavity. (Courtesy University of California–Davis.)

panel in conjunction with the anamnesis, physical exam findings, and the results of other diagnostic tests. Reference intervals for various chinchilla biochemical parameters can be found in Box 18-2.

Urinalysis

A urinalysis is an important diagnostic test in chinchilla medicine and should be considered in any case with signs of upper or lower urinary tract disease. Urine samples may be obtained by free catch, floor catch, or cystocentesis. If urine is to be cultured, it should be collected by cystocentesis. The cystocentesis procedure for chinchillas is similar to that described for cats. The animal should be placed in dorsal recumbency for the procedure. Sedation may or may not be necessary. A 25-gauge needle fastened to a 3-ml syringe can be used to collect the sample. The ventral abdomen should be disinfected before needle insertion using standard techniques. Ultrasound can also be used to guide the needle into the bladder.

The urine of chinchillas is typically yellow to amber in color, although the color may be darker and more orange in color depending on the diet. Pigments (e.g., porphyrins) in the urine can sometimes be mistaken for hematuria and must be ruled out by the absence or presence of blood cells on a direct smear. Because chinchillas are herbivores, the pH of chinchilla urine should be alkaline (pH 8.0-9.0).

Diagnostic Imaging

Whole body radiographs can provide a significant amount of information regarding the status of a chinchilla patient. A

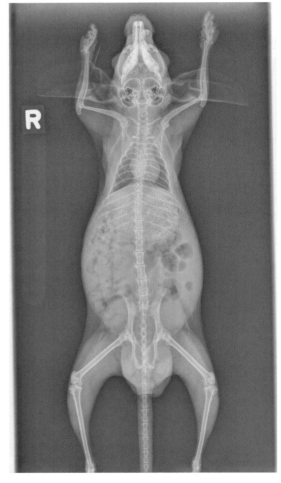

Figure 18-5 A ventrodorsal radiographic view of a chinchilla. Again, note the small size of the thorax and large size of the abdomen in this species. (Courtesy University of California–Davis.)

minimum of two radiographic views should be taken. Our preferences are for lateral and ventrodorsal (or dorsoventral) views (Figures 18-4 and 18-5). Care should be taken to extend the limbs when positioning the patient, to minimize rotation and the superimposition of the limbs over the abdomen or thorax. Chinchillas typically resent aggressive restraint, so sedation or anesthesia is helpful in obtaining diagnostic

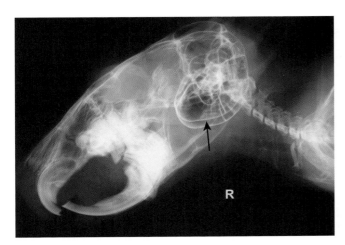

Figure 18-6 Right lateral radiographic view of a chinchilla skull. Note the severe elongation of the crowns and apicies of the premolars and molars as well as the abnormal occlusal angle of the incisors. The large tympanic bullae of the chinchilla are also easily seen *(arrow)*. (Courtesy University of California–Davis.)

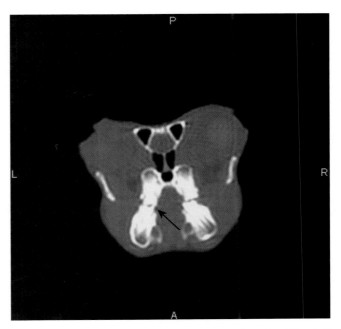

Figure 18-7 Computed tomography image of a chinchilla skull in saggital section. There is mild malocclusion of the cheek teeth visible *(arrow)*. (Courtesy University of California–Davis.)

TABLE 18-1	Guidelines for Radiographic Techniques for Selected Radiographic Studies in Chinchillas	
Anatomic location	**mA**	**kVp**
Whole body	5.0	44
Extremities	6.0	54-56
Skull	6.0	48-52

Data from Silverman S, Tell LA: Radiology equipment and positioning techniques. In Silverman S, Tell LA, editors: *Radiology of Rodents, Rabbits, and Ferrets: An Atlas of Normal Anatomy and Positioning,* St Louis, 2005, WB Saunders. *kVp,* kilovolt peak; *mA,* milliampere.

radiographs as well as in reducing the stress on the patient. Table 18-1 is intended as a general guideline for the techniques used for chinchilla radiographic studies.

Dental malocclusion is a common problem in chinchillas. Skull radiographs can be used to fully assess the degree of malocclusion and secondary bony involvement (Figure 18-6). When taking skull radiographs, it may be necessary to take 3 to 4 different views. In addition to the standard lateral and dorsoventral (or ventrodorsal) views, right and lateral oblique views can be used to more specifically localize lesions. Magnified views of the skull can be obtained by placing the patient on an elevated platform under the x-ray beam without changing the distance between the x-ray cassette and the beam.

Ultrasound is another imaging modality that can be used to diagnose various disease processes in chinchillas. As with radiographs, sedation or anesthesia may be required to reduce patient stress, minimize movement, and improve the overall quality of images that are acquired. The approach to the chinchilla ultrasound exam is similar to that described for domestic species, although there are some exceptions. Chinchillas have a large cecum. If the cecum contains a large quantity of gas, it

may limit the value of an abdominal ultrasound exam. Ultrasound can also be used to assist with the collection of various aspirates (e.g., cystocentesis) or biopsies (e.g., liver biopsy).

Advanced imaging techniques, such as computed tomography (CT) and magnetic resonance imaging (MRI), can also be used to assist in the diagnosis of disease in chinchillas. CT imaging is particularly useful in diagnosing dental problems, such as apical abscesses, osteomyelitis, and minor malocclusions not readily seen on oral examination or radiographs (Figure 18-7). The primary limitations associated with these imaging modalities include limited availability to the general practitioner, the expense associated with the collection and interpretation of the image, and reduced image quality in comparison with that of larger patients. MRI has the added limitation of requiring a significant amount of time (often >45 min) to collect the image.

Regardless of the present limitations associated with these advanced imaging modalities, veterinarians should be made aware that these techniques are available and that reference material exists that depicts normal anatomy for comparison.[5] As chinchilla owners continue to demand high-quality care for their pets, these imaging techniques will likely become more commonplace in exotic small mammal practice.

Microbiology

Chinchillas are susceptible to many of the same pathogens that affect domestic species. The primary pathogens isolated from chinchillas include Gram-negative bacilli (e.g., *Bordetella* spp., *E. coli, Klebsiella* spp., *Salmonella* spp., *Pseudomonas* spp.) and Gram-positive cocci (*Staphylococcus aureus, Streptococcus* spp.). Many of these organisms are opportunists and can be routinely isolated from healthy animals. Samples being submitted for bacterial culture should be collected using sterile swabs and submitted to a diagnostic laboratory capable of isolating and characterizing a range of organisms. The majority of the samples being submitted from chinchillas are for aerobic isolates and require no special attention regarding collection or submission. However, if an anaerobic infection is suspected, it is important to contact the local laboratory to obtain the appropriate materials to collect and submit the samples.

A positive bacterial culture does not necessarily confirm that an organism is responsible for a disease, so it is important to always use the data obtained from the culture, in combination with information obtained from the clinical examination (e.g., elevated body temperature) and additional diagnostic tests (e.g., elevated complete blood count, biopsy, etc.), to confirm a disease. This is especially important in chinchillas, as they are susceptible to antibiotic-induced enteritis and should only be treated with (appropriate) antibiotics when a bacterial infection is highly suspected.

Fungal infections are not common in chinchillas. However, if a fungal infection is suspected (e.g., no response to antibiotics, biopsy results), then standard techniques may be used to isolate the fungus.

Parasitology

Chinchillas may become infested with a variety of endoparasites and ectoparasites. Fortunately, because these animals are bred in captivity, parasites are uncommon. Protozoa (e.g., coccidian) are the most commonly encountered parasites in captive chinchillas. Fecal flotation and/or direct fecal smears mixed with saline can be used to diagnose these infections. These same techniques can be used to diagnose other endoparasites, such as nematodes. Diagnosing ectoparasites in these animals can be done using the same techniques used in domestic animals. Fleas may be identified by closely inspecting the animal hair coat and combing through the fur. Most mites can be identified by using tape preparations or skin scrapes. All of these samples, once collected, should be evaluated under light microscopy.

■ COMMON DISEASE PRESENTATIONS
Infectious
BACTERIAL
Enterotoxemia

One of the most difficult presentations to manage in chinchilla medicine is enterotoxemia. In many of the cases, the animals are presented in severe distress. Lethargy, lateral recumbency, diarrhea, respiratory distress, and fever are all common findings in end-stage disease, whereas in other cases there may be no clinical course of disease and the patients die acutely. *Clostridium perfringens* is commonly associated with this disease.[6,7] In one described outbreak, chinchillas between the ages of 2 and 4 months were most commonly affected.[6] Most of the

affected chinchillas died without showing clinical signs, but some showed signs of colic or diarrhea. This disease reinforces the importance of maintaining the microflora of the chinchilla intestine. The intestinal microflora of the chinchilla is a dynamic mixture of bacteria, protozoa, nematodes, and fungi. In clinically healthy animals, the microflora establish a balance. Alterations to this balance (e.g., administration of inappropriate antibiotics, stress, dietary changes) can result in the overgrowth of certain pathogenic organisms. A number of the bacteria of the microflora produce toxins as a natural defense mechanism against other bacteria and a host's immune response. When these toxins are produced in excess, as is seen with the overgrowth of certain microbes, the host can suffer the consequences. Diagnosing enterotoxemia can be difficult and is generally a postmortem diagnosis. Serial antemortem fecal/rectal cultures may provide insight as to the causative agent. Hematologic results are often consistent with a toxic inflammatory response. Radiographs frequently reveal significant gas within the intestinal tract and an ileus. Treating these patients is difficult. Supportive care, including intravenous fluids and caloric support, should be instituted. Nonsteroidal antiinflammatories may provide some protection against the toxins. If a positive culture is made, an antibiotic sensitivity profile can be performed to determine the most appropriate antibiotic to use for treatment. Because treating enterotoxemia is difficult, it is best to focus on prevention. Judicious use of antibiotics by veterinarians and breeders, as well as providing a balanced, consistent diet, washing all fresh food products thoroughly, practicing strict sanitary practices, and minimizing environmental stress, are practices that can reduce the likelihood of enterotoxemia in a patient.

Enteritis

Enteritis is a common disease in chinchillas and can occur from numerous underlying causes, including diet change or inappropriate diet, improper antibiotic use, stress, and various infectious organisms (e.g., coccidia, *Giardia* spp., *Cryptosporidium* spp., *E. coli, Clostridium* spp., *Proteus* spp., *Pseudomonas* spp., *Staphylococcus* spp., and *Salmonella* spp.).[2,8,9]

Clinical signs associated with enteritis are variable but can include abdominal pain, diarrhea, decreased fecal output, intussusception, intestinal impaction, and rectal prolapse.[8,10] Treatment of enteritis should focus on identifying the underlying cause and treating the presenting signs. Further diagnostics that may be necessary to identify an underlying cause are radiographs, abdominal ultrasound, fecal examinations for parasites and bacteria, and fecal cultures. If a condition such as intestinal intussusception or impaction occurs and requires surgery, the patient should be stabilized first. Nutritional supplementation, fluid replenishment, pain management, and appropriate antibiotic therapy (ideally based on fecal culture and sensitivity) are facets of stabilization in these patients.

Salmonella

Salmonella sp. is a Gram-negative rod from the family Enterobacteriaceae. All members of this genus are considered pathogenic and have been associated with disease in all of the different classes of vertebrates. In chinchillas, infections with this bacterium have been associated with acute death. In an epizootic in Australia involving five chinchilla farms, both *Salmonella* Enteritidis and *Salmonella* Sofia were isolated at necropsy.[11] Affected animals were found to have gastritis, enteritis, splenomegaly, and hepatitis. *Salmonella* sp. was not isolated from any of the fecal samples collected from the affected herds following a course of treatment with enrofloxacin. Isolates were found to be resistant to sulfamethoxazole, but this was attributed to the fact that this drug was routinely added to the chinchillas' feed.

Salmonella sp. may be occasionally isolated from clinically healthy chinchillas. We do not recommend treating unaffected animals, as the risk of antibiotic resistance increases with exposure to antibiotics. In cases where a *Salmonella* sp. is isolated from a clinically diseased animal, the antibiotic selected for treatment should be based on the antibiotic sensitivity profile. If this profile is pending, fluoroquinolones are an excellent first choice antibiotic. Many of the *Salmonella* spp. isolated from chinchillas can be directly attributed to human environments. Because of this, it is important that clients thoroughly wash the fresh foods that they provide their pets and always practice strict hygiene when cleaning their pet's environment.

Listeriosis

Chinchillas appear to be highly susceptible to infections caused by *Listeria monocytogenes*. Ranched chinchillas, which are often fed silage as a portion of their diet, are most commonly affected. This increased risk is primarily attributed to the fact that *L. monocytogenes* thrives in decaying organic matter. Signs of infection can originate from the gastrointestinal or central nervous systems. Clinical signs are usually vague but may include depression, anorexia, weight loss, and diarrhea.[2] In one outbreak, 47 animals from seven ranches were diagnosed with listeriosis. Contaminated food was the suspected source. The course of disease in these animals was short, with the animals primarily displaying gastrointestinal disease and succumbing within 24 hours.[12] *L. ivanovii* has also been described in a single chinchilla.[13] This chinchilla died shortly after purchase. At necropsy, multifocal areas of necrosis and suppurative inflammation were found in the liver. *L. ivanovii* was isolated from these lesions. These cases reaffirm the importance of providing these animals high-quality forage. Clients should request only fresh grass hays for their chinchillas. Grass hay with signs of mold or necrosis should be discarded. Diagnosing listeriosis using antemortem tests can be difficult. Hematology and radiographs are generally suggestive of an inflammatory response of an infectious nature and a corresponding enteritis. Cultures can be attempted, but veterinarians should contact the laboratory to ensure that the samples are collected and processed appropriately. Treatment for this disease is generally based on the provision of supportive care.

FUNGAL

Dermatophytes

Because of the extremely dense nature of the chinchilla's hair coat (up to 90,000 fibers per square inch),[14] ectoparasite infes-

tations are uncommon compared with other mammalian species. Dermatophytosis, however, is not uncommon. *Trichophyton mentagrophytes* is the most commonly isolated dermatophyte in chinchillas, although *Microsporum canis* and *M. gypseum* infections have also been reported.[2,8,9] Dermatophyte lesions can occur on any surface of the body but are most often found on the head and face. The lesions associated with these parasites are similar to those described for domestic species and are typically scaly and alopecic. Diagnosis is based on the results of a dermatophyte culture. Treatment with oral antifungal medications and or topical antifungals is required to resolve the lesions.[8,9] Eliminating the infections can require several weeks of treatment. Because of the zoonotic potential associated with these infections, owners should be educated about handling their chinchillas during the treatment period. We recommend that clients wear latex or nonlatex exam gloves when treating their pets and that children not handle the chinchilla during the treatment period. Clients should also be directed to contact their personal physician if they develop dermatologic conditions consistent with a dermatophyte infection.

Parasitic

ENDOPARASITES

Several parasitic diseases have been reported as causes of gastrointestinal disease in chinchillas; however, most of the reports have been in farm-ranched chinchillas. The incidence of parasitism in pet chinchillas is relatively low and is most likely due to the fact that these animals are housed indoors. *Giardia* spp. are often found in low numbers in normal chinchillas.[15] These parasites can cause problems when, combined with housing stress and poor hygiene, they develop into active infections with severe diarrhea and even death.[16] One report of *Cryptosporidium* spp. infection has been reported in a young chinchilla.[17] This chinchilla had a severe diarrhea that was not responsive to supportive therapy and ultimately succumbed to the infection. Diagnosing endoparasites of the intestinal tract can be done using standard techniques (see Diagnostic Testing: Parasitology).

Larval Migrans

Baylisascaris procyonis, the raccoon roundworm, has been associated with larval migrans in a number of different vertebrates. The raccoon is the definitive host of this parasite. In nonraccoon hosts, this parasite has a predilection for ophthalmic and neural tissue. Once an animal is infected, the prognosis for the animal is guarded to grave. This parasite has been associated with disease in a group of farmed chinchillas.[18] Affected animals were found to have clinical signs associated with neurologic disease, including ataxia, incoordination, and paralysis. Malacic tracts consistent with parasitic migration were identified in the brains of five animals presented for necropsy, and *Baylisascaris procyonis* larvae were identified in two of these animals. The chinchillas were exposed to the parasite after being fed hay that had been contaminated with raccoon feces. Although not described in pet chinchillas, *B. procyonis* should be included on any differential list for chinchillas displaying neurologic signs, especially those given access to the outdoors where they could potentially come in contact with raccoon droppings.

ECTOPARASITES

Chinchillas are susceptible to various ectoparasites, including fleas, mites, and ticks. Ectoparasites are not common in pet animals, because they are generally housed in limited numbers and housed indoors. When chinchillas present with a history of crusting and scaling that is consistent with ectoparasitism, it is important for the veterinarian to pursue the case using standard diagnostics. Skin scrapes and tape preparations are the most common initial tests. The majority of ectoparasites found on chinchillas, excluding fleas, are responsive to ivermectin (0.2-0.4 mg/kg). The course of treatment will depend on the life cycle of the parasite. In most cases, 2 to 3 treatments every 14 days will eliminate most ectoparasites. During the ivermectin treatment, it is also important that the owner clean the animal's enclosure daily to remove any adult organisms or eggs that fall into the substrate.

Neoplasia

Neoplastic disease processes are relatively uncommon, or at least uncommonly described in the literature, in chinchillas. However, several tumor types have been documented as occurring in chinchillas, including neuroblastoma, carcinoma, lipoma, and hemangiosarcoma. Unfortunately, because many of these diagnoses are associated with farmed chinchillas from the 1950s, there are no detailed pathologic descriptions or even descriptions of the organ(s) involved.[14] The Animal Medical Center in New York conducted a 5-year retrospective study of chinchillas and found only one neoplasm, a uterine lyomyosarcoma, among all of the chinchillas examined. The tumor was an incidental finding at necropsy.[14] One case of malignant lymphoma in a chinchilla is described in the literature.[19] This chinchilla displayed marked lymphadenopathy and evidence of metastases to the liver, spleen, and kidneys.

Even though descriptions of neoplastic diseases are not well reported in chinchillas, as owners begin seeking more routine care for their pets and as appropriate care results in longer lives, veterinarians caring for these animals are more likely to encounter such geriatric diseases as neoplasia.

Miscellaneous
GASTROINTESTINAL

To reinforce the importance of the gastrointestinal tract to the inner workings of a chinchilla, one of us (Mitchell) often states that the "chinchilla is basically a bowel wrapped in fur." Although this may seem rather simplistic, it is the gastrointestinal tract that serves as the major site of complications for these animals. Veterinarians working with these animals should always reinforce to their clients the importance of maintaining the function of the gastrointestinal tract to ensure the good health of their pet.

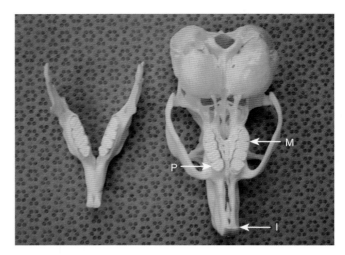

Figure 18-8 Open view of a chinchilla skull. (*I*, incisor; *P*, premolar; *M*, molar.)

DENTAL DISEASE

The dentition of the chinchilla is *aradicular hypsodont,* meaning all teeth are continuously growing and open-rooted.[20] This is an important concept, as any damage to the teeth or inherent (e.g., genetic) changes to the growth of the teeth can result in malocclusion. The dental formula of the chinchilla is similar to that found in the guinea pig: I 1/1, C 0/0, P 1/1, M 3/3 (Figure 18-8). As in other rodent species but differing from lagomorphs, the mandible is wider than the maxilla and has an occlusal angle that is lowest at the lingual surface. The normal occlusal angle of the chinchilla is very slight, only 5 to 10 degrees from flat. The enamel on the cranial surface of the incisors of chinchillas is normally orange in color and should not be mistaken for a pathologic condition (see Figure 18-3).

The clinical signs associated with dental disease in chinchillas are similar to those seen in guinea pigs and rabbits, including decreased appetite or dysphagia, weight loss, ptyalism, decreased fecal output, and poor coat quality.[21-24] Abscessation of the molar and premolar apices can also occur with the overgrowth of these teeth. Ocular and/or nasal discharge is another common clinical sign seen in chinchilla patients with dental disease. Because the premolars and molars are elodont (open-rooted), it is possible that the apical surfaces of these teeth can overgrow and impinge on the nasolacrimal duct, causing ocular discharge. The apicies can also overgrow into the nasal cavity, which could result in the seeding of the sinuses with bacteria from the oral cavity.

Diagnosing dental disease in chinchillas requires a thorough evaluation of the animal's history and close inspection of the animal's oral cavity. Animals with a genetic history of malocclusion, or that are maintained on an inappropriate diet, should be examined regularly to prevent severe dental disease. Careful palpation of the ventral mandible and maxilla may reveal bony protuberances that correspond to the overgrowth of the apical surfaces of the cheek teeth. To thoroughly examine the oral cavity, it is important to have the appropriate

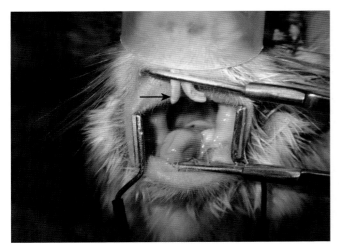

Figure 18-9 Severe incisor malocclusion *(arrow)* in a chinchilla.

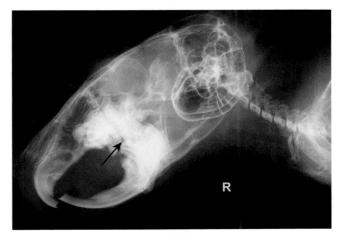

Figure 18-11 Lateral view of a chinchilla skull showing severe malocclusion of the cheek teeth *(arrow)*, with overgrowth of the apices of the molars and premolars. (Courtesy University of California–Davis.)

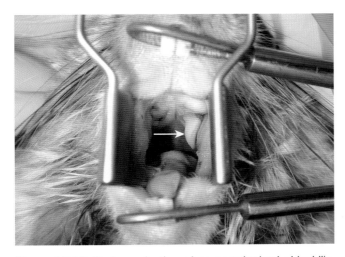

Figure 18-10 Oral examination of an anesthetized chinchilla, demonstrating a large buccal point on a left maxillary premolar *(arrow)*. Note the use of incisor dilators and pouch dilators to improve visualization of the oral cavity.

equipment. Dental specula and pouch dilators are invaluable aids in obtaining an adequate view of the molars and premolars; however, many abnormalities can be overlooked in a conscious animal, and anesthesia is often required to obtain a thorough oral examination. Abnormal oral examination findings that are commonly seen in chinchillas may include an uneven occlusal surface or angle of the incisors and/or cheek teeth (Figure 18-9), formation of sharp points (Figure 18-10) with or without associated ulceration of the oral mucosa, food impaction, and abnormal spaces (diastema) between teeth.

Imaging modalities, including whole body radiographs, magnified skull radiographs, and CT, can be incorporated to better evaluate the extent and seriousness of the process. Radiographic studies should include dorsoventral, lateral (Figure 18-11), and right and left oblique views.

Treatment of dental malocclusion in chinchillas centers on restoring a normal occlusal plane to the teeth. This is a procedure that must be performed under general anesthesia to allow adequate visualization of the oral cavity and to minimize stress to the patient. Patients that are dehydrated have altered gastrointestinal motility, or other potentially complicating symptoms and should be provided with supportive care before undergoing the anesthetic event.

Utilizing the right tools is important to ensure the best outcome of treatment. A high-speed surgical dental handpiece can be used to restore a normal occlusal plane and to reduce any sharp points that have formed because of improper wear. Handheld trimmers, such as canine nail trimmers, are not acceptable, as they tend to crush teeth and can cause fractures and pulp exposure.[23] Dremel tools are not acceptable either because the small size of the chinchilla's oral cavity will not allow for appropriate trimming. With any dental instruments, care should be observed to minimize oral soft tissue trauma.

Dental malocclusion is a disease that can be managed but rarely cured. The owners of chinchillas diagnosed with malocclusion must be made aware that this will be a lifelong problem for their pets; it will require repeated anesthetic procedures, which could result in significant cost. With many cases, routine occlusal adjustments will be necessary for the remainder of the animal's life.

One of the most significant differences seen with malocclusions in chinchillas—as compared with other rodent species and rabbits—is that it is not infrequent for a chinchilla's oral exam to be normal while significant disease is present in the portions of the tooth that are not visible. For this reason, imaging, such as skull radiographs or CT, is especially useful in these patients to determine the extent of the disease as well as the presence of apical abscesses or osteomyelitis, which may complicate treatment. Chinchillas normally have very short clinical crowns, limiting the amount of correction that may be performed during occlusal adjustments.

Because dental disease appears to have a heritable component, animals with dental disease should not be allowed to breed.[21,22] A dietary component is also considered likely.[23,25] Owners of chinchillas with malocclusion should be advised to increase the amount of roughage in the animal's diet to increase the grinding motion of the teeth and increase wear.

CHOKE/BLOAT

Like other rodent species, chinchillas do not have the ability to vomit. Because of this, small pieces of food can become lodged in the esophagus. When this occurs, it is generally referred to as "choke." The most common food items that become lodged in the esophagus are small treat items (e.g., raisins and nuts) that are not thoroughly chewed. Choke can also occur in chinchillas with dental malocclusion and often results from the animal's inability to chew their food properly. The clinical signs most commonly observed in a chinchilla with choke include retching, ptyalism, pawing at the mouth, anorexia, and respiratory distress.[9] If left untreated, a chinchilla with choke will die. Diagnosing choke in chinchillas should follow the same standard protocol as for any gastrointestinal foreign body. Hematologic testing should be done to evaluate the patient's physiologic status. Radiographs should be taken to determine the location of the foreign body. In many cases, the foreign material can be retrieved using an endoscope. Supportive care, including fluids and caloric support, should be provided to the patient to ensure that the gastrointestinal tract continues to function. However, caloric support should not be instituted until after the foreign material is removed or after a feeding tube has been placed that is distal to the foreign body.

Bloat, often a common sequela to choke, occurs because the obstruction of the esophagus does not allow the animal to eructate and release the gas that accumulates in the stomach. Animals with bloat are often depressed, painful on palpation, and lethargic. A diagnosis of gastric tympany can be confirmed via radiographs. Removing the foreign material from the esophagus will resolve the bloat. In an emergency situation, the gas within the stomach can be relieved via aspiration through a needle. The prognosis for chinchillas with bloat is guarded to grave.

UROGENITAL
Fur Ring

Fur ring is a generic name used to describe a common condition in male chinchillas, in which the fur surrounding the base of the penis can accumulate and form a restrictive ring. This is often a subclinical problem, but it can progress into causing paraphimosis or inflammation of the penis. To prevent this from occurring, clients should be shown how to routinely examine the prepuce for the accumulation of fur and how to extract the penis from the prepuce to inspect it for signs of inflammation.

Clinical signs associated with fur ring can include stranguria, excessive grooming of the prepucial area, lethargy, and decreased appetite. This condition can be resolved by removing the fur ring. Sedation or anesthesia may be required for those animals that cannot be restrained manually. If paraphimosis has occurred, a hypertonic solution (e.g., 50% dextrose) can be applied to the penis to reduce the edema and facilitate replacement of the organ. A sterile, water-based lubricant can also be used to aid in replacing the penis into the prepuce.

DERMATOLOGIC CONDITIONS
Fur Slip

Because chinchillas have evolved as a prey species, it was important for them to develop protective measures against predators. As it is common for predators to grab or bite the skin of a prey species when they attempt to capture them, it would seem logical that to have a mechanism to prevent this from occurring would increase the likelihood of survival for a species. Chinchillas have developed an adaptive process that allows for a clump of fur that is grabbed roughly to easily epilate. This is known as *fur slip,* and can be problematic in both ranched and pet populations. Large areas of fur can be easily epilated when a chinchilla is handled roughly or is fighting with another chinchilla. While the underlying skin is usually not damaged, regrowth of the missing fur can take up to 4 to 6 months.[2] For ranched animals this is associated with a significant loss of money. In captive pet animals, this can lead to a decrease in aesthetics. Fortunately, fur slip can be avoided in captive situations by teaching support staff and clients how to properly handle a chinchilla. In cases where this is associated with combat between male chinchillas, it is important to separate animals to prevent contact.

Fur Chewing (Barbering)

Chinchillas occasionally develop a tendency to overgroom or barber their own fur or the fur of a cagemate. This can result in an animal having an unkempt or uneven hair coat quality. The underlying cause for this negative behavior is not known, but there are a number of suspected causes, including boredom or housing stress, poor diet (e.g., low fiber), or hereditary factors.[1,2] Histopathologic examination and testing of the adrenal and thyroid glands of fur-chewing chinchillas have demonstrated increased hormone activity in these glands that is consistent with stress-induced changes.[26,27] Histopathologic changes consistent with Cushing's disease (e.g., cutaneous calcinosis, comedone formation) have also been described in fur-chewing chinchillas, suggesting that stress and genetics may both play roles in the development of this problem.[27]

MUSCULOSKELETAL

Fractures of the long bones of the pelvic and thoracic limbs are relatively common in chinchillas. Improper caging, such as wire flooring with spaces large enough for a limb to become entrapped, and improper handling are common causes. Chinchillas are likely more prone to fractures of the distal limbs because of the relatively long, delicate construction of the limbs in comparison with the stocky body (Figures 18-12 and 18-13).

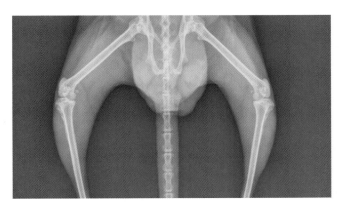

Figure 18-12 A ventrodorsal radiograph of the pelvic limbs of a chinchilla, demonstrating the delicate structure of the long bones, particularly the tibia. (Courtesy University of California–Davis.)

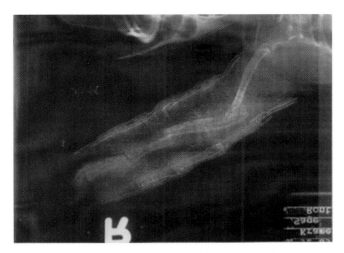

Figure 18-14 A lateral radiograph of the forelimb of a chinchilla demonstrating the use of external coaptation for stabilization of mid-diaphyseal fractures of the radius and ulna. (Courtesy University of California–Davis.)

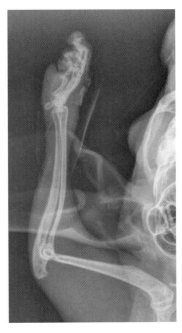

Figure 18-13 A ventrodorsal radiograph of the right forelimb of a chinchilla. (Courtesy University of California–Davis.)

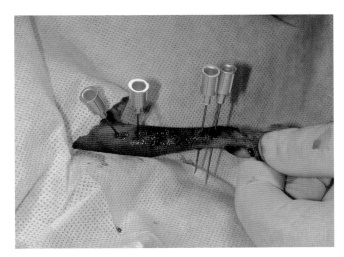

Figure 8-15 Application of a Type-II external skeletal fixator using hypodermic needles as cross bars. (Courtesy Paul M. Gibbons, DVM, MS, DABVP [Avian].)

The cortices of the long bones of chinchillas are rather thin and brittle and are covered with little soft tissue.[14,28] For these reasons, fractures of the limbs are often comminuted and open, complicating repair. External coaptation (Figure 18-14) is typically not adequate for stabilization of these fractures, and surgical repair is often necessary. Because these bones are so thin and fragile, most orthopedic equipment available for use in domestic animals is too large, and the veterinarian must be creative in developing fixators using such components as small K-wires and hypodermic or spinal needles (Figure 18-15). Chinchillas are rather active animals, and strict cage rest is extremely important for a positive outcome of any fracture repair.

Unfortunately, despite the type of fracture fixation, malunion fractures are common in chinchillas. Degree of commi-

nution, contamination of the fracture site, and poor soft tissue coverage are all contributing factors. Because malunion occurs frequently, owners should be made aware of this possibility from the beginning of treatment. Fortunately, chinchillas typically adapt well to the loss of a limb, so amputation does not affect them negatively in the long run.

HEART DISEASE

Heart murmurs are relatively common physical exam findings in chinchillas. Anecdotal reports suggest cardiomyopathy as a possible underlying cause.[14] One report exists of a heart murmur in a young, male chinchilla that was found to be caused by a ventricular septal defect and tricuspid valve regurgitation on echocardiography,[29] but cardiomyopathy has not been reported as a significant cause of cardiac disease in chinchillas.

Chinchilla patients with cardiac murmurs should be treated as any domestic pet with a heart murmur. Thoracic radiographs, electrocardiography, and echocardiography may be necessary to achieve a diagnosis. As more chinchilla owners begin seeking a higher level of veterinary care for their pets, cardiac disease may become more commonly reported and better described.

LEAD TOXICOSIS

There have been a few cases of lead toxicosis in chinchillas reported in the literature. Blood concentrations of lead higher than 15µg/dl are considered suspicious for lead toxicosis, and levels higher than 25µg/dl are considered definitive.[14] Chinchillas affected with lead toxicosis display primarily neurologic signs, including seizures and blindness.[8,30] These cases were successfully treated with calcium disodium edentate (25 mg/kg SC q6h × 5 days,[30] 30 mg/kg SC q12h × 5 days[8]). Interestingly, in the reported cases of lead toxicosis in chinchillas, the affected animals were housed in older apartments in urban neighborhoods. Because of the tendency of rodents to gnaw on different surfaces, lead toxicosis should be included on any differential list for animals with neurologic disease and exposure to lead-based paints.

HEATSTROKE

Chinchillas are native to the cool mountainous regions of South America and are therefore rather intolerant to temperatures higher than 80° F.[10,14,31] Ideally, chinchillas should be housed in well-ventilated enclosures at temperatures between 65° F and 75° F. Animals that are exposed to excess heat can develop life-threatening heatstroke. Clinical signs in affected animals include panting, lethargy, poor peripheral perfusion, and ptyalism.[10] Treatment includes reducing the animal's core body temperature with cool water baths or the application of alcohol to the feet and ears and fluid therapy (either intravenously or subcutaneously) to improve perfusion. It is important to cool the animal gradually, as a rapid decrease in body temperature can induce a life-threatening hypothermia. Nonsteroidal antiinflammatories and antibiotics are often recommended to minimize endotoxemia and overgrowth of opportunistic pathogens, respectively. The prognosis for this condition is guarded to grave.

DIABETES MELLITUS

Diabetes mellitus has been reported in a single obese female chinchilla.[32] Clinical signs in this chinchilla were similar to those seen in domestic animals and included polydipsia, polyuria, weight loss, lethargy, and bilateral cataracts.[22,32] This chinchilla had a blood glucose of higher than 400 mg/dl, glucosuria, and ketonuria. Treatment with insulin, 2 to 12 IU daily, did not succeed in controlling the hyperglycemia, and the chinchilla was eventually euthanized. Histopathologically, the pancreas was found to have marked vacuolation of the islet cells, consistent with diabetes mellitus.

■ THERAPEUTICS

Fluids

Chinchillas, like other rodents, are highly dependent on the function of their gastrointestinal tract to provide essential calories in the form of volatile fatty acids. Any changes to the function of the intestinal tract can be catastrophic to the animal. Unfortunately, when these animals become dehydrated, it is often the gastrointestinal tract that suffers. The shift of the fluid balance to maintain the function of the brain and heart often comes at the expense of the gastrointestinal tract. As the shift in the fluid balance occurs, gastrointestinal motility diminishes, microflora changes occur, and the animals reduce their dietary intake and production of calories. If left untreated, these patients die. To minimize the likelihood of this occurring, it is essential that these patients receive parenteral fluids. Replacement of a fluid deficit, and the maintenance of normal hydration, can be achieved by administering crystalloid substances via the subcutaneous, intravenous, intraperitoneal, or intraosseous routes. In cases of severe dehydration, the intravenous and intraosseous routes are preferred. For mild dehydration, or when the animal cannot be catheterized, the oral, subcutaneous, or intraperitoneal routes can be used.

In those cases where the gastrointestinal tract is functioning normally, and the patient is only mildly dehydrated, replacement fluids can be delivered per os. The simplest method of delivering fluids per os is via a syringe. Some chinchillas will tolerate this, whereas other will not. Mixing the water with food or using fruit-flavored electrolyte solutions may increase success. Chinchillas can also be provided per os fluids via a feeding tube; however, this is often difficult to do in these animals because of their narrow, long oral cavity. In those cases where a chinchilla will not accept fluids via a syringe, we rely on the other techniques of providing fluids (e.g., subcutaneous fluids).

Subcutaneous fluid administration is generally well tolerated by chinchillas. Fluids can be administered into the subcutaneous space of the dorsal or lateral thorax, similar to that described for domestic species. When grasping the skin to introduce the needle, care should be taken to avoid causing fur slip. Butterfly catheters can be used to deliver fluids via the subcutaneous space; these catheters allow the patient to move around without pulling out the injection needle. The quantity of fluids that can be administered in a single space should be based on the size of the animal and elasticity of the skin. Fluids should be administered only to a point where the skin is mildly stretched, not taut. In many cases, veterinarians should use their best judgement when determining a maximum volume to deliver. Veterinarians should remember that they can deliver the fluids into multiple subcutaneous sites or increase the frequency of fluid administration over the course of a day to diminish the volume that needs to be delivered at a single point in time. The primary disadvantage associated with the delivery of drugs via the subcutaneous route is that fluid absorption is not as rapid as with the other routes. Another disadvantage is that there are certain types of fluids that should not be delivered via this route, such as 5% or higher dextrose. This type of fluid can be irritating to the subcutaneous space. However, we have delivered lower concentrations of dextrose (2.5%) via this route without concern.

The intraperitoneal cavity is an underutilized route of fluid administration in chinchillas. We prefer this route for moderately to severely dehydrated juvenile animals and adult animals that have collapsed peripheral veins. Fluids administered via the intraperitoneal route are presumed to be absorbed via the serosal surfaces of the viscera and the peritoneal membrane. Because of the large surface area of the peritoneal membrane and visceral surfaces, larger boluses of fluids can be provided via this route. However, care should be taken to avoid inducing an ascites. This is best prevented by monitoring the hydration status of the animal closely during treatment and routinely inspecting the size (direct visualization) and fluid status (ultrasonography) of the abdomen. The chinchilla should be placed into dorsal recumbency for the procedure, as this will allow gravity to displace the organs away from the injection site. The injection site should be disinfected using standard protocols. The needle should be inserted at a 20- to 30-degree angle off the abdominal wall. A sharper angle will increase the likelihood of inserting the needle into the viscera. Veterinarians should always aspirate the syringe before delivering the fluids to ensure that the fluids are not going to be delivered into an organ. The fluids being inserted into the abdomen should always be prepared at body temperature, as the provision of cool fluids into the abdomen can be painful to the animal and require additional energy from the animal to maintain its core temperature.

When chinchillas are severely dehydrated and the peripheral vessels are collapsed, fluids can be administered via the intraosseous route. The proximal femur and tibia are the preferred sites for catheter placement. We suggest clipping the fur surrounding the proximal femur to increase the likelihood of visualizing the insertion landmarks. The injection site should be disinfected using standard sterile techniques to limit the likelihood of inducing an osteomyelitis. For a catheter being placed into the proximal femur, the space between the neck of the femur and the greater trochanter should be used as the insertion landmarks. For catheters being placed into the proximal tibia, the tibial crest is the insertion landmark. A spinal needle with a stylet should be used for the procedure to limit the likelihood of coring the needle. We secure the catheters into place using butterfly tape and suture, and we generally leave the catheters in place for 72 to 96 hours.

Intravenous catheters remain the preferred route of delivering fluids in severely dehydrated chinchillas. The primary vessels used for intravenous fluids are the cephalic, lateral and medial saphenous, and jugular veins. To ensure the patency of the smaller peripheral vessels, we tend to use only the jugular veins for venipuncture. The peripheral vessels in these animals tend to be very moveable under the skin in comparison with those in other domestic mammals. We find that the likelihood of inserting an intravenous catheter increases significantly when the animal is sedated. Once a catheter is placed, it should be secured using standard bandaging techniques. In some cases, a distasteful substance may need to be placed on the bandage to prevent the chinchilla from extracting the catheter. An Elizabethan collar constructed out of exposed radiograph film may also be used to prevent a chinchilla from tampering with its catheter.

Antimicrobial Therapy

Because many of the diseases diagnosed in chinchillas have a bacterial origin, the use of antibiotics in the captive management of this species is common. It is important to remember, however, that the indigenous microflora of these animals is predominantly Gram positive and that certain antibiotics can cause severe changes (antibiotic induced dysbiosis) in the bacterial population of the chinchilla gastrointestinal tract. Enteral administration of penicillins (e.g., amoxicillin, ampicillin), macrolides (e.g., erythromycin, lincomycin), and first-generation cephalosporins are most commonly associated with these changes.[8] A list of common antibiotics used in these animals can be found in Table 18-2. As fungal disease can also occur in these animals, in some cases as a direct result of the misuse of antibiotics, it is important to be familiar with dosages for these compounds too (see Table 18-2).

TABLE 18-2   Common Antimicrobials Used in Chinchilla Medicine

Drug	Route(s) of administration	Dosage(s)[33-35]	Dose frequency
Chloramphenicol	PO, SC, IM, IV	30-50 mg/kg	q12h
Ciprofloxacin	PO	5-20 mg/kg	q12h
Enrofloxacin	PO, SC, IM	5-15 mg/kg	q12h
Metronidazole*	PO	10-20 mg/kg	q12h
Trimethoprim-sulfa	PO, SC, IM	15-30 mg/kg	q12h
Anti-fungal agents			
Griseofulvin	PO	25 mg/kg	q24h
Ketoconazole	PO	10-40 mg/kg	q24h
Itraconazole	PO	5 mg/kg	q24h

*Use with caution.
IM, intramuscular; *IV*, intravenous; *PO*, per os; *SC*, subcutaneous.

TABLE 18-3	Antiparasitic Drugs Commonly Used in Chinchilla Medicine		
Drug	**Route(s) of administration**	**Dosage(s)[33-35]**	**Dose frequency**
Fenbendazole	PO	20 mg/kg	q24h
Ivermectin	SC	0.2-0.4 mg/kg	q7-14days
Lime-sulfur dip	Topical	–	q7days
Metronidazole*	PO	10-30 mg/kg	q12h
Praziquantel	PO, SC, IM	5-10 mg/kg	q10-14days
Sulfadimethoxine	PO	25-50 mg/kg	q24h

*Use with caution.
IM, intramuscular; *PO,* per os; *SC,* subcutaneous.

TABLE 18-4	Common Emergency Drugs Used in Chinchilla Medicine		
Drug	**Route(s) of administration**	**Dose(s)[33-35]**	**Dose frequency**
Epinephrine	IV, IT, IO, IC	0.2 mg/kg	prn
Dopram	IV, IT, IO, IC	20 mg/kg	prn
Furosemide	PO, SC, IM, IV (low dose)	2-10 mg/kg	q12h
Atropine	IM, IT, IC	0.1-0.2 mg/kg	prn

IC, intracardiac; *IO,* intraosseous; *IT,* intratracheal; *IV,* intravenous, *prn,* as needed; *SC,* subcutaneous.

Antiparasitic Therapy

Chinchillas that present with parasites should be treated promptly to limit the spread of disease between conspecifics. In a previous section of this chapter we reviewed the most common parasites identified in captive chinchillas. Table 18-3 represents a list of the compounds that can be used to treat these parasites.

Emergency Drugs

Because of their ability to mask illness, chinchillas routinely present to veterinary clinics in emergency situations. It is also not uncommon for these animals to become emergencies during their stay in a hospital (e.g., enterotoxemia) or as a result of an anesthetic event. Although the prognosis for these cases is guarded to grave, attempts to provide emergency care should be made. A list of common emergency drugs used in chinchilla medicine can be found in Table 18-4.

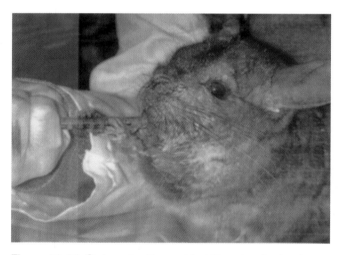

Figure 18-16 Syringe feeding a chinchilla using 1-ml syringes.

Nutritional Support

Nutritional support should be considered for any chinchilla that is not eating. Anorexic chinchillas can experience a significant change in their gastrointestinal microflora in as little as 8 to 12 hours. This change in the microflora can lead to ileus, colic, overgrowth of pathogenic bacteria, and enterotoxemia. To minimize the likelihood of the gastrointestinal tract from slowing or stopping, it is important to provide these animals calories. Oxbow Critical Care for herbivores (Oxbow Hay Company, Murdock, NE) is a commercial product that we have used with good success. This enteral provides essential calories and contains bacteria that can be used to refaunate the gastrointestinal microflora. It is important to follow the manufacturer's feeding recommendations to ensure that the desired quantity of calories is provided. Patients will often eat the enteral directly from a dish or can be force-fed via a 60-ml catheter tip syringe. For patients that are more resistant to eating, a technique that we have used is to remove the plungers from 1-ml or 3-ml syringes and fill them individually using a catheter tip syringe (Figure 18-16). Although this method may seem tedious, it allows the delivery of small boluses of food to be incrementally dispensed.

TABLE 18-5	Common Therapeutic Agents Used to Treat Chinchillas		
Drug	**Route(s) of administration**	**Dosage(s)[33-35]**	**Dose frequency**
Cimetidine	PO, SC, IM, IV	5-10 mg/kg	q6-12h
Cisapride	PO	0.1-0.5 mg/kg	q8-12h
Diphenhydramine	PO, SC	1-2 mg/kg	q12h
Furosemide	PO, SC	2-10 mg/kg	q12h
Lactated Ringer's	SC, IV	50-100 ml/kg	q24h
Metoclopramide	PO, SC, IM	0.2-1.0 mg/kg	q12h
Sucralfate	PO	25-100 mg/kg	q8-12h

IM, intramuscular; *IV,* intravenous; *PO,* per os; *SC,* subcutaneous.

Miscellaneous Drugs

Chinchillas, like domestic pets, can present to a veterinary hospital for a variety of different disease conditions. Because of this, it is important to consider treating these animals with the same compounds used to manage domestic pets. Unfortunately, the drugs used in small animal medicine are untested in chinchillas. To limit liability, it is important for the veterinarian to explain and document to their clients the limitations associated with the use of any therapeutic when treating their chinchilla patients. In our opinion, however, it is better to treat and accept a smaller risk than to not treat and accept certain patient loss. A list of common therapeutics used, at least anecdotally, in chinchilla medicine can be found in Table 18-5.

■SURGERY

Preoperative and Postoperative Considerations

CATHETERIZATION

As with venipuncture, catheterization for fluid or drug administration in chinchillas can be a challenge. Peripheral vessels typically used for catheterization in dogs and cats, such as the cephalic and lateral saphenous veins, are very small in chinchillas. Because of their small size, 24- to 26-gauge intravenous catheters are considered the most useful in these patients (Figure 18-17). However, small-gauge catheters tend to bend when piercing the skin. Catheter failure can be prevented by making a small puncture in the skin using a 22-gauge needle before placing the catheter. Care should be taken to avoid lacerating the vein before introducing the catheter.[36] In some cases, sedating the chinchilla may reduce the stress and ease catheter of placement.

Intraosseous catheters can be used as an alternative to intravenous catheters. The most common sites for intraosseous catheterization in the chinchilla are the proximal femur and the proximal tibia.[36] A spinal needle with a stylet is preferred. Because intraosseous catheterization is a painful procedure, patients should be placed under general anesthesia and topical anesthetic (e.g., lidocaine) used to reduce the pain at the insertion site. If the patient is debilitated and general anesthesia is a risk, then the local is generally sufficient to place the catheter. The catheter insertion site should be disinfected using standard

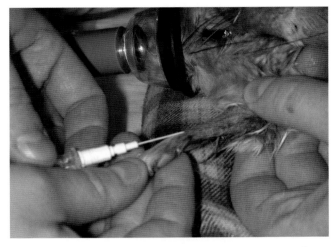

Figure 18-17 Placement of a 26-gauge intravenous catheter into the cephalic vein of a chinchilla.

aseptic techniques to minimize the risk associated with introducing pathogens. After placement, the catheter should be secured with a butterfly (tape) placed around the catheter hub and then sutured to the skin.

INTUBATION

Intubating chinchillas is generally considered a difficult procedure. The long, narrow oral cavity of these animals makes the visualization of the glottis difficult. As in dogs and cats, laryngoscopes may be used to visualize the glottis, but extreme care should be taken to avoid damaging the soft tissues of the oral cavity or even fracturing the mandible. Even with the use of a laryngoscope, direct visualization of the glottis is very difficult. Another technique that may be used for intubating chinchillas is to affix an endotracheal tube to a stethoscope and place the tube via auditory cues. To place the tube, the anesthetist should listen through the ear pieces of the stethoscope for when the animal expires, and then gently insert the tube into the trachea. This technique requires practice to perfect, but once the procedure has been performed several times, can be a reliable method for intubating chinchillas. Application of a small amount of lidocaine to the *rima glottis* can also ease intubation by decreasing laryngospasm. One of the most productive methods of intubating chinchillas is to use a rigid endoscope. We have found that a 2.7-mm rigid endoscope can be used to visualize both the glottis and the endotracheal tube as it is passed into the airway.

Anesthesia

Anesthesia should be provided to any chinchilla undergoing a painful or stressful procedure. Inhalant anesthetics are by far the most common way of anesthetizing these patients. Chinchillas can be induced using isoflurane or sevoflurane administered by face mask or induction chamber (Figure 18-18). Induction is generally done at 3% to 5% isoflurane (per 1 L oxygen) or 5% to 7% sevoflurane (per 1 L oxygen). Once anesthetized, patients can be maintained at 1% to 3% isoflurane and 2% to 4% sevoflurane, respectively. Sevoflurane is generally better tolerated by chinchillas, because they tend to object less to its odor than to the odor of isoflurane. This also reduces the amount of breath-holding that occurs during induction, which expedites induction and reduces the potential for complications. Chinchillas should not be fasted more

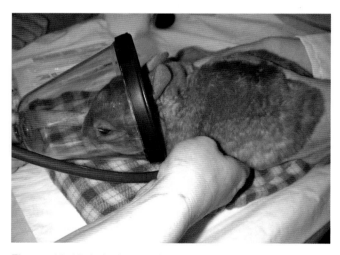

Figure 18-18 Inducing a chinchilla using a gas anesthetic agent.

than 2 to 3 hours before anesthesia. Disruption of intestinal microflora can occur if food is withheld for longer periods of time, potentially resulting in negative sequelae such as enterotoxemia. Water does not need to be withdrawn before an anesthetic event.

Preanesthetic agents can be used to reduce the anxiety associated with a procedure and decrease the amount of inhalant required for induction and maintenance of anesthesia. A combination of intramuscular midazolam (0.2-0.5 mg/kg) and butorphanol (0.2-0.5 mg/kg) has been used with good success. A list of other anesthetic and analgesic agents can be found in Table 18-6.

Careful monitoring of the patient during anesthesia is essential. Respirations should be visually monitored for depth and character. Heart rate and rhythm should also be monitored continuously using a pediatric stethoscope or Doppler unit, placing the transducer on a peripheral artery (Figure 18-19). Changes in heart rate or respiratory rate can occur rapidly, so it is advantageous to have pre-calculated doses of emergency drugs (e.g., glycopyrrolate, epinephrine, atropine, doxopram) drawn and available for use prior to anesthetic induction.

Monitoring a chinchilla's body temperature is also very important during an anesthetic procedure. In chinchillas, as in other small animals, hypothermia often occurs when anesthetized animals are not provided thermal support. Supplemental heat should always be provided through water-circulating heating pads, heat lamps, or forced air blankets. Body temperature should be monitored closely to ensure that the patient is not overheated, which could lead to hyperthermia and death if not corrected.

Common Surgical Procedures

Chinchillas may present for a variety of potential surgical procedures, including fractures, trichobezoar/foreign body, and cystic calculi. The majority of these procedures can be performed using the same basic practices described for domestic mammals. The only primary difference between chinchilla surgery and that for domestic pets is that chinchilla tissues are

TABLE 18-6	Common Analgesic and Anesthetic Agents Used in Chinchilla Medicine		
Drug	**Route(s) of administration**	**Dosage(s)[33-35]**	**Dose frequency**
Atropine	IM	0.1-0.2 mg/kg	–
Buprenorphine	SC, IV	0.05 mg/kg	q8-12h
Butorphanol	SC, IM	0.2-2.0 mg/kg	q4h
Carprofen	SC	4 mg/kg	q24h
Glycopyrrolate	SC, IM	0.01-0.02 mg/kg	–
Ketamine	IM	20-40 mg/kg	–
Ketamine/diazepam	IM	20-40 mg/kg(K)/1-2 mg/kg(D)	–
Ketamine/midazolam	IM	5-10 mg/kg(K)/0.5-1.0 mg/kg(M)	–
Ketoprofen	SC, IM	1 mg/kg	q12-24h
Midazolam	IM	1-2 mg/kg	–

IM, intramuscular; *IV*, intravenous; *SC*, subcutaneous.

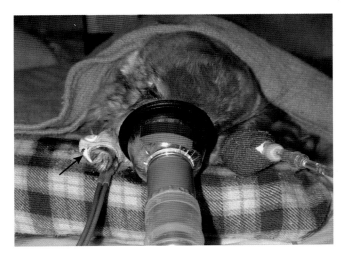

Figure 18-19 An anesthetized chinchilla. Oxygen and anesthetic gas are being provided via a face mask. An intravenous catheter is being used to deliver fluids via the cephalic vein. The heart rate is being monitored via a Doppler unit *(arrow)*.

generally more fragile. Therefore, when working with chinchillas, it is important to take extra care when manipulating the tissues (e.g., intestines, bones, bladder).

Reproductive Surgery
OVARIOHYSTERECTOMY

The indications for ovariohysterectomy in chinchillas are similar to those in domestic species, and include routine sterilization, dystocia, and reproductive tract disease (e.g., neoplasia, muco/hydro/pyometra). The surgical approach and techniques for this procedure in chinchillas are also similar to that of domestic species. The patient should be placed in dorsal recumbency and a ventral midline incision made through the *linea alba.* Care must be taken upon entering the abdomen to avoid incising the large cecum, which is often situated along the ventral body wall. Using forceps to lift the linea alba when incising the body wall can help reduce the risk of complication. The body of the uterus can be located dorsal to the urinary bladder. Manual expression of the urinary bladder before beginning the surgery will increase the visualization of the uterine body. The ovaries lie caudally and laterally to the kidneys and are 6 to 8 mm in length.[37] The ovarian vessels are short, which does not allow for exteriorization of the ovaries for ligation of vessels.[38] Care must be taken to avoid tearing these vessels when removing the ovaries. Once the ovaries are removed, the uterus is ligated and transected in a manner similar to that used with other mammals.

ORCHIECTOMY

An orchiectomy is typically performed to prevent reproduction, decrease undesirable sexual behavior, and reduce the likelihood for reproductive tract disease. The orchiectomy procedure in chinchillas is performed by making an incision through the scrotum over each testicle. A closed technique or open technique, whereby the vaginal tunic is incised, may be performed. Although herniation of abdominal contents through the inguinal canal does not commonly occur with open castration, it is still advisable to close the inguinal ring if this technique is used. The incisions may be closed with either an intradermal suture pattern or with tissue glue.

■ ZOONOSES

Many of the opportunistic bacterial pathogens (e.g., *E. coli, Salmonella* spp.), fungi (e.g., dermatophytes), and protozoal infections (e.g., *Giardia* spp., *Cryptosporidium parvum*) found in chinchillas can be infective to humans. To minimize the likelihood of transmitting these agents, young children should not handle these animals during their treatment period. When adults handle these animals to apply treatment, they should wear protective gloves. Gloves should also be worn when cleaning the animal's enclosure. Overall, chinchillas represent a low potential zoonotic risk for pet owners; however, clients should always be advised to follow standard disinfection and hygiene practices when working with these animals.

REFERENCES

1. Merry CJ: An introduction to chinchillas, *Vet Tech* 11(5):315-322, 1990.
2. Webb RA: Chinchillas. In Beynon PH, Cooper JE, editors: *Manual of Exotic Pets,* Cheltenham, Gloucestershire, 1991, British Small Animal Veterinary Association.
3. Quesenberry KE, Donnelly TM, Hillyer EV: Biology, husbandry, and clinical techniques of guinea pigs and chinchillas. In Quesenberry KE, Carpenter JW, editors: *Ferrets, Rabbits, and Rodents: Clinical Medicine and Surgery,* ed 2, St Louis, 2003, WB Saunders.
4. de Oliveria Silva T, Kruetz LC, Barcellos LJG et al: Reference values for chinchilla *(Chinchilla laniger)* blood cells and serum biochemical parameters, *Ciência Rural,* 35(3):602-606, 2005.
5. Silverman S, Tell LA: Radiology equipment and positioning techniques. In Silverman S, Tell LA, editors: *Radiology of Rodents, Rabbits, and Ferrets: An Atlas of Normal Anatomy and Positioning,* St Louis, 2005, WB Saunders.
6. Moore RW, Greenlee HH: Enterotoxaemia in chinchillas, *Lab Anim* 9:153-154, 1975.
7. Bartoszcze M, Nowakowski M, Roszkowski J et al: Chinchilla deaths due to *Clostridium perfringens* a enterotoxin, *Vet Rec* 126:341, 1990.
8. Hoefer HL: Chinchillas. *Vet Clin North Am Small Anim Pract* 24(1):113-120, 1994.
9. Kraft H: *Diseases of Chinchillas,* Neptune City, NJ, 1987, TFH.
10. Jenkins JR: Husbandry and common diseases of the chinchilla *(Chinchilla laniger), J Small Exot Anim Med* 2(1):15-17, 1992.
11. Naglić T, Šeol B, Bedeković Ž et al: Outbreak of *Salmonella enteritidis* and isolation of *Salmonella sofia* in chinchillas *(Chinchilla laniger), Vet Rec* 152:719-720, 2003.
12. Finley GG, Long JR: An epizootic of listeriosis in chinchillas, *Can Vet J* 18(6):164-167, 1977.
13. Kimpe A, Decostere A, Hermans K et al: Isolation of *Listeria ivanovii* from a septicaemic chinchilla *(Chinchilla lanigera), Vet Rec* 154:791-792, 2004.
14. Donnelly TM: Disease problems of chinchillas. In Quesenberry KE, Carpenter JW, editors: *Ferrets, Rabbits, and Rodents: Clinical Medicine and Surgery,* ed 2, St Louis, 2003, WB Saunders.
15. Eidman S: Studies on the etiology and pathogenesis of fur damage in the chinchilla. Hannover, Germany, *Tierarztliche Hochschule* 61:163, 1992.
16. Newberne PM: An outbreak of bacterial gastro-enteritis in the South American chinchilla, *North Am Vet,* 34:187-188, 191, 1953.
17. Yamini B, Raju NR: Gastroenteritis associated with a *Cryptosporidium* sp. in a chinchilla, *JAVMA* 189:1158-1159, 1986.

18. Sanford SE: Cerebrospinal nematodiasis caused by *Baylisascaris procyonis* in chinchillas, *J Vet Diagn Invest* 3:77-79, 1991.

19. Newberne PM, Siebold HR: Malignant lymphoma in a chinchilla, *Vet Med* 48:428-429, 1953.

20. Osofsky A, Verstraete FJM: Dentistry in pet rodents, *Compend Contin Educ Dent* Jan:61-74, 2006.

21. Crossley DA: Dental disease in chinchillas in the UK, *J Small Anim Pract* 42:12-19, 2001.

22. Richardson VCG: Chinchillas: systems and diseases. In Richardson VCG, editor: *Diseases of Small Domestic Rodents,* Oxford, UK, 2003, Blackwell.

23. Verstraete FJM: Advances in diagnosis and treatment of small exotic mammal dental disease, *Semin Av Exotic Pet Med* 12(1):37-48, 2003.

24. Legendre LFJ: Malocclusions in guinea pigs, chinchillas, and rabbits, *Can Vet J* 43:385-390, 2002.

25. Crossley DA, Jackson A, Yates J et al: Use of computed tomography to investigate cheek tooth abnormalities in chinchillas *(Chinchilla lanigera), J Small Anim Pract* 39:385-389, 1998.

26. Varonjack WJ, Johnson HD: Relationship of thyroid and adrenal function to "fur-chewing" in the chinchilla, *Comp Biochem Physiol* 45:115-120, 1973.

27. Tišljar M, Janić D, Grabarević Ž et al: Stress-induced Cushing's syndrome in fur-chewing chinchillas, *ACTA Vet Hung* 50(2):133-142, 2002.

28. Williams J: Orthopedic radiography in exotic animal practice. In Tully TN, editor: *Vet Clin North Am Exot Anim Pract* 5(1):1-22, 2002.

29. Hoefer HL, Crossley DA: Chinchillas. In Meredith A, Redrobe S, editors: *BSAVA Manual of Exotic Pets,* ed 4, Quedgeley, Gloucester, 2005, British Small Animal Veterinary Association.

30. Morgan RV, Moore FM, Pearce LK et al: Clinical and laboratory findings in small companion animals with lead poisoning: 347 cases (1977-1986), *JAVMA* 199:93-97, 1991.

31. Cousens PJ: The chinchilla in veterinary practice, *J Small Anim Pract* 4:199-205, 1963.

32. Marlow C: Diabetes in a chinchilla, *Vet Record* 136:595-596, 1995 (letter).

33. Plumb DC: *Veterinary Drug Handbook,* ed 5, Ames, Iowa, 2005, Blackwell.

34. Morrisey JK, Carpenter JW: Formulary. In Quesenberry KE, Carpenter JW, editors: *Ferrets, Rabbits, and Rodents: Clinical Medicine and Surgery,* ed 2, St Louis, 2003, WB Saunders.

35. Carpenter JW: *Exotic Animal Formulary,* ed 3, St Louis, 2005, WB Saunders.

36. Briscoe JA: Techniques for emergency airway and vascular access in special species, *Semin Av Exot Pet Med* 13(3):118-131, 2004.

37. Bennett RA, Mullen HS: Soft tissue surgery. In Quesenberry KE, Carpenter JW, editors: *Ferrets, Rabbits, and Rodents: Clinical Medicine and Surgery,* ed 2, St Louis, 2003, WB Saunders.

38. Jenkins JR: Surgical sterilization in small mammals. In Bennett RA, editor: *Vet Clin North Am Exot Anim Pract* 3(3):617-627, 2000.

Maya Bewig
Mark A. Mitchell

CHAPTER 19

WILDLIFE

IMPORTANCE OF VETERINARIAN PARTICIPATION IN WILDLIFE CARE

As humans continue to encroach on previously undisturbed and pristine wild habitats, the frequency of wildlife-human encounters has increased. These increased encounters have led to an increased need for veterinary participation in managing sick and injured animals. For much of the public, veterinarians are still held in reverence because of the James Herriott stories. We believe that it is important for veterinarians to maintain this image. This does not necessarily suggest that veterinarians should consider themselves experts on all animal species, but that as professionals, they should develop an infrastructure of resources that enables them to provide medical and surgical care for those animals in need. In addition, because many of these animals can serve as reservoirs for zoonotic diseases, veterinarians can play an important role in minimizing the risk of disease transmission between wildlife and concerned citizens. For some veterinarians, their role may require them to maintain a current list of veterinarians or wildlife rehabilitators capable of managing an injured wildlife patient and refer clients to these professionals. For others with a more invested interest, it may mean that they will pursue available resources to develop the knowledge and skill for managing these animals in their hospital. The last thing clients, or prospective clients, want to hear from veterinarians is "We don't work with those animals." Instead, if veterinarians can, at a minimum, direct clients to the most appropriate resource, veterinarians maintain (and justify) their image among the professions.

DECIDING WHETHER OR NOT TO TREAT WILDLIFE

There are many financial, ethical, and emotional issues for veterinarians to consider when deciding whether to accept wildlife cases to their practice. Wildlife is not owned and therefore do not come with paying caretakers. In many cases, the hospital will be expected to absorb the cost of treatment, although avenues for monetary compensation, including grants and public donations, do exist. Accepting wildlife cases is often perceived by (prospective) clients as a positive reinforcement of a veterinarian's compassion toward animals and can serve, directly or indirectly, as a method of increasing a veterinarian's domestic and exotic pet caseload. One ethical consideration to make with these cases is deciding when intervention may interfere with a natural process occurring in a population. In some cases, euthanasia will certainly end suffering, whereas in others treatment may interfere with both natural selection and the disease status in a population. However, because the lives of humans have become so enmeshed with populations of wild animals, it is unavoidable that some, if not most, of the injuries or disease processes occurring in wildlife populations are the direct result of human contact. In these cases, there may be a strong moral (ethical) obligation to repair damage caused by the human species. An early and rational assessment of the likely return to function for a patient is imperative to conserve the available resources for treatment and prevent undue suffering in the patient. Animals who are considered poor candidates for release or placement should be considered for euthanasia as soon as an assessment is made. Release candidates should be able to function appropriately within their natural habitat (including reproduction) and with conspecifics; otherwise, a disservice is rendered to both the animal and its population.

Certain factors should be weighed before deciding to accept wildlife cases to a practice. These factors should be considered with every case as well. The potential costs include those welfare expenses associated with captivity, treatment, release, and failure to reestablish the animal in the wild, as well as the welfare risks to conspecifics and other species through the possible introduction of infection or competition for resources and the upset in natural selection (e.g., treating animals that have increased susceptibility to disease may inadvertently select for less fit animals). The potential benefits associated with working with these animals include the emotional pleasure humans derive from helping a "lesser" species, the potential to educate the public, and the opportunities this type of medicine provides for monitoring threats to wildlife and human populations.

Assessing the balance or inherent value between welfare costs and benefits is often difficult. In addition to the unpredictability of responses between individual cases to treatment, there are few robust yardsticks for use in judging, for example, whether any stress or pain associated with captivity and treatment does or does not outweigh the potential welfare benefit to the animal. The task is not made easier by the scarcity of information on outcomes of wildlife rehabilitation cases, although more studies are being done. Veterinarians have an important role in these ethical assessments and in helping to design protocols that will best manage the welfare of these animals in both captive and wild settings.

KNOWING THE REGULATIONS

Veterinarians working with wildlife should become familiar with the regulations addressing the handling, transport, and treatment of these animals. These regulations have been enacted at the federal and state levels to ensure the protection of these animals against individuals that would otherwise exploit them (e.g., meat or fur). Historically, veterinarians were perceived as "good Samaritans," and it was just accepted that veterinarians would or could provide any medical and surgical care that a particular wildlife patient required. Unfortunately, some veterinarians, like many unlicensed wildlife rehabilitators, will attempt to complete the rehabilitation process for their wildlife patients, even though they cannot meet their patient's husbandry, nutritional, or posttreatment rehabilitation needs. Currently, federal and state governments are committed to maintaining veterinarians as an integral component to the care of injured wildlife and consider veterinarians to be the experts for providing medical and surgical care for these animals. However, these agencies also realize that most veterinarians do not have the time or facilities to fully rehabilitate injured wildlife. Because of this, federal and state agencies require veterinarians (without state and/or federal rehabilitation permits) to transfer these animals to licensed rehabilitators to complete the rehabilitation process. It is expected that a veterinarian will transfer any wildlife patient to a licensed wildlife rehabilitator within 24 hours of stabilizing the patient. A stabilized patient is one that is no longer in dire need of

veterinary medical care. Patients that require medical treatment that can be administered via an experienced (trained) rehabilitator should be transferred.

The federal government is primarily invested in the protection of migratory birds and all other species that are listed federally as species of special concern, threatened, or endangered. State agencies also require rehabilitators to maintain permits to cover these same species, as well as mammals and other species (reptiles, amphibians, and fish) considered threatened or endangered at the state level. Veterinarians interested in obtaining federal permits can find information regarding the permits on the United States Fish and Wildlife Service website (www.fws.gov). Veterinarians interested in obtaining state rehabilitation licensure should contact their state wildlife and fisheries service.

BECOMING MORE INVOLVED

Wildlife medicine is in its infancy. Because of this, much of what veterinarians do is based on anecdotal or subjective recommendations. With this knowledge, it is important for those veterinarians working with these animals to document their work and disseminate it to others. This information can be disseminated through presentations at local, state, or national wildlife rehabilitation meetings, or published in appropriate bulletins or journals. In our opinion, the knowledge base regarding wildlife medicine, more so than any other aspect of veterinary medicine, would benefit from more active participation by veterinarians.

COMMON SPECIES PRESENTATIONS

Veterinarians that publicize an interest in accepting wildlife cases may be surprised by the diversity of cases being presented to their hospitals. In our practices, amphibians, reptiles, birds, and mammals are all routinely presented. Such a diverse caseload requires veterinarians to be adaptive to the different needs of these animals, both in their medical and surgical knowledge and in their ability to meet the rehabilitation needs (e.g., diet, environment) of the patient. Many veterinarians will limit the types of cases presented to their hospitals. Some of the veterinarians we consult with only accept chelonians, whereas others may accept only avian cases. It is important that veterinarians inform wildlife rehabilitators and clients of particular species they exclude from their practices. It would also be helpful to have a list of other veterinarians on hand that do accept those species, so that those individuals can be referred to an appropriate facility.

PREPARING FOR WILDLIFE IN VETERINARY HOSPITALS
Staff Preparedness

When veterinarians accept wildlife cases into their hospitals, it is important that they have buy-in from their staff. Wildlife cases can require a significant amount of time and effort, especially orphaned animals. Therefore, it is often the veterinary staff that will have the most contact with the wildlife cases. Veterinarians that accept these types of cases on a moderate to large scale would certainly benefit from providing at least some of their staff an opportunity to obtain continuing education in wildlife rehabilitation. Many of these opportunities can be obtained from local or state meetings, although the large national meetings (e.g., the annual conferences of the National Wildlife Rehabilitators Association and the International Wildlife Rehabilitators Association) provide the most diverse training opportunities. Membership in these organizations is also highly recommended, as they publish regular bulletins or journals and provide a real resource of potential personal contacts.

It is important that veterinarians train their staff to avoid becoming emotionally attached to their wildlife patients. In our opinion, this is the single most controversial issue that can arise in a hospital. If staff members (and veterinarians) become emotionally attached to their cases, they are less likely to maintain an objective outlook on their cases. It is important to always approach these cases with a triage mentality (Figure 19-1). The time spent treating these patients should also be limited to necessary contact only. Animals that become habituated to humans in captivity may be at greater risk of reinjury or death after release if they lose their fear of humans. For orphaned animals, imprinting is a major concern. Imprinting occurs when an animal recognizes a human as the "parent" animal. Imprinting can potentially lead to dangerous encounters for humans and wildlife, especially with mesopredators, carnivores, and raptors. For this reason, it is important that only trained staff manage orphaned animals.

When accepting wildlife patients into a hospital, veterinarians must maintain a complete record for each patient. We have found that staff can prove invaluable for this task. The following information should be collected for each patient: the species, age (if known or adult/juvenile), gender (if known),

date of presentation, location and date found, type of injury, medical treatment provided (if any), diet and husbandry provided (if any), and name and contact information of the person(s) presenting the animal. Each patient should also be thoroughly evaluated daily and the data recorded using a standard format (SOAP: subjective, objective, assessment, plan). Maintaining this information in a computer database will allow for routine review and analysis of the data. This information can then be used to develop reference ranges for a particular species or area and can be published and presented to a wider audience.

Equipment

Most of the medical and surgical equipment required for wildlife patients is already available in veterinary hospitals that treat domestic species. However, if a practice is primarily based on domestic species, there may be some specialty equipment that needs to be obtained. A list of different equipment we consider important can be found in Box 19-1.

BOX 19-1 **Specialty Equipment Required to Manage Wildlife at a Veterinary Hospital**

Incubators
Incubators are thermostat-controlled microhabitats for small mammals, birds, reptiles, and amphibians. These enclosures should be capable of providing a range of environmental temperatures (80°-100° F).

Oxygen Cage
Both orphaned animals that aspirate during feeding and avian species with respiratory disease may benefit from placement in an oxygen cage.

Ophthalmic Loupe
A loupe can be used to provide better definition to small structures (e.g., blood vessels).

Endoscopic Equipment
A 2.7-mm rigid endoscope can be used to perform exploratory coeliotomies in birds. Sexing birds can also be done using this equipment.

Radiosurgery
A radiosurgery unit can be used to control hemostasis. This can be especially important in small patients.

Restraint Materials
Leather gloves are required to restrain raptors and mesopredators. Body wraps can be used for birds. A rabies pole or pole-syringe can be used to handle mesopredators.

Digital Scale
A scale or scales capable of measuring the variety of animals being presented to the facility are needed. We suggest a scale capable of measuring 1-g increments.

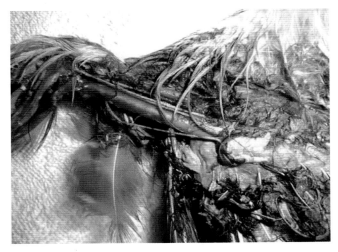

Figure 19-1 This barred owl presented with a degloving injury over the entire antebrachium. Although the animal was alert, responsive, and eating, it was euthanized because of the extensive tissue necrosis associated with the wound.

■ HOUSING

Veterinarians that accept wildlife cases into their practices must be prepared to house a variety of species. It is always best to house wildlife separately from domestic species, to minimize the likelihood of interspecies disease dissemination; however, when this is not possible, all attempts should be made to minimize transmission (e.g., wear gloves, clean cages with separate sponges). The following are some recommendations for housing different wildlife species.

Avian
PASSERINES

The most difficult aspects of providing housing for small birds is preventing escape and providing security. Using a room that can be darkened will facilitate capture of escapees. Mesh or metal used to cover a cage must have a small diameter to prevent escape. It can also be important to have the enclosure open into a room that will allow for ease of capture (e.g., low ceilings, few hiding spots) should the bird escape the primary cage. The setup of feeding and water stations will vary greatly depending on the species.

PIGEONS AND DOVES

For short-term housing, any container, such as a dog or cat kennel, is sufficient. Because pigeons and doves are reservoirs for various avian pathogens, it is always best to isolate them from other species to limit the potential for disease transmission. For longer periods in captivity, these birds may be best housed in an aviary.

GAMEBIRDS

Principles of short-term and long-term housing are the same for these birds as was described for pigeons and doves, although the size of the cage may need to be increased for larger specimens. No perching materials need to be provided for short-term housing but should be provided if the bird is kept for a longer period of time to allow roosting at night.[1] Substrate should be easily disinfected, to prevent foot disease (e.g., Astroturf is a good substrate).

WATERFOWL

For short-term waterfowl care, the principles are the same as with those previously mentioned, with the exception of providing water in a container large enough for the bird to stand in. For long-term care, adequate housing will require the addition of a large pool or pond, which may not be feasible in a general practice setting.

WADERS

Short-term housing for waders should be tall enough to enable the animal to stand naturally. The cage should also be kept dark and quiet with moist, nonslip flooring (e.g., moist sand or newspaper).[2] Water should be provided in a shallow container. For long-term housing, a shallow pond or pool and suitable natural cover should be provided. As with waterfowl, this may be difficult for general practitioners to provide.

SEABIRDS

Seabirds have special requirements in captivity that may make rehabilitation difficult, especially for beginners. Some species of seabird are gregarious and do better when housed in groups. Seabirds are sensitive to sudden noises and should be kept in a quiet environment. A soft substrate that is easy to clean, such as Astroturf, rubber mats, or deep layers of wood shavings, should be used. Animals left on firm substrates (metal flooring or concrete) can develop pododermatitis. Straw or hay bedding should never be used, as they can be a source of fungal spores. It is important to provide ample ventilation to minimize the risk of respiratory disease. For stable patients in medium- to long-term captivity, a water source (e.g., pool or pond) must be provided. This water source should be cleaned regularly to prevent autoinfection.

RAPTORS

All of the general principles for housing apply to raptors. In addition, it is extremely important to provide an environment that will prevent any self-induced trauma. Raptors are prone to damaging their feathers, wings, talons, and cere in captivity. Injuries to any of these body parts can delay the rehabilitation process and should be avoided at all costs. The best cage materials to use for housing raptors are those that do not bend or damage the feathers. Because most veterinary hospitals maintain chain-link fence kennels or stainless steel cages, housing for raptors may be limited. Covering the cage with a soft mesh can help diminish the amount of feather damage done to hospitalized raptors. Tailguards made out of old radiograph film can be used to reduce tail feather damage. Perches can also be used to help limit the amount of damage done to the tail feathers. The perch should be positioned so that the tail feathers do not touch the base of the cage and the flight feathers have minimal contact with the sides of the cage. For extended hospitalization, raptors should be housed in an appropriately sized aviary. Whereas groups of some species can be housed together, mixing raptors is not recommended. As with short-term housing, care must be taken that the animal cannot injure itself. An easily disinfected substrate, such as Astroturf or gravel, can be used for the aviary. Multiple perches should be provided. If the bird is not a solid flier, the perches should be maintained close to the ground. Covering the perches with a rough surface (e.g., Astroturf) will minimize the likelihood of a bird developing pododermatitis. Multiple diameter and textured perches should be placed in the cage; however, the diameter should not be so small that the talons puncture the plantar surface of the foot.[3] The perches should be cleaned regularly to minimize the likelihood of fecal contamination. As with other species, hay or straw should not be used because of the potential for exposure to *Aspergillus* spp. spores. Certain species, such as owls, will benefit from shelter.

Mammals

SMALL RODENTS

Housing for small rodents must be constructed to withstand aggressive chewing and escape. For adult rodents, wood, some plastics, and aluminum caging materials are not recommended. Galvanized or stainless steel are more appropriate, as they can handle chewing and are easier to disinfect. For short-term housing, adult rodents can be housed in stainless steel hospital kennels. It is important, of course, that the width of the bars be narrow enough to prevent escape. Within the enclosure, a nest box should be provided, which can be made from wood or cardboard. Recycled newspaper is a suitable substrate. Tree limbs and other natural substances are also recommended and will provide the animals a surface to chew on. Orphaned animals or nonchewing species (e.g., bats) can be housed in clip-top plastic containers. It is important to drill a sufficient number of holes in the container to provide ventilation. Newspaper or towels can be used as a substrate for these cages. For long-term rehabilitation, larger portable cages are recommended. Galvanized wire is probably the least expensive material for constructing these cages. It is best to secure these cages to protect against predation.

LAGOMORPHS

Lagomorphs are extremely sensitive and prone to stress, so maintaining a quiet, predator-free environment is essential. Care must be taken to make the enclosure escape-proof. Covering the cage will increase the feeling of security for the animal. Attention to the flooring is also important, as these animals like to dig. A hay bedding or false floor can be used to simulate a burrow. The cage types described for rodents can also be used for lagomorphs.

MESOPREDATORS

Mesopredators can be housed in standard domestic animals stainless steel cages; however, this is not without its limitations. Because these cages have swing-doors, it can be difficult to work with these animals if they are fractious. For animals that are difficult to manage, anesthesia is highly recommended. A pole-syringe capable of being inserted between the cage bars can be used to safely deliver an appropriate anesthetic. Shifting these animals to outdoor cages is highly recommended. Chain-link cages can be used to house these animals, but they must be constructed to be escape-proof. Whether inside or outside, the cage should be provided with a shelter box and an area for a latrine.

DEER

For short-term hospitalization, fawns can be kept in an isolation area or any area that is away from the noise of humans and other animals. Large deer can be kept for short periods of time in a stable or outhouse with a deep layer of straw. As for the size of the enclosure, a maximum of 1.5 × 1.8 m and 2 × 3 m for fawns and adult deer, respectively, is recommended.[4] The enclosure should not have windows, and ventilation should be provided through slats at the top of the walls or ceiling. A door that is divided into a stable-door arrangement, with the top portion only 0.5 m high, is preferred. It is best if the door can be swung inward, so that it can be used as a restraint device for the deer. The top portion of the door should be opened for access only from above. Deer will leap toward light when the door is opened, making other arrangements dangerous. Deer who will be kept in captivity for longer periods of time should be transferred to an experienced rehabilitator who has appropriate pens.

Reptiles and Amphibians

The housing needs of reptiles and amphibians will vary greatly depending on species. Some examples of reptile groupings by environment include those that are aquatic, semiaquatic, arboreal, or terrestrial. Of the terrestrial reptiles, subgroups include those that are fossorial (burrowing), thigmotactic (prefer to wedge themselves into rocky crevices when not basking), and those that live on the surface of the soil. Reptiles can also be grouped according to the time of day that they are active: diurnal, nocturnal, and crepuscular (active during dusk or dawn). Species habits must be known before appropriate housing can be provided. Reptiles kept in inappropriate environments can develop a variety of conditions that will delay the rehabilitation process. For example, terrestrial species kept in moist cages may develop integumentary disease, whereas aquatic species housed in dry habitats will become dehydrated. Arboreal reptiles must be provided with branches, reptiles adapted to saline or brackish water should be furnished with water of the appropriate salinity, fossorial species must be provided substrate to burrow in, and secretive reptiles must be provided hiding places. Water should be provided in the form in which the animal is used to imbibing it. Many lizards drink from rain or dewdrops on foliage and will not drink from dishes. Tortoises should be provided with a shallow bowl of water. For additional information regarding the specific husbandry needs of reptiles, see the appropriate chapters in this text.

■QUARANTINE

Quarantine is an important consideration when practicing wildlife medicine in a domestic species veterinary hospital. Unfortunately, most veterinary hospitals are not built with quarantine in mind. Because wildlife can harbor various bacterial, fungal, viral, and parasitic diseases that can be transmitted to domestic pets, it is important to minimize and restrict both direct and indirect contact between these animals. Wildlife should be housed in a separate room from domestic species. A room with its own ventilation system is preferred. The traffic through the wildlife ward should be one-way. A foot bath with a disinfectant (e.g., sodium hypochlorite) should be placed outside the doorway and used after exiting the room to minimize the likelihood of tracking infectious diseases throughout the hospital. The disinfectant should be changed daily, or as often as needed, to minimize the amount of organic debris in the solution. Organic debris renders many disinfectants useless. Laboratory coats, or preferably jumpsuits that totally cover clothing, should be placed in the wildlife ward and worn when working with the animals. These clothing materials should be taken out of the room only for washing. Any materials being removed from the ward should be placed in a garbage bag and carried through the hospital in these bags to minimize the likelihood of disseminating disease through the hospital. A hand-washing station should be placed within the room. Signs should be posted on the wildlife ward door to alert staff and clients about the presence of wildlife and the need to maintain a strict quarantine protocol.

ZOONOSES

Zoonotic diseases should always be a concern for those individuals working with wildlife, as many of these animals can harbor a variety of bacterial, viral, fungal and parasitic zoonotic agents (Box 19-2). Because of this, children and individuals with compromised immune systems should not be allowed to work with wildlife. Staff should not be allowed to eat, drink, or smoke near any wildlife patients, and food and drink items should not be allowed near any of the places where diagnostic samples are held. We strongly recommend wearing examination gloves when handling wildlife. Wearing gloves will help minimize the likelihood of introducing pathogens into cuts or abrasions on practitioners' and staff's hands. For those cases where an aerosolized pathogen is suspected, a protective mask and eyeglasses should be worn. Individuals who develop an illness after working with wildlife should be examined by a health care specialist immediately. *Zoonoses and Communicable Diseases Common to Man and Animals* (ed 3), coedited by P. N. Acha and B. Szyfres and published by the Pan American Health Organization (Washington DC), is an excellent reference for obtaining additional information on zoonotic diseases associated with wildlife.

EMERGENCY CARE
General Concepts

When wildlife cases are presented to a veterinary hospital, they should be considered an emergency. Most of these patients will have injuries that are hours to days old that have limited their ability to obtain food, water, or shelter. Because of these limitations, many of these animals will be dehydrated, cachectic, and possibly hypo- or hyperthermic (seasonally dependent). To increase the likelihood of success with these cases, it is vital that the veterinarian stabilize these patients before pursuing a case diagnosis.

Cardiopulmonary Resuscitation

In some emergency situations an animal may present with or develop cardiac or respiratory failure during a course of treatment. Veterinary staff should determine beforehand the level of response they will provide in these cases. If the clinic adheres

---

| BOX 19-2 | A Partial List of Common Zoonotic Diseases Associated with Wildlife |

Bacterial
Chlamydophila psittaci
Salmonella spp.
Campylobacter spp.
Escherichia coli
Staphylococcus aureus
Bacillus anthracis
Streptococcus spp.
Mycobacterium spp.
Leptospira interrogans
Clostridium spp.
Francisella tularensis
Yersinia pestis
Yersinia pseudotuberculosis

Fungal
Aspergillus spp.
Histoplasma spp.
Blastomyces spp.

Viral
Rabies
West Nile virus
St. Louis encephalitis
Eastern equine encephalitis
Influenza

Parasitic
Giardia spp.
Cryptosporidium parvum
Baylisascaris procyonis
Ancylostoma spp.
Sarcoptes spp.
Encephalocytozoon cuniculi

---

to a strict triage protocol, then most cases of cardiac or respiratory failure will not be treated. If the clinic does attempt to resuscitate these animals, then the staff should be prepared for a low success rate (<5%).

The first steps to performing cardiopulmonary resuscitation are to intubate the patient and initiate cardiac compressions. In most birds and reptiles, the glottis is located at the base of the tongue and can be easily visualized and intubated (Figure 19-2). The choice of endotracheal tube should be commensurate with the animal's tracheal diameter. For small species, intravenous catheters (14- to 16-gauge) may be modified into an endotracheal tube. Because birds, crocodilians, and chelonians have complete tracheal rings, the cuff on their endotracheal tube should not be insufflated. In mammals, the intubation procedure can be more difficult, especially in rabbits; however, a laryngoscope or endoscope can be used to assist with intubation. In those cases where intubation is difficult, if not impossible, the animal should be masked and a high flow of oxygen provided. The success rate for animals that

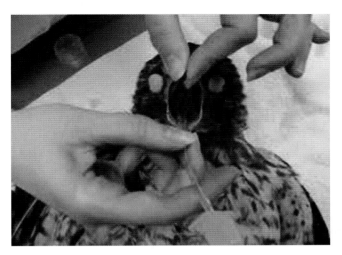

Figure 19-2 Intubating birds, such as this red-shouldered hawk, is straightforward. Once the glottis is located at the base of the tongue, the endotracheal tube can be inserted.

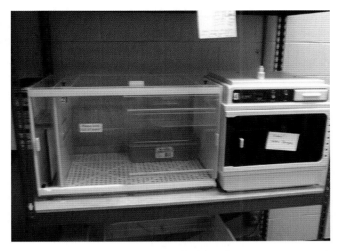

Figure 19-3 Temperature-controlled incubators are an excellent method for warming hypothermic wildlife.

cannot be intubated will be less than 1%. Respirations can be given every 5 to 30 cardiac compressions.

Cardiac compressions in wild mammals can be done using the same technique described for domestic mammals. The animal should be placed into lateral recumbency for the procedure. In mammals, the heart is generally located at the point of the elbow. Mustelids are an exception to this rule, with the heart being located more caudally in the thorax. Cardiac compressions can be done by placing the palm of the hand on the lateral surface of the rib cage and compressing ventrally or by grasping the ventral thorax in between the fingers and thumb (fingers on the down side and thumb on the upside of the thorax) and compressing the heart. Cardiac compressions should be done continuously. In birds, chest compressions can be done by pressing the keel. This technique allows for the heart to be compressed by being trapped between the spine and keel. For snakes and lizards, the heart can be directly massaged between an index finger and thumb. In chelonians, cardiac compressions are not possible.

Emergency drugs are an important component of the treatment of cardiac and respiratory failure. Epinephrine should be given when the animal has asystole. The drug can be delivered via a central line, the trachea, or directly into the heart. Multiple doses may be required. In cases where the heart begins beating but remains bradycardic, atropine can be given. Atropine can also be given via a central line, the trachea, or the heart. Doxapram is generally given to stimulate breathing. Different groups of animals appear to respond differently to this drug. The same injection routes may be used for this drug, and it may need to be administered multiple times.

Hemostasis

The first step in stabilizing emergency cases with acute hemorrhage is to provide hemostasis. Sutures, radiosurgery, tissue glue, and bandages can all be used to control hemorrhage in the wildlife patient. Once the patient is stabilized, the veteri-

narian should estimate the volume of blood lost and provide an appropriate replacement fluid. Evaluating a packed cell volume immediately after an acute hemorrhaging event may have limited value. In most cases, it is best to evaluate the packed cell volume 18 to 24 hours after presentation.

Respiratory Distress

Animals presenting with respiratory distress represent a true emergency. In many cases, animals will go into respiratory arrest after only minimal handling. To increase success with these cases, it is often best to restrict handling and allow the animal time to compensate. Placement of the animal into a covered oxygen cage will allow the patient time to stabilize its oxygen levels (if it is going to stabilize). Animals can also be given oxygen directly through a mask, although restraining the animal to deliver the oxygen may be stressful. Once the animal has compensated, then an exam and series of diagnostic tests can be pursued.

Thermoregulation

The body temperature of a patient can provide a significant amount of information regarding its physiologic status. Although birds are endotherms, there are times when the provision of supplemental heat is important. Birds that fluff their feathers do so to maintain body heat. Birds displaying this behavior must convert energy to maintain their core body temperature. To confirm this, the animal's body temperature should be taken. Birds naturally maintain a higher body temperature than mammals, with most birds falling between 104° F and 108° F. Because birds with an illness must conserve energy, it is important that veterinarians provide supplemental heat to minimize the energy expenditure associated with heat conservation. Temperature-controlled incubators provide an excellent method of providing a consistent environmental temperature (Figure 19-3). Heating pads, hot water bottles, and incandescent lights can also be used to provide supplemental heat, but all should be monitored closely. Adult birds that are hypothermic can be maintained in an environmental temperature of 82° F to 88° F, whereas juvenile birds may need to be kept warmer depending on the extent of their feather coverage (e.g., nestling vs. fledgling). Mammals, like birds, are also endothermic, and although they can control their own body temperature, they may require supplemental heat on occasion. Mammals that are hypothermic may shiver, have cold extremities, and have a body temperature below the acceptable reference range. Most mammalian body temperatures are between 100° F and 104° F. Opossums are an exception, generally having a body temperature between 92° F and 96° F. Reptiles are ectotherms and depend on their environmental temperature to regulate their core body temperature. For North American reptiles, a temperature range of 80° F to 90° F is appropriate.

Fluid Therapy

Fluid therapy should be provided next. The volume of replacement fluids required for a patient can be calculated by determining the maintenance rate of fluids for a day and degree of dehydration. A list of maintenance fluid rates for different types of wildlife is found in Table 19-1. The techniques used to assess dehydration can be found in Table 19-2. Fluids should always be warmed to the patient's physiologic temperature before being administered. Identifying which fluid is most appropriate will be based on the type of dehydration. Most wildlife cases present with isotonic dehydration, so a balanced fluid (e.g., 0.9% saline, lactated Ringer's solution) can be used. Calculating the patient's osmolality is the best method for estimating the type of dehydration. Laboratories using osmometers can calculate this number; however, if submitting a sample is not possible, then an estimate can be made using the following mathematical formula: OsM = 2(sodium + potassium) + urea + glucose. For reptiles and birds, uric acid can be used as a substitute for urea; however, it may underestimate the true osmolality. A fluid deficit in a mammalian patient can be corrected within 24 to 36 hours, whereas in birds and reptiles, it may take 48 and 96 hours, respectively.

Fluids can be delivered to wildlife using the same basic techniques described for domestic pets. Animals that are only mildly dehydrated and have a functional gastrointestinal tract can have fluids delivered per os. Subcutaneous fluids can be used for those patients that are mildly dehydrated but have some gastrointestinal disease (e.g., diarrhea, vomiting). For moderately dehydrated reptile and mammalian patients, fluids can be given intracoelomically or intraperitoneally, respectively. Because birds have air sacs, they should never be given fluids intracoelomically. For moderate to severe dehydration, fluids should be given intravenously (Figure 19-4) or intraosseously.

Fracture and Wound Management

Fractures should be stabilized to minimize the risk of further injury to the patient and to control pain. Depending on the site and nature of the fracture, various emergency bandaging methods can be employed. We generally immobilize wing fractures with a figure-of-eight splint (Figure 19-5) or a body wrap. The figure-of-eight splint is appropriate for fractures distal to

TABLE 19-1	Maintenance Fluid Rates for Wildlife Patients	
Group	**Suggested maintenance fluids**
Avian	75-100 ml/kg/day
Mammals	80-100 ml/kg/day
Reptiles	10-30 ml/kg/day

TABLE 19-2	Estimating Dehydration in Wildlife
Percentage dehydrated	**Clinical signs**
5%	Some loss of skin turgor Skin slow to return after tenting (2-3 sec) Some tackiness in mucous membranes Capillary refill time (<2 sec)
7%-8%	Moderate loss of skin turgor Skin slow to return after tenting (3-5 sec) Ropy mucus in oral cavity, dry mucous membranes Capillary refill time (<3 sec)
>10%	Significant loss of skin turgor Skin very slow to return after tenting (>5 sec) Significant ropy mucus in oral cavity Capillary refill time (>3 sec) Sunken eyes (loss of retroorbital fat pads)

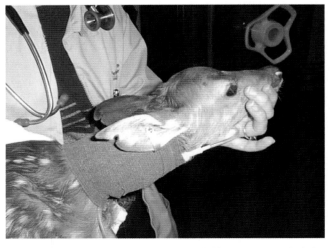

Figure 19-4 Intravenous fluids are highly recommended for those patients that are severely dehydrated. In this white-tailed deer fawn, a jugular catheter was placed.

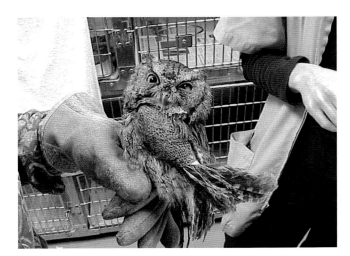

Figure 19-5 This screech owl presented with a radial fracture. Because the fracture was reduced, the wing was splinted using a figure-of-eight bandage.

the elbow, and a body wrap is recommended when the fracture includes the humerus. Vet-wrap (3M Corp., St. Paul, MN), or another comparable bandage material, can be used. For small birds (e.g., hummingbirds), placing the wings in a normal position and taping the primaries where they cross can provide an adequate splint. When immobilizing the wings of a bird, it is important to change the bandage and provide physical therapy every 3 to 4 days. This will prevent excessive contraction of the patagial tendon and atrophy of the muscles. We prefer to replace the bandage under anesthesia, as this minimizes the likelihood of the animal reinjuring itself and controls the pain associated with the procedure. In birds, fractures of the legs can be immobilized with modified syringe-case splints, tape splints, a ball bandage, or a Robert Jones–type splint. Syringe case splints are best suited for fractures distal to the stifle. Tape splints can be used to stabilize toes or the distal leg of a passerine or other lightweight bird. We generally use white, porous tape for these splints. For mammals, limbs can be splinted using the standard techniques described for domestic mammals. Fractures of the reptile limb can be immobilized by taping the limb to the animal's body. In lizards, a forelimb can be secured against the body wall using porous tape while the rear leg can be immobilized against the tail. In chelonians, the limb can be reduced into a normal position within the shell and taped into place. When splinting any limb, it is important to always immobilize the joint above and below the fracture site.

Wound management should be initiated to limit the amount of fluid or moisture lost from the break in the integument and to limit wound contamination. There are a variety of methods that can be used to manage a skin wound in a wildlife patient. The first and most important step to managing a wound is to remove any necrotic tissue. If necrotic tissue is left behind, it will delay the healing process. Sharp dissection of the wound should be done to remove all of the necrotic tissue. Wound disinfection can be done by irrigating the

wound with dilute chlorhexidine, Betadine, or 50% dextrose. We have used the hyperosmotic dextrose, with excellent results. Others report similar results with honey. After disinfection, the wound should be rinsed with a warmed sterile saline. Once disinfected, the wound should be protected against additional contamination. Silver sulfadiazine, or another topical antimicrobial, can be applied to the wound to protect it against opportunistic pathogens and to maintain the hydration of the exposed tissues. Bandage material can be applied to the wound if additional protection is required. A wet-to-dry bandage can be applied to any wound that requires decontamination. Depending on the size of the wound, either 2″ × 2″ or 4″ × 4″ gauze pads can be used for the bandage. The first 4 to 5 gauze pads should be irrigated with sterile saline or a disinfectant, such as chlorhexidine. The gauze pads should be wrung out before being applied to the wound. An additional 4 to 5 dry gauze pads should be placed on top of the moistened pads. All of the gauze should be secured to the wound with Vet-wrap. The bandage should be changed daily. Any necrotic tissue should be removed in between bandage changes. While uncovered, the wound should be disinfected using the technique described previously. The wet-to-dry bandage should be used only until the wound is considered disinfected. Prolonged use of this bandage can lead to tissue desiccation.

■ THERAPEUTICS

Once fluid therapy is initiated, chemotherapeutics can be given. It is important to wait on certain drugs until after fluid therapy has been instituted. For example, the administration of steroidal antiinflammatories could have a negative response if given to a dehydrated patient. A variety of chemotherapeutics are available to the veterinarian, including antiinflammatories (steroidal and nonsteroidal), analgesics, antibiotics, antifungals, antivirals, anesthetics, antiemetics, chelating agents, vitamins, and minerals. A list of common drugs used to treat wildlife can be found in Table 19-3.

■ CAPTURE AND TRANSPORT

Most injured wildlife cases will be transported to a veterinary clinic by the public, but there may be times when veterinarians are in a situation that requires them or their staff to capture an animal or give counsel on appropriate capture and transport to a member of the public. The techniques vary according to the species being approached, but some generalities apply. If observing the animal before capture, it is best to evaluate its posture and attitude from a distance (e.g., alert, depressed, lethargic). This information can be used to develop a capture strategy. Animals that are depressed and lethargic should be approached cautiously, as they may be more susceptible to sudden death or capture myopathy. When developing a capture strategy, it is also imperative to consider the humans involved with the procedure, to ensure no harm comes to those involved. Before capture, identify the major "weapons" an animal will use to defend itself. Raptors, for example, may use their talons and beak as weapons.

TABLE 19-3	Drugs Commonly Used to Treat Wildlife	
Drug	**Dose**	**Comments**
Emergency drugs		
Atropine	0.5 mg/kg	IV, IO, IT
Diazepam	0.5-1.0 mg/kg	IV, IO
Doxapram	20 mg/kg	IV, IO, IT
Epinephrine	0.5-1.0 mg/kg	1 : 1,000; IV, IO, IT
Antibiotics		
Amikacin	3-5 mg/kg	Reptiles: IM, q72h
	15-20 mg/kg	Birds: IM, q24h
	2.5-10 mg/kg	Mammals: IM, q12-24h
Amoxicillin	10-30 mg/kg	Reptiles: PO, IM, q12-24h
	100 mg/kg	Birds, PO, q12h
	10-20 mg/kg	Mammals: PO, q12h; NOT recommended for rodents or lagomorphs
Cephalexin	20-40 mg/kg	Reptiles: PO, q12h
	100 mg/kg	Birds, PO, q12h
	15-30 mg/kg	Mammals: PO, q12h; NOT recommended for rodents or lagomorphs
Ceftazidime	20 mg/kg	Reptiles: IM, q72h
Ciprofloxacin	10 mg/kg	Reptiles: PO, q24h
	15 mg/kg	Birds: PO, q12h
	15 mg/kg	Mammals: PO, q12h
Doxycycline	5-10 mg/kg	Reptiles: PO, q24h
	25-100 mg/kg	Birds: PO, q24h
Enrofloxacin	5-10 mg/kg	Reptiles: PO, q24h
	10-15 mg/kg	Birds: PO, q12h
	5-10 mg/kg	Mammals: PO, q12h
Tetracycline	200 mg/kg	Birds: PO, q12-24h
	20 mg/kg	Mammals: PO, q12h; use with caution in lagomorphs and rodents
Trimethoprim-sulfadiazine	15-30 mg/kg	Reptiles: PO, q24h
	50-75 mg/kg	Birds: PO, q12-24h
	5-25 mg/kg	Mammals: PO, q12-24h
Antifungals		
Itraconazole	5-10 mg/kg	Reptiles: PO, q24-48h; monitor for neurologic disease
	2.5-10 mg/kg	Birds: PO, q24h; monitor for neurologic disease
	2.5-5 mg/kg	Mammals: PO, q24h; monitor for neurologic disease
Ketoconazole	25-50 mg/kg	Reptiles: PO, q24h
	20-50 mg/kg	Birds: PO, q12-24h
	20-50 mg/kg	Mammals: PO, q24h
Nystatin	100,000 IU/kg	Reptiles: PO, q24h
	100,000-300, 000 IU/kg	Birds: PO, q12h
Antiparasitics		
Fenbendazole	25-100 mg/kg	Avian, reptiles: PO, once, repeat 10-14 days
	5-10 mg/kg	Mammals: PO, q24h × 3-5 days
Ivermectin	0.2-0.4 mg/kg	All wildlife: IM, PO; Do not use in chelonians
Metronidazole	25-50 mg/kg	Reptiles: PO, q24-48h
	20-40 mg/kg	Birds: PO, q12-24h
	15-25 mg/kg	Mammals: PO, q12-24h
Praziquantel	5-8 mg/kg	Reptiles: IM, repeat 10-14 days
	20-40 mg/kg	Birds: PO, q12-24h
	5-10 mg/kg	Mammals: IM, repeat 10-14 days

IM, Intramuscular; *IO,* intraosseous; *IT,* intratracheal; *IV,* intravenous; *PO,* per os.

An appropriate-sized, darkened cardboard box (with ventilation holes cut in) or pet carrier that opens from the top can be used to transport wildlife. The cardboard box is an excellent transport carrier because it can be discarded after use; the pet carrier can be disinfected between uses. Homemade wooden boxes may also be used but are more difficult to disinfect. It is important to include a nonslip floor covering in the transport container to ensure proper footing in the transport box. Noncovered cardboard surfaces have been associated with the development of splay leg and bilateral partial paresis in some bird species.[5] When transporting birds, it is imperative that the box be large enough that the bird can turn without damaging its feathers. When flight or tail feathers are damaged, it can increase the rehabilitation time for a patient.

Avian Species

SMALL AND MEDIUM-SIZED BIRDS

Small and medium-sized birds, including songbirds, pigeons, doves, and crows, pose few physical risks to humans, although the larger birds in this group can deliver painful bites or scratches. These animals are best captured using a small diameter hole net or cloth. A cloth sack may be used if no box is available for transport.

GAMEBIRDS

Gamebirds are notorious for biting and scratching. These birds are generally good runners and will often run toward the thickest cover available, making capture difficult. Because gamebirds are generally high-strung, they may be injured by the inexperienced handler. Several people may be needed to flush a bird under cover. A net or towel is preferred for capturing these animals. Once the bird is captured, it is best to keep the box covered (darkened) to minimize the stress associated with transport.

WATERFOWL

Waterfowl, including ducks, geese, and swans, can deliver very painful bites and scratches. In addition, swans can also cause injury by striking with their wings. During the capture process, it is important to prevent these animals from reentering the water. Some form of water transportation and expert assistance may be necessary if the birds are in the water. Specialized equipment, such as swan hooks and bags, may also aid in capture and transport. The easiest method for transporting these animals is to place them in a transport carrier or blanket or sack.

WADERS

Many of the wading species have razor-sharp pointed beaks, and they will use them to stab at the faces of any perceived predators (including humans). Appropriate eye protection, such as safety goggles, should always be worn when handling these birds. Capture is similar to that of waterfowl. Transport boxes should be tall enough that the bird can stand comfortably. If such a box is not available, short trips can be made with the bird wrapped in a towel or blanket and the legs extended behind the bird. Care must be taken that the head is always sufficiently restrained.

SEABIRDS

The main danger posed by seabirds is from their beaks, which they may use to bite or stab at the face. Some seabirds also have sharp claws, which are capable of causing deep lacerations. As with waders, safety goggles should be worn and the bird never restrained close to the face. If the species in hand has internal nares, be careful not to hold the beak closed because it can affect normal respiration. These birds will also attempt to return to the water when they sense danger, so care must be taken to block this route of escape. A net is usually necessary for capture, but a towel or blanket may also be used. The beak can be kept closed by using tape or a rubber band. The head of these animals should be restrained and covered at all times, to prevent injury to the handler and reduce the stress on the animal. A towel can be wrapped around the body of these birds to restrain the wings; however, the towel should not be held so tight that it affects respiration (e.g., keel excursions). Because seabirds commonly regurgitate, it is important to remove any beak restraint before transporting the animal, to prevent aspiration.[5] The transportation carrier must be large enough to prevent damage to the flight and tail feathers.

RAPTORS

Although the beaks of raptors may look formidable, the biggest threat associated with these birds is their talons. Thick leather gloves, such as welding gloves, should be worn when handling medium to larger-sized specimens. Small raptors may be handled using outdoor work gloves (e.g., cotton or leather). When approached, most raptors roll backward and present their talons. When presented with a bird in this position, it is possible to offer them a towel or blanket to grasp before restraining the legs. The legs should always be grasped as close to the body wall as possible, as this will reduce the likelihood of causing a tibiotarsal fracture or injuries associated with self-taloning. The head of the raptor should be grasped using the same techniques to restrain other birds, with the index finger and thumb positioned under the mandible (Figure 19-6). For animals that are free-ranging, a bal chatri trap may be used. These traps can be built out of wire mesh (e.g., chicken wire) and fishing line. The wire mesh is first used to construct a wire cage to hold a live prey species (e.g., pigeon or rodent). A second piece of chicken wire is then placed over the prey cage, thus preventing injury to the prey species. The fishing line is then cut into small pieces (6-8 cm) and tied into small nooses. These nooses are secured over the entire surface of the trap. When the raptor attacks the trap, it becomes entangled in the trap and cannot lift off the ground with the trap.

Mammals

Unconscious mammals must be approached and handled with caution, as they may suddenly regain consciousness. Mammals should only be carried in an appropriate transport container and should never be captured or handled with

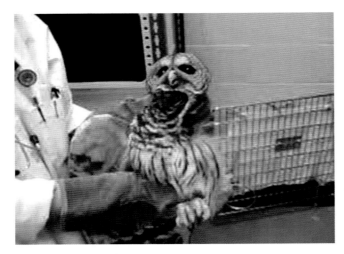

Figure 19-6 The talons and head of a raptor should be securely restrained to prevent injury to the handler.

unprotected hands. For capture, a towel or blanket may be placed over the animal to reduce its vision. Large and potentially dangerous mammals should always be sedated before being transported.

RODENTS

These animals frequently bite when handled. Leather gloves should always be worn by the individual capturing the animal to reduce the risk of injury and disease transmission. Small wild mammals may be caught with small nets or by covering them with a towel or blanket. Transport boxes for these animals should be escape-proof. Because of their ability to chew through cardboard, sturdy plastic or fine-meshed wire carriers are strongly recommended.

LAGOMORPHS

Although considered docile by many, lagomorphs may bite and scratch during capture and handling. Leather gloves should be worn to reduce the risk of injury. Rabbits and hares are more susceptible to the effects of stress than most other species. The short-term effects associated with stress may be manifested in sudden death due to heart failure or fatal oliguria.[6] Over longer periods of time, stress may be manifested as reduced gut motility and the disrupted carbohydrate metabolism, leading to diarrhea, hepatic lipidosis, liver failure, and death. In these cases, the cecal microflora are also disrupted, leading to enterotoxemia and gut stasis. Lagomorphs are also prone to spinal injury during capture and handling.[6] Blankets, towels, or nets may be used to capture animals that are free-ranging.

MESOPREDATORS: OPOSSUMS, RACCOONS, AND FOXES

Mesopredators have very sharp teeth and can deliver a painful bite, even through leather gloves. Animals that are severely ill or in shock may appear tame but can still inflict a serious injury. It is important to know that opossums can climb upward when held by their tail. Mesopredators may be caught

in a net and then pinned using a soft-headed broom. Once pinned safely, they can be scruffed. If this method does not work, a quick-release rabies pole can be used. It is preferable to use one with a rubber end to prevent fracturing an animal's teeth as is bites the pole.[7] Inexperienced individuals should not attempt to capture these animals, as they are likely to injure both the animal and themselves. A live animal trap, plastic domestic pet travel carrier, or sturdy plastic trash can with a tight-fitting lid can be used to transport mesopredators.

DEER

Yearling and adult deer can pose a special danger. These animals are capable of gouging with their antlers or kicking with their feet. Only trained professionals should attempt to capture an injured subadult or adult deer. A deer that is severely injured or in shock may appear tame when approached; however, they are still capable of quick bursts of speed and energy and can injure an inexperienced handler. Before approaching an injured deer, it should be evaluated from a distance to determine its general status. The equipment generally used to capture deer include dark towels or drapes for covering the head, thick blankets, soft ropes, soft cargo or freight netting, and possibly a dart gun or pole-syringe.[4] Anesthetics appropriate for sedating deer and a euthanasia solution should be kept on hand. If the deer is trapped in fencing or some other physical structure, it should be sedated remotely to prevent further injury to the deer. Expert assistance should also be sought for transport of injured deer. Individual deer should never be transported loose within a trailer without restraint. Large deer can best be transported wrapped up in cargo nets with the eyes blindfolded and the feet hobbled. Small deer can be wrapped in blankets. Trussed-up deer can be transported in a vehicle or trailer.

Fawns should be captured by hand and restrained manually. The deer should be approached from behind, and if recumbent, covered with a blanket, net, or coat. Many fawns do not display any resistance to capture. Once restrained, the animal should be blindfolded to reduce its stress levels. Once masked, these deer will lie quietly if they are undisturbed. The animal's legs can be tied together at the level of the metacarpi and metatarsi (cannons) using a soft rope; however, hobbling an animal in this way must be done carefully so that the soft ropes are not too tight. To prevent further struggling, the deer should then be trussed up in a blanket or cargo net and secured with additional ropes. Some deer are very vocal when caught, injured, or handled.

Reptiles and Amphibians

Expert assistance should be sought before attempting to capture and transport venomous snakes. For nonvenomous snakes and other reptiles, a cloth or canvas bag placed in a solid box makes an ideal transportation container. Amphibians can be moved in a similar manner, although the transport bag should be kept moist to prevent desiccation. This can be achieved by placing damp vegetation, such as sphagnum moss, in the bag or frequently misting the bag with dechlorinated water.

RESTRAINT AND HANDLING
Manual

Once the animal is transported to the clinic, the veterinary staff should be prepared to restrain and handle the animal for the physical examination and any diagnostic testing procedures. It is essential that the staff be trained properly to minimize the likelihood of injury to the human handler and patient. Restraint and handling is a stressful time for the patient, often leading to elevated cortisol or corticosterone production. Over time, this physiologic stress could have detrimental effects on the patient, including a reduction in metabolism, immune function, and normal behaviors.

GENERAL AVIAN

For most simple procedures, physical restraint alone can be used. Most species are easier to catch and handle in low light conditions and can be calmed by covering their head. At our hospitals, a towel is often used to support the body, restrain the wings, and cover the head. If the animal is not stable enough for chemical anesthesia during radiography, tape and a plexiglass board can be used to restrain the animals. In all cases of restraint, special care must be taken to ensure that the animal can have normal keel excursions that allow for adequate ventilation, as birds lack a diaphragm. Most birds will attempt to beat their wings during restraint, and this must be prevented for several reasons: They (1) risk damaging their flight and tail feathers, (2) can fracture the bones of their wings, (3) can worsen any injury, and (4) risk expending valuable energy in the process. When the wings are immobilized, they should be placed into their normal resting position.

Passerines

The simplest and most effective method of restraint is to place the bird in one hand with the dorsum of the bird in the palm and the neck held gently between the forefinger and second finger. It is especially important in the handling of small birds that undue pressure is not exerted that may inhibit respiration.

Pigeons and doves

Smaller species can be held with the keel resting in the palm and the head toward the wrist, using the fingers to secure the feet, tail, and wings.

Gamebirds

Smaller gamebirds may be held using the same technique described previously for small passerines; however, because larger gamebirds are both muscular and powerful, they must be held using two hands. When handling these animals, care must be taken to prevent them from losing excessive amounts of feathers, as they are "loosely feathered" and feather loss may delay release. Wrapping these birds in a towel will minimize wing-flapping and feather loss. Sufficient space should be maintained between the legs, as these animals can injure themselves by kicking their legs. Male gamebirds may have danger-ous spurs on their legs, and care should be taken to secure the legs firmly to avoid injury to the handler or bird.

Waterfowl

Smaller waterfowl can be restrained by folding the wings against the body and then holding both the wings and the body in both hands. A wing hold can also be used by grasping the wings near the point of the shoulders, with the index finger between the wings and the other hand supporting the sternum. The wing hold can be used only for short periods of time; otherwise, brachial plexus paralysis may result. Larger waterfowl can be restrained by tucking the body under the arm and against the restrainer's body. The bird's legs can also be tucked up against the body and the beak held with the free hand. For larger waterfowl, multiple individuals may be needed to properly restrain a patient. Both the handler and the animal may incur serious wounds by the calloused carpal joints of waterfowl. Appropriately sized towels or commercial body wraps can be used to limit wing flapping. The ends of the towel can be wrapped diagonally across the bird's body, leaving the head and neck exposed. The towel can be held in place with tape or bandage material. In those species without external nares, it is important to allow the beak to remain slightly open to ensure adequate ventilation.

Waders

A variety of challenges are present in the restraint and handling of waders. The smaller species are very delicate, and damage to the extremities and beak tips can easily be incurred. If waders are restrained with their legs flexed, permanent paralysis may occur due to impeded circulation. Some waders, such as herons and egrets, have very sharp beaks, and will make lightening-fast stabbing movements at the face and eyes of their captors. Safety goggles should be worn at all times when handling these birds. The head should be secured first. As with other birds, placement of the index finger and thumb under the mandible will provide adequate head restraint. The body can be restrained using the techniques described for larger waterfowl. Rubber tubing can be used to keep the beak closed during examinations, but it should never be left on while the bird is unattended, as regurgitation and aspiration may occur.[2] Impaling a cork on the end of the beak has also been used as a safety precaution, but we do not recommend it.

Seabirds

Seabirds can also deliver dangerous blows to the face and body with their beak and should therefore be restrained using the techniques described for waders.

Raptors

Raptors can pose a serious injury risk to any handler, experienced or inexperienced. Therefore, it is important to always remain vigilant around these animals. Raptors will use two primary defenses against their human handlers: their talons and their beak. To protect against injury, leather gloves should always be worn. When approached, raptors generally roll into a dorsal recumbent position and present their talons. The legs should be grasped as close to the body as possible to prevent self-taloning and iatrogenic tibiotarsal fracture. Once the legs are secured, the wings should be secured against the body to prevent feather damage. A towel or body wrap can be used to maintain the wings against the body. Always restrain these animals in an open area in a room, as the animal's feathers may become damaged if the wings strike a counter or table surface. The head of the raptor should be grasped using the same techniques described to restrain other birds, with the index finger and thumb positioned under the mandible. In our experience, owls, eagles, and accipiters are the most prone to bite. Wearing leather gloves will protect the handler against bite injuries. Most medium to large raptors require a minimum of two people to safely restrain them.

MAMMALS
Squirrels
Adult squirrels can inflict deep bite wounds using their incisors. Because of this, it is important to always restrain these animals while wearing a pair of thick leather gloves. The index finger and thumb of one hand can be placed underneath the mandible to control the head, while the free hand can be used to support the body. We strongly recommend wearing gloves when handling these animals, because if they bite a member of the staff they need to be, by law, euthanized. Orphaned squirrels can generally be handled using a single hand.

Bats
Injured bats pose a special risk to veterinarians and their staff. In most states, these animals remain an important vector of the rabies virus. Because these animals have special requirements regarding their care, they should only be handled by individuals with a significant amount of chiropteran experience. When working with these animals, gloves should be worn at all times. Bats are escape artists, and great care must be taken during handling to prevent accidental escape. One method of restraint is to position the bat dorsoventrally across its thorax and use the thumb and forefingers in apposition.[8] Care should be taken not to restrict the animal's ability to breathe. Scruffing appears to be stressful to many chiropteran species and should be avoided. It is important to always support the body of a bat while handling its wings to prevent iatrogenic fractures of the appendicular skeleton.

Lagomorphs
Finding a balance between gentle and secure restraint is essential when handling lagomorphs. These animals may react to any perceived danger by either becoming motionless or fleeing. In those cases where they remain motionless for an extended period of time, the handler should be prepared for them to mount a sudden escape response. Rabbits can be restrained by grasping (scruffing) the skin over the nape of the neck with one hand and using the free hand to support the hindquarters. The skeleton of these animals is lighter than comparable mammals, whereas the musculature associated with the rearlimbs is massive and strong. If the hindquarters are not supported, one quick kick of the rear legs could result in a vertebral fracture. Rabbits can also be restrained by wrapping a towel around the body of the animal ("bunny burrito"), leaving the head exposed. If this technique is used, again, it is important to support the hindquarters of the animal. Another method to assist in the restraint of rabbits is that of "hypnosis," or "trancing."[6] The technique is described as an immobility response that occurs after placing the animal on its dorsum, resulting in a cessation of spontaneous movement and a failure to respond to external stimuli for several minutes.

Mesopredators
Restraining adult mesopredators requires some background knowledge of these animals and is generally best done under sedation. If these animals are presented in a cage or carrier, we prefer to anesthetize them for removal from the cage: Ketamine (5-10 mg/kg IM) (Ketaset, Ft. Dodge Animal Health, Ft. Dodge, IA) or Telazol (tiletamine-zolazepam; 3-5 mg/kg IM) (Ft. Dodge Animal Health). Some individuals recommend removing the animals using a rabies pole, but this method is very stressful to the animal. Once anesthetized, the animals can be examined and sampled for various diagnostic tests. The animals can be moved by scruffing them at the nape and supporting the body with the free hand. For larger specimens, two or more handlers are recommended. Juvenile mesopredators can be restrained manually. Leather gloves should be used to reduce the risk of bite injuries. The juveniles can be handled using the same technique described for the adults. The tail of the opossum can also be used when manipulating or moving an opossum, although we do not believe the entire weight of the animal should be supported by the tail.

Deer
Adult deer should be anesthetized for a physical examination to minimize the stress and risk of injury to the patient and the handler. Anesthetic agents commonly used for deer are found in Table 19-4. Fawns can be restrained by supporting the head and body. Placing a hand under the thorax or abdomen when the animal is in a standing position will minimize the likelihood of the animal falling into a down position. In some cases, however, it is easier to examine a fawn while it is lying down.

Reptiles
Reptiles should be handled carefully to prevent injury to the patient. These animals have only a single occipital condyle supporting the skull and cervical spine, so the head and neck should always be supported to ensure that the cervical spine is not bearing the weight of the animal's body. It should also be taken into account that during times of shedding, reptiles are more susceptible to skin damage.

In the past, hypothermia was considered an appropriate manner of restraint for reptiles; however, this primitive technique is no longer considered appropriate. There are several possible disadvantages associated with this technique: (1) There

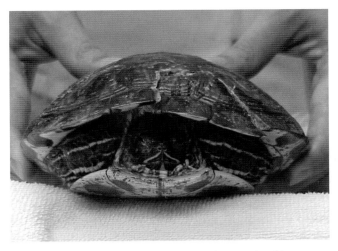

Figure 19-7 Chelonians can be securely restrained by grasping the lateral surfaces of the plastron and carapace.

is no published evidence that suggests that lowering a reptile's body temperature until it no longer responds to external stimuli abolishes the perception of pain, (2) as the animal warms it may suddenly awaken, which can cause danger to the handlers if it is a hazardous species, (3) the animal may die if the hypothermic state is extended, (4) stress and immunodeficiency may result from hypothermic states because immunoglobulin synthesis is temperature dependent, and (5) several safe chemical restraint agents exist for those times when manual restraint is not considered sufficient.[9]

Many noninvasive, short procedures can be done using manual restraint alone, but it should be remembered that although reptiles may not react to painful or stressful stimuli in a manner similar to mammals, they do feel pain and experience stress. Confinement and reduction of vision can minimize the stress experienced by the animal. For example, a reptile can be placed into a dark bag for radiographs because they will generally remain motionless for the procedure. Placing a nonocclusive bandage material over the animal's eyes may also be used to reduce motion for a diagnostic procedure such as radiographs.

Chelonians can be restrained by grasping the lateral surfaces of the shell in the area of the bridges (Figure 19-7). For chelonians that are capable of extending their neck and biting (e.g., snapping turtle: *Chelydra serpentina*), grasping the shell more caudally is recommended. When the head of a chelonian needs to be restrained, the index finger and thumb can be placed behind the points of the ramus of the mandible. It is important that the handler does not exert excessive pressure when extracting the head and neck, as this can lead to cervical injury. For those species that can completely enclose themselves within their shell (e.g., box turtle: *Terrapene carolina*), chemical anesthesia is recommended. Placing the animal in a shallow volume of water may stimulate them to exit their shell, but waiting for this to occur can be time consuming.

Small lizards may be held in one hand, with the index finger under the throat and the thumb on the head or neck. Larger lizards can be held by grasping them behind the head with an index finger and thumb, while securing the rear legs against the base of the tail. It is important to be gentle when manipulating the tail of a lizard capable of tail autonomy. Applying gentle pressure on the eyes of some species of lizards may induce a vagal response (e.g., bradycardia, lethargy).

Large snakes and venomous snakes require at least two experienced handlers for restraint. Specialized equipment is recommended to manage these animals, including snake hooks, clear tubes, and pinning sticks. The snake can be placed on a foam mat, and a rod or hook may be used to pin the head. Once pinned, the head should be grasped behind the angles of the jaw with the thumb and forefinger, taking care not to apply too much pressure. A second person should assist the primary handler by supporting the body of the snake. Clear plastic tubes, either commercial or homemade and slightly larger in diameter than the snake, can be used to restrain venomous snakes. The snake should be placed on the ground with the tube directly in front of it, and the snake encouraged to enter the tube. When one third of the snake is in the tube, the snake and tube are grasped together to immobilize the snake. Preplaced holes in the tube can be used to allow for sampling and injections.

AMPHIBIANS

Restraint and handling of amphibians should be kept to a minimum. Because amphibians are susceptible to skin damage and desiccation, they should be handled with moistened gloves. Larval amphibians can succumb to hypoxia if they are removed from their aquatic habitat for an extended period, and they should only be removed from the water for short periods of time. Some toad species, such as the marine toad *(Bufo marinus)*, can present a danger to the handler by releasing bufotoxin from the parotid glands. Wearing exam gloves can minimize the likelihood of toxin exposure to the handler. Anurans (frogs and toads) can be restrained by placing an index finger and thumb into the axillae or wrapping these fingers around the forelimbs. For small specimens, cupping them in a hand is also recommended. Most salamanders and newts require minimal restraint and can be held in an open hand. The head of caecilians and amphiumas should be restrained because they can bite.

Chemical

While many procedures can be carried out with manual restraint, there will be instances where the patient is too difficult to restrain, the procedure too painful, or the stress associated with the procedure too great for manual restraint to be used alone. When this is the case, it is advisable to use chemical restraint. Although the expense associated with managing the case using anesthesia is greater, the reduced stress and time saved to try to carry out the procedure will outweigh this disadvantage. Both injectable and inhalant anesthetics are available for use in a multitude of wildlife patients, and a list of commonly used anesthetics can be found in Table 19-4. When selecting an anesthetic(s) for a wildlife case, it is important to consider the patient's status and the procedure being performed. Some of the points to consider include the the animal's weight, age, reproductive status, stress level, type of injury, length of procedure, and need for analgesia.

■ PHYSICAL EXAMINATION AND COMMON ABNORMALITIES

The overall aim of wildlife rehabilitation is to return animals to the wild in a condition that allows them to compete with members of its own and other species and to successfully reproduce and behave in a species-appropriate way, with no physical or mental impediments that would affect their chances of performing normally in their environment. The physical

TABLE 19-4 **Anesthetic Agents Used to Anesthetize Wildlife Patients**

Agent	Dose	Comments
Avian		
Isoflurane	3%-5% induction, 1%-3% maintenance	Safe, mask or intubate, low cardiopulmonary risk
Sevoflurane	5%-8% induction, 2%-5% maintenance	Safe, mask or intubate, low cardiopulmonary risk
Propofol	10 mg/kg IV, to effect	Must be given IV or IO, rapid recovery
Xylazine		Not recommended, rough recovery
Ketamine		Not recommended, rough recovery
Mammals		
Isoflurane	3%-5% induction, 1%-3% maintenance	Safe, mask or intubate, low cardiopulmonary risk
Sevoflurane	5%-8% induction, 2%-5% maintenance	Safe, mask or intubate, low cardiopulmonary risk
Propofol	5-10 mg/kg IV, to effect	Must be given IV or IO, rapid recovery
Xylazine	1-5 mg/kg	Deer (combine with ketamine)
Medetomidine	0.15-0.25 mg/kg	
	0.5-0.1 mg/kg	Deer (combine with ketamine)
Ketamine	5-10 mg/kg	Mesopredators
	10-40 mg/kg	Lagomorphs
	80-100 mg/kg	Rodents
	5-15 mg/kg	Deer (combine with xylazine)
	3-5 mg/kg	Deer (combine with medetomidine)
Tiletamine-Zolazepam	5 mg/kg	Mesopredators; not recommended for lagomorphs
Reptiles		
Isoflurane	3%-5% induction, 1%-3% maintenance	Safe, mask or intubate, low cardiopulmonary risk
Sevoflurane	5%-8% induction, 2%-5% maintenance	Safe, mask or intubate, low cardiopulmonary risk
Propofol	10-15 mg/kg IV, to effect	Must be given IV or IO, rapid recovery
Medetomidine	0.15 mg/kg IM	Alligators: reverse atipamezole (equal volume)
	0.75-0.15 mg/kg IM	Chelonians: in combination with ketamine (5-15 mg/kg IM)
Ketamine	5-15 mg/kg	Snakes, lizards: induction
	10-25 mg/kg	Chelonians: induction; not recommended for surgical procedures without additional coverage (inhalant, medetomidine)
Telazol	3-5 mg/kg	Snakes: induction
	5-8 mg/kg	Lizards: induction
	5-10 mg/kg	Chelonians: induction
Amphibians		
MS-222	200-5000 mg/L	Lower doses for larvae
Clove oil	300-350 mg/L	Anurans
	400-450 mg/L	Salamanders
Propofol	35-45 mg/kg ICe	Salamanders
	5-15 mg/kg IV	All

MS-222, tricaine methane sulfonate; *ICe,* intracoelomic; *IM,* intramuscular; *IV,* intravenous.

examination represents the first opportunity the veterinarian has at determining the likelihood an animal can be rehabilitated and released. In some cases, the injury will be life-threatening or not correctable, and humane euthanasia will be warranted. In other cases, the ultimate outcome will be based on the veterinarian's ability to provide medical and surgical assistance. For these reasons, it is important that the veterinarian fully evaluate these animals at the time of presentation to ensure that he or she identifies all of the problems an animal presents with, as well as make a determination as to the value of pursuing or not pursuing a case.

The first, and most important, step in performing a physical examination is to correctly identify the presenting species and its age group. For those with limited knowledge regarding species characterization, we recommend maintaining a library of field guides (both national and state) to assist with species identification. Maintaining friendships with local ornithologists, mammalogists, and herpetologists might also be helpful when attempting to identify resources to assist with species identification. The Internet can also be a valuable resource for identifying species too. If the identification of the actual species is not possible, it would still be useful to be able to characterize the animal to family or generic level. Correctly identifying the animal will allow the veterinarian to determine the (1) natural diet (e.g., carnivore, omnivore, herbivore), (2) habitat and feeding strategy (e.g., aerial feeder, arboreal, ground dwelling), (3) social behavior (e.g., gregarious and nonterritorial, solitary and territorial), (4) movements (e.g., resident, partial migrant, summer or winter visitor), (5) approximate age (e.g., dependent/independent juvenile, or adult) (Figure 19-8), and (6) gender. This information will aid in determining the care an animal should receive and may also determine its release potential. If the animal is being presented from an outside source, a thorough history should be obtained. Unfortunately, the opportunity to obtain a thorough history from these animals is often limited because the individuals presenting the animals may have only recently encountered the animals. Those historical questions that can generally be answered include: (1) Where was the animal found? (2) Under what conditions was the animal found? (3) What day and time was the animal found? (4) How long has the rescuer had the animal? (5) Has the rescuer fed, watered, or medicated the animal? (6) What has the animal been doing while in captivity? (7) Were there any obvious lesions on the animal?

Once an adequate history is obtained, the animal should be observed from a distance to gauge the severity of the illness and determine whether to proceed with the physical exam or allow the animal to recuperate. Avian and reptilian species will attempt to mask any signs of illness when a perceived predator approaches. If the animal is unable to do this, and appears obviously ill, the condition is likely extremely serious. During the observation period, information can be gathered about the animal's posture, conformation, respiratory and neurologic status, and gastrointestinal output (e.g., feces, vomitus).

As with the physical examination of companion animals, it is extremely important to follow the same routine for each examination so that no body system is missed. An example of a standard wildlife physical examination can be found in Box 19-3, and a list of the most common findings during an examination in Table 19-5.

Avian General Examination

Birds that present in shock should be stabilized. Overmanipulating these animals can result in acute cardiopulmonary arrest. Once the bird is stable, a thorough and systematic approach to the physical examination is essential. In addition to the previously described exam protocol, an examination of the pectoral area should be done. Evaluating the condition of the large pectoralis muscles lying over the keel will aid in the assessment of the animal's body condition. A bird can be presumed to be in good body condition when the muscles form an "A" off of the keel. If the pectoralis muscles are concave and the keel is prominent, then the animal is in poor condition. This is generally indicative of chronic disease.[10] An animal that has bulging pectoralis muscles, making the palpation of the keel difficult, can be presumed to be overconditioned. A distended abdominal wall (coelomic cavity) may be indicative of ascites, neoplasia, egg binding peritonitis, bowel distension, or hepatomegaly. In all but laying hens, the abdominal muscles associated with the coelomic cavity should be slightly concave. Both wings and legs should be extended and examined. Feather quality, muscle mass, and bone integrity should be assessed. Special care should be taken to evaluate joint function.

The most common reasons that wild birds are presented to veterinary hospitals are traumatic injuries, poisonings, and infectious diseases. Traumatic injuries most commonly result from collisions with vehicles or windows, predation by domestic animals (e.g., dogs and cats), or gunshot wounds. Traumatic injuries frequently result in fractures, soft tissue injury, ruptured air sacs, nervous system damage (e.g., con-

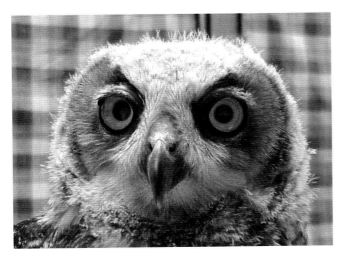

Figure 19-8 It is important for veterinarians to be able to identify the general age of their patients. In the case of this great-horned owl, the downy feathers on the head confirm that it is a juvenile.

Standard Protocol for Performing a Physical Examination on a Wildlife Patient

1. Identify species to determine diet, housing needs, and restraint techniques. A geographically appropriate field guide is essential.
2. Observe the animal from a distance for alertness, aggression, mental status, body condition, and gastrointestinal and respiratory functions.
3. Restrain animal using appropriate techniques for that species.
4. Observe the eyes for pupil size and symmetry, pupillary light responses, menace reflexes, corneal disease, and the presence of hyphema or hypopyon. Perform fundic examination.
5. Examine the ears for injury and ectoparasites.
6. Examine the mouth for abscesses, mucous membrane tackiness, capillary refill time, and presence of parasitism.
7. Examine the nares for discharge.
8. Palpate the head for traumatic injuries or abnormal masses.
9. Palpate the lymph nodes (mammals only).
10. Thoroughly inspect the integument for signs of dermatitis, ectoparasitism, and abnormal masses.
11. Palpate the abdomen or coelomic cavity.
12. Palpate the extremities for obvious injury, asymmetry, muscle atrophy, and loss of feathers or fur.
13. Check anus or vent for abnormalities, diarrhea, or hemorrhage.
14. Auscult the heart and lungs.
15. Weigh the animal.

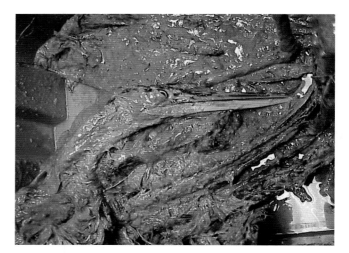

Figure 19-9 This great blue heron presented after falling into an industrial pond full of liquefied plastic.

cussion, paralysis), and damaged plumage and beaks. Poisonings may be intentional or unintentional (Figure 19-9). It is important to attempt to identify the source of the poisoning, if at all possible, to prevent exposure to children, domestic pets, and other wildlife. Rodenticides, insecticides, herbicides, and heavy metals are the most common poisons reported in wildlife. Infectious disease in wild birds may be associated with an individual bird's exposure and immune status, or it may be related to a disease outbreak. *Chlamydophila psittaci,* poxviruses, mycoplasmosis, and trichomoniasis represent diseases that commonly circulate through wild bird populations, while aspergillosis is more often an individual bird disease that occurs as a result of a single direct exposure or the stress associated with captivity. Endoparasites and ectoparasites are frequently found in wild birds, but they are rarely the primary cause of disease.

PASSERINES

Small passerines commonly present as a direct result of a traumatic injury associated with predation or an in-flight collision (e.g., window, automobile). Soft tissue and orthopedic injuries are the most common result. If the trauma results in closed fractures of the ulna, radius, or carpometacarpus, the fracture(s)

may be stabilized by taping the flight feathers together and supporting the wing. Because of their high metabolism, passerines can potentially heal these fractures in 2 to 4 weeks. Unfortunately, fractures of the humerus or fractures of both the radius and ulna have a guarded to grave prognosis. If healing does occur with these fractures, normal flight is often compromised. Closed fractures of the femur with the fragments in near alignment will usually heal with cage rest; however, if the fracture occurs distal to the femur, light splints can be placed to align fracture segments. Small passerines will generally tolerate supporting their weight on one leg while the other heals. There is some debate about the long-term survival rates of one-legged small birds in the wild.

Cat predation of passerines is a major concern in the United States. It has been estimated that these animals are responsible for killing millions of birds every year. In our practices, fledglings are the most commonly presented. The severity of wounds will vary greatly, from minor soft-tissue wounds to severe lacerations, punctures, and fractures. In most cases, feather loss is apparent as well. The wounds are often contaminated with mixed Gram-positive (e.g., *Staphylococcus* spp. and *Streptococcus* spp.) and Gram-negative bacteria (e.g., *Pasteurella multocida* and *E. coli*). Euthanasia is appropriate in severe cases. Superficial wounds carry a better prognosis and can be managed with appropriate antibiotic therapy and wound management.

Passerines are also susceptible to the previously mentioned infectious diseases, especially poxvirus, mycoplasmosis, and ectoparasites. A higher prevalence of disease may be expected in these birds because they often congregate at high densities in feeding stations (e.g., suburban bird feeders). Starlings and members of the Corvidae family are susceptible to infection by the nematode *Syngamus trachea* (gapeworm), which can cause severe pulmonary disease and respiratory distress.

Anesthesia may be required to facilitate an examination for the following circumstances: nervous or stressed birds, fractious birds, dyspneic birds (e.g., allows direct delivery of oxygen

TABLE 19-5   Common Species Presentations for North American Wildlife

Species	Common presentations
Squirrels	Orphaned: fallen out of nest
	Traumatic injuries: automobile, domestic predators
	Viral disease: West Nile virus, papilloma virus
	Bacterial disease: Gram-negative opportunists
	Ectoparasites: mites, ticks, fleas
	Endoparasites: coccidians, nematodes
Bats	Traumatic: fractures, wing tears, entanglement
	Poisoning: rodenticides, oil contamination
	Viral disease: rabies virus
	Bacterial disease
	Fungal disease
	Ectoparasites
	Endoparasites[8]
Rabbits and hares	Orphaned: abandoned and kidnapped
	Traumatic injuries: automobile, domestic predators
	Ectoparasites: mites, fleas
	Endoparasites: coccidians, nematodes
	Colic: Bacterial dysbiosis
Otters	Orphaned: parent trapped/killed
	Traumatic injuries: automobile, domestic predators
	Bacterial disease: Gram-negative opportunists, septic bite wounds
	Poisoning
	Ectoparasites: mites, fleas
	Endoparasites: protozoa, cestodes, nematodes
Foxes, raccoons, coyotes	Orphaned: parent trapped/killed
	Traumatic injuries: automobile, domestic predators
	Viral disease: canine distemper virus, parvovirus, rabies
	Bacterial disease: Gram-negative opportunists, leptospirosis
	Poisoning
	Ectoparasites: mites, ticks, fleas
	Endoparasites: coccidians, nematodes
Opossums	Orphaned: parent trapped/killed
	Poisoning
	Traumatic injuries: automobile, domestic predators
	Bacterial disease: Gram-negative opportunists, leptospirosis
	Ectoparasites: mites, ticks, fleas
	Endoparasites: coccidians, nematodes
Deer	Orphaned: kidnapped
	Traumatic injuries: automobile, domestic predators, fire ants
	Viral disease: epizootic hemorrhagic disease, rotavirus, coronavirus
	Bacterial disease: Gram-negative opportunists *(E. coli)*
	Ectoparasites: mites, ticks, fleas
	Endoparasites: coccidians, nematodes
Birds	Orphaned: fallen from nest, parent killed
	Traumatic injuries: automobile, domestic predators, electric wires, fishing hooks
	Poisoning: heavy metal, mercury, organophosphates
	Viral disease: West Nile virus, paramyxovirus, herpesvirus, poxvirus
	Bacterial disease: Gram-negative opportunists
	Ectoparasites: mites, ticks, lice
	Endoparasites: coccidians, nematodes
Reptiles	Traumatic injuries: automobile, domestic predator, lawn equipment
	Viral disease: herpesvirus, iridovirus, paramyxovirus
	Bacterial disease: Gram-negative opportunists, mycoplasmosis
	Ectoparasites: mites, ticks
	Endoparasites: protozoa, nematodes

and reduces stress), musculoskeletal examinations where there is a fracture, and an ophthalmic examination when a fundic exam is required. An ophthalmic examination should be done any time a bird suffers head trauma, as the disease of the posterior chamber is common in these birds.

PIGEONS AND DOVES

As with passerines, pigeons and doves often present to veterinary hospitals after sustaining a traumatic injury. These birds rely heavily on flight to evade predators and reach roosts and should not be released with impaired flight. Euthanasia should be considered for birds with open or comminuted fractures or fractures with extensive joint involvement. Neurologic disorders are commonly seen with traumatic injuries, and the physical examination should include a thorough examination of the animal's posture, demeanor, mentation, and reflexes. Traumatic wounds secondary to strike by raptors usually present as wounds on the bird's dorsum. Ruptured crops are commonly seen in these species, likely because their crops are usually more heavily filled than those of other avian species. These cases will present as a necrotic granulating wound and associated crop fistula.

Pigeons and doves are susceptible to a range of infectious diseases. Trichomoniasis commonly causes white plaques in the oral cavity. This organism is extremely contagious in these birds. Mild cases can be simple to treat, but advanced cases carry a poor prognosis. Many of the severe cases show some improvement with treatment, only to succumb before the completion of the treatment and elimination of the signs. For this reason, we generally recommend euthanasia for the severe cases. Bacterial and fungal infections of the crop (ingluvitis) are common, especially in young birds. A foul smell in the oral cavity can be an indication of a crop infection. The crop itself may appear thickened, enlarged, and have a decreased emptying time. Septic arthritis, often the result of infection with *Salmonella* sp. or *E. coli,* is common in these birds and may resolve with broad-spectrum antibiotic therapy; however, some authors advise against treatment because of the chronic joint problems that may arise after treatment and the zoonotic potential for the handlers.[1] Pigeons and doves can serve as reservoirs for pathogens that are highly infectious to other birds, including paramyxovirus (Newcastle disease—a reportable disease) and poxvirus. Pigeons or doves presenting with clinical signs consistent with these diseases should be euthanized to minimize the likelihood of disease transmission to other birds. A bird with a paramyxovirus infection may display a range of clinical signs, including head tremors, diarrhea, deformed eggs, torticollis, polyuria, polydipsia, and anorexia. Birds with pox lesions generally have multiple masses in their featherless areas (e.g., legs and surrounding the oral cavity and eyes). When these lesions are draining, they are contagious to other birds. *Mycoplasma* spp. infections are commonly associated with upper respiratory tract disease, resulting in swollen sinuses and ocular or nasal discharge. Other than ticks or lice, external parasites are rarely seen. Various species of coccidians can cause wasting and diarrhea. Pigeons and doves are commonly infected with *Capillaria* spp. and ascarids.

GAMEBIRDS

Common reasons for presentation include trauma (e.g., hit by automobile) and infectious disease. Gamebirds who have been traumatized may present with orthopedic injuries, ocular hemorrhage, or neurologic disease. Infectious diseases seen in gamebirds include viral disease, bacterial infection, fungal disease, and parasitic disease. Paramyxovirus (Newcastle disease) and pheasant coronavirus, which causes multiple masses around the head and limbs, are the most common viral diseases. These birds are susceptible to a variety of opportunistic bacterial pathogens. Some of the more common pathogens are *E. coli, Salmonella* sp., and *Mycobacterium avium.* Birds with *E. coli* infections generally present in critical condition and often appear hypothermic (fluffed) and depressed. *Salmonella* sp. is usually associated with hemorrhagic enteritis, and animals often succumb to this disease acutely. Mycobacteriosis is generally associated with general body wasting, sinusitis, and tenosynovitis. This pathogen is zoonotic, so appropriate precautions should be taken when handling and disposing an animal. Fungal infections with *Aspergillus* spp. can result from spore inhalation, and affected animals develop clinical signs associated with the respiratory tract, including coughing and dyspnea. The parasitic diseases reported in gamebirds are similar to those seen in pigeons and doves. *Capillaria* sp. is a common finding in both wild and captive gamebirds. This endoparasite can cause severe loss of body condition, and it is not uncommon for animals to succumb to infection. Commonly, gamebirds are semi-intensively farmed before release and may be prone to parasitic infections. A soiled vent and diarrhea are common findings in gamebirds with endoparasitic infections. Ectoparasites such as feather lice, hippoboscid flies, and mites may be present in large numbers on debilitated birds.

WATERFOWL

Waterfowl are commonly presented to the veterinary hospital because of traumatic injury (e.g., vehicle collision, fishing line injuries), poisoning (e.g., lead ingestion), and infectious disease. Traumatic injury often results in both soft tissue and orthopedic injuries. Loss of the use of one or both legs or feet, an inability to fly, and open fractures or fractures involving joints are all indications for euthanasia. Injury due to fishing line and hooks may be obvious at presentation, or it may be unknown until further diagnostics are pursued (e.g., radiographs).

The ingestion of lead shot or lead sinkers has been a major problem for wild waterfowl. Lead toxicity can result in a range of clinical signs, including acute, asymptomatic death or bright green diarrhea, progressive weight loss, anorexia, anemia, kinking of the neck, neurologic symptoms, muscle weakness, dehydration, and poor feathering. Birds with a more chronic presentation may shows signs consistent with starvation and severe anemia. Lead becomes toxic to the waterfowl when the gastric acid ionizes the lead, allowing it to become absorbed and affect various organ systems (e.g., liver). Botulism *(Clostridium botulinum)* is a common seasonal problem in waterfowl. Affected animals present with a flaccid paralysis of the muscles, commonly known as *limberneck.* Three grades of paralysis have been described: (1) cannot fly but can walk and swim, (2) cannot fly or walk but can swim and move by a flopping motion when assisted by the wings and unable to lift head out of water or off the ground, and (3) almost completely paralyzed.[11] The prognosis for grade 1 is generally fair to poor, whereas the prognoses for grades 2 and 3 are poor to guarded and grave, respectively. Oil contamination and blue green algae toxicity can also affect wild waterfowl.

Infectious diseases of waterfowl are generally divided into two categories: individual and flock. Any individual suffering from stress (e.g., low food source, stress of predators, habitat loss) can develop opportunistic infections. Aspergillosis is an example of this. On the other hand, there are also those diseases that primarily affect entire flocks. Fortunately, many of these are rare. Duck viral enteritis, which is caused by a herpesvirus, can result in hemorrhagic gastroenteritis, neurologic abnormalities, polydipsia, and signs associated with all other body systems. Duck plague, *Pasteurella multocida* infections, can occur in flocks at certain times of the year. Avian tuberculosis can also be disseminated through flocks that are in close association.

WADERS

The most common reasons that waders present to the veterinary hospital are trauma due to fishing lines and hooks, entanglement in telephone cables, poisoning by ingestion of mollusks that have accumulated the phytoplanktons that cause red tides, poor condition after hard seasons, and oil contamination. When working with wading birds, it is important to closely examine the commissures of the mouth and frenulum of the tongue for fishing line. Some waders, especially herons, have prominent keels even when they are considered to be in good health. It is important that these animals are not misdiagnosed as being in poor body condition and oversupplemented with supportive care.

SEABIRDS

As with waders, it is important to carefully examine the oral cavity of seabirds for fishing lines or hooks. The body condition of these animals can be assessed by palpating pectoral muscle mass.[5] The plumage should be closely inspected for signs of oil contamination. Common reasons that seabirds present to veterinary hospitals include fishing line and hook entanglement, wing and leg fractures, aspergillosis, and oil contamination. Euthanasia should be considered with complicated or open wing or leg fractures, or those with joint involvement. Animals that have heavy ectoparasite burdens or present in extremely poor condition often carry a guarded prognosis. When considering the long-term management of these animals in captivity, it is important to minimize stress and maximize nutritional support, as these animals generally do poorly in captivity.

RAPTORS

The most common reasons that raptors present to a veterinary hospital are traumatic injuries (e.g., automobile, gunshot, entanglement in high wires), pesticide toxicity, infectious diseases, and maladapted starvation. Trauma may result in ocular,

aural, orthopedic, and soft tissue injuries. Pesticide toxicity may be a result of intentional or accidental poisoning. Organophosphate toxicity is commonly seen. Viral, fungal, and bacterial infections can cause severe disease. Many raptors are extremely susceptible to West Nile virus infections. Falcon and owl herpesvirus infections are occasionally observed in animals with neurologic disease. Raptors are also susceptible to paramyxovirus. Many raptors become infected with poxvirus when they prey on Columbiformes (e.g., pigeons and doves). Because raptors ingest prey species, the potential for them to become exposed to a variety of opportunistic bacterial pathogens exists. *E. coli*, *Salmonella* spp., *Klebsiella* spp., *Pseudomonas* spp., and *Staphylococcus aureus* infections are commonly reported in raptors. Hippoboscid flies and lice are commonly found on raptors at the time of presentation. In addition to being exposed to poxvirus with columbiformes, many raptors are also exposed to trichomonads. Affected animals often have large white plaques in the oral cavity. Euthanasia should be considered for any of the following presentations: loss of an eye or reduced vision (owls may be an exception), an inability to feed naturally, loss of the function of one or both wings or legs, damage or amputation of the toes or talons that prevents normal hunting and perching, any bird that has become habituated or imprinted on humans and would be dangerous if released, and inability to relate naturally to conspecifics.

Mammalian General Examination

The physical examination of all mammalian patients should be thorough and consistent; this will minimize the likelihood of missing species-based problems. Most orphaned mammals can be examined using standard restraint, whereas adult animals need to be anesthetized. We always recommend wearing gloves, a surgical mask, and goggles when working with rabies vector species. The general body condition of most mammals can be determined by evaluating the epaxial muscles along the spine and the large muscles along the long bones. The amount of subcutaneous adipose tissue, as determined by pinching the skin, can also be used to assess body condition.

SQUIRRELS

The gender of an orphaned squirrel can be determined by identifying the prepuce of the male on the ventral abdomen or the elongate vulva of a female. Sexually mature squirrels are easy to confirm, as the males have large external testicles. Squirrels commonly present to the veterinary hospital for traumatic injuries (e.g., hit by automobile, gunshot, domestic species predation), poisonings, and infectious diseases. Animals that present for traumatic injuries may have unilateral or bilateral epistaxis, musculoskeletal injuries (e.g., fractures), deep puncture wounds, or degloving injuries, or they may be in shock. A decision as to the long-term potential for releasing the animal should be made at the time of presentation. Although some rehabilitators do not advocate this, at times a decision to not pursue a case in which the species is more plentiful (e.g., squirrel vs. bald eagle) must be made. This is the basis for triage, especially when financial and personnel resources are limited. Most squirrel poisonings are associated with rodenticides or pesticides and are, unfortunately, intentional. It is important to identify and pursue potential poison cases to minimize the risk for poisoning of children, domestic animals, or other wildlife. A poxvirus is occasionally observed in wild squirrel populations. Squirrels are susceptible to West Nile virus infections. Many of the infectious agents recovered from squirrels at the time of presentation are presumed to be related to a bite injury sustained from a predator. Because the predator (e.g., dog or cat) has a mixed microflora, a broad-spectrum antibiotic should be used to manage the squirrel's injury.

BATS

Species determination is critical, and field guides are highly recommended to assist with identification. Determining the animal's gender and age is also important. Male bats have an obvious prepuce on the ventral abdomen and can easily be differentiated from a female. Juvenile bats are smaller than their adult counterparts, are dependent, and have underdeveloped wings. Once a bat becomes independent, aging becomes more difficult. Transillumination of the phalanges should reveal still developing bones, and a magnifying lens can be used to visualize small digits.

Gloves should always be worn when handling bats. Body condition score can be used as a general health assessment; extremely underweight bats will have a concave abdomen. A very thorough examination of the wings should be performed. Even minor injuries will impair flight. The body should be supported while examining each wing. The bones, joints, and soft tissue elements of each wing should be examined for fractures, tears, and joint mobility. Common reasons that chiropterans present to veterinary hospitals are traumatic injuries (e.g., hit by automobile, gunshot), fishing line entanglement, oil contamination, poisoning, and neurologic symptoms secondary to lyssavirus infection. Again, because these animals are important rabies virus vectors throughout much of the United States, all animals should be considered positive until proven otherwise and should be handled accordingly.

LAGOMORPHS

Gender determination of lagomorphs can be difficult in juvenile animals. In adult rabbits, an examination of the external genitalia will often reveal the gender. It is important to note that male rabbits do have open external rings, which allows them to draw their testicles into their body cavity. If the testicles have ascended into the abdomen, it should still be possible to extract the penis.

Careful examination of the head and limbs, abdomen, and perineum should be performed on every lagomorph case. The most common reasons that rabbits present to a veterinary hospital are traumatic injury, fly strike, dental disorders, viral disease, bacterial disease, and parasitism. Traumatic injuries for presenting cases can range from minor soft tissue wounds to severe fractures or spinal injury. Fly strike may result from open wounds or viral disease. Myxomatosis is a common viral disease causing skin and respiratory disease. Rabbits are susceptible to a range of bacterial diseases, including pasteurellosis, which can colonize wounds or cause respiratory disease; infection with *Treponema cuniculi*, a spirochete that is sexually transmitted and causes lesions on the face, external genitalia, and perineum; infection with *Yersinia pseudotuberculosis*, which can cause internal abscesses and septicemia; and infection with *Francisella tularemia*, which causes an acute septicemic disease. Because some of these diseases are zoonotic, it is important that the veterinarian and staff wear gloves and take appropriate precautions. As with most mammals, lagomorphs are susceptible to ectoparasites and endoparasites.

MESOPREDATORS

The most common reasons that mesopredators (e.g., opossums, raccoons, foxes, coyotes) present to the veterinary hospital are traumatic injuries (e.g., hit by automobile, gunshot, trapping), intentional poisonings, and infectious diseases. Raccoons, opossums, foxes and coyotes are frequently the victims of gunshots or trapping attempts, which may result in severe orthopedic and soft-tissue injuries. They may also present with infected bite wounds from other animals.

Poisoning is generally from organophosphates or vitamin K antagonist rodenticides (e.g., warfarin), although antifreeze poisonings are also occasionally reported. To characterize the type of poison, it is important to examine the animal closely. Animals with organophosphate toxicity often present with miotic pupils, excessive salivation, and ataxia. Animals poisoned with warfarin or another vitamin K antagonist, generally present with coagulopathy, hemorrhage from different orifices, weakness, and acute death. Animals with antifreeze toxicity generally succumb to renal failure. Treatment for organophosphates and vitamin K antagonists are supportive care and atropine/2-pam and vitamin K, respectively.

Mesopredators are susceptible to a variety of viral, bacterial, fungal and parasitic diseases. Viral infections are common. Animals that are febrile (reference temperatures: opossum 92°-95° F; raccoon, fox, coyote, 100°-104° F) should be quarantined and handled with care. Certain viral diseases may cause a lymphopenia or lymphocytosis. Raccoons, coyotes, and foxes are all susceptible to canine distemper, parvovirus, adenovirus, and rabies. Opossums should also be considered to be susceptible to rabies, although infection is rare. Sarcoptic mange and ringworm are also common in these animals and may cause extreme pruritus, dermatologic disease, and eventually emaciation and death. Some may not exhibit signs but instead serve as reservoirs for the mites. Because both sarcoptes and ringworm are zoonotic, the veterinary staff should wear gloves and change their laboratory coats (and clothes) in between handling these animals and other animals.

DEER

Adult deer presented to a veterinary hospital pose a special risk because injured deer will make every attempt to evade capture. In most cases, these animals must be sedated the entire time they are hospitalized, or they will worsen their injuries. For some facilities, euthanasia is considered the most humane option for these cases. Common reasons deer are presented to veterinary hospitals include traumatic injury (e.g., automobile, entanglement, dog attack, gunshot), myopathy, healthy fawns mistaken for orphans, and fawns suffering from starvation after hard winters. Traumatic injury commonly results in limb, pelvic, or facial fractures, or spinal injury. Deer can survive with a missing limb, and some authors believe amputation is a viable alternative to euthanasia. Myopathy may occur following attempts to evade predators (including humans) and may be evidenced by recumbent, hyperthermic, hyperventilating deer with hindlimb paralysis. Irreversible metabolic changes usually result.[4] Johne's disease, epizootic hemorrhagic disease, coronavirus diarrhea, rotavirus diarrhea, colibacillosis, salmonellosis, and mycobacteriosis represent common infectious disease presentations for deer. Because of chronic wasting disease, many state wildlife and fisheries departments have discontinued deer rehabilitation. Veterinarians can obtain state regulations from their state wildlife agents.

Reptiles

Reptiles in the process of shedding, especially snakes, should be handled gently. Overmanipulation of the animal can result in damage to the new underlying skin. Lizards, snakes, and crocodilians can be examined using manual restraint. We recommend taping a crocodilian's mouth closed to minimize the likelihood of injury to the handler. As a group, chelonians are difficult animals to evaluate clinically. Many chelonians are capable of withdrawing into the margins of their shells when threatened, becoming "bony boxes." Clinicians experienced in evaluating chelonians have devised methods for coaxing them out of their shells. For medium to small sized chelonians, gently touching the hindlimbs will often lead to the animal extending its head. Slow, deliberate movements can also help reduce fearful responses by the animal and retraction into its shell. Many tortoises extend their forelimbs and head if tilted slightly downward, perhaps in an effort to avoid falling. Above all, an examination of a chelonian requires patience. In the end, many chelonian patients require sedation or anesthesia to perform an exam (see Table 19-4). In those cases where the animal can be examined without anesthesia, it is important to minimize the amount of stress placed on the head and neck when extracting the animal from its shell. Excessive force can lead to cervical injury.

A thorough exam should be done on every patient, and the outline found in Box 19-3 can be used for reptiles too. With the exception of obvious traumatic injuries, reptiles show few or subtle signs of disease. A magnification lens will aid in detection of lesions in smaller reptiles. From a distance, lizards should ambulate normally and resist handling. An undisturbed, healthy snake should be coiled or partially coiled, and when approached, it should explore the air with its head and flick its tongue to detect any new odors.

The hydration status of a reptile can be assessed by examining skin turgor (e.g., increased skin turgor will result in "wrinkles" on the animal's body), the oral cavity (e.g., excessive ropy saliva indicates dehydration), and the eyes (in snakes, an opaque, wrinkled spectacle is an indication of dehydration; in lizards, snakes, and chelonians, sunken eyes indicate dehydration). Hematologic data can be used to confirm that a patient is dehydrated.

A standard ophthalmic exam should be done. Retrobulbar abscesses, tumors, or injury can cause unilateral exophthalmos. Unilateral enophthalmos may indicate injury, whereas bilateral enophthalmos can result from microphthalmia, inanition, or dehydration. Edema or vascular obstruction can cause bilateral exophthalmos. The cornea and lens should appear clear. One exception is a snake during ecdysis, when its spectacle may appear a gray-blue color. Corneal ulcers may be obvious or covered with plaques that are protecting healing tissue.

The oral cavity and glottis should be examined for discharge, signs of injury, broken teeth, and signs of necrotic stomatitis (caseous plaques, ulcers, inflammation). A rubber or plastic spatula can be used to open the mouth of snakes and lizards to examine the oral cavity. Although these can also be used for chelonians too, a metal paperclip or dental scaler is often more appropriate. The paperclip or dental scaler can be inserted at the most rostral point of the mandible and used to draw the mandible down. In lizards that are acrodonts, care should be taken to avoid injuring the nonreplaceable teeth. The beak of a chelonian should be examined for any flaking, malocclusion, or fractures. Nares should be examined for ulceration or discharge. Tympanic membranes should be examined for the presence of ectoparasites (e.g., lizards) or aural abscesses (e.g., chelonians).

The entire body should be palpated to determine the animal's body condition and identify any abnormal masses or fractures. A snake should appear rounded, with prominent epaxial muscles running the length of the spine. If the animal is emaciated and/or dehydrated, the animal will assume a more triangular shape on cross-section as the epaxial muscle mass atrophies. In lizards, the pelvic bones and spine are more prominent in emaciated animals. Chelonian body condition can be assessed by examining the temporal muscles and the muscles covering the long bones. A chelonian's carapace should be convex and even, and the scutes should be without lesions. Measurement of the carapace at midline should be taken.

General guidelines for respiratory rate in reptiles are 10 to 30 breaths per minute, with variations according to age, temperature, and species. Thoracic auscultation has limited use but can be facilitated with the placement of a damp cloth between the stethoscope and the animal. In this way, breath sounds may be heard; however, cardiac evaluation is still difficult. Thoracic percussion can be used in chelonians to check for lung field abnormalities. The animal should be resting on the palm of one hand or platform, and then the carapace tapped with the index finger of the other hand. The sound should be symmetric. If the tone is dull, this denotes fluid or increased soft tissue mass. A "tinny" sound is generally produced if there are superficial carapacial scute or dermal bone plate lesions. Aquatic species with pulmonary disease can be placed in water and checked for inconsistencies in buoyancy (e.g., one side floating higher than the other). An ultrasonic Doppler can be used to assess the heart rate.

Wounds, abnormal patterns of keratinization, and swelling of the integument should be noted. In terrestrial species, asymmetric patterns of toenail wear can be associated with lameness. All limbs should be examined for swellings, muscle atrophy, pain, and abnormal movement. The contralateral limb can be used to help discern the extent of abnormalities if the condition is not bilateral.

Urates and feces should be examined. The urate portion should be chalky and should vary from white to yellow in color. Terrestrial reptiles may pass colorless liquid urine with the stool. Urates and urine may appear green if colored by biliverdin, the major bile pigment in reptiles. The appearance of green urates and urine can be an indication of chronic anorexia or liver disease.

The most common reason reptiles present to a veterinary hospital are traumatic injuries (e.g., hit by automobile or landscaping equipment, domestic pet predation), poisonings, and infectious diseases. Animals suffering from a traumatic injury may present with both soft tissue and orthopedic injuries. Many of these injuries are contaminated with opportunistic Gram-negative bacteria and should be managed accordingly.[10] Chemical spills or chemical run-off can cause a large number of reptile deaths, especially in aquatic species. Mycoplasmosis, iridovirus infections, and herpesvirus infections have all been associated with mortality events in wild chelonians. Other reasons for presentation include necrotic stomatitis, pneumonia, epidermal disorders, septicemia, cellulitis, parasitism, and organochlorine toxicity (a potential cause of aural abscesses in chelonian species). A thorough diagnostic work-up is required to identify a specific etiology for a reptile case.

REASONS FOR EUTHANASIA

The practice of wildlife medicine should follow standard triage protocols. Animals that cannot be rehabilitated and released into the wild should be considered for either euthanasia or permanent captive placement. There are restrictions associated with captive placement, and questions regarding placement should be directed to state and federal wildlife agencies. A final decision on a patient's outcome should be made only after careful assessment of the patient's condition, likelihood for rehabilitation and release, and potential for placement.

In assessing the significance of a physical disability or abnormal behavior pattern, the possibility must be considered that, although the condition may not be immediately life-threatening, it would by its nature permanently prevent the animal from surviving in the wild. In such cases the alternative to euthanasia would be permanent placement in captivity. This should only be pursued if, for the foreseeable future, it could be determined that the animal would maintain a reasonable quality of life in captivity and there is a sound justification for this action. Justifications for retaining permanently disabled wildlife cases in captivity include captive breeding programs, education programs, and imprint models.[12] Permanently disabled adult animals have long been used to produce offspring for both endangered species and falconry programs. Much of the conservation success associated with the bald eagle and

peregrine falcon in the United States was based on this type of model. Many of the education programs provided by wildlife hospitals and rehabilitators use permanently injured wildlife. These types of education presentations allow children and adults to observe these animals up close and, in many cases, display the negative impact humans have on these animals. Rehabilitators that work with orphaned animals can benefit from using imprint models. Imprint models are used to teach an orphaned animal what it should do in the wild to survive.

When a decision is made to euthanize a wildlife patient, a standard domestic species euthanasia protocol can be followed. We prefer to sedate or anesthetize a wildlife patient before delivering the final euthanasia solution. Birds can be masked down with isoflurane (5%, 1 L oxygen). The euthanasia solution (barbiturate overdose) can then be delivered into the basiocciptal sinus, heart, available blood vessel, intraosseous catheter, or coelomic cavity. Euthanasia dosing may vary among different solutions and manufacturers. Delivery of the drug into the heart, a blood vessel, or an intraosseous catheter will result in an almost immediate cessation of cardiac function. If the euthanasia solution is delivered into the coelomic cavity, the animal may require 5 to 20 minutes to expire. Additional doses of euthanasia solution can be given if needed. Mammals can also be masked down, although for larger specimens, an injectable anesthetic is generally used (e.g., ketamine). Again, the euthanasia solution can be given intravenously, intracardiacally, intraosseously, or intrathoracically/intra-abdominally. It is also recommended that reptiles be pre-anesthetized before being euthanized. Again, dissociative agents are preferred. Freezing reptiles is not considered an appropriate euthanasia method.

ORPHAN CARE

Orphaned animals are one of the most common wildlife presentations to the veterinary hospital. The fact that concerned citizens take the time out of their schedules to collect and present these animals is a sign that humans have great compassion for animals. In many of these cases, the citizen presenting the animal becomes emotionally attached and has a desire to monitor its progress. It is important for veterinarians to show compassion to these individuals while also explaining to them how nature works. For some of the presentations, the animals will surely be orphaned. A bird that was blown from its nest after a thunderstorm and cannot be safely replaced or juvenile opossums found on a dead female that was hit by a car represent are orphaned truly. However, a fawn or rabbit kidnapped from its nest is not. We believe that the encounters with these citizens represent a great opportunity to discuss wildlife conservation and educate the public on the importance of protecting wildlife.

All orphaned wildlife presentations should be considered emergencies. Juvenile animals have limited hydration and energy stores, and after a short period of time (hours), they may develop negative energy and fluid levels. Correcting for these deficits is essential to patient survival. As with other presentations, it is imperative to have proper species identification and a complete history when accepting orphaned animals. Many orphaned wildlife cases may have been cared for by the public before being presented to the veterinary hospital, and in almost all cases the care was inappropriate or insufficient. The natural history of the species will ultimately determine the care it should receive in captivity. As reptiles are born precocial, they do not require any special attention as juveniles and will not be discussed in this section.

Avian

If a baby bird is found on the ground, every attempt should be made to locate the nest and replace the bird; however, if replacement of the animal into the nest places a human at risk, it should not be done. In most cases, the orphaned bird will be accepted by the parents, giving it the best chance for survival. It is important to realize that some orphaned animals are intentionally orphaned by the parents because of limited food resources. Although this may appear harsh to the public, it is natural selection.

Most baby birds presented to veterinarians will have a subnormal body temperature, and warming the bird to an appropriate temperature to maximize the animal's metabolic rate should be done first. A heating pad under the "nest" (nest substitutes will be discussed later) is the easiest method of providing heat, but bottles or bags of warmed fluids can be used as well. If access to an incubator is available, the nest should be placed in a temperature between 85° F and 95° F (29° C and 35° C). Ultimately, the temperature selected should be based on the age and plumage of the animal. In general, the highest temperatures are reserved for the hatchlings, moderate temperatures for the nestlings, and lowest for the fledglings. Placing baby birds in direct sunlight is not recommended, as heat prostration is likely. Being able to recognize hyperthermia or hypothermia in an orphaned bird is essential to correcting the problem. In general, hyperthermic birds will pant, extend their necks, and hold their feathers tightly against their bodies. Birds with a subnormal body temperature will be depressed, feel cool to the touch, and elevate their feathers in an attempt to trap heat.

The provision of a nest is important to maintain a bird in a specific area for heating purposes and to encourage normal development. Nest substitutes can be made in a variety of ways. Used natural nests should not be provided, as they are a source of various parasites and bacterial and fungal pathogens. The nest must be constructed to assure that the nestling rests in a natural position. In the wild, the nest provides an environment that supports the bird with it legs under its body, feet under the chest, and body weight centered in the back, knees, and lower coelomic cavity. The curved sides of the nest give the body this support and allow the nestling to push against the side of the nest for balance while feeding. Inappropriate nest construction can result in a bird's developing skeletal anomalies (e.g., splay leg) that limit the potential for release.[13] Suitable nest substitutes can be made from small plastic tubs (e.g., margarine containers or flower pots) that are

perforated for air flow, or plastic berry boxes. The nest should be filled with crumpled paper, paper towels, or cloth (e.g., towel, old T-shirt). Occasionally a bird's toenails may become caught in the cloth or paper substrate, so the animal should be monitored closely. Trimming the nails will prevent this from occurring. While the bird should be secure and supported in its nest, it should never be wrapped so that it cannot move.

Orphaned birds can be categorized into one of two groups, altricial or precocial, and each has its distinct needs. Altricial species hatch in a helpless state (e.g., blind and featherless). They are unable to feed or care for themselves in any way. Precocial species are down-covered and ambulatory and can feed themselves soon after hatching. Examples of precocial species include ducks, chickens, geese, and quail. Most other species are altricial and require intensive care in captivity.

Feeding regimes will vary greatly with species, but general principles do apply. A bird should be warmed before it is fed. This will maximize the metabolic rate and gastrointestinal tract motility. If the bird is dehydrated, then fluids should be given next. Animals that are dehydrated will have decreased gastrointestinal times, which can lead to obstipation or constipation. Avoid physical contact during the feedings whenever possible. Hatchling birds are prone to imprint. Feeding the birds using a surrogate (e.g., puppet look-a-like) or by hiding behind a blanket or towel will ensure the animal does not imprint onto humans. Placing a mirror in front of the animal so that its own reflection is the only animal it can see may also be done. Feeding intervals for birds should be consistent to promote regular gastrointestinal transit times. If the bird does not gape to be fed, its beak can be gently opened by pressure on the base at each side. The beaks are really delicate, and care must be taken to avoid damaging them. Most baby birds will gape when the nest is slightly disturbed, as this mimics the parent landing on the side of the nest. The bird will usually stop gaping when it is satiated. It is generally difficult to overfeed these animals, although there may be some instances when birds will continue to gape with a full crop. Feeding should be discontinued in these birds until their crop is emptied; otherwise, they may develop crop stasis. Sharp metal objects (e.g., tweezers) should not be used to feed these birds, as these objects can damage delicate mouth and crop tissues.

The type of food being offered will vary with species, but many will present having been fed on bread and cow's milk, which is not a natural diet in any species and can result in secondary complications. After each meal, the bird will pass dropping in a sac, which should be removed immediately. As the nestlings mature, they will be able to void over the side of their nest.

Many species of juvenile birds benefit from placement in nests containing conspecifics of the same age. This will encourage natural behaviors and help minimize the chance of imprinting. It is ideal to place orphaned birds with a rehabilitator who may have more of the same species (as long as no injuries have been sustained). For orphaned nestlings to develop normal social behavior, they must be exposed to a conspecific during the critical period (within 36 hours after hatching for precocial species, variable for altricial species).[14] In the absence of an appropriate adult, a surrogate should be provided. The order of preference for surrogates is juvenile or fledgling conspecifics, sibling conspecifics with a bird-skin puppet, and finally a puppet alone. Hand-rearing orphaned birds is very time consuming and has a high mortality rate. It is important to consider all of these factors when deciding to accept this challenge.

When working with orphaned birds, it is important to estimate the age of the animal in order to develop a management plan for the bird. Hatchlings are naked, have closed eyes, and need to be hand-reared. Nestlings are partially feathered, will gape and call when disturbed, and will also need to be hand-reared. Fledglings are fully feathered, but they retain down feathers on the head and back and have less intensive rearing needs. Fledglings can leave the nest, but they still depend on their parents for feeding and protection. They may present to a practice as orphaned when they are displaced from their parents and should be returned near the area found under the cover of vegetation if no predators are present.

Emaciated orphans should be fed every 15 minutes for 1 or 2 hours until they have regained their strength. Feedings should then be extended to half-hour intervals and eventually hourly intervals. Diurnal orphans can be fed from 7 AM until 7 PM. Nocturnal species are generally fed on a similar basis, but with the room darkened.

In general, small bird nestlings will consume 10% to 20% of their body weight in food daily. Body weight should be measured daily to ensure that the nestling is gaining an appropriate amount of weight. The frequency of feeding will vary with the age and species of the bird (Table 19-6). In the wild, diurnal species are fed only during the day and are brooded overnight. Crepuscular and nocturnal species are likewise primarily fed during their peak activity periods. Once a bird fledges, it should be encouraged to feed independently on appropriate foods. The foods can initially be presented in a shallow bowl but then ideally presented in more natural ways that encourage foraging.

For nestlings less than 2 weeks old, a substitute nest, as described previously, should be provided. Branches, natural vegetation, and shallow water containers should also be provided. Once the bird has fledged, it should be placed in an outdoor aviary. By 3 or 4 weeks, most small birds will be independent and can be released using soft-release methods. A soft-release program is one in which the birds are housed in an outdoor aviary that allows for natural foraging for about 2 weeks before release.

The choice of food used for hand-rearing orphans will vary with species, but it should be as varied as possible to ensure the proper balance of carbohydrates, fats, proteins, vitamins, and minerals. The food should also be readily available, affordable, and easily prepared. The nestling feeding experience will affect the feeding success later in the bird's life; thus, it is important to provide as natural a diet as possible.

Other important considerations to include when developing an orphaned animal rehabilitation program are the need to expose the animal to conspecifics to develop its normal song, lessons on predator avoidance, and migratory function (if appropriate). For some birds, exposure to their own species' song must occur within 50 days after hatching. This can be provided with tape recordings if no adults are available. It is imperative that orphaned animals not be exposed to mammalian or avian predators; otherwise they may become habituated to their presence and lose their natural protective response to avoid these animals. For nocturnal migratory species, a full view of the setting sun and night sky must be provided (especially in the second month posthatch) for development of migratory function.[14]

PIGEONS AND DOVES

In the wild, squabs (hatchling pigeons and doves) differ from other altricial chicks, requiring less than six feedings per day.[3] The primary reason for this is associated with the type of nutrition (crop milk) these animals receive from their parents. For these birds, crop milk provides the sole source of nutrients during the first few days of life and remains the primary food for the first week to 10 days after hatching. Gradually, crop milk is mixed with the adult diet and fed to hatchlings by both adult parents. Crop milk is crucial for the survival of squabs, as they hatch in a relatively undeveloped state. Squabs are unable to use food found in their environment, cannot digest an adult bird's diet, hatch with their eyes unopened, and do not possess feathering for thermoregulation after hatching. The composition of crop milk is similar to that found in mammals; it contains water, fat, protein, and ash. The primary difference between the avian milk and mammalian milk is in the carbohydrate and protein fractions. Pigeon milk is devoid of lactose. It does, however, contain high levels of crude protein and fat. When working with these animals, attempts to mimic this formula should be made. The following formula (for a day's feeding) has been recommended: Mix one hard-boiled egg yolk (mashed), 3 tablespoons mixed baby cereal, 3 tablespoons oatmeal, and 3 tablespoons cornmeal.[13] We have used both a

TABLE 19-6	Recommended Feeding Schedule for Orphaned Birds Based on Age	
Age	Appearance	Feeding regime
1-4 days	Egg tooth evident, naked, eyelids fused	q15 min for 12 h/day
5-7 days	Naked, early development of pin feathers	q30-60 min for 12 h/day
8-14 days	Feathers covering the body, complete feathers on wings and tail	q60-90 min for 12 h/day
15-21 days	Wing and tail feathers fully grown	q2h for 12 h/day, encourage self-feeding
22-28 days	Fledged	q2-3h for 12 h/day, encourage self-feeding
29-42 days	Capable of flight	Should be self-feeding

commercial critical care psittacine formula and a psittacine neonatal formula (Lafeber Company, Cornell, IL) with good success in these animals too.

Pigeons and doves also feed differently than other birds. A squab gets its food by thrusting its beak far down either side of its parents' esophagus, where it can have access to the crop milk. *Squeakers,* or nestling pigeons and doves, will feed the same way but instead take seeds from the parents' crops. To compensate for this feeding technique, we tube the squab or squeaker or cut the tip off of a 1-ml or 3-ml syringe, fill the syringe with gruel, and place the beak of the bird in the open-ended syringe. This technique can be used to simulate the normal strategy of having the beak inserted into the esophagus of the parent bird. Once the beak is inserted into the syringe, the bird will thrust its head and start imbibing the gruel. Squeakers that are free-feeding can be offered water-soaked gamebird chow.

PRECOCIAL YOUNG

There are two different feeding strategies among the precocial birds: free-feeding birds (e.g., gamebirds, waterfowl, and plovers) and those fed by their parents (e.g., grebes, divers, rails, terns, and gulls). A variety of homemade diets may be made that are similar to the diet described for doves and pigeons, but fortunately many of these animals readily accept chicken or turkey starter diets. To further diversify these diets, live insect pupae (e.g., mealworms) can be added. All precocial birds should have a shallow dish of water near their food.

GAMEBIRDS

Orphaned gamebirds are not commonly presented to veterinary hospitals because the chicks are precocial, and social imprinting is uncommon. Soon after birth, these birds leave their nest and maintain a close relationship with their nestmates and parents. When the parent birds denote danger, they set a decoy for a predator to protect their juveniles. Even truly orphaned chicks are more capable of caring for themselves than other avian species. If a chick is in immediate danger, hand-rearing can be attempted; however, certain species, such as quail, are especially difficult to hand-raise because they require a diverse diet comprised of various insects and weed seeds.[13] Orphaned gamebirds should be offered a quiet, secure cage. Most of these birds will accept chick crumb or poultry pellet and fresh water in a shallow dish. Artificial heat, as discussed in the general avian section, should be provided. A suspended clean feather duster can be used as a synthetic parent.

WATERFOWL

Whereas certain species of orphaned waterfowl are easy to care for, others are not. Mallard ducks and Canada geese will readily adapt to captive care and accept a gamebird chow or chicken starter soaked in water. Supplementing the starter diet with invertebrates (e.g., mealworms) is also highly recommended. On the other hand, orphaned wood ducks do not adapt well to captivity and often experience high mortalities. To limit these losses, every attempt should be made to transfer these cases to a specialized facility for care.

WADERS

Wader chicks are rarely seen in captivity but may present if the parents are killed or they have been displaced from their nest. Once stabilized with supportive care, healthy orphans can be offered an adult appropriate diet (in smaller amounts). Once fully fledged (about 3 weeks of age for smaller species, 6 weeks for larger species), the chicks are independent. Immediately after fledging is the optimal time for release.[2]

SEABIRDS

Other than gulls, seabird orphans are rarely presented to veterinary hospitals, as they usually migrate out to sea soon after fledging. Orphaned gulls, on the other hand, commonly present as orphans after being displaced from nests. They must be reared in groups of conspecifics to avoid imprinting. Chopped fish, day-old chicks, or fish-flavored cat foods can be offered. An avian-specific multivitamin and mineral supplement should also be added to the diet.[5]

RAPTORS

Although it is important to limit human contact with all orphaned avian wildlife, this is considered most important with raptors. Imprinted raptors pose a risk not only to themselves but also to humans. Raptors that have lost their fear of humans have been known to attack humans that enter their territory. Veterinarians and wildlife rehabilitators have a duty to the animals in their care, and to the community in which these animals are released, to minimize the potential for imprinting. Orphaned raptors should be raised with similar aged conspecifics if it is at all possible, as this will minimize the likelihood of imprinting. If no similar aged orphans are available in the immediate vicinity, every effort should be made to contact local rehabilitators to find a companion, or at a minimum, a surrogate adult from the same species. Surrogate raptors can be an invaluable resource to those who are rehabilitating orphaned raptors. A surrogate puppet can also be used as a last resort.

When preparing a diet and feeding regime for a particular raptor, it is important to correctly identify the species and have a realistic age estimate. Food choices should mimic the natural diet of the species as closely as possible. Rodents (e.g., mice, rats, gerbils, guinea pigs, rabbits), chickens (chicks), and invertebrates (e.g., crickets and mealworms) are the most commonly available commercially raised prey items for raptors. Some facilities recommend feeding wild squirrels and songbirds that die of noninfectious causes (e.g., traumatic injury), as this is economical and a natural process for many of the opportunistic feeding raptors. Unfortunately, these types of prey items may still serve as a source of parasites or other latent infectious disease for the raptors. Raptors should never be offered a wild prey item that was euthanized using a barbiturate overdose.

To elicit a feeding response in a raptor, the food item should be placed in front of the beak or touched to the tactile bristles at the base of the beak. Newly hatched raptors should be fed every 2 to 3 hours for 2 to 3 days. It is important not to overfeed these animals, as constipation can occur. For the first 2 to 3 days of life, no bone, fur, or feathers should be offered. At 3 days to 1 week of age, mice, pinky rats, or smaller songbirds can be offered every 3 to 5 hours, with no large bones or bone splinters and no fur or feathers. After the first week, the amount of fur and feathers offered, as well as the size of morsel, should be gradually increased until the raptor chick is eating the entire contents of the prey item. Raptor chicks will generally eat more food than an adult of the same species, reaching a peak at 2 to 3 weeks when they will eat more than double an adult.[3] Downy raptors should be fed every 4 to 6 hours and fed as much as they will take at one feeding. Do not offer artificial casting materials (e.g., dog fur, cotton), as they have been implicated in causing intestinal blockage and crop impaction.[15] Once the chick's eyes are open and they are investigating with their beaks, fresh carcasses should be left in the environment. The body weight of these animals should be monitored closely and the diet adjusted accordingly. At 2 to 3 weeks of age, various sized perches and branches should be offered. Once the chick is fully feathered and attempting to use its wings, it can be moved to an outdoor aviary to begin learning to fly and build strength.

Mammals
GENERAL

All orphaned mammals should be provided an enclosure that is dry and warm and has an appropriate nesting material (e.g., shredded paper, towels). Excessive humidity often leads to the development of severe dermatitis. The patient's body temperature and hydration status should be monitored closely. Orphaned mammals that are dehydrated or hypothermic will reduce their caloric intake. Because these animals do not have a ready source of energy reserves, anorexia or cachexia can be fatal. The fecal output of each orphan should be monitored closely. A reduction in fecal output may be suggestive of a decreased gastrointestinal transit time and should be corrected immediately. Orphaned mammals do not need to be bathed or washed. All feeding utensils should be cleaned thoroughly before being used to limit the transfer of infectious diseases between patients. Orphans should be weighed daily and their diet altered if necessary.

SQUIRRELS

With squirrels, it is important to, first, determine whether the animal is actually an orphan. Juvenile squirrels are frequently displaced from their nest after a major weather event (e.g., periods of high winds), but the parent(s) will later retrieve them and return to the nest. If this appears to be the case with a recent presentation, then the animal should be returned to where it was found and placed in a protected area (e.g., shrubs) until the parents return.

In general, orphaned squirrels are easy to care for. These animals should be housed in a secure, warmed enclosure. An electric heating pad or warmed water bottle can provide supplemental heat. A nest substitute can be placed in the enclosure to mimic an animal's natural setting. A small open cardboard box with tissue paper, paper towels, or a cotton blanket will serve as an appropriate nest substitute. A squirrel's eyes open between 19 and 21 days of age. Males and females may need to be separated; sibling penis suckling is common as the penis can be mistaken for a teat. Omnivore (e.g., canine) or carnivore (e.g., feline) milk replacers most closely represent the natural composition of a squirrel's milk. The formula should be made daily, refrigerated between feedings, and warmed to body temperature before each feeding. A small syringe (e.g., 1-ml or 3-ml) can be used to nurse the squirrel. For feeding, the animal can either be placed in lateral recumbency or sternal recumbency. We prefer positioning the animals in sternal recumbency. The formula should be delivered at a pace found acceptable to the squirrel, as feeding the animal too quickly can lead to the aspiration of the milk. Neonates should be fed every 2 hours, with a total volume of 3 ml/day. Anogenital stimulation should be performed after each feeding until the squirrel has urinated and defecated. Dehydrated orphans should be fed a balanced electrolyte solution for one or two feedings and gradually introduced to the milk formula over the following three to four feedings. Diarrhea and bloat commonly occur in animals that have reduced or hypermotile gastrointestinal transit times. When these problems occur, the volume of formula should be decreased.[16] Neonates are messy feeders, and excess formula should be cleaned from their face after each feeding with a warm washcloth. After being fed, neonatal squirrels will sleep until their next feeding. Once a squirrel's eyes have been open for about a week (25-28 days old), begin offering formula from a shallow dish (<0.5 inches deep) every other feeding. When a squirrel readily drinks formula from the dish, discontinue syringe feeding. At the same time, begin to offer other natural foods (e.g., nuts and pine cones) and rodent chow. Rodent chow is the preferred food type to offer, as it is a balanced rodent diet. At 2 months of age, the animal should begin to be acclimated for release. Squirrels received during the late fall should be overwintered until the spring, and spring-born orphans should be released in the early summer to ensure that they will have the time to develop the skills necessary to survive in the weather.

LAGOMORPHS

Orphaned rabbits are a common presentation to veterinary hospitals. Most of the animals are encountered accidently when an individual is doing yard work or their domestic pet uncovers a nest. If it is at all possible, the animals should be returned to their nest. Wild rabbits only return to their nest once a day, so citizens should not be concerned if they do not see the doe return. Orphaned rabbits that present as a result of a domestic pet attack carry a guarded prognosis.

Orphaned rabbits are one of the most difficult animals to raise in captivity. These animals have a very sensitive digestive system and are prone to developing life-threatening diarrhea. In addition, the stress caused by the routine handling needed to care for these animals can lead to sudden death. To minimize the stress level of these animals, they should be housed in a room that is quiet and dimly lit. It is also best to limit the number of individuals feeding the rabbits.

The primary problems encountered with orphaned rabbits are hypothermia and hypoglycemia. In general, it is thought that the glucose reserve of neonatal rabbits is approximately 6 hours postpartum.[17] Because these animals have minimal energy reserves, a hypoglycemic episode can quickly result in ketosis and death.[17] A common mistake made with these animals is to give fluids or milk replacer per os to hypothermic animals. Because the gastrointestinal tracts of these animals are often static, the energy and fluids provided will remain in the intestinal tract and potentially become overgrown with opportunistic bacteria. To prevent this, these animals should be warmed and provided fluids with dextrose. Because the placement of an intravenous catheter is difficult in these animals, fluids are generally given subcutaneously or intraperitoneally. Once warmed and rehydrated, additional per os calories can be provided.

In the wild, rabbits suckle their young only once a day, and their milk is concentrated to have a high nutritional value and a low lactose content.[6] The composition of the milk changes toward the end of lactation, when protein and fat levels increase. Orphaned lagomorphs can be reared on powdered milk replacers (e.g., Esbilac; PetAg, Hampshire, IL) or goat's milk. As milk replacers are a nutritional compromise, hand-reared lagomorphs need to be fed more than one time per day and the milk replacer should not be dilute beyond a 2 : 1 (formula-to-water) ratio. In captivity, most young lagomorphs will accept two to four feedings a day, depending on their weight, appetite and general condition. The volume consumed per feeding will also vary based on age and general condition, with animals accepting between 2 and 30 ml of milk per feeding. Orphaned rabbits should be weighed daily using an accurate digital scale. The most common problem encountered with these animals is aspiration of the milk replacer and the development of diarrhea. Aspiration can occur when tubing these animals or forcing the fluids through the tube so fast that they backflow up the esophagus and enter the trachea. Affected animals should immediately be given furosemide and broad-spectrum antibiotics (e.g., trimethoprim-sulfadimethoxine). Rabbits that develop enteritis should also be given antibiotics. In the wild, such a problem does not generally occur because of the rabbit's unique physiology. Juvenile rabbits are unusual among mammals in that they naturally have very few micro-organisms in their stomach and small intestine while suckling. A natural antimicrobial fatty acid, or "milk oil," is present in the stomach of a suckling rabbit, which is produced by an enzymatic reaction in the doe's milk.[6] This milk oil gives some protection against enteric infection. Orphaned rabbits that are fed a milk replacer do not develop this antimicrobial factor and are therefore susceptible to developing an enteric bacterial infection during nursing.

Most suckling rabbits are stimulated to urinate and defecate when the doe grooms their perineum and lower abdomen. There is a debate as to whether this is the case in all wild lagomorphs; however, to be safe, we recommend cleaning/stimulating the perineum of captive, orphaned rabbits to stimulate urination and defecation. Between feedings, the animals should be returned to their nest and left alone.

Rabbits are born naked, blind, and helpless. Birth weights for these animals range between 40 and 100 g. In the wild, neonatal rabbits are totally dependent on milk for approximately 10 to 15 days, at which time they start eating small amounts of solid food.[17] Neonatal rabbits begin to leave their nest and are weaned between 3 and 4 weeks of age. For captive animals, it is important to provide grass hay and assorted vegetables. At the same time, fresh cecotrophs from healthy adult rabbits should be provided to ensure the intestinal tract is transfaunated with the appropriate bacteria. These fecal pellets can be offered either with the grass hay or mixed into a gruel and offered per os. Commercial probiotics can also be used, but they will not provide the same diverse microflora that a rabbit fecal pellet will provide.

MESOPREDATORS

Mesopredators are routinely presented to veterinarians as orphans. These animals should be transferred to an experienced licensed wildlife rehabilitator as soon as possible to minimize the likelihood of imprinting. It is important that these animals are not maintained in veterinary hospitals for extended periods of time because of the risk of disease transmission. In addition to these health concerns, the mesopredators also need to be raised with conspecifics to ensure proper behavioral development. Opossums, foxes, and raccoons can be raised on canine formulas, whereas bobcats should be raised using a feline formula. Veterinarians can use domestic puppy and kitten feeding regimens to manage these animals. The mesopredators can generally be weaned by 6 to 8 weeks of age. Weaned mesopredators can be offered canine or feline kibble diets that are supplemented with other natural foods. For example, bobcats and foxes can also be offered prekilled rodent prey, and raccoons and opossums can be offered fruits, vegetables, and invertebrates.

DEER

Fawns are generally left unattended by their doe for long periods of time during a day. This primarily serves as a protective measure against predation on the fawn. Unfortunately, humans often come upon these nested fawns and believe that they are abandoned. Although they believe they are rescuing the fawn, they are, for all practical purposes, kidnapping it instead. Citizens should be instructed to return the fawn to its nest even if the doe is not in sight. The doe will not approach her fawn in the presence of humans. Neonates can be successfully returned to their nest for up to 24 hours after removal. Human handling will not prevent the return and maternal care of the doe.

Fawns that cannot be returned to the wild pose a real dilemma for the veterinarian. In some states (e.g., Louisiana), fawns cannot be rehabilitated and released back to the wild because of the concern associated with chronic wasting disease. Therefore, veterinarians should contact their state wildlife and fisheries office for the regulations on rehabilitating fawns. Animals that cannot be released should either be placed in an appropriate institution or euthanized. Male deer in particular can become unpredictably violent and dangerous once imprinted. In our opinion, castration and captivity are more inhumane alternatives to euthanasia for male deer.

Deer milk is considerably higher in protein and fat than cow's milk but has lower lactose content. A suitable deer milk replacer can be created by adding one whole egg, 5 ml cod liver oil, and 20 g glucose to 1 L full cream cow's milk. Commercial deer and goat milk formulas can also be used for orphaned fawns. The formula should be offered every 3 to 4 hours at 37° C. Fawns can be fed from a lamb's bottle (e.g., larger animals) or a human baby bottle (e.g., smaller animals). A cross-slit in the nipple on the bottle will ensure a good flow rate of milk.[4] Some deer will only accept milk when the bottle has a dark (e.g., black) nipple. After each feeding, the anal region of the fawn should be massaged with a wet warm tissue to stimulate defecation. If the young deer is obstinate, dehydrated, or collapsed, intravenous fluids should be given to correct any deficits. Because many of these animals will not suckle, they should also be offered their milk replacer directly via a stomach tube. Healthy young deer will nibble succulent foods from 1 week of age but will not be fully weaned from the milk until they are at least 10 weeks old. Deer should be transferred to an experienced licensed wildlife rehabilitator as soon as possible to minimize the likelihood of imprinting.

DIAGNOSTIC TESTING
Clinical Pathology

Clinical pathology is an important diagnostic method for assessing the health of a wildlife patient. Many of these animals have evolved to mask their illness and may appear nondiseased even when they are near death. Hematology and plasma biochemistry screens can provide the veterinarian with a wealth of information regarding the physiologic status of their patients.

In some cases, the greatest challenge to performing these tests is collecting the blood samples (Figure 19-10). Animals that are fractious or pose a danger to the veterinary staff should be anesthetized. A list of venipuncture sites can be found in Table 19-7. When collecting a blood sample, it is important to consider the total sample volume to be collected. For larger patients this is not as important, but for a 100-g avian, reptile, or rodent patient, this becomes very important. In general, 1 ml blood/100 g of body weight can be collected from mammals or birds, and 0.5-0.8 ml blood/100 g of body weight can be collected from reptiles and amphibians. If a patient has experienced acute of chronic blood loss, the sample volume should be decreased.

Hematologic samples from mammals can be processed using standard domestic mammal techniques. Because the red blood cells and thrombocytes of avian, reptile, and amphibian patients are nucleated, the samples are processed using hand

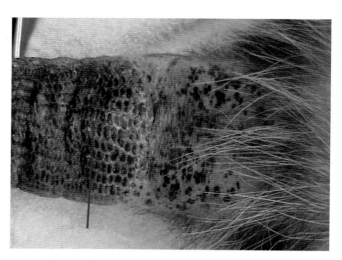

Figure 19-10 The ventral tail vein can be used to collect blood from opossums. The sampling technique is similar to that described for tail venipuncture in lizards and cows. The needle can be inserted anywhere along the ventral midline (arrow).

TABLE 19-7	Common Venipuncture Sites in Wildlife
Group	**Venipuncture sites**
Avian	Jugular
	Cutaneous ulnar/basilic
	Medial metatarsal
	Basioccipital (Columbiformes)
Mammal	Jugular
	Cephalic
	Lateral/Medial Saphenous
	Femoral
	Lateral tail (rodents)
	Ventral tail (opossums)
Reptile	Jugular (chelonians, snakes, lizards)
	Cardiac (snakes)
	Brachial (chelonians)
	Subcarapacial (chelonians)
	Femoral (chelonians)
	Cephalic (lizards)
	Ventral tail (lizards, crocodilians, snakes)
	Dorsal tail (chelonians)
	Ventral abdominal (lizards)
	Supravertebral (crocodilians)
Amphibian	Ventral abdominal vein (anurans)
	Femoral
	Ventral tail (urodelans)

counts. There has been some work to show that the blood samples from these animals can be analyzed using specialized equipment, but these machines were not readily available at the time of this writing. Most hand counts are done using the eosinophil unopette technique. The eosinophil unopette method enables the technician or veterinarian to count stained heterophils and eosinophils. Once this count has been done, a differential is read (high dry/oil magnification) using a stained blood-smear slide. Inserting the numbers from the eosinophil unopette estimate and the differential into the following formula will provide an estimated total white blood cell count: (# cells counted) × 1.1 × 16/(% heterophils + % eosinophils). Once the estimated total number of cells has been determined, the percentages generated from the differential count can be applied to the total number to derive the estimated absolute numbers for each cell type.

Plasma biochemistries can be analyzed using any of the commercially available analyzers. However, the Abaxis Vet Scan is a favorite of ours, as it can provide a complete plasma biochemistry profile from 0.1 ml of whole blood. Because of this system, blood samples can be processed from animals as small as 10 to 20 g.

Interpreting blood samples from wildlife can be difficult, as there are few references. Because of this, one of us (Mitchell) has developed a general set of rules for evaluating hematologic and plasma biochemistry results for wildlife. Regardless of the species, white blood cell counts are generally between 5000 and 15,000 cells/μl in clinically healthy patients. By establishing a basic range of values, the veterinarian can develop a comfort zone for what is or is not acceptable. It is important, however, to realize that animals with white blood cell counts within this range can be suffering from disease. This would be no different if there was an established "normal" reference range for a particular species based on a rigorous study. There can always be abnormal patients within a normal distribution and normal patients that fall out of a mean ±2 standard deviations. The way to ultimately determine healthy versus nonhealthy is to evaluate the entire white blood cell count (e.g., differential) and examine the patient. There are two generic reasons that white blood cell counts can be elevated: inflammation and stress. Many veterinarians want to naturally label the elevation as infection or stress, but this would not be appropriate. If veterinarians always consider a white blood cell count to be associated with an infection, they will miss other potential causes of inflammation (e.g., trauma, neoplasia, toxins) and overprescribe antibiotics. When interpreting the differential it is important to first identify the predominant cell (neutrophil/heterophil or the lymphocyte). In most species, the heterophil (e.g., reptile, amphibian, avian) or neutrophil (e.g., mammal) will be the predominant cell, whereas within certain groups (e.g., chelonians, deer) the lymphocyte is the predominant cell. In general, the ratio of the predominant cell to the secondary cell will be 1 : 1 to 3 : 1. Therefore, in a clinically healthy raptor the ratio of heterophils to lymphocytes may be as low 1 : 1 or as high as 3 : 1, whereas the inverse may be said for a chelonian. If the ratio is outside of these parameters, the veterinarian must decide if one cell is elevated, the other decreased, or both. Lymphocyte counts in wildlife less than 1500 cells/μl are consistent with lymphopenia. Monocyte, basophil, and eosinophil counts are generally less than 500 cells/μl. Monocyte counts between 500-1200 cells/μl are generally associated with stress, while counts greater than 1200 cells/μl are strongly suggestive of chronic inflammation.

TABLE 19-8 General Reference Estimates for Plasma Biochemistries for Wildlife

Parameter	Group	Range
Glucose (mg/dl)	Birds	80-200
	Mammals	80-150
	Reptiles	60-150
Sodium (mEq/L)	General	140-160
	Marine species	150-170
	Chelonians	135-150
Chloride (mEq/L)	General	90-120
	Marine species	100-130
Potassium (mEq/L)	General	3-6
Calcium (mg/dl)	General	8-12
	Gravid reptiles, birds	15-50
Phosphorus (mg/dl)	General	4-8
	Gravid reptiles, birds	6-15
Total protein (g/dl)	Birds	3-6
	Mammals, reptiles	4-8
Albumin	Birds	1-2.5
	Mammals, reptiles	2-3
Urea (mg/dl)	Mammals	<30
Creatinine (mg/dl)	Mammals	<2
Uric acid (mg/dl)	Birds, reptiles	<10
	Postprandial: carnivorous reptiles, birds	<25
AST (IU/L)	General	<250
ALT (IU/L)	General	<250
CK (IU/L)	General	<500
ALP (IU/L)	General	<250

ALT, alanine aminotransferase; *ALP*, alkaline phosphatase; *AST*, aspartate aminotransferase; *CK*, creatine kinase.

For a review of general references for the plasma biochemistries, see Table 19-8.

Diagnostic Imaging

Diagnostic imaging is an important component of the thorough work-up of a wildlife case. Many wildlife veterinary hospitals utilize radiographs as a parallel component to the physical examination. Survey radiographs are often invaluable for assessing musculoskeletal injuries and the presence of foreign bodies (e.g., fish hooks, lead shot) (Figure 19-11). Radiographs can even be used to characterize infectious disease. For example, raptors with systemic aspergillosis often have an increased radiopacity associated with their air sacs. Those types of radiographic findings direct us to perform coelioscopy. When pursuing radiographs, it is important to always take at least two different images (e.g., lateral and dorsoventral). Attempts to interpret a single radiograph can lead to misclassification. Animals that are fractious should be anesthetized. Any movement during the procedure will result in less than diagnostic images.

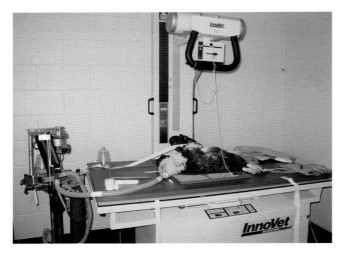

Figure 19-11 Survey radiographs can prove invaluable to diagnosing disease in wildlife. The standard equipment found in small animal veterinary hospitals can be used for wildlife too.

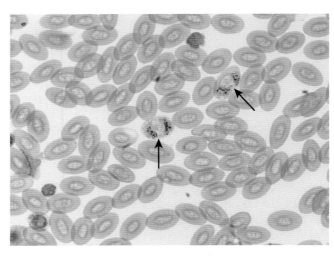

Figure 19-12 Hemoparasites *(arrows)* are a common finding in wild bird patients. To determine whether these organisms are detrimental to the patient, a thorough exam and blood profile (e.g., hematocrit) are needed.

Ultrasound is generally reserved for mammals and reptiles; it can also be used with birds, but their large bony keel and extensive ribs can limit the amount of imaging that can be done on the viscera. When selecting an ultrasound, it is best to use transducers that are capable of providing the detail needed for the depth of tissue being examined. For example, 7.5- to 12-MHz transducers should be used for small patients (e.g., mink), while 5- to 7.5-MHz units can be used for larger animals (e.g., bear). To become proficient with an ultrasound, it is important to pursue continuing education opportunities in the field.

Microbiology

Wildlife are susceptible to a variety of microbial pathogens. The microbiologic cultures collected from wildlife can be processed using the same techniques described for domestic species. More species-specific information regarding culture techniques is available in other chapters of this book. It is important for veterinarians to establish a relationship with a microbiology laboratory. The laboratory scientists should be made aware of the different types of patients the veterinarians are working with, as the isolation of certain organisms requires more specialized techniques (e.g., *Pasteurella multocida*, *Salmonella* spp.). Interpreting the results of a culture should be done carefully. Just because an organism was isolated from an animal does not necessarily infer that it is causing disease. Cytologic examination or histopathologic testing of a wound that confirms the presence of a uniform population of organisms consistent with an isolate would certainly lend more strength to the association. Discussing the findings with the laboratory can also be beneficial. The laboratory may be able to provide insight into the growth and density of the organism on the plate or growth of secondary organisms that might be useful for case management.

Parasitic Testing

Wildlife are routinely presented to veterinary hospitals with both endo- and ectoparasite infestations. Each animal should be examined closely for the presence of ectoparasites. Close inspection of a patient may reveal fleas, flies, mites, ticks, or lice. Confirmation of the type or types of ectoparasites present on the patient can be made by examining the organism(s) under a light microscope. Veterinarians should always wear gloves when working with wildlife to minimize the likelihood of being infested with these organisms. Animals infested with ectoparasites should be treated with an appropriate antiparasitic. Fipronil can be used to eliminate ectoparasites on reptiles and birds. It is best, however, to be cautious when applying the drug to a species for the first time. This topical spray can be used for mesopredators. Firponil is not recommended for lagomorphs or rodents, as it can be associated with neurologic disease and death. Ivermectin can also be used to control ectoparasites but should never be used with chelonians.

Determining the endoparasite status of a wildlife case can be done using standard techniques, such as a blood smear, fecal float, and direct smear. Most wildlife cases will present with some degree of endoparasitism (Figure 19-12). The question generally asked is whether or not to treat a patient. If the parasite burden does not appear to be associated with clinical disease in the patient, and also does not pose a health risk to the veterinary staff, then treatment may be postponed. However, if the patient presents in a compromised state, then it should be treated because the parasites will only add to the animal's burden.

Miscellaneous Testing

In the past, most diseases were considered to be bacterial in origin because microbiological culture was the primary infectious disease–based assay available. With the advancement of diagnostic assays, veterinarians can now identify and confirm the presence of viral, parasitic, and fungal pathogens too. There are a variety of serologic and molecular-based assays available to the wildlife veterinarian, and a review of those most commonly used is found in Table 19-9.

TABLE 19-9	Diagnostic Tests Available to the Wildlife Veterinarian	
Agent	**Test**	**Laboratory**
Reptile		
Chelonian herpesvirus	ELISA, PCR	UF-CVM*
Chelonian mycoplasmosis	ELISA, PCR	UF-CVM†
Chelonian iridovirus	PCR	UF-CVM*
Cryptosporidium	Serology	UM‡
Snake paramyxovirus	HI	UF-CVM*
Alligator West Nile virus	ELISA	UF-CVM*
Salmonella spp.	PCR	UG-CVM§
Adenovirus	PCR	UF-CVM*
Protein electrophoresis		UM‡
Histopathology		NWZP¶¶
Avian		
Aspergillus	ELISA	RC,¶ UM‡
Chlamydophila	Serology	UM‡
	PCR	UG§
Herpesvirus	Serology	NVSL#
Influenza	Serology	NVSL#
Mycoplasma	Serology/PCR	NVSL#
Mycobacterium	Serology/PCR	NVSL#
Newcastle disease	Serology/PCR	NVSL#
Salmonella	Serology/culture	NVSL#
Protein electrophoresis		UM‡
Histopathology		NWZP¶¶

*UF-CVM: Dr. Elliott Jacobson, University of Florida, College of Veterinary Medicine, Department of Small Animal Clinical Sciences, PO Box 100126, Gainesville, FL 32610, (352) 392-4700 ext 5700.

†UF-CVM: Dr. Mary Brown, University of Florida, College of Veterinary Medicine, Department of Small Animal Clinical Sciences, PO Box 100126, Gainesville, FL 32610, (352) 392-4700 ext 5700.

‡UM: University of Miami, School of Medicine, Division of Comparative Pathology, PO Box 016960 (R-46), Miami, FL 33101, (305) 243-6928.

§UG: University of Georgia, College of Veterinary Medicine, Department of Medical Microbiology, Athens, GA, 30602, (706) 542-5812.

¶¶NWZP: Northwest Zoo Path, 18210 Waverly Drive, Snohomish, WA 98296 (360) 668-6003.

¶RC: The Raptor Center, University of Minnesota, College of Veterinary Medicine, 1920 Fitch Avenue, St. Paul, MN 55108, (612) 624-4745.

#NVSL: National Veterinary Services Laboratory, APHIS, USDA, PO Box 844, 1800 Dayton St., Ames, IA, 50010, (515)-239-8266.

ELISA, enzyme-linked immunosorbent assay; *HI,* hemagglutination inhibition; *PCR,* polymerase chain reaction.

■ DISEASES

Wildlife may present to a veterinary hospital for a variety of different reasons. Although traumatic injuries represent the most common presentation at most hospitals, there are certainly infectious, parasitic, and toxic diseases that lead to illness in these animals. Lists of the most common infectious, parasitic, and toxic causes of illness in wildlife are presented in Tables 19-10, 19-11, and 19-12, respectively.

■ RELEASING WILDLIFE
Preparing for Release

Before attempting to release a wildlife case, an in-depth assessment of their suitability for release must be made (Figure 19-16). An animal's ability not only to survive in the wild but also to normally reproduce and interact with conspecifics and other species must be evaluated. Returning an animal that is fit but unable to reproduce may displace a normally functioning member of its species in that environment, whether it be through prey, territory, or mate competition. This can have an overall deleterious effect on the population. The criteria for release vary slightly according to each species, but in general, the animal must be able to locate and kill prey or food items, withstand normal climatic conditions, avoid predation, breed normally, and perform any other specific activites related to their species-particular performance in the wild. Animals kept in captivity for long periods of time or juveniles raised in captivity may have difficulties in performing some or all of these functions. Loss of muscle or feather condition, abnormal socialization, and imprinting are common problems preventing suitable performance in their natural habitat.

A thorough knowledge of the natural history and behavior of an animal in the wild is necessary before an assessment for release can be made. Both mental and physical fitness must be evaluated. The use of a remote monitoring device, such as a closed circuit television, can be very helpful in assessing normal behavior, as many animals will not behave as they would in the wild in the presence of humans. In the absence of such technology, attempts can be made to monitor the animal from a concealed area. It is also imperative to consider any ongoing infectious disease that may pose a threat to the animal or the population into which it is released. Attempts to gradually bring the animal to an acceptable state of fitness can be made in large aviaries or pens, with techniques that mimic as closely as possible the conditions they will meet on their return to the wild. Conditions that may preclude an animal's return to the wild include, but are not limited to, anything that may prevent normal hunting activity, migration, or avoidance of predation, abnormal feather or fur condition (which also affects their ability to regulate their body temperature), amputation, any cause of restricted mobility, loss of senses commonly used for normal behavior, pelvic fractures (in females) that may predispose them to dystocia, and any animal that is imprinted

TABLE 19-10	Infectious Diseases Commonly Encountered in Wildlife		
Group	**Agent**	**Clinical signs**	**Treatment**
Reptiles			
Chelonians	*Mycoplasma* spp.	Upper and lower respiratory tract infections, sinusitis, blepharoedema, conjunctivitis	Release not recommended, doxycycline, azithromycin, fluoroquinolones
Snakes	Paramyxovirus	Upper and lower respiratory tract infections, hemorrhage, neurologic disease	No treatment, release not recommended
Crocodilians	West Nile virus	Neurologic disease	Supportive care
Chelonians	Iridovirus	Necrotic stomatitis, pneumonia	Supportive care, release not recommended
Chelonians	Herpesvirus	Upper and lower respiratory tract infections, glossitis, pneumonia, enteritis, fibropapillomas, hepatitis, neurologic disease	No treatment, release not recommended, acyclovir reduces clinical signs
Avian			
	West Nile virus	Asymptomatic, muscle weakness, torticollis, opisthotonos	Supportive care
	Paramyxovirus	Paresis, muscle tremors, death	Quarantine, euthanasia
	Influenza	Asymptomatic, pneumonia, neurologic disease	Supportive care, zoonotic forms-euthanasia
	Equine encephalitis	Anorexia, weakness, neurologic disease, acute death	Preventive vaccine, supportive care
	Poxvirus (Figure 19-13)	Dry form: masses on featherless areas; wet form: mucous membranes	Supportive care, antibiotics, quarantine
	Chlamydophila psittaci	Anorexia, depression, enteritis, splenitis, hepatitis, pneumonia, rhinitis, conjunctivitis	Doxycycline
	Mycobacterium avium (Figure 19-14)	Emaciation, weakness, increased appetite, osteomyelitis (tibiotarsus), pneumonia, multifocal granulomas	Not recommended
	Pasteurella multocida	Peracute death, neurologic disease	Supportive care, antibiotics
	Salmonellosis	Diarrhea, peracute death, osteomyelitis, sepsis, neurologic disease	Supportive care, antibiotics
	Aspergillus spp.	Pneumonia, tracheal granulomas, air sacculitis, multifocal granulomas	Itraconazole, amphotericin B
Mammals			
	Canine distemper virus	Weakness, depression, hyperkeratosis on the foot pads, diarrhea, pneumonia, paresis, death	No treatment
	Infectious canine hepatitis (adenovirus)	Diarrhea, hepatitis, paralysis, death	Supportive care
	Influenza	Sneezing, coughing, fever, pneumonia	Supportive care
	Parvovirus	Anorexia, diarrhea, myocarditis, leukopenia	Supportive care
	Rabies	Dumb form: depression Rabid form: aggressive	Euthanize and confirm
	Leptospirosis (*Leptospira interrogans*)	Asymptomatic, fever, weakness, jaundice, hemorrhage, diarrhea	Tetracyclines
	Tyzzer's disease (*Clostridium piliforme*)	Diarrhea, depression, peracute death	Tetracyclines

TABLE 19-11	Parasites Commonly Encountered in Wildlife		
Agent	**Group**	**Clinical signs**	**Treatment**
Angiostrongylus cantonensis	Mammals	Depression, circling, paresis, paralysis	No treatment
Baylisascaris procyonis	Mammals, birds	Non-raccoons: neurologic disease	No treatment
Cestodes	All	Asymptomatic, diarrhea	Praziquantel
Coccidia	All	Asymptomatic, diarrhea	Sulfa-based antibiotics
Cryptosporidium serpentis	Snakes	Regurgitation, diarrhea, weakness, death	No treatment
Cryptosporidium parvum	Mammals	Regurgitation, diarrhea, weakness, death	No treatment, supportive care
Entamoeba invadens	Reptiles	Hemorrhagic diarrhea, dehydration, death	Metronidazole
Fly larvae (Figure 19-15)	All	Mass with breathing hole, discharge	Surgically remove, ivermectin
Giardia spp.	All	Hemorrhagic diarrhea, dehydration	Metronidazole
Pinworms	All	Asymptomatic, diarrhea	± Fenbendazole
Toxoplasma gondii	Mammals, birds	Asymptomatic, reproductive anomalies, blindness	Supportive care

TABLE 19-12	Toxins Commonly Encountered in Wildlife	
Agent	**Clinical signs**	**Treatment**
Botulism *(Clostridium perfringens)*	Paresis, paralysis, difficulty holding head (limberneck)	Supportive care, antitoxin
Heavy metals (zinc, lead)	Weakness, lethargy, ataxia, paresis, anemia, diarrhea (hemorrhagic)	Remove metal, administer chelating agent (calcium EDTA)
Mycotoxins	Ataxia, death	Supportive care, spore-free diet
Oil contamination	Hypothermia, anemia, oil contamination on feathers, hepatitis, death	Supportive care, oil removal with Dawn dish soap
Organophosphates	Hypersalivation, miosis, lethargy, weakness, paresis, death	Atropine, 2-pam

EDTA, ethylenediaminetetraacetic acid.

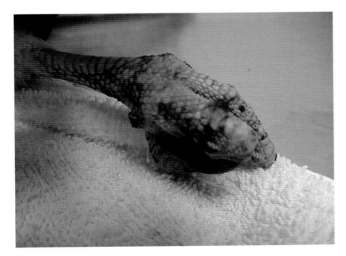

Figure 19-13 Dry forms of pox are a common finding in raptors. These animals generally become exposed when feeding on infected prey.

or improperly socialized to humans or domestic animals. These animals may displace others in their breeding territories, pose a threat to humans, or be less likely to recognize humans or domestic animals as threats and be injured or killed as a result.

General Principles of Release

There are many different factors that must be considered when developing a release strategy. A thorough knowledge of the natural history of the animal is imperative. Some species will have a better chance of survival in the wild if the time of day or season is considered in their release. It is ideal to release the animal to an area near where it was found, unless this area is unsuitable for release (e.g., near a busy highway). Release methods will also depend on the fitness, time in captivity, and age of the animal. Migratory animals must be released during an appropriate season.

The following points should be considered when selecting a release site:[19]

1. The habitat must have foraging areas for the species, with available prey or other food resources.
2. No resident members of the individual's own species or genus or of conflicting species should be present.
3. The site should be secure from public interference.
4. The site should not be located near an area where there is extensive use of herbicides, insecticides, or rodenticides.
5. The site would be, preferably, at least one mile or more from any major roads.

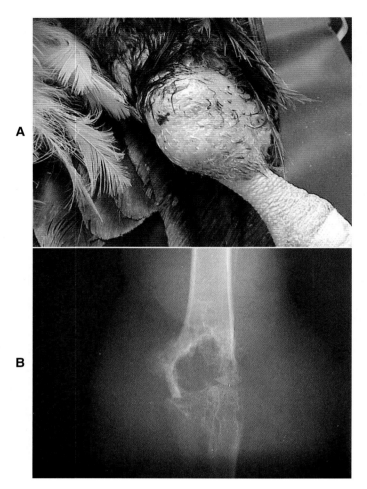

Figure 19-14 **A,** *Mycobacterium avium* is an important pathogen of wild birds. This bald eagle presented with systemic lesions. **B,** Most notable was the classic distal tibiotarsal osteomyelitis.

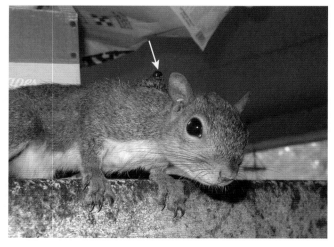

Figure 19-15 Fly larvae, such as this bot *(arrow)*, are a common finding in wild mammals. They should be surgically removed.

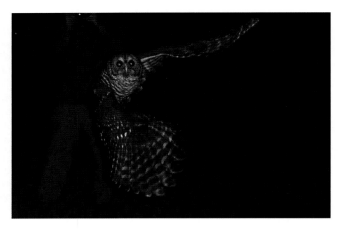

Figure 19-16 Releasing wildlife is very satisfying; however, to ensure that the patient has the best chance for survival, it is important to consider whether the animal will be able to re-adapt to its environment. (Courtesy Jessica Enes.)

Postrelease Monitoring

One of the most important questions asked of those who rehabilitate wildlife is whether the animals survive after being released. Unfortunately, there have been very few studies done to evaluate survival postrelease. Veterinarians interested in pursuing these issues may partner with wildlife rehabilitation facilities or biologists to assess postrelease survival. There are a number of monitoring techniques that can be used to answer these questions, but they are rarely pursued because of the personnel and monetary expenses associated with such programs. This is certainly one aspect of the rehabilitation process where veterinarians could become more involved.

REFERENCES

1. Chitty JR: Gamebirds, pigeons and doves. In Mullineaux E, Best D, Cooper JE, editors: *BSAVA Manual of Wildlife Casualties,* Quedgeley, Gloucester, 2003, British Small Animal Veterinary Association.
2. Best D, Lawson L: Wading birds, including herons. In Mullineaux E, Best D, Cooper JE, editors: *BSAVA Manual of Wildlife Casualties,* Quedgeley, Gloucester, 2003, British Small Animal Veterinary Association.
3. Martin RM: *First Aid and Care of Wildlife,* North Pomfret, Vt, 1984, David and Charles.
4. Green P: Deer. In Mullineaux E, Best D, Cooper JE, editors: *BSAVA Manual of Wildlife Casualties,* Quedgeley, Gloucester, 2003, British Small Animal Veterinary Association.
5. Keeble E: Seabirds: gulls, auks, gannets, petrels. In Mullineaux E, Best D, Cooper JE, editors: *BSAVA Manual of Wildlife Casualties,* Quedgeley, Gloucester, 2003, British Small Animal Veterinary Association.
6. Harcourt-Brown F, Whitwell K: Rabbits and hares. In Mullineaux E, Best D, Cooper JE, editors: *BSAVA Manual of Wildlife Casualties,* Quedgeley, Gloucester, 2003, British Small Animal Veterinary Association.
7. Brash MGI: Foxes. In Mullineaux E, Best D, Cooper JE, editors: *BSAVA Manual of Wildlife Casualties,* Quedgeley, Gloucester, 2003, British Small Animal Veterinary Association.
8. Routh A: Bats. In Mullineaux E, Best D, Cooper JE, editors: *BSAVA Manual of Wildlife Casualties,* Quedgeley, Gloucester, 2003, British Small Animal Veterinary Association.
9. Frye FL: *Reptile Clinician's Handbook: A Compact Clinical and Surgical Reference,* Malabar, Fla, 1994, Krieger.
10. Vogelnest L: Birds and reptiles. In Vogelnest L, Spielman D, Bellamy T et al: *Urban Wildlife, Proc 2004,* Postgraduate Committee in Veterinary Science, University of Sydney, Australia, 1994.

11. Cooke SW: Waterfowl: swans, geese, ducks, grebes and divers. In Mullineaux E, Best D, Cooper JE, editors: *BSAVA Manual of Wildlife Casualties,* Quedgeley, Gloucester, 2003, British Small Animal Veterinary Association.

12. Best D, Mullineaux E: Basic principles of treating wildlife casualties. In Mullineaux E, Best D, Cooper JE, editors: *BSAVA Manual of Wildlife Casualties,* Quedgeley, Gloucester, 2003, British Small Animal Veterinary Association.

13. Hickman M, Guy M: *Care of the Wild Feathered and Furred, A Guide to Wildlife Handling and Care,* Santa Cruz, Calif, 1973, University Press.

14. Beaver P: Behavioral requirements in rearing orphan birds and maintenance and feeding of orphaned songbirds, *Introduction to Wildlife Rehabilitation,* St. Cloud, Minn, 1986, National Wildlife Rehabilitators Association.

15. Garcelon D, Bogue GL: *Raptor Care and Rehabilitation,* Walnut Creek, Calif, 1977, Night Owl Press.

16. Sainsbury AW: Squirrels. In Mullineaux E, Best D, Cooper JE, editors: *BSAVA Manual of Wildlife Casualties,* Quedgeley, Gloucester, 2003, British Small Animal Veterinary Association.

17. Kraus A, Weisbroth SH, Flatt RE et al: Biology and diseases of rabbits. In JG Fox, BJ Cohen, FM Loew, editors, *Laboratory Animal Medicine,* New York, 1984, Academic Press.

18. Evans AT: *Introduction to wildlife rehabilitation,* St. Cloud, Minn, 1986, NWRA.

19. Llewellyn P: Rehabilitation and release. In Mullineaux E, Best D, Cooper JE, editors: *BSAVA Manual of Wildlife Casualties,* Quedgeley, Gloucester, 2003, British Small Animal Veterinary Association.

Note: Page numbers followed by *f* indicate figures; *t*, tables; and *b*, boxes.